UNDERWATER MEDICINE AND RELATED SCIENCES

A Guide to the Literature

Volume 2

An Annotated Bibliography,
Key Word Index, and Microthesaurus

UNDERWATER MEDICINE AND RELATED SCIENCES

A Guide to the Literature

Volume 2

An Annotated Bibliography, Key Word Index, and Microthesaurus

Margaret F. Werts and Charles W. Shilling

Undersea Medical Society, Inc.
9650 Rockville Pike
Bethesda, Maryland

IFI/PLENUM • NEW YORK-WASHINGTON-LONDON

Library of Congress Cataloging in Publication Data

Shilling, Charles Wesley, 1901-
Underwater medicine and related sciences.

"Supported jointly by the Bureau of Medicine and Surgery and the Office of Naval Research under ONR Contract N-00014-67-A-0214-0009."
Authors' names in reverse order in v. 2
Published in 1971 under title: An annotated bibliography on diving and submarine medicine.
1. Diving, Submarine—Physiological aspects—Abstracts. I. Werts, Margaret F., joint author. II. Title.
RC1220.D5S48 1973 616.9'8022'08 73-80326

The preparation of this bibliography was supported jointly by the Bureau of Medicine and Surgery and the Office of Naval Research, United States Department of the Navy, under ONR Contract N-00014-67-A-0214-0009.

ISBN 978-1-4684-6188-6 ISBN 978-1-4684-6186-2 (eBook)
DOI 10.1007/978-1-4684-6186-2

IFI/Plenum Data Company is a division of
Plenum Publishing Corporation
227 West 17th Street, New York, N.Y. 10011

United Kingdom edition published by Plenum Press, London
A Division of Plenum Publishing Company, Ltd.
Davis House (4th Floor), 8 Scrubs Lane, Harlesden, London, NW10 6SE, England
Softcover reprint of the hardcover 1st edition 1973

CONTENTS

ACKNOWLEDGMENTS

The authors wish to thank the individuals, other than themselves, who prepared the abstracts in instances where no adequate abstract was furnished. These individuals are identified by initials; they are Oscar L. Casarella, Mary Ellen Hashmall, and Arthur Turner. The initials BSCP and SCD indicate that the abstracts were written during the period in which the contract existed between the Office of Naval Research and The George Washington University. The initials UMS signify the Undersea Medical Society, with which the contract now is held.

The final copy of the abstracts was prepared by Robinson Graphics, Inc. The indexes were prepared by Cathleen Coppola, Britta de Mello, Yvette Desautels, Rosemary Mathias, Sally McAllister, Patty Podolak, and Darlene Sadler.

FOREWORD

This volume is the third annotated bibliography on this subject area to be compiled by these authors. The first, published by Gordon and Breach, Science Publishers, in 1971, was entitled AN ANNOTATED BIBLIOGRAPHY ON DIVING AND SUBMARINE MEDICINE. It covered material published during the 1960's. The second volume, entitled UNDERWATER MEDICINE AND RELATED SCIENCES: A GUIDE TO THE LITERATURE, published in 1973 by Plenum Press, covered primarily material published during 1970 and 1971, with some material from 1968 and 1969. The present volume covers material published during 1972 and 1973, but here again some earlier material has been included.

The purpose of these annotated bibliographies is to make available a large proportion of the published material, in abstract form, indexed in such a manner as to make it possible to compile a reasonably complete annotated bibliography on any specific subject area in the field. It is possible thus to learn where the work is being done, by whom, and how extensively. Also, it becomes obvious what areas of research are lacking or inadequate. These specific searches can also form a background of reference material on which to base further research, or from which to write monographs or state-of-the-art surveys. Papers, articles and reports listed here are in most cases readily available.

With the increasing need for knowledge of the underwater environment and the medical, physiological, psychological, and technological problems posed thereby, this ongoing bibliographic effort should prove invaluable to the professional diving community, from the aspect of practical considerations as well as that of research.

The Undersea Medical Society is grateful to the U.S. Navy for supporting the production of this valuable tool for use by the hyperbaric community.

Dennis N Walder

Professor Dennis N. Walder
President
Undersea Medical Society, Inc.

EXPLANATORY NOTE

In a great majority of cases, the complete article was seen and the citation verified. If a satisfactory abstract was available, it was used and credit given to the author. Abstracts otherwise prepared are identified by initials, as explained in ACKNOWLEDGMENTS.

In cases where abstracts have been taken directly from abstracting journals, appropriate credit has been given, as follows: Material taken from the abstract section of Aerospace Medicine is identified as (Aerosp. Med.); from Biological Abstracts (© BA); from Engineering Index (Eng.Ind.); from Government Report Announcements (GRA); from International Aerospace Abstracts (IAA); from the Library of Congress Federal Research Division, (S & T Alert); from Scientific and Technical Aerospace Reports (STAR). In the case of some government reports, the abstracts furnished by Document Control Data (DCD) were used.

The citations and abstracts are arranged alphabetically by the surname of the senior author, and chronologically within the works of an author. They are numbered sequentially. Anonymous articles are listed chronologically and alphabetically by title. It will be noted that in a few instances, numbers are omitted, and in one instance an item has been inserted by adding .1 to the preceding number. These changes were due to rearrangement found to be necessary upon revision.

Documents bearing AD numbers, JPRS numbers, and N numbers are usually available from the National Technical Information Service, U.S. Department of Commerce, Springfield, Virginia 22151. Prices vary according to the length of the document. Government reports for which no number is given may often be obtained from NTIS, by giving such bibliographic information as is furnished in this bibliography.

In the preceding bibliography, a microthesaurus of key terms was presented. This word list has been considerably condensed, to the point where it is a convenient and manageable tool for the retrieval of documents. The permuted index of this volume is based entirely upon this list. The condensed microthesaurus is presented before the permuted index, in order to enable the reader to make the most effective possible use of the index.

UNDERWATER MEDICINE AND RELATED SCIENCES

A Guide to the Literature

1.
AARON, A.L. Jr.

A unique approach to environmental control in a 1000-ft commercial saturation diving system.
In: 1973 Offshore technology Conference, April-May 1973, Houston, Texas. Preprints, Vol. I, p. 505-509. Published by the conference.

A 1000-ft saturation diving system was designed specifically for installation aboard a semisubmersible drilling vessel. Operational requirements and space restrictions made it necessary to develop modular explosion-proof external environmental control units for the deck chamber complex. These units use a special pumping system to circulate chamber breathing gas. Humidity is controlled without refrigeration equipment, and contaminants and odors are removed by means of regenerable chemicals. (Author's abstract)

2.
ABBOTT, R.T.

Mollusks dangerous to scuba divers.
Del. Med. J. 45:161-164;June 1973.

Severe stings sometimes resulting in death are inflicted by fish- and mollusk-eating cones. The severe symptoms are generally similar in most cases. Most potent of the venomous mollusks are the cone snails, a group of attractive tropical seashells of worldwide distribution, which are avidly sought by shell-collecting divers. To date, over 30 cases of human injury from cone snail stings have been recorded in the medical literature. Ten of these resulted in the death of the victim. All fatal cases have occurred in the southwest Pacific. Two non-fatal stings have been reported from the western Atlantic, the most recent being in St. Petersburg, Florida, in 1970, when a collector was stung by the common Alphabet Cone, Conus spurius. After the initial sharp and painful sting, numbness and paralysis of the limb occur, which finally spread to all parts of the body. There are usually speech difficulty and difficulty in swallowing. Of equal virulence are the bites of octopuses. Fifteen cases are known, but only one fatality has occurred. The latter, in 1954, resulted from a bite from the polka-dotted Australian octopus, Hapalochlaena lunulata. Characteristically, there was no pain felt from the initial bite of this species. The bitten victim, an adult Australian man, had a dry feeling in his mouth, difficulty in swallowing, a trickling of blood from the small puncture wound, vomiting, rapid loss of coordination, failure of the limbs, semiconsciousness, cessation of breathing and cyanosis. Death occurred within two hours of being bitten. (Author)

3.
ABERNETHY, J.D.

Inert gases in the kidney; influence of the countercurrent multiplication of sodium.
Aust. J. Exp. Biol. Med. Sci. 50(3):375-388;1972

Small but significant partial pressure differences between urine and blood can be detected [in a dog and humans], indicating that in passage through the kidney, N_2 tension is reduced by 1.35% (7mmHg) whereas Ar tension is increased by 0.77%. This differential behavior is an inevitable side effect of the countercurrent multiplication of Na in the [renal] medulla, given the known propensity of electrolytes for increasing the chemical potential of non-polar solutes (the salting-out effect). The primary event in Na multiplication, removal of Na from the ascending limb of Henle's loop is then of necessity accompanied by a local reduction in partial pressure of dissolved gas. This initiates a chain of events culminating in active countercurrent attenuation of partial pressure, the effect being greater for the gas with the greater diffusivity (N_2). The multiplication of Na which parallels this attenuation tends also to offset it: increased salt concentration potentiates partial pressure through a direct salting-out effect. The net result is a dynamic balance, determined for each gas by its diffusivity and salting-out factor. Because there is an equilibrium between inner medulla and urine (verified by He gas) these changes in the inner medulla are also reflected in the urine. This analysis is supported by a single-loop model which predicts a value for maximal Na concentration in the inner medulla reasonably close to physiological values (particularly if the contribution of urea to salting-out is included). Low values of He in urine, found during inhalation experiments, were also consistent with the model, although there were indications that attenuation takes several hours longer than potentiation for completion. The implications for acute (non-steady state) experiments are that urine concentrations of non-electrolytes tend to be elevated with respect to blood. A probable example of this is the ethanol concentration of urine in forensic studies. (© BA)

4.
ABERNETHY, J.D.

The mechanism of secretion of inert gases into the fish swimbladder.
Aust. J. Exp. Biol. Med. Sci. 50(3):365-374;1972.

Gases customarily viewed as biologically inert may, like their biologically active counterparts, O_2 and CO_2, be secreted into the swimbladder at high pressure. Werner Kohn proposed that the mechanism for all gases was counter-current multiplication of small changes in partial pressure, initiated by secretions of the gas gland situated near the bend of the multiplier loop. An analysis of swimbladder data on Ar/N_2 ratios confirms the hypothesis for inert gas. The nature of the secretory agent relevant to inert gas is also discussed. Kuhn postulated the secretion of an electrolyte to salt out dissolved gas, in addition to lactic acid secretion known to operate in the release of O_2 and CO_2. This postulate may be redundant:lactic acid releases N_2 from fish red cells, perhaps by a pH-related change in Hb polar groups. Countercurrent multiplication of all gases would thus be controlled by a single agent. Interspecies variations in swimbladder gas content would not be inconsistent with this unitary theory, since these may merely reflect interspecies variations in the development of the multiplier apparatus and probably variations in the pH-effect. (© BA)

5.
ABIDIN, B.I., V.I. Belkin, A.N. Mal'kuta and G.D. Yukhnovskiy.
Effect of hyperoxic atmosphere on rat tolerance to acute carbon monoxide exposure.
Space Biol. Med. 6:40-42;Aug. 1972.
(JPRS 56675)

It is demonstrated that the 30-day exposure of white male rats to a hyperoxic atmosphere (45% O_2) at normal barometric pressure caused a delay in their body weight increment and a decrease in their oxygen consumption. This exposure exerts no real influence on animal tolerance of acute exposure to carbon monoxide. (Authors' abstract)

6.
ABIDIN, B.I., V.V. Kustov, T.A. Lekareva, K.P. Bugar', L.T. Poddubnaya and V.I. Belkin.
Effect of a high oxygen content on the intensity of formation and elimination of some gaseous products of vital functions by rats.
Space Med. Biol. 6:7-11;Sept. 1972.
(JPRS 57139)

In experiments on albino male rats it was demonstrated that a two-day exposure of the animals to a hyperoxic atmosphere (PO_2 = 729.6 mm Hg) at normal barometric pressure increased the formation and elimination of carbon monoxide and decreased the elimination of ammonia. (Authors' abstract)

7.
ABRAHAM, A.
Oxygen poisoning.
J. Indian Med. Assoc. 57:228-231;Sept. 1971.

The aim of the discussion is only to bring out the toxic manifestations of the disease and hence treatment and prophylaxis are not dealt with. Both the 'Paul Bert' effect and 'Lorrain Smith' effect are dealt with in detail. Many of the clinical features have been demonstrated in experimental animals by the author. The early manifestations of the disease, so important for the diver, are enumerated. They are: (a) narrowing of the visual field, (b) increase in diastolic blood pressure, (c) pallor of the face, (d) giddiness, vertigo and syncope, (e) nausea and vomiting, (f) sensation of the approach of loss of consciousness, (g) numbness of the terminal phalanx, (h) numbness of the upper lip, (j) burning sensation in retrosternal region, (k) tremors of lips and fingers, (l) twitching of small groups of muscles, (m) facial twitching and (n) respiratory difficulty. Mechanisms of oxygen poisoning are described. Lastly, the present position as regards hyperbaric oxygen therapy are briefly reviewed. (From author's summary and text)

8.
ACKER, H., D.W. Luebbers and M.J. Purves.
Local oxygen tension field in the glomus caroticum of the cat and its change at changing arterial PO_2.
Pfluegers Arch. 329(2):136-155;1971.

The distribution of O_2 tension [PO_2] was measured in the carotid body of 97 cats using Pt microelectrodes. In only 7 cats was there evidence from measurement of chemoreceptor afferent discharge in the sinus nerve of damage to carotid body tissue or blood vessel. Eleven carotid bodies were histologically controlled, 2 showed obvious damages of the puncture. The distribution of PO_2 in carotid body tissue was consistent with a few exceptions and consisted of a relatively high PO_2 (ca. 25-90 mmHg) at the greatest distance from the surface progressively falling toward the surface where there was a zone of low PO_2, 0-15 mm Hg, and then a barrier to the inward diffusion of O_2. This pattern of PO_2 distribution was altered to the point of reversal following death of the animal and following injections of antimycin into the common carotid artery. The surface barrier to O_2 could also be reduced or abolished with antimycin and local destruction of tissue by electrolysis. The frequency distribution of tissue PO_2 showed that 79% of all values obtained were less than 40 mmHg. The local tissue PO_2 and the distribution of PO_2 was systematically altered by changes in PaO_2 [arterial O_2 tension], the alterations being least conspicuous in the outer zone of low PO_2. Blood flow through the carotid body is probably far from homogeneous. The various mechanisms which may be involved are discussed. (© BA)

9.
ACKERMAN, M.J.
Effects of diving on reticular and thalamic biopotentials in rats.
In: Aerospace Medical Association. 1973 annual scientific meeting, Las Vegas, Nevada, May 1973. Preprints, p. 267-268. Published by the Association, 1973.

This study was undertaken to investigate the depressing effect of nitrogen on the central nervous system (CNS), specifically the midbrain reticular formation and the reticular nucleus of the thalamus. . . These results indicate a depression of the CNS under nitrogen narcosis and a recovery corresponding to an adaptation to the nitrogen environment. They also indicate a possible disruption of the reticular nucleus outflow. Further studies with subjects breathing helium-oxygen are recommended to separate pressure effects from nitrogen narcosis effects. (Author)

10.
ACKLES, K.N., L.A. Kuehn and R.A. Stubbs.
Pneumatic analogue decompression computer calculations for submarine escape.
Downsview Ontario, Def. Civ. Inst. Environ. Med., Def. Res. Board, Rep. DCIEM 808 (revised), 21 p. July 1971.

Great progress has been made by the Royal Navy in the technique of submarine escape since the end of World War II. The dangers of multi-man compartmental escape were realized at an early date and in recent years much study has been devoted to single man-tower escapes. The most recent man escapes in the sea were from a depth of 600 feet. These escapes involved a pressurization time of 20 sec. bottom time of 1.5 sec. and a free ascent at approximately 8.5 ft/sec directly to the surface. No decompression problems were reported. Since these time-depth exposure profiles are outside the practical experience gained thus far with our pneumatic decompression computer, the computer's response to them, and more particularly its predictions in regard to the possible extension of the RN submarine escape technique to greater depths, is of considerable interest. In this paper RN experience is related to theoretical considerations underlying the computer, and the factors critical to successful escape are identified and discussed. . . . The assumptions and equations discussed are applied to determine optimum safe ascent profiles for submarine escape under a variety of conditions. A summary of the predictions made by the pneumatic analogue decompression computer is presented in Table 4, and examples of complete computer print-outs are shown in Appendix 1. Table 4 is arranged so that the effects of changing one variable at a time can be examined. . . . An examination of Table 4 shows that the most inportant factor in a successful escape is the ascent rate. A compression time of 20 seconds appears to be acceptable because the decompression time is not much affected by shortening it to 15 seconds. A practical minimum time on bottom appears to be 1.5 seconds. The most recent escapes had an ascent rate of 8.5 ft/sec or 510 ft/min. As shown in Profile 14, safe escape from 700 feet would probably be possible if an ascent rate of 10 ft/sec could be maintained. . . . One possibility exists for extending the capability of the escape system to 1000 feet. This involves the construction of a semi-rigid submarine escape garment which would maintain 5-10 psig over ambient pressure. Such suits are used in space programs, but the submarine escape requirements would be easier to meet, since limb mobility would not be required. A collapsible escape capsule constructed of rubberized canvas with circular reinforcing rings which would assume a streamlined rocket-like appearance when inflated is probably technically and economically feasible. Reduction of hydro-dynamic drag, achieved by streamlining, would be necessary to attain an ascent rate of about 900 ft/min. The escapee would float on the surface in his inflated capsule until rescued, or he might himself release the pressure by an internal valve after an appropriate decompression interval. With such a system escape from depths up to 1000 feet would probably be feasible. (Author)

11.
ACKLES, K.N.
Submarine escape — additional considerations on when to escape.
Downsview, Ontario, Def. Civ. Inst. Environ. Med., Def. Res. Board, Rep. DCIEM 830, 5 p. Feb. 1972.

One of the many problems involved in submarine escape is knowledge of the best time to commence escape procedures. All tests of the adequacy of the R.N. single-man escape tower system for depths to 600 ft have assumed that the escapee is in equilibrium with air at 1 atmosphere absolute (ATA). In a disabled submarine there is a strong possibility that this condition would not be fulfilled: pressure would be higher than 1 ATA due to partial flooding or the release of high-pressure air. Accordingly, using our pneumatic analogue decompression model, a computed graph is presented which relates the safe waiting period before escape to external and internal pressures. (Author's abstract)

12.
ACKLES, K.N., ed.
Blood-bubble interaction in decompression sickness. Proceedings of an international symposium held at Defence and Civil Institute of Environmental Medicine, Downsview, Ontario, Canada.
Published by the Institute, December 1973. 302p. (DCIEM 73-CP-960).

Many aspects of blood-bubble interaction are discussed in the papers presented: sludging, coagulation, platelet activity, humoral factors, effects of drug therapy, etc. Specific papers will be found under the following author entries: Ackles, K.N., R.B. Philip and M.J. Inwood; Chryssanthou, C.P.; Elliott, D.H.; Hallenbeck, J.M., A.A. Bove and D.H. Elliott; Heimbecker, R.O., I. Koven and K. Richards; Holland, J.A., W.E. Davis, W.G. Wolfe and J.A. Kylstra; Inwood, M.J.; Kindwall, E.P.; Kinlough-Rathbone, R.L.; Lee, W.H., Jr.; Martin, K.J.; McCormick, J.G., T. Philbrick and W. Holland; Philip, R.B.; Powell, M.R., R.W. Hamilton, Jr. and G.F. Doebblen; Ricci, G.C. and E. Massa; Smith, K.H., P.J. Stegall, L.A. Harker and S.J. Clichter; Vroman, L., A.L. Adams, M. Klings and G. Fischer; Warren, B.A. (MFW/UMS)

13.
ACKLES, K.N., R.B. Philp and M.J. Inwood.
Effects of orally-administered pyrimido-pyrimidine derivatives (RA233 and VK744) on platelet functions in human subjects decompressed from a hyperbaric environment.
In: Ackles, K.N. ed. Blood bubble interaction in decompression sickness. Proceedings of an international symposium held at Defence and Civil Institute of Environmental Medicine, Downsview, Ontario, Canada, p. 201-210. Published by the Institute, December 1973. (DCIEM Conference Proceedings 73-CP-960)

It has been confirmed in two separate experiments that the platelet count is depressed 24-48 hours following dives in which there have been no evidence of decompression sickness. The decrease in platelet count has been successfully prevented by the administration of two different platelet active drugs, RA233 and VK744. (Authors' summary)

14.
ADAMS, G.M.
The role of lipids in etiology of decompression sickness.
In: Abstracts of BuMed-ONR sponsored Navywide research in high pressure biomedical research, U.S. Submarine Base, Groton, Conn., May 1971, p. 41. Published by the Naval Submarine Medical Research Laboratories, 1971.

Abstract only. Excerpt quoted: Using the male rat as a model animal we have investigated the source of potentially embolic lipid in some detail. In vitro studies with liver slices suggest that lipid biosynthesis is not affected by pressure and remains unaffected unless the partial pressure of oxygen is increased. As the liver is the principle site of lipid biosynthesis, these results suggest that lipid synthesis is probably not involved in the etiology of decompression sickness at normal partial pressures of oxygen. Detailed in vitro lipolysis studies utilizing pre-labeled (C-14) epididymal fat pad slices suggest that the lipolytic process and its hormonal regulatory processes are not affected by pressure. Therefore, altered lipolysis would not seem a contributing factor in vivo unless physiological activation occurs under conditions leading to decompression sickness. At the present time in vivo experiments utilizing various agents to inhibit or activate either synthesis or lipolysis are being carried out to ascertain the contributions of the observed in vitro results in decompression sickness.

15.
ADAMS, J.R., J.F. Manuel and R.W. Cook.
New offshore recovery advancement for deep water completions.
In: 1973 Offshore Technology Conference, April/May 1973, Houston, Texas. Preprints Vol. II, p.133-148. Published by the conference.

This paper presents a review of the development status of three subsea oil production systems under development by Subsea Equipment Associates Limited (SEAL). The SEAL Intermediate System (SIS) is described with particular emphasis on utilization of a Manned Working Enclosure (MWE) to permit men to perform maintenance operations in a dry environment at the sea floor. The MWE concept involves lowering the structure over the well-head, expelling the water and transferring personnel by the use of a Personnel Transfer Bell (PTB). . . The SEAL Shallow System is similar to the MWE with the exception that the maintenance personnel are carried in the SEAL Bell. Once the bell is pulled to the subsea wellhead, water is expelled and the atmospheric pressure reduced to sea level to permit the men to enter the work chamber and perform the necessary operations. . . . The SEAL Atmospheric System is. . . based on the use of a large habitat-type structure permanently installed on the sea floor to house oil field equipment. Future applications of this concept would be as a manifold center, a test separator center, or a complete oil production system. In a similar manner to the other systems, men are transported to and from the Subsea Work Enclosure (SWE) through the use of a Personnel Transfer Bell. . . A common element in each of the three systems being developed by SEAL is the use of a Personnel Transfer Bell to transport maintenance workers to the subsea structure in a safe and efficient manner. A prototype Personnel Transfer Bell has been built for SEAL by Perry Oceanographics. Details concerning the construction of the vehicle and its operation are presented in this paper. (Authors)

16.
ADEBAHR, G.
Morphologische Schokaquivalinte bei Luftembolie Taucherunfall und Decompressionskrankheit.
[Morphologic shock equivalents in air embolism, diving accidents and decompression sickness].
Beitr. Gerichtl. Med. 29:87-91;1972.

In normovolemic shock in air embolism, diving accidents and decompression sickness common morphologic factors can be demonstrated: aggregation of platelets, leukocytes, and red blood cells at the sites of gas bubbles, and also independently of bubbles, especially in capillaries and venoles. These findings are to be seen after five minutes. Complete intravascular blood coagulation is only seldom recorded. This may be related to the short survival time, particularly in air embolism. But probably the gas bubbles in the blood vessels, the little ruptures in the tissue and fat embolism (in decompression sickness), are present in normovolemic shock as additional factors that are inadequate to induce more complete coagulation of the blood. (English summary)

17.
ADOLFSON, J.A., K. Bjerver, E. Fluur and L. Goldberg.
Vestibular reactions during hyperbaric conditions.
Forsvarmedicin 6:234-238;1970.

Ten experienced divers were compressed to 10 ATA in two minutes, kept there from 16-19 minutes, then decompressed to 1 ATA in 185 minutes. The reaction pattern of the entire vestibulo-ocular reflex arc was studied. Changes were extremely slight. There were also no significant differences in activity between the left and right labyrinths. The authors suggest that subjectively felt dizziness and severe postural disturbances found at increased pressure at a steady level is of a CNS origin. (MFW/SCD)

18.
ADOLFSON, J.A. and T. Berghage
Effects of increased ambient air pressures on standing steadiness in man.
In: Abstracts of the Twenty-fifth Congress of Physiological Sciences Satellite Symposium. Recent progress in fundamental physiology of diving. Marseille, France, July 1971, p.46-49. (Proceedings unpublished)

Abstract only. The authors investigated the relationship between increased air pressure and vestibular function under the following conditions: eyes open, eyes closed, and in sagittal and lateral direction. The subjects were ten experienced divers and pressures were 2.2, 4, 7, and 10 ATA. It was found (1) that there is a strong relationship between balance and depth; (2) balance deteriorates much more rapidly in the eyes closed condition than in the eyes open condition, and (3) performance at depth is related to performance at surface. These findings indicate that the diver would have much trouble with orientation underwater. Individual differences among the subjects were great. The authors conclude that the postural disturbances that occurred during this experiment consitute a symptom of nitrogen narcosis. Studies of the influence of carbon dioxide on balance are at present carried out. (MFW/BSCP)

19.
ADOLFSON, J.A., L. Goldberg and T.E. Berghage
Effects of increased ambient air pressures on standing steadiness in man
Aerosp. Med. 43:520-524;May 1972

The effects of increased ambient air pressures on standing steadiness at 2.2 ATA, 4 ATA, 7 ATA and 10 ATA as compared with results obtained in two control situations at ambient air pressure (1 ata) were studied in ten experienced divers. Body sway was recorded quantitatively by statometry and in four different conditions; with open and closed eyes and in sagittal and lateral directions. The device used — Statometer IV — allowed analog and digital recording and evaluation of variations in frequency and amplitude of the pattern of body sway, and an advanced statistical analysis was made by using a randomized block factorial analysis of variance design. The results indicated that (1) there is a strong quadratic relationship between balance and depth, (2) deterioration in balance increases at a much faster rate for the eyes closed condition than for the eyes open condition as depth is increased, (3) there are highly significant individual differences, (4) the performance at depth is related to the performance at the surface, (5) there seems to be no habituation or other adaptation to the test device and (6) there seem to be no essential after-effects to the exposure to increased ambient air pressure under the present conditions. It was concluded that the postural disturbances at increased ambient air pressure might be related to the effect of the breathing medium on the central nervous system as one symptom of nitrogen narcosis in man. (Authors' abstract)

20.
ADOLFSON, J.A., L. Fagraeus and C.M. Hesser.
Deterioration of standing steadiness in hyperbaric environment.
In: Hesser, C.M. and D. Linnarsson, eds. Proceedings of the first annual scientific meeting of the European Undersea Biomedical Society, Stockholm, 13-15 June 1973. Forsvarsmedicin 9:253-256;July 1973.

It was concluded that the postural disturbances at high ambient air pressures are mainly due to the rise in N_2 pressure and, in conditions associated with hypoventilation, also to the rise in alveolar CO_2 tension, whereas the rise in O_2 pressure is only of minor importance. (From author's abstract)

21.
ADOLFSON, J.A. and C. Lindemark.
Pulmonary and neurological complications in free escape.
In: Hesser, C.M. and D. Linnarsson, eds. Proceedings of the first annual scientific meeting of the European Undersea Biomedical Society, Stockholm, 13-15 June 1973. Forsvarsmedicin 9:244-246;July 1973.

Since complications with signs of lung rupture occasionally also show signs of air embolism to CNS, 112 subjects were studied by means of EEG in order to: (1) Investigate the incidence of lung rupture and to study whether lung rupture always is followed by neurological symptoms during training in free ascent, and (2) to study the time course of the symptoms of lung rupture with or without neurological symptoms. It was found that free escape as such affects the EEG only slightly by giving rise to a moderate increase of the slow wave content in many cases. In some subjects without neurological symptoms the increase was, however, so marked that the records following the diving were classified as abnormal. The complication frequency during the years 1966 through 1971 was 0.9% of the number of trainees who started the practice in free ascent. The EEG-study shows a complication frequency of 3.5%. This strengthened diagnostics includes thorax X-ray and was confirmed during 1973 by a complication frequency of 3.1%. (From authors' abstract)

22.
AEROSPACE MEDICAL ASSOCIATION.
1971 annual scientific meeting, Houston, Texas, April, 1971. Preprints. Published by the Association, 1971. 263p.

Most of the papers read at this meeting deal with aviation or aerospace subjects. The following sessions contained material related to the hyperbaric environment: Hyperoxia (Hematology); Oxygen toxicity; Hyperbarics (pulmonary; Toxicology I Hyperbarics (operational); Hyperbarics (clinical); Undersea-aerospace symposium (papers not made available); An international open decompression data bank (papers not made available). Specific papers will be found under the following author entries: Bassett, B.E. and J.M. Dunn; Bennett, P.B. and A.N. Dossett; Coler, C.R., R.M. Patton and E.C. Lampkin; Feld, J.N., H. Bardin and C.J. Lambertsen; Houlihan, R.T. and B. LaLone; Johnson, W.P., D. Jefferson and C.E. Mengel; Popovic, V.P. and J.E. Baughman; Serrill, W.S., C.E. Mengel and D. Jefferson; Uhl, R.R., C. Van Dyke, R.B. Cook, R.A. Horst and J.M. Merz; Van Dyke, C., R.R. Uhl, R.B. Cook, R.A. Horst and J.M. Merz; Waller, J.R. and C.A. Zogg; Wilks, S.S.; Wright, W.B., A.B. Fisher, P.L. Hendricks, J.S. Brody and C.J. Lambertsen. Preprint of the paper by Sass, D.J., E.L. Pitman, P.E. Caskey, W. Van Norman and E.H. Wood appears as entry 1386 in our second bibliography. Papers by Chryssanthou, C., F. Teichner and W. Antapol, by Gaume, J.G., P. Bartek and H.J. Rostami, By Hills, B.A., and by Zogg, C.A. were subsequently published in Aerospace Medicine and appear in our second bibliography as entries 389, 627, 781 and 1761 respectively. The paper by Reeves, E., A.E. McKee, J.A. Stunkard and P.W. Schilling was subsequently published in Aerospace Medicine and will be found in this bibliography. (MFW/BSCP)

23.
AEROSPACE MEDICAL ASSOCIATION
1972 annual scientific meeting, Bal Harbour, Florida, May, 1972. Preprints. Published by the Association, 1972. 275p.

Most of the papers read at this meeting deal with aviation or aerospace subjects. The following sessions contained material related to the hyperbaric environment: Physiology—hyperbaric biochemistry; Physiology—cardiopulmonary (hyperbaric); Physiology—decompression; Underseas. Specific papers will be found under the following author entires: Akers, T.K. and D.K. MacCarter; Antopol, W. and C.P. Chryssanthou; Beckman, D.L. and R.T. Houlihan; Cockett, A.T.K., S.M. Pauley, A. Pilmanis and A.P. Roberts; Feld, J.N. and C.J. Lambertsen; Gelfand, R. and C.J. Lambertsen; Hall, P.; Pauley, S.M., N. Alazraki and J. Chandler; Ricci, G.C.; Richardson, B., S.R. Jaskunas and E.J. Stork; Roberts, A.J., T.F. Bobbitt and S.R. Jaskunas; Schaefer, K.E. and R.D. Allison; Uhl, R.R., P.L. Hendricks, J. Merz, D.B. Arlin and E.L. Miller; Wilks, S.S.; Wright, W.B., Y. Seki and C.J. Lambertsen. (MFW/BSCP)

24.
AEROSPACE MEDICAL ASSOCIATION.
1973 annual scientific meeting, Las Vegas, Nevada, May, 1973. Preprints. Published by the Association, 1973. 304p.

Most of the papers read at this meeting deal with aviation or aerospace subjects. The following sessions contained material related to the hyperbaric environment: Thermal physiology, Cardiopulmonary physiology; Hypoxia/other stress; Oxygen toxicity; Decompression; Environmental physiology. Specific papers will be found under the following author entries: Ackerman, M.J.; Feinstein, R., B.A. Gooden and H.R. Skutt; Hamilton, R.W., Jr., D.J. Kenyon, H.R. Schreiner and P.O. Edel; Hammond, R.E. and T.K. Akers; Henderson, J.V. and E.H. Lamphier; Jacey, M.J., D.V. Tappan and K.R. Ritzler; Langley, T.D. and R.W. Hamilton, Jr.; Michaelson, E.D. and B. O'Byrne; Narahara, K.A., F.W. Booth and C.L. Giannetta; Perkins, G.F. and C.D. Wood; Powell, M.E.; Schaefer, K.E. and J.H. Dougherty, Jr.; Sinclair, R.D.; Spaur, W.H., W.R. Braithwaite and W.B. Wright; Strauss, M.D., W.S. Lee and R.W. Cantrell; Walsh, J.M.; Webb, P.; Wilcox, R.W.; Williamson, R., R. Liebelt and K. Doener; Wright, W.B. and J.E. Crothers; Zehl, D.N., A.T.K. Cockett, J. Hanley, W.R. Adey, A.P. Roberts and R. Zweizig. (MFW/BSCP)

25.
AFANASJEV, Yu. I., V.P. Derevyanko, V.V. Korolev, E.E. Kotovsky and K.K. Rogazhinskaya.
Gisto-strukturnye izmeniya gemato-parenkhimatoznogo bar'era magistral'nykh sosudov v eksperimente.
[Experimental histo-structural changes in the hemato-parenchymatous barrier and major vessels].
Arkh. Anat. Gistol Embriol. 63:53-60;Dec. 1972.

The work has shown that under different experimental conditions (hypergravitation effect 100% and 70% hyperoxia) inducing hypoxic state of the tissue there occur regular changes in the hemato-parenchymal barrier consisting of the endothelium, basal membrane, surrounding cells and intercellular substance as well as the membranes of parenchymatous cells. In the endothelium of the fine vessels of different organs pinocytotic vesicles appeared and the amount of microvilli increased. Subendothelial space widened. Permeability of the basal membrane and the pattern of tissue respiration in parenchymatous cells changes. Thus, morphological manifestations of the changes of the hemato-parenchymal barrier were not varied and reflected functional state of the organs under investigation. (English summary)

26.
AGADZHANYAN, N.A. and A.V. Sepgienko.
Perenosimost' ostroi gipoksii posle razlichnyakh srokov prebyavaniyav srede s porschennym soderzhaniem uglekisloty.
[The resistance to acute hypoxia following various periods of exposure to an environment with high carbon dioxide content].
Akad. Nauk SSSR (Ser. Biol.) 2:487-489, 1970.

The effect of concentrated CO_2 breathing on resistance to subsequent hypoxia has been studied in white mice. The animals were kept for seven days in a chamber containing air with 6% CO_2 under normal atm pressure, average temperature of 25°C and humidity of 89%. Following prolonged breathing of air containing a high percent of CO_2, the resistance of the animals to subsequently induced hypoxia varied in degree depending on the CO_2 concentration, as well as the duration of exposure to CO_2. CO_2 is known to slow down metabolic processes thus reducing the requirement for O_2 and the danger of acute hypoxia. This beneficial effect of CO_2 was observed by the authors during the first days of their experiment, that is after short-time exposure of the animals to CO_2. Prolonged hypercapnia, however, significantly lowered the resistance of the mice to hypoxia by inhibiting the compensatory adaptational reactivity of the organism. The authors conclude that the resistance to hypoxia depends not so much on the CO_2 concentration as on the length of time of exposure. (OLC/BSCP)

27.
AGADZHANYAN, N.A. and B.K. Rybakov.
Effects of hyperoxia on coagulating and anticoagulating systems in blood.
Eksp. Khir. Anest. 6:66-70;Dec. 1971.
(Translation JPRS 55553)

The results of this investigation demonstrate that during a prolonged stay in a hyperoxic environment, blood coagulability changes in the direction of hypocoagulability. The degree to which the coagulating activity of the blood changes depends not only on PO_2 but also on the duration of the exposure to the hyperoxic atmosphere. This experimental data can be used for a scientifically based use of oxygen in clinical practice and for adjusting the gas medium in inhabited closed spaces. Some indexes of the coagulating activity of the blood were determined in 24 experimental subjects exposed to hyperoxia (40,54,60, and 94% of oxygen) at a normal barometric pressure for longer (10-14 days) and briefer (24 hours) periods. The coagulating activity of the blood was reduced, and the degree of this hypocoagulability was determined by both the partial pressure of oxygen and the duration of hyperoxia. (Authors) (GRA)

28.
AGARATE, C.A. and A.J. Jegou.
A simulated dive at 2001 feet.
In: 1973 Offshore Technology Conference, April/May 1973, Houston, Texas. Preprints, Vol. I, p.511-513. Published by the conference.

The deep simulated dive was carried out as part of the C.N.E.X.O.-COMEX research program in COMEX from May 18 to June 2, 1972. Two professional divers were progressively pressurized with an oxy-helium mixture to 2001 feet which they reached on May 24 at 1.20 A.M. where they stayed for 80 min before decompression. The various physiological results obtained during this experimental dive permit optimism with regard to the feasibility of industrial underwater work in the 1500 foot range. The important amount of data gathered during this operation is still under processing and interpretation. But it can be stated right away that the High Pressure Nervous Syndrome which appeared on arrival in the 1100 ft range and disappeared at the end of the stay at this depth, was more marked at 1750 and 1850 feet after sleeping at constant depth than during the compression phases. At these depths, an undeniable respiratory insufficiency appeared at rest which was somewhat different from that which we had already observed and measured under effort in the 1700 ft range. It seems that this maladjustment of the pulmonary ventilation has played a role in the reinforcement of the HPNS which, thanks to the compression schedule, was perfectly controlled throughout the experiment thus permitting the maximum depth to be reached in complete safety. (Authors)

29.
AIBULATOV, N.A.
Okeanologicheskie issledovaniya iz obitarmykh podvodnykh laboratorii.
[Oceanographic research from the manned underwater laboratories].
Okeanologiya 12(1):144-154;Jan./Feb. 1972

A review of hydrophysical, geological and biological research conducted from the manned underwater laboratories of different countries is given. Advantages and disadvantages of the new method of ocean research are discussed, and a conclusion is made that a long stay of man underwater enables him to get unique information that is not obtainable by the methods used so far. (English summary)

30.
AJIKI, H., J. Wada, K. Ikeda, S. Sugii, K. Karino and T. Iwa.
Our collapsible hyperbaric bag.
In: Wada, J. and I. Takashi, eds. Proceedings of the fourth international congress of hyperbaric medicine, Sapporo, Japan, Sept. 1969, p.500-504. Baltimore, Williams and Wilkins, 1970.

The authors have developed a small, lightweight, collapsible, hyperbaric bag for emergency use under conditions in which a chamber would be impracticable. The bag is easily portable and can be installed in an ambulance. One of the uses mentioned for this equipment is the treatment of decompression sickness. The bag could be installed as standard equipment on small boats used in support of working divers. (MFW/BSCP)

31.
AKERS, T.K. and D.K. MacCarter.
The effects of hyperbaric $He\text{-}O_2$ on the interaction of norepinephrine on alpha and beta sympathetic receptors.
In: Aerospace Medical Association. 1972 annual scientific meeting, Bal Harbour, Florida, May 1972. Preprints, p.126. Published by the Association.

The present study examines the effect of pressure on adrenergic receptor activity. Isolated rabbit duodenum was suspended in Tyrodes solution in a standard Casella automated drug assay apparatus. The entire apparatus was placed in a pressure vessel at 1 Atm of air and pressurized with He up to 30 ATA. The O_2 levels were kept constant at 160 ± 10 mmHg. The temperature was maintained at $37 \pm 2°$ C. The muscle was washed at one-minute intervals. Norepinephrine (10^{-7}gm/cc) was injected and followed by several washes. The results indicate that the norepinephrine latency varies directly and linearly with the increase in pressure. It would appear from the data that pressure has a physical effect on the cell membrane where alpha blockers and norepinephrine are acting. (Authors)

32.
AKERS, T.K. and D.K. MacCarter.
Effects of high pressure on alpha and beta adrenergic receptors of the rabbit duodenum.
Aerosp. Med. 44:60-62;Jan. 1973.

In analyzing the effects of hyperbaric helium-oxygen on alpha and beta adrenergic receptors of rabbit duodenum, norepinephrine latency was found to vary directly and linearly with the increase in pressure. This relationship is described by the equation $Y = 9.114 + .905\ x$. Increasing pressure had no significant effect upon the drug induced change in magnitude of smooth muscle contractions. Pressure does not effect contractile depression by norepinephrine or phentolamine. Alpha receptor blockade by phentolamine was optimal at 10 ATA. Beta receptor blockade with propranolol was maximal at 30 ATA. (Authors' abstract)

33.
AKERS, T.K.
Temporal characteristics of the simple muscle twitch under hyperbaric O_2, N_2, He, and Ar conditions.
Physiologist 16:250;Aug. 1973.

Abstract only. Entire item quoted: The purpose of these experiments was to measure the effect of non-narcotic gases on the temporal characteristics of compound action potentials, synaptic delay, muscle membrane potentials, and contraction of the frog sciatic nerve-gastrocnemius muscle preparation. The sciatic nerve, including spinal cell bodies and associated gastrocnemius muscles, was carefully dissected out from pithed *Rana Pipiens* and mounted in a plastic moist chamber with appropriate stimulating and pick-up electrodes in place. A Statham U-2 universal transducer was used for muscle tension recordings. The preparation was placed at 25° C into a Bethlehem pressure chamber and appropriate mixtures of gases added. Pressurizing with N_2 to 10 ATA above room air decreased synaptic delay and coupling time. He and O_2 to 10 ATA also decreased these times significantly. Argon produced a slight increase in these times. Increased pressure and substitution of other gases for N_2 produced a reduction in contraction time. These results point towards the interaction of these gas mixtures with the physico-dynamics of the membrane.

34.
AKIMOV, G.A.
Disorders of the nervous system in decompression disease.
Zh. Nevropat. Psikhiat. 69:979-984;1969.
(Translation, Orpington, U.K., Def. Res. Inf. Cent., Rep. Nos. DRIC-2788, DRIC-BR-30159, 12 p. May 1972)
(AD 744 298)

On the basis of a clinical study of 56 cases with neurological symptoms in decompression sickness (caisson disease), the authors distinguished the following varieties: cerebral forms, spinal, neural and obliterated. In two cases which were attributed to the cerebral (with comatose conditions) and spinal forms of decompression sickness, pathomorphological studies were also performed. It was established that the main significance should be connected with circulatory disturbances and the peculiarities of vascularization in the pathogenesis of nervous-system lesions. (Author) (GRA)

35.
ALBANESE, R.A.
On microelectrode distortion of tissue oxygen tensions.
J. Theor. Biol. 38(1):143-154;1973.

The gentlest insertion of an O_2 measuring electrode into living tissue may distort the normal distribution of O_2 in the tissue, and thereby cause the electrode to determine erroneous O_2-tensions. A model tissue is studied. An electrode inserted into this tissue distorts tissue O_2 tensions and measures incorrect values. The effect can be minimized by using the smallest electrodes. (© BA)

36.
ALBANO, G. and P.M. Criscuoli.
Electroencefalograma del ratto libero ad estreme pressioni ambientali.
[EEG of unrestrained rats at extreme ambient pressures].
Boll. Soc. Ital. Biol. Sper. 47(23):787-790;1971.

Male albino rats bearing permanent electrodes underwent compression to 100 or 125 bar in a helium-oxygen (O_2 pressure 450-550 mb) atmosphere while EEG changes were noted. Base rhythm changes were first noted at 60-70 bar, accompanied by trembling. At 100-125 bar a slow base rhythm of unstable voltage and high voltage paroxystic bursts were noted, accompanied by brief hyperkinetic crises. An increase in O_2 pressure to 2.5 bar led to the disappearance of these symptoms, and EEG traces became normal as decompression was completed. When the experiment was repeated with O_2 pressure at 1000 mb, the first EEG anomalies appeared around 75-80 bars, the tremor at 85 bars. An increase in the O_2 pressure to 3.4 bar was followed almost immediately by typical grand mal seizures. It has, therefore, been shown that an increase in O_2 pressure tends to postpone the moderate neuronal disturbance caused by extreme ambient pressure. But the increased sensitivity of the organism to oxygen under these conditions has also been demonstrated. (MEMH/SCD)

37.
ALBANO, G., G.M. Burrano, M. Mazzone, G. La Monaca and G.S. Scaglione.
Indagini istopatologiche sulle neuropatie disbariche autoctone da heliox nella cavia.
[Histopathological investigation on the autochthonous dysbaric neuropathy of heliox in the guinea pig].
Folia Med. (Napoli) 54:217-232;1971.

Histologic cross-section series was developed on cerebro-spinal axis of guinea pigs killed at first phase of primary disbaric neuropathies due to air or heliox. In both cases the basal lesion resulted in the miliary and autochthonous gas embolism of capillary vessels in the white matter of thoracic spinal cord or brain stem, sometimes with gas bubbles outside the vessels (only in white bundles of cord). Disseminated intravascular coagulation, secondary thrombosis and occasionally hemorrhagic areas were also observed. No qualitative differences between pathological lesions due to two aetiologic agents were noted, but only the slight quantitative variations that are discussed. The interpretation of present data further confirms the theory of gas nucleus. (English summary)

38.
ALBANO, G., P.M. Criscuoli, G.C. Scaglione, M. Mazzone, G. La Monaca and G. Gurruano.
La sindrome da estreme pressioni ambientali, rilievi EEG ed ECG su ratti liberi con elettrodi a dimora.
[The syndrome of extreme ambient pressure: EEG and ECG recordings in free rats with electrodes implanted].
Ann. Med. Nav. (Roma) 78:11-28;Jan/Mar. 1972.

The authors exposed 36 white rats at pressures between 100 and 150 bar in atmosphere of helium and oxygen. EEG and EKG were drawn by stationary electrodes. The authors observed a "syndrome of extra-high environmental pressure" for white rats, that consist in serious troubles of the CNS and of the heart. This syndrome has five phases and the last two are irreversible because the atrioventricular conduction is irreparably compromised. At present the pathogenesis is uncertain, but the precociousness of the autonomic system involvement and the beneficial effect of a moderately high dose of oxygen are impressive. (English summary)

41.
ALBANO, G.
Il trattamento con ossigeno iperbarico delle neuropatie da decompressione e degli infarti ossei epifisari. Considerazioni su 27 casi di embolia gassosa.
[Hyperbaric oxygen therapy of decompression neuropathies and epiphyseal bone infarcts. Twenty-seven cases of gas embolism].
Ann. Med. Nav. (Roma) 77:497-534;Oct./Dec. 1972.

The author describes the technique of "mixed" recompression which he has used successfully in the treatment of 27 cases of decompression sickness in the last four years. Oxygen and air are given alternately during the recompression procedure, low-molecular-weight dextran is also used in some cases. Details of the symptoms and treatment of the case material are given, as are three schedules of "mixed" recompression; one is for "bends", the other two for other neuropathies. The physiological justification of the "mixed" therapy is discussed, and the author calls attention to the recently increasing incidence of decompression accidents. (MEMH/BSCP)

42.
ALBERTSEN, N.D.
Influence of compressive strength and wall thickness on behavior of concrete cylindrical hulls under hydrostatic loading.
U.S. Nav. Civil Eng. Lab., Rep. NCEL-TR-790, 32 p. June 1973.
(AD 764 054)

Sixteen unreinforced, cylindrical concrete hull models of 16-inch outside diameter were subjected to external hydrostatic loading to determine the effect of concrete strength and wall thickness on implosion and strain behavior. The test results showed that an increase in concrete strength of 70% produced an average increase in implosion pressure of 87% while increases in hull wall thickness by factors of 2 and 6 produced increases in implosion pressure by factors of approximately 2 and 11, respectively. Changes in concrete strength had little effect on strain behavior; however, strain magnitudes generally increased with increasing wall thickness when comparisons were made at a constant percentage of P (im). Design recommendations are presented to aid in the design of cylindrical concrete hulls for underwater use. (Author) (GRA)

43.
ALBRIGHT, L.J. and J.F. Henigman.
Seawater salts — hydrostatic pressure effects upon cell division of several bacteria.
Can. J. Microbiol. 17:1246-1248;1971.

An increased concentration of seawater salts increased the maximum hydrostatic pressure allowing cell division of the marine bacteria Achromobacter aquamarinus, Micrococcus sedentarius, Serratia marinorubra, and Vibrio adaptatus. Increased concentrations of these salts did not have as great an influence on the maximum hydrostatic pressure for cell division of Escherichia coli and Micrococcus luteus, which were isolated from a terrestrial environment. (Authors' abstract)

44.
ALDERMAN, J.L., B. Culver and M.K. Shellenberger.
The interaction of increased brain gamma-aminobutyric acid with hyperbaric oxygen induced seizures.
Fed. Proc. 32(3,pt.1):304;Mar. 1973.

Abstract only. Entire item quoted: It has been proposed that seizures induced by hyperbaric oxygen (OHP) result from a reduction in brain gamma-aminobutyric acid (GABA) levels. Furthermore, it has been suggested that increases in the endogenous GABA may be responsible for the protection against OHP seizures afforded by pargyline. In order to evaluate the possible role of GABA in OHP seizures, female Holtzman rats weighing 200 ± 10g were pretreated with the relatively specific GABA-transaminase inhibitor, hydrazino propionic acid (HPA), in doses which increase whole brain GABA levels from 25 to 150% above normal. These animals and their saline treated controls were subsequently exposed to OHP at a pressure of 5A (60psi) for a period of 90 minutes. This caused 70% of the controls to convulse while 100% of the drug treated animals over the entire dose range showed convulsions. The mean time to onset in those controls that convulsed was 73 ± 3.9 (S.E.) min while HPA animals had seizure onset in 27 ± 2.0 and 44 ± 9.0 min for the high and low doses. Amino-oxyacetic acid was administered to another group of animals in a dose known to protect against electroconvulsive seizures gave similar results. These data indicate that drug induced increases in GABA were not only unable to protect against OHP seizures but in fact caused potentiation.

45.
ALDRICH, T.C., R.D. Ballard, C.O. Bowin, F.R. Hess and B.P. Luyendyk.
Advanced marine technology.
Woods Hole, Mass., Woods Hole Oceanog. Inst., Dept. Geophys., Rep. WHOI-73-37, 56 p. June 1, 1973.
(AD 763 372)

This is a progress report for the period 1 August 1972 — 31 January 1973 on the following projects in advanced marine technology (a) submerged navigation and submersible instrumentation, (b) handling and transfer at sea, (c) bottom reconnaisance and detailed site survey by research submersible, (d) near bottom magnetics studies using a deep submersible, (e) near bottom gravity studies from a deep submersible, (f) a self-contained deep sea rock drill, (g) self-contained ancillary modular platform (SCAMP), (h) modular acoustic system, (i) air-seas system (Long Range Echo Ranging). (Authors) (GRA)

46.
ALEXANDER, C.W., C.S. Leach, C.L. Fischer, C.J. Lambertsen, and P.C. Johnson.
Hematological, biochemical, and immunological studies during a 14-day continuous exposure to 5.2% O_2 in N_2 at pressure equivalent to 100 fsw (4 ata).
Aerosp. Med. 44(7, Sec. II):850-854;July 1973.

Measurements of blood cellular, protein, and chemical characteristics were performed in conjunction with studies of urine composition on subjects exposed to nitrogen-oxygen breathing at 4 ata. No gross or evidently hazardous effects were observed either for the acute exposure or during the 14 days of sustained pressurization at 4 ata of nitrogen partial pressure. Evidence of hemoconcentration was found, with slight elevation of hemoglobin concentration, hematocrit, red cell count, plasma protein and cholesterol. These findings relate qualitatively to the increase in plasma volume also observed, and to the prominent diuresis. Several measurements indicated the probable occurrence of a tissue loss, which may have been largely related to change in muscle mass and red cell mass. (Authors' abstract)

47.
ALEKSANDROV, V.N. and V.A. Mozin.
Apparatus for determining expired carbon dioxide and device for dynamic sampling of inspired air.
Voennomed. Zh. (9):82-83;Sept. 1973.

A piece of equipment is described for sampling and analyzing inspired air in a confined space contaminated by short-duration but concentrated chemical factors. (S&T Alert).

48.
ALFONSO, P.J. and J.D. Harris.
The use of circumaural earphones for attenuating ambient noise in bone conduction audiometry.
U.S. Nav. Submar. Med. Res. Lab., Rep. NSMRL 728, 12p. Oct. 16, 1972.

Auditory sensitivity to a bone-conducted (BC) acoustic stimulus is increased when the ear canal is plugged ("occlusion effect"), thus increasing the eardrum-ossicle component. It is desirable to plug the ear against extraneous ambient sound during BC testing, but it is not desirable at the same time to affect the BC threshold. It is found that one of the new circumaural earmuffs does a superior job of insulating the ear from ambient sounds, thus allowing BC testing in otherwise unsatisfactorily noise audiometric workspaces, while at the same time creating so large a volume of air connected to the ear canal that the occlusion effect is negligible at autiometric frequencies as low as 250 Hz. It is recommended that in some audiometric workspaces such earmuffs be used for BC audiometry. (Authors' abstract)

49.
ALINIAZEE, M.T.
Oxygen toxicity in Tribolium species.
Environ. Entomol. 2(2):293-295;1973.

Studies were conducted with the adult and immature stages of T. confusum Jacquelin du Val and T. castaneum (Herbst) by exposing them to atmosphere containing 100% O_2 for varied lengths of time. Immature stages were more susceptible to O_2 poisoning than adults. Increasing exposure temperature from 15.6° to 26.7°C usually increased the susceptibility of insects, however, exceptions were noticed with the adults of T. castaneum and larvae of both species. (© BA)

50.
ALLEN, J.E., D.B.P. Goodman, A. Besaral and H. Rasmussen.
Studies on the biochemical basis of oxygen toxicity.
Biochim. Biophys. Acta 320(3):708-728;1973.

The toxic effects of high pressure O_2 on the isolated toad urinary bladder were studied. Na transport in this system is reversibly inhibited by high pressure O_2. This inhibition is potentiated by adrenal steroid hormones and occurs despite increased glycolytic and Kreb's cycle flux and tissue ATP content. High pressure O_2 leads to increased pyruvate/lactate and pyruvate/malate redox couples, as well as to a decrease in the weight percentage of phospholipid long-chain unsaturated fatty acids and [2-^{14}C] pyruvate incorporation into tissue lipid. During recovery from high pressure O_2 treatment, [2-^{14}C] Pyruvate incorporation into lipid is increased and the weight percentage of long-chain unsaturated fatty acids increases. These data indicate that high pressure O_2 poisoning in this tissue does not result from an inhibition of carbohydrate metabolism, but may result from the formation of toxic lipid peroxides. (© BA)

51.
ALLNUTT, R.B.
Deep sea simulation facilities: present status 1972.
U.S. Nav. Ship Res. Devel. Cent., Rep. NSRDC-3825, 54 p. Sept. 1972.
(AD 761 899) (Supersedes AN 751 026)

The report lists the deep sea simulation facilities presently available in the United States. It indicates the possible needs for additional facilities and gives some insight into the conditions that require updating of existing facilities. Background material on types and frequencies of failures will be helpful to those concerned with design and certification. (Author) (GRA)

52.
ALTOSE, M.D., S.G. Kensen, N.N. Stanley and N.S. Cherniack.
The effect of hypercapnia on inspiratory and expiratory muscle EMG.
Fed. Proc. 33(3,Pt.1):437;Mar. 1974.

Abstract only. Entire item quoted: To determine whether CO_2 affects inspiratory and expiratory muscles similarly, we compared the effect of progressive hypercapnia on the electromyogram (EMG) of inspiratory muscles (the diaphragm and the external intercostals) and on the EMG of an expiratory muscle (the external oblique) in 10 anesthetized dogs; the EMG was detected with surgically implanted bipolar platinum electrodes. Two aspects of the EMG were assessed: (1) the total integrated EMG per breath (E_D E_{IC} and F_{AB}) and (2) the average EMG per breath (A_D, A_{IC} and A_{AB}) determined by dividing E by the duration of the EMG burst. Progressive hypercapnia without hypoxia was produced by rebreathing 6% CO_2 in O_2. E_D and E_{IC} increased in all studies but E_{AB} increased in only 6 of the 10 animals. However, hypercapnia shortened the duration of the EMG in all muscles and the average EMG of both inspiratory and expiratory muscles regularly increased. Since tidal volume always increased with hypercapnia, vagal reflexes caused by the lung volume changes may have contributed to the increase in average EMG. The EMG effects of such vagal reflexes were separated from those of hypercapnia as follows: In 6 animals the airway was intermittently occluded during rebreathing for a single breath to prevent a lung volume change and the EMG of the occluded breath measured. In these 6 animals the average EM ; of both the inspiratory and expiratory muscle measured during occlusion rose with hypercapnia. Additionally, in 2 of 6 animals vagal section abolished all abdominal muscle electrical activity, but in the 4 remaining animals A_D, A_{IC} and A_{AB} continued to increase with hypercapnia. The results suggest that hypercapnia affects inspiratory and expiratory muscles in the same way by producing an increase of average EMG.

53.
ALVIS, H.J.
Editorial comment on decompression sickness treatment.
Hyperbaric Med. Newsletter 9:3;Jan./Feb. 1973.

The author makes four comments on the article on decompression sickness therapy by Dr. Eric P. Kindwall: (1) While more nitrogen may be dissolved into the tissues during treatment with compressed air, higher oxygen partial pressures are also present; the oxygen is probably beneficial, and the additional nitrogen is taken care of because of the slowness of the decompression. (2) It should be emphasized that the patient should never be taken to a shallower stop until his condition is stable, regardless of the time allotted on the schedule. (3) The use of oxygen to shorten the extremely long decompression schedule developed by Dr. Hempleman for treatment of decompression sickness incurred at great depth is approved. (4) Use of steroids in cases presenting CNS symptoms, and of heparin in cases of decompression shock are considered still debatable. (MFW/BSCP)

54.
ANAGNOSTAKIS, J.P. and A. Kyriakou.
The effect of breathing 100% and 10% oxygen on airway resistance.
Eur. J. Clin. Invest. 3(3):208-209;1973.

Abstract only. Entire item quoted: In 20 asthmatic or normal subjects (mean age: 12.5 years) the effect of breathing 100% and 10% oxygen on airway resistance was studied. Vital capacity, forced expiratory Volume in 1" and maximum mid-expiratory flow were measured from vitalograph records on each subject after breathing 100% oxygen, room air and 10% oxygen in nitrogen.

Table 1. Airway resistance (No. of subject)

	Decreased	Unchanged	Increased	Total
10% O_2	13	7	0	20
100% O_2	5	9	4	18

The results (table) showed that breathing 10% oxygen decreased airway resistance and that breathing 100% oxygen did not produce any change. It is not possible to conclude that this effect of 10% oxygen is due to hypoxia, since hypoxia would be expected to cause hyperventilation, which would decrease PCO_2, which itself might decrease (or increase) airway resistance. These results have produced no evidence in favour of Overholt's hypothesis that hypoxia reflexly increases airway resistance in asthmatic or normal subjects.

55.
ANDERSEN, B. and J. Madsen.
Gas permeability of the alveolo-pleural wall in the mouse lung.
Acta Physiol. Scand. 84:382-392;1972.

Transpulmonary pressure was recorded in isolated mouse lungs during and after step increases in volume. The concomitant sudden increase in transpulmonary pressure was immediately followed by a sharp pressure fall, indicative of stress relaxation. This fall passed into a less pronounced, continuing decline, which appeared to decrease monoexponentially with time. Time constants for this monoexponential pressure fall scattered between 0.005 and 0.017 min^{-1} with a tendency to highest values in small animals. In similar experiments, where the lungs were filled and surrounded with N_2, time constants were found of the same order of magnitude. In these experiments diffusion capacities for N_2 between 0.1 and 0.2 1 — min^{-1} cm H_2O^{-1} were found. The volumes of gas disappearing from the lungs per unit time and pressure were slightly larger, when the experiments were conducted in air than when done in N_2. This difference is probably due mainly to oxygen consumption by surviving lung tissue. Xe passed the alveolo-pleural wall at a rate 3 times that of N_2, while O_2 passed the wall at a rate twice that of N_2. These figures are consistent with gas diffusion through the intact lung wall. (Authors' abstract)

56.
ANDERSEN, B.G.
Test plan: operational capabilities of a manual impact wrench in an underwater environment.
Alexandria, Va., Whittenburg, Vaughan Ass., Inc., Rep. on contract N00014-70-C-0070, 5 p. May 1970.

The underwater tool performance tests described herein are the second in a series of field tests designed to provide operational performance data on the capabilities of powered and manual hand tools operating in an underwater environment, and to develop user oriented design criteria for the development of tools specifically designed to operate underwater. The initial field tests conducted as part of this research program investigated the use of pneumatic and hydraulic powered impact wrenches and conventional manual wrenches in performing a diver work task on an underwater well head assembly. The current tests will be carried out to study the feasibility of using a manual impact wrench to perform operational wrenching and torqueing tasks underwater. A second purpose of these tests will be to determine if the manual impact wrench is suitable for tightening nuts and bolts on a repetitive basis to within specific torque values. Quantitative measures of performance will be taken to determine the maximum torque value which can be achieved, to degree of accuracy with which a diver can achieve a specific torque value, and time required to operate the impact wrench. Subjective data will also be recorded with respect to ease of handling and operation, most effective operating techniques, and the ability of the tool to withstand the deleterious effects of prolonged and repeated immersions in salt water. (Author's introduction)

57.
ANDERSEN, B.G.
Human factors guide for the design of diver-operated hand and power tools.
Landover, Md., Oceanautics, Rep. 01-TR-72/2-Sk, 150 p. July 1972.

This final technical report describes the results of a research study directed toward expanding the available data base of man's ability to work underwater, by providing human factors data on man's requirements and capabilities as an undersea worker. The report is a basic human factors criteria guide for the design of diver-operated tools and work systems. Data included were developed and compiled through evaluation of operational diver work tasks, in-the-field observation of diving operations, and survey and review of existing human factors research data. The document is organized into five major sections: (1) anthropometry and biomechanics, (2) Body restraint and tethering systems, (3) Underwater visibility, (4) Control/Display criteria, and (5) Human engineering considerations for specific underwater tools. The appendix contains detailed specifications for a selected number of frequently used power tools. (Author's abstract)

58.
ANDERSEN, B.G.
Arctic III expedition: diving equipment and human performance during operations in the high Arctic.
Landover, Md., Oceanautics, Inc., Rep. 01-TR-73-1-Ch, 71 p. Mar. 1973.
(AD 759 051)

The report describes the research findings of the underwater human performance program which was conducted in the high Arctic during the Arctic III Expedition. A primary objective of the human performance program was to add to the limited body of knowledge regarding diver performance in Arctic waters. Focus of the program was an evaluation of the underwater construction of the manned underwater work station Sub-Igloo which was assembled at a depth of 40 feet in Resolute Bay. During the period of the project, ice cover over Resolute Bay was 37 inches, with a constant water temperature of 28.5F. Surface temperatures ranged between -5F and -45F., with wind velocities of up to 35 mph. The performance program also examined the effects of physiological stress on the divers working under the ice. Measures of diver ECG/heart rates and deep body temperatures were obtained using an acoustical telemetry system. An evaluation was also made of the diver and support equipment used during the expedition, including diver apparel, communications equipment, life support systems, ice cutting apparatus and portable surface structures. (Author's abstract modified by GRA)

59.
ANDERSON, G.L., G.E. Resch and X.J. Musacchia.
Hypoxia, an adjunct in helium-cold hypothermia:sparing effect on hepatic and cardiac metabolites.
Amer. J. Physiol. 224:144-147;Jan. 1973.

Depletion of carbohydrate stores has been related to hypothermic induction and survival times. Of interest in this regard is the role hypoxia may have on induction time and metabolite depletion. Induction of hypothermia (T_{re} 7 C) by the helium cold technique, i.e., with gas mixtures containing 20% of oxygen and 80% helium at T_a o-7 C, results in severe depletion of hepatic glycogen, cardiac glycogen, and cardiac norepinephrine. Reducing the oxygen tension in the induction medium to 10% oxygen results in a marked sparing of these metabolites. There appear to be at least two factors that account for the sparing effect of hypoxia. First, hypoxia reduces induction time, i.e., the time required to reduce rectal temperature from 37 to 7 C, which markedly reduces depletion of metabolites. Second, hamsters exposed simultaneously to hypoxia and cold (T_a = 0-7) exhibit a bradycardia. This slowing of the pulse apparently affords a further sparing of metabolites, viz., hamsters inducted with a hypoxic gas mixture have significantly higher metabolite levels than shaven hamsters inducted with normoxic mixtures, even though induction times in the two groups do not differ. An explanation of these results is that hypoxia limits the energy expenditure by the heart during induction. (Authors' abstract)

60.
ANDERSON, V.C.
The first twenty years of acoustic signal processing.
San Diego, Cal., Scripps Inst. Oceanog. Mar. Phys. Lab., Rep. MPL-U-69/70, 6p. May 11, 1971.
(AD 751,710)
(Also published in J. Acoust. Soc. Amer. 51(3, Pt.2):1062-1065;1972)

The decade of the 1950s marks the beginning of acoustic signal processing as a subfield of underwater acoustics. The forerunner, signal recognition, gradually evolved into a unified class of spatial and temporal processing techniques and theory which came to stand on its own. The doctrines that emerged in that decade, such as spectrum analysis, correlation, and multiple beamforming, have continued to grow in sophistication, until one now finds methods used such as the fast Fourier transform, sequential detection, and adaptive beamforming. The milestones of signal processing over the past 20 years present a striking record of progress in that field. (Author) (GRA)

61.
ANDREW, G.M., M.R. Becklake, J.S. Guleria and D.V. Bates.
Heart and lung functions in swimmers and nonathletes during growth.
J. Appl. Physiol. 32:245-251;Feb. 1972.

Lung and heart function were studied over a 3-year period in children engaged in swim training. Resting lung volumes, expiratory flow rates, and diffusing capacity (Dl) on exercise have been measured annually, and cardiac output (Qc) and related functions during graded exercise have been measured on one occasion. These results were compared with similar measurements in a group of children who were not undergoing any specific athletic training. In general, swimmers were taller at a given age and the difference between groups became greater in older children. Swimmers also had larger lung volumes (TLC) as a consequence of larger values for vital capacity, as well as higher expiratory flow rates for any given height; these differences were apparent even in the youngest swimmers. Absolute Dl was significantly higher in swimmers, a difference consistent throughout the height range studied, but the difference disappeared if Dl was expressed per unit volume of TLC. Qc in relation to VO_2 was lower in swimmers, a difference attributable to a lower heart rate, since no group difference in stroke volume was found. Although endowment may have contributed to the superior measurements in swimmers, the data do suggest that training between ages of 8 and 18 has effects on physical growth rate, as well as on heart and lung function. (Authors' abstract)

62.
ANONYMOUS
Diving simulator for simulation of a water depth of 1000 m. by Drager.
Lubeck, West Germany, Dragerwerk, Press release, n.d.

Diving and breathing apparatus can soon be tested with utmost security under similar pressure conditions to which the diver is subjected in great water depths. A novel diving simulator which is absolutely unique throughout the Federal Republic of Germany will soon be taken into operation in the diving technics centre of Dragerwerk A.G., Lubeck. This consists of a spherical steel chamber with a diameter of 2 m, which is completely filled with water and subjected to pressure. The divers enter the chamber with their novel diving apparatus, by way of a lock system. The entire system comprises another large pressure chamber which is cylindrical in shape. This has a pressure tight connection to the spherical chamber and it is comfortably equipped, since decompression periods may amount to several days, until the divers are decompressed to normal atmospheric pressures. The entire volume of the decompression chamber amounts to 11 m^3. Among other equipment it carries a complete life support system, a television device, WC, supply lock, as well as several comfortable beds. (Author)

63.
ANONYMOUS
Deep submergence systems terminology and usage.
Silver Spring, Md., Northrop Corp., Elec.-Mech. Div., Rep DSSP-TD-19-Rev-B, 77p. June 30, 1970.
(AD 750,736)

The report presents terminology and usage peculiar to the Deep Submergence Systems Project. The document is intended to serve as a reference and guide for government and contractor organizations engaged in the preparation of manuals, technical documents, drawings, and other material for DSSP. (Author) (GRA)

64.
ANONYMOUS
Novel submersible design from Dutch company.
Hydrospace 3:38-39;June 1970.

A small Dutch company is at present engaged on an ambitious programme for building submersibles, submarine crew rescue craft and diver transport vehicles. All aspects of the programme incorporate some novel design features. The company, Nereid N.V., has a six-phase programme the first part of which is the development, construction and testing of the manned Undersea Work Vehicle (UWV), the Nereid 330. . . The Nereid 300 UWV is a two-man (pilot and observer) vehicle with a depth capability of 330 ft., and is intended as a prototype vehicle on which to base a design for a 2,000 ft. vehicle. It is 29 ft. long, 11 ft. wide and 12 ft. deep and weighs 24,000 lb. in air. A feature is the deadweight to payload ratio of 24,000/5,500 lb. This is achieved by having a large seawater ballast tank. This feature means that in addition to being able to lift an object weighing 5,500 lb. from the seabed and take it to the surface the craft can also use the considerable negative buoyancy to fasten itself to a ship, submarine or the seabed and carry out heavy work. Nereid NV point out that most small submersibles have a negative buoyancy of about only 300 lb. The large payload can also be used to enable the craft to carry an extra power pack-up to 100 kWh. (Author)

65.
ANONYMOUS
SBV rethink.
Hydrospace 3:26-27;June 1970.

A very detailed drawing, showing 48 numbered parts, of the Cammell Laird Sea Bed Vehicle is presented. In the accompanying text, it is stated that the first seatrials of the vehicle were to begin in June, 1970. The main features of the design include: a two-section pressure hull with diver lookout and support to 600 feet; a sea-bed implacement mechanism employing a sinker and winch system; power and communications umbilicals from the surface; conversion of electric to hydraulic power on board, providing propulsion to the four wheels; life support for two operators and two or three divers adequate for 20 man-days of normal work, and additional 40 days in emergency. (MFW/BSCP)

66.
ANONYMOUS
Abstracts of the Twenty-fifth Congress of Physiological Sciences Satellite Symposium, Recent progress in fundamental physiology of diving, Marseille, France, July 1971.
Published by the Congress, 1971. 68p.

This symposium was made up of the following sessions: Diving bradycardia; Limiting factors in breath hold diving; Effects of pressure on living structures: physical and cellular mechanisms; Effects of increased pressure on respiration; Effects of increased pressure on performance; Inert gas exchanges; The nitrogen problem. As of the summer of 1972, the proceedings had not been made available. Abstracts were furnished through the courtesy of Dr. K.E. Schaefer. Individual abstracts will be found under the following author entries: Adolfson, J.A. and T. Berghage; Balldin, U. and C. Lundgren; Bennett, P.B.; Berghage, T.E.; Broussolle, B., E. Belnet-Bensimon, J. Chouteau, D. Bouteille and H. Burnet; Chouteau, J., R. Guillerm, J. Hee and J.C. LePechon; Chouteau, J., J.M. Ocana de Sentuary and L. Pironti; Chouteau, J., J. Parc, Y. Berry and G. Imbert; Doell, D., N.R. Anthonisen and M. Zutter; Dubois, A.A., Y. Kawakami and B.H. Natelson; Elsner, R., B.A. Goden and S.M. Robinson; Fagraeus, L.; Fructus, X., E. Agarate, J.P. Charpy, A. Gosset, R. Naquet and J.C. Rostain; Goodman, M.W. and T.E. Berghage; Greenbaum, L.J. and D.E. Evans; Hamilton, R.W., Jr. and T.D. Langley; Hills, B.A.; Hong, S.K., Y.C. Lin, D.A. Lally and T.O. Moore; Hugon, M., J. Chouteau, J.P. Roll, M. Bonnet and G. Imbert; Imbert, G., J. Chouteau, C. Roman and J. Corriol; Krekeler, H., W. Liese and G. Von Nieding; Martin, R.R., N.R. Anthonisen and M. Zutter; Miller K.W.; Moore, T.O., D.A. Lally and S.K. Hong; Muyers, K. and J. Smidt; Pilmanis, A.A. and J.P. Meehan; Proctor, L.D., C. Casey, E. Lee, H. Van Den Ende and K.E. Schaefer; Salzano, J.V., H.A. Saltzman and J.A. Kylstra; Sciarli, R., J.M. Feliciano, J. Mayol, H. Regis, C. Andrac and P. Laval; Sterk, W.; Stromme, S.B., M.W. Kalland and H.D. Meen; Van Liew, H.D.; Von Nieding, G., H. Krekeler, W. Liese and H. Oser; Vorosmarti, J., Jr., M.E. Bradley and N. Anthonisen; Yayanos, A.A.; Yokoma, T.; Zimmerman, A.M. (MFW/BSCP)

67.
ANONYMOUS
Canada lock-out sub completed.
Hydrospace 5:36;Apr. 1971.

The Canadian Armed Services diver lock-out submersible SDL-1, built by International Hydrodynamics, Vancouver, is now in service. With an operating depth of 2,000 ft. and lockout to 1,000 ft. the vehicle has maximum dimensions of 20.5 x 9.8 x 10.8 ft. and maximum reducible dimensions of 19.7 x 8.5 x 8.3 ft. Maximum weight is 28,600 lb. The HY-100 steel pressure hull consists of two spheres connected by a tunnel. The forward 7 ft. dia. sphere serves as the main control centre. The after, 5 1/2 ft. dia. sphere is used for diver lockout. The exostructure consists of tubular steel framework and glass fibre fairing. . . The life support system is based on an average mission length of 10 hours for a crew of six. Allowing for a 24-hour emergency period (ABS requirement) this totals 204 man-hours of life support. (Author)

68.
ANONYMOUS
Four men at 330 feet for a month.
Hydrospace 4:46;Aug. 1971.

The habitat to be used in the Japanese "Seatopia" project has been completed by Mitsubishi Heavy Industries, Ltd. The plan is to start saturation diving experiments at 100 feet in 1971, and to work up to a month-long sojourn for four divers at 330 feet by 1973. The complex includes a habitat, a surface support vessel, a deck decompression chamber and a personnel transfer capsule. The habitat is approximately 39 by 15 by 21 feet. It has an automatically controlled helium-oxygen heating mixture, CO_2 scrubber and charcoal filter. To maintain 30°C temperature, the pressure hull is lined with cork and fitted with six radiant heaters, the wires of which are embedded in the concrete floor. Dehumidifiers will maintain 70% or less humidity. Electric power is supplied from the support vessel, communication is by telephone with helium speech unscrambler, an electrowriter and an ultrasonic telephone link. There are four TV cameras in the habitat for monitoring purposes. (MFW/BSCP)

69.
ANONYMOUS
Hakuyo for Ocean Systems Japan.
Hydrospace 4:43;Aug. 1971.

Hakuyo has been built by Kawasaki Heavy Industries, Ltd., with the Japan Ship's Machinery Development Association. The six-ton submersible is 21 feet long, 5 feet wide and 6.5 feet deep. It has 14 viewports. The battery-driven motor has a speed of 3.5 knots and an endurance of five hours at one knot. It has a detachable hydraulic manipulator, sonar, echo sounder, underwater telephone, depth gauge, inclinometer, batometer, wireless system, flash lamp, still camera and a means for detaching the battery in an emergency. It operates to a depth of 984 feet and carries a crew of three. (MFW/BSCP)

70.
ANONYMOUS
How Shelf Diver and South Shore recovered the ELF platform.
Hydrospace 4:38-41;Oct. 1971.

A British offshore supply vessel, a French offshore contracting company and a diver lockout submersible have recently worked successfully together to recover the Elf Experimental Oscillating Platform (POE) in the Bay of Biscay and tow it back to shore. The supply vessel was the 462 grt. 1,600 hp South Shore, on charter from Cunard subsidiary Offshore Marine Ltd. to Cocean of France. The ship acted as surface support vessel to the Perry diver lockout submersible Shelf Diver which is now permanently stationed in Europe in association with Cocean. The operation involved using the submersible and a team of divers to inspect the 400 ft. high x 40 ft. dia. platform which was moored in 325 ft. of water, to disconnect it from its base plate, to tip it over to the horizontal ("de-basculing") and to tow it to La Pallice—a journey of 125 miles. (Author)

71.
ANONYMOUS
Two new submersibles.
Hydrospace 5:22;Dec. 1971.

The first of the submersibles described in this brief news item is Nekton Gamma, of General Oceanographics, Inc., recently launched at Long Beach, California. Similar to Nekton Alpha and Nekton Beta, the submersible is 15.5 feet long, weighs 2.5 tons, carries radio, voice communication equipment, sonar, magnetic compass, directional gyro, manipulator, exterior strobe and sonic tracking system. It will operate at 1000 feet, and carries a crew of two. The second is the West German Mermaid, of Bruker-Physik AG, which weighs 6.3 tons, is approximately 17 feet long, operates at 1000 feet. It has a speed of two knots, and endurance of between five and ten hours depending on battery load. (MFW/BSCP)

72.
ANONYMOUS
Underwater lighting.
Hydrospace 5:45,50;Dec. 1971.

A range of modular underwater lighting equipment has been introduced by the AquaTek Division of Electronic Control and Surveillance Ltd., UK. . . All units in the system are capable of operation wet, dry and at great depths without pressure enclosure or protection against thermal shock. Known as the AquaBeam system, the range of supporting equipment follows, wherever possible, the free-flooding trend set by the lamp and includes lampholders, reflectors, independent high power divers' lanterns, buoyancy jackets, battery recharging units, mains-fed submersible power supply units, surface power units and multiple lamp arays. Each is designed to meet specification suggested or laid down by the Ministry of Defence (Navy). The system uses 24v supply and the lamp itself can be used to 24,000 ft. without protection and can be replaced underwater. (Author)

73.
ANONYMOUS
Asthme et plongee
[Asthma and diving]
Maroc Med. 52:453-456;1972

The possible physiopathological effects of sport diving on the asthmatic subject are considered. Scuba diving is not recommended for the asthmatic. However, the effects of apnea diving on asthma and certain types of respiratory insufficiency appear clearly positive, in the author's opinion. "The most important factors are: psychic motivation, physical training, respiratory re-education, cardiovascular adaptation, and in the air on the surface of the ocean, the purity, the absence of allergens, the presence of oligo-elements and tensio-active substances." Depth is also reported to play a favorable role. (Author's conclusion and MEMH/SCD)

74.
ANONYMOUS
1972 Offshore Technology Conference, May 1-3, Houston, Texas.
Preprints, Volumes I and II. Published by the Conference, 1971, 1856 pp.

These preprints contain several papers dealing with aspects of diving technology and physiology. Specific papers will be found under the following author entries: Baccaglini, R. and J. Irgon; Bailey, V.R., J. La Cerda and J.F. Manuel; Benton, R.D., F.G. Bartlett, G.D. Bryant and H.B. Killen; Black, S.A. and R.L. Brackett; Black, S.A. and C.A. Sellars; Collipp,

B.G. and C.A. Sellars; Delauze, H.G. and A. Jejou; Long, R.W. and N.E. Smith; Myrick, J.A.; Reuter, S.H.; Schreiner, H.R., R.W. Hamilton Jr., and T.D. Langley, (MFW/BSCP)

75.
ANONYMOUS
NOAA initiates three-month Project FLARE.
Oceanol. Int. 7:13;Feb. 1972

Project FLARE (Florida aquanaut research expedition) is "intended to demonstrate the scientific value of an easily movable habitat/vessel combination." Edalhab II, built by students at the University of New Hampshire, will be used in combination with Lulu, normally Alvin's support vessel. Ten dives will be made for the purpose of collecting marine environmental data. John G. VanDerwalker of Project Tektite, and William Rainnie of Woods Hole Oceanographic Institution will be directors of the program. In addition to Edalhab II and Lulu, an undersea instrument chamber (USIC) constructed under the direction of Dr. J. Morgan Wells at the University of North Carolina. Dives will be at 50 feet, making possible the use of compressed air as the breathing mixture; excursion dives to 100 ft will be made. A limitation of five days has been put on all dives, to avoid the possible danger of oxygen toxicity. Decompression lasting 19 hrs will be carried out in a two-compartment chamber aboard Lulu; the chamber was built at the University of New Hampshire. The overall funding of the program is from NOAA's MUST (Manned undersea science and technology) program. (MFW/BSCP)

76.
ANONYMOUS
Normal speech possible at 2,000-ft depths.
Oceanol. Int. 7:43;Feb. 1972.

A helium speech unscrambler permits communication between a tender and one or two divers, and allows two divers to talk clearly to each other. The Model WP-12H Hellephone, developed by Helle Engineering, compresses the diver's voice to normal baritone range as it is translated, eliminating scrambled talk normally associated with diving gas mixtures. There is no time lag in the transmission, and every word is clear and distinct to a depth of 2000 ft. The Hellephone comes equipped with a rechargeable battery pack, built-in charger, headset with noise-cancelling boom microphone, and switch to turn off speaker. Any inexpensive speaker with an impedance of bewteen 3.2 and 16 Ω may be used as the diver's speaker microphone. (Entire item quoted.)

77.
ANONYMOUS
McDermott tests new deep-diving mini system in Gulf.
Oceanol. Int. 7:10-11;Mar. 1972.

A new deep-diving mini-habitat system, developed by J. Ray McDermott & Co. has been successfully tested in 285 feet of water in the Gulf of Mexico. The system consists of a cylindrical diving bell, two decompression chambers connected by a transfer sphere, and a control house. This system is used mainly for lowering divers to a work site, in contrast to McDermott's larger system, in which the work is done within the habitat. The diving bell can accommodate two men, and has a depth capability of 650 feet. Because of having 2 DDCs the system can handle three pairs of divers in a constantly rotating cycle. (MFW/BSCP)

78.
ANONYMOUS
Taylor Diving gets Navy salvage contract.
Oceanol. Int. 7:9-10;Mar. 1972.

The Navy has contracted with Taylor Diving and Salvage Co. for use of its diving system aboard Navy salvage vessels. A test was made to determine whether the 41-ton system could be mounted on an ARS, and if so, whether the divers could work from such an installation. The divers were first pressurized to 365 feet for 15 hours to check all systems and interfaces. Later they were compressed to 400 feet in the evening, and made the dive in the morning. The working time in the water was 90 min. Decompression took 104 hours. A unique feature of the Taylor system is that no crane is needed to lift the SDC out of the water and on to the top of the DDC. The Taylor SDC is large enough to rescue six men at one time. It has been used in conjunction with the Makai Range habitat. The Taylor diving system has a capability of 600 feet. The systems now being designed will have a depth capability of 2,000 feet. Taylor expects to accomplish this within two years. (MFW/BSCP)

79.
ANONYMOUS
Diver death inquiry verdict.
Hydrospace 5:42;Apr. 1972.

An account is given of a diver's death from air embolism. The diver disregarded the recommendation of his company to wait at least 24 hours between dives. He dove after an interval of 17 hours, and went to 250 feet, where he stayed about 40 minutes. As he entered the cage and was about to ascend, his line became fouled. He got out of the cage to disengage his line, then surfaced very rapidly because of the fact that his suit was inflated. He died shortly after being placed in the pressure chamber. It was concluded that the immediate cause of the rapid ascent was the inflation of his suit — a condition that can be controlled only by the diver himself. (MFW/BSCP)

80.
ANONYMOUS
Lockout submarine in action.
Meerestechnik 3:50;Apr. 1972.

The Perry diver lockout submersible "Shelf Diver" has completed a series of dives inspecting platforms in French and Libyan waters, in association with the French firm Cocean. This mission marked the completion of the total lockout system assembly, including the submersible, the launch and retrieval system from a 149-foot supply boat, and the deck chamber system which mates to the lockout compartment. The gas shortage sphere, with a capacity of 4500 ft^3 of premix, supplied the divers' umbilicals and also pressurized the compartment. The lights are detachable, and all tools are mounted outside the vehicle or in the lockout compartment. (MFW/BSCP)

81.
ANONYMOUS
Navy awards contract for robot research to new MIT laboratory.
ONR News Release 11-72, 2 p. Apr. 13, 1972.

An Artificial Intelligence Laboratory has been established at the Massachusetts Institute of Technology under a contract with the Office of Naval Research, with initial funding of $1 million provided by the Advanced Research Projects Agency. The immediate goal for the new laboratory is to conduct research on techniques that will endow robot-like devices with human-like learning, viewing and manipulative capabilities. It is intended that the robots will be able to survey their environment, move about in it, and also understand natural English instructions in relation to performing tasks within that environment. The robots would not only see (via television) and hear, but would also have a sense of touch. Such devices, which would be remotely controlled by computer, are expected to be able to supplant or supplement man in performing essential military tasks in hostile or stressful environments. Examples of application are deep sea exploration, bomb demolition and intelligence data collection. Work at MIT under a previous ONR contract resulted in a machine with an arm and handlike manipulator that can distinguish blocks of various sizes and shapes in sight and feel. When instructed the manipulator can pile several blocks one on top of another according to their exact order of descending size. The machine system can also interpret statements and commands even when language is used that might be ambiguous, incomplete or ungrammatical. (From author)

82.
ANONYMOUS.
Encouraging underwater developments outlined at Oceans Ontario.
Can. Petroleum 13:52-55;June 1972.

One of the recent underwater developments in Canada is the completion of a 9400-lb. submerisble with a "hinged transparent nose, nickel-cadmium batteries to give her a 15-mile operating range cruising at 2 knots plus a 50% reserve, a dual-motor propulsion system, new navigational and positioning systems working under ice, a removable conning tower and modular constructions." Other developments described at this conference include a cryogenic stainless steel diving bell, built by Foundation-Comex, to work at 1350 ft. depths; communication, power and breathing gases are supplied by two umbilicals. On board the drilling boat are two decompression chambers, equipped for saturation diving. Heat loss was prevented by electrically heated undergarments worn inside constant-volume dry suits; the garments create a thermal barrier between the diver and the water. Respiratory heat loss was prevented by a heater also designed by Comex, worn on the divers' backs and supplied by power through the umbilical. This heater maintains breathing mixture (oxygen-helium) at $37 \pm 2°C$. Recent operations by Tenneco, using this equipment, have demonstrated that work at great depths in cold water with durations of up to 120 minutes will be possible in the future. (MFW/BSCP)

83.
ANONYMOUS
Oceanology International '72: conference reports.
Underwater J. 4:98-109;June 1972.

The first session on instrumentation was concerned mainly with sensors and measurement systems, but instrumentation in submersibles was covered in a review paper by K.R. Haigh. There was a session on underwater vehicle operation, which covered manned and unmanned, tethered and free-swimming vehicles; the towed sensor equipment of Mizar was discussed, as a search and rescue technique. There were sessions dealing with industry and with purely technological, non-diver-oriented subjects. There was a session devoted to safety in underwater work, attended by eight countries. In the discussion, it was agreed that international standardization was important to achieve; warranties should be given by manufacturers; mixed gases should be used only from a submersible compression chamber with a transfer under pressure facility; one-man chambers should be used only in emergencies, where transportation to more adequate facilities may take a long time; combatting of heat loss is a serious and unsolved problem; only closed-circuit breathing apparatus should be used; Navy diving manuals are not satisfactory guides for commercial operations; individual medical and experience records of individuals should be compulsory. In the session on diving and diving technology, a paper was read on Taylor's 670m chamber complex, on the activities of Comex in developing equipment, evolving diving routines and testing decompression schedules. The problem of the safety depth limit (now tentatively set at 600 m) was discussed. The success of the German habitat Helgoland, from which diving tasks are successfully performed in cold turbid waters, was noted. In an unpresented Russian paper, the author definitely saw a higher "coefficient of relative productivity" in saturation diving as opposed to diving from the surface. New submarine escape techniques for 200 m depths were described. Dramatic improvements in helium speech unscrambling were evidenced by recordings of the ARL/Marconi unscrambler at work. Discussion of the desirability of hydrogen in deep diving breathing mixtures led to the conclusion of some that the danger of explosion outweighed its physiological advantages. (MFW/BSCP)

84.
ANONYMOUS
Oceanology International '72: exhibition review.
Underwater J. 4:92-97;June 1972.

Seventy exhibits are briefly described, and the addresses of the manufacturers are given. Ten countries were represented, with the host country, the United Kingdom, having by far the greatest number of exhibits (35). The countries next in line were West Germany (nine), and France and the United States with seven each. Comex exhibited new diving equipment; Drass, Italy, exhibited simulated diving systems for training and testing divers; Emerson and Cuming, Inc., USA, exhibited new material for diving suits; Galeazzi, Italy, exhibited a one-man recompression chamber and a saturation diving system; Kawasaki, Japan, exhibited a three-man submersible; Rolex, UK, a new underwater watch; Slingsby Sailplanes, UK, a lightweight buoyancy material and a submersible of glass reinforced plastic; Strongwork, UK, a new diving system; Underwater Security, UK has developed an underwater training and equipment center; Maschinenblau Gabler, West Germany, two submersibles; Partech, UK, a diving school; Dragerwerk, West Germany, a wide range of diving equipment; Thomson-CSF, France, hand-held sonars and underwater television and telephones; Laird, UK, a ten-man compression chamber; Dornier, West Germany, an unmanned submersible; Deutsche Babcock and Wilcox Aktiegesellschaft, West Germany, recompression chambers and deep diving systems; ACB, France, manipulators for handling of radioactive materials, for use on submersibles or habitats; Graseby Instruments, UK, a diver-to-diver communication set; Fort Bovisand, UK, training in underwater techniques; Bauer, West Germany, compressors; Bruker, West Germany, a battery-operated submersible; Marconi Space and Defence Systems, a helium speech converter as well as oceanographic equipment; Siebe Gorman, UK, a wide range of diving equipment; Flip Schulke Enterprises, Inc., diving accessories and photographic equipment; Nereid NV, the Netherlands, submersibles and habitats. (MFW/BSCP).

85.
ANONYMOUS
Performance factors in underwater environment.
Def. Doc. Cent., Rep. DDC-TAS-72-42, 193p. Aug. 1972.
(AD-748 000)

The 156 references in this bibliography include information on the effects of underwater environment on divers, on tools and equipment, and on human factors aspects of underwater performance. Corporate Author-Monitoring Agency and Subject Indexes are included. (Author) (GRA)

86.
ANONYMOUS
World's first permanent underwater wellhead chamber is installed.
Offshore 32:32-33;Aug. 1972.

World's first permanent, underwater wellhead chamber has been installed on a "live" oil well in the Gulf of Mexico. Installation of the 30-foot tall, 10-foot diameter steel chamber was made in a record 375 feet of water offshore Louisiana by Shell Oil Company and Lockheed Petroleum Services Ltd. of Vancouver, Canada. The chamber, positioned atop a well recently drilled by Shell, will permit oilmen to work in a dry, normal atmospheric environment on the ocean floor. It contains wellhead valves and equipment which will be assembled into a conventional wellhead "Christmas tree" later this summer. Completion of the Shell well will be accomplished at that time in the wellhead chamber through use of a manned service capsule, developed by Lockheed. This capsule also operates under normal atmospheric pressure and will carry a crew of up to four workmen from the surface to the wellhead chamber. (Author)

87.
ANONYMOUS
Puerto Rico International Undersea Laboratory.
Undersea Technol. 13:35-37;Sept. 1972.

Perry Oceanographics, Inc., has completed a habitat for the Puerto Rico International Undersea Laboratory (PRINUL). Based on the concept of Tektite, the habitat, "La Chalupa" will house "the biggest continuing undersea program ever undertaken, as well as being first full-fledged computer equipped undersea laboratory representing a generation state-of-the-art leap over Tektite." The habitat consists of two cylinders, 20 feet long by 8 feet in diameter, mounted inside an airtight barge, with a 9-ft wet room, thus making the unit buoyant and easily towed. It will support four saturated divers, and has its own decompression chamber. The habitat will be raised at the end of each mission and towed to shore with the divers in the pressure chamber. There the decompression will be carried out under medical supervision. Support is from an unmanned craft, via umbilical. A wet submersible, Reef Hunter, will be carried in the wet room and used for diver transport. (MFW/BSCP)

88.
ANONYMOUS
Unmanned Arctic research submersible successfully tested by Navy.
Nav. Res. Rev. 25:31;Sept. 1972.

An Unmanned Arctic Research Submarine (UARS) has been successfully tested by the Navy under Arctic ice. Special ice-cutting techniques have been developed to make it possible to launch the vehicle, which is later retrieved through the hole by a net. The remote-controlled sub has a fiberglass hull, a speed of three knots, endurance of ten hours, a range of 9000 feet and a depth capability of 1500 feet. It is equipped with an acoustic command control subsystem for navigation and data telemetry. During the tests, an under ice profile of a one-mile diameter area was made. The UARS can be fitted with instrumentation that will enable it to carry out surveys which previously could have been done only by fleet submarines or divers. (MFW/BSCP)

89.
ANONYMOUS
DSRV-2
Nav. Res. Rev. 25:32-33;Oct. 1972.

DSRV-2 is the second Deep Submergence Rescue Vehicle completed and successfully tested by the Navy. It has been submerged to a depth of 5,280 feet, although its operating depth is considered to be 3,500 feet. It is 49 feet long, 8 feet in diameter and propelled by electric motors and batteries. The outer hull is made of fiberglass; three interconnected spheres of HY-140 steel form the manned pressure capsule. The forward sphere contains the control equipment and two crew members; the two other spheres can accommodate 24 passengers and another crewman. The DSRV-2 will be available for international emergencies. Information as to modifications that will enable any submarine in the world to be aided by the DSRV is readily available to all nations. (MFW/BSCP)

90.
ANONYMOUS
Hypoxia, gas narcosis and metabolic response to argon and nitrous oxide.
Cincinnati, O., Cincinnati Univ., Rep. on contract NGR-06-002-075 (NASA CR 133214), 55 p. Oct. 31, 1972.
(N73 25120)

Studies of the mechanism of inert gas influence on metabolism are reported. The studies reported include: metabolic response of hamsters to argon and nitrous oxide, membrane fatty acids and susceptibility to narcotic gas influence, narcosis induced histotoxic hypoxia, biochemical study of inert gas narcosis, hypoxia-induced protection against cardiovascular deterioration in the weightless state, and acute metabolic and physiologic response of goats to narcosis. (FOS) (STAR)

91.
ANONYMOUS
Navy successfully tests large object salvage system.
Nav. Res. Rev. 25:28-29;Oct. 1972.

The Navy has recently completed three weeks of successful open sea testing of a newly developed Large Object Salvage System (LOSS) which lifted a 100-ton object from 100 feet of water in the Gulf of Mexico off Panama City, Florida. Termed "LOSS" the system now consists of a large pontoon which is lowered over the sunken object, attaches arms to the object by firing explosive studs and through new buoyant gas generating techniques raises the object to the surface. The latter two steps are accomplished by remote control, from a surface support ship. When development is complete, LOSS will have a self-positioning pontoon and, through use of multiple pontoons, will be albe to lift aircraft and medium hull ships from depths of 1000 feet. Presently a single pontoon can lift 100 tons. Though divers are now required to attach guidelines from the support ship to the pontoon to the sunken object, the completed system will eliminate use of divers. (Author)

92.
ANONYMOUS
New diving system for Sedco-135F.
Offshore Serv., p. 33; Oct. 1972.

A diving system developed by K.D. Marine Ltd., UK, is briefly described. The entire system weighs over 40 tons and is transportable from rig to rig. After a dive the 7-ton bell is winched up then lowered onto a trolley which carries it to a position over the transfer lock, through which the divers pass to the deck decompression chamber. The system also includes a control unit, an oxygen-helium mixing system, and remote underwater TV systems. (MFW/BSCP)

93.
ANONYMOUS
Table ronde sur "La therapeutique de la maladie de la decompression."
[Round table on "Therapy of decompression sickness"].
Bull. Medsubhyp 7:37-44;Oct. 1972.

This paper consists of a summary of a discussion by Drs. Chouteau, Du Cailar, Maestracci, Ohresser, and Michaud, moderated by Dr. Joly, dealing primarily with the treatment of Type II decompression sickness. Recompression in pure oxygen for such cases is recommended, because of its additional efficacy in denitrogenation, and its ability to supply oxygen to ischemic, weakly vascularized tissues. Twelve cases presenting such symptoms as motor function disruption, sensory disorders, and even convulsions, were successfully treated in this manner; some were subjected to as many as 28 compressions. (Dr. Du Cailar). In any type of decompression accident, the breathing of normobaric oxygen during transportation to a therapeutic chamber, and the simultaneous administration of Rheomacrodex, Hydergine, and corticoids is recommended. Speed in administering recompression is imperative when central nervous system symptoms are present; Dextran of low molecular weight, injectable aspirin, and heparin are recommended, in addition to the previously mentioned drugs. (Dr. Maestracci). A brief mention is made of pulmonary barotrauma, frequently indistinguishable in its symptoms from decompression accidents; even the most severe cases generally respond to recompression and hyperoxygenation. Because of the increasing frequency of dives at depths of more than 40m, the incidence of Type II decompression sickness is becoming much greater. If it is impossible to recompress immediately, an autonomous illness sets in regardless of the fact that the bubbles have been dissolved. For this illness, which presents vasomotor and edematous symptoms, no effective treatment exists at present. In this connection, the need for numerous and widespread monoplace chambers is urged; however, cases presenting unconsciousness or respiratory difficulties should preferably be transported, under normobaric oxygen, to a multiplace chamber. It is noted that really inexplicable decompression accidents are rare, and are probably due to some physical idiosyncracy. Some brief comments are made regarding the modification of therapeutic recompression-decompression schedules, with reference to both American and French methods. (Dr. Michaud) (MFW/BSCP)

94.
ANONYMOUS
Transceiver ends "helium speech".
Electronics, p.55;Nov. 6, 1972.

The West German AEG-Telefunken laboratories have developed a small inexpensive unit that renders helium speech as intelligible as telephone speech. The equipment "uses delta pulse-code modulation, where only the difference values between two subsequent signals are processed, obviating the need to handle individual signal content as a whole. The difference values are quantized and coded before transmission." It is claimed that the finished product will be reduced to the size of a cigarette pack. (MFW/BSCP)

95.
ANONYMOUS
U.S. and French submersibles to explore mid-Atlantic depths.
Nav. Res. Rev. 25:30-32;Nov. 1972.

Deep diving research submersibles from France and the United States will plumb the depths of the mid-Atlantic Ocean for the first time, in a three-year international scientific program announced today by the Commerce Department's National Oceanic and Atmospheric Administration (NOAA) and the Woods Hole Oceanographic Institution (WHOI). . . Following two years of site surveys and training, a fleet will assemble at the site selected, in the summer of 1974. The French bathyscaphe Archimede and French submersible SP-3000, the American submersible Alvin and four surface ships will carry out the most extensive deep ocean manned submersible study ever undertaken. Some 40 dives will be made at that time, with special missions for each submersible. The submersibles will do detailed mapping of the area, collect special bottom samples and place instruments on the seafloor. Each of the deep-diving research vehicles will have special assignments to make best use of their differing capabilities. The SP-3000 which has a high degree of maneuverability will be used for rapid visual reconnaissance and for studies within the rift valley of the midocean range. Archimede, a bathyscaphe designed for maximum depths and heavy payloads, but in relatively gentle terrain, will explore the fracture zones of the seafloor. The highly maneuverable Alvin, owned by the Office of Naval Research and operated by WHOI will explore both terrains as well as the rift valley wall. (Author)

96.
ANONYMOUS
1973 Offshore Technology Conference, April/May 1973, Houston, Texas. Preprints, Volumes I and II.
Published by the conference, 1973.

Papers dealing with diving physiology or technology will be found under the following author entries: Aaron, A.L., Jr.; Adams, J.R., J.F. Manuel and Roger W. Cook; Agarate, C.A. and A.J. Jegou; Corwin, R.F. and U. Conti; Davidson, A.R., Jr. and L.E. Lesster; Haye, E.F.; Haynes, H.H.; LePage, A. and Peter Wide; Lewis, J.W.; Munton, S.V. and J.R. Buck; Nuytten, P.; Polvani, D.G.; Sheffield, J.R. and R.A. Masonheimer; Sherwood, W.G. (MFW/SCD)

97.
ANONYMOUS
New 300 m diving system under construction.
Underwater J. 5:3;Feb. 1973.

Oceaneering International, Inc., has recently contracted to the Continental Oil Company to provide diving support to depths of 300 m for the 1973 drilling programme in the North Sea. The 300 m saturation diving complex will allow divers to live for days, or even weeks at a time, under pressure as did the aquanauts in the US Navy Sea Lab programme. The living chambers will be equipped with hot showers, sanitary facilities, a library, a dining area, and even piped music. The saturation complex is made up of a 1.67 m diameter spherical diving bell which is used to transport divers to the underwater site and back, two 2.4 m diameter living chambers, and a back-up chamber which can be used to evacuate pressurized divers from the rig should the need arise. (Author)

98.
ANONYMOUS
Navy submersible pot bubbling.
UnderSea Technol. 14:37;Mar. 1973.

Although the NRZ and the Deep Submergence Search Vehicle (DSSV) with a 20,000 foot depth capability will not be funded in 1974, component development for 20,000 foot depths continues under the Advanced Development Submersible-2 (ADS-20) program. An authoritative book on submersible development since 1960 is being written under the sponsorship of the Naval Oceanographic Office. SUBTRAP, the Submersible Training Platform, is now in operation. It is towed at a depth of 100 feet, and is used in diver training. Alvin is being improved; Beaver Mk IV may be given an emergency rescue capability. (MFW/BSCP)

99.
ANONYMOUS
1000-foot experimental dives completed at Duke University.
UnderSea Technol. 14:13, 16;Mar. 1973.

The divers made five 1000-foot excursion dives from a saturated depth of 870 feet, over a period of four days. The water into which they made the excursions from the chamber was of freezing temperature. Performance and physiological experiments were carried out while the divers were submerged. Some of the objectives of the various groups participating in this dive were: to evaluate performance under conditions similar to cold water oil field diving; to complete training in the use of saturation diving equipment and techniques; to develop the capability for scientists to work under these conditions from lockout submersibles and to study problems related to helium speech. Tests were made to learn more about hpns. Measurements were made of manual dexterity, mental function, and physical work capability. Heart rates, respiratory rates, core temperatures and other parameters were measured, with satisfactory results. The new equipment, developed by Oceaneering International, included a deep-water fiberglass diving helmet, and a breathing gas heater. This equipment will be used with the new Oceaneer 1000 saturation diving system in the North Sea this summer. (MFW/BSCP)

100.
ANONYMOUS
Nitrogen-oxygen saturated excursion dive tables produced.
UnderSea Technol. 14:11;Apr. 1973.

Entire item quoted: A somehow neglected area of diving decompression tables is being filled in. Diving scientists, living saturated in oxygen-nitrogen mixtures in habitats on the continental shelf, like to make excursion, or bounce, dives to greater depths. Until now they have had no tables to tell them how long they can stay deeper without decompression stops or how long to decompress at what levels if they stay too long. The Navy and commercial companies developed such tables for helium-oxygen atmospheres for use at greater depths from 300 to 1000 feet. A series of dry chamber dives made by divers of Ocean Systems, Inc., led by Craig Jennings, at the company's research facility at Tarrytown, N.Y. has produced the tables. The work was done under a contract for $74,712 let by the Manned Undersea Science and Technology (MUS&T) office of the National Oceanic and Atmospheric Administration (NOAA). Principal investigator was Dr. R. William Hamilton, a physiologist, working under laboratory director Dr. Heinz Schreiner. Downward dives were made from 30 feet and downward and upward dives from 60, 90 and 120 feet. Maximum bounces were made to 250 feet from 90 and 120 feet. It was discovered, for instance, that a diver could go from 100 to 200 feet for 135 minutes without the need for a decompression stop on the way back. Practical tests are being conducted this month at the Puerto Rico National Underwater Laboratory (PRINUL) by a five man team led by Dr. James Miller of MUS&T and Ian Koblick of PRINUL.

101.
ANONYMOUS
Survey of ocean waste-disposal sites by manned submersible.
Meerestechnik 4:58;Apr. 1973.

An inspection of three sites was made recently [Southern California ocean dumping] for NOAA, using the submersible 'Deep Quest'. . . Direct observation by submersible can provide valuable results that would otherwise be difficult or impossible to obtain using surface techniques. . . For the ocean dumping dives, 'Deep Quest' was fitted with film cameras, a salinity/temperature/depth measuring system manufactured by Plessey Environmental Systems, a transmissometer, a six-core sampler, and a multirosette water sampler supplied by the General Oceanics Company. . . 'Deep Quest', which has descended to 8310 ft is owned by the Lockheed Missiles and Space Company and operated by Lockheed Ocean Laboratory, San Diego. (Author)

102.
ANONYMOUS
Navy initiates diving program using hydrogen as breathing gas.
Off. Nav. Res. News Release 3/73, 3p. May 7, 1973.

This news release describes briefly Project Hydrox II, which is a series of dives made for the purpose of studying the characteristics of hydrogen as a breathing gas. The series consists of eight dives using hydrogen, eight using helium, and eight using nitrogen. Special decompression tables for the hydrogen dives have been calculated. The costliness of helium, its greater density, and the possibility that its use contributes to hpns, are among the reasons for considering the possibility of substituting hydrogen as a breathing gas for deep diving. (MFW/BSCP)

103.
ANONYMOUS
Drowning and the diving reflex.
Can Med. As. J. 108:1209;May 19, 1973.

In this editorial, the author reviews briefly some of the literature on the diving reflex in marine mammals such as seals, and the similar but less pronounced cardiovascular responses that occur in man. It has been observed in man that blood flow in the arm and leg, while the subject is undergoing face immersion diminish to an extremely marked degree, thus indicating that the reason for the cardiovascular reflex is the conservation of oxygen for the heart and brain. These findings are important in relation to cases of near drowning, in which an individual may have cyanotic limbs and appear to be dead, and still have a supply of oxygen available to heart and brain. In such cases, the carotid pulse or the pupillary reactions must serve as guides to the state of the central circulation, and vigorous efforts must be made to revive the apparently drowned. (MFW/SCD)

104.
ANONYMOUS
Perry completes new super-submarine.
Offshore 33:148;May 1973.

A new "super submarine," having a transparent nose and able to lock out divers for seabottom work-tasks, has been completed for use primarily in offshore petroleum operations. The submarine, originally called PC-15 and rechristened VOL 1, was built in Florida by Perry Oceanographics, Inc., for Vickers Oceanics Ltd. of Great Britain, which will use the sub initially in the North Sea. The submarine is of modular construction. With it was built a deck decompression chamber complex capable of simulating depths of 1,200 ft. (Author)

105.
ANONYMOUS
Bones problem.
Skin Diver 22:56;June 1973.

Entire item quoted: Divers who spend a lot of time underwater for long periods tend to develop bone disorders says Dr. Hiroshi Hayashi (chief of high pressure medical treatment research division of Kyushu Labor Accident Hospital). According to Ocean Science News, 135 divers were studied; 72 had abnormalities with 25 suffering osteonecrosis, 47 others unknowingly had calcification of thigh bones and upper arms. Hyashi found the abnormalities to be related to depths. Those working less than 10 meters down didn't suffer, 12% at 20 to 30 meters were affected, 14% were affected below 30 meters and 43% were affected at depths of more than 51 meters. The osteonecrosis was thought to occur due to too-rapid ascents (not necessarily causing bends, but nitrogen bubbles all the same).

106.
ANONYMOUS
Bone-wasting dives.
Med. World News 14:17-18;July 13, 1973.

The general discussion of osteonecrosis resulting from diving or compressed air work starts with an account of the very inadequate decompression methods employed in the sewer tunnels of Milwaukee. Dr. Eric Kindwall discovered, by means of X-ray, that these workers had a 41% incidence of osteonecrosis as a result of too-rapid decompression. The most generally accepted theory of the etiology of osteonecrosis — lack of blood supply to the bone caused by bubbles, is presented. Case histories are cited which indicate the disease can follow brief exposure, minimal repetitions and moderate pressure and need not be related to a history of decompression sickness. Recent surveys in the U.S. Navy, following similar surveys in the British Navy, have revealed a surprisingly high incidence of osteonecrosis. Although the study has just begun, 76 cases have been discovered, in the majority of which joints were affected. The insurance aspects of the problem are discussed, and the high cost to the diving industry is noted. It is most essential that divers and compressed air workers should be X-rayed before being taken on a job, and the X-rays should be read by a radiologist trained in the detection of early signs of osteonecrosis. (MFW/SCD)

107.
ANONYMOUS
50-Ft. reinforced epoxy vehicle carries acoustic test equipment.
Sea Technol. 14:23;Aug. 1973.

The Shamu, a unique epoxy underwater test vehicle named for the killer whale it resembles, was recently used by the Navy to successfully test the ability of an acoustic lens to pick up the sound of distant subs. The vehicle, thought to be the largest marine vehicle made of epoxy, simulates a submarine's movement without the associated noise. Marine experts generally agree that the successful evaluation of the lens was possible largely because of the epoxy test vehicle which had to be extremely buoyant and have acoustical properties close to those of water so the sound signals would not be distorted as they traveled through the material. (Author)

108.
ANONYMOUS
Submarine escape and rescue.
Alexandria, Va., Def. Doc. Cent., Rep. DDC-TAS-73-39, 52 p. Aug. 1973.
(AD 764 950/2)

The bibliography comprises citations of unclassified reports dealing with submarine escape and rescue, deep submergence vessels, search techniques and exploration. The following references are on some of the topics dealing with the subject: submarine escape, sea rescue, submarine personnel, naval training, underwater vehicles, and sea rescue equipment. (GRA)

109.
ANONYMOUS
Diving decompression data.
Pressure Med. Physiol. 2 (Spec. Insert 2):1-4;Sept./Oct. 1973.

The Decompression Data Bank Committee of The Undersea Medical Society presents summaries of the scope and function of 13 data centers. They are: The Integrated Diving Computation System, of Ocean Systems, Inc; The U.S. Air Force School of Aerospace Medicine at Brooks Air Force Base record of hyperbaric chamber treatment in U.S. Air Force facilities; Canadian Diving Data (decompression information); National Underwater Accidents Data Center at the University of California at Davis (human physical performance under environmental stress); Naval Safety Center, Norfolk, Va. (hyperbaric chamber exposures and associated accidents or injuries); International Diving Accident Reporting System, NAVI headquarters, Grand Terrace, California (statistical analysis of safety improvements in recreational diving); Directory of World-wide Shore-based Hyperbaric Chambers, Naval Ships Systems Command (to be updated annually); Diver Equipment Information Center, Battelle Columbus Laboratories; Computerized Diving Literature File, U.S. Navy Experimental Diving Unit; International Decompression Data Bank at the Institute for Environmental Medicine, University of Pennsylvania (experimental decompression studies, human and animal); Bibliographical Material on Diving and Submarine Medicine (semi-monthly abstracting service, published biennially in book form, formerly under the George Washington University Medical Center and now under The Undersea Medical Society); Decompression Sickness Central Registry, Newcastle-upon-Tyne, United Kingdom (principally devoted to data on compressed air workers with emphasis on radiological data on osteonecrosis); in recent years, commercial divers have been included (MFW/UMS)

110.
ANONYMOUS
COMEX 620 ft. North Sea dive profile.
Offshore Services 6:18;Oct. 1973.

Further details are given regarding the 621 ft. saturation dive made by COMEX in the North Sea on 10 September 1973. The dive was one of a series of proving dives for a 1000 ft. diving system. The divers were pressurized slowly to their living depth in the deck decompression chamber (DDC). Working depth was 30 feet below living depth. Water temperature was 10°C (50°F), but temperature control was adequately maintained by means of heating in the bell (type of heat not specified) plus electrically heated diving suits and breathing gas. After 30 minutes work, the diver returned to the bell, where he was decompressed to living depth, then transferred to the DDC for hot shower and food. The same operation was repeated, with one of the other divers in the water. Following the second dive, decompression to surface in the DDC took 3½ days. The type of bell used has an internal volume of 160 ft^3 and 8 ft of headroom. Entry and exit through the bottom is facilitated by 2 ft. 7 in. trunking. (MFW/SCD)

111.
ANONYMOUS
New TV sled.
Offshore Services 6:34;Oct. 1973.

At the interocean 73 Exhibition in Dusseldorf (November 13-18) IBAK, Kiel, are showing, for the first time in Germany, a deep sea photo and TV towing system (TFF) which will be used in 1974 on a German expedition to explore for manganese nodules in the Pacific. Trials of the TFF system have already taken place on the research vessel Valdivia off Hawaii. The development of the system was sponsored by the German Federal Ministry for Research and Technology. The system will allow systematic mapping of nodule deposits to depths of 6000m. It keeps a constant, pre-fixed distance from the seabed and the TV picture content is analyzed automatically, with results being fed into a computer, along with positioning data. Towing speeds up to six knots are planned, and impulse lights, as used in high speed photography, will reduce blur. (Author)

112.
ANONYMOUS
Wireless diver communication (Subcom 130).
Underwater J. 5:235;Oct. 1973.

The Subcom 130 is wireless, and intended primarily for free swimming divers, but can be used as 'back-up' with umbilical systems, especially in critical diving operations, where communications are essential. It can be used with most self-contained diving equipment as well as modern lightweight surface supplied systems. Any number of units can be used together for diver to diver, and diver to surface communication. Operation is on an acoustic principle with "Single Sideband Suppressed Carrier" modulation. The self-contained, battery power-supplies in the surface and diver sets make the units easily portable, regardless of boat size or diver platform configuration. The power supplies provide up to 15 hours of normal operation between battery recharges on the diver unit. The Subcom 130 is designed for medium range diver communication (in excess of 500 ft under normal conditions), but will operate over greater distances under favourable conditions. (Author)

113.
ANONYMOUS
Drug used to treat alcoholism may allow divers greater use of oxygen.
Off. Nav. Res., News release ONR 15-73;Nov. 23, 1973.

Disulfiram, also known as Antabuse, has been found to delay onset of both pulmonary and CNS forms of oxygen toxicity. Protection varies with different species and different strains. It is not known whether similar protection would exist for humans, nor is it known whether or not the large doses of disulfiram required to give protection might in themselves have toxic effects. If it is found feasible to use the drug on divers undergoing decompression, decompression time would be considerably shortened by the increase of the tolerance to oxygen, since oxygen breathing during decompression is known to speed up the removal of inert gas from tissues. (MFW/SCD)

114.
ANONYMOUS
New technology report.
Berkeley, Cal., Andros Inc., Rep. on Contract N00014-73-0185, 15p. Nov. 1, 1973.
(AD-769,133/OGA)

The report discusses work concerned with demonstrating the feasibility of using a gas density modulation technique to determine the concentration of CO_2 in hyperbaric gaseous environments, in which the total pressure could range between 15 and 1200 psia. This was done by subjecting a sample of gas to a constant fractional change in volume, and measuring the fractional change in the infrared radiation transmitted through the sample. (GRA)

115.
ANONYMOUS
Man-in-the-sea project in North Dakota.
Nav. Res. Rev. 26:10-14;Dec. 1973.

This facility at the University of North Dakota, supported by The Office of Naval Research, consists primarily of two seven-foot spheres, each of which is surrounded by seven small animal chambers. The animals can be transferred to the main spheres while under constant pressure, so that the small chambers can be decompressed, cleaned, and resupplied. The pressure capacity is equal to 1300 fsw. The facility was five years in the building, but during this time, research was carried out as various components came into being. Among areas of investigation have been the toxic effects of inert gas breathing mixtures, and various pressure effects such as modification of brain wave patterns during decompression, change in eye movements brought on by vertigo, and the learning behavior of small rodents. Other areas of study are nutrition, thermal balance, and microbiological changes brought on by the hyperbaric environment. Most of the experiments have been of short duration, but now that the facility is complete, studies of six weeks to two years are planned. (MFW/UMS)

116.
ANTANOVICH, A.A. and M.A. Plotnikov.
Apparatus used for the experimental study of the thermodynamic properties of gases at pressures of up to 10-12 kilobars and at temperatures up to 3000K.
In: Thermophysical properties of gases, p. 156-159. 1970. Translation, Wright-Patterson AFB, Foreign Technology Division, Rep. FTD-HT-23-1266-72, 11 p. Aug. 30, 1972.
(AD 749 653)

Special apparatus has been developed for the study of the thermodynamic properties of gases at high temperatures. The apparatus consists of a thick walled power cylinder with internal pressure amounting to 10-12 kilobars. Channels of a water cooling system are located in the power cylinder wall. The internal space of the thermal chamber is heated by an electric coil on which short ceramic tubes have been placed. A pyrolitic graphite bushing is used. (Author) (GRA)

117.
ANTONOV, I.I.
O pushkovykh i neir okhimicheskikh mekhanizmakh termor equliastsii v usloviiakh giperoksii.
[Triggering and neurochemical mechanisms of thermoregulation under conditions of hyperoxia].
Dokl. Akad. Nauk. SSR 199:245-247;July 1, 1971.

Experiments on intact rabbits exposed to hyperoxia under increased ambient pressures showed temperature increases in various sections of the cerebrum during the initial four to five minutes of exposure, follcwed by temperature decreases in the cortical and subcortical formations at later stages of the exposure period. In rabbits with inactivated respiratory tract acceptors these temperature reactions had similar but slower developing trends. (Aerosp. Med.)

118.
ANTOPOL, W. and C.P. Chryssanthou.
Experimental production of aseptic bone necrosis in mice.
In: Aerospace Medical Association. 1972 annual scientific meeting, Bal Harbour, Florida, May 1972. Preprints, p. 255-256. Published by the Association.

The findings of this preliminary investigation reveal that exposure to compression-decompression produces aseptic bone necrosis in thin mice and increases the incidence of this lesion in the obese animals. The former observation suggests that development of aseptic bone necrosis after exposure to compression-decompression is independent of decompression sickness since thin mice are not "susceptible" to this disease. Supporting this hypothesis is the fact that PPCH and bradykinin, which were previously reported to influence the incidence and severity of decompression sickness in obese mice did not alter the frequency of aseptic bone necrosis in the present investigation. The occurrence of necrotic bone alterations in control obese mice may indicate that this species is subject to the lesion *ab initio* and exposure to compression-decompression precipitates aseptic bone necrosis in these predisposed animals. This study also indicates that the bone lesion is manifest after a latent period of at least five months following the initial treatment, and that with multiple exposures to compression-decompression the incidence is greater than with single exposure. (From author's discussion).

119.
APPAIX, A. and F. Demard.
Notre experience des complications O.R.L. au cours de la therapeutique hyperbare.
[Our experience of ENT complications in hyperbaric therapy].
In: Fructus, X., ed. Third international conference on hyperbaric and underwater physiology p. 178-181. Paris, Doin, 1972.

The authors report on the nature and frequency of ENT complications of hyperbaric oxygen therapy in 495 patients treated over the past seven years. These patients were treated for cardiovascular conditions, injuries, and ophthalmologic and dermatologic diseases. Patients undergoing hyperbaric therapy for ENT conditions were excluded from the study. An overall incidence of 9% (44 cases) of ENT complications was noted; most of these involved the middle ear. Of these complications, however, only 11 could be considered serious, leading to cessation of hyperbaric therapy. The use of the transtympanic drain in the treatment of these complications is recommended. (MEMH/UMS).

120.
APPAIX, A. and F. Demard.
Etude audiometrique et electro-nystagmographique chez l'homme normal — en plongee tres profonde.
[Audiometric and electronystagmographic study in normal man during very deep diving].
Acta Otolaryng. (Stockholm) 73:141-147;Feb./Mar. 1972.

The auditory and vestibular functions of four divers, previously selected and tested, were examined. The auditory study showed, at different pressures, an elevation of the airway thresholds; bone conduction remained unchanged. The vestibular examination with ENG [electronystagmogram] remained normal. Comprehension difficulties related to phonetic disturbances were eliminated thanks to the utilization of a vocodar (Bathyphone IBM). (Author's abstract translated by MFW/BSCP)

121.
APRIGLIANO, L.F. and C.A. Zanis.
Diffusion bonding of alloy titanium for pressure hull fabrication.
U.S. Nav. Ship Res Devel. Cent., Rep. NSRDC-4177, NSRDC-28-787, 33p. Nov. 1973.
(AD 770,128/7GA)

A diffusion bonding investigation of alph-beta forged and alpha-beta rolled Ti-6A1-2Cb-1Ta-0.8Mo alloy titanium was undertaken as a first step in determining the feasibility of using out-of-chamber diffusion bonding for pressure hull fabrication. It was found that the mill processing history significantly affected the parameters necessary for bonding. The higher creep rate of the rolled material was primarily responsible for obtaining quality bonding at lower temperatures. It was also found that a total sample compression of more than 0.7% was necessary to obtain quality diffusion bonds. (Modified author abstract) (GRA)

123.
ARBORELIUS, M. Jr., U.I. Balldin, B. Lilja and C.E.G. Lundgren.
Hemodynamic changes in man during immersion with the head above water.
Aerosp. Med. 43:592-598;June 1972.

Cardiac output (dye dilution method) right atrial and brachial arterial pressures were recorded in ten subjects sitting in neutral temperatures in air (28°C) or immersed with the head above water (35°C). Measurements were made both during air and oxygen breathing. In three air breathing subjects the central blood volume and the pulmonary arterial pressure were also measured. During immersion and air breathing, cardiac output increased by 1.8 l/min or 32% and stroke volume by 26 ml or 35%, while heart rate was almost unchanged. Right atrial and pulmonary arterial transmural pressure gradients increased in the immersed subjects by about 13 mm Hg. Systemic vascular resistance decreased by 30%. The central blood volume increased during immersion by about 0.7 l. Extra systoles were sometimes seen during the first minutes of immersion. The relative changes in circulatory parameters measured during air and oxygen breathing were essentially the same. (Authors' abstract)

124.
ARDASHNIKOVA, L.I. and G.N. Evstropova.
On the circulation in man at muscular work under hyperbaric conditions.
In: Hesser, C.M. and D. Linnarsson eds. Proceedings of the first annual scientific meeting of the European Undersea Biomedical Society, Stockholm, 13-15 June 1973. Forsvarsmedicin 9:337-345;July 1973.

In men staying during 7 days at 5 ATA in N_2-O_2 medium (N_2 =4.5 ATA=0.5 ATA) in resting state the ECG data showed bradycardia, increase in systolic index, increase in systolic index, increase in amplitude of the P-wave; according to rheographic data there arose changes in regulation of the peripheral vascular tone. Under these conditions at work in most cases there occurred an increase in heart rate. The increase in pulsatory blood flow and the systolic index were more pronounced than at work under normal conditions. In some subjects electrocardiographic and rheographic indications of the increase in pulmonary vascular resistance were observed. The role of various factors in circulatory changes in hyperbaria is discussed. (Authors' summary)

125.
ARDISSON, J.L., C. Dolisi and M. Gastaud.
Les effets ventilatoires de l'hyperoxie normobare.
[The respiratory effects of increased oxygen concentrations at normal atmospheric pressure].
Pathol. Biol. 20(3/4):195-203;1972.

A review of all work published since 1945 on the respiratory effects of inhalation of pure O_2 at normal atmospheric pressure is given. In healthy man, there is an immediate brief hypo-ventilation followed, in most cases, by relative hyper-ventilation or, more often, persistence of the hypo-ventilation. The mechanisms of these reactions are very complex. A sudden increase in PIO_2 [inspired air O_2 pressure] causes suppression of O_2 stimulation by the chemoreceptors. This produces hypo-ventilation. During a second stage, a humoral phenomenon intervenes: CO_2 transport is disturbed by the Haldane effect, and CO_2 thus accumulates in the tissues (Gesell effect). The consequence is a hyperventilation. This conflict partly explains the delay and the nature of the respiratory response observed secondarily. In chronic respiratory insufficiency, this course of events if modified by the state of preexisting chemical equilibria. This is why the observed effects are variable depending on the patients studied. Only hypoxemic subjects with a high degree of hypercapnia react with persistent severe hypo-ventilation. (DRL) (© BA)

126.
ARMSTRONG, B.W.
Traumatic perforations of the tympanic membrane: observe or repair?
Laryngoscope 82:1822-1830;1972.

Traumatic perforations of the tympanic membrane deserve the same careful attention as any other injury, and healing should not invariably be left to chance. Sometimes early repair is clearly indicated. A foreign object rupturing the postero-superior quadrant may cause obscure damage to the ossicular chain, a perilymphatic leak, or leave an unsuspected foreign body in the middle ear. All very large traumatic perforations and all perforations in the posterosuperior quadrant should be repaired promptly to reduce the incidence of permanent impairment. Small perforations in less vulnerable quadrants can be treated in the traditional expectant manner. Steroid-containing ear drops inhibit healing and are contraindicated in the treatment of traumatic perforations. (Author's abstract)

127.
ARNDT, W.R.
Holographic acoustic imaging for underwater viewing.
In: IEEE international conference on engineering in the ocean environment, Panama City, Florida, September 1970. Digest of technical papers, p.82-84. Published by the conference.

Ultrasonic holograms of objects as small as 0.25 in. in diam. have been made in water at 5 ft using 5 MH_z. High-resolution images have been constructed from such holograms using optical and computer techniques. (Eng. Ind.)

128.
ARNOLD, G.
Physiologische Grundlagen einer Hyperoxie.
[Physiological basis of hyperoxia].
Pneumonologie 149:39-48;Oct. 31, 1973.

During hyperoxia the O_2 consumption of the tissues can be covered by the physically dissolved oxygen. The O_2 supply to high-metabolic tissues by means of high PO_2 is dangerous as it could lead to O_2 intoxication. Breakdown of tissue CO_2 transport in the brain increases central venous PCO_2 and thus also respiration. This is followed by a decrease in arterial PCO_2 and vasoconstriction (protection of the tissue against high PO_2). Addition of CO_2 accelerates the beginning of O_2 intoxication. Under hyperoxic conditions the vital capacity is decreased in proportion to pressure and duration of exposure. Lung-tolerance curves show early alterations in ventilation. The effects on heart and circulation are slight, except for bradycardia and vasoconstriction. (English abstract)

129.
ARNOLD, R.M. and L.J. Albright.
Hydrostatic pressure effects on the translation stages of protein synthesis in a cell-free system from Escherichia coli.
Biochim. Biophys. Acta 238:347-354;1971.

Hydrostatic pressure inhibits the binding of aminoacyl transfer RNA to ribosomes in a cell-free system from Escherichia coli, and has an ever greater inhibitory effect on peptide bond formation. Evidence that pressure decreases the stability of the messenger RNA-ribosome complex is also presented. (Authors' summary)

130.
ASHBAUGH, D.G.
Oxygen toxicity in normal and hypoxemic dogs.
J. Appl. Physiol. 31:664-668;1971.

Normal and chronically hypoxemic dogs were exposed to oxygen at 1 atm until death or an arbitrary 2-week limit terminated the experiment. No differences were seen in the response of normal and hypoxemic animals to oxygen exposure. Within each group, striking differences were observed between individual animals. The lung was equally damaged in both groups of dogs while other organs did not demonstrate pathological changes in either group. Changes in serum enzymes were noted in both groups but were probably related more to dehydration than to oxygen toxicity. This study has shown that hypoxemia does not protect animals exposed to oxygen. (Author's abstract)

131.
ASHTON, N., B. Tripathi and G. Knight.
Effect of oxygen on the developing retinal vessels of the rabbit. I. Anatomy and development of the retinal vessels of the rabbit.
Exp. Eye. Res. 14:214-220;1972.

This paper is the first of a series providing a detailed account of in vivo and in vitro investigations of the effect of hyperoxia on the growing retinal vessels of the rabbit and reports the findings in our preliminary study of the anatomy and development of the retinal vessels in the normal rabbit as seen by injection methods, histology and electron microscopy. (Authors' abstract)

132.
ASHTON, N., B. Tripathi and G. Knight.
Effect of oxygen on the developing retinal vessels of the rabbit. II. In vivo experiments.
Exp. Eye. Res. 14:221-232;1972.

This paper is the second in a series reporting studies on the effect of hyperoxia on the developing retinal vessels of the rabbit and gives an account of in vivo experiments. The effects of hyperoxia, with and without air survival, were studied by exposing young rabbits in incubators to hyperoxia for several days, and the vessels were then examined by injection methods, whole mounts, histology and electron microscopy. The oxygen effect was also studied directly by observing the reaction of the vessels through a window inserted in the anterior segment of the eye. It was found that the immature retinal vessels of the rabbit were as readily destroyed by hyperoxia as those of other mammals examined and that the vessels similarly proliferate abnormally on transfer to air. There are, however features peculiar to the reactions of the rabbit and these are described and discussed. Electron microscopy revealed that the vessels are destroyed through disintegration of their endothelial cells and that this is preceded by the appearance of prominent autophagic vacuoles in the cytoplasm in the presence of normal mitochondria. The significance of these findings is considered and reasons are given for believing the changes to be due to a selective cytocidal action of oxygen, rather than secondary to vessel closure. [See Tripathi et al. Exp. Eye Research 15:321-351; Mar. 1973]. (Authors)

133.
ASKEROV, A.A. and V.I. Kronshtadskii-Karev.
Medical supervision in the pursuit of underwater sports.
Arlington, Va., Joint Publication Research Service, Nov. 7, 1972. 250p.
(JPRS — 57439)

The report contains a review of the development of various aspects of underwater sports in the USSR. Results are cited of a clinico-experimental study of the effect of underwater sport activity on the body and the use of medical safeguards for this sport. An extensive bibliography is included. (GRA)

134.
ATTWOOD, D.A. and C. McCann.
Human engineering evaluation of the SDL-1.
Downsview, Ontario, Def. Civ. Inst. Environ. Med., Def. Res. Board, Rep. DCIEM 73-R-994, 96p. Dec. 1973.

The results of a human engineering evaluation of the Canadian Forces Submersible Diver Lockout (SDL-1) are presented. Modifications are suggested to improve the design of operator and diver seating and the design and layout of the controls and displays associated with most aspects of vehicle operation. Conclusions and recommendations are illustrated with the aid of a full-scale static mock-up of the SDL-1. (Authors' abstract)

135.
AUDET, N.F.
Hydrospace simulator facility for materials testing.
U.S. Navy Clothing Textile Res. Unit, Rep. TR-99, 10-71, 34 p. Feb. 1972.
(AD 739 695)

The Navy Clothing and Textile Research Unit (NCTRU) developed a hydrospace simulator facility for testing material properties at sea depths to 1,000 FSW. The facility contains three testers to study material thickness, stretch-flex, and thermal conductance properties from normal ambient pressures to 1,000 FSW. The equipment complex also integrates the gas control and instrumentation hardware, testers and pressure chamber equipment necessary for studying the material properties outlined. The material properties which can be studied with this facility are of significant importance in the development and/or screening of materials suitable for deep sea swimmers' suits. (Author) (GRA)

136.
AUDET, N.F. and M.N. Larrivee.
Development and evaluation of deep-sea swimsuit materials.
U.S. Navy Clothing Text. Res. Unit, Rep. TR-108-5-72, 59 p. June 1973.
(AD 763 378)

The Navy Clothing and Textile Research Unit (NCTRU) has developed a swimsuit material that meets the requirements of Navy personnel who operate at great sea depths for long periods of time. Two chemically distinct, flexible, syntactic foams — Unit-developed, polyurethane, hollow-glass-microsphere composite and a proprietary polyvinylchloride, hollow-glass-microsphere composite — have been produced which may prove useful for swimsuit applications in deep-sea environments down to 1000 FSW. Tests showed that both materials were essentially incompressible to depths of 1000 FSW (less than 3%) and provided more insulation than currently used Neoprene-foam materials at depths greater than 20 FSW. The materials, however, were considerably heavier than the foam although significantly less dense than sea water. Standard wet-style swimsuits were fabricated from these experimental materials for verification of sample thermal-conductivity data. (Authors' abstract modified by GRA)

137.
AYERS, L. and D.F. Tierney.
Pulmonary tolerance to 1 atmosphere oxygen.
Clin. Res. 21:221;Feb. 1973.

Abstract only. Excerpt quoted: Pulmonary tolerance to 1 atm. of O_2 can be produced by several agents which produce alveolar injury. A nonspecific cellular response to injury may enable the lung to tolerate injury from oxygen. An increased capacity to synthesize cell components would permit rapid replacement of injured parts. Increased synthesis by cells is generally associated with increased glucose-6- phosphate dehydrogenase (G6PD) activity. Finder, La Force, and Huber (Clin. Res. 20:577, 1972) have reported that O_2 tolerance can be reproduced after lung injury by alpha naphthyl thiourea (ANTU) in a strain of mice. We have produced O_2 tolerance in rats by prior injection ANTU (4 mg./Kg.) and by prior exposure to 85% O_2 (1 atm.) for 7 days. These procedures increased G6PD activity of rat lung. However these procedures did not produce tolerance in a strain of Swiss Webster mice and no significant increase in G6PD activity in the mouse lung occurred. These results are consistent with the hypothesis that sublethal injury to the alveolar tissue may subsequently result in tolerance to lung injury including exposure to O_2 (1 atm.).

138.
BACCAGLINI R. and J. Irgon.
The use of command buoyancy systems with submersibles in the recovery or manipulation of subsea equipment.
In: 1972 Offshore Technology Conference, May 1-3, Houston, Texas. Preprints, Vol. II, p.181-190. Published by the Conference, 1972.

The most practical command buoyancy system is a compact unit with almost no submerged weight which releases an uncommonly large quantity of latent gas into an attached lift bag or flooded ballast tank when the buoyancy device is actuated either for chance emergencies or programmed purposes. Its design simplicity permits use of the device for object recovery and a variety of load support functions in almost any desired combination of lift capacity, operating depth and actuation sequence. It can be made an integral part of the load whenever desired, such as emergency buoyancy for the submersible per se. The command buoyancy technique can significantly improve the safety and economy of submersible operations involving manipulation or retrieval of submerged equipment. (Authors' abstract)

139.
BACHRACH, A.J.
"Signatures" Project.
In: Abstracts of BuMed-ONR sponsored Navywide workshop in high pressure biomedical research, U.S. Submarine Base, Groton, Conn., May 1971, p. 30. Published by the Naval Submarine Medical Research Laboratory, 1971.

Abstract only. Entire item quoted: A major emphasis of the Department's research has been on the "Signature" project in which standards for microtremor and speech are being developed, using power spectral density analysis. Work reported on tremor measurement taken during the 620-foot Makai Range saturation dive in June 1970, indicated that, among three divers recorded during compression and decompression all had normal tremor with individual characteristics sufficiently different as to constitute a tremor signature for each person. The measurements were made with a muscle-force transducer. Similar work reported on speech, also using power spectral density analysis techniques, suggested that individual vocal rhythm analysis can provide a speech signature for a person. Helium speech samples recorded systematically during the Makai dive are currently being analyzed by power spectral methods to demonstrate that individual speech characteristics of divers can be used, along with microtremor, as recorded standards against which on-line monitoring samples may be compared to detect and quantify behavioral and physiological change.

140.
BACHRACH, A.J. and P.B. Bennett.
Tremor in diving.
U.S. Nav. Med. Res. Inst., and Roy. Nav. Physiol. Lab., Alverstoke, Joint Rep., 1, 39p. Dec. 1972.
(Also published in Aerospace Med. 44:613-623;June 1973).

The problem of tremor in diving as part of the High Pressure Nervous Syndrome has been recognized since the mid-1960s. The authors review reports of tremor in diving and discuss methods of objective measurement of tremor. The etiology of tremor is also discussed with specific attention to the question of compression rate and neurophysiological factors which constitute a sketch of needed research. A matrix of deep dives in which tremor was observed and measured is presented, as well as data from dives in which objective measurement of tremor was accomplished. (Authors' abstract)

141.
BACHRACH, A.J.
Never mind the diver's mind.
Skin Diver 22: March 1973

The author takes issue with an earlier article written for Skin Diver, entitled "Mind beneath the sea," in which the author adopts the psychodynamic viewpoint which emphasizes inner states of mind, rather than the behavioral viewpoint, with its emphasis on observable responses. In the former article, the author had put forth, as a method of overcoming panic, verbal self-reassurance by the diver. This suggestion, it is stated here, is unrealistic. This author believes that thorough training is the most effective means of preventing panic. The hpns, and techniques of behavioral research and performance measurements are discussed briefly. (MFW/SCD)

142.
BACHRACH, A.J. and P.B. Bennett.
The high pressure nervous syndrome during human deep saturation and excursion diving.
In: Hesser, C.M. and D. Linnarsson eds. Proceedings of the first annual scientific meeting of the European Undersea Biomedical Society, Stockholm 13-15 June 1973. Forsvarsmedicin 9:490-495;July 1973.

A short review is given of the development of knowledge regarding the high pressure nervous syndrome (hpns), beginning with the observation of tremor in 1965 during a chamber dive to 600 and 800 feet, observation of EEG anomalies during a chamber dive to 1500 feet, and motor function detriment, chiefly in the ball bearing test, and mental impairment in instances of rapid compression. Compression rate has been slowed down in recent dives, on one occasion (Saggittaire II), to 14 ft./hr. Rapid compression excursions have been made from saturation depths arrived at by slow compression without serious hpns effects. In January, 1973, at Duke University, divers were slowly compressed to 870 feet, then compressed at different rates (16.7 ft./min., 50 ft./min., and 100 ft./min.) to 1000 feet. The impaired motor function of hpns did not occur at any compression rate, nor did the rise in theta activity of the EEG. There was, however, a depression of the EEG due to hydrostatic pressure. (MFW/UMS)

143.
BACKTEMAN, O., N.A. Nelsson, S. Soderqvist and M. Weibull.
Proposed noise specifications for the hyperbaric installations at Sjodal.
Stockholm, Sweden, Akustikbyran AB, Tech. Rep. 869.02, 28p. Apr. 1973.

Limiting curves for allowable noise during different working conditions have been suggested. The limit is set by the hearing damage risk during fast compression and decompression and by the demands for good speech communications in the stationary case. At the control panels speech communication between two operators should always be possible. Some measurements on Swedish installations and some flownoise calculations are also reported. They show that the actual levels inside the chambers will be far above the proposed limits unless means for noise reduction are introduced. These means are also discussed. (Authors' summary)

144.
BADDELEY, A.D.
Diver performance.
In: Woods, J.D. and J.N. Lythgoe, eds. Underwater science: An introduction to experiments by diver, p. 33-67. London, Oxford University Press, 1971.

The author concentrates on the effects of inert gas narcosis and on visual performance. It is emphasized that studies of narcosis in simulated conditions have limited applicability. First the author discusses the difficulties of experimental design, the chief of which is the effect of practice and transfer, since performance will always improve with practice. Some of the more or less unsatisfactory methods of combating practice effects — reversing the pressures of testing, or balancing the order in which various tests are presented — are described. Placebo effects are useful in testing the effects of a drug. When possible, experienced divers should be used as subjects. Next, the author considers test design; the two basic requirements are sensitivity and validity. A brief review is given of the results of pressure-chamber studies of diver performance. There is no indication that oxygen toxicity affects performance until the actual convulsive stage is reached. The studies using oxy-nitrogen mixtures include those to determine minimum depth (generally considered to be 30m), those to determine time at depth (the rate of onset is in doubt) and the nature of the task. (narcosis is more readily detected in more complex tasks, such as reasoning tasks). The narcotic effects of oxy-helium mixtures are negligible at depths of less than 100 m. and there is some evidence that there is an adaptation factor involved at greater depths. The possibility of using neon or hydrogen as diluents is noted. In open-sea studies, it appears that the narcotic effect of the breathing mixture at pressure interacts with other stresses to produce a far greater performance decrement than that observed in chamber studies. The crucial variable seems to be the level of anxiety of the subject. In discussing visual performance, the effects of refraction, the reduction of light intensity, brightness contrast and color contrast are mentioned as important factors. Drawings and diagrams illustrate the effects of distortion. The problem of visual field, and its limitation by the face mask, is discussed. The greatest visual field is given by the recessed kidney-shaped mask. Diagrams and drawings show the median visual fields for various face masks. In addition to the optical limitations of a diver's visual field, there is an attentional narrowing which affects performance of peripheral tasks. Numerous experiments with visual acuity are reviewed. The loss of visual acuity underwater is probably due to the absorption and scattering of light. The loss of acuity is greater at longer distances. In concluding, the author discusses the relationship between the ergonomist and the diver and poses two possible solutions to the problem. First, is to train the equipment engineer as an ergonomist; the second lies in cooperation between the engineer and the ergonomist. (MFW/BSCP)

145.
BADDELEY, A.D.
Selective attention and performance in dangerous environments.
Br. J. Psychol. 63:537-546;1972.

Evidence on human performance in dangerous environments is reviewed and suggests that danger reduces efficiency, except in the case of experienced subjects. Perceptual narrowing is shown to be one source of decrement. It is suggested that danger increases the subject's arousal level which influences performance by producing a narrowing of attention. The nature of the performance decrement and of the performance decrement and of adaptation to danger are discussed in this context. (Author)

146.
BAEYENS, D.A., J.R. Hoffert and P.O. Fromm.
A comparative study of oxygen toxicity in the retina, brain and liver of the teleost, amphibian and mammal.
Comp. Biochem. Physiol [A] 45:925-932;Aug. 1973.

1. Teleost retinas showed increased oxygen consumption after 4 and 24 hr exposures to hyperbaric oxygen. This is interpreted as indicating that the availability of oxygen is rate limiting and that oxygen does not inhibit any essential respiratory enzymes in this tissue. 2. Exposure of amphibian retinas to high oxygen tensions resulted in no change in oxygen consumption which is consistent with the hypothesis that the rate of oxidative retinal metabolism is not limited by availability of oxygen or the inhibition of any associated enzymes. 3. Mammalian retinas exposed to similar elevated oxygen tensions demonstrated marked decreases in oxidative metabolism mediated through inhibition of one or more essential enzymes of carbohydrate metabolism. 4. In the three species studied both hepatic and brain tissue showed marked deleterious metabolic effects upon exposure to elevated oxygen tension for 24 hr. 5. In general it was noted that the higher the metabolic rate of the tissue the more susceptible it is to oxygen toxicity. When the temperature is decreased there is a lowered susceptibility to oxygen toxicity mediated through the decreased metabolism. (Authors' summary)

147.
BAILEY, V.R., J. LaCerda and J.F. Manuel.
Diver lockout and observation submersibles: a perspective of participation in offshore operations.
In: 1972 Offshore Technology Conference, May 1-3, Houston, Texas. Preprints, Vol I, p.548-556. Published by the conference, 1972.

This paper presents a perspective of the developing capabilities and participation of diver lockout and observation submersibles in offshore oil operations. The basic submarine capabilities that were available in 1968 when Perry submersibles were first offered for services to the offshore industry is established. Operations in the Gulf of Mexico are reviewed and the shortcomings, as well as the advantages, that were revealed in these first operations discussed. Subjects covered include low visibility operational problems, logistic and handling, and submarine maneuverability requirements. The capabilities and problems are all related to actual operations performed, including inspection of 30" pipe, initial training of diving companies in diver lockout operations, and the first commercial submarine lockout mission. (Author)

148.
BAIN, E.C., III and T.E. Berghage.
Diver first class reading ability.
U.S. Navy Exp. Diving Unit, Rep. NEDU-3-73, 7p. Jan. 1, 1973.

The Nelson-Denny Reading Test was administered to thirty Navy first class diver candidates to evaluate the group's vocabulary, reading comprehension, reading rate and overall reading ability. The findings showed the Navy divers to have an overall reading ability equivalent to the college freshman norm. Reading rate and comprehension were at the twelfth grade level, while vocabulary ability was equal to the college freshman norm. (Authors' abstract)

149.
BAIN, E.C., III and T.E. Berghage.
Preliminary evaluation of SINDBAD tests.
U.S. Navy Exp. Diving Unit., Oct. 3, 1973.

This informal report gives a brief description of each of the tests which can be administered by SINDBAD (System for Investigation of Diver Behavior at Depth), which was installed at the U.S. Navy Experimental Diving Unit in 1968. Results of tests as undergone by 27 subjects for the first 14 tests, and 16 subjects for the remaining eight tests, are given and analyzed statistically. Tests are designed to measure the following abilities: flexibility of closure; perceptual speed; spatial orientation; finger dexterity; manual dexterity; reaction time; time interval estimation; wrist-finger speed; associative memory; induction; number facility; spatial scanning; visualization; control precision; multilimb coordination; response orientation; system equalization; vigilance; memory span; time sharing; visual monitoring. (MFW/UMS)

150.
BAKEMAN, R. and R. Helmreich.
Time effects on behavior.
In: Miller, J.W., J.G. Van Derwalker, and R.A. Waller, eds. Tektite 2: Scientists-in-the-sea, p. VIII-46 — VIII-49. Washington, D.C., U.S. Department of the Interior, August, 1971.

The effects of time on behavior was studied with regard to the following variables: total work, habit maintenance, total marine science, direct marine science, total leisure, co-recreation, solitary recreation, sleep, and gregariousness. In the short missions there was more of a tendency to work very hard at the beginning, then to slack to a greater degree, than in the long missions. The authors believe that the three-week missions are probably long enough to serve as analogues for long-term missions. (MFW/BSCP)

151.
BAKKE, D.R.
Russian industry calls on own divers.
Offshore 33:49-52;Aug. 1973.

The Expeditionary Division for Underwater Technical Work of the USSR Ministry of the Oil Industry's Main Transport Administration, established in 1971 and based in Kiev, USSR, consists of seven teams of highly trained divers and support personnel. They not only build, inspect, and repair existing installations but help to design new ones, both in the Caspian Sea and in Siberia, where gas pipelines have to be laid across rivers a mile or more wide. The chief task of the divers is pipeline inspection. Improvements in suits and other equipment are briefly discussed. One important development is an underwater radio telephone communication system which is operative over distances of 300-600 feet. (MFW/UMS)

152.
BALDRIDGE, H.D.
Shark attack against man: a program of data reduction and analysis.
Sarasota, Fla., Mote Marine Lab., 135p. Oct. 31, 1973.
(AD 771, 465/2GA)

Data from 1165 case histories of shark attack against man were reduced to a form handleable by automatic data retrieval systems. Numerous probes by computer were made to provide statistical significance to the existence or absence of common factors associated with known instances of predaceous shark behavior, and evaluate the present approach of gathering meaningful data on shark attack and thereby determine requirements for maintaining such an effort in the future. Although information was carefully screened for correlations between occurrence of shark attack and a number of environmental and behavioral parameters, it was considered of greater importance that patterns or relationships be identified that distinguished victims from non-victims among exposed populations. Points of interest were examined in the light of previously accepted correlations and popular beliefs. (Modified author abstract) (GRA)

153.
BALLDIN, U.I. and C. Lundgren.
Nitrogen elimination in man during immersion, shifts in temperature and body position.
In: Abstracts of the Twenty-fifth Congress of Physiological Science Satellite Symposium. Recent progress in fundamental physiology of diving, Marseille, France, July 1971, p.59-60. (Proceedings unpublished)

Abstract only. Excerpt quoted: The increased nitrogen elimination rate during immersion appears to be due to an enhanced circulation. Thus, in a separate study, the hydrostatic forces during immersion have been found to increase cardiac output by about 25%. Similar mechanisms come into play when shifting from sitting to supine body position. Changes in environmental temperature probably also influence the nitrogen elimination by inducing circulatory changes. It appears that some of the experimental conditions described above have a rather profound effect on nitrogen elimination and presumably also on nitrogen uptake. They probably should be taken into consideration when planning certain pressure exposures.

154.
BALLDIN, U.I.
Effects of ambient temperature and body position on tissue nitrogen elimination in man.
Aerosp. Med. 44:365-370;Apr. 1973.

The influence of ambient temperature (25°, 28° and 37°C) and different body positions (sitting and supine) on tissue nitrogen elimination during (two hours) oxygen breathing was studied in six subjects. A persistently larger volume of oxygen breathing was studied in six subjects. A persistently larger volume of eliminated nitrogen was recorded under warm (37°C) conditions compared to thermally neutral (28°C) conditions. The difference was particularly marked towards the end of the experiments, the mean nitrogen yield then being about 17% larger in 37°C. In cool temperature (25°C) there was a tendency for a slight increase in nitrogen elimination compared to neutral temperature conditions. During supine body position there was a prompt increase in nitrogen elimination when compared to the sitting position, the nitrogen yield being 24% larger after 30 min and 15% larger after two hours (in neutral temperature). The most pronounced and sustained gain in nitrogen elimination was observed during the supine body position in warm environment, the nitrogen yield being about 30% larger than in sitting position and at a neutral temperature both after 30 min. and two hours. It is suggested that the increased nitrogen elimination induced both by supine body position and warm environment was due to enhanced blood circulation. The present observations may bear on decompression routines. (Author's abstract)

155.
BALLDIN, U.I.
The preventive effect of denitrogenation during warm water immersion on decompression sickness in man.
In: Hesser, C.M. and D. Linnarsson, eds. Proceedings of the first annual scientific meeting of the European Undersea Biomedical Society, Stockholm, 13-15 June 1973. Forsvarsmedicin 9:239-243;July 1973.

Tissue nitrogen elimination during oxygen breathing is enhanced when human subjects are immersed in water, particularly in warm water. The effect of this procedure on the occurrence of decompression sickness was tested by immersing 10 oxygen breathing subjects to their neck in water of 37°C for 25 min before experimental decompression.

Control experiments involved oxygen breathing without immersion. Provocation of decompression sickness was made by decompression to an ambient pressure of 155 mm Hg (corresponding to 38,000 feet altitude) and standardized leg exercise. The subjects were observed for a maximum of 2 hr before recompression. Three subjects were resistant to the ordinary exposures and got an extra nitrogen loading with air-breathing at 2 ata before denitrogenation. In 9 out of 10 of the non-immersion experiments and 2 out of 10 of the immersion experiments bends developed after decompression. All symptoms disappeared upon recompression to the surface level. This preventive effect on decompression sickness obtained by denitrogenation during immersion in warm water might bear on the decompression procedures for divers and compressed air workers. (Author's abstract)

156.
BALOUET, G., L. Barthelemy, J.P. Leroy, A. Michaud and J. Parc.
Etude des lesions provoquees par l'utilsation de melanges respiratoires oxygene-hydrogene dans des conditions hyperbares.
[Study of lesions induced by the use of respiratory oxygen-hydrogen mixtures under hyperbaric conditions. Animal experiments].
C.R. Soc. Biol. (Paris) 165:1750-1753;1971.

The authors' first experimental findings concerning the use of oxygen-hydrogen mixtures in saturation diving indicated the necessity for great prudence. Recent results reported, following the breathing of O_2-H_2 mixtures at 29 Bars, for about one hour, indicate, even at such short intervals, the necessity of the same reservations (at least as far as the rabbit is concerned, since only one animal of six survived the experiment). Histological examinations demonstrated, in addition to nonspecific vascular lesions, signs of cellular damage, particularly neuronal, which seemed to be the result of anoxia. It is interesting to note that the animal whose stay at 29 Bars was reduced to 50 minutes presented no cellular signs, a fact all the more interesting as it was noted, during recent experiments carried out at GERS (Groupe d'Etudes et de Recherches Sous-Marines), that rabbits survived stays of 30 minutes in the same conditions of pressure and breathing mixture (O_2-H_2, 41.6 of O_2, 29 Bars). These findings make it possible to state precisely the period of onset of irreversible toxicity from O_2-H_2 mixtures. The authors intend to continue experimentation with O_2-H_2 mixtures employing histoenzymological techniques. These studies should permit them to define the risks incurred during the respiration of O_2-H_2 mixtures and the mechanism of the observed disorders that are perhaps due to disturbances at the level of the respiratory pattern and of the process of oxydo-reduction. (Authors' conclusion, translated by MFW/BSCP)

157.
BALOUET, G., L. Barthelemy, J. Chouteau, J. Corriol, E. Girin, J. LeChuiton, A. Michaud and J. Parc.
Bilan d'une experimentation animale de plongees aux melanges hydrogene-oxygene.
[Report of an animal experiment in dives with hydrogen-oxygen mixtures].
In: Hesser, C.M. and D. Linnarsson eds. Proceedings of the first annual scientific meeting of the European Undersea Biomedical Society, Stockholm, 13-15 June 1973. Forsvarsmedicin 9:301-309;July 1973.

This paper is a somewhat condensed version of a report carrying a similar title that was issued as Rep. 01/73/GERS. (See preceding entry). Rabbits and white rats were the experimental animals. EEG and ECG recordings, histological examinations of all principal organs, and some histoenzymological examinations were made. All animals exposed several days to hydrogen died presenting the same EEG, ECG, and clinical symptoms. Animals subjected to short exposures were often brought back to surface pressure alive. This suggests that there might be a limit to the use of hydrogen in human diving. Histological and histoenzymological results suggest histotoxic hypoxia. (From authors' abstract, translated by MFW/UMS)

158.
BALOUET, G., L. Barthelemy and A. Belaud.
Etude, a partir d' un vertebre aquatique, des effets specifiques de la pression per se.
[Study, by means of an aquatic vertebrate, of the specific effects of pressure per se].
In: Hesser, C.M. and D. Linnarsson eds. Proceedings of the first annual scientific meeting of the European Undersea Biomedical Society, Stockholm, 13-15 June 1973. Forsvarsmedicin 9:483-489;July 1973.

An aquatic animal (Anguilla anguilla L.) was chosen for an experiment to determine specific pressure effects, dissociated from gas effects. The eels were placed in a rubber container filled with water within a hyperbaric chamber, and subjected to various degrees of pressure. Respiratory and circulatory parameters were measured; EEG's were also recorded. Tachycardia was noted, followed at higher pressure by EEG anomalies and a strong hyperventilatory reaction. After a time the hyperventilation diminished, the EEG returned to normal, and the tachycardia persisted. The disorders appeared more quickly and were more intense when the compression rate was faster. Mean oxygen consumption at 101 ATA was 1.31 ml. $mn.^{-1}$ kg^{-1} as compared to 0.54 in normal conditions. Hyperoxia and hypothermia reduced hyperventilation without stopping it completely. Decompression brought on no pathological phenomena and the physiological parameters became normal in a few minutes. Examination of the brain, kidney, heart, and liver revealed a significant vasoconstriction and a moderate degree of edema in the white matter of the encephalon. Because of the EEG anomalies, a neurological mechanism is hypothesized. It is also noted that the onset of these reactions might be the result of a transitory imbalance between arterial and venous blood pressure. (MFW/UMS)

159.
BANGE, C., R. Bange-Barnoud and L.T. Nghia.
Modifications de l'alanine-amino-transferase, d l'aspartate amino-transferase et de certains substrats dans le plasma et les tissus de rat au cours de l'hypercapnia.
[Changes in alanine aminotransferase, aspartate aminotransferase, and certain substrates in the plasma and tissues of rats during hypercapnia].
J. Physiol. (Paris) 65 (Suppl. 3):432A;1972.

Aspartate amino transferase (GOT) and alinine aminotransferase (GPT) levels were measured in arterial blood, plasma, and liver, muscle, and kidney tissues of fasting male rats subjected to a CO_2-rich atmosphere for one hour. (A group of similar rats served as controls.) As compared with the controls, a clear rise in plasmatic and hepatic GOT activity was observed, while muscle GPT activity was decreased. A significant decrease of renal and muscular glutamate was also observed. The phenomena noted in this experimentation correlate well with the observations of other experiments. (MEMH/UMS)

160.
BANGE, C.
Correlations des acides amines plasmatiques du rat au cours de l'hypercapnia.
[Correlations of plasma amino acids in the rat during hypercapnia].
J. Physiol. (Paris) 65 (Suppl. 3):341A;1972.

Blood amino acid levels in rats were studied with ion-exchange chromatography. The animals, fasting for 18 hours, breathed an atmosphere rich in carbon dioxide for one hour; samples of arterial plasma were collected after decapitation. Covariance and the Bravais-Pearson correlation coefficient r were calculated for individual levels. In control animals, significant correlations existed only for the indispensible amino acids. In experimental animals the correlations among the indispensible amino acids were much less marked, and other correlations appeared. These changes are thought to explain some of the metabolic and enzymatic changes previously observed in hypercapnia. (MEMH/UMS)

161.
BANGEN, P.
Haematologische Untersuchungen nach "kritischer" Dekompression aus Uberdruck.
[Hematologic studies after rapid decompression].
Deutsche Luft-und Raumfahrt, Rep. DLR-FB 73-63, 55p. 1973.

The purpose of these studies was the quest for the mode of behavior of several hematologic values after rapid decompression. After specification of the normal physiological values, eighty miniature-pigs were exposed ten times in weekly intervals to a rapid decompression. The following tests in blood on fifteen animals, each time showed prevailing significant changes in the field of cellmorphology, albumin-chemistry and physiology of coagulation. In a discussion of the results, it has been attempted to explain the causing factors which may have affected the process of experiments. (English summary)

162.
BANISTER, E.W., A.J. Davison, N.M.G. Bhakthan and C. Asmundson.
Biochemical effects of oxygen at high pressure in rats.
Can. J. Physiol. Pharmacol. 51(9):673-678;1973.

Changes in brain and muscle lactate dehydrogenase, cytochrome oxidase and NADH dehydrogenase (cytochrome c reductase) were measured in rats convulsed by exposure to O_2 at high pressure 6 ATA (OHP). Blood glucose levels and some plasma and serum enzymes (lactate dehydrogenase, alkaline phosphatase, aspartate transaminase and creatine kinase) were measured simultaneously. The lack of widespread inhibition of several markers for the glycolytic sequence, the Krebs cycle or the cytochrome chain, together with elevated blood glucose levels in hyperoxia and increased blood alkaline phosphatase and lactate dehydrogenase in all hyperbaric conditions (and as well as O_2), suggests tissue damage and a generalized etiology for the convulsive state. (© BA)

163.
BANKS, R.H.
Electrical-electronic equipment in high-pressure HeO_2 environments.
In: The working diver, 1972. Symposium proceedings, February 1972, Columbus, Ohio, p. 197-213. Washington, D.C., Marine Technology Society, 1972.

Unique problems encountered when electrical and electronic equipment is used in a high-pressure, helium-oxygen environment will be discussed. Solutions, as well as some of the problems that remain to be solved are explored. Among the problems are: the high thermal conductivity of the helium environment; the greater density of a hyperbaric environment, humidity; the tendency of helium to permeate all materials; the destructive effect of pressure on materials; the danger of fire due to a high concentration of oxygen. Solutions require that equipment be placed in helium-purged containers, or in pressure-proof containers. Various methods of accomplishing this are discussed. Numerous photographs of types of electronic equipment before and after pressure tests are shown. Another safety factor that is noted is the out-gassing of noxious vapors from materials such as paints, adhesives, lubricants and plastics; vapors which would be harmless in an open environment may become harmful in a closed one. (MFW/BSCP)

164.
BARACH, A.L. and M.S. Segal.
Oxygen therapy in cardiopulmonary disease with a review of oxygen toxicity.
Ann. Allerg. 30(3):113-121;1972.

A review of some of the pertinent literature on O_2 toxicity is presented. An O_2 enriched atmosphere of 40%, 50% and probably 60%, may be continuously inhaled, for months if necessary, without irritant effects on the lungs. When hypercapnia develops gradually during controlled O_2 administration, without acid shift in arterial pH, a lower volume of ventilation is made possible. An increased CO_2 tension in the alveolar air under these circumstances is utilized as a valuable adaptive response required for the continuous relief of dyspnea in breathless subjects with pulmonary emphysema. O_2 administration is regulated according to needs of the patient for O_2, without arbitrary limit to the degree of hypercapnia. Clinical evidence indicates that moderately high O_2 concentrations, 45% — 50%, may be effectively administered in the treatment of cardiopulmonary failure. The relation of so-called hyperoxia and hypercapnia to renal flow is considered applicable to short-term experiments rather than to therapy of acute cardiac insufficiency. (JFL) (© BA)

165.
BARADA, B.
Tomorrow 2500 ft.
Skin Diver 21:30-33;87;June 1972.

The author gives a resume of the development of the man-in-the-sea program from Genesis through Sealabs I, II and III, when the U.S. Navy's saturation diving program was indefinitely suspended. He then describes the Ocean Simulation Facility (OSF) at the Naval Coastal Systems Laboratory in Panama City, Florida. This facility will be capable of testing divers and equipment to 2250 feet simulated depth. Basic problems of deep diving such as heat loss, communication and navigation have not yet been solved. The difficulty of breathing gas of the density it attains at 2000 feet is one of the problems being tackled. Speech unintelligibility is another. The OSF will give a systems approach to underwater technology that has never before existed. Closed-circuit breathing apparatus is expected to be the type used in Navy deep diving in the future, but at present no completely satisfactory equipment has been developed that will permit a diver to swim free at great depths with safety. It is thought that at the present state of development, the band mask with hose and gas from the surface is the most satisfactory apparatus for a deep working dive. The oxygen sensors and the warning buzzers that indicate when the oxygen supply gets out of balance are among the crucial factors of the closed circuit scuba which are still dangerously unreliable, putting the diver in peril of either oxygen starvation or oxygen toxicity if the oxygen percentage goes as much as .1% below or .3% above the acceptable level. The new cryogenic equipment for storing, supplying and purifying breathing gas is promising, but in very early stages of development. Semi-closed circuit units are deemed completely unacceptable. The OSF consists of the largest (47 feet long) wet pot in the world, with five dry chambers attached to it. Any ocean condition can be simulated and the chamber can accomodate a small submersible. Each dry chamber has its own life support system, and a standby gas loop can be instantly cut into any one of them. Each chamber is connected to a separate console, with TV monitor and computer. The computer can be locked into any component, and programmed to ring a warning bell under certain conditions. Sensors can be installed on components and a readout obtained. All consoles are tied to a central control panel. The facility will be available for use by universities and by industry as well as by the services. A look is given into the future of saturation diving at 3000 feet, with fixed habitats and small nuclear powered submersibles, that would berth underwater. (MFW/BSCP)

166.
BARATS, Y.M., S.A. Gulyar and Y.N. Kiklevich.
O nekotorykh voprosakh pitaniya akvanavtov v podvodnykh laboratoriyakh i vodnoi srede.
[Some problems of aquanaut nutrition in submarine laboratories and in aqueous environment].
Vopr. Pitan 30(2):17-22;1971.
(Translation JPRS 53161)

Caloric requirements for divers are 5,000 to 5,500 Kcal daily. Aquanauts living in underwater habitats should not be given such large amounts of food. It is believed that emphasis should be placed on meats, fruits and vegetables; fats, sauces and starches are likely to be rejected. Liquid intake is small. Stressful conditions cause excretion of potassium, sodium, calcium, phosphorous, and products of nitrogen metabolism. Supplementary vitamins are needed. In the Russian Ikhtiandr 68 experiment, aquanauts were given 4,000 kcal per day. It is important to remember that man must receive substances which cannot be synthesized in his body, i.e. irreplaceable amino acids, vitamins, unsaturated fatty acids and trace elements. It is possible to live on cold food entirely for 10-14 days. Dehydrated foods are highly practical. In the Chibis experiment, the divers ate underwater. A device was developed (not clearly described here) which allowed the divers to ingest liquid and semi-liquid food through a tube. It was found that foods that were neutral in flavor were preferable, because the mucous membranes of the mouth and throat did not become irritated and excessive thirst was avoided. In the Chibis 2 experiment the special suits with individual life support systems made it possible for the divers to remain submerged for 27 to 38 hours. (MFW/BSSCP)

167.
BARER, G.R., T.W. Astin, J.W. Shaw and P.M. Warren.
Bronchomotor effects of respired gases.
Bull. Physiopathol. Resp. 8:459-466;May/June 1972.

Hypoxia and hypercapnia cause bronchoconstriction or bronchodilatation in different circumstances. There are also differences between findings in man and animals. In dogs hypoxia and hypercapnia cause bronchoconstriction through mechanisms involving the vagus nerve. The vagally mediated hypoxic bronchoconstriction may be active in patients with chronic bronchitis, but a bronchoconstrictor action of hypoxia in normal man appears not to involve a nervous mechanism. In both man and animals hypocapnia caused by hyperventilation or occluding a pulmonary artery lead to bronchoconstriction. In animals this is a local action; on man some reports implicate a vagal and others a local mechanism. In animals ventilation with high CO_2 concentrations causes dilatation of bronchi previously constricted by a variety of stimuli. These include pulmonary artery occlusion, 5-hydroxytryptamine, acetylcholine, histamine and vagal stimuli. Dilatation is greater during some stimuli than others. The local action of CO_2 has probably been demonstrated in man. Hypoxia also dilates the constricted airway in animals by a local mechanism. (Authors' abstract)

168.
BARES, W.A.
Direct digital control of a high pressure life research laboratory.
In: IEEE international conference on engineering in the ocean environment, Panama City, Florida, September 1970. Digest of technical papers, p.172-175. Published by the conference.

This report describes planning, selection, and incorporation of a digital computer operating in the direct digital mode (DDC) for complete computer management of a large High Pressure Life Laboratory (HPLL) for deep submergence simulation to 40 atm. (Eng. Ind.)

169.
BARET, Le Guenedal, Broussolle, Legeron, Burnet and Morcellet.
Incorporation du ^{32}P dans les phospholipides alveolaires chez le rat au cours de l'hyperoxie normobare.
[Incorporation of ^{32}P in alveolar phospholipids in rats during normobaric hyperoxia].
Cent. Etud. Rech. Biophysiol. Appl. Mar., Rep. 73-06, 9p. plus illustr. 1973.

Five hundred microcuries of $^{32}PO_4HNa_2$ were injected intravenously into rats which spent 5 days in a pure oxygen atmosphere at normal pressure. (Control animals did not breath the pure oxygen atmosphere.) Two to twenty hours after injection, the rats were killed and pulmonary lavage was done in order to study the incorporation of ^{32}P into alveolary phospholipids. ^{32}P was incorporated into dipalmitoyl lecithins at a much greater rate than into phosphatidyl ethanolamines and lysolecithins. But the beginning of the incorporation process is later (8h) in experimental rats for all classes of phospholipids than in control rats (6h). Times of peak incorporation of the various phospholipids vary only slightly in control rats, but much more widely in experimental animals. And in control rats, a decline in radioactivity between 12 and 16 h, followed by a rise at about 18 h, is observed; this phenomenon tends to disappear in experimental rats. (MEMH/SCD)

170.
BARKHINA, T.J.
O vzaimootnoshenii ekzokrinnoi i endokrinnoi parenkhimy podzheludocnoi ghelezy u uslovyakh giperoksii na submikroskopicheskom urovne.
[Interrelationship between exocrine and endocrine pancreatic parenchyma on submicroscopic level during hyperoxia].
Arkh. Anat. Gistol. Embriol. 63(1):48-52;1972.

Male Wistar rats were given pure O_2 during 12 hour in an altitude chamber at normal barometric pressure. Shortly after exposure of 12 hr an electron microscopic examination of the pancreas revealed acinar-island cells characterized by two types of granules: zymogenic and island granules. In such transitional cells there occurred organelles characteristic of both the achinar cells and islet cells. Two kinds of mitochondria and two structural types of granular endoplasmic reticulum occurred in these organelles. The appearance of acinar-island cells suggested transformation of acinar and island parenchyma. (SGB) (© BA)

171.
BARNARD, E.E.P.
Submarine escape from 600 feet (183 metres).
Proc. Roy. Soc. Med. 64:1271-1273;Dec. 1971.

The USS Squalus and the HMS Thetis both sank in the summer of 1939. The 33 Squalus survivors were rescued by means of the McCann Rescue Bell carried on the submarine salvage ship USS Falcon. The method of escape from the British submarine was via an escape chamber designed to take two men at a time. Unfortunately only four men escaped although the escape chamber was only about 10 feet below the surface, due to the angle at which the boat was lying. Free escape was used extensively, both experimentally and in training by both countries, but hooded ascent was extensively used in training by the British and proved satisfactory. (CWS/BSCP)

172.
BARNARD, E.E.P.
Some problems of human diving.
In: The effect of pressure on organisms. Symposia of the Society for Experimental Biology, No. 26, p.343-353. London, Cambridge University Press, 1972.

The author first briefly discusses sensory impairment and the effects of cold, then breath-hold diving, with its problems of equalization of pressure in the ear, of squeeze, hypoxia, carbon dioxide, and the possibility (rare in breath-hold diving) of decompression sickness. Compressed air diving brings the dangers of decompression sickness, carbon dioxide build-up, nitrogen narcosis, and oxygen toxicity (rare in compressed-air diving, because of the depth limitations imposed by nitrogen narcosis). Passing to deeper diving, and breathing mixtures other than air, the author compares helium, neon, and hydrogen. The fire danger of hydrogen, and the expense of neon, leave helium the currently most widely used breathing gas for deep diving. A characteristic of helium is that it diffuses more rapidly than nitrogen and might therefore form bubbles more quickly, reducing the onset time of decompression sickness symptoms. The high pressure nervous syndrome (hpns) is discussed, and it is noted that slow compression delays symptoms and holding pressure constant at long intervals has an ameliorating effect. The syndrome would appear to be primarily pressure-related, and may well be the first true pressure effect noted in man, since previously observed effects of hyperbaric environments have been related to the gases present in the breathing mixture. (MWF/SCD)

173.
BARNARD, E.E.P.
Formula and fashion in the treatment of decompression sickness in divers.
J. Roy. Nav. Med. Serv. 58:4-8;Spring 1972.

The author discusses the recompression method of treating decompression sickness. It is his belief that relief of symptoms should be the criterion for degree of pressure. In acute cases, 30 minutes should suffice; in chronic cases six hours is the minimum requirement. Decompression following therapeutic recompression usually follows the stage method, but a gradual and continuous decompression is sometimes used in cases at extreme depths. The table preferred here is the oxygen/air table of Goodman and Workman. If recompression at 60 feet does not bring relief in 10 minutes, the pateint should be taken to 165 feet for 30 minutes. If relief is complete, return to 1ATA is made in accordance with the table. If relief is not complete, time can be extended to 120 minutes. Where hypovolemic shock is present, such agents as plasma and dextran should be used, possibly combined with heparin. Hypothermia may be used in cases where paralysis is present. The value of urea or mannitol to reduce edema is uncertain, but a possibility. Widespread education both of divers and doctors is essential. (MFW/BSCP)

174.
BARNARD, E.E.P. and R. de G. Hanson.
The relation of therapeutic to causative pressure in decompression sickness in mice.
In: Hesser, C.M. and D. Linnarsson eds. Proceedings of the first annual scientific meeting of the European Undersea Biomedical Society, Stockholm, 13-15 June 1973. Forsvarsmedicin 9:507-513;July 1973.

The results showed that there was a relationship between the survival of the mice and the depth of recompression. The depth at which a statistically significant improvement compared with those not recompressed, varied with the depth of the original dive. The exposures to 125 m and 150 m showed an improvement at 5 m ($P < .05$ and $P < .01$ respectively). The 175 m exposure showed no significant improvement at 5 m but there was an improvement at 10 m ($P < .001$). After the 225 m there was no significant improvement following 5 m or 10 m recompression but an improvement at 15 m ($P < .001$). No mice died after recompression to 40 m or 80 m except for six which had become moribund on the surface. A similar relationship was shown with regard to the prevention of serious symptoms; only one mouse developed serious symptoms after being recompressed to 80 m and none after being recompressed to 40 m. It would appear that the depth of the original exposure may have a slight bearing on the results of shallower recompressions but there appears to be an optimum depth for recompression between 15 m and 50 m, probably around 20 m, which for all practical purposes would be the same for all four exposures. These experiments indicated that there was no need to return to the original depth of exposure to obtain optimal results. (Authors' abstract)

175.
BARNARD, E.E.P., R. de G. Hanson, B.J. Reid and J. Williams.
Studies in nitrogen elimination.
In: Hesser, D.M. and D. Linnarsson eds. Proceedings of the first annual scientific meeting of the European Undersea Biomedical Society, Stockholm, 13-15 June 1973. Forsvarsmedicin 9:496-501;July 1973.

The rate of nitrogen elimination during the first five minutes appears to depend upon frequency of respiration. Investigations into the effect of pure oxygen breathing upon respiratory rate have revealed that at higher pressures a fall in the rate is seen. This fall was observed in these experiments. It was noted that after about 50 minutes of the denitrogenation period, oxygen breathing became more effective than helium-oxygen breathing. After 100 minutes, the difference became marked. The findings of this experiment support the generally held belief that pure oxygen breathing accelerates nitrogen elimination, and disproves the hypothesis that oxygen breathing brings on vasoconstriction, thereby reducing tissue perfusion and interfering with nitrogen elimination. (MFW/UMS)

176.
BARTHELEMY, L., A. Belaud, M. Bellett and C. Peyraud.
Etude, chez le poisson, des effets de la pression soit en tant que force appliquee, soit associee a une augmentation de la mass des gaz dissous.
[Study, in fish, of the effect of pressure either as an applied force, or associated with an increase in mass of dissolved gases].
C.R. Soc. Biol. (Paris) 165:1754-1756;1971.

Pathological nervous and respiratory phenomena in mammals during deep dives have been attributed both to pressure per se and to the increase in gas partial pressure. Some twenty experiments on six eels were undertaken in an attempt to dissociate the effects of these two parameters. The eels were subjected to pressure singly, either in a closed aquarium, in which the quantity of gas dissolved in the water remained constant (technique A) or in an open container, in which compression causes an increase in mass of dissolved gases. ECG readings were recorded throughout the experiments. Under technique A, fish reacted to compression and decompression with bradycardia and brief periods of apnea. These transitory effects disappeared when variations in pressure ceased. Under technique B, the same inhibitory cardio-respiratory reactions appeared. In addition, during the period of constant pressure, there appeared phases of tachycardia accompanied by increases in the size of ECG fluctuations. After successive dives, fibrillation may be observed. Three deaths occurred within 24 hours of decompression, and autopsies revealed the presence of embolisms and intra-tissular bubbles. Reactions occurred during the constant-pressure phase only with technique B, and are therefore attributed to the increase in the mass of the dissolved gases. The effects of change of the gaseous content of the environment seem more important than those of pressure per se, but further experimentation is clearly called for. (MEMH/BSCP)

177.
BARTHELEMY, L. and A. Belaud.
Constatations physiologiques et physiopathologiques faites sur un poisson (Anguilla Anguilla L.) en conditions hyperbares.
[Physiological and physiopathological findings during compression in the eel (Anguilla anguilla L.) in hyperbaric conditions].
Bull. Medsubhyp 8:33;Nov. 1972.

Compression of eels (Anguilla anguilla L) was carried out with the following experimental conditions: (1) in a rubber membrane stoppered container filled with water and enclosed in an hyperbaric chamber where the eels are submitted to pressure only, (2) in an open tank placed in the hyperbaric chamber where the fishes are submitted to both pressure and dissolved gaseous mass. Condition 1: 15 ATA resulted in no appreciable behavioral and physiological changes. Condition 2: various physiological reactions were recorded and related to gas mixtures, pressure and duration of the experiments. OHP and inert gases (He and N_2) were specially investigated. OHP toxic threshold is greatly increased in fishes as compared with mammals. Decompression sickness occurred in condition 2 only. (English abstract).

178.
BARTON, R.
Making diving safer.
Hydrospace 4:30-32;Mar. 1971.

The author reports on a discussion held following the publication of "Principles of safe diving practice", by the Underwater Engineering Group. The discussion was informal and inconclusive, and dealt with such subjects as the legal implementation of the safe diving code, the present inadequacy of diver training courses, the lack of an accurate diver classification system, the need for more definite specifications regarding medical examinations for divers. There is a need for a national standard of medical data and of treatment, and a national record center. A start has been made toward the last named with the Medical Research Council Decompression Sickness Central Registry at Newcastle. It was suggested that the diving code should not at present include decompression tables, since these are still in the experimental stage. It is noted that there is a lack of diver statistics — how many working divers there are, what depths they work at, what the accident rate is, and so on. (MFW/BSCP)

179.
BARTON R.
Armoured suit has 1000 ft capability.
Offshore Services 6:18-21;May 1973.

One answer to the problem of the high cost of employing divers using current methods lies in the development of the armored, one-atmosphere diving suit. Interest in this type of equipment lapsed after World War II, but increased activity in the offshore oil industry has revived it. The suit described here has been developed by a British company, DHB Construction Ltd. It is made of magnesium alloy, weighs 1100 lbs in air with diver, is supplied with general purpose hand-like manipulators at the end of each arm enclosure, which can be changed for special purpose devices. Buoyancy is infinitely adjustable. The life support system carries 800 liters of oxygen and 12 lb of soda lime, which allows for work missions of four hours with an emergency reserve of from 8-16 hours. Oxygen partial pressure is monitored by a Beckman Minos instrument. Obvious advantages are the elimination of compression and decompression delays, greater bottom time, comfort, security, and ease of surface communication for the diver. Depth changes become unimportant. A dive can be immediately repeated. The suit is transportable by helicopter. The advantages over the manned submersible lie in its capability of closer contact with the job, and of access to places impossible of access to a submersible (MFW/SCD)

180.
BARTUS, R.T.
Evidence for a possible memory impairment resulting from nitrogen narcosis in the rhesus monkey.
U.S. Nav. Submar. Med. Res. Lab., Rep. NSMRL 751, 5p. Aug. 30, 1973.

Three Rhesus monkeys were maintained at 200 FSW equivalent and tested on the reversal of a previously trained visual discrimination problem. All three monkeys displayed a higher percent of errors on this reversal problem than on another reversal problem tested on the surface. These data, supplemented by changes in the monkeys' post-response stimulus observation time, are interpreted as possible evidence for memory impairments resulting from nitrogen narcosis. (Author's abstract)

181.
BARTUS, R.T. and S.H. Ferris.
A modified method of implanting monopolar cortical electrodes in large laboratory animals.
U.S. Nav. Submar. Med. Res. Lab., Rep. NSMRL 750, 4p. Aug. 1973.

[The problem was] to modify the electrode implantation technique developed for recording visual evoked responses from rats, so that it can be used with larger animals. [It was found that] the general technique was successfully adapted for use with cats, providing an electrode assembly as inexpensive, durable, and reliable as that previously developed for the rat. A very simple technique is now available for chronically implanting monopolar brain electrodes in laboratory animals of all sizes. Because of its simplicity, as well as generality and inexpense, laboratories interested in studying neural effects of hazardous environments (such as high compression atmosphere) should have little trouble adapting this technique to their research program. (Authors' summary)

182.
BARTUS, R.T.
Behavioral effects of nitrogen narcosis in the rhesus monkey.
U.S. Nav. Submar. Med. Res. Lab., Rep. NSMRL 755, 9p., Sept. 12, 1973.

Rhesus monkeys performed highly trained visual discrimination problems while breathing air at normal pressure or the sea water equivalent of 200 feet. A significant drop in performance was observed at 200 feet depth with greatest deficits occurring on the most difficult discrimination problems. This impairment was partially alleviated by allowing the monkeys to view the stimuli longer before making their choice responses. These deficits were interpreted as specific impairments in mechanisms necessary for processing visual information. (Author's abstract)

183.
BARTUS, R.T.
Nitrogen narcosis and visual evoked responses in the unanesthetized cat.
U.S. Nav. Submar. Med. Res. Lab., Rep. NSMRL 757, 10p. Sept. 12, 1973.

Four cats were implanted with gross, unipolar electrodes in the lateral geniculate nucleus (LGN), pretectum-superior colliculus (P-SC), primary visual cortex (VI), and secondary visual cortex (VII). After an adequate recovery period, and following preliminary testing the cats were exposed to the sea water equivalent depth of 340 feet in a dry pressure chamber. It was found that no decrements in the amplitude of the visual evoked response occurred at the LGN, but that significant decreases did occur at all other sites. These data were interpreted as evidence that the effects of inert gas narcosis on the visual system are primarily central, and not simply peripheral in nature; that these effects are not limited to the visual cortical mantle; and that the narcosis apparently influences the neural activity of the brain structures involving several anatomical levels of the brain which mediate several types of visual processes. On the basis of these conclusions, one can expect performance on almost any type of task requiring visual processing to be affected by various degrees of inert gas narcosis. (Author's abstract)

184.
BASSETT, B.E. and J.M. Dunn.
U.S. Air Force compression therapy experience — 1965 through 1970.
In: Aerospace Medical Association. 1971 annual scientific meeting. Houston, Texas, April 1971. Preprints, p.158-159. Published by the Association, 1971.

During the period from January 1965 through December 1970, 37 treatment dives were conducted at 7 USAF compression facilities for 25 military and 9 civilian patients with decompression sickness or air embolism. There were a total of 89 treatment dives conducted for 27 patients with suspected or confirmed gas gangrene. Only 3 of these 27 patients were military members. There were also 62 treatment dives conducted for 8 patients with other disorders. Five of these patients, with systemic coccidioidomycosis, received 29 treatments. The total caseload for this period therefore consisted of 188 treatment dives for 33 military and 36 civilian patients. While the hyperbaric therapy experience does not represent a large contribution to the overall USAF medical mission, the compression training and therapy program as conducted and monitored by the USAF School of Aerospace Medicine certainly represents a unique fraction of the overall mission. For the specific disorders of decompression sickness, air embolism, selected cases of gas gangrene and carbon monoxide poisoning, this mode of therapy has no equal, and the majority of patients treated represented true medical emergencies that would have had a dire outcome had such therapy not been available or administered. (Authors' summary)

185.
BATTELLE COLUMBUS LABORATORIES
U.S. Navy diving-gas manual. Second edition Washington, D.C., United States Navy Supervisor of Diving, 1971.
(NAVSHIPS 0994-003-7010)

The principal objective of this manual is to provide the best available information on gas properties in a form convenient for use in diving research, engineering, and operations. All of the data in this manual are based upon calculation from theoretical relationships, substantiated where experimental information can be found in the literature (as for pure gases), and unsubstantiated where such information does not exist (as for helium-oxygen mixtures). It is felt that the data presented are the best that can be generated today, and that they will be generally satisfactory in the pressure range up to about 500 psi. For the higher pressures used in storing of diving gases, errors are indeterminate and may be significant. Future experimental research is needed to improve the state of knowledge of mixture properties at very high pressures, and to explore the properties of helium-oxygen-nitrogen mixtures. (From authors' introduction).

186.
BATTELLE COLUMBUS LABORATORIES
Proceedings, 1973 divers' gas purity symposium, November 27-28, 1973.
U.S. Navy Supervisor Diving, Nav. Ships Syst. Comm., Rep. 2-73, 1973.

The papers presented in this symposium deal with numerous aspects of maintaining the quality of divers' breathing mixtures, of detecting contaminants, of techniques employed in analyzing the mixing gases, and of purity standards and toxicological limits. Specific papers will be found under the following author entries: Bishop, R.P.; Clark, J.M.; Devel, C.L.; Gilardi, R.C.; Gillen, H.W. and R.W. Brauer; Hazard, H.R.; Joyce, J.W. and R.L. Woods; Lewis, W.F., R.J. Lee and B.M. Hoffert; Melka, L.A. and J.A. Henkener; Padden, J.B. and M.G. Jacko; Purer, A.; St. Clair, J.C.; Schmidt, T.C., D.J. Kenyon, M. Freitag and R.W. Hamilton, Jr.; Smith, J.G.; Thalman, E.D.; Thomas, C.; Trigger, A.W.; Vind, H.P., C. Mathews and O.R. Hansen; Wischhoeffer, L.L. (MFW/UMS)

187.
BAUER, B.B., L.A. Abbagnaro and J. Schumann.
Wide-range calibration system for pressure-gradient hydrophones.
J. Acoust. Soc. Amer. 51(5, pt. 2):1717-1724;1972.

A gradient hydrophone calibrator consists of a precisely made water-filled tank, with ports to receive the hydrophones to be calibrated and the reference pressure hydrophones, which is set into axial oscillation with suitable drivers to develop a standing wave of sound in the water. An improved calibrator is described, which, by using a very rigid tank, covers a range of 3-2500Hz. Measurements are simplified through use of electrical feedback, which maintains a constant pressure-gradient versus frequency function. The applications and limitations of this system to the measurement of sensitivity, frequency response, and phase response of pressure-gradient and pressure hydrophones, and for obtaining the polar patterns of gradient hydrophones are described. (Authors' abstract)

188.
BAUME, A.D.
Underwater habitats—a review.
Meerestechnik 3:239-242;Dec. 1972.

This is a rather comprehensive review of the state of the art in underwater habitats as bases for working divers, and the comparative usefulness of diving systems, submersibles, and habitats. Where a platform is involved and the tasks are localized, the diving system is the ideal choice. When a large area need to be covered, the lock-out submersible is better able to meet the requirements. With the development of saturation diving techniques, the habitat is becoming more desirable as a base for scientific operation, permitting a more continuous and flexible approach to the research project. Habitats have not yet been used widely in commercial operations, because in their present state of development they are uneconomical. As they become more mobile, they will doubtless become more practicable for commercial use. Specific habitats such as SeaLab III, Aegir and Helgoland are discussed. Jobs of longer durations will eventually be more efficiently carried out from habitats. It is stated that "the ideal diving system is one which can make its way from base to site and back, with crew aboard but with no external help. Habitats and lockout submersibles are converging on this point. It will no doubt be reached in some form." (MFW/BSCP)

189.
BAYLES, J.J.
Salvage work projects — SeaLab III.
U.S. Nav. Civ. Eng. Lab., Tech. Rep. R-684, 135 p., June 1970.

The Navy is authorized by public statute to provide salvage facilities to assist both public and private vessels. In keeping with this responsibility, the Supervisor of Salvage, U.S. Navy, is prosecuting a vigorous program to incorporate the latest techniques and equipments into the Navy's salvage forces. The SeaLab III Program under the direction of the Ocean Engineering Branch, Deep Submergence Systems Project Office, was initiated to advance the state-of-the-art of man's capability to live and work in the deep ocean environment. It was the goal of the Salvage Projects for SeaLab III to demonstrate and field test some of the more important new salvage devices and techniques. This report discusses the aquanaut familiarization and training phases associated with the Salvage Projects planned for Team Two — SeaLab III, and the modifications to both equipments and procedures as suggested by the divers. Preliminary results are included with recommendations regarding future plans. Human factors studies were conducted in conjunction with the training phases in preparation for SeaLab III. Goals included assessment of divers performance, the development of improved underwater work procedures and improvement of underwater equipment design through development of design criteria. (Author's abstract)

190.
BEAN, J.W., J. Lignell and D.W. Burgess.
Cerebral O_2, CO_2, regional cerebral vascular control, and hyperbaric oxygenation.
J. Appl. Physiol. 32:650-657;May 1972.

The influence of O_2 and CO_2 on regional cerebral vascular control and tissue PO_2, EEG, and the occurrence of epileptiform convulsions was studied by implanted O_2-thermoflow probes built to monitor simultaneous changes in blood flow, tissue PO_2 and neural activity at the same cellular site in two regions of unanesthetized rat brains. It is concluded that O_2-sensitive vascular controls contribute with individual and regional variation, to the regulation of regional cerebral blood flow. In O_2 at high pressure this frequently fails, due in part to precapillary escape of O_2 under high arterial transmural O_2 diffusion gradient. In prolonged exposure this control breaks down due in part to the toxic action of O_2 on the vascular smooth muscle. The resultant abrupt shift in regional flow patterns to large parallel increases throughout the brain precipitously further elevates tissue PO_2 above the toxic level for the CNS, triggering the convulsive EEG discharge, disrupting neurogenic regional vascular controls, and precipitating overt epileptiform convulsions. The effects of CO_2 are presented and discussed in relation to O_2 cerebral vascular control. (Authors' abstract)

191.
BEATTY, H.T. and T.E. Berghage.
Diver anthropometrics.
U.S. Navy Exp. Diving Unit, Rep. NEDU-10-72, 155 p. June 1, 1972.

To aid the design engineer in the development of future U.S. Navy diving systems and equipment a comprehensive anthropometric study was undertaken. Fifty-four anthropometric measures, two pulmonary function measures, and three derived body measures were obtained on 100, 41 and 100 U.S. Navy divers respectively. Descriptive statistics and measures of interrelationship are given for each measured and derived variable. The minimum number of anthropometric variables needed was determined by factor analysis. The measures obtained on the U.S. Navy divers were compared with anthropometric data available for the male aviation populations. (Authors' abstract)

192.
BEAUBIEN, L.A., I. Wolock, C.L. Buchanan and C.L. Whitman.
Behavior of materials in a subsurface ocean environment.
U.S. Nav. Res. Lab., Rep. NRL-7447, 111 p. July 14, 1972.
(AD 747 245)

Information is presented on the deterioration in sea water of materials and undersea-system components, based on published and unpublished studies, and on authoritative opinions. The items chosen for evaluation are primarily those likely to be used in deep-ocean structure and systems. Materials included are photographic materials, magnetic tape, electronic components and propellants and explosives. Marine corrosion of metals is represented in the form of an annotated bibliography; the remaining entries consist of summaries of material and component behavior coupled with pertinent bibliographies. The form and scope of these summaries run from comprehensive evaluations in the areas of plastics and propellants to relatively brief opinions of authorities for items of lesser marine utility or occurrence. (Author) (GRA)

193.
BECKMAN, D.L., R.T. Houlihan and J. Saha.
Sympathetics surfactants and hyperbaric oxygen.
Fed. Proc. 31:823;Mar./Apr. 1972.

Abstract only. Entire item quoted: Sympathetic stimulation via the stellate ganglion and mechanical CNS injury produced alveolar surfactant changes and decreased lung compliance (Proc. Int. Cong. Physiol. Sci. p.47, 1971).

Unlike the situation found in rats, these changes occurred in monkeys in the absence of gross lung damage. The lung changes from CNS injury were blocked by sympatholytic agents (J.A.P. 29:631; 1970). In the present study seven adult cats exposed to 5 atm oxygen (OHP) unitl overt epileptiform seizures had occurred showed similar surfactant changes (min. surface tension 22 dynes/cm). These surfactant changes occurred in the absence of the gross lung damage or increase in lung weight as previously reported in rats exposed to OHP. In addition to the species difference, our findings may suggest that at least part of the toxicity of OHP on the lungs is a result of a centrally mediated sympathetic influence on the alveolar surfactants. These results support the previous conclusion (J.A.P. 30:394; 1971) that alveolar surfactants are under sympathetic control.

194.
BECKMAN, D.L. and R.T. Houlihan.
Surfactant changes from OHP in the absence of gross lung damage.
In: Aerospace Medical Association. 1972 annual scientific meeting, Bal Harbour, Florida, May 1971. Preprints, p.179-180. Published by the Association.

The present experiments were performed in order to determine whether OHP could alter the alveolar surfactants without causing any attendant gross lung damage. The results showed that rats exposed to OHP had both altered surfactants and hemorrhagic edema of the lungs; however, cats which were similarly exposed to OHP had altered surfactants without this attendant gross lung damage. The lung weight/body weight ratios in cats were normal. The results from this and previous work suggest that in addition to a sepcies difference at least part of the toxicity of OHP on the lungs is a result of a centrally mediated sympathetic influence on the alveolar surfactants. (Authors' summary)

195.
BECKMAN, D.L. and R.T. Houlihan.
Hyperbaric oxygen and alveolar surfactants.
Aerosp. Med. 44:422-424;Apr. 1973.

Gross lung damage was previously found in rats exposed to mechanical head injury similar to that which occurs during exposure of rats to oxygen at high pressure (OHP). The pulmonary effects from this CNS injury and OPH exposure were blocked by sympatholytic and antiepinephrine agents. In monkeys CNS injury altered the alveolar surfactants in the absence of any immediate gross lung damage. Surfactant changes were also produced by electrical stimulation of the pulmonary sympathetics in monkeys and cats. The present experiments were performed in order to determine whether OHP also could alter the alveolar surfactants before the occurrence of any gross lung damage. The results indicate that while rats exposed to minimal OHP have both altered surfactants and gross lung damage, that cats had altered surfactants without the attendant gross lung damage; lung weight/body weight ratios were normal in the cat. In addition to the species differences, our results suggest that at least part of the toxicity of OHP on the lungs is a result of a centrally mediated sympathetic influence on the alveolar surfactants. (Authors' abstract)

196.
BECKMAN, E.L., R.G. Masson and E.M. Smith.
Medical support program.
In: Miller, J.W., J.G. Van Derwalker, and R.A. Waller, eds. Tektite 2: Scientists-in-the-sea, p. IX-1 — IX-24. Washington, D.C., U.S. Department of the Interior, August 1971.

This report describes the organization, responsibilities, observations, and conclusions of the medical program. Included are descriptions of the staff, training requirements, physical facilities, examination and decompression procedures, the development of new decompression tables, and a review of some problems faced. In general it can be said that no serious medical problems were encountered. Of 915 man-days in the habitat, only 13 man-days in the water were lost because of medical reasons. A brief discussion of non-diving medical problems is included. [Appendix A gives Tektite 1 decompression table, Appendix B, the revised table for Tektite 2 (more oxygen breathing and more stops), Appendix C, the table for Minitat, and Appendix D, the treatment schedule for emergency or accidental decompression from 100 feet]. (Authors' abstract)

197.
BECKMAN, E.L.
Diving standards.
In: United States-Japan conference on natural resources development. Proceedings of the first joint meeting of the U.S.-Japan panel on diving and technology, Tokyo, 1972, p. 104-115. Japan, Ministry of Agriculture and Forestry, 1972.

The author discusses the economic and safety problems of the diving industry in the United States, and emphasizes the difficulties of agreeing on regulations for decompression tables, for medical certification of divers, and for standards regarding equipment and procedure. The necessity of developing new decompression tables for industrial diving is noted. The U.S. Navy decompression tables are so conservative as to be prohibitive in cost, due to the extremely high wages received by divers. In spite of the conservatism of the Navy tables, there is a large incidence of osteonecrosis in former Navy divers who are now working in the industry. The author has been assigned the task of developing commercial decompression tables, and requests the cooperation of Japan in the testing of these tables. (MFW/UMS)

198.
BECKMAN, E.L. and E.M. Smith.
Tektite II. Medical supervision of the scientists in the sea.
Texas Rep. Biol. Med. 30:1-204;Fall 1972.

This report constitutes an entire special issue of the journal. The contents are as follows: I. Introduction; II. Saturation diving; III. Tektite I; IV. Evolution of project Tektite II; V. Medical staff and responsibilities, psychological monitoring; VI. The spectrum of medical supervision of the aquanauts; VII. Other medical and biological objectives; VIII. Tektite logistics; IX. Mission-by-mission experiences; X. The aborted 100-FSW (Minitat) Program; XI. Decompression tables; XII. General medical observations; XIII. Some preliminary psychological observations; XIV. Biochemical, hematological, and endocrine studies; XV. Conclusions. (MFW/BSCP)

199.
BEHAN, F.L., R.A. Behan and H.W. Wendhausen.
Color perception underwater.
Hum. Factors 14:41-44;Feb. 1972.

Twelve scuba divers were assigned in groups of four to depths of 30, 60 and 90 feet in the ocean to examine 13 plates of a standard diagnostic color perception test. In clear water, under conditions of low illumination, colors in the full range of the visible spectrum were detectable at 90 feet. In a few instances, low saturation greens and reds were not identified. All colors seemed somewhat faded due to reduced contrast and low illumination. (Authors' abstract)

200.
BELAUD, A. and L. Barthelemy.
Modifications de quelques parametres physiologiques chez le poisson en conditions hyperbares. [Changes in some physiological parameters in fish under hyperbaric conditions].
J. Physiol. (Paris) 65 (Suppl. 3):346A;1972.

Abstract only: Eels (Anguilla anguilla L.) were subjected to pressure (with or without a change in the mass of gas dissolved in the water) below or equal to 16 ATA. Parameters observed were: EKG, arterial pressure, opercular mechanics, telencephalic electrical activity, and motor activity. Pressure per se does not materially affect these parameters, but changes in pressure are followed by reflex bradycardia and bradypnea. Rapid decompression (15 ata/min) is not reflected in any symptoms, including aeroembolism. An increase in the mass of dissolved gases gives rise to physiological reactions related to the gas or gases involved, test pressure, and length of time. Hyperbaric hyperoxia gives rise to a hypoventilatory effect proportional to oxygen partial pressure and unrelated to the diluent gas. The eel's particular resistance to decompression accidents and to the toxic effects of hyperbaric oxygen may be partly explained by the important role which anaerobic metabolism and the pentose pathways may play in fish. (Transl. MEMH/UMS)

201.
BELL, C.F.
Advanced biotechnology for underwater operations.
J. Hydronautics 5:91-96;July 1971.

Within the past two decades an up-surge has been witnessed in the universal interest in the oceans. This results from the sophistication of submarines, the development of small diving vehicles and increased diving activities by commercial, military, and sportsmen groups. In the development of the undersea vehicle and of new diving techniques, the biotechnological requirements for these must be continuously brought up to date and resolved. New submarines are under water from 50 to 75 days, and their environmental problems both in relation to biomedical sciences and behavioral sciences are continually being evaluated for the safety and well-being of submarine personnel. New diving techniques require extensive hyperbaric chamber testing, especially in respect to those dives of a saturation nature and at great depth. (Eng. Ind.)

202.
BELL, J.D.
Preliminary evaluation of the Battelle Memorial Institute prototype one-man recompression chamber.
Downsview, Ontario, Def. Civ. Inst. Environ. Med., Def. Res. Board, Rep. DCIEM 73-OR-982, 74p. Dec. 1973.

A preliminary evaluation of the Battelle Memorial Institute's one-man portable recompression chamber was conducted at the U.S. Navy Experimental Diving Unit, Washington, D.C. The objective was to assess the suitability of the prototype chamber as a replacement for those presently in service within the Canadian Forces. The chamber provides for patient treatment using the air treatment tables; however, incorporation of a built-in breathing system for O_2 therapy treatment is feasible if required. The chamber internal diameter is only 21 11/16 inches. This is due to a U.S. Navy requirement that the chamber be able to pass through a 24-inch hatch. The findings, based on a theoretical analysis, laboratory test data, and subjective assessments, are summarized in Table 1. Subject to implementation of the suggested component modifications, and acceptance of the limitations imposed by the chamber diameter, it is concluded the prototype one-man chamber is suitable for service within the Canadian forces. (Author's summary)

203.
BELLAMY, D.
Diving information and inshore biology.
In: Diving applications in marine research. Proceedings of a seminar, National Institute of Oceanography, Godalming, Surrey, U.K., December 1971, p.45-47. Published by the Institute. 1972.

Scuba divers then have three main roles to play: (1) As watchdogs within the hydrosphere. (2) As active participants in gathering the scientific data needed to conserve and develop the resources. (3) As teachers of matters environmental to the cross-section of the world, from which they are drawn and with which they have contact. To this end it is planned to consolidate the work described above, by setting up three environmental monitoring stations. . . The first monitoring site in the Mediterranean was surveyed during the summer of 1971, and it is hoped to develop a world matrix through the world federation of divers (Committee Mondiale des Activites Subsquatique). At the first Scientific Congress of CMAS, held in 1970 in Havana, plans were laid for a marine information centre organised by the Cuban Academy of Sciençes. This is now in operation. The main requirement is for recognized courses in Proficiency in Diving Biology; plans and details of such a course will be presented. (Author)

204.
BELLES, F.E.
High pressure oxygen utilization by NASA.
NASA, Lewis Res. Cent. NASA-TM-X-68203 18p. Mar. 1973.
(N 73 20276)

Although NASA is not one of the country's major oxygen consumers, it uses oxygen under severe conditions including very high flow rates and pressure. Materials for such applications must be carefully selected for compatibility, because susceptibility to ignition increases as operating pressure is raised. Much work is needed, however, to define the selection criteria. Some of the work in this area that is being performed under sponsorship of NASA's Aerospace Safety Research and Data Institute (ASRDI) is described. (Author) (STAR)

205.
BENATAR, S.R., A.M. Hewlett and J.F. Nunn.
The use of iso-shunt lines for control of oxygen therapy.
Br. J. Anaesth. 45:711-718;July 1973.

The concept of "virtual shunt" is presented as a practical means for determining the optimal inspired oxygen concentration for patients with hypoxaemia due to pulmonary venous admixture. The approach permits a reduction in the number of blood-gas analyses needed. Its limitations have been explored and its validity assessed from a series of 44 observations made on 4 patients. (Authors' abstract)

206.
BENITEZ, S.
Annual report in support of hyperbaric physiology research.
Frederick, Md., Automation Counselors Inc., Rep. ACI-1009-4, 18p. June 1973.
(AD 763 474)

The report describes the progress made in the development of a physiological monitoring system for use in hyperbaric research. The system, designed around a mini-computer configuration, is able to monitor up to 16 channels of analog data and 5 channels of data from radioisotope detectors. Both real-time and non real-time data analysis is included as part of the operational system. During the period covered by the report the system was used to: monitor physiological response of divers subject to various hyperbaric environments and workloads; test the effectiveness of electronically heated suits; and monitor inert gas uptake and distribution in anesthetized dogs under hyperbaric conditions. (Author) (GRA)

207.
BENNETT, P.B. and K.N. Ackles.
The narcotic effects of hyperbaric oxygen.
In: Wada, J. and I. Takashi, eds. Proceedings of the fourth international congress on hyperbaric medicine, Sapporo, Japan, Sept. 1969, p. 74-79. Baltimore, Williams and Wilkins, 1970.

Five subjects were each exposed to 3 different pressures of oxygen and the amplitude of the averaged evoked responses together with arithmetic efficiency compared with that at atmospheric pressure. The results (Table I) indicate that hyperbaric oxygen will indeed depress the auditory evoked response without affecting arithmetic performance, except at 3 ATA O_2 (66 ft.) when the sums were significantly depressed (sums correct $P < 0.05$, sums attempted $P < 0.01$). However, at this pressure the evoked response is lower than at 2 ATA O_2 (33 ft.), where arithmetic efficiency appeared unaffected. This may be due to the small number of subjects studied or because of a balancing increase in excitability as one approaches pressure causing convulsions. It is relevant that Frankenhaeuser, Graff-Loggevig and Hesser using simple choice reaction times and mirror drawing found no significant impairment in 10 men exposed to oxygen at 3 ATA

(66 ft.). More experiments are therefore required to verify the relationship between evoked response and arithmetic or other performance tests at 3 ATA. Nevertheless, hyperbaric oxygen does depress auditory responses in the brain without unduly affecting mental performance and this indicates a depression of the central nervous system by oxygen at pressures not sufficient to produce convulsions but enough to cause minimal narcosis. Before the narcosis is sufficient to materially depress performance, some other factor probably is affected by this gas which is very active, when compared with the inert gases. This factor is most probably enzyme inhibition. Wood has shown that the central inhibitory enzyme gamma-aminobutyric falls in the brain of animals exposed to hyperbaric oxygen and suggests convulsions are due to the decrease in its modulating action on nerve transmission. It is significant that unpublished data by Wood and the author did not show a similar fall in this enzyme in animals exposed to narcotic pressures of nitrogen and argon. (Authors)

208.
BENNETT, P.B. and A.N. Dossett.
Studies of cationic and anionic compounds on the effects of high pressures of nitrogen and oxygen.
In: Aerospace Medical Association. 1971 annual scientific meeting. Houston, Texas, April 1971. Preprints, p.69-70. Published by the Association, 1971.

Intraperitoneal administration of cationic and anionic detergents in rats exposed to $0.9O_2/6.41\ N_2$ ats abs have shown that narcosis, as measured by a reduction of photically induced averaged cortical evoked potentials, is prevented by the cationic detergents stearylamine and cetyl trimethyl ammonium bromide but not by the anionic compounds sodium hexadecyl sulphate and soidum dodecyl sulphate. Since certain antipyretic compounds such as acetylsalicylic acid, also will stabilise membranes, this too was investigated and found effective in preventing the depression of evoked potentials due to inert gas narcosis. . . The present study was to determine whether, cationic detergents also would be effective in ameliorating oxygen convulsions. Accordingly 50 wistar rats were exposed to 6.44 ats abs oxygen applied at a rate of 3.4 ats/min, and their times to convulsions measured. . . The results indicate that the anionic detergents sodium hexadecyl sulphate and sodium dodecyl sulphate caused decreases in the mean time to convulsions of 34.7% and 7.2% respectively. On the other hand the cationic compounds stearlyamine and cetyl trimethyl ammonium bromide caused significant increases in the mean time to convulsions of 18.3% and 75.5% respectively. . . It is suggested, therefore, that stabilisation of cell membranes by cationic detergents as with inert gas narcosis may ameliorate oxygen toxicity by prevention of an increased permeability to cell electrolytes. That convulsions eventually do still occur may be due to the action of HBO on other factors such as gamma aminobutyric acid metabolism. (Authors)

209.
BENNETT, P.B.
Changes in the EEG during exposure to inert gases at high pressures.
In: Abstracts of the Twenty-fifth Congress of Physiological Sciences Satellite Symposium. Recent progress in fundamental physiology of diving, Marseille, France, July 1971, p.52-53. (Proceedings unpublished)

Abstract only. The author reviews experiments on EEG changes made with inert gases from 1951. Effects of nitrogen, argon, helium and xenon have been observed with various experimental animals, as well as with surgical patients and normal human subjects are described. In general, helium has been found to have the least effect on the amplitude or frequencies until depths of 1300 feet are attained. Helium differs from other inert gases in that it produces increased theta activity. The author plans to compare previous findings with similar studies carried out with men at depths to 300 feet, breathing air or oxygen-helium, applied at a rate of 100 feet/min., and to consider their importance with relation to deep diving and nitrogen narcosis. (MFW/BSCP)

210.
BENNETT, P.B. and E.J. Towse.
Electroencephalogram, tremors and mental performance during exposure to air or oxygen-helium at 100 ft., 200 ft. and 300 ft.
Alverstoke, U.K., Roy. Nav. Physiol. Lab., Rep. 3/72, 29 p. 1972.

The effects of a rate of compression of 100 ft/min are compared in men breathing either air or oxygen-helium at depths equivalent to 100 ft, 200 ft. and 300 ft., from measurement of EEG with frequency analysis, tremors and cognitive function, to ascertain the presence, if any, of the High Pressure Nervous Syndrome (HPNS). An arithmetic test indicated a decrement breathing air at all depths and a very small decrement with oxygen-helium. The Wechsler Bellevue Digit Symbol test indicated a decrement with air only at 200 ft and 300 ft and no effect with oxygen-helium. The EEG measurement indicated a depression of alpha activity on compression regardless of the gas breathed, and at depth, in the subjects breathing compressed air, an increase in the alpha and fast beta frequencies. Oxygen-helium had no effect at depth. Measurements of tremor by transducer indicated that there were no tremors present. It is concluded there are no significant signs and symptoms of the HPNS at this rapid rate of compression to a maximum depth of 300 ft. However, this rate does exert a measurable action on the brain. The relationship of these findings to the HPNS is discussed. (Authors' summary)

211.
BENNETT, P.B.
Review of protective pharmacological agents in diving.
Aerosp. Med. 43:184-192;Feb. 1972.

From 89 references the effects of a large number of pharmacological agents capable of ameliorating or preventing the major physiological hazards in diving of decompression sickness, oxygen toxicity and inert gas narcosis are reviewed. The indications, which the use of these compounds give, of the possible mechanisms for the production of these hazards is discussed and the direction of contemporary research on the use of drugs indicated. (Author's abstract)

212.
BENNETT, P.B.
Physiological problems of deep-sea diving.
Meerestechnik 3:177-185;Oct. 1972.

This is an excellent survey of the subject. The gas pressure and volume relationship in diving is explained and illustrated. The major physiological hazards of diving are listed, and a diagram is presented which indicates at what depth each type of trauma or disorder is likely to occur; oxygen toxicity, lung damage, nitrogen narcosis, hpns, decompression sickness, air embolism, aseptic bone necrosis, labyrinth syndrome, carbon dioxide retention, respiratory difficulty and the effects of cold are included. The importance of substituting helium for nitrogen at depths of more than 60 m is emphasized; even though an experienced and adapted diver might be able to perform a routine task in spite of mild narcosis, he would not be capable of dealing with emergencies. The two types of oxygen toxicity are discussed — the first, which can occur at a PO_2 of 0.6 to 1.0 ATA causes lung damage which can lead to death from hypoxia. In deep saturation dives, PO_2 of 0.45 ATA should be safe. It has been found in animal experiments (citing Chouteau's goats) that the normal oxygen level of 0.21 ATA is insufficient in helium breathing at great depths (488 m); behavioral disturbances and partial paralysis necessitate an increase of oxygen to 0.25 ATA. Subsequent simulated dives with human subjects contradicted these findings to some extent, but in the latter case the pressure effect was achieved by a simulated density, which might account for the difference. Diver's arthralgia, also known as the "no joint juice" syndrome can be brought on by moderate pressures of less than 200m. This varies with individuals, and also with rates of compression. Also associated with rapid compression is hpns. Diagrams from the 457 m dive at Alverstoke show EEG effects and finger tremor as recorded by a transducer. Compression was carried out in stages; after each compression, theta activity rose sharply, then gradually returned to normal during the 24 hour period at that depth. A deeper dive (518 m) was conducted by COMEX, also using stage compression but a slower compression between stages. These deep helium dives have proved conclusively that helium is not a narcotic gas; no decrement in mental performance has occurred. The tremors which are part of the hpns, once called helium tremors, are now known to be due to pressure; these can occur at depths of only 100 m, if the compression is rapid enough. The problems of heat loss and communication are briefly discussed; a helium speech processor tested during the Alverstoke dive has proved satisfactory and is now in production. The dangers of ascent—air embolism, decompression sickness and aseptic bone necrosis are explained. It is pointed out that entirely successful decompression tables have not yet been worked out, and that decompression sickness is an ever-present danger. Research into aseptic bone necrosis which may or may not be related to decompression sickness has been greatly intensified recently. (MFW/BSCP)

213.
BENNETT, P.B.
Experiments in human work capabilities under pressure, now being conducted at the Royal Naval Physiological Laboratory.
Ind. Med. Surg. 41:10-20;Dec. 1972.

The author presents general and specific data relating to the physiological and medical limitations of man in a hyperbaric environment. The problems dealt with are: respiratory resistance, carbon dioxide retention and intoxication; narcosis; oxygen toxicity; pressure; cold; decompression sickness; psychological problems (in saturation diving); nutrition (in saturation diving); helium speech distortion; action of drugs. Following this overview is an account of some of the research projects being carried on at the Royal Naval Physiological Laboratory at Alverstoke, the facilities of which are described in some detail. The effects of inert gas under pressure are discussed, and it is noted that at moderate depths, using compressed air, mental efficiency is more impaired than manual dexterity, while with helium oxygen at great depths, the reverse is true. Some degree of adaptation to high inert gas partial pressures has been demonstrated. Decompression tables for air dives to 300 feet are at present very unreliable. The theories concerning the mechanism of inert gas narcosis are discussed. The chief factor is the solubility in oil, which indicates the relative narcotic strength of the gas. In descending order of narcotic potency, the inert gases are xenon, krypton, argon, nitrogen; helium and neon are not narcotic. The dives of the mid-sixties, in which the hpns was first observed, are discussed. The symptoms are described. The dive to 1,500 feet in 1970 was undertaken chiefly to investigate this problem, and to determine whether or not there actually is a helium barrier. The most important incident of this dive was a rather severe vestibular dysbarism which occurred in one subject during decompression. This type of decompression problem, referred to here as "vestibular bends" is becoming much more common, and is receiving much current attention. This 1,500 ft dive which has been previously covered in this bibliography, is discussed at some length, and EEG auditory evoked response and tremor recordings are shown, as are charts of manual dexterity and cognitive function. It is believed that the tremors are not due to helium, but to pressure. The author believes that 2,000 feet is a perfectly feasible working depth, provided compression is carried out slowly and in stages, and precautions are taken to circumvent convulsions. (MFW/BSCP)

214.
BENNETT, P.B. and A.N. Dossett.
EEG activity of rats compressed by inert gases to 700 feet and oxygen-helium to 4000 feet.
Aerosp. Med. 44:239-244;Mar. 1973.
(Also published Alverstoke, U.K., Roy. Nav. Physiol. Lab., Rep. 5/72)

Twenty Wistar rats were exposed to increased air pressures of argon, nitrogen, helium, or oxygen at 100 ft/min in the presence of 2 ats abs. oxygen to 700 feet (22 ats abs). Two rats were compressed also at 10 ft/min to 4000 feet (122 ats abs) helium. Five rats were exposed without change of pressure. Spontaneous EEG was recorded with on-line analysis of the activity bands delta (2-4 c/sec), theta (4-8 c/sec), alpha (8-13 c/sec), beta 1 (13-20 c/sec) and beta 2 (20-30 c/sec). At 100 feet (4 ats abs) activities were augmented except for argon-oxygen and oxygen alone. Compressed air, argon-oxygen and oxygen alone, on compression to 700 feet, reduced all activity bands whereas helium-oxygen and nitrogen-oxygen caused little effect, except for a marked rise of delta with helium. Compression to 4000 feet (122 ats abs) with oxygen-helium caused a progressive reduction of all EEG activities. The results suggest that such neurophysiological changes may set the limit to deep diving and further confirms narcotic properties for oxygen. (Authors' abstract)

215.
BENNETT, P.B.oand D.G. Blenkarn.
Arterial blood gases in man during inert gas narcosis.
In: Hesser, C.M. and D. Linnarsson eds. Proceedings of the first annual scientific meeting of the European Undersea Biomedical Society, Stockholm, 13-15 June 1973. Forsvarsmedicin 9:447-451;July 1973.

Narcosis brought on by breathing air at increased pressure is generally attributed to increased nitrogen partial pressure. Another theory attributes the narcosis to hypercapnia and hypoxia, caused by increased airway resistance brought on by increased density of the breathing mixture, resulting in subsequent bronchial collapse. An attempt was made to test this theory during the decompression phase of a 1,000-ft. oxygen-helium dive. Measurements of Pa CO_2, Pa O_2, and pH were correlated with performance efficiency at 286 feet and 190 feet, with both air and oxygen-helium. Narcosis was observed at 286 feet, and to a lesser degree at 190 feet, breathing air. All subjects, at both depths, and using both breathing mixtures, demonstrated hypocapnia, alkalosis, a positive base excess, and hyperoxemia. Thus, the carbon dioxide theory was not supported by direct experimental measurement. (MFW/UMS)

216.
BENNETT, P.B. and J.A. Kylstra.
Hyperbaric research at Duke University: ethical considerations.
In: Hesser, C.M. and D. Linnarsson eds. Proceedings of the first annual scientific meeting of the European Undersea Biomedical Society, Stockholm, 13-15 June 1973. Forsvarsmedicin 9:373-378;July 1973.

All research activities supported through grants, awards or contracts by the United States Public Health Services must provide for the safety, health and welfare of the research subject according to specific guidelines. His rights include rights of privacy, voluntary participation and most important of all, that the direct or potential benefits of the research must outweigh the inherent risks to the individual. Responsibility for assuring this protection rests with the recipient of the Federal funds. The procedures and organization for ensuring that the provision of the Public Health Service are complied with at Duke Medical Center are discussed with particular emphasis on the guidelines for obtaining informed consent of subjects and the submission of protocols to the Committee for Clinical Investigations. Some of the philosophical considerations that suggest the need for such restraints are considered together with the moral problems of who should be responsible for ethical considerations of the use of human subjects in diving experiments and the role of the experimenter in such decisions. A distinction is made for ethical considerations where patients are involved and where the subjects are healthy volunteers. (MFW/UMS)

217.
BENTON, R.D., F.G. Bartlett, G.D. Bryant and H.B. Killen.
A towed observation system for remote assessment of underwater resources to 400 fathoms.
In: 1972 Offshore Technology Conference, May 1-3, Houston, Texas. Preprints. Vol I, p.297-309. Published by the conference, 1972.

This paper describes the development of a remotely controlled towed vehicle system designed to operate to a depth of 2400 feet. The system consists of three basic parts: 1. The underwater remote observation vehicle. This assembly includes control surfaces — with a loop to maintain either a constant height above bottom or a constant depth. It also includes a television camera with a pan and tilt mechanism and lighting, a data camera and lighting, a forward looking sonar for obstacles avoidance, and provisions for additional underwater instrumentation. 2. The control console on board a ship. The control console includes sled attitude controls, television monitors, video tape recorders, depth and attitude monitors, control signal coders, and telemetry tranducers. 3. The interconnecting cable. The underwater vehicle is connected to the control console by an armored four conductor cable with two power conductors and two coaxial conductors. One coax is used for the television and one for the telemetry commands and data signals up and down the cable. A slip ring winch is employed. The development of this system follows the successful design, development, and operation of a shallow water (50 fathoms) Remote underwater fisheries system (RUFAS) by the National Marine Fisheries Service. This project is funded by the Mississippi Universities Marine Center with Sea Grants funds. The work is divided into three phases: (a) design study, (b) design and fabrication of the vehicle system, and (c) final instrumentation and sea test. This paper reports the first phases as Final Instrumentation and Sea Tests are scheduled for the Fall of 1972. (Authors' abstract)

218.
BENTZ, R.L.
A study of approaches for supplying a diver with warm breathing gas.
In: The working diver, 1972. Symposium proceedings, February 1972, Columbus, Ohio, p.271-291. Washington, D.C., Marine Technology Society, 1972.
(Also published as U.S. Nav. Coastal Syst. Lab., Rep. NCSL-105-72, 60p. Apr. 1972)

Recent investigations have shown that a diver working in cold water below 500 feet for extended periods of time must be provided with a warm breathing gas. This paper investigates various practical approaches for supplying the diver with a warm breathing gas. The approaches investigated were influenced by their applicability to the U.S. Navy SCUBA Mark 11 Mod. 0 (Mark 11). This system uses warm water to heat the diver, and therefore, is the only heat source considered. A thermal analysis of the Mark II yields theoretical temperatures throughout the system for an arbitrarily chosen helium-oxygen gas mixture at 1000 feet and for air at surface pressure. The same analysis is made considering the system components insulated. The other approaches investigated were a heat exchanger, heated breathing hose and a heated back pack. (Author's abstract)

219.
BERGEL'SON, M.N. and L.A. Bokeriya.
Matematicheskaya model' saturatsii i desaturatsii organizma kislorodom pop povyshennym davleniem v usloviyakh sbrosa krovi spava nalevo.
[A mathematical model of oxygen saturation and desaturation of the body under increased pressure in a right to left blood shunt].
Eksp. Khir. Anesteziol. 17:59-64;May/June 1972.

A mathematical model of body saturation under increased pressure is offered. The system lungs-blood-tissues is described by a differential equation of the first order, which takes into account the oxygen consumption by tissues, the minute heart volume, the volume of tissues in the body, the magnitude of the right to left blood shunt. An electrical model has been constructed for the solution of a non-linear equation which has enabled to study non-stationary processes of oxygen saturation of the body in a blue type defect of the heart. A nomogram for computing regimes of hyperbaric oxygenation during surgical treatment of blue type heart defects is appended. (English summary)

220.
BERGEL'SON, M.N. and A.G. Rybalov.
Fiziko-kimi cheskii mekhanizm gemoliza v usloviyakh povyshennogo barometricheskogo davleniya.
[Physico-chemical mechanism of hemolysis under increased barometric pressure].
Probl. Gematol. Perelv. Krovi 17:11-16;Nov. 1972.

The paper is devoted to the explanation of causes of blood hemolysis under conditions of hyperbaric oxygenation. The authors suggest a theory of destruction of an erythrocyte under increase of partial pressure of inhaled gases based on the change of osmotic pressure of gases in a solution. Calculations of osmotic pressure values are presented; it is shown that for various gases hemolysis should occur at various pressures. (English summary)

221.
BERGER, A.J., J.A. Krasney and R.E. Dutton.
Respiratory recovery from CO_2 breathing in intact and chemodenervated awake dogs.
J. Appl. Physiol. 35:35-41;July 1973.

The transient respiratory recovery from hypercapnia (end tidal = 8% CO_2) in five awake dogs before and after peripheral chemoreceptor denervation was studied. These experiments demonstrate and quantify the contributions of the fast acting peripheral and slower acting central chemoreceptors. Three time constants are identified. Only the first short time constant appears to be associated with the peripheral chemoreceptors. The second and third time constants appear to be centrally mediated. The data indicate that the peripheral contribution to the dynamic response is variable. Based upon means from 31 intact runs and 31 denervated runs it appears that the peripheral chemoreceptors contribute 18% (range of values 8-35%) to the dynamic ventilatory response, have a mean response time constant of 4 sec., and rapidly initiate a decline in ventilation. The peripherally chemodenervated, and hence only centrally mediated, transient ventilatory recovery can be modeled as two time constants of 20 and 118 sec., with contributions of 56% and 44% respectively of the total central contribution. This response has a 4-sec. greater latency than the intact response. (Authors' abstract)

222.
BERGER, L.R.
Effects of hydrostatic pressure on photosynthesis and growth of unicellular marine algae and diatoms.
Honolulu, Univ. Hawaii, Dept. Microbiol., Final Rep. on contract N00014-67-A-0387-0008, 41p. June 1, 1972.
(AD 742 509)

Carbon dioxide assimilation and light-dependent oxygen evolution has been measured at 25C with a variety of algae under various conditions of light intensity, bicarbonate concentration, oxygen tension and hydrostatic pressure. Unicellular green, and blue-green algae, diatoms and filamentous algae have been studied. A new device which permits the measurement of oxygen evolution in closed culture at fixed oxygen tension is described. The apparatus may also be used at hydrostatic pressures up to 1000 atmospheres. It permits growth of algae in closed containers without gas phase at constant PO_2. A pressure vessel was also designed which permits enzyme kinetics to be done rapidly at increased hydrostatic pressures up to 1000 atmospheres and 40C. The system can be brought to the desired pressure and monitored spectrophotometrically about 10 seconds after reaction components are mixed. This permits studies of enzyme kinetics at limited substrate concentrations, on a time scale commensurate with in vivo reactions. (Author) (GRA)

223.
BERGHAGE, T.E.
An integrated measurement system for testing human performance in hyperbaric environments.
In: Abstracts of BuMed-ONR sponsored Navywide workshop in high pressure biomedical research, U.S. Submarine Base, Groton, Conn., May 1971, p. 29. Published by the Naval Submarine Medical Research Laboratory, 1971.
(Also presented at the Twenty-fifth Congress of Physiological Science Satellite Symposium: Recent progress in fundamental physiology of diving, Marseille, France, July 1971.)

Abstract only. Entire item quoted: This paper describes an integrated measurement system that has been developed for the U.S. Navy Experimental Diving Unit for testing diver performance. The system can be used in a wet or dry environment at pressures up to 445 psi, equivalent to a depth of 1000 feet of sea water. The 26 tests included in the system were selected to measure man's cognitive and perceptual-motor abilities. Their inclusion in the system was based upon: (1) their factorial purity, (2) test reliability and validity, (3) anticipated future diver activities, and (4) engineering constraints. As the divers perform the experimental tasks their responses are automatically scored and punched into computer data cards. This measurement system provides a flexible new tool for research related to human performance in hyperbaric environments.

224.
BERGHAGE, T.E.
The use of standard Navy classification test scores for the selection of diver first class candidates.
U.S. Navy Exp. Diving Unit, Rep. NEDU-20-72; 65p. Aug. 15, 1972.

Training records at the Naval School of Diving and Salvage for the years 1965 to 1970 were surveyed. Four hundred and sixty-four complete records for diver first class students were found. These records were used to evaluate existing, readily available aptitude tests as predictors of success in diver training. Scores on the four subtests (GCT-General Classification test, MECH-Mechanical test, ARI-Arithmetic test, and CLER-Clerical test) of the standard navy enlisted classification battery along with age were evaluated statistically. Results also indicate that even the best combination of scores on the Navy's standard classification test will only account for about 15 percent of the variance in trainee performance. (Author's abstract)

225.
BERGHAGE, T.E., K.J. Conda and F.W. Armstrong.
The synergistic effect of pressure and oxygen and its relationship to decompression sickness in mice.
U.S. Nav. Med. Res. Inst. and U.S. Navy Exp. Diving Unit, Res. Rep. 22-73, 18 p., Dec. 31, 1973.

This study was undertaken to explore the possibility of an interaction between total pressure and oxygen partial pressure and its possible effects on decompression. Four hundred and eighty male albino mice were given a 30-minute hyperbaric exposure at pressures of 14.1, 14.6, and 15.2 ata. At each of these pressures 40 mice, eight at a time, were exposed to one of four oxygen partial pressures: 0.5, 1.0, 1.5, or 2.0 ata. Following the pressure exposure the mice were rapidly decompressed to the surface, where they were observed for five minutes. Manifestations of decompression sickness were graded while the mice were exercised in a rotating cage. The results suggest that the oxygen partial pressure interacts with total pressure to affect decompression outcome. Reduction in the incidence of decompression sickness associated with increased oxygen partial pressures changes with the exposure pressure. Decompression results appear to be affected by nitrogen partial pressure, oxygen partial pressure, and the relative concentration of these gases in the breathing medium. The mechanism of this effect is yet to be delineated. (Authors' abstract)

226.
BERGMAN, S.A. Jr., J.K. Campbell and K. Wildenthal.
"Diving reflex" in man: its relation to isometric and dynamic exercise.
J. Appl. Physiol. 33:27-31; July 1972.

To test the influence of physical activity on the "diving reflex", ten normal men held their breath with their faces immersed in 15C water during rest, bicycle exercise, and sustained isometric handgrip contraction. At all conditions, a slight but statistically significant elevation of blood pressure and a marked decrease in heart rate occurred during each "dive". During moderate bicycle exercise heart rate fell more rapidly than at rest and the final level of bradycardia approached that achieved at rest, despite the fact that predive heart rates were much higher during exercise. When diving occurred in combination with isometric exercise, bradycardia was less severe than during resting dives and final heart rates could be represented as the sum of the expected responses to each intervention alone. In all conditions apnea without face immersion caused bradycardia that was less severe than during "wet dives". The results indicate that the diving reflex in man during dynamic and static activity persists. Decreases in heart rate are more marked during dynamic exercise than during rest or isometric exercise. (Authors' abstract)

227.
BERGONZI, M.
Etude du comportment de l'appareil cardio vasculaire dans la plongee profonde a saturation reactions au travail musculaire de l'homme soumis a ces conditions.
[Behavior of the cardiovascular system during deep saturation dives. Reactions to muscular exertion of man under these conditions].
Paris, France, Univ. Paris VI, Fac. Med., Thesis 120p., Nov. 1973.

Human cardiovascular behavior was observed in a series of simulated dives to between 300 and 600 metres, using a helium-oxygen breathing mixture. In resting subjects under continuous ECG observation, no bradycardia was noted; the authors suggest that observations of bradycardia reported by others may be due to factors other than high ambient pressure. The physical exertion of the step test and bicycle exercise was very well tolerated by the four subjects at 300m. No great variations of cardiac behavior could be correlated with variations of O_2 partial pressure of 300, 450, and 600 millibars, but systolic pressure increased when the oxygen content of the breathing mixture was increased. Bicycle tests were carried out down to depths of 565m with a ventilation rate similar to that observed at atmospheric pressure. But at greater depths this rate decreased alarmingly. It may be that at these depths the increased density of the gases constitutes the limiting factor on ventilatory performance. (MEMH/UMS)

228.
BERJU, K.K., E.L. Daniels and E.M. Strohlein.
Engineering the storage battery as an underwater power supply.
In: Ocean 73. 1973 IEEE international conference on engineering in the ocean environment, p.279-283. IEEE publication 73-CHO-7740-OCC.

Engineering of the storage battery into an integrated oceanographic power system has been successfully accomplished. This is evidenced by the scores of systems in operation below the seas today. This accomplishment was made possible by the development of a sophisticated pressure compensation system and applying it to existing electrochemical couples. Comprehensive studies of lead-acid and silver zinc cell operating characteristics at temperatures as low as 30°F and pressures up to 10,000 psi have led to the use of these batteries in systems ranging from small underwater vehicles to mobile sea floor equipment to large stationary habitats. From laboratory evaluations, it was determined that the advantageous effect of elevated pressures on the performance of lead-acid batteries is offset by the deleterious effect of cold temperature. The net effect of these same environs on the silver zinc cell is a decrease of 10% in discharge performance. (Authors' abstract)

229.
BERNSTEIN, H. and M. Krenske.
Lightweight syntactic foam as buoyancy material for a 20,000-ft deep-sea vehicle.
Soc. Nav. Architecht. Mar. Eng. 9:1-16; n.d.
(AD 734 582)

Present investigations of syntactic foam, (hollow glass microspheres dispersed in a resin matrix) are the result of extensive tradeoff studies of candidate buoyancy systems for a small manned vehicle capable of operating to ocean depths of 20,000 ft. Early studies indicated that the use of highly packed binary mixtures of microspheres held promise for reducing the density of high-strength foams without sacrificing desirable 'fail-safe' characteristics. Subsequently, fine and coarse microspheres manufactured specifically for this purpose were combined with various resin systems to produce experimental foams. These were then subjected to extensive testing under simulated service conditions. Results indicate that this approach should reduce the present density of 42 pcf to at least 34 pcf, with a consequent saving of more than 30 percent in overall vehicle weight. (Author) (GRA)

230.
BERRY
Animal tests on a small hog at depth: 1100 meters.
Groupe Etud. Rech. Sous-marines, Rep. GERS 07-71, 20p. May 1972.
(Navships Transl. 1337)

A minihog was compressed to 1100 meters at the following rate: 100m/3 min to 500m, 50m/3 min to 850m; stages were of one half hour duration. At 1000m, hyperexcitability was evident. The bottom time was 17 1/2 hours, during which time the hyperexcitability decreased. Decompression took three days and three hours. The only incidents were modification of the breathing rate. At four points, breathing became abnormally rapid, and decompression was halted until breathing rate returned to normal. The author believes that the success of the experiment was due chiefly to the careful regulation of the oxygen partial pressure, particularly during the transition from helium-oxygen to air. It is concluded that 1000 meter dives will be well within the realm of possibility for divers using helium-oxygen. The incidents of breathing irregularity and of hyperexcitability can probably be avoided by lengthening the stages. (MFW/BSCP)

231.
BERTHARION, G., H. Burnet and B. Broussolle.
Action de la lysolecithine sur l'electrocorticogramme du rat blanc.
[Effect of lysolecithin on the electrocorticogram of the white rat].
Cent. Etud. Rech. Biophysiol. Appl. Mar., Rep. 73-01 bis, 10p. 1973.

It had been theorized that lysolecithin, found in increased quantities in the pulmonary lavage fluid obtained from rats exposed to normobaric hyperoxia, might be responsible for the electrocorticographic changes observed in rats injected with the pulmonary lavage fluid. White rats received intraperitoneal injections of lysolecithin in doses of 1000 g/kg in a test of this hypothesis. About ten minutes after the injections, definite electrocorticographic disturbances were noted in most of the subject rats. But the electrocorticographic changes due to lysolecithin differed from those provoked by injections of pulmonary lavage fluid. The above-mentioned theory must therefore be abandoned, and another neurotoxic component of the pulmonary lavage fluid must be sought. (MEMH/UMS)

232.
BERTHARION, G., H. Burnet and B. Broussolle.
Action sur l'electrocorticogramme de liquide de lavage pulmonaire de rats ayant ete soumis a une hyperoxie normobare de 5 jours.
[Effect on the electrocorticogram of the liquid of pulmonary lavage of rats exposed to normobaric hyperoxia for 5 days].
Cent. Etud. Rech. Biophysiol. Appl. Mar., Rep. 73-01, 3p. plus illustr. 1973.

Rats wearing permanent electrodes were injected with liquid from the pulmonary lavage of rats which had spent 5 days in normobaric hyperoxia. Twenty to forty minutes after injection there appeared a slow cortical activity of 5-6 cycles/sec., frequently interrupted by paroxystic anomalies. In some recordings, periods of repeated, sometimes total, depression alternated with discharges of generalized synchronous paroxystic activity. The authors suggest that the neurological effects observed may be due both to an increase in the quantity of pulmonary surfactant and to a change in its composition, most probably a change in the fatty-acid composition of lecithin. (MEMH/SCD)

233.
BEUTTENMULLER, R.A. and H.A. Perry.
Biomarine resistance of surface-compression strengthened glasses.
U.S. Nav. Ordn. Lab., Rep. NOLTR 71-57, 13p. Oct. 13, 1971.

A study was made to determine what effect, if any, extended periods of stress and strain during exposure to the chemical and biological environments of the ocean had on the structural properties of surface-compression strengthened (SCS) glasses. Exposures for as long as 504 days, while under constant strain up to 60% of ultimate, and the growth and subsequent removal of marine organisms did not deform the specimens and increased the bending strengths of the SCS glasses. An exposure test program of longer duration is recommended. The further development of processes for deeper compression treatment of SCS glasses is also recommended. (DCD abstract)

234.
BEVAN, J.
Many lessons for commercial divers from Bahamas symposium.
Offshore Serv., p. 28-30,31;Oct. 1972.

This article summarizes the ten sessions of the Fifth Symposium on Underwater Physiology, held at Freeport in the Bahamas, in August, 1972: Session 1: Comprehensive studies of pressure and decompression (Chairman, Dr. Peter Bennett, UK); "Limitations to future deep diving in the sea would be due to the joint interaction of the so-called "High Pressure Nervous Syndrome" (HPNS) and respiratory difficulties associated with breathing very dense gas mistures." Session 2: Ventilation and gas exchange (Chairman, Dr. J.A. Kylstra, USA). "Breathing problems are among the greatest besetting a diver and the importance of a complete understanding of the mechanics and physiology

of hyperbaric respiration cannot be overstressed." Session 3: Pathophysiology of bone (Chairman, Professor D.N. Walder, UK). "The cause of [osteonecrosis], which has been somewhat of an enigma for so long, was defined concisely by Stegall and Smith (USA) as an obstruction of bone blood flow due to bubble induced coagulation of blood (anemic infarction). It was stressed that better decompression schedules are the answer and indeed these already exist." Session 4: Dysbarism (Chairman, C.M. Hesser, Sweden). "Perhaps the most impressive [paper] was that of Hallenbeck, Elliott and Bove (USA) who demonstrated magnificently using X-ray cinematography, the closing of certain strategic veins associated with the spinal cord caused by inadequate decompression, [thus illustrating] factors leading to typical spinal bends, which previously could only have been conjectured by intuitive guessing at best." Session 5: Inert gas exchange and bubble formation (Chairman, Capt. R.C. Bornman, USA). "Lambertsen's group. . . provided cinefilm unequivocably demonstrating the massive formation of bubbles in living tissues. . . without any change whatsoever in ambient pressure. . . If two different gases existed each side of a multilayered tissue, such as a human being breathing neon but surrounded by helium, then the counterdiffusion of the gases across the tissues can under certain circumstances produce areas of super-saturation and consequential evolution of bubbles." Session 6: Hydrostatic pressure (Chairman, Dr. E.B. Smith, UK). "The old concept that liquids and solids such as make up the human body are sufficiently incompressible as to be totally unaffected under the orders of pressures encountered in diving, is crumbling slowly but surely under a hail of experimental evidence." Session 7 and 8: Oxygen, inert gases and hydrogen, (Chairman, Dr. J.D. Wood, Canada and Dr. H.R. Schreiner, USA). "On the subject of hydrogen, Bennett proposed that it was most unlikely that it would ever be used in operational diving since it has little advantage over helium in the 0-2000 ft. range." Session 9: Perception, performance and communications (Chairman, Dr. A. Bachrach, USA). "The findings indicated that neon was very similar to helium at least in the depth range its density allows it to be used. . . It certainly has some advantage over helium inasmuch as it is a better thermal insulator and does not mutilate the human voice." Session 10: Thermal balance (Chairman Dr. E.L. Beckman, USA). "The problem of maintaining divers in reasonable thermal comfort is now clearly understood to be. . . an absolute necessity for the safety of the divers." (MFW/BSCP)
Editors' note: A somewhat fuller summary of the symposium, by the same author, is found in Underwater J. 4:256-259;Dec. 1972.

235.
BEVAN, J.
Instrumentation course for the professional diver.
Underwater J. 5:196-197;Aug. 1973.

The Society for Underwater Technology conducted its second Diver Instrumentation Course at the Fort Bovisand Underwater Centre at Plymouth. The course was directed at professional divers; its purpose was to "provide a sufficient working familiarisation in order to allow the candidates to assess for themselves the usefulness or otherwise of the equipment," rather than to completely qualify the individual in the use of any of the equipment. Fifteen organizations both governmental and industrial were represented by divers. The first week was devoted to methods of surveying, and to the use of metal detectors and hydraulic cutting tools. Lectures and films dealt with electric hazards, habitats, codes of practice, and drilling and coring devices. The second week was devoted largely to acoustic devices of communication and navigation. Wet submersibles were discussed and demonstrated. Helmets and suits were tested. Lectures and films were presented on such subjects as thermal limitations, heated suits, heated breathing gas, decompression procedures, helium speech processors, and future instrumentation. A film was made of the entire proceedings, which will constitute a record of the state-of-the-art of diving technology at present. (MFW/SCD)

236.
BIANCHI, L.
Le attivita' bioelettriche cerebrali nei conigli sottoposti a 6 ata di O_2.
[Cerebral bioelectric activity in rabbits subjected to 6 ATA of O_2].
Boll. Soc. Ital. Biol. Sper. 48:196-199;Apr. 30, 1972.

The electroencephalographic symptomatology of ten male rabbits subjected to 6 ATA of oxygen was studied. The atmosphere of the chamber was replaced by pure oxygen five minutes before compression was begun. Compression to 6 ATA was accomplished in about 15 minutes; humidity in the chamber was maintained at about 80%. From the beginning of exposure EEG patterns showed the effects of hyperbaric oxygen on the central nervous system in the form of generalized bilateral convulsions beginning usually around 6 ATA but sometimes at much lower pressures. These convulsions are of the epileptic "grand mal" type. Blood tests taken simultaneously demonstrate that blood chemistry values were affected more slowly, showing changes of increasing severity throughout the exposure period. (MEH/BSCP)

237.
BICHER, H.I., D.F. Broley, D.D. Reneau and M.H. Knisely.
Autoregulation of oxygen supply to microareas of brain tissue under hypoxic and hyperbaric conditions.
Bibl. Anat. 11:526-531; 1973.

The availability of oxygen throughout the brain is far from homogeneous, oxygen tensions varying 30 or 40 mm Hg within a distance of few microns. However, the pO_2 at a given microarea of cerebral tissue is remarkably constant, and can be changed only through major alterations in blood supply or the composition of respiratory gases. The present experiments represent an attempt to determine some of the mechanisms responsible for keeping pO_2 constant in microareas of cortical tissue. Using our oxygen ultramicroelectrode, pO_2 and neuronal electrical activity were determined simultaneously with other pertinent physiological parameters, as the oxygen availability was changed using different experimental procedures. PO_2 was also determined in kidney and arterial blood to compare the responses of different organs. (Authors' summary)

238.
BIEBER, M.M., M.G. Cogan, T.C. Durbridge and R.C. Rosan.
Oxygen toxicity in the new-born guinea pig lung. The incorporation of tritiated uridine into monoribosomes.
Biol. Neonate 17(1/2):35-43; 1971.

Newborn guinea pigs, poisoned in flowing 100% O_2 for four days were studied for monoribosome synthesis by their lungs. Results obtained by sucrose gradient isolation technique showed that T-uridine incorporation into monoribosomes was not inhibited, when tests were compared to littermate controls. Combined biochemical and morphological experience suggested that the production of new monoribosomes by single cells outweighed or equalled tissue necrosis. When four-day controls were compared to newborn controls or four day O_2 intoxicated animals to newborn ones, there was an unequivocal and inexplicable decrease in net synthesis of monoribosomes by the lung. (CMM) (© BA)

239.
BIERNACKI, P.S. and J.J. Kalvinskas.
Carbon dioxide monitoring.
Anaheim, Cal., Rockwell Int. Corp., Electron. Res. Div., Rep. C73-447.1/501, 11 p. May 7, 1973.
(AD 760059)

The progress of a program involving Investigation into Applications of Bioluminescent Technology to Swimmer Life Support Systems, Office of Naval Research, is reported. Results of early tests have been most encouraging. Characterized bacteria responses to varying levels of carbon dioxide have been sharp — with excellent signal-to-noise ratio. A collection of 32 cultures of luminescent microorganisms are currently under cultivation. This collection will be used to a source of selection of biosensors suitable for CO_2 detection tests. (GRA)

240.
BIERNACKI, P.S. and J.J. Kalvinskas.
Carbon dioxide monitoring.
Anaheim, Cal., Rockwell Int. Corp., Electron Res. Div. Rep. C73-447-501, 91p. Aug. 1973.
(AD 765 342/1)

The program was initiated to establish the feasibility of applying bioluminescent technology for monitoring of carbon dioxide (CO_2) in life-support systems for divers, swimmers, and underwater habitats. Experiments were performed to obtain bioluminescent cultures which are sensitive to levels of carbon dioxide as low as 81 ppm, in an 80% helium and 20% oxygen (life support) gas mixture — at hydrostatic pressures up to 1000 psig. Fourteen luminescent cultures were tested under conditions of varying pressures, gas proportions, sample sizes, and flow rates. Strong responses to low concentrations of CO_2 were exhibited by five cultures — thereby demonstrating the feasibility of employing a luminescent detection system in the environments of interest. The luminescent responses were sensed by a photomultiplier tube. The photomultiplier output was fed through a log amplifier to a strip-chart recorder. This detection system was more than adequate for laboratory measurements; however, the requirements for a more compact system were also examined. It appears that — by using a solid-state sensor and integrated-circuit electronics — a small, low-power, portable unit can be developed and constructed. This unit would provide "fail safe" monitoring of CO_2 in underwater life-support systems. (Author) (GRA)

241.
BIERSNER, R.J.
Selective performance effects of nitrous oxide.
Hum. Factors 14:187-194;Apr. 1972.

Twenty-one U.S. Navy divers were given several standard visual tests, the Purdue Pegboard, the Bennett Hand Tool Dexterity Test, and the Wechsler Memory Scale while breathing air of 30% nitrous oxide. The results showed that visual function, fine and gross motor performance, and long-term memory were normal under nitrous oxide, while learning and short-term memory were significantly impaired. The subjective effects of breathing nitrous oxide were similar to those experienced during compressed air narcosis. The selective impairment of short-term memory suggests that divers might be able to perform useful work at depths deeper than those currently authorized, provided the tasks were well learned and practiced. (Author's abstract)

242.
BIERSNER, R.J., E.K.E. Gunderson, D.H. Ryman and R.H. Rahe.
Correlations of physical fitness, perceived health status, and dispensary visits with performance in stressful training.
U.S. Nav. Med. Neuropsychiat. Res. Unit, Rep. NMNRU-71-30, 8p. June 1972
(Also published in J. Sports Med. Physical Fitness 12:107-110;June 1972.
(AD 763 306)

Physical fitness tests and a health status index were correlated with dispensary visits and training success in stressful underwater demolition team (UDT) training. Subjects were 329 Navy enlisted volunteers for UDT training. A composite physical fitness-health index scale was correlated with the training success cirterion. The results suggested that physical fitness and self-perceived health status are important factors in successful completion of an extremely rigorous training program. (GRA)

243.
BIERSNER, R.J., E.K.E. Gunderson and R.H. Rahe.
Relationships of sports interests and smoking to physical fitness.
U.S. Navy Neuropsychiat. Res. Unit., Rep. NMNRU-71-36, 8 p. June 1972.
(Also published in J. Sports Med. 12:124-127;June 1972)
(AD 764,330)

Subjects were 241 Navy enlisted volunteers for UDT training. Sports interest and smoking were correlated with the Physical Fitness Scale (PFS) and with each other. Interest in sports was positively correlated with PFS scores. Smoking correlated negatively with both the PFS and sports interest. The results suggest that habits, such as smoking, and attitudes toward sports can be used to specify some of the behaviors associated with physical fitness. (Author) (GRA)

244.
BIERSNER, R.J.
Social development of Navy divers.
Aerosp. Med. 44:761-763;July 1973.

Ninety-five U.S. Navy divers and 93 fleet controls, matched for age, rate, pay grade, and the age at which they joined the Navy, were compared for several important biographical characteristics. The divers were found to be similar to controls in education, present marital status, educational level of parents, marital status of parents, number of brothers and sisters, number of moves made before joining the Navy, and size of hometown. The divers were significantly different from the fleet controls in running away from home, playing hookey, receiving traffic tickets and being arrested for nontraffic violations. These results show that divers rebelled early against the restrictions of formal social institutions, and were successful in directing this activity and aggression toward an occupation in which these characteristics may not only be useful, but necessary. (Author's abstract)

245.
BILODEAU, D.E.
Development of advanced deep sea diving equipment for the Navy hard hat diver.
In: The working diver, 1972. Symposium proceedings, February 1972, Columbus, Ohio, p. 175-189. Washington, D.C., Marine Technology Society, 1972.

As a result of this survey, a preliminary hard hat diving system design was completed. This system consisted of a lightweight helmet, scrubber/recirculator, undergarment, breastplate, dry suit, overgarment, weighted boots and gloves. The system incorporated design improvement in the following areas: lightweight helmet, improved recirculation, acoustic noise reduction, self donning, positive reserve gas, linear controls, combined air or mixed gas capability, improved weight matrices, materials, integrated dress. A phase II program was defined consisting of critical component testing of the helmet and control valves, scrubber/recirculator, and some noise reduction components. The overall results of critical component tests on the advanced surface supplied deep dive system were excellent. Phase III of this program will provide three prototype systems which will allow Navy technical evaluation testing. The results of those tests will determine which of the prốposed design features will prove worthy of incorporation into a replacement system for the old reliable Mark V Hard Hat. (From author's abstract and conclusions)

246.
BINGMAN, D.
Responses of chemoreceptor fibre units of the cat carotid body to slow and rapid changes in arterial PCO_2.
Pfluegers Arch. (Suppl.) 343:R10; 1973.

Abstract only. Entire item quoted: In previous experiments slow changes of PCO_2 compared with hypoxic stimuli, exerted only a small excitatory effect upon the discharge rate of chemoreceptor fibre potentials led from microstrands of the carotid sinus nerve. When $\Delta PCO_2/\Delta t$ was increased the excitatory effect of hypercapnic stimuli was markedly enhanced. To analyse this phenomenon in more detail chemoreceptor responses to steep changes of the arterial PCO_2 ($PaCO_2$) were tested. Using two gas exchangers and a roller pump for an artificial perfusion of the carotid sinus region in vivo, nearly rectangular hypercapnic stimuli could be achieved. Under these conditions abrupt increases of $PaCO_2$ were followed by a steep enhancement of chemoreceptor activity. The amplitude of this initial excitation was closely related to the steepness of changes in PCO_2. After reaching a peak the discharge rate declined to a steady state, the level of which was now determined by the absolute PCO_2. An abrupt decrease of PCO_2 correspondingly induced a steep decline of receptor activity with a subsequent rerise. Simultaneous recordings of tissue PO_2 (PTO_2) in the carotid body showed that these receptor responses cannot be due to shifts of PTO_2 at the receptor site. Since rectangular changes of PaO_2 under the same conditions induced proportional reactions of chemoreceptor activity, it has to be concluded that chemoreceptor units of the cat carotid body adapt considerably to changes in PCO_2.

247.
BISHOP, R.P.
OSHA breathing gas purity standards.
In: Battelle Columbus Laboratories. Proceedings, 1973 divers' gas purity symposium November 27-28, 1973, p.V-1-V-10. U.S. Navy Supervisor Diving, Nav. Ships Syst. Comm., Rep 2-73, 1973.

The Occupational Safety and Health Administration (OSHA) has developed standards for exposure to atmospheric contaminants which may have a significant impact on the diving industry. The results of a study of the applicability of OSHA standards of diving activities, recently completed for the U.S. Navy Supervisor of Diving, indicate a number of areas in which accepted diving practice conflicts with OSHA standards. OSHA and Department of Defense regulations permit the Navy to use diving practices which do not comply with OSHA regulations, but this option is not available in commercial diving. Compliance with all applicable OSHA standards may result in increased diving costs, a need for expensive systems to ensure compliance, and reduced efficiency in diving operations. In order to prevent these problems a standard specifically directed towards the diving industry should be incorporated into OSHA regulations which will ensure safe and healthful working conditions for divers while reflecting the needs and proven technology of the industry. If such a standard is not quickly enacted, existing OSHA regulations may be applied to commercial diving despite the problems that will result. (Author's abstract)

248.
BITTER, R.A. and T.W. Nielsen.
Urinary corticosterone excretion in laboratory rats exposed to pressures of 10, 20 and 30 ATA ($He-O_2$).
Physiologist 13:150; 1970.

Abstract only. Entire item quoted: It is generally accepted that corticosterone is the major adrenal corticosteroid excreted in response to stress in the laboratory rat. The purpose of this study was to investigate some of the possible relationships between high pressure and adrenal cortical activity. Adult male Sprague-Dawley rats (250-300 gm) were exposed in a high pressure chamber to $He-O_2$ (80-20% at 1 atm) while control urine samples were collected. Animals were then exposed to $He-O_2$ mixtures at 10, 20 and 30 Ata. The partial pressure of O_2 was kept between 150 and 250 mmHg during experimental periods. Animals were exposed to the high pressure $He-O_2$ mixture for 24 hours and then stage decompressed in 8 to 12 hours. Excreted corticosterone levels were measured along with appropriate standards according to the method of Mattingly (1964). Urinary corticosterone, expressed as ug/24 hour sample, was found to be 0.95 $\pm$ 0.27 (S.D.) for room air (N_2-O_2), and 1.83 $\pm$ 0.29 (S.D.) for $He-O_2$ at normal pressure. At 10, 20 and 30 Ata, the urinary steroid levels were 3.04 $\pm$ 0.87; 3.95 $\pm$ 0.75; and 2.79 $\pm$ 0.39; respectively. Urinary corticosterone excretion returned to normal levels during the 24 hour period following exposure. Unexplained but statistically significant differences were found between the N_2-O_2 and $He-O_2$ control samples. Significant increases over control values were noted in the groups of animals treated at 10, 20 and 30 Ata.

249.
BITTER, R.A. and T.W. Nielsen.
Unconjugated urinary corticosterone excretion in laboratory rats exposed to high pressure helium-oxygen environments.
Aerosp. Med. 43:984-988;Sept. 1972.
(Also published by N. Dak. Univ., Sch. Med., Rep. on Contract N00014-68-A-0499, 5p. 1972)
(AD 750,859)

The excretion rate of unconjugated urinary corticosterone collected from male Sprague-Dawley rats (250-400 gm) was used as an index of stress. 24-hour urine samples were collected during control periods in room air (N_2-O_2) and during exposure to a mixture (80-20% of helium-oxygen ($He-O_2$) at one atmosphere absolute (ATA). The animals were then exposed to $He-O_2$ mixtures at 5, 10, 20 or 30 ATA for 14 hours and then stage decompressed. Food and water were available ad lib., and chamber temperature was maintained at 30 $\pm$ 0.5°C at 1 ATA $He-O_2$. Chamber temperature was increased with pressure up to 33°C at 30 ATA $He-O_2$. Unconjugated urinary corticosterone was analyzed fluro-metrically and expressed as ng/100 gm body weight/24 hours. Statistically significant increases in corticosterone excretion rates were found in $He-O_2$ control samples above those excretion rates collected in N_2-O_2 samples. Excretion values of corticosterone were increased as much as three-fold over basal values upon exposure to pressure. Urine volume and creatinine excretion both showed general increases with a change of $He-O_2$ and to increased pressures. Loss of body weight was observed with pressures greater than 5 ATA $He-O_2$. (Authors' abstract)

250.
BITTER, R.A., J. Hootman and T.W. Nielsen.
Fast Fourier transform analysis of the circadian rhythm of urinary 11-hydroxycorticosteroids in laboratory rats exposed to high environmental pressures of helium and oxygen.
Aerosp. Med. 44:1261-1263;Nov. 1973.

Fast Fourier transform (FFT) analysis was performed on levels of 11-hydroxycorticosteroids (11-OHCS) in urinary samples collected from laboratory rats. The control animals were exposed to ambient conditions. The experimental animals were exposed in an experimental pressure chamber in 20 atmospheres absolute of helium and oxygen (20 ata He-O_2). Four 6-hr urine samples were obtained daily and analyzed for the free 11-OHCS content according to the method of Mattingly. The animals were given food and water ad libitum. Marked increases were noted in the excretion rates of the animals subjected to the 20 ata He-O_2 pressure. Using the FFT to calculate the modified power spectrum, a change in periodicity from diurnal 24-hr cycle to one of 28.4 hr was obtained. (Authors' abstract)

251.
BLACK, S.A. and R.L. Brackett.
Design, fabrication and evaluation of an experimental diver-operated construction assistance vehicle.
In: 1972 Offshore Technology Conference, May 1-3, Houston, Texas. Preprints, Vol II, p. 158-168. Published by the conference, 1972.

An experimental diver-operated Construction Assistance Vehicle (CAV) was designed, fabricated and evaluated to determine the utility and general specifications for a prototype diver work vehicle. The CAV fabricated from off-the-shelf components, is capable of carrying 1300 pounds of wet-weight cargo between the surface and the ocean bottom work site. The craft's pneumatic and hydraulic power is available to operate hand power tools. Over one hundred test dives were conducted in the ocean. During these tests, a maximum depth of 110 feet was reached. Operational testing proved the CAV to be a safe and effective means for both delivering cargo and powering diver tools. (Authors' abstract)

252.
BLEAKLEY, W.B.
New subsea deep production technique unveiled.
Oil Gas J. 71:86-90;Oct. 29, 1973.

An ocean floor system now under construction by Transworld Drilling Co. is described. The system consists of a wet wellhead installed in a face up hemisphere, with which an underwater work chamber can mate, providing a one-atmosphere environment at the wellhead. A personnel transfer capsule enables crew members to be changed without removing the chamber to the surface. A flow line transports crude to surface storage. Unique pipe-laying and connecting techniques have been developed electric and/or hydraulic systems have made a great degree of automation possible. (MFW/UMS)

253.
BLIX, A.S. and S.H. From.
Lactate dehydrogenase in diving animals: A comparative study with special reference to the eider (Somateria mollissima).
Comp. Biochem. Physiol. (B):40(3):579-584; 1971.

The isoenzyme pattern in brain, heart and skeletal muscle of some diving animals, the seal and the eider, were compared to a non-diving animal, the sheep, by disc electrophoresis. The quantitation of the isoenzymes were made by densitometry. In contrast to the sheep which showed an isoenzyme pattern similar to the usual findings on non-diving animals all isoenzymes were relatively abundant in all tissues examined in the seal. The enzyme from the same tissues of the eider did not separate either at pH 8.3 or at pH 7.4 and 9.3. Only one "band" coinciding with that of LDH_5 (lactate dehydrogenase) of the seal and sheep was obtained. Biochemical adaptations on enzyme level are taking place as response to the hypoxic conditions induced upon prolonged diving. (© BA)

254.
BLIX, A.S.
Fysiologiske tilpasninger til dykkende sevevis: Sirkulatoriske forandringer.
[Physiological adaptations to diving habit: Cardiovascular responses].
Fauna (Oslo) 25(2):97-104; 1972.

Studies on the physiological adaptation to diving in diving vertebrates such as *Phoca titulina, Pagophilua groenlandicus,* goose and duck are reviewed. Compared to non-diving animals, divers have considerably higher blood volume and blood Hb concentration, while the lung capacity is largely the same. As the amount of O_2 available during diving is insufficient, cardiovascular and circulatory changes (bradycardia, and preferred blood supply to heart and brain at the expense of most other organs) occur during diving. (MDS) (© BA)

255.
BLIX, A.S., R. Hol and O. Iversen.
Equipment for use in angiographic examinations of animals during diving.
Acta Physiol. Scand. 87(1):3A; 1973.

Abstract only. Entire item quoted: It has for long been known, that submersion causes great alterations in the cardiovascular system of diving animals. Only recently, however, by the development of angiographic techniques has it been possible to visualize how, and to what extent, these phenomena are developed. Preliminary studies by use of the above mentioned technique, have in fact been carried out on head-immersed animals. Although, this condition is known to initiate the diving reflex, it seems obvious that the methods used so far are inferior to one involving a fully submerged animal. This condition may be obtained by the setup indicated in the figure, where the animal (a seal) is enclosed in a plexiglass tube, shown in cross section. This tube should have a slightly greater diameter than the animal, ensuring a minimum quantity of water, and preventing the animal to move. While at surface position the tube should therefore be aerated. Diving, on the other hand, may be performed by filling the tube with water from the hydraulically operated reservoir. By this setup, which may be incorporated into any modern X-ray equipment, any diving animal may be examined for periods only limited by the diving capacity of the animal itself. [The abstract is accompanied by a schematic drawing of the equipment].

256.
BLIX, A.S. and R. Hol.
Ventricular dilation in the diving seal.
Acta Physiol. Scand. 87(3):431-432; 1973.

During diving the cardiac output of seals decreases as a result of conspicuous bradycardia combined with a constant stroke volume. The O_2 content of the arterial blood diminishes linearly from 22 to about 5 volume % during a 15 min. dive. Thus, insufficient oxygenation of the heart of the seal during a prolonged dive is imminent, and although an elevated myocardial O_2 extraction during the increased diastolic periods (10-20s) must be considered, this animal may provide an interesting model for the study of coronary insufficiency in man. Information on the functional properties of the heart of the diving seal was obtained during an angiographic examination of a Harp seal (Papophilus groenlandicus) during 10-18 min. dives. The right ventricle was strikingly dilated with a large end systolic volume, after only 6 min. of submersion, closely resembling that of humans during acute cardiac infarction. Thus, contrary to man, where the above described effects indicates severe cardiac failure, the reversible ventricular dilation in the seal may represent an important life-securing mechanism in this diving species (HTS) (© BA)

257.
BLUM, J.W. and D.S. Cohen.
Acoustic wave propagation in an underwater sound channel. I. Qualitative theory.
Pasadena, Cal., Cal. Inst. Tech., Rep. TR-19, 17p. Sept. 1970.
(AD 735 030)

The report gives a qualitative study of wave propagation in an inhomogeneous medium principally by geometrical optics and ray theory. The inhomogeneity is represented by a sound/speed profile which is dependent upon one coordinate, namely the depth; and we discuss the general characteristics of wave propagation which result from a source placed on the sound channel axis. We show that our mathematical model of the sound/speed in the ocean actually predicts some of the behaviour of the observed physical phenomena in the underwater sound channel. Using ray theoretic techniques an investigation is made on the implications of the profile on the following characteristics of SOFAR propagation. (Author) (GRA)

258.
BLUM, J.W. and D.S. Cohen.
Acoustic wave propagation in an underwater sound channel. II Quantitative theory.
Pasadena, Cal., Cal. Inst. Techno., Rep. 19, 24p. Sept. 1970.
(AD 735 031)
(Also published in J. Inst. Math. Appl. 8:199-200; 1971)

By using ray-theoretic-techniques as developed in our previous paper: "Acoustic Wave Propagation in an Underwater Sound Channel. 1. Qualitative Theory" a certain qualitative understanding of several features of SOFAR propagation in an underwater sound channel. In the present paper a more penetrating quantitative study is done by means of analytical techniques on the governing equations. A study is made of transient problems for the Epstein profile by employing a double transform to formally derive an integral representation, and several alternative representations are obtained which are needed for asymptotic results. (Author) (GRA)

259.
BOBBER, R.J.
Underwater electroacoustic measurements.
Washington, D.C., U.S. Government Printing Office, 1970. 333p.

As man explores and uses the ocean depths, whether for military, commercial, or scientific purposes, he faces sensory and communication problems unlike those met in any other environment. The medium is hostile to man and equipment. It is essentially opaque to visible light, infrared, radio, radar — to all the familiar forms of electromagnetic radiation used for sensing and communicating in the atmosphere and in space. Because acoustic signals are, and probably will remain, the only feasible general method of transmitting information with waves through water at distances beyond a few yards, electroacoustic transducers are the only practicable means for sensing underwater sounds, and in most cases, for producing them as controlled signals. The electrical and acoustical measurements described in this book are those required to calibrate, test, or evaluate an underwater electroacoustic transducer and to enable one, indirectly, to produce or detect and measure an underwater acoustic signal, usually in terms of its acoustic pressure. (From author's introduction)

260.
BODROV, V.A., A.S. Yegorov and B.N. Yakovets.
Study of some psychic functions of aquanauts during prolonged exposure to increased pressure.
Voennomed. Zh. (8):71-73;Aug. 1972.
(Translation JPRS 57541)

The purpose of this study was to evaluate man's mental function both during prolonged (up to 30 days) exposures to hyperbaric environments, and after emergence. Tests were made at 5 and at 40 meters on nitrogen-oxygen mixtures, and at 40, 100, 130, and 160 meters on helium-oxygen mixtures. Attention, memory, and cogitation functions were tested. Diaries were kept to record subjective reactions, and behavior during the experiments was observed. Comparison of results obtained at the outset of the experiments and those obtained subsequently indicate a degree of adaptation. At 40 meters, results obtained when helium-oxygen mixtures were used were superior to those obtained when nitrogen-oxygen mixtures were used. Stability of attention decreased when the oxygen partial pressure of the nitrogen-oxygen mixture was increased. In general, results indicate that prolonged stays at pressures of up to 16 atm by trained men can be undergone without significant impairment of mental function. (MFW/BSCP)

261.
BOEGEMAN, D.E., G.J. Miller and W.R. Normark.
Precise positioning for near-bottom equipment using a relay transponder.
Mar. Geophys. Res. 1(4):381-396; 1972.

The Marine Physical Laboratory of the Scripps Institution of Oceanography has developed an acoustic relay transponder for precise relative positioning of near-bottom instruments and geologic sampling devices. Although specifically designed to position equipment lowered on standard wire ropes without a need to maintain direct electrical contact with the surface ship, the relay transponder may be used to track free vehicles, such as deep submersibles, from the surface. The relay transponder is positioned relative to an array of bottom-anchored acoustic transponders. It is interrogated acoustically from the surface ship; it then sequentially interrogates the bottom transponders which, in turn, reply to the ship. From the measurement of the total travel time (ship to relay transponder to bottom transponder to ship) and assuming, or knowing, the sound velocity of the water, we obtain a relayed range measurement. These relayed ranges, used in conjunction with ship to bottom-transponder ranges, allow us to calculate the position of the relay transponder. A recent application of this technique is described in which several gravity core samples from the crest of the Horizon Guyot were positioned with respect to the detailed bathmetry and the geology within the area. The estimated error in positioning the samples is less than 20 m inside a navigational net extending over 100 km. (Authors' abstract)

262.
BOENING, D., H.-V. Ulmer, U. Meier, W. Skipka and J. Stegemann.
Effects of a multi-hour immersion on trained and untrained subjects: I. Renal function and plasma volume.
Aerosp. Med. 43:300-305;Mar. 1972.

In 30 experiments the effects of 8-hr recumbency and 4- to 8-hr immersion in thermo-indifferent water on renal function and plasma volume of trained and untrained persons were consecutively followed. Recumbency led to an increased diuresis and sodium excretion. With immersion the diuresis rose even more. For the trained subjects the urine excretion increased more slowly than in the case of the untrained. No reproduceable difference of electrolyte excretion between both groups could be substantiated. The plasma volume was diminished after recumbency and immersion. No difference between trained and untrained persons could be substantiated. The decrease of plasma volume depended mainly on the amount of urine excreted. The later rise of diuresis for trained persons may exhibit an adaptation of the volume regulating reflexes to blood volume fluctuations during frequent work. (Authors' abstract)

263.
BOENING, D., H.-V. Ulmer, U. Meier and J. Stegemann.
Effects of a multi-hour immersion on trained and untrained subjects: II. Blood protein and electrolyte concentrations.
Aerosp. Med. 43:415-418;Apr. 1972.

Serial measurements on blood protein and electrolyte content were carried out during four to eight hour immersion of trained and untrained human subjects. After an initial drop the hemotocrit value and the hemoglobin concentration showed a general increase, which could be accounted for by water-displacement. There was no significant change in total protein and albumin content in plasma. The sodium concentration fluctuated and the potassium concentration increased temporarily. Inorganic phosphate concentration, probably because of a change in metabolism, increased steadily. In the erythrocytes the potassium concentration fluctuated and the chloride concentration decreased. No important differences could be ascertained between trained and untrained subjects. (Authors' abstract)

264.
BOGGS, J.M. and J.C. Hsia.
Spin label studies on the mechanism of pressure reversal of anesthesia.
Proc. Can Fed. Biol. Sci. 16:13;1973.

Abstract only. Entire item quoted. The effects of anesthetics in luminous bacteria, newts, tadpoles, and mice and on isolated nerves can be reversed by application of 150-200 atmospheres pressure. Any theory of anesthesia must account for this phenomenon. We investigated the effect of pressure on the membrane partition coefficient and location of a water soluble lipophilic spin label TEMPO (1-oxyl-2,2,6,6-tetramethyl-piperidine) which was found to reversibly block the action potential of rat phrenic nerve with an ED_{50} of 6.4 x 10^{-3} M (A. Staiman and P. Seeman, unpublished results). TEMPO binds to a hydrophobic site in the phrenic nerve membrane and synaptosomal membranes similar to that in egg lechithin vesicles. The partition of TEMPO between egg lecithin or egg lecithin-cholesterol and aqueous phase is not significantly affected by 150 atmospheres of helium. However, pressure has a dramatic effect on the distribution of TEMPO in both synaptosomal vesicles and the intact phrenic nerve. We interpret the results to mean that pressure reversibly induces a new, more polar binding site which has very high affinity for TEMPO, effectively removing it from the hydrophobic site is the primary site of action, removal of the anesthetic from this site could account for the reversal of anesthesia by pressure.

265.
BOGOSLOVOV, G.B.
Pathogenesis of some respiratory and circulatory reactions accompanying drops in barometric pressure.
Space Biol. Med. 6:38-42;Jan. 18, 1973.
(JPRS 58010)

Decompression disease continues to remain a timely problem in high-altitude and space flights. In 44 experiments on dogs the author studied the reactions of respiration, blood circulation, gas composition of the blood and a number of other indices in response to embolism in the pulmonary artery induced by different quantities of nitrogen introduced at different rates (as a model of a decompression gas embolism). Some of the animals were first intravenously injected with novocaine. A satisfactory tolerance of the animals to a gas embolism was established. In the reactions to gas injection it is not so much the quantity which is of importance as the rate of entry into the lesser circulatory system. The deactivation of vascular interoceptors by novacaine depresses the adaptive compensatory reactions of respiration and circulation developing after injection of the gas and leads to a predominance of symptoms of mechanical impairment of pulmonary circulation. (Author's abstract)

266.
BOKERIIA, L.A. and R.A. Kovaneva.
Giperbaricheskaya Oksigenatsiya pri Kessonnoi Bolezni.
[Hyperbaric oxygenation in caisson disease].
Klin. Med. 51:50-53;Feb. 1973.

A detailed description is given of possibilities and advantages of hyperbaric oxygenation in caisson disease. The authors describe a case of successful use of this method in the moderate spinal form of acute caisson disease in patients who were admitted to the hospital on the fifth day following the onset of the disease. After two seances of hyperbaric oxygenation recovery came. (English summary)

267.
BONDI, K.R. and H.D. Van Liew.
Fluxes of CO_2 in the lung gas studied by continuously recorded arterial pH.
J. Appl. Physiol. 35:42-46;July 1973.

Arterial blood pH, measured continuously in anesthetized, paralyzed dogs, was used to investigate time-dependent factors in gas exchange. When the ventilatory pump was stopped at the end of inspiration, there was often a rise of pH before the fall brought on by CO_2 accumulation. The rise or "hump" was more pronounced when the animal breathed a helium-oxygen mixture. When the ventilation was changed from the usual end-expiratory pause pattern to a pattern with end-inspiratory pauses, the hump phenomenon could no longer be elicited by a breath hold and there was a gradual rise of mean pH of the blood, indicating better clearance of CO_2. Apparently the effectiveness of a breath, so far as CO_2 exchange is concerned, can be improved upon because of better mixing if the breath remains in the lung for a time, rather than being immediately expelled as in ordinary expiratory-pause breathing. (Authors' abstract)

269.
BONIN, B., P.W. Straub, R. Schibli and A.A. Buhlmann.
Blood coagulation during critical decompression following diving experiments with oxygen/helium.
Aerosp. Med. 44:508-512;May 1973.

Healthy male volunteers were exposed during two hours to 10 ATA in a pressure chamber and were then subjected to a border-line sufficient decompression regimen. Analysis of blood coagulation and fibrinolysis was performed before and at the end of the experiments. The observed changes were usually minor and did not exceed those observed in stressful situations. There was notably no evidence for clinically significant intravascular coagulation, even in subjects complaining of decompression symptoms. (Authors' abstract)

279.
BONNET, M., J. Chouteau, M. Hugon, G. Imbert and J.P. Roll.
Activites motrices reflexe et spontanee chez le singe sous heliox (99 ATA).
[Spontaneous and reflex motor activities in the monkey under heliox (99 ATA)].
In: Hesser, C.M. and D. Linnarsson eds. Proceedings of the first annual scientific meeting of the European Undersea Biomedical Society, Stockholm, 13-15 June 1973. Forvarsmedicin 9:314-317;July 1973.

In extreme diving conditions in helium, Papio papio did not demonstrate peripheral electrophysiological disorders. Central disorders existed, expressed by a certain tonic hyperactivity, a sensorimotor hyperreactivity, a tremor of central origin. These disorders appeared to originate in a disturbance of the interneurones rather than an alteration of the motoneurone activity, the excitability of which varied little. (Authors' conclusion translated by MFW/BSCP)

280.
BOODA, L.L.
Concrete: excellent undersea material.
UnderSea Technol. 13:21;Sept. 1970.

Entire item quoted: Engineers from the Naval Civil Engineering Laboratory, Port Hueneme, Calif., recently recovered and tested six concrete blocks which had been in the Los Angeles breakwater for 67 years. Compressive strength tests of the blocks (5.75' x 5.75' x 3' in size) made from six different brands of commercial cement in 1905, showed some blocks have actualy increased in strength since previously tested in 1932. Four-inch diameter cores were taken from each block. They have been replaced in the breakwater — perhaps to be raised again in 40 years. In a related project, NCEL recently launched a 60-ton semi-submersible ocean platform model made of concrete (except the deck). The one-tenth scale model consists of two cylindrical hulls, each 37 ft long by 5 1/2 ft in diameter and 4-in thick walls. The steel deck is supported by eight vertical columns 7 ft long by 3 1/2 ft in diameter and with 3-in. thick walls. The model is undergoing a series of structural and hydrodynamic tests this summer. The proposed full scale platform would have a 300 ft x 300 ft deck. The excellence of concrete as an undersea construction material was demonstrated by the performance of a 100,000 lb concrete cylinder placed at a depth of 600 ft for one year. When recovered recently there were not major malfunctions or failures. The cylinder contained a 42-inch acrylic window, high voltage electrical connectors, television and test instrumentation.

281.
BOODA, L.L.
The Navy must continue to lead in undersea technology.
UnderSea Technol. 13:32-33;Sept. 1972.

In the course of this discussion of the Navy's hydrographic and oceanographic programs, based on an interview with the Oceanographer of the Navy, Rear Adm. J. E. Snyder, Jr. it is noted that the Navy plans to put money into the budget to increase the use of submersibles, many of which now lie idle for lack of funds. Also mentioned are DSRV-1 and DSRV-2, which have the capability of mating, not only with U.S. submarines, but also with those of other nations if the hulls are modified to conform to our plans, which are now available. (MFW/BSCP)

282.
BOODA, L.L.
Protecting marine equipment from fouling, erosion, corrosion and cavitation.
Undersea Technol. 13:16-17;Dec. 1972.

B.F. Godrich Company has developed a coating called "nofoul" which is believed to offer much longer life and much greater protection than any anti-fouling coatings known to date. The basic idea behind the development of this product is the dissolving of an effective anti-fouling toxicant in an elastomeric material. It is important that the toxicant not be soluble in sea water, and also that it not materially alter the basic coating. The materials used are the toxin bis-n-tributyltin oxide, and the polymer neoprine. The product has been in limited use since 1965, and apparently performs satisfactorily. (MFW/BSCP)

283.
BOODA, L.L.
Alvin's familiar appearance only skin deep.
UnderSea Technol. 14:39;Jan. 1973.

Alvin's new titanium pressure hull is nearing completion. The first sphere is due this month for testing in a pressure chamber at the U.S. Naval Ship Research and Development Command Laboratories, and will probably be installed in April. The second will be ready about one month later. A unique variable sea water ballasting system and new, improved sensors will also be installed. The titanium spheres have been constructed as part of the Naval Ship System Command's Project Titanus. They are designed to withstand pressures of 12,000 feet in depth. (MFW/BSCP)

284.
BOODA, L.L.
Navy has new unmanned deep ocean vehicle.
UnderSea Technol. 14:11;Feb. 1973.

The Remote Unmanned Work System (RUWS), designed to operate at 20,000 feet, has passed its first tests at the Naval Undersea Center's Hawaii Laboratory. It is an improved version of CURV. Its important features include: control through a 4 1/6 mile coaxial synthetic cable; high accuracy navigation; advanced sonar; head coupled TV; advanced manipulator. It is designed in modules for easy air transportation. Final tests are scheduled for 1975. (MFW/BSCP)

285.
BOODA, L.L.
Tragedy in the Johnson-Sea-Link.
Sea Technol. 14:17,28,58;July 1973.

An account is given of the disaster of the Johnson-Sea-Link, in which two lives were lost after the submersible had become jammed against a sunken destroyer. The cause of the accident appeared to be an underestimation of the strength of the current, or a failure to appreciate the possible consequences of operating under such conditions. The current also hampered rescue attempts, and the delay resulted in the death of the two men who were in the lock-out ambient pressure compartment. The cause of death is not discussed here, but from the facts given, it would seem to be either carbon dioxide poisoning due to the Baralyme scrubbers becoming less effective as the temperature decreased, or cold exposure, or a combination of both. An investigating board has been convened. (MFW/SCD)

286.
BORNMANN, R.C.
Proposed instructions for use of tables for repetitive, no decompression helium-oxygen, saturation-excursion dives.
In: Fructus, X., Ed. Third international conference on hyperbaric and underwater physiology, p.63-68. Paris, Doin, 1972.

The author gives no-decompression limits tables, repetitive group designations tables, and repetitive excursion timetables for depths of 150 to 300 fsw, and for depths of 300 to 600 fsw, along with instructions for their use. Another table gives habitat interval credit for saturation exposure at depths from 150-600 fsw. Any dive following another dive by less than 24 hours is considered a repetitive dive, since that is the length of time generally required for the body to lose its excess of helium. These tables are limited to depth and bottom time combinations which enable return to habitat pressure at the rate of 60 feet per minute, with no need for intermediate stops. Atmosphere control requirements for both habitat and personnel transfer capsule are specified. (MFW/UMS)

287.
BORNMANN, R.C.
Underwater research and military medicine in certain European countries: Part I — Norway, Germany, and Sweden.
U.S. Off. Nav. Res. London, Rep. 21-73, 23p. Sept. 5, 1973.
(AD 789,653)

This report is not intended as a scientific document, but rather as a sort of news letter summarizing the research recently being conducted in the countries concerned. The Norwegian Navy is developing a deep diving capability in order to exploit the North Sea oil deposits. Surgeon Commander Smith-Sivertsen has undergone education and training at New London and at Alverstoke. Dr. Sem-Jacobsen has worked largely in electrography, and particularly in miniaturizing monitoring equipment. He is also attempting to develop a program by which saturation diving habitats will be constructed within coastal mountains, by drilling tunnels. In Germany, the Ship Travel Medical Institute has conducted a recent symposium on naval human engineering and occupational medicine. Its present director, Captain Wandel, and its future director, Dr. Seemann, have both received training in New London and in Washington. The development of deep diving techniques in Germany is necessarily limited by the shortness of the Coastline and the shallowness of the national waters. Emphasis is on submarine escape techniques, and submarine design. The Physiology Division of the Institute has a small animal hyperbaric chamber where a great variety of experiments has been carried out. In Sweden, the Naval Diving Office is run by Drs. Muren and Adolfson. The latter has spent a year at the Naval Medical Research Institute in Bethesda. The Diving Center has a chamber complex with a depth capability of 40 atm, a wet pot, an igloo, and two decompression chambers. Small animal chambers exist, and work in saturation diving is active. Special studies have been made recently in diver selection. The Navy's diving training ship and submarine rescue vessel Belos is described. In the Department of Naval Medicine at the Karolinska Institutet, experiments have centered largely around breathing mixtures, with particular interest in hydrogen mixtures. Drs. Hesser, Fagraeus, and Linnarsson are active in these experiments. At the University of Lund, Professor Lundgren is head of the Laboratory of Aviation and Naval Physiology. Research has recently been concerned chiefly with the effect of immersion on pulmonary dynamics. Subclinical air embolism after ascent is another object of study. (MFW/UMS)

288.
BORNMANN, R.C.
Underwater research and military medicine in certain European countries: Part II — France. U.S. Off. Nav. Res. London, Rep. R-22-73, 17p. Sept. 5, 1973.
(AD 769,654)

At time of writing, work on the large lock-out submersible Argyronete had been temporarily discontinued, and the thinking was in favor of smaller 10-20 ton research submersibles similar to that recently developed by COMEX. The non-profit research company of Jacques Cousteau, CEMA, has largely sold out to the commercial company COCEAN. For this reason, the high pressure research that Professor Jacques Chouteau had been carrying on was temporarily interrupted. Means will probably be found to continue this important work. The Centre d'Etudes et de Recherches Biophysiologigues Appliquees a la Marine (CERB) at Toulon is under the actual direction of Commander Broussolle, since its titular director, Captain Joly, is occupied primarily with the Reanimation Department at the Ste. Anne Hospital there. Studies at CERB include ventilatory response to CO_2, mechanics of ventilation, and gas exchange in hyperbaric environments. In conjunction with COMEX, studies of the effects of hyperbaric oxygen on the lung have been carried out. Other areas of experimentation are inert gas narcosis and platelet changes in decompression sickness. The Groupe d'Etudes et Recherches Sous-Marines (GERS), under Commander Berry, is also at Toulon. Studies have been made by Dr. Michaud of oxygen effects at 1200 m, using minipigs. The diving ship Triton has made 140 and 200 m saturation dives. The Centre d'Etudes et Recherches Techniques des Sous-Marins (CERTSM) is primarily technical rather than medical, but it does have a biomedical research program, and its director is an M.D., Dr. Guillerm. It has an extensive contaminant control program. Mercury, hydrocarbons, and tobacco smoke are among the contaminants under study, as well as carbon dioxide. Submarine escape techniques are discussed. Temperature and humidity control and various aspects of design and technology are under study. The Centre d'Etudes et de Recherches Service de Psychologie Appliquee (CERPA) is under the direction of Captain Caille. Problems of training and selection are studied, and extensive personality inventories have been compiled. Effects of chronic hypercapnia on vigilance have also been studied. (MFW/UMS)

289.
BORNSIDE, G.H., G.W. Cherry and M.B. Meyers.
Introcolonic oxygen tension and in vivo bactericidal effect of hyperbaric oxygen on rat colonic flora.
Aerosp. Med. 44:1282-1286;Nov. 1973.

Intracolonic P_{O_2} and P_{CO_2} were measured in germfree and conventional rats breathing 100% O_2 at 3 ata. A gas sampling cannula was passed 8 cm into the colon. Intracolonic gaseous tensions were measured by mass spectrometry. Conventional rats had a lower intracolonic P_{O_2} (7 mm Hg) than germfree rats (15 mm Hg), and a higher P_{CO_2} (73 mm Hg versus 40 mm Hg) because of the presence of a microflora. During exposure to HPO, the mean intracolonic P_{O_2} increased to peaks of 400 to 450 mm Hg. After exposure the rat was killed, and the sampled segment of colon was resected and cultured. An antibacterial effect against anaerobes was discernible after 30 min exposure. Neither anaerobes nor coliforms were isolated after exposure for 4 hr. However, aerobic lactobacilli and gram-positive cocci, particularly enterococci, were but partially diminished in number. Hence, an in vivo antibacterial effect on colonic flora was produced by breathing HPO and increased with duration of exposure. (Authors' abstract)

290.
BOROWIKOW, P.A.
Untersuchung der Atemluftveranderung in "Tschernomor"
[Investigation of breathing-air changes in "Tschernomor"].
Meerestechnik 4:37-38;Apr. 1973.

During the tests with the underwater laboratory "Tschernomor" (Black Sea) in the years 1968 and 1969, the changes of the breathing-air composition in the manned station were investigated. The dynamic of the change determines, for instance, the lay-out of the regeneration system. With the found parameters, the state of the gas, thereby, the processing installations of closed underwater systems can be determined by calculation. (Authors' abstract)

291.
BOUSHEY, H.A. and P.S. Richardson.
The reflex effects of intralaryngeal carbon dioxide on the pattern of breathing.
J. Physiol. (London) 228:181-192;1973.

The reflex effects on the pattern of breathing and total lung resistance of introducing 30, 10 and 5% CO_2 in air into the larynx have been studied in anaesthetized and decerebrate cats breathing through a tracheostomy tube. Flowing 30% CO_2 into the larynx caused a two-phased response. First, respiratory frequency and tidal volume decreased, with a consequent fall in minute ventilation. After two to ten breaths, frequency remained slow, but tidal volume increased beyond the control level, so that minute ventilation was restored to control levels. Flowing 5 or 10% CO_2 into the larynx caused slowing of breathing with small and inconsistent changes in tidal volume. Minute ventilation was significantly diminished. Off effects, on re-introducing air into the larynx, after 2 and 10 min of CO_2 exposure, suggested that the reflex response diminishes with increased duration of exposure to CO_2. None of the concentrations of intralaryngeal CO_2 changed total lung resistance or compliance. CO_2 mixtures in the larynx generally caused no change in blood pressure or pulse rate of the cats. The reflex effects of intralaryngeal CO_2 were abolished by denervating the larynx. Hypoxic mixtures introduced into the larynx did not change breathing. (Authors' summary)

292.
BOUTELIER, C., J. Colin and J. Timbal.
Determination de la zone de neutralite thermique dans l'eau.
[Determination of the zone of thermal neutrality in water].
Rev. Med. Aeronaut. Spatiale 10:25-29;1st quart. 1971.

Study of heat exchange between the human body and water, in order to determine the zone of thermal neutrality. Knowledge of this zone and the laws of reduction of body temperature as a function of ambient temperature and metabolism make it possible to determine limits of tolerance in cold water and to devise protective equipment. Many experiments are reported which were carried out on nude subjects almost totally immersed in rough water. (Aerosp. Med.)

293.
BOUTELIER, C., J. Colin and J. Timbal.
Determination du coefficient d'echange thermique dans l'eau en ecoulement turbulent.
[Determination of the coefficient of thermal exchange in turbulent water].
J. Physiol. (Paris) 63:207-209;May 1971.

The authors have attempted to determine the coefficient of heat exchange by convection, using the method of fractional calorimetry. Thirty-six experiments, involving nine male subjects, were carried out in a 3 m^3 tank of water maintained at a constant temperature of 32.5-33.5°C. The subjects, clad in swimming trunks and equipped with thermocouples, were almost totally immersed in turbulent water for 90 to 180 minutes. Ten cutaneous and one rectal temperature readings were taken every minute, and the metabolisms of the subjects were regularly monitored. The coefficient of transfer h_c was calculated as:

$$h_c = 53.3 + 0.8\,K\,Ca/m^2h.°C.$$

or

$$62.9 + 0.93\,W/m^2.\ °C.$$

The calculations are given in detail on pp. 208-209. (MEMH/BSCP)

294.
BOVE, A.A., J.M. Hallenbeck and D.H. Elliott.
Changes in blood plasma volumes during decompression sickness in dogs.
Fed. Proc. 32 (3,pt.1):396;Mar. 1973.

Abstract only. Entire item quoted: Decompression sickness (DCS) was produced in 8 conscious dogs by a 220 foot air dive in a hyperbaric chamber. A mild lesion (limb bend) was produced in 4 animals with a dive of 30 minutes or less while in 4 others, a spinal cord lesion (paresis) occurred with dives of 40 to 45 minutes. Ascent from depth was continuous at 60 ft per minute. Plasma and RBC volumes were measured with I^{125} albumin and Cr^{51} labelled red cells. Blood volume was calculated from peripheral hematocrit (HCT), plasma, and RBC volumes. No change in HCT occurred in control or limb bend animals, while a rise from 39 to 46% occurred with spinal cord lesions. While RBC volume remained constant, blood volume using Cr^{51} RBC's showed a fall only in paretic dives. However, no change was noted with I^{125} albumin. Plasma volume measured from Cr^{51} RBC data showed a 30% fall after paretic dives and no change in control or limb bend dives. Serious CNS lesions in acute DCS are associated with loss of plasma from the vascular space, producing hemoconcentration and hypovolemia. Mild peripheral DCS is not associated with significant loss of the plasma from the vascular space. The opinions contained herein are the private ones of the authors and are not to be construed as reflecting the views of the Navy Dept.

295.
BOVE, A.A., A.L. Pierce, F. Barrera, G.A. Amsbaugh and P.R. Lynch.
Diving bradycardia as a factor in underwater blackout.
Aerosp. Med. 44:245-248;Mar. 1973.

Heart rate was studied during prolonged breath holding with face immersion in 45 men. A diving bradycardia manifested by a fall in heart rate immediately after facial immersion occurred in all subjects. In four subjects a second decline in heart rate occurred after about 140 seconds of breath holding and continued until breathing was resumed. This secondary decline is thought to be due to hypoxia developing during prolonged apnea in individuals who are more tolerant to hypoxia and hypercapnia. These particular individuals may be more prone to sudden underwater blackout during breath hold dives because the initial diving bradycardia is later potentiated by progressive hypoxia which further reduces cardiac output and blood flow to vital tissues. (Authors' abstract)

296.
BOYD, E.
Navy divers — pride of the fleet.
Skin Diver 22:13-19;July 1973.

The overall Navy diving program is described. There are seven classes of divers: deep sea air divers, deep sea helium divers, (both surface supplied), scuba divers, SEAL (sea, air, land) teams, explosive ordnance disposal (EOD) dives, underwater demolition teams (UDT) and saturation divers. The deep sea divers work to a depth of 300 feet, the scuba divers to 130 feet; the SEAL teams are similar to green berets or commandos; EOD and UDT functions are self-explanatory. The latter have the additional duty of assisting at Apollo splashdowns. The saturation diver is the deepest diver (a recent open water working saturation dive was carried out successfully at 1010 feet). This is considered the dive of the future. The U.S. Navy Experimental Diving Unit is described. The Unit's function is not only to develop, test and evaluate diving equipment but also to develop saturation diving techniques. The training schools at Indian Head, Maryland give the very rigorous courses that turn out the EOD divers. The Second Class Diver's school in San Diego qualifies divers in scuba and deep sea techniques. It is noted that hard-hat diving retains some advantages over scuba: the diver can go deeper and stay longer, he has better protection, and he has communication with the surface. The Ocean Simulation Facility at the Naval Ship Research Development Laboratory at Panama City, Florida is described. This facility will make it possible to predict the performance of man and machine prior to actual ocean trials. Also at Panama City is the Scientist-in-the-Sea training program, which is jointly sponsored by the Navy, NOAA, Sea Grant, and the Florida State University system. This ten week course includes training in night diving, saturation diving technology, diving medicine, underwater communication, navigation, search and recovery, advanced umbilical techniques, engineering and photography. Students take qualification dives to 110 feet. The Underwater Swimmers School at Key West, in addition to giving rigorous physical training geared toward UDT work, also places emphasis on psychological factors involved in diving. The Naval Civil Engineering Laboratory at Port Hueneme, California, tests and evaluates underwater tools and power systems; the laboratory is also developing hydraulic tools for use at great depths. (MFW/SCD)

297.
BOYLAN, L.H.
Recent Soviet developments in undersea technology.
Mar. Technol. Soc. J. 6:41-43;Sept./Oct. 1972.

The USSR's most advanced underwater research vehicle Sever-2, has been tested and has carried out operations, together with its support ship, Odissey, consisting of four months of dives in the Black Sea during the winter of 1971-1972. During these operations, a Soviet submersible depth record of 2020 meters was reached. The purpose of the dives was the study of fish behavior, as well as the testing of various maneuvers of the vehicle itself. Safety measures include an extensive check list inspection before diving; the check list includes emergency surfacing systems, fire-suppression devices, power and seal-integrity checks of the outboard equipment, etc. There are more than 1000 cable leads through the hull penetrators. Another safety measure is the requirement that Sever 2 communicate (by hydroacoustic means) with Odissey every 20 minutes; if communication cannot be made, Sever-2 must surface immediately. The submersible carries four men. A small two-man vehicle, the Afalina, has been designed by the students of the Leningrad Shipbuilding Institute, to be used for bottom mapping and other sea-floor studies. An underwater drone, the Skorpena, has been designed by the Underwater Research Laboratory of the all-Union Scientific Research Institute of Fisheries and Oceanography; proposed function is carrying cameras and other research equipment to 1000-meter depths. The hull consists of modules, some of which serve as buoyancy units, others as power and automatic control systems. When the drone reaches a predetermined depth, the camera or other instruments, and the motor, are activated. As the cycle is completed, the unit moves up until it is over the next area to be photographed, then it descends and the cycle begins again. An emergency surfacing system can be activated by water seepage, excessive depth, or submerged time, or certain mechanical failures. The drone has apparently not yet been put into production. (MFW/BSCP)

298.
BOYLE, J., III.
Theoretical trans-respiratory pressures during rapid decompression: II. Animal experiments.
Aerosp. Med. 44:157-162;Feb. 1973.

A theory is developed and an equation derived which provides the maximal trans-respiratory pressure (P_{Dmax}) which is generated during rapid decompression (RD). This theory includes those physical and physiological parameters which affect decompression of the lungs and cabin. Animal experiments are used to test the theory. The correlation coefficient between experimental and theoretic (calculated) pressures was 0.82. Mean theoretic and measured values of P_{Dmax} were 34 and 23 mm Hg, respectively. The time constant of the lung was measured during decompression and found to vary at different altitudes. This effect is felt to be due to alterations in compressibility and airway resistance at altitude due to changes in gas density. Determination of P_{Dmax} generated by RD provides an objective measure of the severity of decompression and should provide a valid means of calculating pulmonary tolerance limits for RD. (Author's abstract)

299.
BRAITHWAITE, W.R.
The calculation of minimum safe inspired gas temperature limits for deep diving.
U.S. Navy Exp. Diving Unit, Rep. NEDU-12-72, 13p. July 1972.

Loss of body heat through the lungs of divers breathing cold gas at depths greater than 600 feet can be lethal; no adequate guidelines to safe inspired gas temperatures are currently available. Review of the recent research in hyperbaric respiratory heat loss has allowed the development of a rational method of calculating the minimum safe inspired gas temperatures for deep diving. In this report, the recent respiratory heat loss research is summarized, the rationale and calculations of safe breathing gas temperatures are presented, and minimum safe inspired gas temperature limits for depths from 600 to 1000 feet are proposed. (Author's abstract)

300.
BRAITHWAITE, W.R.
Systematic guide to decompression schedule calculations.
U.S. Navy Exp. Diving Unit, Rep. NEDU-11-72, 13p. July 15, 1972.

This report is designed to be used in conjunction with Workman's presentation of the theoretical basis for the calculation of decompression schedules, EDU Report No. 6-65, to clarify the definitions and simplify the calculation procedure. An attempt has been made to explain verbally and graphically the basic concepts in areas known to be difficult for students of Workman's method. The report includes a step-by-step program designed to lead one through the calculations with a minimum of confusion, and a discussion of methods for shortening the time involved. The necessary tables and worksheet used in the calculations are also included. (Author's abstract)

301.
BRAMHAM, E., J.L. Dineley and B. Wharmby.
Heat loss compensation in deep diving.
Hydrospace 5:20;Aug. 1972.

Laboratory tests have proved that the standard neoprene wet suit compresses in thickness at increased depths, to the extent that heat loss at 100m increases by 300 percent. A compensated cellular pressure material has been developed which uses automatic pressure control supplied by the diver's breathing mixture to maintain a constant thickness in the heat insulating layer. The thickness of this layer is monitored electrically and the cellular pressure adjusted to maintain a constant thickness. In order to maintain the diver's temperature at 100 m, the standard suit requires a heat supply of 2.6 kw, as contrasted with 300 w for the compensated suit. (MFW/BSCP)

302.
BRANDT, L., G. Walther, H. Rothschenk and T. von Lieven.
Enzym histochemische Untersuchungen am Hoden der Ratte nach hyperbarer Sauerstoffirrgiftung.
[Enzyme histochemical studies on rat testicles following hyperbaric oxygen poisoning].
Beitr. Gerichtl. Med. 29:312-320; 1972.

Rats were exposed to high oxygen pressure (3.8 atmospheres absolute, 4 hours) and the testicles were studied histologically and histochemically. The tissue slides were examined for the distribution of the dehydrogenases (lactate-, malic-, isocitrate-, and succinate-dehydrogenase) and 5-nucleotidase. The rats demonstrated the clinical symptoms of O_2 intoxication: hyperesthesia, convulsions, spasms and deep respiration. Histological investigations of the tissue slides show hyperemia of the capillary. The histochemical findings point out a decrease of enzyme activity in the interstitial cells (LEYDIG cells). One explanation of oxygen toxicity is the oxydation of SH dependent enzymes and destruction of membrane permeability. The decrease of histochemical enzyme activity in the interstitial cells suggests another cause, that is, disruption of the neuro-hormonal mechanism, especially with respect to the action of the hypothalamus, the hypophysis and the adrenal glands on the interstitial cells. (English summary)

303.
BRASHEAR, R.E. and R.E. DeAtley.
Decreased pulmonary oxygen toxicity by pretreatment with hypoxia.
Arch. Environ. Health 24:77-81;Feb. 1972.

The effect of 10% or 12% oxygen pretreatment on subsequent mortality as a result of breathing 100% oxygen was studied. Rats exposed to 100% oxygen without prior treatment died after 66 $\pm$ 7 hours. Those pretreated with compressed air for 120 hours died after 61 $\pm$ 10 hours of exposure to 100% oxygen. Those pretreated with 10% oxygen for 120 hours survived exposure to 100% oxygen for 336 hours ($P < .01$) and were killed. Six of 16 rats pretreated with 120 hours of 12% oxygen died after 134 $\pm$ 104 hours of exposure to 100% oxygen and ten were killed after surviving 336 hours of exposure to 100% oxygen. Pretreatment of rats with 10% or 12% oxygen for 120 hours has a significant effect on subsequent survival in an environment of 100% oxygen. (Authors' abstract)

304.
BRASHEAR, R.E., H.M. Sharma and R.E. DeAtley.
Prolonged survival breathing oxygen at ambient pressure.
Amer. Rev. Resp. Dis. 108:701-704;Sept. 1973.

The effect of 5 days of hypoxia on the subsequent mortality of rats breathing 99 per cent oxygen at ambient pressure was studied. Thirty-one of the 32 rats not previously subjected to hypoxia died after 64 $\pm$ 10 (mean $\pm$ SD) hours of breathing oxygen. Five of 32 rats, subjected to 5 days of hypoxia, died after 281 $\pm$ 76 hours of subsequent oxygen. Twenty-seven of the group that was exposed to hypoxia survived after breathing oxygen for 28 days. Microscopy demonstrated delayed perivascular and peribronchial edema in the group subjected to hypoxia, and pulmonary fibrosis was noted after 48 days of breathing oxygen. (Authors' summary)

305.
BRASHEAR, R.E. and J.C. Christian.
Endobronchial lavage phospholipids and protein in rats protected from oxygen toxicity by hypoxia pretreatment.
Metabolism 22:1345-1348;Nov. 1973.

Endobronchial lavage phospholipids and proteins were compared in controls, rats exposed to 99 + % oxygen for 52 hr, and rats exposed to 5 days of hypoxia followed by 52 hr of 99 + % oxygen. The rats exposed to 99 + % oxygen had significantly less phospholipids and more protein in their endobronchial washings than the controls. In contrast, the hypoxia-pretreated rats had comparable levels of phospholipids and protein in endobronchial washings compared to controls. This study indicates that phospholipids and proteins in endobronchial lavage provide a metabolic marker for the study of oxygen toxicity. (Authors' abstract)

306.
BRAUER, R.W.
Untitled.
In: Abstracts of BuMed-ONR sponsored Navywide research in high pressure biomedical research, U.S. Submarine Base, Groton, Conn., May 1971, p.38. Published by the Naval Submarine Medical Research Laboratories, 1971.

Abstract only. Entire item quoted: Data are reported concerning studies on the high pressure hyperexcitability syndrome in Rhesus monkeys and squirrel monkeys. These include blood gas analyses, relations between compression rate and seizure thresholds, observations on the tremor phase of the syndrome, and preliminary observations concerning the events which result in death of primate exposed to pressures between 90 and 110 atm. Some data on the comparative physiology of the syndrome are presented including in particular observations concerning the relation between tremor and convulsion thresholds in different species and under different exposure conditions. Data concerning the protective effect of narcotic gases in admixtures with the basic compression atmosphere are briefly reviewed with particular reference to the difference in effect upon the several phases of the syndrome. Preliminary observations with the Wrightsville Marine Bio-Medical Laboratory high pressure aquarium system are made available for discussion.

307.
BRAUER, R.W., M.R. Jordan and R.O. Way.
The high pressure neurological syndrome in the squirrel monkey, Saimiri sciureus.
In: Fructus, X., Ed. Third international conference on hyperbaric and underwater physiology, p.24-30. Paris, Doin, 1972.

Transition from surface to a high pressure environment entails changes in the excitability of the CNS manifested most dramatically in a greatly increased liability to epileptiform convulsions. These phenomena may either be the expression of the effect of hydrostatic high pressures on living tissues, or more probably they may reflect dislocation in cell composition, cell structure, or cell metabolism as a result of the change from surface to great depths. Some accomodation to these effects appears to take place as time goes on, so that the neurological effects might be expected to decrease in severity as the sojourn in a particular high pressure environment is lengthened. How far this accommodation may go, whether it entails complete restoration of normal function or whether it will merely progress part of the way and leave a seriously stressed subject surviving under distinctly unfavorable conditions, remains to be determined. Studies with various gas mixtures show that the syndrome can indeed be modified and its most severe manifestation can be postponed by inclusion of narcotically active gases. These effects contradict any hypotheses seeking the basis of the syndrome in changes in gas density or respiratory mechanics. Other data support this conclusion. Specific histoxic effects of hydrogen have not been detected. (From authors' conclusions)

308.
BRAUER, R.W.
Studies concerning the high pressure hyperexcitability in the squirrel monkey.
Wilmington, N.C., Wrightsville Mar. Bio-Med. Lab., Final report on contract N00014-69-C-0341, 13p. July 13, 1972.

Development of knowledge on the high pressure neurological syndrome (HPNS) in vertebrates is described on the basis of five years of investigative effort. Besides tracing the historical sequence of events, the report details experimentation aimed at providing a basis for predicting the onset of severe HPNS complications in man at various compression rates ranging from those in current use for cautious descent of subjects seeking to reach maximum depths to the very fast compression rates contemplated in relation with submarine escape techniques. A variety of other data concerning the HPNS are reviewed briefly from the points of view of their bearing upon design of prophylactic or therapeutic procedures, formulation of questions requiring additional clinical exploration, and elucidation of basic biophysical mechanisms. Attention is called to the fact that the underlying mechanisms seem to be common not only to all vertebrates tested, but to a rather similar sequence elicited by high pressures in many invertebrates. Problems of adaptation and of selection for individual variation are touched upon. (DCD abstract)

309.
BRENNAND, R.
Protective interface circuits for use with hyperbaric oxygen chambers.
In: Innes, G.S. ed. The production and hazards of a hyperbaric oxygen environment. Proceedings of a symposium held at University College, London, January 1968, p.107-116. Oxford, Pergamon Press, 1970.

The purpose of this communication is to consider ways in which electrical circuits constitute an ignition risk, to outline the various ways in which electronic apparatus may be rendered safe and, finally, to describe a preferred system which offers an economical solution permitting the use of externally located mains operated patient monitoring and communication equipment. Also included are some considerations of the minimum electrical energy required for ignition. (Author)

310.
BRESLAV, I.S., A.G. Zhironkin, V.N. Salazkin and A.M. Shmeleva.
Mathematicheskii analiz reaktsii dykhatel'noi sistemy cheloveka na gipoksiyu i giperkapniyu. [Mathematical analysis of responses of the respiratory system in man to hypoxia and hypercapnia].
Fiziol. Zh. SSSR 58:1749-1755;Nov. 1972.
(Translation JPRS 58292)

The ventilatory responses of man to inhalation of hypoxic and hypercapnic gas mixtures studied in 300 experiments, were subjected to the mathematical processing by means of multiple correlation and regressive analysis. The equations were obtained characterizing quantitative relations between the minute respiratory volume and the parameters of the gas mixture in inner milieu and environment. The equations make it possible to estimate the relative importance of hypoxic and hypercapnic stimuli in regulation of breathing in man. (English summary)

311.
BREWER, R.D.
1000 foot unmanned certification dive in #5 Chamber Complex.
U.S. Navy Exp. Diving Unit, Rep. NEDU-19-72, 8p. Aug. 14, 1972.

An unmanned dive was made in #5 Chamber Complex at the Navy Experimental Diving Unit on 29 June 1972. The dive's purpose was to demonstrate the operation for the purpose of certification before commencing a manned deep dive program reaching depths of up to 1000 feet seawater. With the exception of the leaking exhaust fitting, and the hot water shower fitting, the complex met all performance requirements satisfactorily. Based on this test, the complex demonstrated that it is capable of supporting life at 1000 feet sea water after correcting the leaks. (Author's abstract)

312.
BREWER, R.D.
1000 foot unmanned certification dive in #6 Chamber Complex.
U.S. Navy Exp. Diving Unit, Rep. NEDU-21-72, 5p. Aug. 25, 1972.

An unmanned dive was made in #6 chamber complex at the Navy Experimental Diving Unit on 7 August 1972. The dive's purpose was to demonstrate the operation for the purpose of certification before commencing a manned deep dive program reaching depths of up to 1000 feet sea water. With the exception of the problem of foulage in the drain valves, and the two false alarms in the fire suppression system, the complex met all performance requirements satisfactorily. Based on this test, the complex demonstrated that it is capable of supporting life at 1000 feet sea water, after removal of foulage in the drain valves. (Author's abstract)

313.
BREWER, R.D.
Report on the 100' saturation dive series for complex system check and personnel training on #5 Chamber Complex.
U.S. Navy Exp. Diving Unit, Rep. NEDU-18-72, 8p. Aug. 10, 1972.

On 5, 9 and 13 June, a series of saturation dives were made to depths of 100 feet. Their purpose was for the training of personnel and equipment checkout prior to commencing a deep dive program reaching depths of up to 1000 feet. With the exception of the equipment not installed, and the refrigerator system, the complex and its associated equipment performed satisfactorily meeting design specifications. The experience gained through the training of the personnel involved was such that the deep dive program can commence according to schedule. (Author's abstract)

314.
BRIGGS, C. and A.R. Howard.
Compressibility data for helium, nitrogen, and helium-nitrogen mixtures at 0, 25, and 50C and at pressures to 1,000 atmospheres.
Washington, D.C., Bu. Mines, Rep. BuMines-R1-7639, 200 p. Sept. 1972.
(PB212,481)

A special-pressure Burnett-type compressibility apparatus was constructed and used to determine compressibility factors for pure helium, pure nitrogen, and nine helium-nitrogen mixtures containing 89.47, 79.04, 69.69, 60.09, 49.24, 41.02, 30.99, 20.53, and 10.67 mole percent helium. A total of 161 runs were made, consisting of 2,355 observed pressures. Data were obtained at 0, 25, and 50C and at pressures to 1,000 atmospheres. A power series in the reciprocal volume (commonly called a Leiden series) is used to represent the compressibility factors. Three parameters in the series are required to represent helium, five parameters for nitrogen, and from three to five parameters for the mixtures. Compressibility factors are believed to be accurate to better than 0.1 percent over the entire pressure, temperature, and composition range. (Authors) (GRA)

315.
BRIGHT, C.V.
Diving under polar ice.
In: The working diver, 1972. Symposium proceedings, February 1972, Columbus, Ohio, p. 145-157, Washington, D.C., Marine Technology Society, 1972.

For the first time, oceanographer/divers from the U.S. Naval Oceanographic Office have conducted a series of dives under the Arctic Ice Cover. This operation was to determine the feasibility of characterizing the underside of the sea ice canopy using scuba equipped divers. It was concluded after a series of 40 dives, ranging in duration from 27 to 115 min that divers can function efficiently and safely under polar ice, and perform tasks of considerable difficulty. It has been adequately demonstrated that it is practical and relatively easy for divers to measure underice features, take still and motion picture photography, and collect biological samples while using off-the-shelf equipment. In the interest of greater safety and efficiency of future ice diving operations, the following recommendations are listed below: (a) Always use a diver safety-line. (b) Always use the buddy system. (c) Always use dual breathing regulators and tanks (this should include a small pressure line between the tanks permitting both tanks to be used with either regulator). (d) Always use a two hose, two-stage regulator for the primary regulator. (e) Attempt to provide a warm dressing area near the diving site. (f) Provide protection for the air compressor in extreme temperatures. (g) Provide a means of heating divers' hands and feet. There is an urgent need for research and development in this area. (h) Use only experienced mature divers. Experience in night diving and cave diving would be desirable. (i) Use only experienced divers as tenders. (Author's abstract and recommendations)

316.
BRIGHT, C.V.
Diving in the Arctic.
Nav. Res. Rev. 25(8):1-11;Aug. 1972.

In November 1970, a group of oceanographer/divers from the Naval Oceanographic Office conducted an investigation on the feasibility of using SCUBA-equipped divers to characterize the bottom surface of the Arctic sea ice. In ten diving days four divers accumulated 39 hours and 2 minutes under the ice in 40 separate dives. The longest single dive was one hour and 55 minutes, and the shortest was 26 minutes. . . . The air temperature averaged 10°F for the three days at Point Barrow with an essentially constant water temperature of 28.9°F. Daylight conditions were minimal — approximately five hours of useful light per day. The presence of longshore current with a maximum velocity of approximately 1/4 knot did not cause any problems. Diver visibility in the water decreased from the first day to the third day; however, the loss of visibility did not affect the operation. The average ice thickness was 12 inches. . . . It is practical and relatively easy for divers to measure under-ice features, take both still and motion pictures, collect biological samples and perform numerous tasks of varying complexity. (Author)

317.
BRITO SUAREZ, M.
Artropatias barotraumaticas.
[Barotraumatic arthropathies].
Rev. Esp. Reum. 13:428-434;July 1970.

Joint lesions among subjects who worked under conditions of increased atmospheric pressure have been observed since 1888. Since the beginning of the century many authors have associated the accidents which they have observed in these workers with the action of a more or less rapid decompression. The conclusion has been drawn that the decompression accidents were due fundamentally to two mechanisms: (A) to the expansion of gases, and (B) to the formation of bubbles. In order to understand the formation of bubbles, as well as other factors which permit explanation of the symptomatology of these patients, it is necessary to study the fundamental laws of gases which explain a fundamental fact: the formation of bubbles. In the first place, thanks to Henry, we know that the concentration of molecules of a gas dissolved in a liquid is proportional to the pressure of the gas to which the liquid was exposed. The influence of temperature on the coefficient of solubility, the diffusion of a gas across a membrane, the rapid interchange of gases in pulmonary alveoli, the length of time during which a subject is exposed to elevated atmospheric pressure, are all discussed. Decompression sickness is a combination of clinical manifestations produced in an individual, upon passing from a high pressure to a lower pressure, that are due to the formation of bubbles and the expansion of the gases. This pressure lowering is able to produce digestive, cutaneous and nervous symptomatology, and so-called asphyxial syndrome, serosinusitis and aerotitis, and arthromyalgic discomfort that is the most frequent manifestation and which is of interest to us. The frequency of decompression accidents and therefore of barotraumatic arthropathies, appears to increase with the time one has remained in the hyperbaric environment, the depth attained, the rhythm of ascent, as well as age, obesity and exercise, which is a very important factor. In the frequency of presentation of the arthropathies, prominent roles are also played by endocrine factors, articular dysplasia, etc. Divers, aviators, and those who work or play under hyperbaric conditions may suffer decompression effects. The role of nitrogen in the formation of bubbles is discussed. Theories are discussed to explain the late-appearing clinical phenomena when there has been no acute decompression sickness. Involvement of the osseous epiphysis and the articular cartilage nourished by fine vascular ramifications, muscular atrophy, limitations of motion, radiologic appearance of the affected joints, and suggested treatment are all discussed briefly. (ART/BSCP)

318.
BROOKLER, K.H.
Otitic barotrauma.
Laryngoscope 83:966-968;June 1973.

Otitic barotrauma occurs upon descent in individuals with a nasopharyngitis, a large basopharyngeal lymphoid mass, and for no apparent reason. A Surface Active Membrane (SAM) was found lining the eustachian tube with surface tension lowering properties similar to pulmonary surfactant SAM. Eustachian SAM allows the lumenal surface of the tube to separate in response to the pull of the musculature. SAM is destroyed by proteolytic enzyme producing bacteria and pulmonary SAM is reduced in cigarette smokers. Reduced or absent eustachian SAM will not allow the lumenal surfaces to separate and pressure equalization to take place. Otitic barotrauma occurs when there is insufficient eustachian SAM resulting in an inability to allow transmission of air from the nasopharynx to the middle ear during descent. A lechithin aerosol used as an effective treatment of hyaline membrane diseases (absent SAM) of the newborn may treat or prevent otitic barotrauma. (Author's Abstract)

319.
BROUSSOLLE, B., E. Belnet-Bensimon, J. Chouteau, D. Bouteille and H. Burnet.
Respiratory gas exchange and partial alveolar pressures of CO_2 and O_2 during simulated divings in condition of saturation at 26 and 41 ATA with helium-oxygen.
In: Abstracts of the Twenty-fifth Congress of Physiological Sciences Satellite Symposium. Recent progress in fundamental physiology of diving, Marseille, France, July 1971 p.32-34. (Proceedings unpublished)

Abstract only. Two separate experiments were conducted. Helium-oxygen was the breathing mixture. In the first, two subjects were compressed to 26 ATA for 24 hr. then decompressed to 21, 16 and 11 ATA each for 24 hr. In the second, two subjects were compressed to 41 ATA followed by two 4-hr periods at 36 and 31 ATA. Parameters were measured at rest and at exercise at all depths. It was found that VO_2 did not increase with pressure, contrary to previous findings of Taunton et al and Salzano et al; findings tallied with those of Hamilton et al and of Schaefer et al. $PACO_2$ did not differ from those recorded at sea level, while these values had previously been found to increase with air breathing at 4 and 7 ATA. No respiratory limitation was found up to 41 ATA (1312.23 ft). (MFW/BSCP)

320.
BROUSSOLLE, B. and E. Belnet-Bensimon.
Etude de la ventilation pulmonaire en milieu hyperbare.
[Study of pulmonary ventilation in a hyperbaric environment].
Cent. Etud. Rech. Bio-Physiol. Appl. Mar., Final Rep. on period of Aug. 1967-Sept. 1971, 137p. 1971.

Ventilatory sensibility to carbon dioxide decreases in highly trained divers; this results in a ventilatory regulation different from that of non-divers in a hyperbaric environment. Mechanical limitation of ventilation brings on a retention of carbon dioxide at 7 ATA, or 70 meters, and muscular exertion of more than 110 volts, when breathing air. With a helium-oxygen mixture, measurements made at 41 ATA (400 meters) did not reveal this phenomenon; it is thus possible to remain and work at this depth. Density is lower than that of air at 7 ATA. It is believed that a helium-oxygen environment of more than 500 meters would present risks. (Authors' abstract translated by MFW/UMS)

321.
BROUSSOLLE, B., E. Bensimon, A. Michaud and C. Vegezzi.
Comparaison des reponses ventilatoires et des pressions partielles alveolaires de CO_2 de plongeurs sous-marins entraines et de temoins non plongeurs au cours de travail musculaire en atmosphere hyperbare.
[Comparison of ventilatory responses and alveolar partial pressure of CO_2 of trained divers and non-diver controls during muscular work in a hyperbaric atmosphere].
In: Fructus, X., ed. Third international conference on hyperbaric and underwater physiology, p. 80-87. Paris, Doin, 1972.

At 7 atm. abs. and a work load of 110 watts, trained divers demonstrated a significant CO_2 retention related to their adaptation to CO_2, while non-divers increased their ventilation and maintained normal CO_2 levels. It must be concluded, first, that when physiological studies are carried out during deep dives, the type of subject must be specified. The second conclusion concerns CO_2 retention. The harmful effects of CO_2 on mental function in diving, on the increased risk of decompression accidents, on potentiation of inert gas narcosis, and on oxygen intoxication. For muscular work during deep diving, subjects not susceptible to CO_2 retention must be chosen; they must also have high maximum ventilation. Under any circumstances, a work load of more than 150 watts at a depth equivalent to 7 atm. abs., should probably be avoided. (Authors' conclusion, translated by MFW/UMS)

322.
BROUSSOLLE, B., H. Burnet, R. Ricci, A. Baret, C. Boutier, S. Plouvier and R. Hyacinthe.
Effet de la toxicite de l'oxygene pur normobare sur le surfactant pulmonaire chez les rats.
[Effect of the toxicity of normobaric pure oxygen on the pulmonary surfactant of rats].
J. Physiol. (Paris)65(Suppl.3):365A; 1972.

[The experiment consisted of exposing a group of rats to 48 hours of pure oxygen followed by five hours of air, over periods of 5, 10, and 20 days]. Pure oxygen under these conditions, led to an augmentation of the pulmonary surfactant accompanied by a decrease in its quality. The degradation is not explained by a difference of chemical composition, but would be related to a modification of the combination of various molecules. Starting with the twentieth day a tendency of the surfactant to return to normal was noted, but anatomo-pathological lesions approaching fibrous alveolitis with angiocapillaritis continued to develop. (Authors' conclusions translated by MFW/SCD)

323.
BROUSSOLLE, B., R. Hyacinthe, H. Burnet, A. Battesti and D. Gresson.
Echanges gazeux respiratoires et mecanique ventilatoire au cours d'une plongee fictive a 51 ATA (500 metres) en melange helium-oxygene).
[Respiratory gas exchange and mechanics of ventilation during the course of a simulated dive at 51 ATA (500 meters) in a mixture of helium and oxygen].
Cent. Etud. Rech. Bio-physiol. Appl. Mar., Rep. 72-1, 44p. 1972.

The chief purpose of this experiment was to observe modifications of gas exchange and problems of alveolar-capillary diffusion during exercise at high pressure, and to investigate mechanical limitations of breathing gas at high density. To determine alveolar-capillary diffusion, divers attempted to measure the alveolar-arterial difference for oxygen and carbon dioxide, but results were not satisfactory due to their inexperience in taking and analyzing blood samples. As to the production of carbon dioxide and the consumption of oxygen, these increased with exercise, owing to increased density. The $PACO_2$ of one subject rose during exercise, while that of the other fell. It never surpassed normal values and there was no carbon dioxide retention at 51 ATA. Heart rate increase at rest was clearly apparent between 3.5 and 51 ATA. During exercise, there was a decrease at 41 ATA. Results of the measurement of ventilatory mechanics indicated that dynamic compliance and vital capacity did not vary significantly while dynamic expiratory resistance rose steadily. The maximum ventilation per minute was greatly lessened at 51 ATA (58% and 54% for the two subjects) due to increased resistance and expiratory flow. The authors discuss their findings, comparing them with those of previous investigators. In this experiment, gas exchange was not affected and there was no mechanical limitation of ventilation. There was a great difference in the work capability of the two divers at high pressure, and the importance of selecting subjects with a low ratio of expiratory flow to maximal ventilation is emphasized. Although further experiments at this depth are necessary it is concluded tentatively that moderate work can be performed at 500 meters by experienced subjects. This is probably the limit of safe depth. (MFW/SCD)

324.
BROUSSOLLE, B. and R. Hyacinthe.
Affinite de l'hemoglobine pour l'oxygene chez l'homme, au cours d'une plongee fictive a 31 ata avec melange helium-oxygene.
[Affinity of hemoglobin for oxygen in human beings during a simulated dive to 31 Ata with a helium-oxygen mixture].
Cent. Etud. Rech. Biophysiol. Appl. Mar., Rep. 73-21, 28p. 1973.

The effect of long-term relative hyperoxia on the affinity of hemoglobin for oxygen was studied during the experiment Sagittaire III, a 29-day simulated dive to 31 Ata. The parameters measured were: erythrocyte 2,3 di-phosphoglycerate, erythrocyte ATP, lactic acid, and P_{50}, the oxygen pressure in mmHg which corresponds to 50% saturation of hemoglobin. The experiment demonstrated an increased affinity of hemoglobin for oxygen. This increase appeared slowly, maximum depth, but was unrelated to PIO_2, which remained constant. During decompression, the affinity slowly returned to normal values, in spite of increased oxygen partial pressure. It is known that hyperoxia alone increases affinity, so total pressure is shown to be a more important factor than hyperoxia in the variation of hemoglobin affinity for oxygen. (MEMH/UMS)

325.
BROUSSOLLE, B., J.F. Stoltz, G. Mainart, R. Hyacinthe and F. Brue.
Plaquettes sanguines et accidents de decompression: comptage et mesure de la pression de filtration du plasma riche en plaquettes (PRP) chez le rat.
[Blood platelets in decompression accidents: count and measurement of filtration pressure of platelet rich plasma (PRP) in the rat].
J. Physiol. 67(Suppl. 1):181A; 1973.

Abstract only. The experiment was made on a rat rapidly decompressed after a sojourn of one hour at 8 atm abs (60% suffered accidents). The filtration pressure was measured (using the method of Swank) and a count was made of the number of platelets in platelet rich plasma obtained from blood taken at the moment of the accident or 30 minutes after decompression (for the rats without accidents). The values were compared with those of the control rats. The filtration pressure did not vary between controls and rats without accidents, but was increased 32% at the moment of the accident. The platelet count was 28% lower in rats without accidents and 51% lower at the moment of the accident. Thus, even without accident, there exists after decompression a fall in platelet count due to the existance of noncirculating microthrombi; this fall is more important at the moment of an accident, with microthrombi present in the circulation. (MFW/SCD)

326.
BROUSSOLLE, B., J.F. Stoltz, G. Mainart, R. Hyacinthe and R. Pietrini.
Modifications des plaquettes sanguines au cours des accidents de decompression chez le rat. II. Mesure de l'agregabilite plaquettaire.
[Changes in blood platelets during decompression accidents in rats. II. Measurement of platelet aggregation].
Cent. Etud. Rech. Bio-physiol. Appl. Mar., Rep. 73-04; 12p. 1973.

This experiment, carried out on 29 male rats, was intended to demonstrate an increase in platelet sensitivity to adenosine diphosphate (ADP) in animals presenting decompression lesions. It was found that after rapid decompression a concentration of 2.4×10^{-6}M of ADP resulted in hypoaggregability of circulating blood platelets. Earlier studies had demonstrated hyperaggregability. The authors explain the apparent inconsistency by suggesting that hyperaggregability of young, reactive platelets in peripheral areas could occur simultaneously with hypoaggregability of older platelets. This poses a problem for the study of platelet aggregability, since a sample of platelet rich plasma taken after a decompression accident would demonstrate a different distribution of platelet populations from one taken from a control. The authors plan to attempt to determine whether platelet distribution changes before and after decompression, using a technique of ultracentrifugation on discontinuous saccharose gradients. (MFW/SCD)

327.
BROUSSOLLE, B., F. Brue, A. Chaumont, R. Hyacinthe, D. Monget and B. Pineau.
Affinite de l'hemoglobine pour l'oxygene chez le rat expose a l'oxygene pur normobare.
[Affinity of hemoglobin for oxygen in rats exposed to pure oxygen at atmospheric pressure].
In: Hesser, C.M. and D. Linnarsson eds. Proceedings of the first annual scientific meeting of the European Undersea Biomedical Society, Stockholm, 13-15 June 1973. Forsvarsmedicin 9:287-292;July 1973.

The rats manifested a significant metabolic disorder, which was indicated by an increase in their lactacidemia explicable perhaps by tissue hypoxia or perhaps by tissue hyperoxic intoxication. There exists an augmentation of the affinity of hemoglobin for oxygen which appeared to be related to the diminution of the erythrocyte concentration. It is possible that the diminution of the concentration in the hemoglobin in rats which had undergone a long exposure in pure oxygen is a reaction of adaptation following a significant diminution of their oxygen consumption. (Author, translated by MFW/UMS)

328.
BROUSSOLLE, B., J.F. Stoltz, G. Mainart, R. Hyacinthe and R. Pietrini.
Etude des modifications des plaquettes sanguines au cours des accidents de decompression chez le rat. III. Essais d'antiagregants plaquettaires, a titre preventif.
[Blood platelet changes in decompression accidents in rats. III. Trials of platelet antiaggregants used preventively].
Cent. Etud. Rech. Biophysiol. Appl. Mar., Rep. 73-14, 15p. July 1973.

Rats were pressurized in a caisson to depths between 3 and 70 metres, and received injections of one of three antiaggregants 20 minutes before staged or rapid decompression. The drugs tested were ASPEGIC, diamicron, and 2574SE. ASPEGIC had a minimal effect on the incidence of decompression accidents and on blood platelet levels. With diamicron, a significant decrease in the number of decompression accidents was noted. Although blood platelet levels fell immediately after decompression, they returned to normal much more quickly than in control rats. 2574SE at the dosage of 100mg/kg completely blocks the post-decompression decrease in blood platelets and significantly reduced the incidence of decompression accidents. Since it does not cause hypoglycemia, it can be administered in large doses. (MEMH/UMS)

329.
BROUSSOLLE, B., R. Hyancinthe, G. Mainart, J.F. Stoltz and F. Streiff.
Plaquettes sanguines et accidents de decompression chez le rat.
[Blood platelets and decompression accidents in the rat].
In: Hesser, C.M. and D. Linnarsson eds. Proceedings of the first annual scientific meeting of the European Undersea Biomedical Society, Stockholm, 13-15 June 1973. Forsvarsmedicin 9:514-519;July 1973.

After rapid decompression a 51% reduction in the platelet count in rats experiencing decompression accidents proves the existence of disseminated platelet aggregates of which only a small number are circulating. After decompressing in accordance with the tables, it was also noted that there was a moderate fall (15%) of platelets; the count did not return to normal until the third day after decompression. To prevent platelet aggregation, the following drugs were injected: aspirin (20 mg/kg), and two non-commercial drugs — 1702 SE (20 and 50 mg/kg) and 2574 SE (50 and 100 mg/kg), before and after decompression and for three days thereafter. The best results were with 100 mg/kg SE, which prevented even the initial platelet fall. At equal doses, 1702 SE was more effective than 2574 SE, but it had an undesirable hypoglycemic effect. If injection was made before rapid decompression, mortality was reduced. These findings confirm the importance of platelets in decompression sickness. The therapeutic experiments project the possibility of the use of these products on humans. (MFW/UMS)

330.
BROUSSOLLE, B., R. Hyacinthe, G. Mainart and J.L. Stoltz.
Utilisation d'antiagregants plaquettaires dans la therapeutique des accidents de decompression chez le rat.
[Utilization of platelet antiaggregants in the treatment of decompression sickness in the rat].
Bull. Medsubhyp 10:40-43;Dec. 1973.

A previous study had shown evidence of disseminated platelet aggregants during induced decompression accidents in rats (Broussolle, Rep. CERB 73-04). It existed even in decompressed rats, which were symptomless as indicated by a fall in the free platelets rates, which did not disappear until the third day. Different antiaggregants were used as preventives to avoid this platelet fall. Aspirin did not give significant results, but an experimental drug, the 2475 SE, completely inhibited the platelet fall. The authors also observed the protective effect against accidents induced by rapid decompression. The number of accidents is not modified but the gravity is. The "serious" symptoms decreased from 76% for controls to 47% in rats protected by the 2574 SE. This interesting antiaggregant has to be assayed as curative first on animals then on human pathology. (English abstract)

331.
BROWDER, L.P.
Experimental system for deep-ocean electroacoustic immittance measurements.
U.S. Nav. Res. Lab., NRL Mem. Rep. 2247, 12p. May 18, 1971.

An experimental, remote-controlled, immittance-measuring bridge with telemetry equipment was used during sea trials to obtain electrical impedance and admittance measurements on electroacoustic transducers at depth in the ocean. This report describes the electronic instrumentation used and the results obtained from measurements on six transducers. Recommendations are made for improving and modifying the system. This is an interim report on the problem. (Author's abstract)

332.
BROWN, O.R.
Correlations between sensitivities to radiation and to hyperoxia in microorganisms.
Radiat. Res. 50:309-318; 1972.

The bactericidal and bacteriostatic effects of hyperoxia from 1 to 15 atm and from 1 to 4 atm, respectively were measured for Escherichia coli strains E-26, B, B/r, and B_{s-1}. Percentage survival was minimal for all strains in oxygen (O_2) at 4.2 atm (E-26, 51%; B, 1.5%; B/r, 60%; and B_{s-1}, 0.25%). O_2 at 1-2 atm produced little killing and O_2 at 6 atm or greater was less bactericidal than was 3-5 atm. Strain B/r survived better in all hyperoxic environments than did strain B or B_{s-1}. Survival of E-26 and Micrococcus radiodurans at 4.2 atm O_2 was similar to B/r. When B_{s-1} was exposed to O_2 at 4.2 atm without organic nutrients, 66% survived. During the first hour of exposure, the growth rate of straing B/r was inhibited 13.2% per atm O_2 with an extrapolated intercept of 100% survival at 0.6 atm; growth inhibition of B_{s-1} was 12.2% per atm with an intercept of 1.2 atm. We concluded that: (1) strains B and B_{s-1}, which are radiation sensitive, were also more sensitive to the bactericidal effect of hyperoxia than was strain B/r, which is radiation resistant; however, strain B/r was not more resistant to O_2 than strain E-26 which has no unusual radiation resistance; (2) growth and synthesis potential in hyperoxia were required for the bactericidal effect. (Author's abstract)

333.
BROWN, O.R.
Mechanisms of oxygen toxicity at the cellular level.
Columbia, Mo., Univ. Mo., Space Sci. Res. Cent., Rep. on Contract N00014-67-A-0287-0002, 36p. Jan. 1972.
(AD 742,443)

Over the preceding year, progress has been achieved in several related lines of research which contribute to the contract objective of delineating basic, cellular mechanisms of oxygen toxicity. Each of the following areas has been previously identified with proposals and reports and progress in each area will be reviewed separately. The areas are: (A) Techniques of measuring the toxicity of gaseous environments for cells, (B) Quantification of the oxygen sensitivities of species and strains, (C) oxygen sensitivity of fatty acid synthetase and its components, and the effects of hyperoxia on (D) pyridine nucleotide coenzymes, (E) oxidative phosphorylation, (F) cellular permeability, (G) respiration, and (H) cellular sulfhydryl. (Author) (GRA)

334.
BROWN, O.R. and D. Peterson.
Sensitivity to oxygen at high pressure of radioresistant and radiosensitive strains of bacteria.
Aerosp. Med. 44:71-73;Jan. 1973.

Radiation strains of bacteria were tested for sensitivity to hyperoxia. Escherichia coli B_{s-1} γ R (resistant to γ-ray, sensitive to UV) had an oxygen sensitivity pattern similar to that previously reported for its parent, B_{s-1} (sensitive to UV and γ-ray). Hence, develoment of selective resistance to γ-rays did not produce resistance to hyperoxia. E. coli K-12 polymerase+(resistant to X-ray) and polymerase-(sensitive to X-ray) strains were both relatively resistant to hyperpoxia but on the average, the strain lacking polymerase was approximately 1.4 times as sensitive to hyperoxia. This suggests that single-stranded breaks in DNA (repairable by polymerase) may have some role in oxygen toxicity. Salmonella typhimurium KSU strains 3845 and 2480 (sensitive to UV and X-rays) showed statistically significant killing at 4.2 atm of oxygen while 3598 and 2484 (sensitive to UV, resistant to X-ray) did not. No strains, whether resistant or sensitive to X-, γ - or UV radiation, approached the sensitivity of B_{s-1} γ R which was at least 100 times as sensitive at 4.2 atm of oxygen. The correlation between sensitivity to radiation and to hyperoxia previously found for B strains of E. coli, does not appear to be a universal property of radiation-sensitive bacteria. (Authors' abstract)

335.
BRUE, F., J.L. Morcelet, P. Revelat and P. Burtin.
Modifications precoces du mode d'oxydation du glucose par l'hyperoxie.
[Early modifications of oxidative pathways of glucose metabolism by hyperoxia].
In: Fructus, X., Ed. Third international conference on hyperbaric and underwater physiology, p.145-153. Paris, Doin, 1972.

Mice were given D-Glucose-1-^{14}C or D-Glucose-6-^{14}C by intraperitoneal injection, and immediately exposed to various oxygen pressures. In air, the more rapid elimination of $^{14}CO_2$ from GLucose-1-^{14}C than from Glucose-6-^{14}C is explained by the tissue pentose-phosphate pathway activity. The maximum of the $^{14}CO_2$ production from Glucose-1-^{14}C is significantly delayed by O_2 - 1 ata, and apparently by O_2 - 3 ata. (English abstract)

336.
BRUE, F., P. Joanny, G. Bertharion, J.L. Morcellet and J. Corriol.
Metabolisme du glucose dans des tissues nerveus isoles sous oxygen hyperbare: stimulation du cycle des pentoses phosphates et de la glycolyse.
[Glucose metabolism in nerve tissues isolated under hyperbaric oxygen: stimulation of the phosphate pentose cycle and of glycolysis].
J. Physiol. (Paris) 65 (Suppl. 3) 366A; 1972.

Glucose metaboism in rat and guinea pig brain and heart sections, and in bovine retinas, was studied under 1, 3, 6, and 10 ata of oxygen using U-^{14}C glucose. Hyperbaric oxygen led to a marked general decrease in the liberation of $^{14}CO_2$, confirming the classical inhibition of glucose oxidation. The inhibition of the Krebs cycle noted in this experimentation confirms the results of earlier work. An increase in phosphate pentose cycle activity was also noted. Glucose consumption increased in retinal tissue, but not in heart tissue, while lactate production increased significantly in all tissues studied. This stimulation of glycolysis and of the phosphate pentose cycle suggests that neither of these can be considered the mechanism of the cellular toxicity of hyperbaric oxygen. (MEMH/UMS)

337.
BRUE, F., R. Guillemenot, D. Berl and B. Broussolle.
Mise en evidence d'un syndrome nerveux de l'intoxication hyperoxique chronique chez la souris soumise a des expositions intermittentes a l'oxygene pur 1 ATA.
[Demonstration of a nervous syndrome of chronic hyperoxic intoxication in the mouse submitted to intermittent exposures of pure oxygen at 1 ATA].
Bull. Medsuphyp 8:709;Nov. 1972.

The purpose of this experiment was to study adaptation to pure oxygen at atmospheric pressure. Thirty mice were exposed to pure oxygen for 58, 86, 117, 120, and 158 hours, with intermittent returns to air of 120 hours. They were returned to air each time when respiratory difficulties became serious. Of the mice who were submitted to a further oxygen exposure, all died within 12-14 days. Some died of respiratory failure, others following paraplegia of the inferior members. In the latter cases, respiratory distress apparently did not occur, and the mice continued to eat until they could no longer move sufficiently to do so. Possible physiopathological mechanisms are suggested. Hypoxia of the nervous cells due to respiratory insufficiency is a possible cause. Also, slowly developing vascular lesions (hypertrophy of the vascular wall, formation of masses of erythrocytes and platelets) might alter the vascular endothelium so as to cause edematous lesions in numerous organs. Heavily vascularized tissues such as the bone marrow at the last dorsal vertebrae would be the first to suffer from progressive vascular obliteration, thus bringing on the type of paraplegia that was observed in this experiment. (MFW/BSCP)

338.
BRUE, F., P. Joanny, J.L. Morcellet, J. Villeville and J. Neveux.
Les voies du metabolisme du glucose dans la retine sous oxygene hyperbare.
[Glucose metabolism pathways in the retina under hyperbaric oxygen].
Bull. Medsubhyp 9:1;Mar. 1973.

$^{14}CO_2$ evolved from (1-^{14}C) or 6-^{14}C glucose in ox retina incubated under various oxygen pressures (0.2, 1.5, and 10 ata) were continuously recorded. At 5 and 10 ata, decreased C_6 evolution and increased (C_1 - C_6) difference showed the inhibition of the KREBS-cycle and the stimulation of the pentose-phosphate pathway. Glycolysis was enhanced as indicated by increased glucose uptake and lactate release. (English abstract)

339.
BUCK, B.M. and A.W. Magnuson.
Measurements of underwater explosive source levels for yields of 0.0012 to 126 pounds.
Santa Barbara, Cal., General Motors Corp., Delco Electronics Div., Rep. TR-73-02, 28p. Apr. 1971.
(AD 756 246)

The equivalence of using energy measurements for explosives and intensity for CW sources in the determination of underwater acoustic transmission loss has been previously investigated by Hasse and Stockhausen for one-pound TNT charges. It was concluded that use of Weston's theoretically derived energy source levels was satisfactory for this size charge. The objective of the present experiment was to investigate the applicability of Weston's predictions of energy source level for a broader range of charge yields in view of estimates by Arons and others that the range at which an explosive signal propagates as an acoustic wave is critically dependent on charge yield. Shot energy source levels were determined by measuring received signal energy and then adding transmission loss values for paths which were using a constant wave projector. It was found that, within the accuracy limits of the experiment, Weston's 'sum' formula is a close representation of the true energy source level of explosives in the yield range of 0.0012 to 126 pounds TNT above frequency equal to about the first bubble pulse frequency and is therefore usable for transmission loss determinations. (Author) (GRA)

340.
BUCKLES, R.G. and E. Hardenbergh.
Hamster mortality from rapid decompression.
In: Wada, J. and I. Takashi, eds. Proceedings of the fourth international congress of hyperbaric medicine, Sapporo, Japan, Sept. 1969, p.109-115. Baltimore, Williams and Wilkins, 1970.

The authors attempt to define the etiology of decompression sickness in hamsters subjected to rapid decompression. It is explained as follows: First bubbles form because of supersaturated tissues; second, the bubbles may then pass through the right heart and lungs to the arterial system; third, if the bubble masses are large, they displace blood in the heart and lung vessels, causing cardiac and respiratory failure. Because in the hamster the disease cannot be identified until it has reached its final fatal stage, this is not considered a suitable experimental animal for the study of decompression sickness in man. (MFW/BSCP)

341.
BUHLMANN, A.A., W.H. Ziegler and J. Muller.
Catecholamine excretion and plasma corticosteriods during deep diving breathing oxygen-helium mixtures.
In: Fructus, X., Ed. Third international conference on hyperbaric and underwater physiology, p.69-73. Paris, Doin, 1972.

Plasma corticosteroids have been estimated in 8 subjects performing a dive at 11 ATA breathing oxy-helium. Catecholamine excretion has been measured in 4 subjects performing a dive at 11 ATA and in 6 subjects performing dives at 31 ATA breathing oxy-helium. Plasma corticosteroids are moderately elevated immediately before compression in 3 out of 8 divers. This parameter decreases in 6 out of 8 divers during isopression. Noradrenalin- and adrenalin excretion is often elevated before compression and during compression and the first hours of isopression. Sometimes the adrenalin excretion increases during the compression. Urinary catecholamines are normal during decompression. All 24 hours values of catecholamine excretion determined during a saturation dive at 31 ATA with excursions to 36 ATA are within normal limits. (Authors' Summary)

342.
BUHLMANN, A.A., R. Schibli and H. Gehring.
Experimentelle Untersuchungen uber die Dekompression nach Tauchgangen in Bergseen bei vermindertem Luftdruck.
[Experimental studies on decompression following diving in mountain lakes at reduced air pressure].
Schweiz. Med. Wochenschr. 103:378-383;Mar. 10, 1973.

Fifty subjects underwent 106 exposures of 17-120 min in a dry pressure chamber at a pressure of 4.2-5.2 ATA. They performed physical work on a bicycle ergometer followed by decompression at a pressure of 0.7 ATA corresponding to an altitude of 3000 meters. 35 of the 106 simulated dives were performed as repeated dives at an interval of 40-45 min and a pressure of 0.7 ATA. In a second series 108 real dives, including 44 repeated, were performed in a lake at 1250 meters altitude without decompression symptoms. Decompression was calculated in the usual laboratory manner, having regard to diminished surface pressure without alteration to the N_2 halflife spectrum of 5-640 min or the oversaturation factors. These experiments without decompression symptoms offer the basis for decompression tables for different altitudes including rules for repeated dives. (English summary)

344.
BUHLMANN, A.A.
Ethical considerations in hyperbaric research. — Situation in Switzerland.
In: Hesser, C.M. and D. Linnarsson, eds. Proceedings of the first annual scientific meeting of the European Undersea Biomedical Society, Stockholm, 13-15 June 1973. Forsvarsmedicin 9:367-368;July 1973.

The author describes three categories of risk in hyperbaric research: (A) Exposures involving entirely new and untested conditions, in which the investigator should act on his own subject. (B) Experiments involving higher than routine risks, in which volunteers selected and trained for experimental work should be used. (C) Trials involving only normal risk, which can be made with untrained volunteers or professional divers. The authors discuss in some detail the requirements governing experiments in category B, among which are the following: The experiment must be supervised by a scientifically qualified medical doctor. Subjects must be real volunteers, informed of the risks and intelligent enough to understand them. Possibility of permanent damage must be very remote. Earlier experimentation must be studied in the evaluation of tests. Only tests which absolutely require human subjects should be performed. Results must be published. Treatment facilities and qualified personnel must be immediately available. Insurance protection must be high. Experiments should be checked by a disinterested group. (MFW/UMS)

345.
BUKHALOVSKIY, I.N. and A.I. Ivanov.
[Effect of increased physical loads on the electrical activity of the heart of a submariner at sea].
Voennomed. Zh. (4):70-71;Apr. 1973.

In order to determine the [effects] of exercises with sports equipment on the body of submarine personnel, special examinations were conducted on a group of ten men who regularly exercised with an expander or average-weight dumbbells before a voyage and continued to exercise while at sea at a slightly reduced rate (20%). The shipboard space limitations were recreated in the microclimate of the building where the tests took place. Before the test and 3 min after completion ECGs were taken using both standard leads, amplified from the extremities, and from six chest leads. . . . The results of these investigations show that after moderate physical exercise, the hearts of those in the group retained excellent functional ability. The results demonstrate the measured physical exercise during a voyage is extremely important in keeping the submariners fit. Exercises should be conducted with strict accounting for the individual physical training of the personnel and the special features of the particular voyage. Such measures should always be under the control of a doctor. (S&T Alert)

346.
BUNT, J.S.
New lab beneath the Bahamian Sea.
Sea Frontiers, 17(3):171-174; 1971.

The author made use of Perry Foundation's Hydro Lab to carry out a study of marine plant life. Hydro Lab is a compact underwater habitat and laboratory. The design incorporates an untended life support buoy at the surface, diver-controlled decompression within the habitat, and dry transfer of personnel to and from the surface. The decompression was supervised by Dr. J.B. MacInnis. This method is most satisfactory in that it eliminates the necessity for long hours spent in the confinements of surface decompression chambers. (MFW/BSCP)

347.
BURCH, G.E. and T.D. Giles.
A digital rheoplethysmographic study of the vasomotor response to "simulated diving" in man.
Cardiology 55:257-271; 1970.

The digital rheoplethysmogram was recorded from ten normal subjects during the act of "simulated diving", i.e. submersion of the face in a pan full of water. Digital vascular responses to various maneuvers and stimuli associated with simulated diving were also studied. In general, digital vasoconstriction was seen after most maneuvers and stimuli associated with the diving phenomenon (other than placing the face in water itself.) The response of the pulse rate was variable, although a decrease was usually seen as much during 'simulated diving' without water in the pan as with water. Decreasing the temperature of the water exaggerated the responses to most stimuli. Digital vasoconstriction was produced by audio stimulation (bell) and deep inspiration, whereas a variable effect on pulse rate was produced. The role of psychic factors and 'orienting reflexes' in the production of the cardiovascular response to diving are discussed. It is concluded that respiratory, thermal and psychic factors all play a role in the physiologic response to 'simulated diving' and that wetness is only a contributing factor. (Authors' abstract)

348.
BURGESS, D.W. and A.N. Dossett.
Oxygen changes in the brain during narcotic air dives.
In: Hesser, C.M. and D. Linnarsson eds. Proceedings of the first annual scientific meeting of the European Undersea Biomedical Society, Stockholm, 13-15 June 1973. Forsvarsmedicin 9:297-300;July 1973.

Rats were implanted with two gold polargraphic electrodes under sodium pentobarbital anaesthetic, care being taken to ensure that two probes were in equal regions of the controlateral hemispheres. One week was then allowed for the animal to recover from surgery. After recovery the rats were connected to a feedback polargraphic recorder and the brain oxygen level monitored. Feedback was used in the polargraphic recorder to minimise the effect of brain potentials changing the reference level and producing a false oxygen reading. The rats were then placed in a small pressure chamber and dived to greater than 100 metres on air, recordings being made on a FM tape recorder of all oxygen changes. On completion of the dive these records were analysed and the changes in brain oxygen at the various depths noted. Previous work (Burgess and Bean, 1970) had shown that the brain oxygen was constant under various levels of perfused oxygen. However, in the records of diving animals it was observed that the oxygen control broke down when the animals became narcotic showing that the effect of narcotic agents is very similar to that of an anaesthetic. (Authors' abstract)

349.
BURKE, R. and J.H. Stuart.
Atmospheric contaminant sensor. Book 3 of 3 addendum.
Pomona, Cal., Perkin-elmer Corp., Aerosp. Div., NASA-CR-128604, 45p. Sept. 1972.
(N73-11395)

The modification of the atmospheric contaminant sensor (ACS) to produce a carbon dioxide measuring capability is discussed. The modified instrument is described and the instructions for its operation and maintenance are included. Schematic diagrams and circuit drawings are included to clarify the text. (Authors) (STAR)

350.
BURNETT, J.W. and R. Goldner.
Partial purification of sea nettle (Chrysaora quinquecirrha) nematocyst toxin.
Annapolis, Md., Md. Fish Wildlife Admin., Rep. NOAA-72091920, 5p.
(COM 72 11234)
(Also published in Proc. Soc. Exp. Biol. Med. 133(3):978-981;Mar. 1970)

Soluble toxin was released from fresh Chrysaora quinquecirrha (sea nettle) nematocysts by gentle grinding or sonic treatment in distilled water. The lethal activity was not decreased by three cycles of freezing and thawing nor by lyophilization. Organic solvents such as acetone, ether, alcohol, and dimethylsilfoxide inactivated the toxin. Passage of the toxin through Sephadex gel results in partial purification and separation of the lethal activity into at least two fractions which are presumably proteinaceous. (Authors) (GRA)

351.
BURNETT, J.W. and R. Goldner.
Some immunological aspects of sea nettle toxins.
Annapolis, Md., Md. Fish Wildlife Admin., Rep. NOAA-72091979, 9p. Dec. 29, 1970.
(COM 72 11188)
(Also published in Toxican 9:271-277; 1971)

Chrysaora venom was antigenic to rabbits with complement fixing antibodies and protective factors against the lethal, hemolytic and dermonecrotic factors being formed. The thermal stabilities of the lethal, hemolytic and dermonecrotic factors of nettle venom were different, suggesting that an identical particle did not produce these three actions. Complement fixing antibodies were demonstrated in guinea pigs repeatedly stung by nettle medusae. The appearance of a cutaneous eruption after contact with nettle tentacles could not be blocked by intradermal injection of hyperimmune sera, however actively immunized animals did not develop an eruption after stinging. (Authors) (GRA)

352.
BURNETT, J.W., W.M. Gould and H. Rubinstein.
Further studies on the purification and physiological actions of sea nettle toxin.
Annapolis, Md., Md. Fish Wildlife Admin., Rep. NOAA-7209181, 5p. July 1, 1971.
(COM-72-11361)
(Also published in Proc. Soc. Exp. Biol. Med. 138:759-762;Dec. 1971).

Isoelectric focusing was applied to separate and define the active components of the toxin of the sea nettle, Chrysaora quinquecirrha. (GRA)

353.
BURNS, J.D.
Concentration-dependent attenuation of hyperbaric oxygen toxicity.
Aerosp. Med. 43:989-992; Sept. 1972.

Ninety male albino mice were exposed to 4, 6, or 8 atm O_2 partial pressure in 100, 50, or 25% dilutions. Tolerance was measured in terms of convulsions and death latencies. Results indicated (a) both convulsion latency and death latency tended to increase with decreases in oxygen concentration, (b) the degree of change in tolerance as a function of concentration was greater for the low partial prssures, and (c) convulsion and death latencies showed significant correlation only at the 4 atm partial pressure condition. The results further indicate a distinct decrease in susceptibility to toxic O_2 effects with increases in absolute pressure at fixed PO_2. (Author's abstract)

354.
BURROWS, D.W. and J.F. Hadwin.
A scanned laser and tracking system for sea floor profiling and precision survey.
In: Ocean 73. 1973 IEEE international conference on engineering in the ocean environment, p.39-43. IEEE publication 73 CHO 774-O OCC.

A feasibility study for a scanned laser to generate a contour map of the sea floor has been completed. Analysis and experimental test results indicate improved horizontal resolution compared to side scan sonar for ranges to approximately 90 meters in clear water ($\alpha \leq .05m^{-1}$) and vertical accuracy to 0.75%. The configuration studied performs best in a side-to-side scan below the vehicle and, therefore, can "fill the gap" for side scan sonar. The Scanned Laser and Tracking System, SLATS, employs a blue-green laser which scans mechanically in a lateral direction about the nadir. Reflected light from the sea floor is sensed by an integrating image tube which is located a fixed distance from the laser. This receiver registers the location of the laser as the beam sweeps the scene, with range to the sea floor determined by triangulation. Lateral scan of the laser provides one dimension of a raster while forward motion produces the second. (Authors' abstract)

355.
BURROWS, M.L. and C.W. Niessen.
ELF communication design.
Lexington, Mass., Mass. Inst. Technol., Lincoln Lab., Rep. MS-3394-ESD-TR-72-220, 16p. Sept. 13, 1972.
(AD 752, 956)

Radio waves of frequency below about 1 kHz propagate around the earth-ionosphere cavity with very little attenuation. These waves also can propagate useful distances down into the ocean. They are attractive therefore, for providing long-range communication to submarines from a single site. By considering the various components of the communication channel in turn, the paper develops the design principles for such a system. (Authors) (GRA)

356.
BURSAUX, E., A. Freminet and C.F. Poyart.
The Bohr effect, the Donnan equilibrium and the estimation of P_{50} in human whole blood.
Bull. Physio-pathol. Resp. 8(4):755-768; 1972.

Much interest has been recently devoted to the measurement of the O_2 Hb affinity in whole blood, estimated by the P_{50} (Hb half saturation O_2 pressure) usually calculated at a plasma pH (pHe) of 7.40. These calculations use a Bohr factor Δ log P_{50}/Δ pHe (Be) -0.48 to compensate for any deviation of pHe from 7.40. In many circumstances P_{50} would be meaningful if expressed at a normal intracellular pH (pHi), 7.20. As the pH difference across the red cell membrane is not constant (Donnan effect), it was of interest to determine the intracellular Bohr factor (Bi): Δ log P_{50}/Δ pHi. According to the Donnan equilibrium the extracellular Bohr factor should be lower than the intracellular Bohr factor as Be = Bi. Δ pHi/ Δ pHe. These 2 factors were measured in fresh human whole blood at constant PCO_2 and 2,3-diphosphoglycerate concentration. The values observed were: Be = -0.392 $\pm$ 0.016 and Bi = 0.546 $\pm$ 0.051. The ratio of Be/Bi is similar to the slope of the regression line of pHi on pHe. These results indicate the inadequacy of using the same Bohr factor for both intra and extracellular compartments. Because of the variations of the Bohr factor, depending upon the origin of the pH disturbance, a single Bohr factor should not be used in all circumstances. (© BA)

357.
BURT, J.F., Jr. and A.J. Dietrich.
Oxygen monitor and control system.
In: Ocean 73. 1973 IEEE international conference on engineering in the ocean environment, p.305-308. IEEE publication 73-CHO-7740-OCC.

Until recently, the limiting parameter in the design of hyperbaric life support systems has been the method of oxygen partial pressure control. This paper describes in detail a control system incorporating a new oxygen sensor especially designed for prolonged exposure to high pressures followed by rapid decompression. The electronics control system incorporates triple redundant oxygen level measurement, output limiting, and system disabling in the event of malfunction. In addition, a sampled data control system for such as a closed cycle diver rebreather, is discussed. (Authors' abstract)

358.
BURTON, R.
Cold-water survival.
Sea Frontiers 19:240-249;July-August 1973.

The author is concerned mainly with shipwreck survival, but there are observations on heat loss in water that apply to any underwater activity. The physiology of heat loss in water is discussed, with emphasis on the importance of protective clothing. It is stated that in dangerously cold water, "the average man should not exercise, otherwise increased blood flow and conductance will lead to greater heat loss." After-drop, which has caused many deaths, is probably due to the return of limb blood to the core following recirculation. Attempts should be made to re-warm the core without stimulating peripheral circulation; the best method is immersion of the trunk in a hot bath. One possible fatal danger of cold water swimming is ventricular fibrillation. (MFW/SCD)

359.
BUSBY, R.F.
Diver, submersible or instrument package?
Underwater J. 4:115-123;June 1972.

The author lists the advantages and disadvantages of each of three methods of working underwater. In the case of the diver, the advantages are rapid mobilization, unlimited manual dexterity, mobility/maneuverability; most rapid response to changing conditions, and unrestricted viewing capability; the disadvantages are low payload, short duration, depth limitation, instrumentation limitation, low power, limited range, vulnerability. In the case of the manned submersible, the advantages are depth, duration, power, no training required, no decompression, high payload, simple life support requirements, wide array of equipment; the disadvantages are dependence on weather conditions, reduced maneuverability, limited viewing, lower manual dexterity, extensive pre-operational preparations, complexity, In the case of the instrumented package (towed and self-propelled vehicles such as Teleprobe, Deep Tow, etc.) the advantages are unlimited power and duration, no human element, least weather dependency, long range, least vulnerability to environmental conditions; the disadvantages are limited maneuverability, cable interference, least manual dexterity, slowest response to changing conditions, total reliance on equipment. The article is well illustrated with photographs and drawings, and much of the data is tabulated. Certain needs that have not yet been met in these systems are noted. The manned submersible has not yet fulfilled its potential because of the very limited dexterity of manipulators; its value at present is chiefly as a support base and decompression chamber for the diver. Another problem is the lack of a simple and inexpensive underwater navigation system. (MFW/BSCP)

360.
BUTCHER, I.R. and T.J. Boller.
Design and fabrication of a composite sandwich shell for operation at 3000 feet depth.
Akron, Ohio, Goodyear Aerospace Corp., Rep. GER-15984, 29p. Aug. 1973.
(AD 769,383/1GA)

A program was conducted in which a 20.875 inches diameter x 100 inches long Composite Sandwich Shell was designed and fabricated to demonstrate the feasibility of applying composite materials to deep submergence structures. The fabricated shell was delivered to the Naval Ordnance Laboratory for hydrotesting. During the course of the program the shell was designed with an objective of operation at 3000 feet depth. The sandwich shell was constructed in a conventional manner with fiberglass/epoxy laminate skins and an aluminum honeycomb core. Aluminum end rings were provided at each end to facilitate pressure testing. A 3.500 inches diameter was also included in the shell. No unusual problems were encountered during the fabrication of the sandwich shell leading to the conclusion that current state of the art composite processing methods can be successfully employed in producing high performance, weight critical hydrospace composite structures. (Authors) (GRA)

361.
BUTYRESKII, L.S. and B.I. Petlenko.
Structural changes in speech uttered in a helium-oxygen medium.
Akust. Zh. 19(5):653-661; 1973.
(Transl. JPRS 60633)

The report contains an evaluation of disturbances in the basic parameters of speech uttered in a helium-oxygen atmosphere at various pressures of the medium. (GRA)

362.
BYRNES, D.T.
Deep submersible logistic support design concept.
U.S. Nav. Postgrad. Sch., Thesis, 129p. Sept. 1972.
(AD-753,609)

The thesis proposes a simplification of the logistic and operational problems of deep submersibles using a support craft-submersible combination. Shown is an improved vehicle launch and recovery method and a means to transfer personnel supplies, and services during sea conditions presently detrimental to such operations. The combination is shown as capable of short range operations close to port as a complete unit, but for distant areas, the combination, which is air transportable, may require tending services of an available larger ship. A scale model of the combination was built to illustrate a method for support craft and submersible bow-to-stern mating concept. Designs for the submersible indicate how the system components can accommodate an elevator to reduce vehicle drag and to make equipment accessible for maintenance. Efficient buoyancy material is important to the idea. Small diameter porcelain spheres were made and tested to show the feasibility of sphere-syntactic foam conglomerate for buoyancy at 20,000 feet. (Author) (GRA)

363.
CABARROU, P., H. Krekeler, G. von Nieding and K. Muysers.
Helium elimination from the tissue after hyperbaric exposition of 4 hours.
Pfluegers Arch. 332(Suppl):R9; 1972.

Abstract only. Entire item quoted: In 6 healthy male subjects (age 30-45 years) the respiratory helium elimination was measured after 4 hours exposition to 80% He and 20% O_2 in 1.8 ata. 15 min after leaving the hyperbaric chamber the alveolar partial pressure of He was less than 7 torr. The further washout was not a single exponential. After 10 hours (in one case still after 24 hours) the alveolar partial pressure of He was still significantly higher (5 - 10 x 10^{-3} torr) than the atmospheric pHe (3.5 x 10^{-3} torr). The total amount of helium eliminated between 15 min and 10 hours after leaving the hyperbaric chamber was 800 to 1200 ml STPD.

364.
CADES, S.B. and M.R. Kagan.
Airway resistance measurement at depth.
Gaithersburg, Md., IBM Corp., Rep. FSC-72-5010, 83p. Jan. 17, 1972.

This report discusses the design and development of a whole body plethysmograph system intended for ultimate use as a means of measuring airway resistance under ambient hyperbaric conditions for normal breathing patterns. A customer-supplied plethysmograph was greatly modified towards achieving this goal. At present, the plethysmograph can be used to make measurements of airway resistance for any breathing patterns at BTPS conditions (37°C, 100% relative humidity). A computer program has been written which provides automatic correction of the data for a pressure/flow lag. In addition, the program includes compensation techniques (requiring additional validation) which should allow data obtained at ambient conditions to be utilized. The hardware design and modifications are discussed with respect to the guidelines used, the approach taken and the design achieved. The operational use of the system is described in the sections concerning installation and calibration, operating procedures, data analysis techniques, and the computer program. Present capabilities, potential error sources, and specific recommendations round out the project description. (Authors' abstract)

365.
CAHILL, R.E.
Diary of the depths.
Philadelphia, Dorrance and Co., 1972. 187p.

A fascinating collection of diving adventure stories that make good leisure reading. Not a text or a scientific treatise but contains a good deal of practical information for the divers, particularly on what not to do. In conclusion the author says: ". . . the world beneath the sea offers man many challenges. It is the last unexplored frontier that can satisfy the dreams of scientists, sportsmen, treasure hunters, adventurers, naturalists and businessmen alike." (CWS/UMS)

366.
CAILLE, E.J. and P. Meyer.
Etude psychophysiologique du stress en plongee reelle.
[Psychophysiological study of stress in real dives].
Cent. Etud. Rech. Serv. Psychol. Appl., Rep. CERPA, 11p. plus illustr. Nov. 1971.

Eleven divers, some well-adapted, and others who failed during training, served as subjects for a series of experiments on psychophysiological responses to stress in simulated and real dives to 6 and 12 meters. The electrophysiological data were handled by computer, and were correlated with the results of psychological testing. Results show "specific, coherent fluctuations in real dives as compared with simulated dives to the same pressure." Several parameters, including heart rate and the frequency of EEG signals, are more noticeably affected in real dives, particularly in anxious subjects. The authors suggest that these results are to be explained by the hypothesis that thymic control is established late by inhibition of the limbic system. Certain EEG characteristics should be considered to indicate a poor prognosis for adaptation to diving conditions; opportunities for relaxation, recreational sports, and adequate sleep should be encouraged in professional divers with a view to preventing the development of neurotic and anxiety symptoms, and efforts should be made to develop anxiolytic drugs which do not affect alertness. (MEMH/SCD)

367.
CAILLE, E.J., Quideau and Francois.
Influence d'un sejour de 48 heures en atmosphere a 4.5% CO_2 sur la vigilance, la psychomotricite, et l'activite mentale.
[Influence of a 48-hour stay in a 4.5% CO_2 atmosphere on alertness, psychomotor parameters, and mental activity].
Cent. Etud. Rech. Serv. Psychol. Appl., Rep. CERPA 1/72, 14p. plus illustr. Jan. 15, 1972.

The effects of a 4.5% CO_2 atmosphere on psychological, psychomotor, and electrophysiological parameters in young volunteers were studied. Five volunteers, naval technicians 18-22 years of age, spent five days in a caisson. The first two days were spent in a normal air atmosphere; for days 3 and 4 the atmosphere contained 4.5% CO_2, and the final day was again spent in an air atmosphere. Before entering the caisson, the volunteers were given a battery of psychological tests. A series of other mental, psychological, and physiological tests were carried out daily during the stay in the caisson, and the results were subjected to computer analysis. Although ECG differences in the CO_2 atmosphere were noted, they were not statistically significant. Nor could any correlations be made between psychological parameters (such as anxiety indices, psychosomatic preoccupations, or intelligence) and the effects observed under CO_2 on auditive and visual reaction times. The activity of CO_2 seems to occur at the physiological level. Spectral analysis of the EEG will help to verify this hypothesis. (MEMH/SCD)

368.
CAKAR, L. and M. Terzioglu.
The ventilatory responses of normal and chemoreceptor-denervated rabbits to the breathing of hypercapnic gas mixtures in normo- and hypothermia.
Bull. Physiopathol. Resp. (Nancy) 9(3):676-684; 1973.

The ventilatory responses of normal and chemoreceptor-denervated rabbits to breathing of 6.4% CO_2 in air in normothermia and in progressive hypothermia were assessed by the recording of the various related parameters. The lower respiratory rates of the chemoreceptor-denervated group in all experimental phases in normothermia as well as their lower magnitudes of response to the breathing of the hypercapnic gas mixtures ceased at a much higher temperature level than in the control group. This finding together with the relatively shorter duration of the inspiratory phase in the denervated group seemed to indicate the diminution of the direct excitability of the center(s) on cooling. The chemoreceptors, therefore, are more rugged in response than the central chemosensitive areas. The gradual prolongation of the phrenic discharge duration and the drop in impulse frequency per unit time during the course of progressive hypothermia was attributed to a slowing of the depolarization-repolarization processes at the center(s). At very low rectal temperatures, the rhythmic, prolonged inspiratory phases gave way to irregular, short outbursts of activity. The simultaneous potential recordings from the phrenic nerve and the diaphragm indicated that neuromuscular transmission was not affected under the present experimental conditions. (Authors' conclusions)

369.
CALCET, J., P. Joanny, J. Corriol and S. Dimov.
The protection against the cerebral and pulmonary effects of hyperbaric oxygen by pharmacological agents and lithium salts in mice.
Resuscitation 2:37-50;Apr. 1973.

The effect of three phenothiazines, a barbiturate, a ureide, two oxazolidine diones, gamma-aminobutyrate, gamma-hydroxybutyrate and n-dipropylacetate, in diminishing the incidence of convulsions and pulmonary oedema induced by hyperbaric oxygen at pressures up to 6 bars was studied in mice. The order of effectiveness in protection was chlorpromazine (6mg/kg) >LiCl (600mg/kg) >gama-hydrozybutyrate (200mg/kg) >prochlorpemazine (5mg/kg) > pehnobarbitone (5mg/kg). If a drug protected the mouse against convulsions, the pulmonary hydration did not increase. The findings generally supported the hypothesis that the protection from hyperbaric oxygen was due to these drugs preventing the fall of gamma-aminobutyrate in the brain caused by hyperbaric oxygen. (Authors' summary)

370.
CAMFIELD, F.E., W.L. Preslan and H. Wang.
A program in ocean engineering education.
In: Applications of marine technology to human needs. Preprints, 8th annual conference and exposition, Marine Technology Society, September 1972, Washington, D.C., p.165-172. Published by the Society, 1972.

During the past four years, the Department of Civil Engineering at the University of Delaware has developed undergraduate and graduate level programs in ocean engineering. These programs allow both the undergraduate and the graduated student to specialize in ocean engineering as a part of their regular degree requirements in civil engineering, and also provide elective courses in ocean engineering for students in other engineering departments. Eight ocean engineering courses are offered within the department at the advanced undergraduate and graduate level. In addition, supporting courses are offered by the Department of Geology and the College of Marine Studies. Along with classroom instruction, these courses provide both laboratory and field experience for the students. Laboratory facilities have been developed for thesis and special problems research. (Authors' abstract)

371.
CANTY, J.M., E.H. Lanphier and R.A. Morin.
Unusual design features for high pressure experimentation.
In: Fructus, X., Ed. Third international conference on hyperbaric and underwater physiology, p.56-62. Paris, Doin, 1972.

The high pressure research chamber of the State University at Buffalo is described. It consists of a spherical entrance lock and a cylindrical test chamber which is divided into dry and wet sections. The pressure rating is 2500 psi (170 atmosphere, or 1700 meters ocean depth). The ASME Unfired Pressure Vessel Code was used for the structural design. A similar facility was being made for The Oceanic Institute in Makapuu Point in Hawaii, to be used in connection with the Makai Range underwater habitat. This facility had the added feature of a bullet-shaped personnel transfer capsule that could transfer divers from the habitat to the chamber. The Buffalo facility was to have been completed by the fall of 1970. (MFW/UMS)

372.
CANTY, J.M., E.H. Lamphier and R.A. Morin.
Engineering evaluation: Study of environmental conditioning systems for high pressure research vessels.
Buffalo, N.Y., State Univ., N.Y., Dept. Physiol., High Pressure Lab., Final Rep. on contract N00014-72-C-0125, 68p. June 28, 1972.

Several systems were reviewed including low temperature condensation and adsorption as well as the use of soda lime. The results indicate that low temperature condensation of CO_2 might be attractive for pressures up to 30 atmospheres. However, the large refrigeration requirement will probably preclude this technique at very high pressures. Adsorption systems seem to be very attractive but require careful design of the adsorbent bed at high pressures due to the low diffusivity of the gas. Although the information is presented in a general way, the main purpose of this investigation was to select a system for the 170 atmosphere High Pressure Research Facility at the Department of Physiology — State University of New York at Buffalo. A combination low temperature dehumidification followed by low temperature adsorption of water then adsorption of carbon dioxide appears to be best suited for this application. Data and references are included in the report to permit the reader to evaluate other design conditions. (DCD abstract)

373.
CARLOTTI, P.F. and G. Plante-Longchamp.
Un accident central apparemment lie a un Valsalva a la remontee.
[An accident of the central nervous system apparently related to a Valsalva maneuver on ascending].
Bull. Medsubhyp 7:19;Oct. 1972.

An account is given of a 38-year-old man of two year's diving experience, who made a brief dive to 40 m followed by an apparently uneventful ascent, with a stop of three minutes at ten meters. On leaving the water the symptoms of sickness, cold, fatigue, anxiety, discomfort in hands and feet, set in immediately, followed quickly by pronounced obnubilation, left hemiplegia, temporary blindness and facial spasm. He was immediately taken to shore and given oxygen, and by the time he arrived at the hospital he had regained his lucidity and the use of his arm. It was learned that the diver had executed numerous Valsalva maneuvers during his ascent, because he felt vertigo and ear pain. Recompression to 30 meters brought about complete reversal of symptoms. The authors believe that the Valsalva maneuver cause a sudden change of the alveolo-capillary gradient, with a shock at the level of the microcirculation causing pathogenic bubbles which passed through the left ventricle by the pulmonary veins, thus causing cerebral embolisms of varied topography. (MFW/BSCP)

374.
CARUTHERS, J.W.
Lectures on marine acoustics. Volume II. Part I. Selected advanced topics in marine acoustics.
College Station, Tex., Tex. A & M. Univ., Dept. Oceanog., Rep. TAMU-SG-73-403, NOAA 73 073102, 221p. Apr. 1973.
(COM-73-11370/6)

The report is the first part of the second volume representing compilations of lectures presented by invited authors who participated in the short course in Marine Acoustics held at the Department of Oceanography of Texas A & M University in 1971. These invited lectures were selected on the basis of their emphasis on the environmental aspect of their application to civil uses. Following the opening address by Richard A. Geyer, the lectures were: Acoustic telemetry and signal processing; Wave theory; Shallow water acoustic propagation; Marine bio-acoustics; The sonar equations; Sound propagation in the sea; Scattering and reverberation; Seismic reflection and refraction; Travel time analysis; Twenty years in underwater acoustics; Generation and reception; Civil uses of underwater acoustics; Arrays and signal processing; and Uses of sound in the ocean. (GRA)

375.
CARUTHERS, J.W.
Lectures on marine acoustics. Volume II, Part II. Selected advanced topics in marine acoustics.
College Station, Tex., Tex. A & M Univ., Dept. Oceanog., Rep. TAMU-SG-73-404, NOAA 730 73103, 69p. Apr. 1973.
(COM-73-11371/4)

The report is the second part of Volume II of the lectures presented by invited authors who participated in the short course in Marine Acoustics held at the Department of Oceanography of Texas A & M University in 1971. The first paper, by T.G. Muir, deals with nonlinear acoustics with applications to underwater sound. The second by Ivor D. Groves, Jr., deals with hydrophones, projectors and calibration. (GRA)

376.
CARUTHERS, J.W.
Lectures on marine acoustics, Volume I. Fundamentals of marine acoustics.
College Station, Tex., Tex. A & M Univ., Dept. of Oceanog., Rep. TAMU-SG-73-402, NOAA-73073101, 165p. June 1973.
(COM 73-11369-8)

The report is the first of two volumes representing compilations of lectures presented at the short course in Marine Acoustics held at the Department of Oceanography of Texas A & M University in 1971. The introduction reviews sound in the sea, nature of the acoustic field, logarithmic units and spectral notions. Subsequent sections deal with the following: electroacoustic and chemical transduction; hydrophones, projectors, and calibration; arrays and systems; sonar equations and parameters; theory of sound propagation; sound propagation in the sea; reverberation; and finally, noise. (GRA)

377.
CASPERS, H. and E.-J. Speckmann.
Cerebral pO_2, pCO_2 and pH: changes during convulsive activity and their significance for spontaneous arrest of seizures.
Epilepsia 13:699-725;Sept. 1972.

The present study on rats and cats aimed to clarify the role played by hypoxia, hypercapnia and acidosis in spontaneous arrest of seizures. 1. In most experiments cortical PO_2 declined during seizure activity, whereas PCO_2 increased. Occasionally, however, reverse reactions occurred. Since the increase in cortical blood flow varied over a wide range, it could account for the fact that gas tension did not always change in the same direction or to the same degree during a seizure. Cessation of seizure activity was independent of the degree and direction of the changes in gas tension. 2. When seizures were arrested by experimentally produced hypoxia, cortical and spinal neurons always showed a distinct depolarization. When convulsive discharges were suppressed by artificial increase in PCO_2 most units were concomitantly hyperpolarized. 3. When seizures ceased spontaneously, both cortical and spinal neurons showed a steep re- and hyperpolarization, independent of concomitant fluctuations in local gas tension. The findings lead to the conclusion that the degree of hypoxia and hypercapnia usually encountered during prolonged seizure activity does not reach the critical level sufficient to depress seizure activity. It must be assumed that spontaneous seizure termination is based, primarily, on neuronal processes. (Authors' summary)

378.
CASTELLI, V.J. and E.C. Fischer.
Deep ocean microbiological studies. Part II — Oxygen metabolism and gas production at high hydrostatic pressure.
U.S. Nav. Ship Res. Develop. Cent., Rep. 9-57, 12p. Apr. 1971.

High hydrostatic compression exerts unusual effects of bacterial physiology and metabolism. Using Escherichia coli as experimental organisms, compressions as great as 140 and 420 kilograms per square centimeter were found to allow survival in seawater with rapidly increasing oxygen utilization. Efficiency of nitrogen and hydrogen production were increased by hydrostatic compression equivalent to an ocean depth of 13,000 feet. The significance of this fact is discussed in relation to deep ocean microbubble production and biocorrosion. (Authors' abstract)

379.
CATHIGNOL, D.M. Roche and M.-L. Grivel.
Formation de bulles intravasculaires.
[Formation of intravascular bubbles].
Nouv. Presse Med. 2:117-118;Jan. 13, 1973.

For sometime it has been thought that the formation of bubbles in blood and tissues is the cause of serious disorders occurring when living organisms are subjected to rapid decompression. More recently, numerous experiments have sought to detect the existence of bubbles and to relate them technically to decompression disorders. Such a hypothesis was confirmed by Spencer and Campbell [Bull. Mason Clin. 1:22; 1968]. These authors were able to demonstrate that bubbles formed at the level of the vena cava during decompression accidents. In most of the detectors now in existence, the presence of a bubble is indicated in one of three ways: (1) by the appearance of an ultrasonic wave reflected by itself (echo), (2) by the attenuation of the transmitted ultrasonic wave, or (3) by the frequency variation of the ultrasonic wave reflected by the moving bubbles (Doppler effect). (Authors' abstract translated by MFW/UMS)

380.
CATLETT, R.H. and B.L. Johnston.
Cardiac response to diving in wild ducks.
Comp. Biochem. Physiol. (A) 47(3):925-931; 1971.

Submersion of the head in water causes bradycardia in the Redhead (*Aythya americana*), Lesser Scaup (*Aythya affinis*), Ruddy Duck (*Oxyura jamaicensis*) and the Pintail (*Ansa acuta*). Differences in development of bradycardia were demonstrated among the four species. Redheads and Ruddy Ducks have the most rapid response and the sharpest decline in heart rate. Pintails and Lesser Scaups showed a lesser decline and rate of development of bradycardia, with Pintails showing the least. Redheads, Lesser Scaups and Ruddy Ducks reached an average decline of 45 heartbeats/min within 5 s after submergence. Pintails reached this average decline after 20 s of submergence. (© BA)

381.
CATTO, M.E.
Pathology of caisson disease of bone.
In: The Association of Clinical Pathologists: 89th general meeting. Symposium II. Decompression sickness.
J. Clin. Pathol. 25:1006;Nov. 1972.

Abstract only. Entire item quoted: While histological examination is of little help in elucidating the pathogenesis of aseptic bone necrosis in compressed air workers, it throws some light on the sequence of events and radiological changes following bone death. Revascularization of both medullary and juxtaarticular lesions may begin but halt short of completion, the revascularization front becoming collagenous. Bone trabeculae adjacent to this fibrous tissue are often greatly thickened and may give rise to a sclerotic line on clinical radiographs. When such a radio-dense line is seen traversing a bone end it is highly probable that the tissue between it and the joint surface is still dead. The necrotic bone trabeculae may later fracture, with collapse of the articular surface associated with pain. Incongruity of the joint surface is often followed by formation of osteophytes at the living joint margins. At first the joint space remains normal and the articular cartilage covering dead bone is relatively well preserved but later it and the underlying dead bone may be ground away, the end result sometimes being difficult to distinguish from primary osteoarthritis. A similar pattern of events and morphological changes may be seen following juxta-articular bone necrosis due to other causes.

382.
CAULFIELD, J.B., R.W. Shelton and J.F. Burke.
Cytotoxic effects of oxygen on striated muscle.
Arch. Path. 94:127-132;Aug. 1972.

Guinea pigs, hamsters, and rabbits were exposed to 100% oxygen at atmospheric pressure, room temperature, and either 70% or 99% relative humidity. All three species showed skeletal and cardiac muscle lesions at a time of minimal pulmonary change, and in the presence of oxygen pressure measurement in excess of 250 mm Hg. The most severe lesions were located on the pleural aspect of the diaphragm and the intercostal muscles, a site that potentially has the highest O_2 concentration. This suggests a direct rather than indirect toxic effect through an altered vascular bed. (Authors' abstract)

383.
CEGLA, U.H.
Zur Form der CO_2 — Antwortkurve unter kuenstlicher Hyperkapnie.
[Form analysis of respiratory response curve to CO_2 during artificial hypercapnia].
Pneumonologie 149:213-218;Dec. 19, 1973.

Rebreathing was tested in 27 healthy young men (rebreathing time 30-40 min). The distribution of the values is statistically normal, so that the approximately 200 values are treated as 1 collective. An iteration program and a computer type pdp 11 were used to calculate tidal volume-increment curve, the frequency-increment curve and the common minute volume-increment. A linear relationship between $PaCO_2$ (arterial CO_2 tension) and frequency and a parabolic one for the tidal volume increment was stated; thus the AMV (average minute volume) increases to the third power of the $PaCO_2$. The difficulty in interpreting the sensitivity of the respiratory center in calculating the gradient of linear rebreathing curves is stressed. (© BA)

384.
CENTRE NATIONAL POUR L'EXPLOITATION DES OCEANS.
Biologie humanie hyperbare: ou en sommes-nous en 1972?
[Hyperbaric human biology: where are we in 1972?].
Centre National pour l'exploitation des Oceans, Rep. 9, 73p. 1972.

This report summarizes the conclusions reached by a working group called by CNEXO to evaluate the state-of-art in hyperbaric biology and to point out the most crucial areas of research for the future. The first part of the discussion dealt with problems posed by the adaptation of man to the underwater environment, and was divided into the following nine sections: (1) Nervous limiting factors; (2) Respiratory limiting factors; (3) Oxygen-hydrogen breathing mixtures; (4) Decompression problems; (5) Thermal balance; (6) Pollution; (7) Psychophysiology, psychometry, sensory physiology and ergonomy; (8) Body chemistry and hemodynamics (9) Nutrition. The second part of the discussion attempted to define the areas of research most urgently needed. These consisted of nervous and respiratory limiting factors, hydrogen breathing mixtures, and the physiology and pathology of decompression. The report concludes with a bibliography of 114 entries. (MFW/BSCP)

385.
CERRATI, A. and C.F. Fornara.
Il coenzima A, quale agente protettore contro i danni da ossigeno iperbarico.
[Coenzyme A as a protective agent against damage by hyperbaric oxygen].
Atti Accad. Med. Lombarda 25(2/3):172-174; 1970.

The protection of experimental animals (mice) by the preventive administration of Co A against the toxic effects of hyperbaric oxygen was investigated. Results show that a very low Co A dose (200-600 μg of pure Co A/kg body weight) administered to mice is able to completely inhibit convulsions and death (as well as the fall of the liver succino-dehydrogenase activity) occurring in control animals submitted to hyperbarism. (JWS) (© BA)

386.
CESTONE, J.A. and E. St. George, Jr.
Hydrospheric navigation.
Navigation 19:199-208;Fall 1972.

To meet the various navigational requirements of underwater activity, navigation by tether, visual navigation, sonic navigation and dead reckoning have been used. The first consists of following a line from one point to another either by holding onto it when necessary or by swimming above it. Another form of navigation by tether is calculation of the position of a towed instrument package or submersible in relation to that of the towing vessel. This calculation is greatly complicated by the need to estimate drag. A current meter on the towed object is helpful. Visual navigation is difficult underwater for obvious reasons, but there are visual aids, such as rolled-up, numbered, plastic sheets which unroll on impact with the bottom. When dropped in a grid pattern, they enable a submersible to search a bottom area as large as 600 feet. Trieste has used this device. One method is sonic navigation by acoustic transponder, which is emplaced on the bottom and interrogated by a hydrophone on the submersible. Three transponders, placed in the position roughly of an equilateral triangle, make three dimensional navigation possible. In deep water, they can be as much as two miles apart; in shallow water, closer spacing is required. A reverse system exists, in which three receiving hydrophones are placed on the ship or submersible, and a single bottom transponder is interrogated. This system is less accurate, but is useful for tracking a towed vessel from the mother vessel, or maintaining position over a wellhead. Bottom mapping can be accomplished with the help of side-scanning or forward scanning high resolution sonar; navigation depends on recognizable bottom features or on artificial benchmarks. Dead reckoning navigation, which depends on measurement of speed and direction, must be used in under-ice conditions, where benchmarks or radio navigation fixes occur only infrequently. The Doppler sonar eliminates one defect of most underwater speed measuring devices, in that it is referenced to the bottom rather than to the surrounding water mass. Navigational and sensing abilities of some fish and marine mammals are discussed, and it is noted that the possible ability of the porpoise to create a three-dimensional acoustic image of underwater objects has exciting applicability to man's requirements, although acute design problems exist with regard to transducers with thousands of elements, and complex signal processing equipment. (MFW/SCD)

387.
CETTA, T.W.
Evaluation of U.S. diver's Calypso III, Calypso J, Conshelf XII, Aquarius, and Royal Aquamaster open circuit scuba regulators.
U.S. Navy Exp. Diving Unit., Rep. NEDU-LR-9-71, 14p. 1972.
(AD 759 822)

The military specifications for open circuit scuba regulators provide a mechanism by which commercial vendors may submit their regulators to the Navy Experimental Diving Unit for testing for possible approval for U.S. Navy use. Accordingly, U.S. Diver's single hose regulators Calypso III, Calypso J, Conshelf XII and Aquarius and double hose regulator Royal Aquamaster were tested in September 1971. Due to the nonavailability of government test chambers, the regulators were tested at U.S. Divers test facility under the supervision of a government engineer. All five regulators were found to meet the requirements of the appropriate military specifications, and all were approved for U.S. Navy use. (Author) (GRA)

388.
CETTA, T.W.
Evaluation of Dacor's R-4 Olympic 400, Olympic 800 open circuit scuba regulators.
U.S. Navy Exp. Diving Unit, Rep. NEDU 8-73, 9p. July 9, 1973.

Dacor Corporation submitted three open circuit scuba regulators, models R-4, Olympic 400 and Olympic 800 for evaluation by the Navy Experimental Diving Unit. The Olympic 400 and Olympic 800 were found acceptable for service use. The R-4 was found unacceptable for service use. (Author's abstract)

389.
CETTA, T.W.
Evaluation of U.S. Diver's Co. modified Conshelf VI and Conshelf XI conversion to Conshelf XII open circuit regulators.
U.S. Navy Exp. Diving Unit, Rep. NEDU 9-73, 11p. July 9, 1973.

U.S. Diver's Co. submitted conversion kits, to convert Conshelf VIoand XI to Conshelf XII, for evaluation and approval for service use. The modified Conshelf VI and Conshelf XI, (conversion to Conshelf XIII) were found acceptable for service use. (Author's abstract)

390.
CHANDEYSSON, P.L.
Data management and mission support.
In: Miller, J.W., J.G. Van Derwalker, and R.A. Waller, eds. Tektite 2: Scientists-in-the-sea, p. VIII-96 - VIII-97. Washington, D.C., U.S. Department of the Interior, August 1971.

Bellcomm provided support to the Tektite 2 human behavioral studies primarily in the form of data management and assistance in developing observational techniques for aquanaut behavioral monitoring. . . Data on hand-punched computer cards were sent to Bellcomm every week by mail from the Tektite operational site in the Virgin Islands. The cards were duplicated on regular computer cards and printed out. A visual check for data errors was made so that the cause could be immediately determined and corrected. The data were then reformatted into a readily interpreted format developed in collaboration with the scientific investigators. These data were then made available to the investigators in printout form; cards were sent to the University of Texas at Austin for computer analysis. The data were also stored on tapes at Bellcomm. These data are accessible via fastrand for future analysis by Bellcomm or other investigators. (Author)

391.
CHARMASSON, R., F. Sicardi and E. Catella.
Etude par la technique osmometrique de l'action su le sang humain de la pression et des gaz comprimes dissous.
[Study of the effect of pressure and dissolved compressed gases on human blood by means of the osmometric technic].
C.R. Acad. Sci. (D) 275:1779-1782;Oct. 16, 1972.

The effects of atmospheric pressure and of the partial pressure of gases dissolved in human blood on the osmotic pressure of the blood were studied. Atmospheric pressure exerted only a slight influence on the osmotic pressure of normal heparinized blood. But the osmotic pressure of the blood of a recently returned diver varied inversely with atmospheric pressure. In an oxygen-helium breathing mixture where the partial pressure of the oxygen was 400 mb the osmotic pressure values recorded were five to seven times greater than normal values. It is suggested that the inert gas itself may exert a certain toxic effect on the organism at lower pressures than was previously thought, since the effects of atmospheric pressure alone do not seem great enough to account for the disturbances noted. (MEMH/BSCP)

392.
CHARPY, J.P., J.P. Deyts and P. Wide.
Etude psychologique sur les travailleurs sous-marins a moyennes et grandes profondeurs.
[Psychological studies of underwater workers at medium and great depths].
In: Hesser, C.M. and D. Linnarsson eds. Proceedings of the first annual scientific meeting of the European Undersea Biomedical Society, Stockholm, 13-15 June 1973. Forsvarsmedicin 9:452-458;July 1973.

The authors discuss variations of mood, problems of isolation, and of habitat habitability — The necessity for privacy and the need of social life. Psychometric studies of six subjects during three chamber dives of 50 to 62 ATA (Physalie V, Sagittaire II, and Physalie VI). In general, it is noted that variations in mental function were not systematic, since many interdependent factors were involved. As to sensory-motor function, however, a systematic diminution of performance was noted. Psychological examinations for selection are discussed. It is noted that individuals who may demonstrate slightly neurotic characteristics in normal life might better adapt to a career of diving and underwater work than those who seem better balanced. Psychological testing is still in the formative stage; actual criteria have not been established. (MFW/UMS)

393.
CHATEAU, G.M.
Janus II — saturation diving to 250 m. depths.
Oil Gas J. 69:60-63;Jan. 1971.

The author recounts the various French experiments in saturation diving, from Precontinent through Ludion, and Janus I and II. The preferred technique is to have the living quarters, at depth pressure, on a surface vessel, and to lower the divers to the sea floor in a pressurized diving chamber. For oil operations this system gives a much greater mobility than does the use of a sea-floor habitat. The exercise described in this article, Janus II, consisted of 14 divers in a period of eight days, to a depth of 250 meters; the longest dive lasted over three hours. Preliminary simulated dives were made at the COMEX hyperbaric facility, for the purpose of physiological and psychological evaluation, and for selection of divers. Various cutting and welding tasks, pipe assembly and running repairs were accomplished, photographs were taken, and equipment was evaluated. Operations such as these will be feasible, the author believes, in about a year's time. This period is required to make improvements in the comfort of the living quarters and the transfer capsule, in the effectiveness of the tools, and in the safety and practicality of the divers' clothing. (MFW/BSCP)

394.
CHEN, S.C.
Caisson disease.
Br. J. Clin. Pract. 26:385-386;Aug. 1972.

This is a case history of a 60-year old man with a lifetime history of tunnel work, who suffered more or less chronic pain in his right hip. Examination revealed a dense, flattened femoral head resulting from avascular necrosis. Four years later he was operated on, and the femoral head was replaced with a Thompson's prosthesis. Three months later, the pain returned, and the hip movement was considerably more limited. X-ray revealed involvement of the roof of the acetabulum. Another operation was performed, replacing the Thompson's arthroplasty with a McKee-Farrar total hip arthroplasty. The case indicates that not all necrotic bone lesions are detectable by radiography in the early stages, and those that are seen may represent only a small part of the necrotic area. The inadequacy of replacing only one component of the joint is demonstrated. (MFW/BSCP)

395.
CHERKASOV, I.S., N.I. Shibinskaya, O.I. Kobozeva, A.J. Radkovskaya and A.P. Hyashenko.
Gidrodinamika glaza i sostoyanie sosudistogo tonusa zdorovogo cheloveka v usloviya giperbaricheskoi oksigenatsii.
[Ocular hydrodynamics and the state of vascular tonus in healthy subjects under conditions of hyperbaric oxygenation].
Oftalmol. Zh. 26:575-577; 1971.

Investigations were performed in a reconstructed diving altitude chamber, 4.5 m^3 volume. The air in the chamber contained 40-60% of oxygen. The chamber was systematically ventilated to maintain air temperature, oxygen and carbonic acid percentage stable. The investigations were performed at the pressure altitude of 215 atc. Observations were carried out over 10 healthy persons (20 eyes) at the age from 18 to 34 years. All subjects underwent tonography, measurements of blood pressure in brachial artery and central artery of the retina as well as average dynamic arterial pressure, retino-brachial coefficient and coefficient of Lobstein were calculated. The data obtained show that hyperbarometric oxygenation produces no remarkable effect on indices of hydro- and hemo-dynamics of the eye in healthy persons. Slight changes in intraocular fluid secretion and tendency to the decrease of intraocular pressure at the altitude of barometric pressure of 2.5 ats as well as the return of these indices to initial values following decompression demonstrate good state of neurovascular factor regulating intraocular pressure. The increase in the production of intraocular fluid following decompression is explained by stronger blood flow. (English summary)

396.
CHERNIACK, N.S., P.G. Tuteur, N.H. Edelman and A.P. Fishman.
Serial changes in CO_2 storage in tissues.
Resp. Physiol. 16(2):127-141; 1972.

Attempts to use the steady state CO_2 storage capacity of tissues to predict the rate of blood PCO_2 rise during acute exposure to CO_2 were unsuccessful. This discrepancy might be explained by the failure of some or all of the body tissues to exert their full capacity to store CO_2 during brief exposures to hypercapnia. This hypothesis was tested in 29 dogs and 10 goats by determining the in vivo CO_2 dissociation slope (Δ tissue CO_2 concentration/ Δ venous PCO_2) in three different tisues (brain spleen and muscle) during transient states of CO_2 retention produced by apneic oxygenation or ventilation with 3% CO_2. By six min of apneic oxygenation, the CO_2 dissociation slope of the brain was 3.8 ml/kg/mm $PvCO_2$; and that of the spleen, 4.3; while the value for muscle was much less (only 1.0) it was unchanged by alteration in the total level of muscle perfusion. Studies with 3% CO_2 indicated that the CO_2 dissociation of brain and spleen was nearly constant from 5 to 20 min of CO_2 exposure but that of muscle gradually increased. Factors other than perfusion limit CO_2 storage in muscle, and reduced ability of muscle to store CO_2 largely accounts for the low storage capacity of the body during brief periods of exposure to CO_2. (© BA)

397.
CHERNIACK, N.S., N.N. Stanley, P.G. Tuteur, M.D. Altose and A.P. Fishman.
Effects of lung volume changes on respiratory drive under hypoxia and hypercapnia.
J. Appl. Physiol. 35:635-641;Nov. 1973.

The interplay of lung volume reflexes and chemical stimuli on respiratory drive was examined by measuring the phrenic activity occurring per minute (Np) in paralyzed, anesthetized, and artificially ventilated dogs during progressive hypercapnia, progressive hypoxia, and steady-state hypercapnia and hypoxia. When the lungs were inflated with a positive end-expiratory pressure of 10 cm H_2O, the response to progressive hypercapnia (Δ Np/ Δ $PaCO_2$) was reduced to 65% of the control response measured at normal FRC: the response to progressive hypoxia (Δ Np/ Δ log

PaO_2) was also reduced to 65% of control. When the lung was deflated by a negative end-expiratory pressure of 10 cm H_2O, the response to hypercapnia increased to 137% and the response to hypoxia to 147%. In steady-state experiments performed at the same levels of end-expiratory pressure, Np was initially reduced by inflation and increased by deflation. However, with sustained volume changes, Np gradually reverted toward control levels. The return to control levels of Np occurred in a shorter period of time when lung volume was changed in animals ventilated with hypercapnic or hypoxic gas mixtures rather than with room air. All lung effects on Np were abolished by bilateral vagotomy. Lung volume reflexes interact with chemical stimuli in determining respiratory drive, but the brevity of these reflex effects suggests that they shape respiratory patterns rather than setting absolute levels of ventilation. (Authors' abstract)

398.
CHIANTA, M.A. and A.M. Stoll.
Fire retardance of mixtures of inert gases and oxygen.
Aerosp. Med. 44:169-173;Feb. 1973.

The relative effectiveness of helium, nitrogen and argon as fire retardants in oxygen mixtures was assessed at atmospheric and hypobaric pressures under carefully controlled flow and ignition conditions. Combustion rate of a standard fabric, ignited and burned in serial concentrations of each gaseous medium, served as the measure of effectivity. It was found that: 1) Combustion rate is directly and linearly related to the log of the mass flow (weight/time) of oxygen in each instance; 2) preignition time varies directly, and fabric destruction rate inversely, with the heat transport capacity of the medium, thus, the mixture with the highest heat transfer coefficient, O_2/He, exerts the greatest retardant effect and the mixture with the lowest coefficient O_2/A, th least; 3) when heat is supplied by the source in contact with the specimen, the destruction rate depends solely on the oxygen mass flow, possibly because contact results in excessive heating sufficient to mask any retardant effect of the diluent gas; 4) at any one concentration throughout the range of gas mixtures used, as pressure decreases, destruction rate decreases even though the mass flow of oxygen is maintained constant from level to level, probably due to the cooling effect of the increased volume flow required to maintain constant mass flow of oxygen. It is concluded that in situations where heat is applied at a sufficiently low rate, the efficiency of the diluent gas is related directly to the heat transport capacity of the gaseous medium; where the heating intensity is sufficient to overwhelm the retardant effect of the inert component only limitation of oxygen content controls combustion rate. In addition to providing basic information concerning fire retardancy effects in inert gases, the present findings are of immediate practical importance in investigations of fabric flammability in general and the development of meaningful test methods in particular. They indicate that the variability of fabric combustion and the delicacy of balance of the accompanying heat transfer mechanism are such that comparability of data from different sources can be achieved only by use of a standardized method in which pressure, flow, ignitor heat and mode of application, as well as sample size, initial temperature and humidity, etc., are very strictly controlled. In this regard, for instance, it is indicated that the limiting oxygen index (LOI) technique recently adopted as an ASTM standard for plastics flammability testing, and currently under consideration for textiles, will require considerable refinement in order to provide comparable reliability in the assessment of fabric flammability. (Authors' abstract)

399.
CHOUTEAU, J., G. Imbert, J.C. Le Pechon and J. Alinat.
Physiological aspect of prolonged exposure at extreme ambient pressure in an oxygen-helium atmosphere.
In: Wada, J. and I. Takashi, eds. Proceedings of the fourth international congress of hyperbaric medicine, Sapporo, Japan, Sept. 1969, p.126-131. Baltimore, Williams, and Wilkins, 1970.

The atuhors review some of their experiments with goats, during which motor disturbances and paralysis occurred at 1600 feet, to be reversed completely when oxygen was raised from 0.20 ATS to 0.25 ATS. The animals appeared normal at 1820 feet with the raised oxygen tension. After effects of anoxic lesions in lungs and muscles were detected. The same sequence of events occurred with an oxygen-nitrogen breathing mixture, at a depth of 320 feet. Further experiments corroberated these results. The authors explain the hypoxic disorders as a disturbance of the alveolar-capillary exchange. They emphasize the importance of humidity control (70%) as a limiting factor. (MFW/BSCP)

400.
CHOUTEAU, J., R. Guillerm, J. Hee and J.C. LePechon.
Arterial hypoxia when breathing normoxic mixtures under hyperbaric conditions.
In: Abstracts of the Twenty-fifth Congress of Physiological Sciences Satellite Symposium. Recent progress in fundamental physiology of diving, Marseille, France, July 1971, p.37-38. (Proceedings unpublished)

Abstract only. Excerpts quoted: In order to corroborate the hypoxic nature of the troubles observed and described by J. Chouteau, et al in goats breathing gas mixtures under pressure, measurements of arterial oxygen partial pressure (PaO_2) were undertaken in anesthetized rabbits. . . . This paper deals with the results recorded with neon and helium as diluents. In both cases, the main physiological data were PIO_2, PaO_2 and total pressure. During helium dives EKG, body temperature, respiratory rate were added to these data. . . . Neon + oxygen mixture: 15% decrease in in PaO_2 is recorded at 35 ATA, and no significant fall occurs at 21 ATA (7 dives). Helium + oxygen mixture above 91 ATA induces a gradual fall in PaO_2, more important than with the other inert gases. In isobaric stay, or during increase of the total pressure up to 151 ATA, this fall reaches 60 to 90% of the initial PaO_2. At 95 ATA reversibility was demonstrated by increasing PIO_2 or by decompression to 71 ATA. During helium dives, all the animals awakened (movements, muscular contractions, some of them coming back to the normal ventral position). This awaking may be related to hypoxia and promoted by the fact that helium is not narcotic at these pressurs (the other inert gases are narcotic at the pressure of the tests).

401.
CHOUTEAU, J., J.M. Ocana de Sentuary and L. Pironti.
A comparative and theoretical study of compression rate in deep diving.
In: Abstracts of the Twenty-fifth Congress of Physiological Sciences Satellite Symposium. Recent progress in fundamental physiology of diving, Marseille, France, July 1971, p.62-64. (Proceedings unpublished)

Abstract only. The authors have for some time believed that various disorders such as helium tremors, "no joint juice", arthralgia and hpns are attributable to the compression schedule. They have devised equations which establish the maximum gradient for a given tissue with relation to the compression rate. By applying these formulas to different tissues and especially to 120-minute half time tissue, it is shown that Δp maximum values under 8 or 10 ATA do not induce symptoms during compression, while any higher values will produce the classical symptoms. The neurological disturbances of hpns must be considered separately. Animals have been taken to 100 ATA without helium tremor, but neurological disorders have developed at 80 ATA. Hypoxic crises or epileptiform convulsions can be avoided or delayed by increasing the PIO_2. The "helium barrier" appears to be beyond 80 ATA. A mathematical formula for computing a continuous compression curve is given. (MFW/BSCP)

402.
CHOUTEAU, J., J. Parc, Y. Berry and G. Imbert.
Relationship between PIO_2 and hygrometry during deep saturation dives.
In: Abstracts of the Twenty-fifth Congress of Physiological Sciences Satellite Sympoisum. Recent progress in fundamental physiology of diving, Marseille, France, July 1971, p.35-36. (Proceedings unpublished)

Abstract only. In experiments conducted with goats and with minipigs, the authors learned that respiratory difficulties, sometimes fatal, could be induced in even mild hyperoxic conditions in introducing a high value of humidity. In conditions of 40-45% relative humidity, three goats were compressed to 81 ATA where they remained for one week with PIO_2 at .43 ATA, and were returned to atmospheric pressure without respiratory disorders. Animals taken to the same pressure with the same PIO_2, but at a humidity of 80-90% suffered fatal respiratory difficulties. Congestive effects in the upper airways, bringing on intensified ventilatory work, are considered responsible. (MFW/BSCP)

403.
CHOUTEAU, J.
Experimentation animale de plongee profonde en melanges synthetiques realisee au CEMA, au GERS, et au CERTSM.
[Animal experiments in deep diving with synthetic breathing mixtures carried out at CEMA, GERS, and CERTSM].
In: Fructus, X., ed. Third international conference on hyperbaric and underwater physiology, p.8-12. Paris, Doin, 1972.

The author briefly surveys the animal experimentation (rabbits, goats, dwarf pigs) carried out by three French groups over the past five years. The experiments involved simulated dives to various depths in hydrogen-oxygen, nitrogen-oxygen and helium-oxygen mixtures. Attention was focused on neurologic disturbances and related phenomena due to pressure hypoxia, and inert-gas narcosis, especially in relation to EEG findings. The harmful effects of hydrogen in hyperbaric conditions are also noted. Most of the work summarized here has been published elsewhere in greater detail. (MEMH/UMS)

404.
CHOUTEAU, J., G. Imbert and J.C. LePechon.
Physiologie comparee de divers mammiferes aux hautes pressions en atmosphere oxygen-helium.
[Comparative physiology of various mammals at high pressure in oxygen-helium atmosphere].
Maroc Med. 52:448-449;July 1972.

The authors summarize the previously-reported results of experimentation with cattle, dwarf pigs, baboons and rabbits in simulated dives in oxygen-helium atmospheres. The neurological symptoms presented by different animals at the same phase of the experiments may be reversed by an increase in PiO_2, and are therefore considered by the author to be of hypoxic origin. (MEMH/BSCP)

405.
CHOY, O.G., D.H. Ford and R.K. Rhines.
The effect of breathing 100% oxygen at 1 and 3 atmospheres absolute on the accumulation of ^{3}H-lysine into different brain regions, plasma, muscle and liver of ethanol-anesthetized and unanesthetized rats.
Acta. Neurol. Scand. 48:359-380; 1972.

The effect of breathing 100% oxygen at 1 and 3 atmospheres absolute was studied in relation to the accumulation of ^{3}H-lysine into different brain regions, plasma, muscle and liver of ethanol-anesthetized and unanesthetized rats, as well as into the TCA-precipitable protein (PCF) of brain, plasma, muscle and liver. It was shown that hyperoxia at 1 and 3 ATA caused a depression of the ^{3}H-lysine accumulation into the hypothalamus and cerebellum of unanesthetized rats two hours after the injection of the amino acid. Hyperoxia at 3 ATA also caused a depression of lysine accumulation into white matter two hours after injection. No changes were noted in the ethanol-anesthetized rats. By group analysis, there was also a depression of ^{3}H-lysine accumulation in the cerebral grey matter in the 1 ATA animals at both levels of anesthesia. Hyperoxia at 1 and 3 ATA caused a depression in the ^{3}H-lysine accumulation into plasma protein at two and three hours in unanesthetized rats and had somewhat more variable effects in the anesthetized animals. In the skeletal muscle, hyperoxia caused an increase in amino acid accumulation in animals breathing 100% O_2 at 3 ATA as compared to those breathing air or 100% oxygen at 1 ATA when compared by group analysis of whole tissue. Analysis of the muscle PCF revealed a depression in lysine uptake associated with anesthesia (group analysis), and changes in all groups related to time elapsed since injection of labelled amino acid. Finally, O_2 at 1 ATA was observed to depress amino acid accumulation while O_2 at 3 ATA had no effect in the unaesthetized rats. In the liver, there was a significant depression of ^{3}H-lysine accumulation in those animals breathing 100% oxygen at 1 ATA as compared to controls in both the ethanol-anesthetized and unaesthetized rats. ^{3}H-lysine accumulation in animals breathing oxygen at 3 ATA did not differ from the controls and were in general significantly higher than the 1 ATA group at both levels of anesthesia. (Authors' abstract)

406.
CHRIST, M.
Un cas d'explosion de caisson monoplace.
[A case of the explosion of a monoplace chamber].
In: Fructus, X., Ed. Third international conference on hyperbaric and underwater physiology, p.182-183. Paris, Doin, 1972.

A patient was undergoing hyperbaric oxygenation in Mexico when the chamber, which was a telescopic one, exploded, with fatal results. It is concluded that telescopic chambers should be used only in exceptional cases, that they should be subjected to intensive examination once a year, that a preregulated pressure reducer should be part of the equipment at all times, that a monoplace chamber should never be made up of more than two parts, that is, the tube and the door, and that the manufacturers should pay particular attention to the reinforcement of the rings, which comprise the most important weakness. (MFW/SCD)

407.
CHRYSSANTHOU, C.P.
Studies on the mechanism and prevention of decompression sickness.
In: Abstracts of BuMed-ONR sponsored Navywide research in high presure biomedical research, U.S. Submarine Base, Groton, Conn., May 1971, p.42. Published by the Naval Submarine Medical Research Laboratories, 1971.

Abstract only. Excerpts quoted: The possibility that Smooth Muscle Acting Factor (SMAF) could render thin mice susceptible to decompression sickness (DS) was explored. The ability of 2-(4-phenyl piperazinyl methyl) cyclohexanone (PPCH) to counteract the effect of SMAF and prevent DS was also investigated. The following results were obtained: A small percentage of thin mice develop DS when decompression to sea level is followed by exposure to altitude. 2. SMAF appreciably increases the susceptibility of thin mice to DS. Clinical manifestations and histologic changes resemble those observed in the susceptible obese mice. 3. PPCH prevents development of DS despite SMAF administration. PPCH possibly blocks the direct effects of SMAF and/or inhibits smooth muscle stimulants, e.g. bradykinin, to which SMAF increases the responsiveness of smooth muscle. These results further support the postulated implication of humeral smooth muscle stimulating factors in the pathogenesis of DS, thus providing a new pharmacological approach for the prevention or amelioration of the syndrome. Furthermore, SMAF provides the means for producing the syndrome in animals with relatively low susceptibility or with small partial pressure gradients.

408.
CHRYSSANTHOU, C.P., F. Teichner, G. Goldstein and W. Antopol.
Newer concepts on the mechanism and prevention of decompression sickness.
In: Abstracts of papers, 20th international congress of aviation and space medicine, Nice, France, September 1972, p.66. Published by the congress.

Abstract only. Entire item quoted: There is evidence suggesting that smooth muscle stimulating substances such as bradykinin (BK), histamine (H), 5-hydroxytryptamine (5HT), etc., are implicated in the pathogenesis of decompression sickness (DS). This hypothesis is based on the following observations: (1) BK intensifies pathologic alterations and increases mortality in DS produced in obese mice by exposure to 90 psi absolute air pressure for six hours followed by decompression to sea level within one minute. (2) Compounds with anti-BK and anti-H activity such as 2-(4-phenylpoperazinylmethyl) cyclohexanone (PPCH) prevent or ameliorate development of DS in mice, hamsters, and rats. (3) Current experiments suggest that dimethothiazine (Migristene) which combines anti-H, anti-5HT and anti-BK activities can also prevent DS in mice. (4) A new humoral Smooth Muscle-Acting Factor (SMAF), capable of increasing vascular permeability and responsiveness of smooth muscle to BK and other stimulants was recently found in blood and tissues of a variety of animal species including humans. (5) SMAF activity increases in DS. (6) Decompression from 90 psi to sea level produces DS in obese but not in thin mice. Even when decompression to sea level is followed by exposure to altitude, only a small percentage of thin mice develop DS. However, when SMAF is administered to these "non-susceptible" thin mice prior to their hypobaric exposure the incidence of DS increases appreciably. (7) PPCH counteracts this effect of SMAF and prevents DS. Smooth muscle stimulating factors released or activated in DS can induce tissue responses that could contribute to the production of the syndrome (e.g. circulatory changes favoring formation of gas bubbles, respiratory changes interfering with nitrogen elimination, production of pain, increased vascular permeability contributing to hemoconcentration and to hypovolemic shock etc.). The postulated implication of such humoral factors in the mechanism of DS, supported by the above findings, brings up new pathogenic considerations and provides the basis for a novel pharmacological approach for the prevention or amelioration of this malady.

409.
CHRYSSANTHOU, C.P.
Humoral factors in the pathogenesis of decompression sickness (DS).
In: Ackles, K.N. ed. Blood-bubble interaction in decompression sickness. Proceedings of an international symposium held at Defence and Civil Institute of Environmental Medicine, Downsview, Ontario, Canada, p.165-170. Published by the Institute, December 1973. (DCIEM Conference Proceedings 73-CP-960)

The results of these investigations on the pathogenesis of DS indicate: 1. Certain pathologic alterations observed in DS exhibit similarities to some of the histologic changes seen in animals treated with bradykinin. 2. Bradykinin increased mortality and intensified some of the pathologic changes produced in DS. 3. The activity of SMAF, a new humoral smooth muscle stimulating agent, increases in DS. 4. Obese mice are more susceptible to DS than their thin siblings. 5. SMAF increases the susceptibility of thin mice to DS. 6. Compounds with activities against bradykinin, histamine and serotonin prevent or ameliorate DS in obese mice and counteract the increased susceptibility induced in thin mice by SMAF. 7. Preliminary observations suggest that in vitro compression-decompression or nitrogen bubbling of blood increase its smooth muscle stimulating activity. The above findings are consistent with the hypothesis that smooth muscle stimulating agents are implicated in the mechanism of DS. This pathogenetic concept and the striking protective effect of compounds which antagonize smooth muscle stimulations provide the basis for a new pharmacologic approach to the prevention or amelioration of the disease. (Author's conclusions)

410.
CHUSID, E.L., G.G. Maher, A. Nicogossian, A. Miller, A. Teirstein, R.A. Bader, M.E. Bader and J. Jacobson, II.
The effect of a pressurized environment (hyperbaric chamber) on pulmonary emphysema.
Amer. J. Med. 53(6):743-747; 1972.

Five patients with silent type emphysema were observed during 5 consecutive days of treatment in the hyperbaric chamber, then during and after 6 wk of intermittent treatment in the chamber. Although hypercapnia and acidosis were noted while the patients were in the chamber, there was no lasting adverse or beneficial effect on lung volumes or dynamics, diffusing capacities, arterial blood gas levels, oxygen consumption, minute ventilation, ventilation equivalent, pulmonary perfusion by scan technique, blood counts, ECGs or blood chemistries. The hyperbaric chamber was not indicated in the treatment of emphysema. However, its use would not be contraindicated if a patient with emphysema required the chamber for another treatable condition. (© BA)

411.
CIFALDI, E., C. Falconi and G. Marone.
Effetto protettivo dell'-idrossimetiltiofene nell'iperbaria da O_2.
[The protective effect of hydroxymethylthiophene in exposure to oxygen under elevated pressure].
Rass. Med. Sper. 19(1):13-17; 1973.

The effect of irradiated and nonirradiated hydroxymethylthiophene, a radioprotective drug, on the convulsion appearance time was studied in 180 rats submitted to 6 atm absolute of O_2. The maximum effect in preventing and delaying the appearance of the convulsion was observed when the irradiated drug was used for 40 hr. The results obtained were critically discussed. (CMM) (© BA)

412.
CIRIA UNDERWATER ENGINEERING GROUP.
The principles of safe diving practice 1972.
London, CIRIA Underwater Engineering Group, 1972.

This handbook is intended to minimize the dangers of diving. The contents are as follows: Personnel-responsibilities, qualification and classification; General operating and safety instructions; Compression chambers; Decompression;

Equipment; Accidents and incidents; First aid. The subjects are all rather briefly dealt with. Appendixes cover such subjects as the location of emergency chambers; lists of reference publication in the field; a glossary of terms; a list of locations where qualified doctors can be found; samples of forms for registers, certificates, records, examinations, etc.; pamphlets of concise advice for divers, for diving contractors, and for the users of diving services. (MFW/BSCP)

413.
CIZMIC, M., A. Frankio and R. Skarica.
X-ray bone changes in caisson disease.
Med. J. 94(9):23-27; 1972.
(Translation of Lijec. Vjesn. 94(9):449-452; 1972.)

The authors report here on data gathered from examination of 54 sponge and coral divers. After discussing the pathogenesis of decompression sickness, he describes the radiological changes observed in men of long diving experience. The bone changes were of two main types: rarefaction, which is not specific to decompression sickness, and condensation, which is. The condensation is of two types: (1) compact foci, usually located on the head of the humerus or femur, and (2) the less common trabecular type, which appears as small, stringy and dense shadows. Infarctions of the diaphysis are fairly common, sequestrations, usually on the humeral head, are less so. The disease does not appear to be age-connected, but rather to be related to length of diving experience. (MFW/UMS)

414.
CLARK, J.M., R.D. Sinclair and J.B. Lenox.
Tolerance of normal man to the interacting stresses.
Physiologist 14:123; 1971.

Abstract only. Entire item quoted: During exposure to inspired PCO_2 ($PICO_2$) levels of 0, 10, 20, 30 and 40 mm Hg, 9 volunteers in excellent physical condition ran at 4 different speeds on a treadmill at a 10% grade for a total time of 24 minutes. Treadmill speed was increased every 6 minutes and measurements were made during the last 2 minutes of each period. Average values of oxygen consumption (VO_2), which were not altered by changes in $PICO_2$, were 1.08, 1.78, 3.00 and 3.57 L/min at the 4 speeds. Maximum VO_2 measured during air breathing in the same group of subjects was 4.43 L/min or 63 ml-kg min. Ventilation, arterial PCO_2 and arterial pH were altered smoothly and progressively in response to increasing severity of the interacting stresses of exercise and hypercarbia. Average values of these parameters for the highest VO_2-$PICO_2$ combination were 169 L/min, 64 mm Hg and 7.12, respectively. Severe symptoms and ventilatory measurements indicated that physiological limits were approached during exercise at a $PICO_2$ of 40 mm Hg. Two of the subjects collapsed while running at the highest speed in this atmosphere, but both were able to complete the entire run on subsequent attempts. Cardiac arrhythmias were not observed during exercise except for the random occurrence of occasional premature ventricular contractions. The data obtained from these experiments permit the derivation of predictive curves which describe physiological responses to any combination of exercise and $PICO_2$ over the ranges that were studied.

415.
CLARK, J.M.
Ventilatory response to combined exercise and hypercapnia in man.
Fed. Proc. 32(3,pt.1):385;Mar. 1973.

Abstract only. Entire item quoted: Nine well-conditioned subjects were exposed to inspired CO_2 ($PICO_2$) levels of 0, 10, 20, 30 and 40 mm Hg at rest and at 4 exercise work loads which produced average O_2 uptake (VO_2) values of 1.08, 1.78, 3.00 and 3.57 L/min. At the most extreme $PICO_2$-VO_2 combination, ventilation (VE) was nearly maximal and average tidal volume was more than 61% of the vital capacity. Configuration of the VE-VO_2 relationship was altered progressively from curvilinear with upward concavity at 0 mm Hg $PICO_2$ to nearly linear at 20 mm Hg $PICO_2$ to curvilinear with downward concavity at 40 mm Hg $PICO_2$. These data are consistent with increasingly severe mechanical influences upon ventilation as maximal limits are approached. The average slopes of the VE-arterial PCO_2 ($PaCO_2$) relationships at rest and at the 4 incremental work loads were 3.59, 4.70, 4.05, 2.40 and 1.34 L/min/mm Hg, respectively. Both the increase in the VE-$PaCO_2$ slope at the lowest work load and the progressive decrease at higher work loads were statistically significant. It is concluded that the ventilatory response to hypercapnia during exercise differs from that observed at rest. The increased ventilatory response during light exercise may be related to stimulation of the reticular activating system, while the progressive reduction in response during the transition from light to heavy exercise is probably associated with negative mechanical influences.

416.
CLARK, J.M.
Tolerance and adaptation to acute and chronic hypercapnia in man.
In: Battelle Columbus Laboratories. Proceedings, 1973 divers' gas purity symposium, November 27-28, 1973, p. I-1-I-20. U.S. Navy Supervisor Diving, Nav. Ships Syst. Comm., Rep. 2-73, 1973.

Symptomatic and ventilatory responses to acute and chronic hypercapnia are described. Although these effects are barely detectable at inspired PCO_2 levels of 15 mm Hg or less, they are severe, incapacitating and even lethal at inspired partial pressures which exceed 100 mm Hg. Tolerable levels of inspired PCO_2 in man are reduced by exercise and can be increased by the compensatory changes which accompany chronic exposure to hypercapnia. Two sets of criteria which should be applied to the selection of acceptable inspired PCO_2 limits in the design of life-support systems are described. (Author's abstract)

417.
CLARKE, G.M., A.T. Sandison and I.McA. Ledingham.
Acute pulmonary oxygen toxicity — a pathophysiological study in spontaneously breathing anaesthetised dogs.
In: Wada, J. and I. Takashi, eds. Proceedings of the fourth international congress on hyperbaric medicine, Sapporo, Japan, Sept. 1969, p.1-4. Baltimore, Williams and Wilkins, 1970.

A direct toxic action on lung tissue is suggested by the marked respiratory distress observed in animals and humans exposed to increased pressure of oxygen, particularly when supported by the sort of autopsy evidence which has been described in the past. Much of the pulmonary pathology reported by previous workers, however, may reflect mainly terminal and post-mortem changes. By the time that shunting was demonstrable in the present study there was already evidence of considerable central nervous system involvement, as indicated by the altered respiratory patterns, and almost certainly, myocardial deterioration. (Authors' conclusions)

418.
CLARKE, G.M., G. Smith, A.T. Sandison and I. McA. Ledingham.
Acute pulmonary oxygen toxicity in spontaneously breathing anesthetized dogs.
Amer. J. Physiol. 224:248-255;Feb. 1973.

A pathophysiological study of pulmonary oxygen toxicity was performed using 12 pure-bred anesthetized beagle hounds. Six control animals, breathing a mixture of 40% oxygen-60% nitrogen at normal atmospheric pressure (1 atmosphere absolute (Ata)), survived 24 hr without significant change in the measured physiological variables. Six animals breathing 100% oxygen at twice atmospheric pressure (2 Ata) became apneic and died between 16 and 21 hr. The latter group showed a consistent sequence of change in breathing pattern, but the alveolar-arterial oxygen tension gradient ($(A\text{-}a)DO_2$) did not rise until shortly before apnea occurred. Macroscopic and light microscopic study of the lungs in all six animals breathing 100% oxygen showed little difference from the control group. Thus the concept that progressive lung damage was the principal cause of death in dogs dying from acute oxygen toxicity at 2 atmospheres was difficult to substantiate. In six additional beagle hounds breathing 66% oxygen-33% nitrogen at 3 Ata, nitrogen was found to lengthen survival time and abolish respiratory irregularities. Pulmonary histological changes were again minimal. (Authors' abstract)

419.
CLARKSON, D.P., C.L. Schatte and J.P. Jordan.
Thermal neutral temperature of rats in helium-oxygen, argon-oxygen and air.
Amer. J. Physiol. 222:1494-1498;June 1972.

Recent attempts to define a nonthermal component of inert gas effects on metabolic rate have necessitated the adjustment of the ambient temperature such that thermal conductive influence was negligible. Accordingly, an attempt was made to determine the thermal neutral temperature of fed rats exposed to 80% mixtures of helium, nitrogen, or argon with oxygen at ambient pressure. Adult male Holtzman rats were exposed to these mixtures for up to four hours at temperatures ranging from 25 to 35C. Oxygen consumption, tail surface, and deep-body temperature were continuously monitored. An experimentally determined thermal neutral range of 26-28C in air and 31-33C in helium corresponded to the relationship empirically predicted for these mixtures. Although not as clearly defined, the thermal neutral range for the argon-oxygen mixture appeared to be 27-29C, which is slightly higher than predicted. Significant depression of the three parameters in argon relative to air measured at the respective thermal neutral points implied that there was a nonthermal influence in argon. Although the metabolic effect of helium was largely thermal in nature, the possibility of a direct effect could not be ruled out. (Authors' abstract)

420.
CLAUSNER, E., Jr. and W.J. Greenert.
The status of the Navy's undersea technology program.
Mar. Technol. Soc. J. 7:38-45;Jan./Feb. 1973.

The authors discuss operational and developmental systems that fall into three categories: manned submersible vehicles, unmanned search and recovery, and diver/swimmer equipment. Operational manned submersibles are Alvin 6,000, NR-1, Dolphin, Trieste, Turtle and Seacliff. Developmental manned submersibles are: Alvin 12,000 (the present vehicle redesigned to a 12,000 foot depth capability), DSRV-1 and 2, ADDS-20, and Makakai. DSRV is designed to rescue submarine personnel. Makakai is a transparent hull two-man vehicle with a depth capability of 600 feet and a life support capability of 12 hours, with an emergency capability of 36 hours. Alvin, is primarily used as a research submersible. The similar, but larger, Sea Cliff and Turtle are used for training, for search and recovery, and for ocean engineering. The launch and recovery platforms LARP and BALARE are described. The ADDS-20 is in the thinking stage; it will have 20,000 foot depth capability. In the operational unmanned search-recovery system category are CURV III, NRL Towed Fish, Teleprobe, Scripps Towed Fish, Quickfind, Deep Ops and Lift Cable Transfer; developmental are RUW-20, LOSS, and Semi-submerged Platform. Navy diving systems are: (operational) DDS MK I

MOD 0, DDS MK II MOD 0, SDS 450, standard scuba, MARK V Hardhat, Diver Equipment System, MK 10 MOD 4 UBA, U.S. Navy MK I Diver Mask, and EX 8/9 SDV. The first two are saturation diving systems for two and eight divers respectively. A record open ocean dive of 1,010 feet was carried out by the MK II in June 1972. The aspect of the Diver Equipment System currently receiving concentrated effort is the development of a physiological monitoring system. Underlying all these programs is the Deep Submergence Bio-Medical Development Project, which is the only existing coordinated program for research into the physiology, microbiology, pharmacology, toxicology, psychology and bioengineering to further diver capability. Expanded decompression tables, establishment of a decompression data bank, and development of a Doppler bubble detector are among recent accomplishments. The Deep Ocean Technology Program functions as a series of inter-related hardware developments integrated into focal projects: for example, Titanes, which has developed heavy plate titanium for hulls, which will be used in the redesigned Alvin-12,000. Other projects include the development of reliable, compensated electric systems, of acoustic imaging systems, for use in conditions unsuitable for optical systems, work systems, including the Remoted Unmanned Work System (RUWS) which will operate at 20,000 feet. This is scheduled for testing in 1975. Ocean engineering construction systems are also part of the program, such as the long-term sea construction demonstration termed SEACON II. Advanced undersea technology is disseminated by the Navy Deep Ocean Technology Handbook. (MFW/BSCP)

421.
CLAUTICE, W.G. and H.E. Sheets.
Submarine tanker navigation in the arctic.
In: Marine industries: problems and opportunities. Ninth annual conference of the Marine Technology Society, p.471-488. Washington, D.C. Marine Technology Society, 1973.

The current concept of a submarine tanker for the transport of Arctic crude oil is discussed. A critical element of this system is underwater navigation which is analyzed considering safety and economics in relation to the hazards involved. A route analysis and vehicle characteristics are presented which define the problem and lead to a recommended optimum navigation system. The general conclusions reached are that due to the hazards involved and relative lack of experience with large submarines, a vessel of moderate tonnage should be built as a prototype for the East Coast Market or a vessel of the proposed 300,000 DWT could be built for the Northern route to European markets. (Authors' abstract)

422.
CNEXO-COMEX
Physalie V. Centre experimental hyperbare de la COMEX. November 1970.
[Physalie V. Experimental hyperbaric center of COMEX, November 1970].
Marseille, France. CNEXO-COMEX, Rep. 71/296, 110p. 1971.

The "Physalie V" experiment was designed to test a new method of pressurization derived from theory concerning saturation gradients. Two divers were able to attain the depth of 520m. and to remain there comfortably for 77 minutes. (Total experiment time, five days) but neurological and electrographic signs were noted simultaneously in the two subjects at 350m. An early "no joint juice syndrome" was noted by both subjects, and a slight nasal obstruction was observed from 300m. At the extreme depth, both subjects felt well, but did not perform well on the exercise test. Trembling and muscular difficulties were noted. Reaction times and manual dexterity were also affected. Changes in EEG activity were also observed after 300m, and disappeared at about that depth during the ascent. Sleep and dream disturbances occurred during the two nights passed at greater depths. In the author's view, this experiment helps to confirm the existence of the High Pressure Nervous Syndrome. (MEMH/UMS)

423.
CNEXO/COMEX
Sagittaire I. Centre experimental hyperbare de la COMEX.
[Sagittaire I. Experimental hyperbaric center of COMEX].
Marseille, France, CNEXO/COMEX, Rep. 71/296, 119p. Nov. 1971.

Thermal variations and blood parameters were studied in four subjects over a period of 24 days at six successive depths and under oxygen partial pressures ranging from near-normoxia to the limits of hyperoxia. Very discreet symptoms of the High Pressure Nervous Syndrome appeared during rapid pressurization from 152 to 300m (maximum experimental depth). Sensorimotor performances were slightly diminished during the experiment, but no effect in intellectual performance was noted. Muscular performance was minimally affected at 300m. Joint discomfort was noted at depths greater than 75m, but was tolerable and did not seem to affect manual dexterity. Blood parameters showed no important changes, except for a decrease in the number of blood platelets during decompression, and increases in haptoglobin levels and in blood osmotic pressure. The authors conclude that the greatest difficulties faced by the divers at these depths are bacterial and mycotic infections; they recommend further investigation of these and of the biophysical parameters. (MEMH/UMS)

424.
COALSON, J.J., J.J. Beller and L.J. Greenfield.
Effects of 100 per cent oxygen ventilation on pulmonary ultrastructure and mechanics.
J. Path. Bact. 104:267-273; 1971.

Comparison of the lungs of dogs exposed to room air with those of dogs exposed to ventilation of one or both lungs with 100 per cent oxygen shows that exposure to 100 per cent oxygen for so short a period as 15-30 min. produces changes in the lungs. Moreover, when one lung was exposed to 100 per cent oxygen, the other, whether ventilated with room air or not, showed morphological alterations comparable with that exposed to 100 per cent oxygen, suggesting that a blood-borne factor may be responsible for the lung damage. (Authors' summary)

425.
COBET, A.B.
Tektite 2: Microbiological aspects.
In: Miller, J.W., J.D. Van Derwalker, R.A. Waller, eds. Tektite 2: Scientists-in-the-sea, p.IX-36 - IX-52. Washington, D.C. Department of the Interior, August 1971.

The relationship between man and his environment is important in maintaining a proper balance among those microorganisms which comprise his indigenous microflora and hence his health and well-being. Slight changes in the environment may reflect themselves as an alteration in this balance. The conditions necessary to sustain the Tektite habitat in the submerged state from an engineering standpoint and the confinement of the aquanauts to the habitat and marine environment, the interactions of the aquanauts, both with each other and the environment, are major factors, each with its myriad of minor interacting elements which can affect man's indigenous microflora. A study of the effect of these conditions in prolonged submergence is necessary to define the effects of such an environment on the microorganisms associated with the aquanauts. . . The entire microbiological study for all missions has not been completed. It would be premature at this point to make further speculations on the basis of this single mission which was not studied to the same extent as the other remaining missions. This mission was used primarily as an opportunity to check the handling of samples and procedures of identification of bacteria; however, meaningful results were obtained. At the completion of the study a separate complete report will be made available. (Author)

426.
COCKETT, A.T.K., J.C. Saunders, F.L. Depenbusch and S.M. Pauley.
Combined treatment in decompression sickness.
In: Wada, J. and I. Takashi, eds. Proceedings of the fourth international congress on hyperbaric medicine, Sapporo, Japan, Sept. 1969, p.89-92. Baltimore, Williams, and Wilkins, 1970.

The authors report on 15 cases of decompression sickness treated by recompression supplemented by dextran as a plasma expander. It is stated that blood volume studies should be made initially. Blood pressure, pulse and respiration must be carefully monitored during the early stages of recompression. Urinary output should be carefully monitored. In three cases, dehydration had apparently been severe before diving, due to the injection of antibiotics for a few days beforehand. In these cases, decompression sickness was rather severe. (MFW/BSCP)

427.
COCKETT, A.T.K., S.M. Pauley and A.P. Roberts.
Advances in treatment of decompression sickness: an evaluation of Heparin.
In: Fructus, X., Ed. Third international conference on hyperbaric and underwater physiology, p.156-159. Paris, Doin, 1972.

Lipid emboli co-exist with gaseous emboli in decompression sickness. Heparin, an antilipemic agent, can reverse the deleterious effects of decompression sickness. We illustrate significant blood pressure changes which are modified by Heparin. (Authors' summary)

428.
COCKETT, A.T.K., S.M. Pauley, A. Pilmanis and A.P. Roberts.
Formation of lipid emboli after significant decompression.
In: Aerospace Medical Association. 1972 annual scientific meeting, Bal Harbour, Florida, May 1972. Preprints, p.219. Published by the Association.

The purpose of this study is to report the lipid profiles obtained in dogs prior to overcompression and 3 hours after resurfacing from depths of 165 feet. The lipid profiles of human volunteers submerging to 200 feet and maintaining depth for 5 minutes are also included. In humans pre- and postdive blood samples were significantly altered for cholesterol and unesterified free fatty acid determinations (Table II). Both increased following the dive, 192 to 203 mg% and 0.51 to 0.69 mEq per liter, ($P = < .02$ and $P = < .005$ respectively). Manifestations of decompression sickness include shock as an accompanying condition and herald the occurrence of gaseous and lipid emboli. (Authors)

429.
COCKETT, A.T.K.
Pathophysiology of shock secondary to underwater decompression sickness.
Bull. Soc. Int. Chir. 32:229-237;Mar./Apr. 1973.

A plasma deficit usually develops after decompression sickness. Gaseous and lipid emboli probably trigger the pathophysiologic mechanisms. Dextran (70) or colloidal replacement will improve survival rates. The lungs are a major target organ. Pulmonary lung scans are a useful means of localizing emboli. The role of heparin is still conjectural. (Author's summary)

430.
COHEN, J.M.
An experimental analysis of the dynamics of a submerged tethered cradle.
Woods Hole, Mass., Woods Hole Oceanog. Inst., Rep. WHOI-72-45, 73p. June 1972.
(AD 745 379)

Submerged recovery of small submersibles by means of surface tethered platforms offers the possibility of operations in sea states higher than is now possible using surface recovery means. The Woods Hole Oceanographic Institution's submersible support catamaran LULU has such a tethered system. The system consisting of cradle, chains, and hoist is designed to recover DSRV Alvin at a depth of 100 feet, and then lift the submersible rapidly through the air-sea interface. A 1/40 scale model of the catamaran chain and cradle was constructed to investigate cradle heave and pitch response in regular sinusoidal waves. Model tests were conducted at the Massachusetts Institute of Technology Tow Tank Facility and data was recorded electronically and photographically. (Author) (GRA)

431.
COLEMAN, R.F.
Intelligibility and perceptual aspects of helium speech.
In: Sergeant, R.L. and T. Murry, eds. Processing helium speech: proceedings of a Navy-sponsored workshop, August 1971, U.S. Nav. Submar. Med. Res. Lab., Rep. NSMRL 708, p.11-12. May 22, 1972.

The author reaches the following conclusions regarding intelligibility testing: (1) No communication lexicon based on phonemic restriction is likely to be successful. (2) Communication devices should be tested with naive listeners, using a closed set of sentences or words. (3) The practice of using multiple forms of the same test is a dubious one, since equivalent word lists might not be equivalent at depth. (4) A restricted lexicon, resulting in increasing familiarity with a given word, is necessary. (5) The lexicon should include certain types of words in specific positions within a transmission. (6) Talker-listener tasks carried out under standardized conditions are the most effective means of achieving operational evaluation. (MFW/BSCP)

432.
COLEMAN, R.F. and H. Hollien.
Standardization of speech materials for underwater research I: comparative intelligibility of monosyllabic word lists.
Gainesville, Fla., Univ. Fla., Commun. Sci. Lab., Rep. CSL/ONR 25, 14p. Sept. 1, 1972.

Two experiments are reported in which the underwater intelligibility scores of four standard word lists were compared. As would be expected, closed-set word lists produced higher scores than did open-ended tests. Alternate forms of two tests were compared and the results indicated that lists which are "equated for difficulty" in normal environments also are reasonably equated underwater. A preliminary analysis of phoneme type distortion was derived from one closed-set test. The results appeared to demonstrate that, for this type of experiment, the most common phoneme error was in place of production and that fricatives were most affected. (DCD abstract)

433.
COLER, C.R., R.M. Patton and E.C. Lampkin.
Effects of prolonged confinement in a hyperbaric environment on short-term memory.
In: Aerospace Medical Association. 1971 annual scientific meeting. Houston, Texas, April 1971. Preprints, p.152-153. Published by the Association, 1971.

This study was part of a physiological and behavioral test program conducted to support the Tektite II Program. . . The Ames Crew Evaluator (ACE), a test device for assessing human performance in a wide variety of stress situations, was used to measure short-term memory, one aspect of higher order functioning. This test was designed to determine the amount of initial performance decrement, and to show whether this decrement increases with continued exposure or decreases due to adaptation. . . Despite performance impairment at the beginning of confinement, the subjects were able to adapt to the adverse effects of nitrogen narcosis and confinement. However, results of previous studies indicate that the actual Tektite undersea environment, involving aquanaut exposure to sea water, strenuous exercise, cramped living quarters, and danger, in addition to the stresses present in this study might be expected to cause greater performance impairment than was recorded in the pressure chamber. (Authors)

434.
COLES, R.R.A.
Labyrinth disorders in British Navy diving.
In: Hesser, C.M. and D. Linnarsson eds. Proceedings of the first annual scientific meeting of the European Undersea Biomedical Society, Stockholm, 13-15 June 1973. Forsvarsmedicin 9:428-433;July 1973.

In 1,000 experimental deep dives, with 10% incidence of decompression sickness, 5% of the cases were of the otological type. Three cases were auditory only, one vestibular only, and one was mixed. These non-barotraumatic cases were not limited to the decompression stages of the dive, and the site of the trouble was not always in the inner ear. The author emphasizes the importance of "comprehensive audiological investigation to distinguish between cochlear and peripheral neural lesion, central auditory tests to detect and distinguish between brainstem and auditory cortex lesions, and electrocochleography. Vestibular function tests, with ENG recording plus and minus visual fixation, can help to distinguish between central and peripheral sites of vestibular disorders." (MFW/UMS)

435.
COLLIPP, B.G. and C.A. Sellars.
The role of one atmosphere chambers in subsea operations.
In: 1972 Offshore Technology Conference, May 1-3, Houston, Texas. Preprints, Vol I, p.209-214. Published by the conference, 1972.

Subsea chambers maintained at one atmosphere internal pressure will find numerous applications in development of underwater producing systems. They permit use of conventional oil field equipment on the sea floor and provide means for on-site maintenance. A chamber designed to contain a wellhead has been built and tested together with a diving bell for personnel access. Concepts have been developed for subsea manifolds and production stations in one atmosphere chambers. This could be expanded to include pipeline pump stations and instrument and control centers. During the development stage, it would be desirable to field test selected prototype designs. This would provide operating experience in current water depths and design information for extension of the concept to deep water. (Authors' abstract)

436.
COLTON, J.S. and A.R. Freeman.
Intracellular measurements in a closed hyperbaric chamber.
J. Appl. Physiol. 35:578-580;Oct. 1973.

A method for intracellular current passage and voltage recording with two glass microelectrodes mounted on one micromanipulator inside a closed hyperbaric chamber is described. Impalement and maintenance of the electrodes within the cell is accomplished with an electronically pulsed microdrive. The technique permits current passage and voltage recordings to be made in high-pressure, pure-oxygen atmospheres without the danger of fire or explosion. (Authors' abstract)

437.
COMAISH, S.
Instantaneous decompression and the skin.
Arch. Dermatol. 108(2):215-217; 1973.

Suction blister formation in human skin is preceded by intraepidermal vacuolation, which regresses as the blister forms. The vacuoles are shown to contain fluid, not gas, and probably represent a reaction to injury by suction accompanied by increased permeability of epidermal structures. (© BA)

438.
COMEX.
100 hours at 500 meters.
CNEXO/COMEX Rep., 8 p. Feb./Mar. 1972.

This is a preliminary report on the results of the simulated heliox dive carried out by COMEX in Marseilles February 21-March 6, 1972. A pre-dive of 6 days at 33 feet was made, during which environmental parameters were evaluated. Average temperature was 89°F, average humidity was 55, oxygen partial pressure was 4 atm during compression and saturation, and 5 atm during decompression. Compression to 1640 feet took 49 hours. The divers remained at this depth for 100 hours. Decompression took 141-1/2 hours. Complete physiological monitoring was carried out during the dive. The first symptoms of hpns appeared at 100-1200 feet, and increased down to 1640 feet, becoming stabilized after the first 40 hours at 1640 feet. Constant polygraphic monitoring made it possible to complete the 100-hour bottom time. Symptoms were identical with those observed during the Physalie dives, i.e., static tremor, muscular jerks, lack of coordination, EEG changes, lessening of awareness. However, a fairly good persistance of motor, psychomotor and intellectual faculties was demonstrated by the satisfactory execution of psychomotor, and local static and dynamic effort tests. Muscular effort tests showed a sharp drop in stamina, associated with a noticeable respiratory limitation. Articular symptoms were greatly reduced by the slow compression, and disappeared during saturation. The hpns symptoms remained stabilized during the decompression period until the 1000-foot depth was reached. It is noted that these disorders were mitigated by the compression curve, which had decreased to 14 feet per hour at maximum depth. Before further depths are attempted, thorough analysis of the data gathered here must be made. Also, experiments at the same depth with other divers must be carried out. The practical conclusions drawn from this experiment are (1) working dives at 1000 feet are safe; (2) selected divers can work safely at 1400 feet; (3) the depth limit for complete physiological safety is probably around 1700 feet. (MFW/BSCP)

439.
COMMITTEE ON UNDERWATER TELECOMMUNICATION.
Present and future civil uses of underwater sound.
Washington, D.C., National Academy of Sciences, 1970, 131p.

The committee specifically turned its attention toward two questions: who is going to be using what kind of underwater acoustic devices during the next 10 years, and what will be the frequency bands in which these devices will be operating. Specific areas covered included acoustic marking devices, submersibles, seismic exploration systems, acoustic telemetry and control systems, survey markers and fishing. As in any report, the conclusions represent a consensus. Sometimes one feels, however, that a better description would be that it represents a collection of differing, unrelated opinions. For example, at one point the report leads one to believe that by 1975 there will be a large number of acoustically controlled deepwater oil fields with a high density of different acoustic devices operating in a rather restricted frequency band. Yet in another section, it is concluded that no real restrictions on frequency allocation are necessary because there will be no really high-density operations. Recommendations of the committee were rather limited. They included the following general ideas. First, there should be no governmental frequency regulation in the foreseeable future, except a band of frequencies with specified codes which should be designated for (a) marking submersibles, (b) marking submerged structures, (c) navigational aids, (d) search and rescue, and (3) recovery of lost objects. Secondly, a "distress signal for use in the common underwater telephone bands" should be designated. Finally, organizations like MTS and manufacturer groups should develop their own voluntary standardization procedures. (From review by S. Riter in Mar. Technol. Soc. J. 6:61; Mar./Apr. 1972)

440.
COMMON, R.P. and M.P. Kettle.
Diver suit heating.
Underwater J. 4:20-29;Feb. 1972.

Divers require thermal protection to conserve body heat. Thermal insulation problems increase with depth and duration of dives. Eventually diver insulation requires supplementing with positive heat input and ultimately the heating of respirable gas as well. Divers' suits may be heated directly or indirectly by electricity, or by hot water produced locally or piped from the sea surface. Electricity is convenient but involves special precautions against electric shock. Problems are common to all diving but three zones emerge with characteristic optimum solutions. 0-20 metres, shallow and oxygen diving, 20-60 metres, general compressed air diving. Beyond 60 metres, oxygen/helium mixtures introduce special problems. Much fundamental and aimed research is proceeding. Several practical suit designs exist, but no perfect solution has emerged. The state of the art advances, and is capable of producing sound practical designs in the near future. (Authors' abstract)

441.
COMMON, R.P.
Diver's progress — an undersea odyssey.
Meerestechnik 4:27-32;Feb. 1973.

The author traces the development of diving equipment. The "flexible diving dress," or hard hat rig designed originally by Augustus Siebe, was the first satisfactory diving suit: it is described in some detail. Some of the mechanics of respiration are discussed, as are oxygen toxicity and nitrogen narcosis. The development of the "integrated diving system in which heated suit and breathing apparatus have been designed to be used together, and the umbilical incorporates gas hose, electric-heating supply cable and telephone cable, was demonstrated at the Oceanology International 1972 exhibition held at Brighton in March of that year. The development of various components such as submersible decompression chambers and deck decompression chambers (here called compression chambers) is discussed, along with the advent of saturation diving techniques and gas-recovery equipment. The closed circuit breathing apparatus March 10, developed by General Electric, consists of a cylinder of oxygen, one of helium, a CO_2 absorbent canister, two breathing bags, oxygen sensors and valves to inject either oxygen or helium according to the PO_2. The sensors are duplicated, and there is also a third independent sensor to be used in case of malfunction. Three successful habitat projects have been Tektite, Helgoland, and Aegir. The heat conduction property of helium has brought about development of methods of heating breathing mixtures as well as the diver's body. Speech problems of helium appear to have been satisfactorily overcome by an electronic system designed by Dr. Gill of the UK Admiralty Research Laboratory. (MFW/SCD)

442.
CONBOY, M.E.
Project Quick Find: A marine mammal system for object recovery.
U.S. Nav. Undersea Res. Dev. Cent., Rep. NUC-TP-268-Rev-1, 37p. June 1972.
(AD 744 232)

Project Quick Find is a recovery system that consists of two men, a rubber boat, a reel of nylon line, a pinger receiver, a grabber device, and a California sea lion. It was developed to provide the Navy with an effective alternative to the use of divers and submersibles for the underwater recovery of small objects. During training sessions four California sea lions demonstrated the ability to locate and recover pinged objects from a depth of 500 feet. In an actual system demonstration they recovered an inert depth charge from 180 feet of water. The depth charge was 6 feet long and weighed approximately 500 pounds, but the breakout force required to pull it out of the ocean bottom was greater than 500 pounds. Recovery hardware was designed and fabricated that can be used by the sea lion to recover objects weighing approximately 2000 pounds (Author) (GRA)

443.
CONDA, K.J. and F.W. Armstrong, Jr.
A self-contained load-handling pontoon.
U.S. Nav. Med. Res. Inst., Rep 4 on Project M4306-03.2040DAC9, 6p. May 1973.

To increase diver safety, endurance, and performance, and to measure dive work in assembly projects, a self-contained load-handling pontoon was developed. The pontoon is light and small enough for one man to handle, yet big enough to carry a good pay-load. It enables a diver to lift a heavy object, move it from point "A" to point "B" in complete safety, and to control the object's up-and-down movement within a matter of inches. Testing results and specifications of the pontoon are discussed; recommendations for improving future models are made. This self-contained load-handling device should significantly extend the performance capability and safety of the working diver. (Authors' abstract)

444.
CONTI, V. and F. Sicardi.
Difficultes d'approche du metabolisme phosphocalique chez les aquanautes.
[Difficulties of the study of the phosphocalcic metabolism in aquanauts].
In: Fructus, X., ed. Third international conference on hyperbaric and underwater physiology, p.50-55, Paris, Doin, 1972.

The evaluation of the phosphocalcic metabolism was made by radiological negatives and biological analysis. These results indicated that the phosphocalcic metabolism was not particularly disturbed in the course of three saturation experiments but it was not possible to conclude that life in a hyperbaric environment is without effect on the skeleton. (Authors' conclusion translated by MFW/UMS)

445.
CONTI, V.
L'appareil locomoteur et la pratique des sports sous-marins.
[The locomotive apparatus and the practice of underwater sport].
Med. Sort 46(3):171-173; 1972.

The osteoarthropathies and muscular disorders related to compression and decompression are not discussed. Specific disorders include pain at the base of the neck, usually related to simple arthritis, pain in the anterior chest wall, aggravated by arm movement, back pain, caused chiefly by equipment, muscular cramp, usually resulting from cold. These disorders are rare, benign and easily treated. People suffering from certain types of chronic rheumatic disabilities can often benefit from underwater activity. However, osteoarticular weaknesses, whether congenital or resulting from trauma, must be kept under clinical and radiological surveillance, since they can constitute a disposition to decompression sickness. (MFW/BSCP)

446.
CONTI, V. and R. Sciarli.
Lesions osseuses chez le plongeur autonome.
[Bone lesions in the autonomous diver].
In: Hesser, D.M. and D. Linnarsson eds. Proceedings of the first annual scientific meeting of the European Undersea Biomedical Society, Stockholm, 13-15 June 1973. Forsvarsmedicin 9:525-527;July 1973.

Medical examinations of divers before hiring revealed clinically latent bone lesions in cases where there was no record of decompression accident. The pictures resembled benign bone islands or lacunae. The authors were struck by their frequent occurrence in compressed-air scuba divers. One case is described in which a diver had pain and difficulty of movement in his shoulder several months after having suffered a decompression accident affecting that area. Bone anomalies were not discovered in divers who performed deep dives with helium-oxygen. It is concluded that nitrogen is the principal cause, by disturbing the circulation in the spherical and hemispherical bone extremities. It is suggested that a diver who should not work with compressed air might be able to dive safely with helium-oxygen. Because of an apparent relationship between hyperlipidemia and osteonecrosis, no applicant with such a tendency should be permitted to dive at all, at least temporarily. Medico-legal questions are brought up here, in relation to occupational disease and damage suits. Radiological records are most important in this connection. (MFW/UMS)

447.
CONTI, V. and G. Segui.
L'alimentation des oceanautes.
[Nutrition of aquanauts].
In: Hesser, C.M. and D. Linnarsson eds. Proceedings of the first annual scientific meeting of the European Undersea Biomedical Society, Stockholm, 13-15 June 1973. Forsvarsmedicin 9:472-474;July 1973.

An underwater diet should be normal, light, balanced, varied, and should consist of about 4,000 calories a day. It is important to bear in mind the texture of foods, since they will be affected by pressure in the process of getting them to the habitat. Lack of appetite on the part of aquanauts seems to be related to fatigue. Conservation is an important problem in a habitat at 300 meters, whether the food is frozen, refrigerated, or in a sealed container. The necessity for giving working divers an education in nutrition is noted. (MFW/BSCP)

448.
COOK, R.B.
Temperature and pressure effects on Sodasorb and Baralyme.
Annapolis, Md., U.S. Nav. Acad., Rep. USNA-TSPR-25, 30p. May 19, 1972.
(AD 749 708)

Baralyme and Sodasorb are used by the U.S. Navy to remove the carbon dioxide in closed and semiclosed respirators. In this experiment, the two absorbents were studied in their effects of changing the temperature and pressure of the breathing apparatus. The inlet gas contained 2.5% surface equivalent carbon dioxide, and passed through the absorbent canister at a constant rate of about 40 liters/minute. The gas was humidified to 100% for all tests. The inlet gas temperatures ranged from 3C to 31C at 1 ata. The pressures ranged from 2 ata to 4 ata at 30C. The canister held 400 grams of absorbent for each test. The efficiency of the absorbent decreased as temperature decreased. The results from pressure tests indicated decreasing efficiency with depth. (Author) (GRA)

449.
COOKER, H.S.
Improvements in underwater voice communication.
Storrs, Conn., Univ. Conn., Dept. Speech, Rep. UCONN-IUVC/ONR-8, 12p. Apr. 1, 1972.
(AD 745 794)

Various methods and techniques were investigated for improving voice communication between diver/swimmers, within closed environments, and under adverse conditions resulting from water immersion. Improvements were sought in the reduction of channel noise, increased signal reception, reduced gas/pressure distortion, expansion of the useful auditory channel, and clearer diver/swimmer articulation. In order to accomplish these tasks, it was necessary to develop methodologies for better assessment of transducers and transmission channels. Furthermore, studies were conducted to determine the effect of word sequencing on message reception and effect of time/frequency distortion on the transmission of prosodic feature information. (Author) (GRA)

450.
COOPER, R.A. and D.J. Scarratt.
Evaluation of lock-out submarine "Deep Diver" for in situ biological work in boreal waters.
Helglander Wiss. Meeresunters. 24:112-119; 1973.
(Com 73-11426/6)

Six scientists and technicians were trained in lockout diving from the submersible "Deep Diver." A planned program of saturation diving on predetermined sites in depths of between 150 and 250 feet (46 and 76 m) was only partially successful because of extreme cold experienced by divers breathing heliox mixtures in 3.5°C in water, and because of inadequacies in the submarine handling system. An alternate system of bounce lock-out dives permitted completion of an abbreviated scientific program in depths down to 287 ft (87.5 m). Divers took photographs, rock and sediment core samples, and made collections of common benthic species for subsequent analysis for environmental contaminants. It was effectively proved that diver scientists can train rapidly for lock-out diving programs and perform effective scientific work. (Author) (GRA)

451.
COPLEY, A.L. and R.M. Jacobs.
Apparent viscosities of whole blood systems at moderate pressure.
Newark, N.J., Newark Coll. Eng. Dept. Mech. Eng., Rep. on contract N00014-71-A-0124, 18p. Apr. 1972.
(AD 740 853)

Experiments are summarized which present evidence that the apparent viscosity of blood is unlikely to vary significantly with hydrostatic pressures to pressures of 775 psi (fifty atmospheres). (GRA)

452.
CORRIOL, J.H.
Le froid et la noyade.
[Cold and drowning].
Med. Sport 46(3):154-162; 1972.
(Also published in Bull. Medsubhyp 7:22-36;Oct. 1972).

It is stated that many deaths attributed to drowning do in actual fact result from cold. The author discusses the physiological mechanisms of heat loss, giving diagrams from various sources which illustrate survival time at different temperatures; heat loss as a function of the thickness of the subcutaneous fat; the role of subcutaneous fat in thermal isolation and in the production of heat; water temperature and basal metabolism as a function of the season of the year; the variation of core temperature with the season of the year; the effects of exercise. The importance of restricting movements as much as possible, and of retaining as much clothing as possible, is emphasized. The only adaptive factor appears to be the seasonal change in thyroid secretion, discovered during studies made with the Korean Amas. (MFW/BSCP)

453.
CORRIOL J., J. Chouteau and J. Catier.
Human simulated diving experiments at saturation under oxygen-helium exposures to 500 meters: electroencephalographic data.
Aerosp. Med. 44:1270-1276;Nov. 1973.

The EEG data recorded during three saturation oxygen-helium simulated dives at depth are reported. In the Saturation III experiment, the depth of 500 m was attained without serious difficulty, owing to the use of compression at decreasing speed, interrupted by two stops (9 hrs at 50 m, and 27 hrs at 400 m). In Saturation I and II the compression was executed with a progressively increasing speed, including no stops. Severe clinical and EEG abnormalities were noted, primarily when attaining maximum depth (400 m) in Saturation II. These were not due to the effects of pressure and helium, as they disappeared in less than 12 hrs. during the stay at maximum depth. Abnormalities were probably linked to osmotic perturbations induced by unequal melting of the inert gas in the various tissues. The abnormalities could have been avoided by an adequate compression method. (Authors' abstract)

454.
CORWIN, R.F. and U. Conti.
Sea-floor electrical resistivity measurement using a diver-operated system.
In: 1973 Offshore Technology Conference, April/May 1973, Houston, Texas. Preprints, Vol. I, p.638-644. Published by the Conference.

The system used to measure bottom resistivity was designed for operation by two scuba-equipped divers and consists of separate current and voltage units, a length of line on which electrode separations are marked, and an underwater slate for recording data. The output of the current source is a 10Hz square wave, with amplitude adjustable between 0 and 500 milliamps in ten steps. Power is supplied by 16-D-size rechargeable nickel-cadmium batteries, in a series-parallel arrangement that provides a nominal 10-v output. Current electrodes are 1/4-in. (0.64 cm) diameter copper rods, 1/2-in. (1.27 cm) long. . . . The tests indicate that it is feasible to measure subbottom resistivity using a horizontal array deployed on the sea floor. The equipment used for this study, although reliable, was not very efficient. An improved system, incorporating prespaced multiple electrodes strung along a single line, along with digital readout for improved precision, would enable readings to be made rapidly from aboard ship and eliminate the need for diver operation. Such a system would provide economical and useful information about the geology and engineering properties of the sea floor. (Authors)

455.
COTNEY, A.D., III, G. Maples and D.F. Dyer.
The development of a computer-aided conceptual submarine design evaluation tool.
Auburn, Ala., Univ. Ala., Dept. Mech. Eng., Final Rep. on Contract N00014-73-A-0061-0001, 154p. Nov. 1973.
(AD 771,448/8GA)

The requirements for evaluating alternative conceptual submarine designs are presented. The morphology of a conceptual design evaluation tool is established and its basic components developed. Digital computer programs are used to facilitate analysis of design parameters. Representative parameters required by the design tool are determined for an existing submarine. A review of current research in the major areas of submarine design is presented. The effects of several of these technological advances are predicted for the example vessel through use of the design tool. (Authors) (GRA)

456.
COVEY, C.W.
Unisuit takes the chill out of diving.
UnderSea Technol. 13:39-42;Sept. 1972.

There has been a great need for a suit that will protect a diver from cold in long-duration shallow water dives. Many divers have found the Poseidon Unisuit, originally designed in Sweden, satisfactory for this purpose. It is a dry suit, made of 1/4 inch foam neoprene with nylon on both sides. The feet are an integral part of the suit. There is an undersuit of nylon fur, with socks attached. The four major advantages of the suit are: (1) warmth, (2) dryness, (3) buoyancy compensation, and (4) elimination of squeezing and chafing. It can be used with any kind of breathing apparatus. When tested with a wet suit and a non-compressible suit, the Unisuit was shown to provide the most protection. It combines the mobility of the wet suit with the warmth of deep diving dress. Unisuit has been proven in the Arctic diving experiments at Pt. Barrow, Alaska, and at Resolute Bay, Canada. It was used in conjunction with the General Electrics Mark X closed-circuit breathing system. (MFW/BSCP)

457.
COVEY, C.W.
X-rays check welds on Navy's deep diving system.
UnderSea Technol. 14:17;Feb. 1973.

Four Mark II Mod I saturation deep diving systems have been completed for the Navy by the Dixie Manufacturing Co. The system consists of a 66,000 pound deck decompression chamber, and a personnel transfer capsule that displaces 10 tons, and can operate at 850 feet. It will support eight men for 12 days. The Reliance Testing Laboratories, Inc., have tested the welding by X-ray, making 10,000 radiographic exposures to prove completely sound welding. (MFW/BSCP)

458.
COWAN, M.J., D.E. Chandler and S.L. Firess.
Biochemical indexes accompanying functional decay of working muscle in hyperbaric helium-oxygen-carbon dioxide environments.
Toxicol. Appl. Pharmacol. 26(4):585-595; 1973.

Innervated rat diaphragm tissues incubated in bicarbonate buffers saturated at high pressure with $He/O_2/CO_2$ gas mixtures were subjected to isometric work stresses. The muscles were then analyzed for content of creatine phosphate (CP), total creatine (TC), ATP, glycogen and lactate, as indicators of biochemical state. At 15.8-18 atm total pressure and at adequate PCO_2 (0.05 atm), PO_2 ($\geq$0.95 atm) and pH (approximately 7.4), the CP content of the stressed tissue rises by a factor of about 2 above control, the TC content falls to about 80% of control and remains constant, and the remaining biochemical indexes are essentially unchanged. At low PO_2 (0.22 atm) the initial increments in CP decay rapidly with extended incubation/work time, and a rise in tissue lactate is noted. Very high levels of PCO_2 (0.54-0.90 atm) in the hyperbaric gas phase accompanied by drops in buffei pH also lead to transient rise and then decay in the CP content of the muscle. At moderate PCO_2 (0.016-0.16 atm) the hyperbarically worked muscle is functionally and biochemically stable to changes in PCO_2 and buffer bicarbonate concentration, within the buffer pH range 7.4-6.9, but loses twitch function capability as the pH falls to 6.4 and below. These findings are interpreted in terms of tissue responses to pressure and work stresses involving anoxia and the direct action of increased acidity on the tissue. (© BA)

459.
COX, P.T.
Simulated caisson disease of bone.
In: Hesser, D.M. and D. Linnarsson eds. Proceedings of the first annual scientific meeting of the European Undersea Biomedical Society, Stockholm, 13-15 June 1973. Forsvarsmedicin 9:520-524;July 1973.

It would appear that the injection of embolic particles into the artery supplying the lower limb of the rabbit indicates that the arterial supply of the femoral head and to a lesser degree the shaft is poor in that it may be relatively easily obstructed. It also produces avascular necrotic bone lesions of the femur in sites that correspond to those that occur in caisson disease of bone and implies that the aetiological agent in caisson disease of bone may be the embolic occlusion of osseous vessels. (Author's conclusion)

460.
COX, P.T.
Caisson disease of bone.
J. Roy. Coll. Surg. 18:290-293;Sept. 1973.

Diagnosis of dysbaric osteonecrosis is performed by radiology, which reveals the existence of a lesion within three months of its inception, at the very least, and usually much longer. Also, radiology fails to predict joint involvement in the case of a juxta-articular lesion. The use of radioisotope scanning revealed that in some cases a positive radiograph coincided with a negative scan, and vice versa. It is explained that strontium is taken up in the area of the lesion during the period of increased activity and bone turnover, thus revealing the formation of a lesion in its early stages, as well as the cessation of activity which occurs when a lesion becomes static. Experiments were made with rabbits. It was concluded that a positive scan with a negative radiograph indicates that the lesion has not progressed enough to be radiologically visible. In the opposite situation, it is probable that the repair process has ceased, and the lesion is unlikely to progress. (MFW/BSCP)

461.
CRAPO, J. and D.F. Tierney.
Superoxide dismutase and oxygen toxicity.
Clin. Res. 21:222;Feb. 1973.

Abstract only. Entire item quoted: The free radical superoxide (O_2^-) is produced as an intermediate in the reduction of O_2 by a family of metalloglavoenzymes. O_2^- is highly reactive but it will dismute $H_2 O_2 + O_2$ in the presence of superoxide dismutase (SOD). Since O_2^- production might be increased by a high PO_2 we related SOD activity of lung to O_2 tolerance by exposing large rats to 86% O_2 (1 atm.) for 1, 3, 7 days. We then measured the SOD activity (Misra and Fridovich, J. Biol. Chem. 247:3170, 1972) in some rats and determined O_2 tolerance in the remaining rats by placing them in 99% O_2 for 72 hrs. The SOD values are expressed as % SOD of matched controls in air.

Days pretreated (85% O_2)	0	1	3	7
SOD/whole lung	100	109	121	146($P < .01$)
SOD/mg. DNA	100	113	118	133($P < .001$)
% survivors — 100% O_2	0	0	70	100

After 7 days of exposure to 85% O_2 SOD activity was also compared to the activity of an unrelated microsomal enzyme, succinate cytochrome c reductase, and showed a 45% increase ($P < .01$). Hemoglobin assays of these saline perfused lungs showed that whole blood contributed less than 1% to the SOD activity. After 7 days exposure to 85% O_2 10 rats were exposed to 99% O_2 for 7 additional days and SOD activity increased to 206%/whole lung and 169%/mg. DNA. SOD may have a role in oxygen tolerance.

462.
CUNNINGHAM, D.J.C., E.S. Petersen, T.G. Pickering and P. Sleight.
The effects of hypoxia, hypercapnia, and asphyxia on the baroreceptor-cardiac reflex at rest and during exercise in man.
Acta Physiol. Scand. 86:456-465;Dec. 1972.

The sensitivity of the baroreceptor-cardiac reflex was tested in 12 healthy subjects by relating changes in pulse interval to pressure changes induced by phenylephrine. Hypercapnia in high oxygen at rest was associated with a significant rise in systolic pressure and a significant fall of baroreflex sensitivity. Pulse interval changed little. The changes in exercise were qualitatively the same but much smaller. Hypoxia with hypocapnia at rest was associated with a substantial tachycardia but no significant change in pressure or in reflex sensitivity. In exercise the changes were similar except that baroreflex sensitivity was depressed more than by exercise itself. Asphyxia (hypercapnia with hypoxia) at rest was associated with a combination of the changes induced by the two stimuli separately. The observed baroreflex sensitivities were compared to values predicted from the previously reported relations of reflex sensitivity to either steady-state pulse interval (I_0) or the ratio of I_0 to systolic pressure (I_0/P_0). Values predicted from I_0/P_0 were in general closest to the observed values. In hypoxia at rest, however, both I_0 and I_0/P_0 changed, but reflex sensitivity remained unaltered, showing that mechanisms exist for influencing baroreflex sensitivity and other circulatory variables independently of one another. (Authors' abstract)

463.
CUNNINGHAM, D.J.C., M.G. Howson and S.B. Pearson.
The respiratory effects in man of altering the time profile of alveolar carbon dioxide and oxygen within each respiratory cycle.
J. Physiol. (London) 234:1-28; 1973.

Breathing hypoxic gas through an external dead space (ca. 1200 c.c.) stimulated ventilation disproportionately. A loop (ca. 250 c.c.) in the inspiratory pathway reduced the effect. The alveolar time patterns of PCO_2 and PO_2 characteristic of tube breathing with or without the loop have been simulated in moderate hypoxia by changing the composition of inspired gas at selected intervals after the beginning of inspiration. Supplying CO_2-free gas in late inspiration usually stimulated ventilation, but less than did real tube breathing. Supplying CO_2-free gas early in inspiration usually depressed ventilation. The difference between the "CO_2-free late" and "CO_2-free early" effects was 20% of the control ventilation ($P < 0.001$), i.e. was nearly the same as between the effects of real tube breathing without and with the loop. Tube-like PAO_2 time patterns had no effects. A-a PCO_2-PO_2 gradients remained constant throughout The VE, f and VT relations were unaltered in tube breathing. The respiratory system can discriminate between small differences in time patterns of $PACO_2$ but not of PAO_2; the signal is amplified by steady hypoxia. The arterial chemoreceptors are probably responsible for these effects. (Authors' summary)

464.
CURRIE, W.D., R.M. Gelein, Jr., and A.P. Sanders.
Comparison of protective agents against hyperbaric oxygen in large animals.
Aerosp. Med. 44:996-998;Sept. 1973.

Protection against the toxicity of hyperbaric oxygen was achieved in large animals using sodium succinate, glutamate, gamma-aminobutyrate, and glutathione intravenously. Less protection was obtained when disulfiram was injected intraperitoneally and its importance is discussed with reference to its solubility and further need for pharmacological studies. All the metabolites used in this study are linked to energy metabolism, thus the mechanism of protection against hyperbaric oxygen toxicity is proposed to be related to reactions yielding a level of adenosine triphosphate necessary to maintenance of normal brain metabolism. The results in this report show that protection in dogs, which are more sensitive to hyperbaric oxygen than mice or rats, exceeds that obtained with the smaller animals. Clinical trials, with human patients are anticipated. (Authors' abstract)

465.
DADAEV, I.M. and N.A. Kryuchkov.
Organizatsiya meditsinskogo obespecheniya lichpogo sostava pri legkovoda laznykh trenirovkakh i vozhdenii tankov pod vodoi.
[Medical training of the crew for light diving exercises and underwater tank diving].
Voennomed. Zh. (12):16-19;Dec. 1971.

The article deals with the training and preparation of the crew of tank units for underwater operations. The training of underwater tank divers is conducted at special training centers for divers, in water the temperature of which is not below 14°C. The training of tank operators and crew is conducted by the physician attached to the unit. Training begins with education in the physical and physiological aspects of underwater activities, as well as with light diving exercises. The crew has to be trained in the use of masks and special underwater breathing equipment. The prevention of specific underwater diseases related to the breathing of oxygen-gas mixtures is part of the training. The crew has to be instructed about the safe use and maintenance of their equipment, especially masks and oxygen tanks. Psychological preparation of the crew is of special importance in order to overcome the stress of the moments of actual submersion. First aid measures in cases of emergencies are also discussed. (OLC/BSCP)

466.
DAENENS, P.
A case of carbon monoxide poisoning during skin diving.
Arch. Toxikol. 31(2):181-184; 1973.

An oil leak resulted in a high concentration of both carbon monoxide and carbon dioxide in the breathing mixture of a scuba diver, who became nauseated during the first two or three minutes of a dive. Nausea was followed by paralysis of the lower limbs and loss of consciousness. The diver was brought to the surface by his companion. Gas chromatography measured the carbon monoxide in the breathing air at 1.6 per cent, and the carbon dioxide at 2.25 percent. It is noted that 1.6 percent CO at 75 feet is equal to 5.6 percent at atmospheric pressure. (MFW/BSCP)

467.
DAHLBACK, G.O. and C.E.G. Lundgren.
Pulmonary air-trapping induced by water immersion.
Aerosp. Med. 43:768-774;July 1972.

Pulmonary air-trapping in 20 subjects immersed up to the mouth was measured with a nitrogen washout and rebreathing technique. The influence of voluntarily controlled changes in end expiratory lung volume were studied. The volume of trapped air when breathing at FRC amounted to 90 ml or 2.0% of VC, when breathing at RV+5% of VC it amounted to 3.3% of VC, at RV+12% of VC to 1.8% of VC and at RV+20% of VC to 1.1% of VC. No statistically significant difference was found between smokers and non-smokers. It is noted that during immersion air-trapping is, on the average, not eliminated until lung volume is increased to between 38% and 43% of the VC. The possibility that airway closure and air-trapping induced by immersion may add to the danger of lung rupture during so-called free ascent is considered. (Authors' abstract)

468.
DAHLBACK, G.O. and C.E.G. Lundgren.
Dynamic factors in pulmonary air-trapping during immersion.
In: Hesser, C.M. and D. Linnarsson, eds. Proceedings of the first annual scientific meeting of the European Undersea Biomedical Society, Stockholm, 13-15 June 1973. Forsvarsmedicin 9:247-250;July 1973.

The present study aimed at investigating the role of [respiratory effort and gas flow] in air-trapping in the lungs during immersion to the mouth. It was concluded that the reduced air-trapping with increased breathing frequency might be ascribed to the larger inspiratory forces required for the higher flow rates. These forces would cause a more efficient filling of otherwise closed off regions. The more efficient filling would place these regions on a more favourable part of their present-volume curves thus facilitating their ventilation. (From authors' abstract)

469.
DAILY, O.P. and N.A. Schlamm.
Effect of hyperbaric atmospheres on β-galactoside transport in Escherichia coli.
Can. J. Microbiol. 18(7):1162-1164; 1972.

The rates of transport of two β-galactosides by whole cells of E. coli were elevated by pressurization to 68 atm with helium-oxygen gases. Kinetic analyses showed that the high atmospheric pressure caused an increase in V_{max} values of some 20-48% whereas K_m values were unchanged. (© BA)

470.
DANILOV, I.
Underwater research in the USSR.
Sea Frontiers 18:274-280;Sept./Oct. 1972.

The author reviews the developments in means of carrying on underwater research that have taken place in Russia in the past few years. The Ichthiander laboratories, which took various forms, were designed for depths of 32 to 40 feet. Physiological and psychological factors were monitored in great detail during these experiments. Two types of diving suits were tested, together with individual life-support systems which include heater, anti-compression system, breathing apparatus, sanitation unit and feeding facilities. These systems enable a diver to stay submerged for 38 hours. The Chernomor four to five man habitat — a 26-ft long cylinder, 10ft in diameter — has been positioned at depths of 46 to 78 feet, with divers going to 295 feet. Geological studies were carried out, but the chief emphasis in the past two years has been on medical and physiological studies of the divers. Other habitats are the Sadko series and the Sprut series. Moving vehicles are the towed Atlant bathysphere, Sever-1 and Sever-2; the last has a depth capability of 6,560 feet, is free-diving, and is transported from point to point by the research ship Odysseus. Another submersible is the Gvidon which can accommodate a crew of three for 72 hours at 820 feet. Also a deep-sea automatic stereo-camera has been developed and successfully tested. Currently under development is the Benthos-300 a self-propelled, autonomous laboratory-habitat; this will combine the advantages of submersible and habitat. (MFW/BSCP)

471.
DANZIGER, R.E.
Lipid alterations in laboratory rats during hyperbaric exposure.
In: Abstracts of BuMed-ONR sponsored Navywide workshop in high pressure biomedical research, U.S. Submarine Base, Groton, Conn., May 1971, p.18 Published by the Naval Submarine Medical Research Laboratory, 1971.

Abstract only. Entire item quoted: Numerous studies are currently being carried out in various Navy laboratories in an attempt to find a biochemical indicator of the presence and extent of decompression sickness in animals and humans exposed to hyperbaric pressure. Previous work from this laboratory has indicated that the percent composition of lipids in serum from human subjects does not vary appreciably during saturation or saturation-excursion dives. Lipids, however, comprise a family of rather complex molecules. In retrospect, for these to change in amount is much less likely than for them to show alterations in molecular structure, i.e., in their fatty acid composition. In laboratory rats, exposed to hyperbaric pressure and decompressed using a schedule that produces a spectrum of decompression sickness symptoms, a number of striking changes in the fatty acid composition of serum neutral lipids have been observed. At this time it is not yet possible to clearly relate these changes to the hyperbaric exposure. Data are still being collected and analyzed for consistent patterns of chain elongation, saturation and desaturation of fatty acids as they may relate to the dive conditions.

472.
DATTA, C.
Effect of pure oxygen environment on various aspects of brain function in vivo.
Indian J. Exp. Biol. 10:274-276;July 1972.

In vivo effect of pure oxygen environment (756-758 mm Hg) on the activities of acetylcholinesterase (AchE) and adenosine triphosphatase (ATPase), and the levels of free γ-aminobutyric acid (GABA), glutamine and glutamate of rat and mouse brains at different intervals of time (5, 10 and 15 min) was studied. The stress caused significant changes in all the parameters of brain function studied within 5 min in both the species; activities of AchE and ATPase were inhibited and activated respectively, and the levels of all the amino acids were elevated. The changes brought about in the enzymic levels were not uniform, but oscillated around control value with time. Amino acid levels also altered with time, though in unspecific manner. The results suggest a relationship between the activity of AchE and the levels of amino acids of the GABA system. The results also suggest that homeostatic mechanisms may, in some way, be related to dynamic antagonism of opposing biochemical forces. (Author's abstract)

473.
DAVIDSON, A.R. Jr. and L.E. Lesster.
AC powered underwater towed vehicles.
In: 1973 Offshore Technology Conference, April/May 1973, Houston, Texas. Preprints, Vol. II, p.881-890. Published by the conference.

Towed vehicle systems in the past have been powered by direct current requiring increasingly high voltages as power requirements have increased. As vehicle capabilities were augmented, more telemetry channels were required. Multi-wire cables capable of transmitting the vehicle power and carrying the telemetry channels are satisfactory for shallow applications, but greatly restrict the operational range of a towed vehicle due to cable size and inherent drag, telemetry channel cross talk, ground isolation, and noise. Powering the vehicle with alternating current via a single coaxial cable, which could also be shared with multiplexed telemetry, is an alternate approach to meet the demand for increased vehicle capability and operational range. A general description of an AC power system which could transmit up to 15 kw of power and multiplexed data over a single coaxial tow cable several miles long to a towed vehicle is presented. Primary power limitations of the system are attributed to the maximum allowable voltages before corona occurs. Telemetry is primarily limited by the frequency attenuation characteristics of the tow cable. (Authors' abstract)

474.
DAVIDSON, J.K. and F.C. Golding.
Aseptic necrosis of bone in compressed air workers: caisson disease of bone.
In: Proceedings of Symposium Ossium, 1970, p.252-256. Edinburgh, E. & S. Livingstone, 1970.

The statement is made, based on the findings of the Decompression Sickness Panel study of aseptic bone necrosis in 1500 compressed air workers, that lesions most commonly occur in the head of the humerus, the head and shaft of the femur, and the shaft of the tibia. Radiographs show the progress of bone lesions in the head of the humerus from their first appearance as a very faint area of increased density which might have passed for normal through structural failure with sequestration of cortex and a definite linear opacity. The author emphasizes the importance of watching out for dense areas at sites where bone necrosis is known to occur. It is said that it is impossible to predict which men are susceptible, and which lesions will progress and which remain static. Once structural failure has occurred, marginal osteophytes tend to develop. (MFW/BSCP)

475.
DAVIDSON, J.K.
Radiology of dysbaric osteonecrosis.
In: The Association of Clinical Pathologists: 89th general meeting, Symposium II. Decompression sickness. J. Clin. Pathol. 25:1005-1006;Nov. 1972.

Abstract only: The author refers to the first attempt to make a study of the incidence of osteonecrosis in compressed air workers, when the entire work force of the Clyde tunnel in Glasgow was examined radiologically. Findings were 19% incidence, and 10% juxta-articular (potentially disabling). The Medical Research Council Decompression Sickness Registry has kept radiographic records of compressed air workers since that time which give substantially the same figures. The head of the humerus is the most frequent site, followed by the distal shaft of the femur. The earliest radiographic fractures, which develop eight months to a year after exposure, are areas of increased density adjacent to the articular surface. In the medulla, the earliest features are small areas of increased density and small foci of calcification. In diagnosing dysbaric osteonecrosis, other causes of osteonecrosis, such as fracture of the femoral neck, dislocation of the hip, and the idiopathic form sometimes associated with steroid dosage, hemoglobinopathies, Gaucher's disease and Schandler's disease, must be kept in mind. Necropsy radiography following diving fatalities is considered very valuable in demonstrating intravascular bubbles or air embolisms, pneumothorax, mediastinal emphysema, or surgical emphysema. A radiograph of both groins may show gas or air in the iliofemoral artery and vein segments. Radiographs of the head of the humerus and of the femur should be coned to show trabecular detail. The author emphasizes that "correlation of the radiographic and pathological findings is of considerable value and importance in identifying the earliest radiographic features of osteonecrosis with confidence and differentiating this from variation in normal trabecular structure." (MFW/BSCP)

476.
DAVIES, D.M.
Medical experience in nuclear submarines.
J. Roy. Nav. Med. Serv. 57:136-141; 1971.

A summary of medical experience gained on long detached patrols by British nuclear submarine medical officers is presented. Comparisons with American experience are made and indications of what the new submarine medical officer may expect to meet in his practice at sea on patrol are given. The picture reflects the good standard of health of the British submariner and the success of the preventive medicine programme. (Author's abstract)

477.
DAVIES, D.M.
The effect of extended hypercapnia.
Proc. Roy. Soc. Med. 65:796,797;Sept. 1972.

The author states that it is unknown at present what lasting effects chronic hypercapnia might have. As a result of extensive studies, K.E. Shaefer et al., predicted the safe level of CO_2 to be .7%. Subsequent findings put this figure in doubt; levels as low as .5% have been seen to result in significant alterations in calcium and phosphorus patterns. Other environmental factors present in nuclear submarines make it difficult to determine with certainty the effects of CO_2. There is now being built, at the Institute of Naval Medicine, an environmental chamber where men will live in a completely controlled environment, thus making possible more accurate investigations. (MFW/BSCP)

478.
DAVIES, D.M.
Sixty days in a submarine: The pathophysiological and metabolic cost.
J. Roy. Coll. Physicians 7:132-144;Jan. 1973.

The human habitability problems associated with the introduction of nuclear power into submarines, and the physiological, biochemical and metabolic changes consequent on long, continuously-submerged patrols are described. The environmental factors contributing to such changes, particularly raised ambient carbon dioxide and carbon monoxide levels, are discussed, together with the disease processes that might arise from such factors. It is concluded that the existing good state of health of the nuclear sumbariner can be maintained by continued investigation of the effects of the environment and by an adequate preventive medicine programme. (Author's summary)

479.
DAVIS, F.M., J.P. Osborne, A.D. Baddeley and I.M.F. Graham.
Diver performance: nitrogen narcosis and anxiety.
Aerosp. Med. 43:1079-1082;Oct. 1972.

In two experiments in British waters 16 divers were tested twice underwater, once at a depth of 3 meters and once at 30 meters. They performed 4 tasks — a sentence comprehension test, a memory test, a simple arithmetic test and a manual dexterity test. All but the memory test show a significant drop in efficiency at depth: in Experiment 1; manual dexterity 22%, sentence comprehension 16% and arithmetic errors from 6% at 3 meters to 14% at 30 meters; in Experiment 2; manual dexterity 18%, sentence comprehension 10% and arithmetic errors from 5% at 3 meters to 12% at 30 meters. In all three tests these changes are similar to those from boat-diving experiments in the Mediterranean, whereas manual dexterity impairment is greater than for equivalent shore diving in the Mediterranean. A tentative relationship between the extent of performance impairment of manual tasks at depth and anxiety in divers is suggested. (Authors' abstract)

480.
DAVIS, F.M., R. Charlier, R. Saumarez and V. Muller.
Some physiological responses to the stress of aqualung diving.
Aerosp. Med. 43:1083-1088;Oct. 1972.

Nine aqualung (SCUBA) dives to a depth of 3 meters and nine dives to 30 meters were made in British coastal waters at an ambient temperature of 12°C. Skin temperatures (calf, loin and back) and core temperature (rectal) were measured at intervals during the dives. Plasma cortisol and urinary adrenalin and nonadrenalin excretion were measured before and after each dive. Plasma cortisol levels were significantly raised before and after 30 meter dives when compared with 3-meter dives. Raised urinary levels of adrenalin, with high adrenalin to nonadrenalin excretion ratios, were seen in several divers. The average decrease in rectal temperature was 0.33°C and mean skin temperatures remained approximately 16°C above ambient water temperature. Cold stress was considered unlikely to contribute to the hormonal changes seen. These changes are probably due to anxiety over deep open water diving in a "stressful" diving situation. (Authors' abstract)

481.
DAVIS, J.C., J.M. Dunn, C.O. Hagood and B.E. Bassett.
Hyperbaric medicine in the U.S. Air Force.
J. Amer. Med. Ass. 224(2):205-209; 1973.

Hyperbaric chambers are used for treatment of the four disorders generally accepted as amenable to recompression or hyperbaric oxygenation. Patients (94) suffering from decompression sickness, air embolism, carbon monoxide intoxication or gas gangrene were treated. Forty-seven were military patients with surgically, bacteriologically proved spreading, diffuse clostridial myonecrosis brings the total of cases treated with hyperbaric oxygenation during the past eleven years to 267. Recognized and treated early with a combined hyperbaric O_2 debridement-antibiotic and supportive program, survival rates of those with gas gangrene should improve significantly. (© BA)

482.
DAWSON, J.
Safety in the sixth continent.
In: Professional diving safety. Second annual symposium, New Orleans, Nov. 1971.
Mar. Technol. Soc. J. 6:28-31;Jan./Feb. 1972.

This paper was presented at a symposium on professional diving safety held in New Orleans in November 1971. The author is an insurance official of Lloyd's of London. He speaks of the need to set up international safety requirements and standards that will enable diving companies to operate under conditions that will make them acceptable risks to insurance underwriters. One hazard he mentions is the use of shiny materials in diving suits and equipment; these materials act as magnets for sharks and barracudas. The absolute necessity of six monthly medical, mental, and dental check-ups is emphasized. Care should be taken to avoid absolutely the use of alcoholics or psychiatric patients in diving. In the area of commercial diving, there is too wide an area of misunderstanding between the engineer on the surface and the diver below, who often has an incomplete or erroneous conception of his task, and for this reason extends his bottom time beyond the safety limits. Commercial diving companies should follow the example of the navies and train the men first as engineers or electricians and then as divers. (MFW/BSCP)

483.
DEAL, C.W., B.P. Fielden and I. Monk.
Haemodynamic effects of pulmonary air embolism.
J. Surg. Res. 11(11):533-538; 1971.

A large bolus of air was injected into the right atrium of sheep. The cardiac output, right ventricular pressure, and arterial PO_2 were studied. It was found that the cardiac output was quickly regained, in less than ten minutes, despite relatively anoxic levels of arterial oxygen saturation. The cardiac output temporarily exceeded the preinjection level before settling back to this level. The right ventricular pressure rose, corresponding to the regained cardiac output, and then settled to its original levels. The arterial PO_2 fell precipitously and slowly started to rise over the period of study. Bubbles were seen in the coronary arteries during these experiments. A bubble trap was placed across the arch of the aorta which demonstrated that there was no major transpulmonary passage of air. (Authors' summary)

484.
DECOMPRESSION SICKNESS PANEL, MEDICAL RESEARCH COUNCIL.
A medical code of practice for work in compressed air.
London, U.K., Construction Industry Research and Information Association, Rep. CIRIA 44, 90p. Feb. 1973.

The Code sets out recommendations for the medical treatment and supervision of compressed air workers. Appendices include the new Decompression (Blackpool) Tables, and also other proposed and existing working documents. An Annexe compares the recommendations in this Code with the Statutory Instruments (1958). (Authors' summary)

485.
DEECKE, L., R.C. Goode, G. Whitehead, W.H. Johnson and D.P. Bryce.
Hearing under respiratory stress: latency changes of the human auditory evoked response during hyperventilation, hypoxia, asphyxia, and hypercapnia.
Aerosp. Med. 44:1106-1111;Oct. 1973.

The cortical auditory evoked responses (AER), recorded at the skull vertex were studied in 56 experiments using 29 healthy subjects with normal breathing and during the following altered respiratory conditions: hyperventilation, hypoxia, asphyxia and hypercapnia. All four conditions approached the limits of physiological tolerance. Since such conditions can occur in air-crew when exposed to malfunction of the aircraft oxygen regulation system or during other emergencies in flight, it was of interest to know, therefore, which of these conditions might impair hearing perception. Under the assumption that AER latency changes correlate with hearing impairment (or raise in auditory threshold), it can be concluded that only those respiratory changes, which include a raised end-tidal PCO_2, are effective in this regard, for these conditions caused significant latency increase of all the auditory evoked response components (P_1, N_1, P_2 and N_2). These conditions involve asphyxia and hypercapnia. With hypercapnia, a positive significant correlation was found between the relative PCO_2 increase and the relative latency increase. The possible implications of these findings to aircrew safety are apparent. (Authors' abstract)

486.
DEITZ, J.L.
A laboratory for evaluation of underwater surveillance systems.
Sea Technol. 14:33-37;Nov. 1973.

For the past four years, the Librascope Division of The Singer Company in Glendale, California, has been designing and implementing a laboratory that provides a unique capability for evaluating new sonar systems in their totality by combining the major elements of the underwater array, and signal/data processor, the information display, and operator performance measurement. The integral signal processing and display laboratory provides the means of operating on a total system basis, in real time, on live, or synthesized signals. It is possible, for example, to vary performance parameters of any part of a hypothesized sonar system — active or passive — and determine the effect on overall performance in quantitative terms for the evaluation of hardware alternatives. It further allows scientific examination of the optimum way to use man's contribution to the machine function. Work done to date has shown that complete man-machine systems can be simulated in a manner which saves time and money in preparation of realistic hardware and software specifications. (Author)

487.
DELAUZE, H.G.
Keynote address.
In: The working diver, 1972. Symposium proceedings, February 1972, Columbus, Ohio, p.1-8. Washington, D.C., Marine Technology Society, 1972.

The author makes four recommendations in this survey of the present state-of-the-art in industrial diving: (1) There is a great need to establish safety procedures and operating regulations; (2) A major hazard is the development of excessively sophisticated equipment; (3) More research and development should be carried on in open-sea conditions; prototypes developed in laboratories are seldom functional in actual operating conditions; (4) deep water capability must be developed, since deep water operations will be a reality by 1980. The only country that has a diving safety code actually in force at present is Norway. England, France, and the United States are making progress in this direction. When all the codes are formulated, they should be combined into one international code. Some thought is given to the future, when the depth of operation will necessitate the development of diverless systems. It is highly likely, however, that even diverless systems will operate only with the help of divers. (MFW/BSCP)

488.
DeLAUZE, H.G.
The present and projected capabilities of the diving industry in the support of offshore petroleum production.
Ind. Med. Surg. 41:12-19;Nov. 1972.

The author touches briefly upon some of the research and achievements of COMEX, as well as those of American and British groups. It is stated that the problem of cold is well on the way to being solved, as was indicated by the Beluga experiment and by the Labrador dives for Tenneco, in which ten dives of more than an hour's duration were made to 600 feet depths in -2°C water. The lack of universally accepted, published decompression tables for deep dives is pointed out. Each company seems to have its own approach to this problem, when international cooperation would probably result in a better solution. There is a question as to whether the oil industry will require saturation diving; the author believes not for drilling exploration, but if diving assistance is to be used in production, saturation would be the most efficient method. Depth limits due to breathing resistance are discussed. For medium to heavy work, requiring 100-200w, the limit for compressed air is 200 feet, for helium-oxygen 1,500 feet and for hydrogen-oxygen, possible 3,000 feet; in the last case, limitations from pressure per se might interfere. For light work, the depth limits would be greater, but it is not yet understood to what extent pressure effects would be limiting. COMEX is planning a dive to 2,000 feet, undertaken with a very slow compression rate and a long stay at 1,500 feet. The large (17-foot) hyperbaric sphere of COMEX, with a pressure limitation of 1,000 feet, is described. It is used for training divers for experiments such as the Janus II open sea saturation dive to 840 feet. The closed-circuit hookah gas recovery system and the preheating unit, which heated the gas to 37°C, both used in Janus II are described. The same heating unit was used successfully in the Labrador exploration. In the eight-day Janus II, divers usually put in three hours bottom excursion working time. Physalie V culminated in about three hours at 1,700 feet, with a very brief jump to 1,706 feet. The profile of this dive is shown. There were stays of about 24 hours at 1,150 and 1,510 feet. The compression rate was fast to 355, slow to 1,150, fast to 1,310, slow to 1,510, fast to 1,610, and slow to 1,700. (MFW/BSCP)

489.
DeMARD, F.
Les accidents labyrinthiques aigus au cours de la plongee sous-marine.
[Acute labyrinth accidents during underwater diving].
In: Hesser, C.M. and D. Linnarsson, eds. Proceedings of the first annual scientific meeting of the European Undersea Biomedical Society, Stockholm, 13-15 June 1973. Forsvarsmedicin 9:416-422;July 1973.

The author has followed 38 cases over a period of seven years, of acute labyrinth attacks following diving. The most common type of lesion is the isolated cochlear hearing loss following breath-hold dives at shallow depths. Two main mechanisms seem to be involved: (1) a vascular factor, related to the presence of bubbles, and (2) a pressure factor, related to lack of pressure equilibration, sometimes following an excessively violent Valsalva maneuver. The therapeutic goal is to ameliorate the circulatory condition while protecting the neurosensory structures. The treatment here recommended includes the intravenous administration of vasodilators and corticoids in combination with hyperbaric oxygen at 2 or 2.5 ATA, once a day for eight to ten days. Specific cases are cited, in which this treatment was successful, even after delays of as much as twelve days. (MFW/UMS)

490.
DeMATOS, A.
Emergencias em medicina submarina.
[Emergencies in underwater medicine].
Brazilian Navy, Submarine Force, 1973. 103p.

This publication of the Brazilian Navy contains chapters on the following subjects: Man in the underwater environment; Physiological changes caused by diving; Physical aspects of diving; Barotrauma; Air embolism; Decompression sickness; Inert gas narcosis; Oxygen toxicity; Carbon dioxide poisoning; Injuries caused by marine life; Drowning; Breath-hold diving. Each subject is dealt with briefly, but well illustrated by diagrams, drawings and tables. It is interesting to note that the treatment tables of Van der Auer and the oxygen treatment tables of Workman and Goodman are given as appendices to the decompression chapter. (MFW/UMS)

491.
DEMBOWSKI, P.V., J. Pepe and T.E. Davidson.
Hydrostatic pressure induced ductility transitions in pure bismuth and tinbismuth alloys.
U.S. Army, Watervliet Arsenal, Rep. R-WV-T-6-20-73, 48p. June 1973.
(AD 764 241)

The mechanical behavior of pure (99.999%) bismuth and tin-bismuth alloys of various compositions has been observed over a range of superimposed hydrostatic pressures. Results indicate that maxima in ductility (as measured by percent reduction in area at the fracture surface) in specimens tested at atmsopheric pressure occur at compositions bordering pure tin and the eutectic composition. At sufficiently high pressures all compositions failed by rupture, i.e. necking to virtually 100% RA. For pure bismuth, pressure was observed to retard failure due to the formation of cracks at twin-grain boundary intersections; this result was consistent with the hypothesis that the effect of pressure is to shift the mode of crack propagation by decreasing the normal tensile component of stress acting on a crack. (Author) (GRA)

492.
DENISON, D.M.
Hazards within the hyperbaric oxygen environment with particular reference to the fire hazard and how it can occur.
In: Innes, G.S. ed. The production and hazards of a hyperbaric oxygen environment. Proceedings of a symposium held at University College, London, January 1968, p.59-106, Oxford, Pergamon Press, 1970.

This paper describes a series of 45 experiments upon the effects of igniting clothing (mounted on a brass dummy, or on dead pigs) in oxygen-rich environments. Fires were studied in gas environments with oxygen partial pressures ranging from 0.2 to 1.0 atmospheres. The effects of variations in the type, fit and proofing of clothing and in the detailed use of the water spray extinguishing system were noted. These experiments strongly suggest that: (a) The risks of igniting a man are greatly increased in these environments. (b) Fires in oxygen-rich environments are of a fundamentally different character to those in air. (c) Igniting a clothed man in these environments may lead to fatal damage within 5 to 20 sec. of onset. (d) A dense local water spray can control this fire but a manually operated system could not hope to arrest it in the few seconds available. (e) The damage to the man is critically dependent upon the type, fit and proofing of his clothing and on the timing, density and distribution of the extinguishing water sprays. (f) Injuries to the man will be reduced if the recommendations in the text are observed. . . 123 denim overalls have been ignited in a range of artificial gas environments of interest to man; pure oxygen pressures from 50 to 750 mm Hg, oxygen-nitrogen and oxygen-helium mixtures of varying concentrations at a pressure of 750 mmHg and similar mixtures at pressures in the range of 150 to 350 mmHg. The influence of contained moisture, normal soiling and gas flow have also been studied. The burning properties of human skin in air and in oxygen at one atmosphere have also been recorded. The practical implications of the findings are outlined. (Author)

493.
DENISON, D.M., D.A. Warrell and J.B. West.
Airway structure and alveolar emptying in the lungs of sea lions and dogs.
Resp. Physiol. 13:253-260;Dec. 1971.

The pressure-volume characteristics of the lungs excised from four California sea lions (Zalophus californianus) and six dogs have been compared by spirometry during cyclic changes in inflation pressure from +30 to -30 cm H_2O and histologically after recompression to atmospheric pressure from an absolute pressure of 112 mm Hg. In comparison with the dog lungs, the sea lion lungs emptied more completely on mild compression and much more completely on severe compression. These findings support Scholander's hypothesis that some marine mammals are protected from decompression sickness by cartilaginous reinforcement of the small airways which permits alveolar emptying during a dive, so isolating compressed gas from pulmonary capillary blood. (Authors' abstract)

494.
DENISON, D.M., P.D. Wagner, G.L. Kingaby and J.B. West.
Cardiorespiratory responses to exercises in air and underwater.
J. Appl. Physiol. 33:426-430;Oct. 1972.

Respiratory gas exchange, end-tidal gas tensions, alveolar ventilation, respiratory frequency, cardiac output, and pulse rate were measured in four healthy adult males at rest and during mild and moderate exercise (VO_2=0.2-2.0 l/min) in air at 18-22°C and underwater at 35.0-35.5°C. Subjects respired at eupneic pressures from the same breathing circuit throughout the 64 determinations of each variable were made in each environment. Immersion was associated with a 10% increase in pulse rate and cardiac output at all levels of exercise. There were no changes in end-tidal CO_2 tensions or alveolar ventilation. It is concluded that horizontal subjects breathing at eupneic pressures and working against mild and moderate loads in warm water show the same responses to exercise as in air. (Authors' abstract)

495.
DENISON, D.M. and G.L. Kooyman.
The structure and function of the small airways in pinniped and sea otter lungs.
Resp. Physiol 17(1):1-10; 1973.

The structure of the small airways from the lungs of 58 marine mammals was studied. Six were from sea otters, the others were from 14 of the 21 pinniped genera. In comparison with the terminal airways of terrestrial mammals all showed reinforcement by muscle and/or cartilage. The small airways of phocid seal lungs were reinforced by a moderately slender tube of oblique muscle. Those of otariid seals were strengthened by very thick pieces of cartilage.

The airways of sea-otter and walrus lungs were of an intermediate pattern. Both types of reinforcement seem to appear late in fetal life rather than by arrest of development. Calculations suggest the reinforcement in otariid lungs may be excessive for limiting nitrogen absorption during deep dives and behavioral observations indicate that strengthened airways may also be required for rapid ventilation at the surface between dives. (© BA)

496.
DENNISON, W.L. Jr.
A review of the pathogenesis of skin bends.
U.S. Nav. Submar. Med. Cent., Rep. NSMRL 660, 15p. Apr. 22, 1971.

The literature concerning cutaneous aspects of caisson disease, "skin bends" was searched, especially as regards the causes of this condition. This investigator found (by evaluation of the theories from the literature and application of physiological and anatomical data) that gases reach the various layers of the skin by diffusion from the blood and by penetration by osmosis through the skin from the external ambient gas concentrate. The route by which the gases reach the skin and the histological area in which they form bubbles is variable, but the site where they form is important in production of the various clinical varieties of "skin bends". (Author's abstract)

497.
DEPPE, A.H.
A study of psychological factors relevant to the selection of scuba divers.
Univ. of South Africa, Ph.D. Thesis, 202p. plus append. Jan. 1971.

The study covers three related topics, viz. an analysis of psychological and psychophysiological factors affecting human performance in the diving context, prediction of success in a diver training course and prediction of success of adaptation in immersion. Four criterion factors were derived for the training course; these were diving skill, intellectual ability, task-orientation and emotional maturity. Multiple regression involving predictors and single criteria yielded weight validities ranging from .22 to .50. Sources of performance decrement in immersion were concluded to comprise sensory and motor restrictions, limitations in the method, speed and cost of underwater work, and psychological stress. Arguments are given to justify a model of underwater adaptation as centering on arousal and rate of information processing capacity. Hypotheses based on this model were not supported; nevertheless the results of experimentation gave a number of leads regarding arousal and cognitive performance in diving. Main conclusions are that arousal is largely a function of training methods, task-proficiency largely a function of spontaneous work-methods, and underwater cognitive performance primarily a consequence of available ability resources and the extent to which they are limited to arousal. [The appendix consists of glossary, a definition of job analysis factors, the assessment exercise by which senior divers rate trainers, the questionnaire on diving given to trainees, and a diver selection interview. The bibliography contains over 200 references]. (Author's summary)

498.
DEPPE, A.H.
Performance criteria in diver training.
Percept. Mot. Skills 32:718;June 1971.

Using a sample of 71 male diver trainees from scuba diving courses, a study was made of 29 behavioral elements, positively and negatively defined. Instructors reported on their own students, and these data were converted to standard scores, which were "subjected to iterative principal factor analysis followed by varimax rotation to simple structure." The four factors which emerged were diving skill, intellectual ability, task-orientation and emotional maturity. It is noted that social compatibility is apparently unimportant; in fact, it is probable that the successful diver would be the type who would shun social activity. Underwater performance and invulnerability to stress are grouped under one factor. (MFW/BSCP)

499.
DE RITIS, G., P. Pietropaoli and L. Sarcinelli.
Studio sperimentale sugli effetti tossici dell'ossigeno iperbarico in animali pretrattati con pargilina, metaraminolo e metanfetamina.
[Experimental study on the toxic effects of hyperbaric oxygen in animals pretreated with pargyline, metaraminol and methamphetamine].
Acta Anaesthesiol. Ital. 23(6):537-545; 1972.

Swiss mice were given pargyline, an inhibitor of the MAO [monomine oxidase], and then exposed to hyperbaric O_2. Activation of the sympathetic-adrenergic system induced in the CNS methomphetamine and in the extra-cerebral nervous system by metharaminol produced an increase of the Bert and Smith effects respectively. This letter phenomenon cannot be considered the only reason for the toxic effects of hyperbaric O_2 but together with the associated metabolic damage and the vasospasm it is still one of the most important pathogenetic factors. (JGS) (© BA)

500.
DEROANNE, R., J. Dujardin, M. Lamy, R. Marechal, J.M. Petit and F. Pirnay.
Effect of hyperbaric oxygenation on maximum aerobic work capacity.
In: Hesser, C.M. and D. Linnarsson, eds. Proceedings of the first annual scientific meeting of the European Undersea Biomedical Society, Stockholm, 13-15 June 1973. Forsvarsmedicin 9:352-356;July 1973.

Physiologic reactions during maximum exercise on a bicycle ergometer were tested under hyperoxic conditions. Five healthy subjects breathed pure O_2 at 1.0, 2.0 and 3.0 ATA. Ventilation and maximal O_2 uptake (VO_2 max) were determined by a special spirometer where CO_2 was absorbed; different controls were continuously made: PO_2 with a paramagnetic analyzer, PCO_2 with an infra-red analyzer and temperature with a thermocouple. . . . VO_2 max increased by 3% when the subjects breathed pure O_2 and 1 ATA. During hyperoxia VO_2 max measured at 2 and 3 ATA did not differ significantly from that measured at 1 ATA. Heart rate showed highly comparable maximum values under the various experimental conditions. During submaximal exercise, heart rate was consistently lower when the subjects breathed O_2; this difference became slighter with every increase in work load. Exercise ventilation and blood lactic acid concentration were invariably reduced in hyperoxic environment. . . . The slight increase of VO_2 max compared with the additional O_2 carried by the arterial blood, suggests that the circulatory system is not the only limitative factor. The muscle cells also seem to be restricted in their use of the O_2 supplied to them. The ceiling of O_2 consumption could be imposed by biochemical limitations in the muscles. (From authors' abstract)

501.
DESAUTELS, S.
Problemes medicaux de la plongee sportive.
[Medical problems of sport diving].
Vie Med. Can. Fr. 1:660-663;July 1972.

This brief article discusses five physiological problems of diving: (1) change in pressure and volume; (2) increase in density; (3) excess of oxygen; (4) excess of nitrogen; (5) effects of decompression. The dangers of hyperventilation before a breath-hold dive are emphasized. Air embolism is explained as the result of ascent without exhaling, and the necessity of immediate recompression followed by stage decompression is noted. Increase in density causes respiratory difficulty, which is not usually dangerous unless the diver is inexperienced and panic ensues. It is important to avoid excessive exertion underwater, and for this reason underwater competitions should be discouraged. The approach of oxygen toxicity is often heralded by muscle twitching, especially around the lips; this is followed by convulsions which can end in drowning. Nitrogen narcosis is described and it is stated that while experienced divers may adapt to this, they should never exceed 300 feet with a mixture containing nitrogen in any quantity. The usual limit is 100 feet. The symptoms of decompression sickness are described and the generally accepted theories of etiology and recompression therapy are put forth. The author concludes with a brief comment on the fact that 75% of diving accidents are caused by inexperience, inadequate training, or careless security measures. Also, he notes, regarding physical examinations for divers, that special attention should be given to the ears and to the respiratory system. Any abnormality or infection in the lung could cause air trapping. All divers should have an annual chest x-ray. (MFW/SCD)

502.
DEUEL, C.L. and R.M. Roberts.
Complete analysis of naval hyperbaric diving gases.
In: Battelle Columbus Laboratories. Proceedings, 1973 divers' gas purity symposium, November 27-28, 1973, p.XII-1-XII-16. U.S. Navy Supervisor Diving, Nav. Ships Syst. Comm. Rep 2-73, 1973.

Because the properties and concentrations of the constituents in diving gases vary widely, comprehensive analysis requires the application, often in combined form, of several different techniques. Mass spectrometry (MS) is ideally suited to the determination of permanent gases, carbon dioxide, and other inorganic constituents present at fractional percentage levels. If cryogenic trapping is employed and the sample is pressurized, measurements to 0.1 ppm can be achieved on condensable inorganics, e.g. CO_2, SO_x, NO_x, etc. CO and CH_4 can be accurately measured to approximately 0.5 ppm by combining chromatographic separation on a molecular sieve column with a Sabatier conversion of CO to CH_4. A flame ionization detector is used. By utilizing a portion of this system, total hydrocarbon (n-hexane equivalent) can be determined. Individual organic constituents are determined by gas chromatography (GC) using multiple columns with both flame ionization and electron capture detectors. Contaminant concentration techniques are utilized to enhance detectability and to facilitate quantitation. Compound identity is established by mass spectrometric analysis of the column effluent and through the comparison of retention volumes with those of known materials. This method permits detectability to 0.01 ppb for most organic compounds. Compound identifications are greatly facilitated through the application of data obtained from spacecraft contaminant characterization studies and by the use of a tandemized GC/MS system. (Authors' abstract)

503.
DEUTSCH, S.
A man-systems integration study of the behavior of crews and habitability in small spaces.
In: Miller, J.W., J.G. Van Derwalker, and R.A. Waller, eds. Tektite 2: Scientists-in-the-sea, p. VIII-1 - VIII-14. Washington, D.C., U.S. Department of the Interior, August 1971.

The curiosity of men leads them to venture further and further away from the benign environment found on the earth's surface. Tektite 2 provided a unique opportunity to advance our scientific knowledge of the behavior of men in small groups operating under conditions of stress and to improve the technology for development of habitable areas for living and working surrounded by a hostile environment. An extensive Man-Systems Integration Program with emphasis on behavioral research and habitability assessment was undertaken to provide meaningful field study data for application to manned exploration under the seas and in space. (Authors' abstract)

504.
DEWAR, K.M.S., G. Smith, A.A. Spence and I.McA. Ledingham.
Effect of hyperoxia on airways resistance in man.
J. Appl. Physiol. 32:488-490;Apr. 1972.

Nine normal subjects breathed either 100% oxygen or 10% oxygen-90% nitrogen at an ambient pressure of 2 Ata for five hr. After breathing oxygen, there was an increase in airways resistance of 30%, an increase in thoracic gas volume of 25%, and a fall in specific airways conductance of 41%; with air equivalent gas, there were no significant changes. There were no changes in vital capacity, forced vital capacity, or $FEV_{1.0}/FVC$ with either air or oxygen. Measurements of cardiac output, alveolar-arterial oxygen tension difference, and blood pressure in three subjects were unaltered during the period of oxygen exposure. (Authors' abstract)

505.
DEXTER, J.D., D.G. Hof and C.E. Mengel.
Effect of sleep-wake reversal and sleep deprivation on the circadian rhythm of oxygen toxicity seizure susceptibility.
Aerosp. Med. 43:1075-1078;Oct. 1972.

The effect of sleep-wake reversal and sleep deprivation on the circadian rhythm of oxygen toxicity seizure susceptibility was investigated in an attempt to more clearly define its nature. Albino Sprague-Dawley rats were exposed in a previously O_2 flushed, CO_2 free chamber. The exposure began with attainment of 60 psi (gauge) and the end point was the first generalized seizure. Part I. Animals were exposed to reversal diurnal conditions since weanlings until their sleep-wake cycles had completely reversed, and then divided into four groups of 20 based on the time of day exposed. The time of exposure to OHP prior to seizure was not significantly longer in the group exposed from 1900-2000 hrs and reversal of the circadian rhythm of oxygen toxicity seizure susceptibility was noted. Part II. Animals maintained on normal diurnal conditions were deprived of sleep on the day of exposure for the 12 hours prior to exposure at 1900 hrs. while controls were allowed to sleep. There was no significant difference in the time prior to seizure between the deprived animals and the controls with an n=40. Thus the inherent threshold in susceptibility to OHP seizures seems not to be a function of sleep itself, but of some biochemical/physiologic event which manifests a circadian rhythm. (Authors' abstract)

506.
DEXTER, S.C.
Handbook of oceanographic engineering materials. Volume I. Metals and alloys. Woodshole, Mass., Woodshole Oceanographic Inst., Rep. WHOI-TM-4-72, 102p. Dec. 1972.
(COM 73-10660)

The volume consists of two sections. Part A is a series of tabulations of metallic materials ranked according to selected mechanical and physical properties, corrosion resistance, and cost. Part B consists of one page of more detailed data on each of the materials covered. Composition, mechanical and physical properties, corrosion resistance, forms available, fabricability, typical uses and base cost are treated for each material. In this section the materials are grouped into alloy classes according to the base metal of the alloy. Details are given for the following: aluminum alloys, copper alloys, nickel alloys, steels, stainless steels, titanium, magnesium and zinc. (GRA)

507.
DEYO, J.N., J.L. Klann and R.S. Bilski.
Integration of an isotope Brayton power system with a life support system.
In: Fifth intersociety energy conversion engineering conference, Las Vegas, Nevada, September 1970, Paper 16.

Results of an analytical study conducted to determine the feasibility of using an isotope Brayton power system to supply both the electrical and thermal needs of an integrated life support system. Emphasis was placed on studying the steady-state and transient interactions that would result from thermal integration of the two systems. Results of the study show that thermal integration can be accomplished most flexibly by extracting heat in the Brayton power system's waste loop through the use of an auxiliary liquid-to-liquid heat exchanger. Thermal transient effects on both systems are within operating tolerances. (From authors) (Aerosp. Med.)

508.
DIACHENKO, J.A.
A study of a cutaneous code applied to the communication needs of the working diver.
U.S. Nav. Med. Res. Inst., Rep. 2 on M4306.03. 5000BAK9, 18p. Aug. 15, 1972.

As an initial study into the applicability of cutaneous communication for divers, a series of sixteen discrete, left-right (L-R) vibrotactile stimulus patterns was delivered to the lower abdomen of six divers whose task it was to correctly identify the spatio-temporal sequence of each pattern. Correlation analysis of the results showed that older subjects made significantly more errors, and complex code patterns containing three L-R changes in direction contributed significantly to subject error. However, the overall design of L-R patterns was found to be basically satisfactory as a framework on which to build an optimal cutaneous code. Further development of code and hardware are suggested. (Author's abstract)

509.
DIANOV, A.G., V.V. Isayenko and G.P. Sviridova.
Physiological effect of the replacement of atmospheric nitrogen by inert gases at high and low temperatures.
Space Biol. Med. 7:1.11;Jan./Feb. 1973.
(JPRS 58620)

The effect of extreme (death causing) temperature exposures on helium-oxygen or argon-oxygen atmospheres was studied in 153 experiments on rats. At high and low ambient temperatures the replacement of nitrogen with helium produced a negative effect, shortening the lifetime of the animals. This effect can be attributed to a substantial change in heat transfer in the helium-oxygen atmosphere which occurs due to the higher heat conductivity of helium in comparison with nitrogen. At high and low ambient temperatures the replacement of nitrogen [with argon] caused no significant changes: the heat conductivity of nitrogen and argon is similar. It is concluded that human tolerance of extreme temperature effects in atmosphere in which nitrogen is replaced by inert gases is dependent only on their thermophysical properties. (Authors' abstract)

510.
DOBOSZYNSKI, T., K. Ulewicz, B. Lokucijewski and P. Michniewski.
Effect of oxygen at high pressure on opsonic index and some haematologic data in rabbits.
Ann. Immunol. 2(4):245-249; 1970.

Fifteen adult rabbits weighing 2.0 - 2.5 kg. were exposed to 1.8 - 3.1 atm O_2 in a pressure chamber for one hour. The opsonic index and hematological data were measured 1 hr., 24 hr, 48 hr. and 10 days after removal from the chamber and compared to initial values. In rabbits exposed to 1.8, 2.4, and 3.1 atm O_2, the opsonic index increased, while changes in the blood were insignificant. The opsonic index should be used for such investigations. (© BA)

511.
DOELL, D., N.R. Anthonisen and M. Zutter.
Control of ventilation at 4 ATA.
In: Abstracts of the Twenty-fifth Congress of Physiological Sciences Satellite Symposium. Recent progress in fundamental physiology of diving. Marseille, France. July 1971. p.25. (Proceedings unpublished)

Abstract only. Entire item quoted: Subjects rebreathed from a spirometer containing various mixtures of O_2 and CO_2 while minute ventilation and alveolar gas tensions were measured at 1 and 4 ATA. By combining data from different rebreathing runs the ventilatory response to increased alveolar CO_2 was evaluated at alveolar O_2 tension ranging from 40 to more than 200 mmHg. The ventilatory response to CO_2 at high O_2 levels was depressed in all subjects at depth, and the amount of depression was related to the strength of the CO_2 stimulus and the level of ventilation. The hypoxic potentiation of the ventilatory response to CO_2 was only depressed at high (>50 mm Hg) PCO_2 at depth. Indeed at PCO_2 <45 mmHg the ventilatory response to hypoxia was unaffected by depth. It would appear that the respiratory control system responds to hypoxia in a different way than it does to CO_2. It has been shown that CO_2 response is proportional to inspiratory power, while the present data indicates that the hypoxic response is related to ventilation and, so long as maximum levels are not approached, is independent of inspiratory power.

512.
DOELL, D., M. Zuter and N.R. Anthonisen.
Ventilatory responses to hypercapnia and hypoxia at 1 and 4 ATA.
Resp. Physiol. 18:338-346; 1973.

Using a rebreathing method, ventilatory responses to CO_2 and hypoxia were examined at 1 and 4 ATA in 6 young men. Ventilatory responses to CO_2 were less than 4 ATA than at 1 ATA; these data were consistent with the hypothesis that a given increment of $PACO_2$ caused the same increase in inspiratory power at both pressures. At normal $PACO_2$ ventillatory responses to hypoxia were the same at 1 and 4 ATA, indicating that hypoxic responses were related more closely to ventilation than inspiratory power. When both hypercapnia and hypoxia were present ventilatory response tended to be depressed at 4 ATA. (Authors' abstract)

513.
DOLEZAL, V., F. Nadvornik, Z. Makoc and F. Vorel.
The effect of hyperbaric oxygen on some metabolic changes in rats.
Acta Univ. Palacki. Olomuc. Fac. Med. 65:299; 1973.

Abstract only: The authors studied the effect of exposing newborn rats to an oxygen atmosphere at normal barometric pressure for 180 hours after birth and the effect of exposing adult female rats to oxygen at 3 ATA for five hours, on enzyme activity. The first group were highly resistant to oxygen; negligible histological changes were observed. LDH, MDH, ICDH, CLDH, glycogen and lactate were measured in the second group, and also in 23-day old rats who had been born in oxygen and had lived in it for 180 hours, who had also been exposed to oxygen at 3 ATA for five hours. Compared to control animals, significant decrease of LDH and increase of lactate in brain tissue were observed. The enzyme activity of 23-day-old rats after the hyperbaric oxygen exposure was less significant in comparison to adults. The 180-hour exposure of newborn rats to oxygen did not produce significant differences from the control rats. No consistent changes were noted in enzyme activity and pathophysiology of the groups. (Modified by MFW/UMS)

514.
DORIS, I., M.G. Harper and J.E.W. Morris.
The significance of fungal growth in nuclear submarines.
J. Roy. Nav. Med. Serv. 58:123-127;Summer 1972.

The visible presence of fungal growth in certain areas of nuclear submarines has given rise to concern amongst the crews. The airborne spore population was investigated to determine the medical significance of such growths and the methods used are described. It is concluded that no medical hazards are associated with the presence of fungal growths, but that action is necessary to deal with the material deterioration caused by the growths. The overall investigation is a good example of how medical, scientific and engineering staff within the Ministry of Defense (Naval) can work closely together to resolve such problems to mutual benefit. (Authors' abstract)

515.
DORR, V.A. and H.R. Schreiner.
Combustion phenomena in oxygen-enriched environments.
In: Wada, J. and I. Takashi, eds. Proceedings of the fourth international congress of hyperbaric medicine, Sapporo, Japan, Sept. 1969, p.121-125. Baltimore, Williams and Wilkins, 1970.

In order to reduce the probability of further accidents in oxygen-enriched environments, one must strive to eliminate any one of the 3 fundamental prerequisites for a fire: an ignition source, a fuel and an atmosphere capable of supporting combustion. In practice, it is often difficult or impossible to remove any one of these requirements with absolute certainty. Attempts should therefore be made to reduce the contributing effects of all 3 essential factors, i.e., electrical items that may serve as potential ignition sources should be avoided, the quantity of flammable materials in the chamber should be reduced, and the absolute oxygen concentration and the oxygen partial pressure within the chamber should be minimized as much as possible. In order to evaluate the influence of the above factors upon combustion in oxygen-enriched environments, a study has been conducted to (1) assess the effects of environmental parameters upon the combustion rate of a standard material, (2) determine the minimum oxygen concentrations required for the combustion of solid flammables in the presence of nitrogen and helium, and (3) categorize the flammability hazards of cloth fabrics, elastomers and insulations in hyperbaric environments. (Authors)

516.
DOSSETT, A.N. and H.V. Hempleman.
Importance for mammals of rate of compression.
In: The effects of pressure on organisms. Symposia of the Society for Experimental Biology, No. 26, p.355-361. London, Cambridge University Press, 1972.

These experiments, using female Wistar rats, were undertaken in order to explore the etiology of helium tremor, and to learn whether or not the effects observed in man could be produced in small animals. In Series I, rats were compressed to 61 atm, with 0.21 ATA O_2, in Series 2, to 61 atm, with 1 ATA O_2, in Series 3 to 92 atm with 1 ATA O_2, and in Series 4, to 138 atm with 3 ATA O_2. It was found that the onset of tremor was considerably delayed by a very slow compression. The experiments were repeated, using mice, with the same results. The delaying effect of a low compression rate appears to indicate that an adaptive response is at work. (MFW/SCD)

517.
DOUGLAS, F.G. and P.Y. Chong.
Influence of obesity on peripheral airways patency.
J. Appl. Physiol. 33(5):559-563; 1972.

In 9 obese subjects, including 8 with diminished expiratory reserve volume, and in 2 normals, static elastic recoil of lung, pulmonary flow resistance and dynamic lung compliance at 3 breathing frequencies were measured. A nitrogen-washout technique was used to detect trapped air. Lung elasticity was normal in all cases, as was resistance in all but 1. All obese subjects with low lung volume had frequency dependence of lung compliance; 2 with very marked reduction in expiratory reserve volume had air trapping. When lung volumes were normal, the static and dynamic mechanical characteristics of the lung were also normal in spite of obesity. Reduction in expiratory reserve volume due to obesity apparently results in a tendency to closure of small peripheral airways ($<$ 2mm) in dependent lung zones. Impaired gas exchange due to regional phase differences in ventilation is a probable result. [These findings might indicate further reasons for negative consideration of obese individuals in the selection of diving trainees]. (© BA)

518.
DRAGERWERK
International Oceanological Equipment and Services Exhibition (20-24 March 1972). Lubeck, Germany, Dragerwerk AG, Press Release, [1972].

This release consists of brief descriptions of the Drager equipment exhibited at Brighton in March 1972. This equipment includes the following: (1) The deep diving system TTA 200 TS, designed for work at depths to 200 meters. (2) The 2-man pressure chamber "Duocom". (3) The oxygen breathing system SAA-1 for use during decompression. (4) The mixed gas swim diving apparatus SMS 1/B, a semi-closed hose-type breathing apparatus which operates for up to three hours. (5) The mixed gas swim diving apparatus FGG III, to be used in working from an underwater structure, both as a self-contained system with a 20-min capacity, and a hose-supplied system with a 3-hour capacity. (6) The constant volume suit 168, a dry suit enabling the diver to maintain the air content in his suit by means of exhaled air, designed for use with double hose demand valve, mixed gas diving apparatus, or demand valves with knuckle thread connection. (7) Sport diving units adaptable to many requirements. (8) Demand valves for sport diving equipment. (9) High pressure breathing air compressor set DK-5, which can charge two six-liter cylinders simultaneously, in 32 minutes. (MFW/BSCP)

519.
DRISCOLL, R.G.
Investigation of a quasi-holographic synthetic-aperture acoustical imaging system.
U.S. Nav. Postgrad. Sch., Thesis, 44p. Dec. 1972.
(AD 757 253)

A side-looking sonar system which uses coherent electrical processing is investigated. Such a system produces a quasi-hologram of the reflected sound field which may be subsequently imaged to give a visual presentation of the insonified region. An actual working laboratory system is constructed and several quasi-holograms are depicted in the Data and Results section. Imaging is not completed, however, an optical processing arrangement to accomplish this task is presented. (Author's abstract) (GRA)

520.
DRUMMOND, P.C. and D.R. Jones.
Initiation of diving bradycardia in muskrats.
J. Physiol. (London) 222:165P-166P;Apr. 1972.

Abstract only. Entire item quoted: Whether water immersion per se affects the development of the cardiac chronotropic response to submergence has been a matter of some dispute. In unanesthetized muskrats full expression of the diving response may occur within 200 msec after submergence, in marked contrast to ducks in which 40 seconds or so may elapse before full bradycardia develops. The present experiments have been performed on anaesthetized (urethane 1500 mg/kg, I.P.) and curarized (Tubocurarine chloride 2 mg/kg, I.V.) muskrats, tracheotomized and maintained on artificial ventilation thereby eliminating any anticipatory or conscious component in the response. Water flow through the nose, while artificial ventilation was maintained constant, caused a marked fall in heart rate after a latent period of some 3-900 msec, even though PaO_2 measured by an oxygen electrode in a carotid artery loop, rose during the one minute trial. Asphyxia alone caused bradycardia but only after a latent period of some 6-12 sec. Asphyxia combined with water flow through the nose also caused bradycardia with a latent period of 3-900 msec. PaO_2 fell more rapidly under the former than latter conditions indicating that water immersion is indispensable for full expression of the oxygen conserving response.

521.
DRYSDALE, D.B.
The effects of corticosterone, adrenalin, phenoxybenzamine and propranolol in intact and adrenalectomized rats exposed to oxygen at high pressure.
Proc. Univ. Otago Med. Sch. 49(2):29-30; 1972.

These results again confirm that adrenalectomy decreases the susceptibility of rats to oxygen poisoning. The results show too that α-adrenergic receptor blockers, already known to protect rats from oxygen-induced lung damage, also prevent or delay the onset of convulsions and that β-receptor blockers also give protection. However, sympathetic blockade did not decrease the variability in protection afforded by adrenalectomy. Adrenalin again reversed the protective effect of adrenalectomy and did not increase significantly the susceptibility to oxygen of intact animals. Physiological doses of corticosterone also reversed the protection given by adrenalectomy, whilst the high dose if anything enhanced the protection, as others have reported. (Author's conclusions)

522.
DRYSDALE, D.B.
Effects of glutathione, ascorbic acid and tocopherol in vitamin-E-deficient rats exposed to oxygen at high pressure.
Proc. Univ. Otago Med. Sch. 50(1):6-8; 1972.

Vitamin-deficient rats were divided into eight groups. One group received no antioxidant; other groups were given glutathione or ascorbic acid in various doses and time patterns; and the final group was given α-tocopherol acetate. Convulsions occurred after a mean time of 22.6 min after arrival at 6 atm., in all tocopherol-treated animals. One vitamin E-deficient animal convulsed; others became prostrate and dyspneic. Time to onset of poisoning was shorter in untreated than in antioxidant-treated animals. Only those treated with ascorbic acid demonstrated in vivo hemolysis. No animals demonstrated gross lung damage. While time to onset of oxygen toxicity differed in treated and untreated animals, the mode of poisoning was the same, and markedly different from that in tocopherol treated animals. (MFW/SCD)

523.
DRYSDALE, D.B.
The effects of CO_2 on the susceptibility to oxygen at high pressure of intact and adrenalectomized rats.
Proc. Univ. Otago Med. Sch. 50:48-49; 1973.

Adrenalectomy protected against oxygen poisoning only in the absence of CO_2 ($P < 0.01$). There was no significant difference in the time to onset of convulsions amongst any of the groups exposed to CO_2. The mean time to onset of convulsions in all animals exposed to CO_2 was 13.3 mins $\pm$ 0.3 (S.E.M.) which was lower than that of intact animals exposed to O_2 alone ($P < 0.01$). (Author)

524.
DRYSDALE, D.B. and L.N.M. Smith.
The relationship between oxygen consumption and susceptibility to oxygen at high pressure in intact and adrenalectomized rats.
Proc. Univ. Otago Med. sch. 50:50-51; 1973.

Direct measurements of $\dot{V}O_2$ [oxygen consumption] at pressure show a correlation between decreased oxygen consumption and decreased susceptibility to oxygen poisoning. It is not clear however whether the protection is due to a primary decrease in $\dot{V}O_2$ preventing the onset of preconvulsive and convulsive activity or is secondary to the decreased activity and hence lower $\dot{V}O_2$ of the adrenalectomized animals. (Author)

525.
DuBOIS, A.B. and A.B. Fisher.
Prolonged exposure to 50 or 100 feet of air pressure upon airways, lungs and chest cage.
In: Abstracts of BuMed—ONR sponsored Navywide Workshop in high pressure biomedical research, U.S. Naval Submarine Base, Groton, Conn., May 1971, p.1. Published by the Naval Submarine Medical Research Laboratory, 1971.

Abstract only. Entire item quoted: The question concerned whether the depth and duration of Tektite I and II could cause adaptive effects owing to the increased air density, at normal oxygen tension. Though the pulmonary resistance changed with air density as expected, this effect did not show adaptation. It was reversed at the end by decompression. Lung compliance did not change. However, some subjects slowly increased their vital capacity. This change probably was caused by physical conditioning which occurred during the weeks of experimentation. No adverse effects on lung function other than those due to density alone were found in either atmosphere.

526.
DuBOIS, A.B., Y. Kawakami and B.H. Natelson.
Respiratory factors affecting diving reflex in man.
In: Abstracts of the Twenty-fifth Congress of Physiological Sciences Satellite Symposium. Recent progress in fundamental physiology of diving. Marseille, France, July 1971, p.7. (Proceedings unpublished).

Abstract only. Entire item quoted: The object was to determine the effects of face immersion and whole body immersion on the circulation, and to ascertain whether respiratory parameters such as larger volume or intrapleural pressure, alveolar oxygen or alveolar CO_2 affected the reflex circulatory changes that accompany face immersion. The degree of bradycardia which accompanied immersion of the face in cold water was independent of whether the breath was held at total lung capacity (TLC) or functional residual capacity. Likewise, negative intraesophageal pressure (glottis open) did not affect the result at TLC. However, cold water was more effective than cool water or an ice bag on the face. Breath holding on 10% O_2, or on 7.5% CO_2 yielded the usual bradycardia during face immersion. 100% O_2 did not affect the response. Pulmonary bloodflow measured with the plethysmographic N_2O uptake method decreased 22%. Later, studies were made during whole body immersion in neutrally warm water, to determine the effect of whole body immerrsion, and apnea, on pulmonary blood flow, oxygen consumption, and CO_2 output. Briefly, these parameters, sitting in water, are almost equal to those measurements made sitting in air, provided compensatory pressure is applied at the breathing tube. The immersion reflex (bradycardia) appears to be attributable to cooling of the face, and not to O_2 or CO_2 tension, lung volume or intrapleural pressure.

527.
DUEKER, C.W.
Danger at any depth. Air embolism.
Skin Diver 20:16-17;56-57;Oct. 1971.

In free diving, lungs cannot overexpand, because they compress upon descent and expand to their original volume on ascent. In scuba diving, lung volumes remain constant, and if there is not normal exhalation during ascent, the lungs will stretch until they actually burst. The torn alveoli allow air to escape into the supporting tissue of the lung. Results can be mediastinal emphysema, subcutaneous emphysema, pneumothorax, or most serious of all, air embolism, which can cause coronary occlusion or impede blood flow to the brain, resulting in unconsciousness and death. Very small changes in pressure — less than ten feet — can cause the lung to rupture; the danger is much greater in shallow water because the air volume changes more rapidly. Symptoms of air embolism usually appear within ten minutes of surfacing; they include collapse, chest pain, weakness, paralysis, disorientation, visual blurring or convulsions. Death is very quick unless treatment is immediately started. Some cases of air embolism have occurred even when the diver has exhaled normally; these result from some localized abnormality in the airways which can cause air to be entrapped. The current treatment for air embolism consists of rapid recompression to 165 feet, where the patient is kept until his symptoms subside; he is then taken to 60 feet, and given oxygen and air alternately, then to 30 feet where alternate oxygen and air are again breathed; he is then slowly and continuously decompressed to the surface. The author emphasizes the need for annual chest X-rays for divers; also, all applicants for scuba training courses should be required to have chest X-rays. The leading training associations approve of the free swimming ascent, in which the diver swims slowly toward the surface with the head held back, allowing air to flow from the lungs. The free ascent, and the buoyant ascent, both practiced by the Navy, are too dangerous for the ordinary sport diver. Ascent training is a very important part of a scuba course, and emphasis on this aspect of training will make the diver less likely to panic should the necessity for emergency ascent arise. (MFW/BSCP)

528.
DUELLMANN, J.
Hirnschaedigung durch hyperbaren Sauerstoff in niedrigen Druckbereichen.
[Central nervous system lesions by hyperbaric oxygen at low pressure.]
Acta Anat. 81(1):113-118; 1972.

Oxygen at high pressure locally impairs the white matter of the brain and spinal cord even in the tolerance range lacking clinical evidence (lack of lung impairment and oxygen convulsions). The extent of the reaction is dependent on the dose administered. Histochemically, demonstrable alterations in carbohydrate metabolism appear after 1 hr exposure to 2 ata [atmospheres absolute] O_2. A 1 hr exposure to 4 ata leaves locally defined lesions throughout almost the total white matter. The lesions are identified histochemically by a strong Hale-reaction, and are also positive for PAS and Alcian Blue. In this experiment, i.v. injected Evans Blue did not invade brain or spinal cord tissue. (JFL) (© BA)

529.
DUFFY, J.R., T.G. Giolas and R.L. Sergeant.
Studies in Navy communication: The effect of word predictability on sentence intelligibility.
U.S. Nav. Submar. Med. Cent., Rep. SMRL 672, 8p. July 8, 1971.

In line with the Naval Submarine Medical Research Laboratory's continuing effort to improve communication in the Navy, this study was instituted to investigate the relationship between word predictability and sentence intelligibility. This relationship was examined by comparing the accuracy of responses by listeners to several lists of sentences. Three methods of scoring used different groups of key words which had previously been judged to represent different degrees of predictability. It was hypothesized that the scores obtained would be a function of the predictability status of the key words used in scoring. Results indicated significant differences between the three scoring procedures for each sentence list under two filtering conditions, and these differences were in the hypothesized direction. The results suggest that the use of easy-to-predict words will increase sentence intelligibility while the use of difficult-to-predict words will depress intelligibility. It was concluded that word predictability is a factor influencing sentence intelligibility and that careful selection of key words, on the basis of predictability may be a way of controlling the intelligibility of sentences. (Authors' abstract)

530.
DUFFY, R.J., T. Giolas, H.S. Cooker and R.L. Sergeant.
Studies in Navy communication: III The effects of time/frequency distortion on the prosodic features of speech.
U.S. Nav. Submar. Med. Cent., Rep. SMRL 680, 8p. Sept. 7, 1971.

In order to study the effects of time/frequency distortion on the prosodic features of speech, content-standard speech messages representing nine different emotions were subjected to reproduce ratios of 1.0, 1.8, 1.95, 2.05 and 2.15. These emotional speech stimuli were then presented to 50 Ss for identification of the intended emotion. The results demonstrated that identification scores were high for all emotions in the non-distortion condition and remained high for eight of the nine emotions under the most severe distortion condition. Compared to intelligibility scores, which are more easily affected by time/frequency distortion, the information carried by the prosodic features of speech was robust and resistant to distortion. Information contained in this report is useful to the design of communication systems which will improve reception of speech produced underwater and in deep submergence chambers. (Authors' abstract and application)

531.
DULING, B.R.
Microvascular responses to alterations in oxygen tension.
Circ. Res. 31(4):481-489; 1972.

The changes in microvascular diameter and perivascular O_2 tension [PO_2] resulting from alterations in suffusion solution PO_2 were investigated in a study of the participation of O_2 in the regulation of blood flow. Diffusion gradients for O_2 were altered by changing the PO_2 of a solution covering the surface of the hamster cheek pouch. As the solution PO_2 was raised from a low of 11 mmHg, perivascular PO_2 of the large arterioles initially decreased to a minimum at about 40 mm Hg and then increased progressively as solution PO_2 was elevated further. Arterial capillary and tissue PO_2 remained relatively constant over a range of solution O_2 tensions of 11-40 mmHg suggesting that either the precapillary sphincters or the terminal arterioles were active in regulating tissue PO_2 as the input of O_2 from the solution was increased. The arterioles constricted as solution PO_2 was elevated. Average arteriolar diameter decreased by 13% as solution PO_2 increased from 11-47 mmHg. A more pronounced constriction of 20% occurred when solution PO_2 was increased from 11-84 mmHg. The response of large and small arterioles was apparently not mediated by a direct effect of O_2 on the vascular smooth muscle, since decreases in perivascular PO_2 were coincident with decreases in vascular diameter in these vessels over a range of solution PO_2 at 11-47 mmHg. The data did not distinguish between a direct and an indirect effect of O_2 on the vascular smooth muscle of the terminal arterioles and precapillary sphincters. However, the PO_2 measured at these sites (18-30 mmHg) required that the vascular smooth muscle cells respond to altered PO_2 at levels higher than those which were demonstrated experimentally. (© BA)

532.
EASTAUGH, R.W.
Diving support for manned submersibles.
In: Diving applications in marine research. Proceedings of a seminar, National Institute of Oceanography, Godalming, Surrey, U.K., December 1971, p.2-12. Published by the Institute. 1972.

The Vickers System of handling is described here as being typical of other submersible systems. The equipment consists basically of a hydraulic A-frame, hydraulic winch, and electric towing capstan. The divers are technicians who can dive; they are trained as pilots, and as maintenance, communications and handling system operators. As divers, their role includes (1) the release of the submersible, (2) hook-up for recovery, (3) systems work-up from dock tests to 120 feet, (4) shallow water assistance, to the limit of compressed-air diving, (5) the attachment and removal of samples, corers, drills, etc., (6) short duration support in scientific projects, (7) installation of equipment and verification of shallow water findings. The author describes, step by step, a typical launch procedure and a typical recovery procedure. Diver qualification and training are discussed. The paper is followed by a discussion of various techniques and problems involved. (MFW/SCD)

533.
EATON, H.G., M.E. Unstead and W.D. Smith.
A total hydrocarbon analyzer for use in nuclear submarines and other closed environments.
J. Chromatogr. Sci. 11(5):275-278; 1973.

A total hydrocarbon analyzer measured the total organic contaminant levels in the atmospheres of nuclear submarines. The detection of low levels of higher molecular weight organic substances was complicated by large quantities of methane and refrigerant gases. The total hydrocarbon analyzer was a specialized gas chromatograph utilizing compressed air as the carrier gas, a H flame ionization detector as its sensor, and employing backflush chromatography to obtain total hydrocarbons. (© BA)

534.
EDEL, P.O.
Mixing hydrox safely.
Oceanol. Int. 7:31-33;Jan. 1972.

Hydrogen-oxygen mixes are receiving more attention as diving gases. Two of the most important reasons are that nitrogen-oxygen mixtures cannot be used safely below 250 ft. because of the narcotic effect, and there are indications that the maximum safe limits for breathing heliox mixtures may be in the 1,000 to 2,000 ft range. Some experts believe hydrox mixtures might extend the diving depth range — provided there are no adverse long-term effects, and provided proper precautions can be instituted to control the amount of oxygen in hydrogen and keep it within the non-explosive range. Experiments by the Bureau of Mines, Ocean Systems Inc., and the Royal Swedish Navy show that mixtures of 3% oxygen in hydrogen are well within safe limits. With respect to the explosive and flammability ranges, a diver is as safe at 200 FSW breathing 3% oxygen 97% hydrogen as in breathing air at sea level. The major difficulty comes in obtaining this mixture safely since in practice a wide range of hydrogen-oxygen will occur during mixing procedures. This coupled with the relative ease of igniting an explosive mixture, and the relatively high explosive energy of hydrox, have discouraged experimentation. . . . The idea of injecting pure oxygen into a hydrogen cylinder at 2,000 psig would appear — at first glance — to be hazardous. However, if controlled safely, it has the desirable features of minimum handling, a short blending time, a small number of fittings required, and simplicity of operation. A hydrogen bottle at 2000 psig is connected to an oxygen bottle having an appreciably greater pressure, when the valves are opened, the oxygen will flow into the hydrogen cylinder. To control the flow rate, a micrometering valve is installed between the two bottles to prevent pressure surges and the resultant heat of compression which could ignite the mixture, and permit accurate control of the flow rate. (The oxygen is added at 5 psig or less per minute to prevent a significant change in cylinder temperature.) (Author)

535.
EDEL, P.O., J.M. Holland, C.L. Fischer and W.B. Fife.
Preliminary studies of hydrogen-oxygen breathing mixtures for deep sea diving.
In: The working diver, 1972. Symposium proceedings, February 1972, Columbus, Ohio, p-257-270. Washington, D.C., Marine Technology Society, 1972.

Experiments using various mixtures of hydrogen and oxygen were conducted with divers down to 200 feet and dogs down to 1000 feet. No contradictory indications to the use of hydrogen-oxygen as a breathing medium were found; no significant changes resulted from exposure of subjects to this mixture under the conditions tested. It is concluded that there is no significant difference between the diver's speech in hydrogen-oxygen and his speech in helium-oxygen where the oxygen percentage and depth are constant. An unscrambler that would work for helium-oxygen should also work for hydrogen-oxygen. The temperature comfort ranges for the two gas mixtures are also similar. Some difficulty is encountered in assessments. However, similar requirements are evidenced in the decompression requirements of helium-oxygen and hydrogen-oxygen. Hydrogen is seen to possibly be the inert gas of choice for exposures to extreme depths. (Authors' abstract)

536.
EDEL, P.O.
On hydrogen diving.
In: Professional diving symposium, New Orleans, Nov. 1972. Mar. Technol. Soc. J. 7:32-35; Mar./Apr. 1973.

It is possible that depth limits may be set for helium-oxygen diving due to hpns. Other breathing mixtures are under consideration as substitutes, among them hydrogen. Its advantage is its low breathing resistance, its explosive quality is its disadvantage. However, if the oxygen percentage is kept within 3 percent, a hydrogen-oxygen mixture should be safe. There is a danger point, where the oxygen is injected into the hydrogen, at which the percentage exceeds the safety limit. The system must be designed so that this point is located at sufficient distance from personnel. Dives using 72-24-4 hydrogen-nitrogen-oxygen mixtures have been made to 360 feet in Sweden. This depth exceeds the safety limit for nitrogen, however, and subsequently a dive was made using 96-4 hydrogen-oxygen. Methods of mixing hydrogen and oxygen are discussed, the most practicable appearing to be the injection of pure oxygen into a hydrogen cylinder at 2000 psig. This, when controlled adequately, affords minimum handling, short blending time, a small number of fittings, and simplicity of operation. This system is described in some detail and illustrated by a diagram. (MFW/BSCP)

537.
EDELMAN, N.H., P.E. Epstein, S. Lahiri and N.S. Cherniack.
Ventilatory responses to transient hypoxia and hypercapnia in man.
Resp. Physiol. 17:302-314;Apr. 1973.

The contribution of the peripheral (arterial) chemoreceptors to the ventilatory response to acute hypoxia and hypercapnia intact unanesthetized man has been evaluated by methods which assume that ventilatory responses to transient stimuli reflect their effects upon the arterial chemoreceptors while responses to steady-state stimuli reflect their effects upon both arterial chemoreceptors and the central nervous system. Transient eucapneic hypoxia was produced by inhalation of several breaths of N_2 while breathing room air; transient hypercapneic hypoxia was produced by inhalation of several breaths of N_2 with CO_2 added while breathing CO_2 enriched air. Transient euoxic hypercapnia was produced by inhalation of single breaths of from 6 to 20% CO_2 in 21% O_2 while the subject breathed air; transient hypoxic hypercapnia was produced by inhalation of single breaths of CO_2 enriched hypoxic gas while the subjects breathed a similarly hypoxic gas mixture. The ventilatory responses to transient hypoxia were qualitatively similar to the responses to steady-state hypoxia although they were quantitatively significantly greater by an average of 18%. The responses to transient euoxic hypercapnia averaged approximately one-third the responses to steady-state euoxic hypercapnia. Responses to transient hypercapnia were much less enhanced by hypoxia than were responses to steady-state hypercapnia. The findings suggest that: (1) A slight, centrally mediated, depressant effect of hypoxia may be present in unanesthetized man; (2) The peripheral chemoreceptors are responsible for approximately one-third of the overall (steady-state) ventilatory response to hypercapnia; (3) The phenomenon of stimulus interaction (enhancement of ventilatory response to hypercapnia by hypoxia) occurs at both the peripheral chemoreceptors and within the central nervous system but the central effect is the predominant one. (Authors' abstract)

538.
EDMONDS, C.
Vertigo in diving.
Balmoral, N.S.W., Aust., Roy. Aust. Navy, Sch. Underwater Med., Rep. 1/71, 34p. 1971.

The aetiology of vertigo with diving has been assessed with reference to the relevant medical literature and case reports. It has been demonstrated that vertigo may occur: due to caloric stimulation, in which case there is either a perforation of the tympanic membrane, unilateral obstruction of the external auditory canal or unequal responses to vestibular stimulus; inner ear barotrauma, due to external ear barotrauma of descent, middle ear barotrauma of descent with forceful Valsalva manoeuvres, or middle ear barotrauma of ascent; decompression sickness; abnormal gas pressures, especially inert gas narcosis, oxygen toxicity and the carbon dioxide "off effect"; unequal vestibular responses; and miscellaneous conditions which include migraine, sensory deprivation and idiopathic vertigo of diving. Methods of differentiating the various aetiological conditions, both on clinical grounds and on laboratory investigation, are discussed. (Author's conclusions)

539.
EDMONDS, C. and F.A. Blackwood.
Investigation of otological disorders in diving.
Balmoral, N.S.W., Aust., Roy. Aust. Navy, Sch. Underwater Med., Rep. 2/71, 19p. Dec. 1971.

This report discusses some isolated aspects of investigations into otological disorders of diving. It combines within the one paper, information on recent investigations into both hearing and vestibular damage, and discusses the possible methods of demonstrating these abnormalities. The basic requirements considered necessary for the initial data, periodical measurements and investigation of otological disorders of diving, include: 1. Full clinical ENT examination. 2. Audiometer with 250-8000 Hz range, bone conduction, masking, SISI and recruitment capability. 3. Electronystagmogram, with caloric positioning and the compression/decompression stimulation, as described in this article. 4. Sonomanometer. 5. [Investigators must be] specialists in otology, who also have a practical appreciation of diving conditions. (Authors' conclusions)

540.
EDMONDS, C. and R.L. Thomas.
Medical aspects of diving. Part I.
Med. J. Aust. 2:1199-1201;Nov. 18, 1972.

In this, the first part of a six part survey, the authors discuss the problems of breathhold diving; those covered in this article include: (1) Consequences of inadequate physical fitness. (2) Psychological disturbances: (a) phobic anxiety state; (b) claustrophobia; (c) over-reactive anxiety state; (d) illusions; (e) psychological responses to physiological abnormalities. (3) Exposure to cold and immersion: (a) cardiovascular system; (b) central nervous system; (c) gastrointestinal system; (d) renal system; (e) limbs; (f) cutaneous reactions. (4) Hypoxia: (a) breathhold diving without hyperventilation; (b) breathhold diving following hyperventilation. In most cases, suggestions are made for treatment or prevention. (MFW/BSCP)

541.
EDMONDS, C. and R.L. Thomas.
Medical aspects of diving. Part 2.
Med. J. Aust. 2:1256-1260;Nov. 25, 1972.

In this continuation of a discussion of the possible dangers of breathhold diving, the following subjects are treated: (1) Near drowning (based on data from animal experiments): (a) biochemical disturbances; (b) circulatory disturbances; respiratory disturbances; (based on data related to human drowning): (a) clinical observation; (b) immediate first aid; (c) hospital treatment. (2) Dangerous marine animals: (a) sharks; (b) the sea wasp; (c) cone shells; (d) blue-ringed octopus; (e) stone fish; (f) sea snakes. Proper treatment for each type of injury is described. (3) Miscellaneous conditions: (a) salt water aspiration; (b) descent barotrauma; (c) decompression sickness (rare in breathhold diving, but possible if many repetitive dives are made in one day). (MFW/BSCP)

542.
EDMONDS, C. and R.L. Thomas.
Medical aspects of diving. Part 3.
Med. J. Aust. 2:1300-1304;Dec. 2, 1972.

In this section, the authors discuss diving with open circuit apparatus. Barotrauma is defined as "tissue damage and its sequelae, resulting from an imbalance between pressures in the physiological gas spaces and body tissue." Medical problems of this type of diving are here divided into barotrauma of descent and barotrauma of ascent. The first include (a) sinus squeeze, (b) lung squeeze, (c) body squeeze, (d) face squeeze, (e) skin barotrauma, (f) dental barotrauma, (g) aural barotrauma, (external ear squeeze, middle ear squeeze and internal ear barotrauma). The second include (a) Pulmonary barotrauma (tissue damage, surgical emphysema, pneumothorax, air embolism, or a combination of these), (b) gastro-intestinal barotrauma, (c) dental barotrauma, (d) sinus barotrauma, (e) aural barotrauma. A succinct discussion of all these conditions is given, with more emphasis and detail regarding aural barotrauma of descent, and pulmonary barotrauma of ascent. (MFW/BSCP)

543.
EDMONDS, C. and R.L. Thomas.
Medical aspects of diving. Part 4.
Med. J. Aust. 2:1367-1370;Dec. 9, 1972.

In this section, the authors discuss decompression sickness, which they believe to be "the major limiting factor for deep and extended duration diving." It is defined as "the result of liberation of gases into body fluids or tissues, during or subsequent to decompression at too fast a rate." The various types include: (1) cutaneous manifestations, (2) bends, (3) peripheral nerve involvement, (4) lymphatic obstruction, (5) generalized manifestations, (6) gastrointestinal manifestations, (7) central nervous system involvement, (8) intravascular manifestations, (9) postdecompression shock. Following a brief discussion of each of these, is a brief discussion of recompression therapy with intermittent oxygen breathing. There is included a discussion of osteonecrosis. It is stated that possibly this occurs in as many as 50 percent of divers. There is some speculation on the etiology of osteonecrosis. It is stated that it "involves infarction of an area of bone, following obstruction of the vascular supply, probably by gas emboli. Other possibilities include: compression, fat emboli; trauma leading to osteochondritis; obliterating endarteritis of nutrient vessels." It is stated that once osteonecrosis is discovered in a diver, he should be restricted to no-decompression diving. Radiological diagnosis and surgical treatment are discussed. (MFW/BSCP)

544.
EDMONDS, C. and R.L. Thomas.
Medical aspects of diving. Part 5.
Med. J. Aust. 2:1416-1419;Dec. 16, 1972.

In this section, miscellaneous problems are discussed: (1) Nitrogen narcosis: Its mechanism is uncertain; various postulations, such as degree of grease solubility of a gas, its molecular weight, the formation of microcrystals which can interfere with the electrical activity of the brain at synaptic junctions, hypoxia and hypercapnia, hyperoxia, and others, cannot be conclusively demonstrated as the causative factors. It usually occurs at depths of more than 100 feet, and becomes incapacitating at more than 340 feet with most divers. Contributing factors include rapid compression, inexperience and fatigue; adaptation occurs with experienced divers. Motivation and emotional stability are involved, as is tolerance to alcohol. (2) Dangers of various breathing mixtures: The effectiveness of high oxygen tensions in increasing inert gas elimination is offset by the danger of oxygen toxicity. The use of helium or hydrogen instead of nitrogen prevents narcosis, and overcomes the problem of pulmonary airway resistance, but causes heat loss and, particularly in the case of helium, speech distortion. The high pressure nervous syndrome may be related to helium, or simply to high pressure per se. (3) Vertigo: It can be caused by caloric stimulation, barotrauma of middle or inner ear, decompression sickness, occupational complications, unequal vestibular responses. (4) Disorientation: This can result from vertigo, reduction of sensory input, impaired state of consciousness, psychological factors. (5) Syncope of ascent: It is caused by inadequate exhalation. (6) Salt water aspiration syndrome: Until recently, this has been confused with pulmonary barotrauma and with decompression sickness. Its symptoms include rigors, tremors or shivering, anorexia, nausea and vomiting, hot and cold sensations, dyspnea, headaches, malaise, aches in limbs, chest, back, and abdomen. It can result from buddy breathing, free ascent or faulty equipment. (7) Carbon monoxide toxicity: It is caused by a faulty compressor, and can be treated by 100% oxygen, hyperbaric if possible. :MFW/BSCP)

545.
EDMONDS, C. and R.L. Thomas.
Medical aspects of diving. Part 6.
Med. J. Aust. 2:1458-1460;Dec. 23, 1972.

The subject of this section is diving with closed or semi-closed circuit apparatus. The advantages of this type of breathing apparatus are: (1) prolonged endurance for a given amount of gas; (2) minimal water disturbance (bubbles); (3) minimal noise. There are different types of rebreathing equipment, according to the different types of carbon dioxide scrubber used. Accidents, often fatal, are frequent in the use of this equipment; and usually involve the loss of consciousness. The causes of loss of consciousness relevant to the use of rebreathing equipment are hypercapnia, hypoxia, and oxygen toxicity. Hypercapnia can result from increased exercise, faulty scrubbing equipment, water contamination, low temperature, excessive functional dead space, and overuse of equipment. In some cases, onset of hypercapnia is so rapid that loss of consciousness comes on without warning symptoms. Otherwise symptoms include headache, dyspnea, facial flushing, light-headedness, muscular dysfunction, visual disturbances, unconsciousness accompanied by convulsions, respiratory and cardiovascular failure. When symptoms appear, the diver should cease all muscular activity and make a buoyant ascent. Adequate respiration and circulation should be maintained until normal $PaCO_2$ and pH are achieved. Hypoxia can result from oxygen-deficient or inadequate gas supply, excessive exercise, or increased density of diluent gas. Symptoms include loss of consciousness if onset is rapid, euphoria, incoordination, apathy, cyanosis, gradual impairment of consciousness, hyperventilation, headache, amblyopia, convulsions, respiratory and cardiac failure. Oxygen must be given, with circulatory and ventilatory assistance when necessary; trismus may interfere with treatment. Oxygen toxicity takes two forms; respiratory (coughing and dyspnea, decreased vital capacity, with possibly irreversible lung damage), and neurological (convulsions). It is unlikely that lasting damage would result from one convulsion, but preventive measures must be taken immediately to prevent repetition of convulsions. Reduction of oxygen pressure can be achieved either by ascent or by changing the breathing mixture. Another danger is the ingestion of a "caustic cocktail", which consists of water mixed with carbon dioxide absorbent, and which can cause mucosal damage. Irrigation of the area should reduce symptoms. (MFW/BSCP)

546.
EDMONDS, C.
The diver.
Balmoral, N.S.W., Aust., Roy. Aust. Navy, Sch. Underwater Med., Rep. 3/73, 1973.

The chapters of this report are as follows: introduction, a review of the relevant literature on the diver, experimental design, subjective impressions of a diving course; the experienced diver, diver selection surveys; an interpretation of results past and present; Conclusion. The appendices consist of (1) compressed air breathing apparatus course syllabus, (2) medical standards for diving, (3) preliminary diver selection survey questionnaire, (4) regression analysis on preliminary diver selection survey (MFW/SCD)

547.
EDMONDS, C., P. Freeman, R. Thomas, J. Tonkin and F.A. Blackwood.
Otological aspects of diving.
Glebe, N.S.W., Aust., Australasian Medical Publishing Co., Ltd., 1973, 101p.

This book consists of the following chapters: (1) Anatomy and physiology of the ear; (2) the eustachian tube and nasal function; (3) diving physics; (4) infections of the ear; (5) decompression sickness; (6) aural barotrauma; (7) hearing loss in divers; (8) vertigo and disorientation in diving; (9) miscellaneous conditions; (10) otological standards for diving. (MFW/SCD)

548.
EDMONDS, C.
Round window rupture in diving.
In: Hesser, C.M. and D. Linnarsson, eds. Proceedings of the first annual scientific meeting of the European Undersea Biomedical Society, Stockholm, 13-15 June 1973.
Forsvarsmedicin 9:404-405;July 1973.

There have now been 7 middle ears explored, to the author's knowledge, demonstrating a fistula of the round window associated with diving, and attributed to middle ear descent barotrauma. There are still many questions to answer. Are there less serious cases of cochlear and vestibular damage associated with less gross round window fistulae? Do these sometimes heal spontaneously? From the current otological research, we must presume that the answer is Yes to both questions. Also, with an appreciation of our present knowledge on this subject hypotheses made by some other workers in diving medicine must be reassessed. Middle ear squeeze may not be the only otological diving accident with this result. Etiologies such as external ear barotrauma of descent, middle ear barotrauma of ascent and even decompression sickness may be complicated by rupture of inner ear membranes: When this does occur, surgery is the only active therapy currently available. (Author)

549.
EGSTROM, G.H., G. Weltman, A.D. Baddeley, W.J. Cuccaro and M.A. Willis.
Underwater work performance and work tolerance.
Los Angeles, Cal., Univ. Cal., Sch. Eng. Rep. UCLA-ENG-7243, 54p. July 1972.

This report presents findings of the research efforts for 1971 in the study of underwater work performance and work tolerance conducted at the University of California, Los Angeles. The studies were directed towards the development of performance decrement curves related to the specific variables which affect underwater work. Experiments designed to add to the body of knowledge necessary to the formation of decrement curves were conducted. The experiments examined: (a) the effect of cold-water exposure upon memory, reasoning ability, and vigilance, (b) the effect of depth upon memory, (c) wet vs dry training for a specific underwater task, and (d) the physiological and performance effects of heliox as a breathing gas in cold water. The corresponding results show that: (a) cold-water exposure impairs memory but not reasoning ability or vigilance, (b) although narcotic impairment to depths of 110 feet are small, material learned underwater is not remembered well on the surface, (c) training underwater for a specific underwater task is preferable to dry-land training, and (d) physiological state changes and performance levels in cold water are not substantially different for heliox as compared to air for a wetsuited diver. These data and the data from the literature are incorporated and presented as framework for the performance decrement curves. (DCD abstract)

550.
EGSTROM, G.H., G. Weltman, W.J. Cuccaro and M.A. Willis.
Underwater work performance and work tolerance.
Los Angeles, Cal., Univ. Cal., Sch. Eng. Appl. Sci., Rep. UCLA-ENG-7318, 65p. Jan. 1973.

Work conducted at the University of California, Los Angeles, in the area of underwater work performance and work tolerance during 1972 has concentrated on two principal areas: the development of a family of curves describing the effects of pertinent environmental variables on underwater work performance and research attempting to fill some of the apparent voids in the literature. The approach utilized in developing the performance curves was to categorize human performance into four general classes, cognitive, psychomotor, sensori-perceptual, and physical, and to determine the known modification of those classes of performance by the primary environmental variables. Research was conducted to examine: (1) the effect of cold water exposure on the ability to remember and follow instructions received before submersion, (2) the isometric strength capabilities of divers during shallow, cold water exposures, and (3) the effects of hyperbaric exposures on memorization of information. Results of this research indicated: (1) cold water exposure significantly degrades underwater recall but not recognition, (2) isometric strength capabilities are unaffected by one-hour exposures to shallow 43°F water when the divers are protected by 1/4" wetsuits and 3/16" diving gloves, although the gloves themselves cause a considerable reduction in grip strength, and (3) free recall of information learned at 6 ATA is significantly worse than observed at 1 ATA while recognition of the same information is unaffected. These findings were utilized in the formulation of the performance curves. (DCD abstract)

551.
EHM, O.F., A. Piechotta and K. Schimpf.
Alterations of coagulation in decompression sickness.
In: Fructus, X., Ed. Third international conference on hyperbaric and underwater physiology, p.169-170. Paris, Doin, 1972.

The authors describe the case of a diver who died of shock following a generalized purpura resulting from a decompression accident, even though recompression was undertaken immediately. It is believed that the purpura indicated a state of "coagulopathia" that was fatal because it could not be treated. The authors have inaugerated a series of experiments with rabbits to investigate physiological alterations from decompression sickness which can lead to shock. So far it has been demonstrated that after decompression all animals showed a reduction of platelets, a lowering of the prothrombin and factor V levels. (MFW/UMS)

552.
EKLUND, B., L. Kaijser and A. Melcher.
The effect of CO_2 retention on physical performance under hyperbaric oxygen conditions.
In: Hesser, C.M. and D. Linnarsson eds. Proceedings of the first annual scientific meeting of the European Undersea Biomedical Society, Stockholm, 13-15 June 1973. Forsvarsmedicin 9:271-274;July 1973.

An increased $PaCO_2$ did not change performance time to fatigue or maximal O_2 extraction in the active muscle during forearm work when pulmonary ventilation could not be a limiting factor, whereas the addition of CO_2 to inspiratory air during leg work decreased performance time [to fatigue] and possibly also O_2 extraction in the active muscles. It is probable that the effect of breathing is normally a more important limiting factor for physical performance under hyperbaric conditions than muscle metabolic effects of the increased PCO_2 and acidity. (From authors' abstract)

553.
ELCOMBE, D.D. and J.H. Teeter.
Nitrogen narcosis during a 14-day continuous exposure to 5.2% O_2 in N_2 at pressure equivalent to 100 fsw (4 ata).
Aerosp. Med. 44(7, Sec. II):864-869;July 1973.

The narcotic effects of nitrogen breathed at 100 ft of sea water with a natural oxygen pressure of 0.21 ata should be equivalent to the effects of breathing air itself at a depth of 126 ft of sea water. The narcosis produced under these circumstances is clearly evident in some individuals. The present study endeavored to quantitate narcotic effects of nitrogen in normal men during acute exposure and during sustained exposure to the increased nitrogen pressure. Quantitative measurement of the subjects' intellectual capabilities, taste, and olfactory sensations showed no gross differences from normal at increased nitrogen pressure. It is recognized that the narcotic influence of nitrogen is expressed to different degrees in different individuals. The highly motivated, skilled and intelligent subjects used in this laboratory study had, for physical, mental and physiological functions, such high reserve and compensatory ability that their performance was superior even in the narcotic atmosphere. Other individuals without those reserves would be expected to be more affected and could be endangered by exposure to severe physical stress in diving or by a requirement for use of fine judgment or a high order of technical skill. (Authors' abstract)

554.
ELDRIDGE, F.L.
Posthyperventilation breathing: different effects of active and passive hyperventilation.
J. Appl. Physiol. 34:422-430;Apr. 1973.

The posthyperventilation breathing patterns after passive (mechanically generated) hyperventilation in anesthetized cats were compared to those after active (neurally generated) hyperventilation produced by carotid sinus nerve stimulation of calf muscle squeezing. Passive hyperventilation (HV) of several minutes duration always showed posthyperventilation apnea followed by a gradual return of ventilation to control levels over the first minute of recovery. Shorter periods of passive HV were followed by hypopnea and a similar recovery course. In contrast, active HV with either type of stimulation was followed by hyperpnea for the first few breaths after the offset of stimulation, apnea never occurred during the first 15 sec of recovery and ventilation was always maintained for the first minute at a higher level than after passive hyperventilation. Carotid sinus nerve and vagal influences were shown not to be responsible for the phenomenon. Changes in blood pressure and heart rate also do not appear to be responsible. The study shows that a process connected with active breathing supplies sufficient neural facilitation to prevent the apnea associated with a simple decrease in chemical stimulation. (Author's abstract)

555.
EL GHAWABI, S.H., M.B. Mansour, F.L. Youssef, M.H. El Ghawabi and M.M. Abd El Latif.
Decompression sickness in caisson workers.
Br. J. Ind. Med. 28:323-329; 1971.

An investigation of 55 bridge construction workers is reported. The overall bends rate was 0.97%. (The term 'bends' as used in this study is defined in the paper.) Chokes were encountered in 67.27% of workers. A clinical, haematological, and radiological study was performed. Definite bony changes were found in 43.6% of all workers: 91.6% of these had lesions around the elbow. The presence of dense areas in the neck of the scapula is reported in two cases for the first time. The relatively high haematocrit value is thought to play a part in the pathogenesis of bone infarction through its relation with blood viscosity. (Authors' abstract)

556.
ELINSKII, M.P.
Lesions of the nervous system in decompression sickness.
Vop. Psikhiat. Nevropat. 13:615-622;n.d.
Orpington, UK, Def. Res. Inf. Cent., Transl. DRIC-2790, 12p. May 1972.
(AD 743,330)

Of all the pathological conditions brought about by the effects of anomalous conditions in the surrounding air media, the most serious is the disease associated with rapid reduction of the atmospheric pressure. Such diseases are termed decompression sickness. Where there is considerable and rapid reduction of pressure, the gases dissolved in the blood and tissue separate out in the form of bubbles and form vascular embolisms and local affection of the tissue. Such sickness is encountered in ascents to high altitudes (above 8000m), caisson work, diving operations, deep diving sport, pressure chamber research, etc. Affection of the nervous system is one of the most serious complications, and is important as a symptom of decompression sickness. Several characteristic features of the clinic course of the illness which is accompanied by affection of the nervous system are described. (GRA)

557.
ELINSKII, M.P.
"Mute" gas bubbles and their role in decompression pathology.
Voennomed. Zh. (1):56-59; 1969.
(Translation: Orpington, UK, Def. Res. Inf. Cent., Rep. DRIC-Trans-2789 and DRIC-BR-30160, 8p. July 1972)
(AD 748,229)

The presented data shows that in the absence of clinically expressed signs of decompression sickness in the nervous system, definite morphological changes can result from gas forming in the body after decompression. From this it follows that the body possesses a definite degree of tolerance in relation to the post-decompression aeroembolism whose excess leads to an expressed disease. When a person feels unwell, or when there is an excess of local sensations of sickness in people subjected the day before to the influence of increased or lowered atmospheric pressure, it is essential that careful and thorough research be carried out to expose effaced forms of decompression sickness, provoked by 'mute' gas bubbles. (GRA)

558.
ELINSKII, M.P.
Decompression disorders after exposure to 'safe pressure' or 'safe altitude'.
Voennomed. Zh. (7):60-63;July 1970.
(Translation U.K., Def. Res. Inform. Cent., Rep. DRIC-3035. Jan. 1973)
(AD 756,263)

From experimental studies and clinical observations cited, it is clear that decompression starting from 2.25 atm abs or less and also ascents to an altitude of less than 8000 m may lead to the appearance of gas bubbles in the blood and sometimes cause severe decompression sickness. Such cases are probably not always spotted because of the widely held view that disorders do not occur with such pressure drops. The problem raised in this paper seems to be of practical importance because if decompression sickness may arise after exposure to a depth of 12.5 m, this points to the formation of gas bubbles large enough to cause embolism. From this it follows that uninterrupted ascent from these depths is not always harmless, particularly as 'occult' gas bubbles may be formed leading to subclinical forms of decompression sickness. In the second place saturation of the organism with nitrogen and other gases at a pressure of 2.25 atm abs may not be taken as an index of safe supersaturation, both now and hitherto calculations of tables for stepwise decompression are based on the assumption that a pressure drop in the ratio of 2.25:1 does not cause disease. It is possible that the need to reduce the factor with increasing depths is primarily due to a false concept of the complete safety of ascending from a depth of 12.5 m. (GRA)

559.
ELIZONDO, R.S., M.R. Banerjee, N.E. Leatherman, S. Mizell and J.R. Hippensteele.
Physiological adjustments to environmental factors.
Bloomington, Ind., Ind. Univ., Dept. Anat. Physiol., Rep. AFOSR-TR-72-1453, 155p. Dec. 13, 1972.
(AD 753 913)

The report covers the entire scientific effort sustained by Project Themis contract F44620-68-C-0014 over the five-year period under the direction of Robert W. Bullard and the year following his death on June 24, 1971. With it are furnished the scientific publications by year, the meetings attended, the abstracts and the review article by Robert W. Bullard. The report also includes the advantages the project has given the department in creating a biophysical approach to physiology and the advantage to general recruitment of physiologists. The forty published scientific journal articles adequately summarize the scientific results of this project. (Author) (GRA)

560.
ELKINS, J.H.
Requirements of the ideal helium speech communications system.
In: Sergeant, R.L. and T. Murry, eds. Processing helium speech: proceedings of a Navy-sponsored workshop, August 1971, U.S. Nav. Submar. Med. Res. Lab., Rep. NSMRL 708, p.13-17. May 22, 1972.

The author believes that the chief reason for the relative lack of success in the development of helium speech processors is the lack of understanding of microphone requirements. He discusses characteristics essential to successful speech communication systems: (1) Experience in the diver is an important factor. (2) Electronics of the first quality are a prerequisite for initially intelligible input data. The recently developed LTV microphone is an important step in this direction. Also, it is important to consider the mask and the microphone together. Bandwidth is an important parameter; an upper limit of at least 10KHZ is required. (3) Real-time conversion is mandatory. (4) Audio levels should be higher than normal and adjustable. (5) The device should be easily portable; if the diver can hear the corrected version of his own voice, he can increase his intelligibility by adaptation. (6) As to methods of measuring intelligibility, the modified rhyme test appears to be the most successful; here, the diver chooses one of the six possible words on his list. (7) Controls should be kept to a minimum, consisting of on-off and volume; depth compensation adjustments should be automatic. (8) Power should be minimal; the speech processor should be combined with other communication equipment. (MFW/BSCP)

561.
ELLIOTT, D.H.
Aseptic bone narcosis in Naval divers.
In: Abstracts of Bu-Med-ONR sponsored Navywide workshop in high pressure biomedical research, U.S. Submarine Base, Groton, Conn., May 1971, p.26. Published by the Naval Submarine Medical Research Laboratory, 1971.

Abstract only. Entire item quoted: A three-year survey of 350 full-time divers of the Royal Navy revealed a 5% incidence of radiological aseptic necrosis of bone. This is compared with the higher incidence in surveys of civilian divers who are found also to have a significant proportion of juxtaarticular lesions causing severe symptoms. The radiological techniques necessary to ensure consistently high quality films are outlined and particular emphasis is placed on the use of internationally accepted criteria for the diagnosis of lesions. Current thoughts on the management and treatment of lesions found are presented. A study of the diving history of these persons reveals a statistically significant association between the presence of a necrotic lesion and a history of decompression inadequacy, either participation in experimental diving or one or more episodes of decompression sickness.

562.
ELLIOTT, D.H.
The role of decompression inadequacy in aseptic bone necrosis of naval divers.
Proc. Roy. Soc. Med. 64:1278-1280;Dec. 1971.

As a result of analyzing the statistics revealed in a radiological survey of 305 naval divers, it is concluded that there is a positive relationship between the presence of radiological lesion and a history of decompression, also between positive lesion and experience of experimental diving with compressed air, and experimental deep diving with helium. ("Experimental" in this case refers to dives in which the decompression schedules used were not of proven adequacy). (MFW/BSCP)

563.
ELLIOTT, D.H.
Clinical problems of decompression sickness relevant to the surface activity of intravascular bubbles.
In: Ackles, K.N. ed. Blood-bubble interaction in decompression sickness. Proceedings of an international symposium held at Defence and Civil Institute of Environmental Medicine, Downsview, Ontario, Canada, p.140-161. Published by the Institute, December 1973. (DCIEM Conference Proceedings 73-CP-960).

The surface activity of the intravascular bubble should be considered in relation to each of these problems: individual susceptibility and adaptation to decompression sickness; the role of pulmonary micro-barotrauma in (1) platelet response to normal diving, and (2) decompression sickness; prolonged latent period of onset; prognostic value of doppler-detected bubbles: dose-response and possible correlation with some haematological index; the relation of both to overt manifestations of acute decompression sickness, as well as to the later development of aseptic bone necrosis; cause of cutaneous vascular stasis — (ideal site for investigation); relative preponderance of spinal cord lesions in divers; significance of migraine-like episodes in divers and aviators; the nature of staggers, and the particular problem of vestibular system disturbance; the consequences of increased capillary permeability ranging from the presence of some haemoconcentration in the mild bends of compressed air workers to the serious shock of aviators' post-descent collapse; paradoxical response to recompression; ineffectiveness of recompression, particularly in cases of spinal cord involvement after a prolonged delay in contrast to other cases in whom headache or vertigo have responded after a delay of several days; and finally, perhaps a limiting factor to commercial diving and a subject on which we touch later, aseptic necrosis of bone, its cause and prevention. (Author's summary)

564.
ELLIS, J.P., Jr., B.E. Welch and J.M. Prescott.
Effects of hypercapnia and physical deconditioning on musculoskeletal protein in man.
Brooks Air Force Base, Sch. Aerosp. Med., Rep. SAM-TR-419, 8p. 1971.
(AD 736,665)

A recently developed automated chromatographic method for quantifying urinary peptides and free amino acids was used to ascertain the effects of confinement, physical deconditioning, and hypercapnia on a group of three healthy male subjects. A four-day control period preceded a 15-day experimental period, during which time the subjects were housed in a small air-tight environmental chamber. The chamber air was the same as room air except for the middle third of the experiment during which time it was adjusted so as to contain 3% CO_2. The following urinary excretion trends were found: (a) a generalized reduction in amino acids and amino-peptides, (b) a sharp rise followed by an abrupt fall in one hydroxyproline peptide, and (c) a less marked but progressive increase in another hydroxyproline peptide. The timing and magnitude of the latter two changes suggest that perhaps two types of body collagen may have been partially degraded by confinement and/or deconditioning. (Authors) (GRA)

565.
ELSNER, R., B.A. Gooden and S.M. Robinson.
Arterial blood gas changes and the diving response in man.
Aust. J. Exp. Biol. Med. Sci. 49(5):435-444; 1971.

Face immersion breath-holds were performed by five seated male subjects after normal breathing of room air, normal breathing of 100% O_2 for 15 min. and hyperventilation of 100% O_2 for 15 min. Heart rate and forearm blood flow were determined in all three procedures and PO_2 [O_2 pressure] PCO_2 [CO_2 pressure] and pH of brachial artery blood were measured in the O_2 breathing experiments. Simulated diving after breathing room air significantly reduced the heart rate and forearm blood flow. After normal breathing and hyperventilation of O_2, PaO_2 was elevated by three and five times respectively. $PaCO_2$ was unchanged by normal breathing but halved by hyperventilation. "Diving" after both O_2 breathing procedures still significantly reduced both heart rate and forearm blood flow below resting control levels and these responses were not significantly different from those after breathing room air. The fall in arterial O_2 tension during "diving" after hyperventilation of oxygen was inversely related to the fall in forearm blood flow ($P < 0.001$) which fits the concept that the diving response may serve an O_2 conserving function in man. Despite arterial hyperoxia with or without hypocapnia, a significant diving response was still evoked by face immersion breath-holding, showing that the response is basically independent of asphyxial blood gas changes. (© BA)

566.
ELSNER, R., B.A. Gooden and S.M. Robinson.
Circulatory effects of human face immersion: Chemoreceptor influences.
IN: Abstracts of the Twenty-fifth Congress of Physiological Sciences Satellite Symposium. Recent progress in fundamental physiology of diving. Marseille, France, July 1971, p.12-13 (Proceedings unpublished)

Abstract only. Entire item quoted: Breath-holding face immersions were performed by four young adult male subjects after normal breathing of room air, normal breathing of 100% oxygen for 15 min and hyperventilation of 100% oxygen for 15 min. Pulse waves and forearm blood flows were recorded in all three procedures and PO_2, PCO_2 and pH of brachial artery blood were determined in the oxygen breathing experiments. Face immersion after normal breathing of room air produced a rapid reduction in heart rate and blood flow during the 60 sec procedure. After normal oxygen breathing and hyperventilation on oxygen, PaO_2 was elevated three and five times respectively. $PaCO_2$ was unchanged by normal breathing but was halved by hyperventilation. Face immersion after both oxygen breathing periods still produced a prompt fall in heart rate and blood flow below resting control levels. These reductions below control values were, however, significantly smaller than those produced by face immersion after breathing room air. Face immersion lasted about 2 min after normal oxygen breathing and 5 min after hyperventilation on oxygen. During both procedures heart rate and blood flow returned towards control levels after about 90 sec. It is concluded that the circulatory responses to face immersion in man are basically neurogenic and occur despite arterial hyperoxia and hypocapnia. Arterial hyperoxia at the moment of face immersion lessens the intensity of these responses probably through the peripheral chemoreceptors.

567.
ELSNER, R.
Comparative circulatory studies of diving and asphyxia.
Adv. Exp. Med. Biol. 22:69-80; 1972.

The difference between the diving time of a trained human diver and that of a seal does not correspond with the differences in oxygen storage. The author has examined the extent of the circulatory changes in the seal that have been known to exist for a number of years. It is demonstrated that the blood flow in major circuits falls to nearly zero during a dive, while the central arterial blood pressure remains constant. The venous system of the seal is discussed, as are also the acid-base consequences (a fall in pH). Experiments were made with dogs and humans. Dogs demonstrated marked bradycardia and a reduction in circulation in certain organs. In face immersion experiments with human subjects, a marked decrease in limb blood flow occurred during immersion, and the response to procedures designed to increase blood flow was reduced. Experiments with Weddell seals of forced prolonged dives demonstrated a tolerance for very low arterial oxygen pressure (10 mmHg as compared with 25 mm Hg for terrestrial animals). This indicates that there may be an additional explanation for their long diving times, beyond enhanced oxygen storage and circulatory redistribution. Further experiments indicated that during advanced hypoxia at the end of a dive part of the brain energy comes from anaerobic mechanisms which produce lactic acid. (MFW/BSCP)

568.
ENGEL, L.A., H. Menkes, L.D.H. Wood, G. Utz, J. Joubert and P.T. Macklem.
Gas mixing during breath holding studied by intrapulmonary gas sampling.
J. Appl. Physiol. 35:9-17;July 1973.

A new method of sampling gases from intrapulmonary airways has been used to study mixing between dead space (V_D) and alveolar gas during breath holding in anesthetized open-chested dogs. Following an inspiration of O_2, N_2 was detected in airways 2.5-16 mm in diameter within 1 sec of breath holding. After 10 sec all airways contained N_2 in excess of 50% of alveolar concentrations. N_2 tracings from all airways showed cardiogenic oscillations resulting in a stepwise increase in N_2. Gas mixing due to molecular diffusion was studied in lungs after death. The time to reach 50% of alveolar concentrations was approximately five times shorter in vivo than postmortem. This difference is attributed to the dynamic component of gas mixing consequent upon cardiac action. It is responsible for about one-fourth of the reduction in V_D volume during the first ten sec of breath holding. Obstruction to blood flow had no effect on the rate or pattern of gas mixing, whereas manual oscillation of the heart post mortem reproduced both the enhanced gas mixing and the N_2 oscillations seen in vivo. The mechanism for the cardiac effect may involve both Taylor diffusion and convective mixing due to eddy currents and secondary motions. By use of some simplifying assumptions the effect of gas density on gas mixing was calculated to be the reverse of that produced from considerations of molecular diffusion alone. (Authors' abstract)

569.
EPSTEIN, M., L.M. Fishman and H.B. Hale.
Dissociation of aldosterone and 17-hydroxycorticosteroid (17-OHCS) release during water immersion in normal man.
Brooks Air Force Base, Sch. Aerosp. Med., Rep. SAM-TR-71-472, 7p. July 30, 1971.
(AD 737,781)
(Also published in Proc. Soc. Exp. Biol. Med. 138(3):939-942; 1971).

Since previous studies have demonstrated a profound suppression of the reninaldosterone system during water immersion in man, the specificity of this suppression of adrenal function was assessed. Urinary aldosterone and 17-OHCS release were simultaneously measured in six normal subjects studied during a control period and during water immersion under identical conditions of diet, posture and time of day. There was a marked decrease in aldosterone excretion during immersion and during the initial two hours of recovery ($P < 0.005$). In contrast, neither urinary nor plasma 17-OHCS were significantly altered by immersion. The dissociation observed between the effects of immersion on aldosterone and 17-OHCS activity suggests that the suppression of the reninaldosterone system is selective and further supports the concept of independent control of adrenal mineralocorticoid and glucocorticoid secretion. (Authors) (GRA)

570.
EPSTEIN, M., D.C. Duncan and L.M. Fishman.
Characterization of the natriuresis caused in normal man by immersion in water.
Clin. Sci. 43(2):275-287; 1972.

The effects of 4-6 h of water immersion on the renal excretion of water and electrolytes were studied in thirteen normal male subjects in balance on a constant diet containing 150 mEq of Na and 100 mEq of K per day. Each subject was studied during a control period, consisting of quiet sitting, and during water immersion to the neck. Immersion resulted in a natriuresis beginning within the first hour, with the rate of sodium excretion eventually exceeding that of the control period by 3-4 fold; potassium excretion also increased. Despite a progressively negative water balance during the immersion studies, urine flow was greater during the first 4 h and free water clearance was greater during the first 2 h of immersion than during the control study. The demonstration of a highly significant increase in fractional excretion of sodium during immersion suggests that the natriuresis of water immersion is not attributable to changes in filtered sodium load. The prompt onset of the natriuresis, the concomitant kaliuresis and the fact that aldosterone secretion under the conditions of study was probably already suppressed make it unlikely that the natriuresis of water immersion is mediated solely by decreases in aldosterone activity. The data suggest that the natriuresis caused by water immersion is the result of decreased fractional reabsorption of sodium proximal to the renal diluting site. The mechanism whereby increased proximal tubular sodium rejection occurs in relation to immersion remains unclear. (Authors' summary)

571.
EPSTEIN, M., J.L. Katsikas and D.C. Duncan.
Role of mineralocortocoids in the natriuresis of water immersion in man.
Circ. Res. 32:228-236;Feb. 1973.

In an attempt to assess the quantitative contribution of aldosterone suppression to the natriuresis of water immersion, renal sodium handling in normal male subjects undergoing water immersion was examined before and after administration of exogenous mineralocortocoid. The study demonstrated that the administration of a potent mineralocorticoid in pharmacological doses failed to abolish the natriuresis of water immersion. (© BA)

572.
ERASMUS, B.D. and H. Rahn.
Effects of inert gases upon the O_2 and CO_2 gradient across the eggshell of the incubating hen's egg.
Physiologist 16:307;Aug. 1973.

Abstract only. Entire item quoted: The gas exchange of the incubating egg depends upon passive diffusion of gases across the pores of the egg shell. For a given metabolic rate the O_2 and CO_2 gradients across the shell are determined by pore geometry and the binary diffusion coefficient between O_2 or CO_2 and the inert gas. By changing the inert gas from N_2 to SF_6 or He one would predict a large change in the diffusion coefficient and an equivalent change in O_2 and CO_2 gradient. This was tested by determining the percent O_2 and percent CO_2 in the air cell when eggs (15-17 d. incubation) were exposed to normal O_2 in N_2, SF_6 and He. In air the percent CO_2 in air cell is about 5%, rises to 9% in SF_6 and falls to 2% in He. The percent O_2 in the air cell is normally about 16%, falls to 11% in SF_6 and rises to 18% in He.

573.
EREMEEV, N.S., G.V. Troshikhin and V.G. Shaliapina.
Vliyanie povyshennogo partsial'nogo davleniya kisloroda na simpato-adrenalovuyu i atsetilkholinovuyu sistemy.
[Effect of the oxygen increased partial pressure on the sympatheticadrenal system and the brain acetylcholinesterase activity in animals].
Fiziol. Zh. SSSR 58:768-772;May 1972.

In white male mice, noradrenaline content (NR) and acetylcholinesterase activity (ACA) in the brain, and corticosteroids level (CS) in the blood were studied after 10-day stay in hyperoxygenated milieu with 60 and 80% concentration of oxygen at atmospheric pressure. The NR and CS were also studied after 2 hr stay in oxygen at 1, 3 and 3.5 atm. pressure. In male rats, the ACA was studied in different brain areas (the cortex, subcortex, brain-stem, medulla oblongata and the cerebellum) after oxygen seizures (6 atm. pressure). Both the prolonged stay in hyperoxygenated milieu and the short exposition to excessive oxygen pressure were followed by decrease in the brain NR and increase in the blood CS. The ACA increases at the atmospheric pressure and decreases at excessive pressure, particularly in the cortex. (English summary)

574.
ERICKSON, R.D., ed.
The Undersea Journal.
Costa Mesa, Calif., Professional Association of Diving Instructors. From 1969.

This quarterly journal is directed toward the sports diver. It deals with problems of training and equipment, safety measures, diving under ice, cave diving, availability of training courses, and any or all subjects that would be of interest to the sports diver or to the diving instructor. Brief articles on such subjects as nitrogen narcosis, decompression sickness, lung rupture and oxygen toxicity are occasionally included. Articles on marine biology and oceanography also appear. (MFW/BSCP)

575.
ERNSTING, J.
Hyperbaric oxygen therapy:physiological considerations.
Proc. Roy. Soc. Med. 64:873;Sept. 1971.

On physiological grounds hyperbaric oxygen therapy would be expected to be most effective in combating local hypoxia in tissues with a high blood flow relative to oxygen consumption such as the skin and kidney. Furthermore, the administration of oxygen at high pressure may tend to defeat the object of the therapy because it induces local vasoconstriction. There are, therefore, good grounds for combining hyperbaric oxygen therapy with an agent which causes dilatation of the arterioles of the part which is suffering from hypoxia. (Author)

576.
EVANS, A., E.E.P. Barnard and D.N. Walder.
Detection of gas bubbles in man at decompression.
Aerosp. Med. 43:1095-1096;Oct. 1972.

Simulated dives by guinea pigs, goats and men have been monitored with a Doppler ultrasonic transducer applied to the chest wall over the heart. With this technique there is no possibility that air is introduced into the animals or men before the start of the dives. During decompression abnormal sounds believed to be due to bubbles are detected. It appears that bubbles may be present in the circulation without giving rise to any symptoms of decompression sickness (silent bubbles) but profuse bubbling is associated with symptoms. As bubbles appear to be a precursor of decompression sickness we suggest that this simple technique should be used to give an objective endpoint when assessing decompression procedures. (Authors' abstract)

577.
EVANS, A. and D.N. Walder.
Ultrasonic surveillance of subatmospheric decompression.
Nature 246:522-523;Dec. 21/28, 1973.

All nine of these experiments were of short duration (one or two minutes) except the last, which was extended to ten minutes. A full Doppler signal was recording during nine runs, which consisted of a two-minute control period at ground level, a gradual ascent to base altitude (in seven instances, to 8,000 feet, in two instances to 25,000 feet), then a rapid ascent to 4,000 feet from 8,000 and to 54,000 feet from 25,000, a gradual descent to ground level and a final period of five minutes at atmospheric pressure. No clear bubble signals were heard in any instance. This may have been because the time was insufficient for bubbles to grow to detectable size. Indistinct abnormal signals were detected during descent in three of the experiments. (MFW/UMS)

578.
EVANS, M.J. and J.D. Hackney.
Cell proliferation in lungs of mice exposed to elevated concentrations of oxygen.
Aerosp. Med. 43:620-622;June 1972.

The purpose of this study was to determine the effects of concentrations of O_2 greater than 21% but less than 100% on cell division in the pulmonary alveoli. To accomplish this mice were exposed to 40, 60, or 80% O_2 and cells preparing to divide were labeled with tritiated thymidine (^{3}H-TdR). Labeled cells were visualized with autoradiographic techniques and labeled cells counted with the light microscope and expressed as a labeling index. In the present study it was shown that DNA synthesis in endothelial cells also was inhibited by exposure to less than 100% oxygen. However, the other cell types were not affected. Inhibition of DNA synthesis lasted about five days and then returned to control levels or above. Since the animals were continuously exposed to oxygen, these results indicated that the cells had adapted to the oxygen environment. Presumably before they adapted to the oxygen, processes associated with cell division (such as tissue repair and cell turnover) would be inhibited. (Authors' abstract)

579.
FAGAN, C.J. and E.L. Beckman.
Survey of Gulf Coast commercial divers for dysbaric osteonecrosis.
In: United States-Japan conference on natural resources development. Proceedings of the first joint meeting of the U.S.-Japan panel on diving and technology, Tokyo, 1972, p.145-160. Japan, Ministry of Agriculture and Forestry, 1972.

Dysbaric osteonecrosis of bone is not an uncommon disease among Gulf Coast divers. A sample survey consisting of a small number of commercial divers had yielded a high incidence (27%) of roentgenographic findings. As a result of this initial work, we are attempting to expand our survey. A comparison of plain film imaging with xeroradiographic imaging in an admittedly limited number of divers, has not helped us sufficiently to accept the additional radiation exposure inherent in the xeroradiographic technique. Fluorine-18 bone scanning probably represents a reasonable and practical modality in an osteonecrosis survey. We suspect that the bone scan probably relates to the osteogenic activity of the disease process and therefore may be helpful in detecting early or active areas of osteonecrosis. (Authors' summary)

580.
FAGRAEUS, L.
Performance of the isolated guinea-pig heart in hyperbaric environment.
In: Abstracts of the Twenty-fifth Congress of Physiological Sciences Satellite Symposium. Recent progress in fundamental physiology of diving. Marseille, France, July 1971, p.39-40. (Proceedings unpublished)

Abstract only. Previous research has revealed that exposure to hyperbaric conditions is accompanied by bradycardia, caused (1) by raised PO_2, and (2) by some factor or factors related to increased nitrogen pressure and/or gas density. The two types of bradycardia apparently involve different mechanisms. The purpose of this experiment was to investigate the mechanisms of the second type of bradycardia. It was found that neither 9 ATA of hydrostatic pressure, or 8 ATA of nitrogen pressure in the perfusion fluid caused any change in heart rate or myocardial contractile force of the isolated guinea pig heart. Also responses to noradrenaline, isoprenaline and electrical stimulation of the sympathetic nerves remained unaffected under increased hydrostatic and nitrogen pressure. (MFW/BSCP)

581.
FAGRAEUS, L., J. Karlsson, D. Linnarsson and B. Saltin.
Oxygen uptake during maximal work at lowered and raised ambient air pressures.
Acta. Physiol. Scand. 87(3):411-421; 1973.

The maximal aerobic power (VO_2 max) was measured in twelve subjects exercising on a bicycle ergometer breathing air at 0.68, 1.0, and 1.40 ATA [atmospheres absolute] ambient pressures. Seven of the subjects were also investigated at 2.0 and 3.0 ATA. VO_2 max averaged 3.67 l min^{-1} STPD [standard temperature and pressure, dry] at 1.0 ATA and was reduced by 14% at 0.68 ATA ($p < 0.001$), while at 1.40 ATA VO_2 max was increased by 9% ($p < 0.001$). The increased PIO_2 at the two highest pressures did not result in any further improvement of VO_2 max compared to 1.40 ATA. At all pressures changes in endurance time paralleled those of VO_2 max. Ventilation decreased markedly as ambient pressure increased with a concomitant rise of $PACO_2$ up to a mean value of 43 mm Hg at 3.0 ATA as compared to 32 mm Hg at 1.0 ATA. Moderate hyperoxia produced by increased ambient air pressure enhances circulatory transport of O_2 in maximal exercise, the working muscles have an aerobic potential exceeding what the circulation normally can offer. (© BA)

582.
FAGRAEUS, L., J. Haggendal and D. Linnarsson.
Heart rate, arterial blood pressure and noradrenaline levels during exercise with hyperbaric oxygen and nitrogen.
In: Hesser, D.M. and D. Linnarsson, eds. Proceedings of the first annual scientific meeting of the European Undersea Biomedical Society, Stockholm, 13-15 June 1973. Forsvarsmedicin 9:265-270;July 1973.

It is concluded that a rise in PO_2 alone during heavy exercise is accompanied by reductions in catecholamines and heart rate which may correspond to the decrease in relative work load. By contrast, a rise in PN_2 to 4.7 ATA seems to provoke only a slight, if any, decrease of catecholamines in relation to relative work load, whereas heart rate was found to be markedly reduced. If the levels of circulating catecholamines reflect the activity of the sympatoadrenal system, it can be concluded that a decrease in this activity may account for the heart rate decrease in heavy exercise at 1.3 ATA O_2. This compared to our earlier finding suggests that the mechanism for the oxygen-dependent heart rate decrease differs between heavy and light exercise. On the other hand, the marked decrease in exercise HR found at 6 ATA, did not seem to be part of any overall decrease in the activity of the sympatoadrenal system. The non-oxygen dependent decrease in heart rate response to exercise must therefore depend on more specific cardioinhibitory influences. (From authors' abstract)

583.
FAGRAEUS, L. and D. Linnarsson.
Heart rate in hyperbaric environment after autonomic blockade.
In: Hesser, C.M. and D. Linnarsson, eds. Proceedings of the first annual scientific meeting of the European Undersea Biomedical Society, Stockholm, 13-15 June 1973. Forsvarsmedicin 9:260-264;July 1973.

In summary it is concluded, that exercise heart rate is markedly depressed in hyperbaric environment. Part of this depression is due to an effect of raised oxygen partial pressure on the heart, both directly and over parasympathetic efferents. In addition other factors such as gas density, the high inert gas pressure or the hydrostatic pressure may interfere with the sympathetic stimulation of the heart. The observed cardiodepressive influences may be of importance to limit the tolerance for severe exercise in hyperbaria, particularly with normoxia. (Authors)

584.
FAGRAEUS, L. and D. Linnarsson.
Maximal voluntary and exercise ventilation at high ambient air pressures.
In: Hesser, C.M. and D. Linnarsson eds. Proceedings of the first annual scientific meeting of the European Undersea Biomedical Society, Stockholm, 13-15 June 1973. Forsvarsmedicin 9:275-278;July 1973.

Maximal voluntary ventilation (MVV) is known to decrease with increasing ambient pressure. On the assumption that pulmonary ventilation during exercise in hyperbaric environment is affected to the same degree, MVV may be used to predict to what extent exercise capacity is limited by ventilatory impairment at depth. The present investigation was undertaken to study the validity of such a prediction and the underlying assumption. The maximal work level used in this study was tolerated only for a few minutes and was accompanied by a severe and progressive CO_2 retention at 3.0 and 6.0 ATA. It is concluded that the highest work load which can be adequately maintained at a given increased air pressure up to and including 6.0 ATA, is the load which at sea level requires a ventilation that does not exceed 60% of the 15 sec MVV observed at the given pressure. (From authors' abstract)

585.
FAIMAN, M.D., R.G. Mehl and F.W. Oehme.
Protection with disulfiram from central and pulmonary oxygen toxicity.
Biochem. Pharmacol. 20(11):3059-3067; 1971.

Disulfiram protected mice from O_2 convulsions and lung damage. The degree of protection from convulsions was dependent upon both the dose of disulfiram administered and the time interval between disulfiram administration and O_2 exposure. Post-exposure survival of disulfiram-treated mice was very good whereas non-disulfiram-treated mice never survived the O_2 exposure period. Disulfiram protection does not appear to be related to dopamine-β-hydroxylase inhibition.It is thought disulfiram's protection may be due to its action on the cytochrome chain and its inhibition of electron transfer. (© BA)

586.
FAIMAN, M.D. and R.J. Nolan.
Effect of high oxygen pressure on brain ATP.
Fed. Proc. 31:604;Mar./Apr. 1972.

Abstract only. Entire item quoted: Oxygen at high pressure (OHP) produces convulsions in man and animals. Although a number of theories have been proposed, the mechanism(s) by which oxygen produces convulsions are unknown. Sanders et al., (Science 150:1830, 1965) reported that OHP decreased brain ATP, that succinate pretreatment prevented this decrease, and suggested that protection afforded by succinate was due to the maintenance of normal brain ATP. We carried out a series of studies in which mice were exposed to OHP in a specially designed hyperbaric chamber. This chamber allowed animals to be sacrificed while still exposed to OHP, thus avoiding problems associated with chamber decompression. We found that OHP had no effect on cerebral cortex ATP levels. Disulfiram, a previously reported potent oxygen protectant (Faiman et al., Biochem. Pharmacol. 20(11) 3059-3067; 1971) similarly had no effect on ATP levels. It is proposed that oxygen convulsions are not the result of reduced brain ATP, and the protection observed with disulfiram is not due to a maintenance of normal ATP levels. Differences between our findings and those of Sanders et al., may be the result of factors other than increased oxygen pressure, such as decompression and hypoxic effects.

587.
FAIMAN, M.D. and R.G. Mehl.
Effect of high oxygen pressure on brain norepinephrine and serotonin turnover.
Eur. J. Pharmacol. 24(2):123-130; 1973.

The effect of high O_2 pressure on the in vivo turnover of NE [norepinephrine] in mouse and rat brain, and the turnover of 5-HT [5-hydroxytryptamine] in mouse brain was investigated. Turnover of NE and 5-HT was determined by steady-state kinetic methods. In mice, synthesis of NE was inhibited by the administration of α-MPT [alpha methyl-p-tyrosine]. In rats NE turnover was determined from the decline in intracisternally administered H^3NE. Steady-state kinetic methods also were used to determine 5-HT turnover in mice, utilizing probenecid to block the transport of 5 hydroxy IAA. O_2 at 1 and 3 atmospheres had no effect on either NE turnover in mice and rats or 5-HT turnover in mice. Changes in NE and 5-HT turnover do not appear to be implicated in the onset of O_2 induced convulsions. (© BA)

588.
FAIMAN, M.D., R.J. Nolan and G.L. Grunewald.
The role of disulfiram in oxygen toxicity.
Fed. Proc. 32(3,pt.1):306;Mar. 1973.

Abstract only. Entire item quoted: Tetraethylthiuram disulfide (disulfiram) (DSF) previously shown to effectively protect mice from oxygen convulsions and lung damage, has now been found to also protect rats and guinea pigs from oxygen toxicity. In addition, DSF (200 mg/kg i.p.) also protected different strains of mice from oxygen toxicity. DSF's anticonvulsant action appears to be oxygen-specific since mice pretreated with DSF were not protected from electroshock (20 mA-0.2 sec) or pentylenetetrazol (90 mg/kg S.C.) induced seizures. The disulfide bridge in the DSF molecule appears to be required for DSF's effectiveness as an oxygen protectant. Neither tetraethylthiuram monosulfide, NNN'N'tetraethylterephthalamide or NNN'N' tetraethylterephthalthionamide protected against oxygen toxicity. After absorption, DSF is reduced to diethyldithiocarbamate (DDTC), and further metabolized to the DDTC-methyl ester (DDT-Me). The DDTC-Me also protected mice from oxygen toxicity, and seemed more potent than DSF or DDTC as an oxygen protectant. The DDTC-Me may be responsible for DSF's protective action against oxygen toxicity.

589.
FAIMAN, M.D. and R.G. Mehl.
Effect of high oxygen pressure on brain norepinephrine and serotonin turnover.
Eur. J. Pharmacol. 24:123-130;Nov. 1973.

The effect of high oxygen pressure on the in vivo turnover of norepinephrine (NE) in mouse and rat brain, and the turnover of serotonin (5HT) in mouse brain was investigated. Turnover of NE and 5 HT was determined by steady-state kinetic methods. In mice, synthesis of NE was inhibited by the administration of α-Methyl-p-tyrosine methylester. In rats NE turnover was determined from the decline in intracisternally administered H^3NE. Steady-state kinetic methods also were used to determine 5-HT turnover in mice, utilizing probenecid to block the transport of 5-HIAA. In these studies, 100% oxygen at 1 and 3 atmospheres had no effect on either NE turnover in mice and rats or 5-HT turnover in mice. These studies suggest that changes in NE and 5-HT turnover do not appear to be implicated in the onset of oxygen-induced convulsions. (Authors' abstract)

590.
FANG, H.S. and C.M. Tang.
Effects and vagotomy and increased blood pressure on the incidence of decompression-induced pulmonary hemorrhage: Research note.
Space Life Sci. 3(3):268-270; 1972.

Male rats (68) were divided into 4 groups. They were rapidly decompressed from 1 atmospheric presure (760 mmHg) to an ambient pressure of 30 mmHg in 0.4 sec. About 1/2 the control animals (47%) revealed mild pulmonary hemorrhage; all of the cervical vagotomized rats (100%) showed mild to severe pulmonary hemorrhage. The differences between control and experimental groups were statistically significant. During rapid decompression, the overexpansion of the alveoli accompanied by an increased pressure in the pulmonary vessels may be responsible for the production of pulmonary hemorrhage. (© BA)

591.
FANT, G.
Acoustic theory of hyperbaric speech.
In: Hesser, C.M. and D. Linnarsson eds. Proceedings of the first annual scientific meeting of the European Undersea Biomedical Society, Stockholm, 13-15 June 1973. Forsvarsmedicin 9:279-283;July 1973.

This paper is a review of the author's previous work on hyperbaric speech. In air as well as in helium-based breathing mixtures speech attains a typical distortion, often described as "nasal", which increases with pressure. This dimension is separable from the "Donald Duck"-effect of linear frequency transposition in helium speech. The "nasal" distortion is not physiological but related to a non-linear shift to speech frequencies increasing towards the low-frequency end of the spectrum. The physical cause is the increased participation of vocal cavity walls in vocal sound production and transmission. It is demonstrated theoretically that this effect may be cancelled by choosing a gas mixture such that the density of the gas under operation is the same as that of air at sea level pressure. Techniques for improving intelligibility of divers' speech are discussed. (Author's abstract)

592.
FARELL, C. and O. Gueven.
On the experimental determination of the resistance components of a submerged spheroid.
Iowa City, Iowa Univ., Dept. Mech. Hydraul., Rep. on Contracts N00014-68-A-0196-0004, Nonr-1611(07), 9p. June 26, 1972.

Towing-tank measurements of the viscous resistance of a spheroid model by means of wake surveys together with total resistance measurements show that the proximity of the free surface greatly influences the viscous resistance, which becomes much larger than the deep-submergence resistance as the spheroid approaches the free surface. Wind tunnel measurements reveal a similar effect of a rigid wall on the viscous drag of a body. The values of the wave resistance obtained as the difference between the measured values of total resistance and viscous resistance are found to be in agreement, for the range of Froude numbers investigated, with the analytical results obtained neglecting viscous effects and linearizing the free-surface boundary condition, but satisfying exactly the boundary condition on the surface of the body. (GRA)

593.
FARHI, L.E.
New laboratory at SUNY, Buffalo.
In: Abstracts of BuMed-ONR sponsored Navywide research in high pressure biomedical research, U.S. Submarine Base, Groton, Conn., May 1971, p.35. Published by the Naval Submarine Medical Research Laboratories, 1971.

Abstract only. Excerpts quoted: Several members of the Department of Physiology, State University of New York at Buffalo, have had a long-standing interest in the field of environmental physiology, with particular emphasis on the effects of pressure, temperature, inspired gas, and gravity on the cardiovascular and pulmonary systems of man. . . . New laboratory facilities include a very high pressure chamber, a man-rated centrifuge, a submergence basin, a running track and a computer facility. The centrifuge will have the capability of generating up to 7 Gs, with a capsule spacious enough to accommodate an observer in addition to a subject who can be studied in a variety of positions, including sitting on a bicycle ergometer. Pressure inside the capsule can be maintained at any level between 0.5 and 1 ATA. Surrounding the area swept by the centrifuge capsule is a ring-shaped submergence basic, 8 feet wide and

8 feet deep, 200 feet in circumfrence, to be used for the study of temperature regulation in swimmers and underwater ergonomics. It will be possible to use equipment in the centrifuge capsule to monitor swimmers speed. A running track has been built around the submergence basis to allow us to study cardiovascular performance, using again the centrifuge as a rotating laboratory. A computer room (analog and digital) will receive the signals from all laboratories and allow us to calculate on-line several physiological parameters (e.g. O_2 uptake, cardiac output, etc.), and these data can be stored and/or transmitted back to the experimenter. The new laboratory will be entirely functional by September 1971.

594.
FARMER, J.C., W.G. Thomas and M.J. Preslar.
Human auditory responses during hyperbaric helium-oxygen exposures.
In: Thomas, W.G. and J.C. Farmer. Psychoacoustic and electrophysiologic studies of hearing under hyperbaric pressure, p.40-45. Chapel Hill, N.C., Univ. N.C. Med. Sch., Auditory Res. Lab., Rep. on Contract N00014-67-A-0321-0005. June 1, 1973.
(Also published in Surg. Forum 22:456-458; 1971).

These studies suggest: (1) Humans with patent eustachian tubes, exposed to hyperbaric helium-oxygen conditions, develop a reversible conductive hearing loss which is related to depth; (2) After six days of such exposure, at a depth of 600 feet, there is less variation in the hearing levels and a greater loss in the lower frequencies; (3) Sensorineural auditory function, as measured by the SAL and FDL methods, is not altered by hyperbaric helium-oxygen exposures to 19.2 ATA. This conductive hearing loss is postulated to be due to an increased impedance of the middle ear transformer in the denser atmosphere plus an upward shift in the ear resonant frequency in a helium atmosphere. (Authors' conclusions)

595.
FARMER, J.C., Jr. and W.G. Thomas.
Vestibular injury during diving.
In: Hesser, C.M. and D. Linnarsson, eds. Proceedings of the first annual scientific meeting of the European Undersea Biomedical Society, Stockholm, 13-15 June 1973. Forsvarsmedicin 9:396-403;July 1973.

Permanent cochlear and vestibular damage can occur during all phases of diving: during compression, at stable deep depths, and during decompression. The exact pathophysiology of permanent inner ear damage is now known. The following are suspected: (a.) Permanent inner ear damage during compression seems to be related to difficulties with middle ear pressure equalization: (b.) Permanent inner ear damage at stable deep depths seems to be related to experimental changes in inspired inert gas composition; (c.) Permanent cochlear and vestibular damage during decompression seems to be a form of decompression sickness and can be the only manifestation of this problem. Excessive background noise is common under the various diving conditions and does seem to contribute to cochlear damage. (Authors' conclusion)

596.
FATI, S. and R. Pennarola.
Osservazioni anatomopatologiche sperimentali sull' embolia traumatica e sulla embolia gassosa. [Experimental observations on the anatomy and pathology of traumatic and gas embolisms]. Folia Med. (Naples) 557(7/8):231-251; 1972.

Anatomo-pathologic aspects of traumatic and gaseous embolism were studied in animals compressed suddenly or slowly at 6 relative atmospheres. Injuries were similar in animals in which either a traumatic embolism of saturation or a gaseous embolism were induced. The pathogenesis of gaseous embolism is discussed. (AS) (© BA)

597.
FEAD, L.
The truth about Mae West.
Skin Diver 21:62-63;May 1972.

The buoyancy vest is most effectively used to offset additional weight picked up during the dive (rock samples, minerals, etc.). It also enables the diver to rest on the surface, and helps him to penetrate a surf zone. Before each dive the following checks should be made: air tightness; gas inflation system check (remove CO_2 cartridge, make sure it is intact, and exercise the mechanism); in the case of air cylinder systems, test valve and relief valve. The vest should be donned before the scuba gear. (MFW/BSCP)

598.
FEAD, L.
Revolutionary flotation device.
Skin Diver 21:64-65,84;June 1972.

The ATPAC combines the features of a buoyancy vest, a back pack and a weight belt. The buoyancy bag can be inflated orally, but is usually inflated by a valve next to the mouth piece on the oral inflator hose. It is deflated by opening the oral inflator. The ATPAC can be adjusted to fit all standard single and double tank designs. The weight chamber is inside the back pack between the diver's back and his tank. Its capacity is 30 lbs, and it has a trap door through which the lead pellets can be ejected. The ATPAC can be easily donned in the water. (MFW/BSCP)

599.
FEINSTEIN, R., B.A. Gooden and H.R. Skutt.
New techniques for measuring cardiorespiratory responses in free-swimming scuba divers.
In: Aerospace Medical Association. 1973 annual scientific meeting, Las Vegas, Nevada, May 1973. Preprints, p.213-214. Published by the Association, 1973.

The aim of this ongoing project is to study the cardiorespiratory responses of free-swimming SCUBA divers in open water to depths down to 200 feet. A unique ultrasonic underwater telemetry transmitter is attached to the diver's air tank and transmits the following parameters for recording on the surface: heart rate, water temperature, skin temperature and water depth. The transmitter is being modified to accept and transmit respiration rate in place of skin temperature. . . Baseline data has been obtained from six divers, five male and one female aged 18 to 35 years, during working dives to a depth of 80-90 feet. . . A marked difference in heart rate was noted between the experienced divers and the well trained but inexperienced divers. . . . [An experienced diver's] heart rate was maintained at a considerably higher level throughout his dive and he also consumed a greater amount of his air supply. (Authors)

600.
FEINSTEIN, S.H.
Human underwater sound localization.
Halifax, Nova Scotia, Dalhousie University, Doct. Dissert. 1971.

Because of the transmission characteristics of sound in water, the binaural cues normally associated with human sound localization in air are drastically altered. The present research demonstrated that the human capacity to localize sound is not eliminated underwater as had been suggestd by many earlier investigators. Tests of the acuity of the underwater localization response indicated that the human observer may achieve approximately the same acuity as the sea lion or the porpoise. In addition, the precision with which a diver may point to a sound source, given no visual cues, approximates his precision when pointing at a visually detectable target. The auditory localization response was shown not to be an artifact of the test procedures or equipment. Finally, some evidence was presented to support the view that binaural rather monaural cues are utilized in underwater sound localization. (Author's abstract)

601.
FEINSTEIN, S.H., H. Hollien and P. Hollien.
Diver auditory sensitivity:another look at bone conduction.
J. Acoust. Soc. Amer. 52(1, Pt.1):170; 1972.

Abstract only. Entire item quoted: Support for the hypothesis that divers hear primarily by bone conduction was obtained by Hollien and Brandt (J. Acoust. Soc. Amer. 46:384-387; 1969). In a further test of that hypothesis, the thresholds of seven submerged listeners were obtained (at frequencies of 0.25, 0.50, 1.0, 4.0, and 8.0 kHz) under three different conditions: (1) Wearing a full 3/16-in. wet suit with no hood; (2) wearing a full 3/16-in. wet suit with a 3/16-in. hood; and (3) wearing a full 3/16-in. wet suit and hood with 1/4-in. rubber tubes passing through the hood to the meatuses. There were no significant differences between conditions two and three but thresholds were significantly lower in condition one. This finding provides further support for the hypothesis that underwater sound energy is transduced by bone conduction rather than by the normal middle-ear linkage.

602.
FEINSTEIN, S.H.
Acuity of the human sound localization response underwater.
J. Acoust. Soc. Amer. 53:393-399;Feb. 1973.

Minimum Audible Angles (MAA) for divers were determined for 3.5 kHz and broadband white-noise pulses having a duration of 100 msec, a rise-decay time of 10 sec., and a repetition rate of 1/sec. In Expt 1 six divers performed the right-left discrimination with no training or feedback and the mean MAAs obtained were 21.5° for the 3.5 kHz signal, 14.5° for the 6.5 kHz signal and 9.8° for the white noise signal. In Expt. 2 four of the original six divers were given feedback from their performance with the white-noise signal at a single small angle. The mean MAAs obtained after training were 11.3° at 3.5 kHz, 11.5° at 6.5 kHz, and 7.3° with white noise. It was concluded that if one assumes that the MAA reflects the general level at which the binaural system operates then it seems likely that man will be an effective sound navigator in the water. (Author's abstract)

603.
FELD, J.N., H. Bardin and C.J. Lambertsen.
Maximal use of O_2 in underwater operations.
In: Aerospace Medical Association. 1971 annual scientific meeting, Houston, Texas, April 1971. Preprints, p.73. Published by the Association, 1971.

The onset of symptoms of O_2 toxicity can be delayed by purposely alternating between high and low O_2 partial pressures. This paper considers only the pulmonary toxic effects. The flexible computerized program has been developed for calculating decompression schedules of varying inspired breathing gas compositions. The inspired O_2 pattern used during a dive and decompression can consist of either a continuous exposure to elevated O_2 pressure or a series of alternating exposures to high and normal or low O_2 tensions. By employing mathematical optimization procedures, the pressures and durations which made up the inspired O_2 exposure pattern can be selected in such a manner as to minimize the overall decompression time and insure that the level of O_2 toxicity does not exceed a specific, acceptable limit. . . The techniques can be extended to handle other forms of O_2 toxicity and can be employed to find optimal O_2 exposures in any situation where the amount of O_2 utilized is limited by its toxic effects. (Authors)

604.
FELD, J.N. and C.J. Lambertsen.
Optimal choice of inert gases to be breathed for minimum-time decompression scheduling.
In: Aerospace Medical Association. 1972 annual scientific meeting, Bal Harbour, Florida, May 1972. Preprints, p.220. Published by the Association.

The time required for decompression after exposure to elevated pressures depends on the properties of the inspired inert gases. It is possible to safely reduce the required decompression time by purposely alternating inert gases and/or using mixtures of inert gases in the breathing media. A flexible computerized program has been developed for calculating decompression schedules of varying inspired breathing gas compositions. The inert gas pattern to be breathed throughout the dive can consist of several inert gas mixtures. By employing mathematical optimization techniques, the amount of time to breathe each of these mixtures and the composition of these mixtures can be optimally chosen so as to minimize decompression time without violating physiological constraints. (Author)

605.
FELL, R.B., A. Hudson and H.R. Skutt.
Two systems for telemetry of physiological data from ocean divers.
In: Twenty-fifth annual ACEMB meeting, Bal Harbour, Florida, October, 1972. Preprints, p.197. Arlington, Va., Alliance for Engineering in Medicine, 1972.

The systems described here monitor heart rate, body temperature, skin temperature and water depth. The first system uses four ultrasonic frequencies to transmit four parameters sequentially, which are recorded on a strip-chart. The second system uses a carrier frequency of 50 kHz, with each channel sampled four times a minute. This system can provide the heart rate within four beats per minute of accuracy, the respiration rate within four breaths per minute, and the body and skin temperature within 0.5 F. (MFW/UMS)

606.
FELLER, D.D., E.D. Neville and K.S. Talarico.
Effects of exposing rats to 100% oxygen at 450 and 600 mm Hg on in vitro liver and adipose tissue lipid synthesis.
Aerosp. Med. 43:310-313;Mar. 1972.

Male rats (260-285 gm) were exposed to 100% oxygen at 450 or 600 mm Hg for 1 to 4 days. Rats maintained at 450 mm Hg ate 92% the amount of food eaten by ad libitum controls maintained at sea level conditions. At 600 mm Hg the food intake was 77% of the ad libitum controls. No difference was found in the plasma level of glucose, free fatty acids and corticosterone between oxygen exposed rats and their respective pair-fed controls. The invitro conversion of acetate into fatty acids by adipose tissue from rats exposed at 450 mm Hg for 2, 3, or 4 days was significantly increased above pair-fed controls and ad libitum controls. Increasing the oxygen pressure to 600 mm Hg abolished this increase, and in fact, reversed the increased synthesis to a significant decrease for the 4-day exposure. (Authors' abstract)

607.
FELLER, D.D. and E.F. Neville.
Increased partial pressures of oxygen at normal barometric pressure on lipogenesis in rat tissues (37371).
Proc. Soc. Exp. Biol. Med. 143:582-588;June 1973.

Male rats, fed ad libitum, were exposed to 30% and 47% oxygen environments (balance, N_2) at 1 atm for periods of time varying from 1 to 4 days. The rats exposed to increased oxygen tensions for three or four days gained more weight than controls. Fatty acid contents of liver and adipose tissue of the experimental group at four days of exposure found in these tissues for the control group. Conversion of acetate to fatty acids was found to be significantly higher in liver and adipose tissue of oxygen enriched animals. The conclusion is drawn that these findings are the result solely of an increase in alveolar oxygen tension. (Authors' summary)

608.
FENNING, P.
Unmanned submersibles. Part one.
Hydrospace 5:49-51;Feb. 1972.

The first part of this article reviews unmanned submersibles of the cable controlled type, which possess the ability to move under the remote control of a surface operator, and the ability to carry out specific tasks via manipulators. Those described here include CURV (I, II, and III), Sperry Worksub, and Subsea workboat, of the USA, Telenaute and Systeme Eric, of France, the Dornier Sondenfahrzeng SF 1 from West Germany, and Shell's MOBOT, country of origin unspecified. In addition to work capability, all of these vehicles carry observational and sensing equipment, such as echo-sounders, magnetometers, sonar and cameras. They are of open-frame design, and operate at low speeds. They are not suitable for survey of extensive areas of the ocean bottom. (MFW/BSCP)

609.
FENNING, P.
Unmanned submersibles. Part two: cable-less vehicles.
Hydrospace 5:44-46;Apr. 1972.

The cable-less submersible is designed to collect oceanographic data along a pre-programmed course. The most thoroughly documented submersible of this type is SPURV, of the Applied Physics Laboratory at the University of Washington. The chief problem with SPURV is the lack of a really efficient method of launch and recovery. Other submersibles of this type are Sea Drone, United States, and P-01 Pinguin and Dornier System SF-3, West Germany. The author, referring back to the first part of this article, states that the cable-controlled vehicle is capable of performing many of the same tasks as a manned submersible, at much reduced cost, and could perform more complex tasks if more advanced manipulators were available. The SPURV-type vehicle is probably not economically competitive with surface vessels in carrying out inspection and survey operations at the continental shelf depths. However, this type of submersible could be useful in collecting "midwater" oceanographic data, and in carrying out seabed search tasks in deep water. (MFW/BSCP)

610.
FENTERS, J.D. and V. Neary.
Studies on respiratory infections and oxygen toxicity.
Chicago, Ill., IIT Res. Inst., Rep. L6064-3, 22p. May 22, 1972.
(PB 222 089)

Swiss-Webster mice were exposed to 60% O_2 for two weeks or 100% O_2 for 6, 24, 48, or 72 hr. Activation of latent murine viruses, resistance to influenza infection, and interferom production were measured. A gradual increase in the number of mice with Sendai virus antibody was seen with increase of exposure time to 100% O_2. Increased mortality was observed in mice given the virus and immediately exposed to 100% O_2 for 48 hr or to 60% O_2 for two weeks. Delay of exposure to O_2 by 24-48 hr after the infectious challenge resulted in increased mortality only in the 60% O_2/2 week group. Reverse O_2-virus sequence resulted in increased mortality only in mice held in 100% O_2 for 6 and 24 hr. A 1-2 day delay in interferon response was noted in mice exposed to O_2 immediately after influenza infection. Much greater inflammatory infiltration was seen in lungs of mice exposed to hyperoxia and challenged with virus, than infected mice held at ambient condition, or those receiving saline and held in O_2. (NTIS abstract)

611.
FERRANTE, F.L. and B.D. Miller.
Respiratory insensitivity to blood gases in nutrias (Myocastor coypus).
J. Appl. Physiol. 31:175-177;Aug. 1971.

The objectives of the present investigation were to determine the changes in blood gases and pH during submersion apnea in a diving mammal, the nutria, and to determine the degree of hypoxia, hypercapnia and acidosis that could be tolerated prior to breakpoint of breath holding. In 14 nutrias, it was found that PaO_2 decreased from its predive control (avg $\pm$ SE) of 90 $\pm$ 3.3 to 24 $\pm$ 2.7 mmHg at the end of 5 min of submersion. $PaCO_2$ increased from 39 $\pm$ 1.4 to 65 $\pm$ 3.5 mmHg and arterial pH decreased from a predive average of 7.37 $\pm$ 0.02 to 7.25 $\pm$ 0.02 mmHg. In 7 nutrias PaO_2 values of 14-17 mmHg were recorded prior to breakpoint of breath hold, whereas $PaCO_2$ increased to a range of 53-82 mmHg and pH decreased to a range of 7.32-7.17. The results suggest an apparent respiratory insensitivity to the combined effects of hypoxia, hypercapnia and acidosis in nutrias. (Authors' abstract)

612.
FERRIS, S.H.
Loss of position constancy underwater.
Psychonom. Sci. Sec. Hum. Exp. Psychol. 27(6):337-338; 1972.

Due to the optical distortion produced by wearing a face mask, the constancy of visual position would not be maintained underwater, i.e., stationary objects would appear to move when the head moved. Subjects (Ss) rotated their heads about a vertical axis and made magnitude estimates of object movement in both air and water. Twice as much movement occurred in water as in air. Two underwater activities, head rotation while observing vertical stripes and practice in hand-eye coordination produced a small reduction in the loss of position constancy. (© BA)

613.
FERRIS, S.H.
Magnitude estimation of absolute distance underwater.
Percept. Motor Skills 35:963-971; 1972.

Direct estimates of absolute distance were obtained in air and in water of varying turbidity. Distance in water was under- or overestimated, depending on the interaction of three factors: (1) a general tendency to underestimate; (2) optical distortion, which causes underestimation; and (3) water turbidity, which increases the magnitude of judgments, and whose effect increases with distance. Also, whereas the power-function exponent for distance estimation in air was slightly less than 1.0, exponents in water were greater than 1.0 and increased with increased turbidity. (Author's summary)

614.
FERRIS, S.H.
Apparent object movement produced by head movement under water.
U.S. Nav. Submar. Med. Cent., Rep. NSMRL 694, 5p. Jan. 14, 1972.

It was predicted that due to the optical distortion produced by wearing a facemask, the constancy of visual position would not be maintained under water, i.e., stationary objects should appear to move when the head is moved. Subjects made magnitude estimates of object movement in both air and water. Twice as much movement occurred in water as in air. Two underwater activities, head rotation while observing vertical stripes, and practice in hand-eye coordination, produced a small reduction in object movement. The results indicate that apparent object movement (loss of position constancy) should be added to the list of visual problems which confront the diver. (Author's abstract)

615.
FERRIS, S.H.
Improving absolute distance estimation in clear and in turbid water.
U.S. Nav. Submar. Med. Cent., Rep. NSMRL 710, 7p. May 25, 1972.
(Also published in Percept. Motor Skills 36:771-776;June 1973).

Since the errors made in estimating distance under water are dependent on the degree of water turbidity, improvement through training in one body of water will not transfer to another body of water if there is a large difference in turbidity. This experiment demonstrated that the transfer problem can be overcome by training divers under different turbidity conditions so that they learn to tailor their corrections to the prevailing conditions. This training procedure would be useful for all diving tasks in which the estimation of object distances is important. (Author's abstract)

616.
FERRIS, S.H.
Improving distance estimation under water: Long-term effectiveness of training.
U.S. Nav. Submar. Med. Cent., Rep. NSMRL 718, 4p. July 10, 1972.
(Also published in Percept. Motor Skills 36:1089-1090;June 1973).

Due to both optical distortion and water turbidity, divers are usually inaccurate when they estimate distances under water. Previous studies have demonstrated that training with feedback improves judgment accuracy. The present study showed that the effect of training diminishes considerably during the nine weeks following training. A more extensive training program is recommended for diving tasks in which distance estimation is important. (Author's abstract)

617.
FERRIS, S.H.
Improvement of absolute distance estimation underwater.
Percept. Mot. Skills 35:299-305;Aug. 1972.

Estimates of absolute distance underwater were obtained before and after training sessions in which observers were informed of the correct distance after each of a series of judgments. Training in water substantially improved performance, whereas training in air improved performance only in clear water. Training in one body of water did not adequately transfer to performance in another body of water if there was a large difference in water turbidity. (Author's summary)

618.
FERRIS, S.H.
Improvement of absolute distance estimation under water: use of monocular motion parallax.
U.S. Nav. Submar. Med. Res. Lab., Rep. NSMRL 740, 6p. Mar. 1, 1973.

The possible value of monocular motion parallax for improving distance perception under water was investigated. Submerged subjects either kept their heads stationary or rotated their heads about a vertical axis while judging the distance of objects placed 4-15 ft. away. Both before and after training with feedback to increase judgment accuracy, head movement did not significantly improve performance. Water turbidity and loss of position constancy are two probable reasons for the failure to replicate the positive results previously obtained in air. (Author's abstract)

619.
FERRIS, S.H. and R.T. Bartus.
A method for recording and analyzing EEGs and VERs from rats under hyperbaric conditions.
U.S. Nav. Submar. Med. Res. Lab., Rep. NSMRL 747, 10p. July 12, 1973.

A technique is described for recording electroencephalograms (EEGs) and visually evoked cortical responses (VERs) from rats during hyperbaric exposure. A reliable and durable chronic electrode implantation procedure is used in which miniature, self-tapping stainless steel screws serve a dual role as cortical electrodes and as anchors for a miniature connecting socket. Sample data are presented which were obtained from implanted rats during exposure to hyperbaric air. The techniques developed are well-suited for studying the neurophysiological effects of hyperbaric environments. (Authors' abstract)

620.
FERRIS, S.H. and S.A. Shaffer.
35 day, 60 foot air saturation dive with rats: effects on EEG and visually evoked cortical response.
U.S. Nav. Submar. Med. Res. Lab., Rep. NSMRL 756, 7p. Sept. 12, 1973.

EEG and visually evoked cortical responses (VERs) were recorded from rats before, during, and after a 35 day exposure to hyperbaric air at a depth of 60 ft. Recordings were obtained from chronically implanted cortical electrodes each week during the course of the dive. Although systematic changes occurred in both the EEG and VER during the experiment, similar changes occurred in a control group which remained at the surface. Thus the hyperbaric saturation exposure produced no significant changes in the EEG or VER. This result implies that a long-term exposure to a depth of 60 feet does not impair the general functioning of the nervous system. (Authors' abstract)

621.
FIFE, W.P., M.L. Edwards, W.W. Schroeder, F.D. Ferrari and L.R. Freeberg.
Effect of the Hydro-Lab environment on pulmonary function.
Hydro-Lab J. 2(1):73-80; 1973.

In the first of two 7-day, 40-45 foot saturation dives, vital capacity was measured before, during, and after the dive; it was found to have increased slightly (from 0.2 to 3.9%, depending upon the individual). During a second similar dive, measurements included forced vital capacity, maximum voluntary ventilation, 0.5 sec. forced expiratory volume, 1.0 sec. forced expiratory volume, all of which were made before, during and after the dive. These measurements indicated that significant reduction in pulmonary function occurred during the first three days, but became stabilized from then on. It is not known whether this indicates adaptation to the denser gas, or whether pulmonary deterioration was being repaired by the respiratory system as fast as it occurred. It is concluded that a saturation dive of these dimensions holds no danger, and that exposure of 14-days or even longer would probably be safe. It is urged that in further tests females be included, since the female hyperbaric pulmonary function values differ from the male to such an extent that data from male subjects cannot be extrapolated. (MFW/UMS)

622.
FIFE, W.P., W.W. Schroeder and L.R. Freeberg.
Measurement of metabolic rate in aquanauts.
Hydro-Lab J. 2(1):81-84; 1973.

An attempt was made to determine whether a 7-day saturation dive at 40-45 feet, in 82° water, would have any effect on the metabolic rate. The habitat temperature ranged from 72° to 82°. No increase in metabolic rate occurred. It was concluded that at this water temperature, cold stress is not sufficient to cause a change in the metabolic rate. Colder temperatures would probably cause enough physiological stress to bring on a change in the metabolic rate. (MFW/UMS)

623.
FINK, F.W. and W.K. Boyd.
The corrosion of metals in marine environments.
Columbus, O., Battelle Mem. Inst., Def. Metals Inf. Cent., Rep. DMIC-244-H, 97p. May 1970.
(AD 712 585)

The ocean environment — factors affecting the corrosivity of seawater; forms of corrosion. Corrosion of metals in the marine environment — carbon steel, low-alloy steels, stainless steels, nickel and nickel-base alloys, cobalt, copper and copper-base alloys, titanium and titanium-base alloys, aluminum and aluminum-base alloys, beryllium, magnesium, special-purpose metals, refractory metals, noble metals, lead zinc, cadmium and tin. Cathodic protection. (GRA)

624.
FISCHER, C.L., C.S. Leach and W.C. Alexander.
Laboratory medicine.
In: Miller, J.W., J.G. Van Derwalker and R.A. Waller, eds. Tektite 2: Scientists-in-the-sea, p.IX-53-IX-56. Washington, D.C., U.S. Department of the Interior, August 1971.

The original purpose of the Laboratory Medicine evaluation was to support the medical team by the documentation of participating crew members' physical qualifications, related to the dive, and to detect problems which could require remedial or preventive action. This was accomplished and the information was made available, on a real time basis, to the medical support team. If the divers are considered as a group, there were no significant changes in any hematologic or biochemical parameter. These findings are entirely consistent with data previously reported for Project Tektite I. The endocrine data indicates varying trends in individuals, suggesting individual reaction to the two week dive and decompression schedule. However, when the data were evaluated for the population of divers, no significant changes were reflected. In summary, it can be unequivocally stated that under the conditions imposed by the Tektite 2 environment, no significant biochemical, hematologic, endocrine changes can be anticipated. More generally, this statement can be extrapolated to at least 60 days. (Authors)

625.
FISCHER, D.B. and S. Kaufman.
The inhibition of phenylalanine and tyrosine hydroxylases by high oxygen levels.
J. Neurochem. 19:1359-1365; 1972.

The K_m for oxygen for rat liver phenylalanine hydroxylase depended on the structure of the reduced pterin cofacter. When the synthetic cofactor, 6, 7-dimethyltetrahydropterin, was employed, the apparent K_m for oxygen was 20%. When the natural cofactor, tetrahydrobiopterin, was used, the apparent K_m for oxygen was 0.35%. Substrate inhibition (40 per cent inhibition at 43% oxygen) was observed with the natural cofactor but not with the synthetic cofactor. Oxygen also caused substrate inhibition with bovine adrenal medulla and brain tyrosine hydroxylases. The inhibition was more dramatic in the presence of the natural cofactor than with the synthetic cofactor. Substrate inhibition by oxygen of brain tyrosine hydroxylase may explain the lowered brain levels of norepinephrine and dopamine observed after treatment of animals with hyperbaric oxygen. (Authors' abstract)

626.
FISCHER, K.H.
Integrated electronics technology and its impact on ocean environment.
In: 1970 IEEE international conference on engineering in the ocean environment, Panama City, Florida, 21 September. Digest of tutorial papers, p.20-28. New York, Lewis Winner, 1970.

The application of integrated electronics to engineering in the ocean environment involves several advantages. First, is the possibility of reducing the size and weight of equipment. Equipment costs are also reduced. Lower power levels are required, and reliability is improved. Proper design criteria would utilize the principle of throwaway modules, thus doing away with the problem of maintenance. Various possible uses of integrated electronics technology in underwater engineering would include remote monitoring, and the improvement of navigation techniques. (MFW/BSCP)

627.
FISHMAN, D.R., R.A. Leonard, D. Gorshein, E.C. Besa, J.H. Jepson and F.H. Gardner.
Stem cell damage induced by hyperoxia.
Biomedicine 19:290-295;July 20, 1973.

The effect of hyperoxia on endogenous and exogenous erythropoietin stimulation in the mice was evaluated. Suppression of ^{59}Fe incorporation into peripheral red blood cells by high oxygen tension produced an assay animal that responded less to an equal erythropoietin dose as compared to the post-hypoxic polycythermic counterparts. Also normal erythropoietic recovery as measured by ^{59}Fe incorporation was not achieved following interruption of hyperoxic suppression as long as 96 hours. However, elevated plasma erythropoietin titers were detected 6 hours following the interruption of hyperoxic exposure. An inhibition to erythropoietin was not found in plasma obtained from mice maintained in hyperoxia. The number of colony-forming units were decreased in hyperoxic animals, both in spleen and in bone marrow. The results are compatible with a damaging effect on high oxygen tension on the hematopoietic stem cell pool. (Authors' summary)

628.
FITZGERALD, J.R.
Statistical study of sound speed in the inhomogeneous upper ocean.
U.S. Nav. Postgrad. Sch., Thesis, 129p. Dec. 1972.
(AD 756 570)

The statistics of the fluctuations of the in-situ speed of sound in the upper ocean have been studied by analyzing the instantaneous phase difference of the output of two hydrophones separated by one meter for sounds of frequency 15 to 151 kHz. The experiment was conducted at 11 ft in water of depth 60 ft in low sea states at night. Comparison of the speed calculated from the time averaged phase difference, with the speed given by velocimeter or empirical relations, yielded differential speeds which deviate by 1 m/sec to 8 m/sec from the accepted values for frequencies less than 100 kHz. Correlation and spectral analysis of the sound phase and height fluctuations has shown the close relation between these two parameters. There is strong evidence of the presence and importance of bubbles in all of the results, particularly of a large population resonant in the frequency range 56.3 to 71.1 kHz (radius 50 to 60 mivrons). (Author's abstract modified by GRA)

629.
FLAHAUT, J., P. Haine, G. Pulinckx and M. Lambert.
Modifications physiologiques observees chez l'homme au cours de plongees simulees.
[Physiological modifications observed in humans during simulated dives.]
Acta Belg. Arte Med. Pharm. Mil. 16(2):259-274; 1970.

Modifications appearing in different functions of the human body under pressurized conditions were investigated. Peak flow rate and vital capacity show variations at about 2-3 ATA [atmospheres of absolute pressure] appearing in succeeding phases, first a reaction then a compensation. The same applies to nervous conduction. Marked changes in achilles reflex action and oscillometric index at 2 to 3 ATA were noticed. Apparently changes occur due to variations in the different enzymatic reactions. (JJC) (© BA)

630.
FLAHERTY, R.J., J.F. Tobin and E.H. Jones.
Electrical insulating materials for deep submergence applications.
IEEE international conference on engineering in the ocean environment, Panama City, Florida, September 1970. Digest of technical papers, p.182-185. Published by the conference.

To reduce the size of the pressure hull of submersibles or to increase the payload, many components of the electrical power system are mounted external to the hull. The concept of protecting electrical equipment by enclosing the equipment in a thin shell filled with a compensating fluid is examined. (Eng. Index)

631.
FLEMMING, N.C.
Diver training and education.
In: Diving applications in marine research. Proceedings of a seminar, National Institute of Oceanography, Godalming, Surrey, U.K., December 1971, p.136-167. Published by the Institute. 1972.

Physical, medical, and psychological tests reveal that divers do not differ significantly from the average for the population, apart from their being rather fitter. This makes it very difficult to identify the qualities which make a good diver. Selection and training of divers is compared with that for RAF and airline pilots in order to examine testing methods and the possible causes of the high failure rate which is normal on diving courses. In spite of the superficial similarity between the combination of physical and intellectual skills in diving and flying, it is harder to predict the success of diving trainees than flying trainees, and failure rates of 35% are experienced in diving compared with 20-30% in flying. A notable behavioural difference on the courses is that pilots fail in examinations or tests set by their instructors, while divers tend to drop out voluntarily. This is clearly related to the discomfort and danger of diving, and it is difficult to design short selection tests which will predict whether a trainee will be able to endure repeated discomfort. The discrepancy between the apparently average qualities of divers and their actual rarity may be accounted for by assuming that they require to combine certain qualities which are on average negatively correlated in the population as a whole. Consideration is given to the question of training research personnel to dive, and the problem of maintaining their diving standards with minimum interference to their normal work. Where routine working diving is not involved, and where frequent practice dives are not feasible or convenient, it is recommended that the divers engaged in a given diving project should undergo a series of work-up practice dives tailored to the work project, and taking account of the time-lapse since previous diving. (Author's abstract)

632.
FLETCHER, B.L. and A.L. Tappel.
Protective effects of dietary alpha-Tocopherol in rats exposed to toxic levels of ozone and nitrogen dioxide.
Environ. Res. 6:165-175;June 1973.

The effect of dietary alpha-tocopherol at various levels, especially in the range 0-45 mg/kg, on the toxicity of O_3 and NO_2 to rats was studied. The highest level of alpha-tocopherol was 1500 mg/kg of diet in combination with ascorbic acid, DL-methionine and butylated hydroxytoluene; the level of O_3 ranged from 0.7 to 16 ppm and NO_2 from 20 to 25 ppm; and various exposure periods were used. Alpha-tocopherol alone and in combination with the other antioxidants exerted a protective effect in rats exposed to O_3 and NO_2 as measured by acute toxicity and animal weight change. During 1 ppm O_3 exposure voluntary activity decreased, while at lower levels of O_3 (0.7 - 0.8 ppm) alpha tocopherol protection against lipid peroxidation in the lung, as measured by endogenous lung thiobarbituric acid reactants, was a reciprocal function of the logarithm of dietary alpha tocopherol. Extracts of lung tissue from animals exposed to O_3 and O_2 showed no increase in fluorescent products associated with lipid peroxidation. (Authors' abstract)

633.
FLORIO, J.T. and J.B. Morrison.
Ventilatory response to exercise and inspired carbon dioxide measured in divers.
J. Physiol. (London) 234:70p-71p;Oct. 1973.

Abstract only. Excerpts quoted: Five divers were studied at rest and while exercising on a bicycle ergometer. Three subjects maintained end tidal PCO_2 at approximately 40 mmHg while in a fourth subject it rose to 47 mmHg at an oxygen consumption of 2·0 l. min^{-1}. In the case of the fifth subject, I.M., end tidal PCO_2 increased with increasing work load to exceed 56 mmHg at an oxygen consumption of 1·4 l. min^{-1}. This was reduced to 53 mmHg at an oxygen consumption of 2·0 l. min^{-1}. The ventilatory response to carbon dioxide was determined for each subject at rest at constant end tidal PO_2. Since four of the subjects exhibited a normal ventilatory response to carbon dioxide this work does not support the theory that divers in general show acclimatization to carbon dioxide. The abnormal response of subject I.M. may represent acclimatization or, particularly in view of his relatively short exposure to diving equipment, may be due to causes entirely unconnected with diving.

634.
FLOWER, R.A.
Helium speech investigations.
Pleasantville, N.Y., Singer Co., Kearfott Div., Final Rep. on Contract N00014-70-C-0387, 63p. Dec. 1971.

The basic objective of the work was to continue evaluations of and achieve further improvements in the Singer-Kearfott unscrambler technique. The report summarizes briefly the work completed. Two major new topics are reported, an investigation of the formant shift in neon-air, and a miniaturization study of the existing unscramble configuration. Functional descriptions and design data are presented on two miniaturization approaches for a helium unscrambler, one using an all-digital circuit and one using a novel analog memory. The analog approach is attractive, requiring fewer circuit elements and less power drain than the digital type. (Author) (GRA)

635.
FLOWER, R.A.
Developmental evaluations of and improvements to a helium-speech unscrambler.
In: Sergeant, R.L. and T. Murry, eds. Processing helium speech: proceedings of a Navy-sponsored workshop, August 1971, U.S. Nav. Sbmar. Med. Res. Lab., Rep. NSMRL 708, p.29-33. May 22, 1972.

The basic objective of this work was to continue evaluations of and achieve further improvements in the Singer-Kearfott unscrambler technique. Investigations show that improvements result from using single polarity rather than bipolar pitch sync detection, and from excluding input signal components above 10 kHz. Simple compensation of the non-linear formant shift, and modification of the glottal wave decay rate produced no apparent improvement. (Author's summary)

636.
FLYNN, E.T., T.E. Berghage and E.F. Coil.
Influence of increased ambient pressure and gas density on cardiac rate in man.
U.S. Navy Exp. Diving Unit, Rep. NEDU-4-72, 40p. Aug. 1972.

Heart rate was measured in ten normal male subjects in a hyperbaric chamber during a two phase study. In phase I graded exercise was performed at ambient pressures of 1.0, 3.27, and 5.45 Ata. At these depths, subjects breathing a gas mixture having a density equal to that of the surface (1.0 Ata.) and then gas mixtures having greater densities. P_IO_2 was maintained constant at 147-150 mm Hg in all instances. Highly significant ($P < .001$) decreases in heart rate occurred at all levels of exercise tested when the inspired gas density was held constant and the ambient pressure alone increased. At constant ambient pressures of 3.27 and 5.45 Ata., however, further significant ($p < .001$) reductions in heart rate were also observed when the gas density was increased above control values. In phase II heart rate was recorded during an extended saturation dive. Graded exercise was performed at pressures of 1, 5.54, 10.09, 19.18, and 26.75 Ata. During all these exposures subjects breathed the ambient oxygen, helium, and nitrogen chamber atmosphere. The results of these studies suggest that both the increase in ambient pressure and the increase in inspired gas density contribute to the development of bradycardia under hyperbaric conditions. The decrement in heart rate due to an increased gas density appears likely to result from reflex changes associated directly or indirectly with the increased airway resistance. An explanation for the apparent effects of ambient pressure cannot be offered at the present time, although in the light of a recent report by Raymond et. al. at least a fraction of the response may eventually prove to be related to the elevated partial pressure of helium in the breathing medium. (Authors' abstract)

637.
FOEX, P. and R.M.M. Fordham.
Intrinsic myocardial recovery from the negative inotropic effects of acute hypercapnia.
Cardiovasc. Res. 6(3):257-262; 1972.

The inotropic effects of hypercapnia were examined in the isometric papillary muscle preparation from the cat. The initial stage of depression which resulted from the acute induction of hypercapnia was followed by a significant degree of spontaneous recovery during the next hour. When the CO_2 concentration was returned to normal, a temporary rebound in performance to above control levels occurred. These findings may be due to slow changes arising in heart muscle which partially compensate for the direct inotropic depressant effect of hypercapnia. (© BA)

638.
FOLBERGROVA, J., V. MacMillan and B.K. Siesjo.
The effect of hypercapnic acidosis upon some glycolytic and Krebs cycle-associated intermediates in the rat brain.
J. Neurochem. 19(11):2507-2517; 1972.

To study the influence of intracellular pH on the carbohydrate metabolism of brain tissue, the concentrations of glucose, glucose-6-phosphate, pyruvate, lactate, citrate, alpha-oxoglutarate and ammonia were measured in rats exposed to 6-40% CO_2 for 45 min. Hypercapnia of increasing severity gave rise to progressive increases in the concentrations of glucose, glucose-6-phosphate and NH_4+ and to progressive decreases in the concentrations of all metabolic acids measured. The results fit with a H+ inhibition of a rate-limiting step between glucose-6-phosphate and pyruvate, and it was assumed that this step was the phosphofructokinase reaction. Since the proportionally largest decrease occurred in an alpha-oxoglutarate, the results might be comparable either with an inhibition of a second rate-limiting step such as isocitrate dehydrogenase, or with a loss of alpha-oxoglutarate through carboxylation to citrate. (© BA)

639.
FOLBERGROVA, J., V. MacMillan and B.K. Siesjo.
The effect of moderate and marked hypercapnia upon the energy state and upon the cytoplasmic NADH/NAD+ ratio of the rat brain.
J. Neurochem. 19(11):2497-2505; 1972.

The energy state of brain tissue was evaluated from the tissue concentrations of ATP, ADP and AMP and the cytoplasmic NADH/NAD+ ratio from the tissue, cerebral spinal fluid and blood concentrations of lactate and pyruvate and from the intracellular pH', in rats exposed to CO_2 concentrations of 6-40%. The hypercapnia had no effect on the energy state of the tissue. Hypercapnia of increasing severity gave rise to a progressive decrease in the pyruvate concentration; the lactate concentration fell at low [CO_2], but no further decrease was observed at [CO_2] 20%. There ws a progressive rise in the intracellular lactate-pyruvate ratio at increasing [CO_2], corresponding to the fall in intracellular pH, i.e. the calculated NADH/NAD+ ratios remained normal. Hypercapnia probably did not affect the cytoplasmic redox state. (© BA)

640.
FOLBERGROVA, J. and B.K. Siesjo.
Regulatory mechanisms affecting carbohydrate substrates in the brain in hypercapnic acidosis.
Acta Physiol. Scand. 88(2):281-382; 1973.

Rats showed no changes in glucose-6-phosphate or in fructose-1,6-diphosphate at any exposure time. Thus, the relative depletion of metabolic acids in moderate hypercapnia is not due to inhibition of phosphofructokinase. At least part of the metabolic pattern seen at these degrees of hypercapnia could be due to loss of pyruvate and α-ketoglutarate by means of CO_2 fixation. Perhaps the level of metabolic acids is regulated at the pyruvic kinase step. (DT) (© BA)

641.
FORCE, L., J. Esvan, L. Barthelemy, A. Michaud, R. Gilly and R. Joly.
Aspects cliniques d'une serie d'accidents neurologiques de la plongee.
[Clinical aspects of a series of neurological diving accidents].
Bull. Medsubhyp 8:10-11;Nov. 1972.

First, in 24 cases of cerebral accidents, the great majority of cases were typical of pulmonary barotrauma. The signs are those well-known as indicative of cerebral air embolism: immediate appearance of symptoms; initial loss of consciousness, either transitory or prolonged; temporary blindness; absence of pulmonary symptoms in half the cases; frequency of convulsions — immediate, delayed, or extremely delayed; symptoms of hemispheric involvement, sometimes amounting to hemiplegia. Five of the 24 cases died. Of those that survived, all were treated by recompression. Second, 50 cases of medullary accidents corresponded to classic decompression accidents. Three most common types were: quadriplegics, paraplegics, and partial medullary accidents (inferior monoplegia, sensory disorders). In most cases, symptoms appeared within a few minutes of leaving the water; in cases of delayed symptoms, the accidents were less serious. Method of manifestation might be motor or sensory symptoms, pain characteristic of an acute medullary ischemia, or transitory signs such as loss of consciousness which confuse the diagnosis and are put down to cerebral embolism. All cases except one were treated with recompression. One case of paraplegia died. The partial medullary accidents evolved favorably. Some paraplegics were cured, some had sequelae. It was found that accidents following shallow dives were of less consequence. Light or moderate cases, even when treated belatedly, were cured. Severe cases, even when treated promptly left sequelae. It is noted that in a few cases, treated by the old tables, aggravation of symptoms was observed. The third group of accidents briefly mentioned were those that combined cerebral and medullary symptoms. One combined a confused state with EEG anomalies and massive paraplegia. In other cases where a mild or transitory symptomatology was associated with a medullary accident, pulmonary rupture was suspected, although the conditions of the dive did not in every case support this conclusion. (MFW/BSCP)

642.
FORD, D.H. and R.K. Rhines.
The effect of multiple exposure to high pressure oxygen on the accumulation of [^{3}H] lysine into spinal cord grey matter, retina and various types of neurons.
J. Neurol. Sci. 19:483-490;Aug. 1973.

Male Wistar strain rats were subjected to repeated exposures to oxygen at high pressure (OHP) at 3 atm absolute for 1 hr each day for 10 days. They were then injected with [^{3}H]DL-lysine while in the awakened state through indwelling intravenous cannulas and compared with appropriate controls in relation to [^{3}H] lysine accumulation in plasma, retina, spinal cord grey matter, Purkinje cells, ventral horn motor neurone and in dorsal root ganglia and supraoptic neurone.

Accumulation of lysine into blocks of tissue was depressed in retina, whole dorsal root ganglia and spinal cord grey matter, but not in Purkinje cells or central horn motor neurons. Accumulation was depressed in cells of the dorsal root ganglia, but elevated in the cells of the supraoptic nucleus. These variations would seem to represent regional differences in response to OHP. (Authors' summary)

643.
FORGAYS, D.G., G. McClure and F.C. Evering, Jr.
Modulated light transmission for electrical isolation in a multichannel physiological monitoring system.
Aerosp. Med. 44:68-70; Jan. 1973.

A system has been developed for subjects undergoing physiological signal monitoring, to provide electrical isolation between the electrode or "ground" leads connected to the subject and those of the recording apparatus. This is accomplished by utilizing a modulated light transmitter-receiver, which has the advantage of being low in cost, relatively simple in design, and able to provide a large number of stable and reliable channels, free from external or cross-channel interference. The present system can accommodate up to 12 chanels. Safety, isolation, and signal-to-noise ratios are enhanced by the use of battery power. By using this isolator in conjunction with ground fault detectors, and other safety measures, a complete fail-safe monitoring system has been constructed and is being utilized in a water environment for psychological studies in sensory deprivation. (Authors' abstract)

644.
FORMAN, W.R.
Kumukahi
Mech. Eng. 93:9-13;Aug. 1971.

The design and development of a transport-hull submersible, capable of submerging to depths of 300 ft with its two-man crew, is described. The spherical hull is fabricated in quadrants which are bolted together. This process allows good control of sphericity and wall thickness. (Eng. Index)

645.
FOSTER, J.J., G. Cameron, C.C. Hemmings and B.B. Parrish.
The case for a towed underwater vehicle for fisheries research.
Trans. Inst. Mar. Eng. 84:218-222; 1972.

Physiological limitations on depth, endurance, and speed of free divers make their employment for investigating fish capture processes impracticable. These limitations are only partly overcome by the use of wet towed vehicles. Self-propelled manned submersibles are too costly for general use. The authors here describe a towed dry vehicle, which consists of two cylinders, side by side, with a hemispherical viewing port in the front of each. The pilot lies face down in one section, the observer in the other. Although the working depth would probably not exceed 300 feet, the vehicle has a depth capability of 600 feet. It has an air supply of 12 hours, although the duration of the mission would probably not exceed one hour. Technical problems are discussed, with emphasis on the difficulty of combining acrylic material with metal. The vehicle, weighing 3700 pounds, would be carried to a 110-foot fisheries research vessel. Launch and recovery systems are described. A full scale model has been successfully tested, with only a few minor design faults coming to light. Seven men, three of whom would normally be part of the crew of the surface vessel, are required for launch and recovery. (MFW/BSCP)

646.
FOWLER, B.
Some comments on "a behavioral approach to nitrogen narcosis".
Psych. Bull. 78:234-240;Sept. 1972.

R.D. Jennings' recent paper, dealing with nitrogen narcosis, (Psych. Bull. 69:216-224, 1968) argued that almost no attention has been paid to the behavioral aspects of this phenomenon and that the problem has been approached only from the physiological and medical viewpoint. The present paper reviews a number of behavioral studies of nitrogen narcosis not covered by Jennings and points out certain inaccuracies in his paper. It is concluded that considerable attention has been paid to the behavioral aspects of nitrogen narcosis involving skilled performance but that there is now a need to apply new analytic approaches to this problem. (Author's abstract)

647.
FOWLER, B. and K.N. Ackles.
Narcotic effects in man of breathing 80-20 argon-oxygen and air under hyperbaric conditions.
Aerosp. Med. 43:1219-1224;Nov. 1972.

The qualitative effects of breathing 80-20 argon-oxygen and air were compared at the surface and at 4 and 7 ATA with 10 subjects using three measures — mental arithmetic, subjective estimates of narcosis and an adjective checklist. Both the mental arithmetic task and the subjective estimates of narcosis indicated that the argon-oxygen mixture was more narcotic than air. The adjective check-list revealed that similar types of adjectives were used to described the subjective effects of both mixtures and that these choices corresponded to previous descriptions of narcosis. There was also evidence that factors other than internal subjective cues influenced the subjects' estimates of narcosis, the major one being feedback from performance on the arithmetic test. It was concluded that the qualitative effects of argon and nitrogen were the same on the various measures of narcosis but the discrepancy between the dose response functions for various measures found by a comparison of the present results and those of other studies of nitrogen narcosis in humans raises questions about the usefulness of quantitative differences between the inert gases as indicators of underlying causal mechanisms of narcosis. (Authors' abstract)

648.
FOWLER, B.
Effect of hyperbaric air on short-term and long-term memory.
Aerosp. Med. 44:1017-1022;Sept. 1973.

Three experiments are reported which investigated the effects of hyperbaric air on STM and LTM (short- and long-term memory). In the first experiment the dichotic stimulation technique was used to examine STM at 1, 4 and 7 ata. The second experiment was similar to the first except that an increased pressure (10 ata) was used. A decrement in performance was found in both experiments but this was attributed to a deficit in auditory perception and it was concluded that STM is not affected by hyperbaric air. In the third experiment a free-recall learning task was used to examine input to, and retrieval from, LTM. A decreased rate of learning was found at 10 ata breathing air. After switching to an 80/20 helium-oxygen mixture midway through the learning task the rate of learning returned to that found at the surface although the relative difference in recall that was established breathing air remained. It was concluded that these results indicate a loss of ability to store information in LTM and may explain the amnesia that has sometimes been observed after breathing hyperbaric air. (Author's abstract)

649.
FRANCOIS, R.E.
The unmanned Arctic research submersible system.
Mar. Technol. Soc. J. 7:46-48;Jan./Feb. 1973.

As part of an ARPA-ONR sponsored arctic technology program at the University of Washington, an Unmanned Arctic Research Submersible System has been developed and successfully employed. This system, known as UARS, comprises two major elements — the submersible which serves as a mobile instrument carrier, and an acoustic tracking, command, and recovery system. The first year of the program was devoted to design, with test hardware limited to breadboard assemblies, while during the second year, the system was fabricated, tested, and its performance demonstrated in an arctic under-ice experimental program. The UARS is a compact vehicle which weighs 900 pounds in air and has a length of approximately 10 feet and a diameter of 19 inches. The hull is fabricated from aluminum forgings and filament wound fiberglass to give a 1500 foot operating depth capability. Its tri-axial control system is designed to accommodate speeds as low as three knots; the speed of the unit operated in the Arctic was 3.7 knots. Higher speeds can be obtained by motor substitution. The main batteries (silver-zinc) supply sufficient energy for run times in excess of 10 hours with an equal propulsion and instrumentation power load. A reserve battery is carried for emergency purposes. At a speed of three knots, the vehicle is operated at 10 pounds positive buoyancy. (Author)

650.
FRATTALI, V. and R. Robertson.
Nutritional evaluation of humans during an oxygen-helium dive to a simulated depth of 1000 feet.
Aerosp. Med. 44:14-21;Jan. 1973.

A biochemical evaluation of the nutritional status of two divers was performed during a saturation helium-oxygen dive to a simulated depth of 850 ft with two excursions to 1000 ft. The experimental protocol included exposure of divers to cold water and cold breathing gases at constant temperatures of 35°, 45°, or 55°F. The subjects consumed airline-type meals throughout the 23-day period in the chamber. Dietary records of food consumption permitted estimation of caloric and nutrient intake based on food composition tables. Physiological samples, blood and urine, were collected on several occasions prior to and during the dive for evaluation of vitamin status and other indicators of nutritional state. Analyses were conducted for plasma levels of vitamins C and A, carotene, protein, sodium, potassium, calcium, magnesium, copper and zinc. Excretion levels of thiamin, folacin, riboflavin, niacin, N^1-methylnicotinamide, and vitamin B_6 were determined. Enzymatic activity of erythrocyte transketolase was also measured. The acitivity of this enzyme is generally accepted as a reflection thiamin nutriture. Most analyses gave normal results. However, marked decreases in thiamin excretion and erythrocyte transketolase activity were observed at depth. These conditions persisted in one diver to the end of the decompression phase. Since thiamin requirement is directly related to energy expenditure, it is possible that hyperbaric stress exacerbates exercise and cold stress, thereby creating a greater thiamin demand. (Authors' abstract)

651.
FRATTALI, V., M. Quesada, R. Robertson and A. Shackelford.
Some observations on proteinase inhibitor therapy for decompression sickness in the rat.
Res. Comm. Chem. Pathol. Pharmacol. 6:1033-1042;Nov. 1973.

Trasylol, a kallikrein-trypsin inhibitor, and 6-amino-n-caproic acid were tested for their ability to reduce the incidence of decompression sickness in male, Sprague-Dawley rats that were subjected to a bends-producing dive using N_2-O_2 gas mixtures. Animals were administered one or the other drug either intraperitoneally or intravenously before being dived. Saline-treated animals served as controls. All animals were observed postdive for symptoms of decompression sickness and scored according to severity of reaction. Other means of assessing incidence and severity of decompression sickness included observations of lung pathology and postdive survival times. Neither drug preparation was found to decrease susceptibility to decompression sickness. From this it was concluded that this study cannot support adjuncts or alternatives to the bubble theory that invoke, for example, disseminated intravascular coagulation in the etiopathology of decompression sickness. (Authors' abstract)

652.
FREEMAN, P. and C. Edmonds.
Inner ear barotrauma.
Arch. Otolaryngol. 95:556-563;June 1972.

Five patients demonstrated a sensorineural hearing defect following aural barotrauma. Preincident and postincident audiograms show the extent of impairment to vary from a high frequency loss to a total sensorineural deafness. The men involved were all Navy divers and they all experienced difficulty in clearing their ears on descent. The terminology recommended for this condition is "inner ear barotrauma," to differentiate it from other forms of barotrauma and from the involvement of the eighth nerve in decompression sickness. (Authors' abstract)

653.
FREEMAN, P.
Inner ear barotrauma.
Arch. Otolaryngol. 97:429;May 1973.

In this letter to the editor, a case of bilateral rupture of the round window membrane following inner ear barotrauma is described. The subject had had difficulty in clearing his ears and noticed progressive hearing loss. The rupture was found to have occurred in both ears, with perilymph pouring from the inner ear. The fistula was plugged with a fat graft from the ear lobe in each case, with the result that the patient's hearing returned nearly to the level existing before the rupture. (MFW/SCD)

654.
FRIDOVICH, I.
Superoxide radical and superoxide dismutase.
Acc. Chem. Res. 5:321-326;Oct. 1972.

The author traces the development of the understanding of the involvement of superoxide radicals (O_2^-) in biologically significant oxidations, and the existence of a defense mechanism (superoxide dismutase) against O_2^- and its potential toxicity within acrobic cells. Because of these discoveries, diverse situations which had been imperfectly understood have become somewhat more clarified. One of these is the etiology of oxygen toxicity. It is now apparent that excessive amounts of O_2^- has a toxic effect. Therefore, any method by which the superoxide dismutase level could be raised would enhance tolerance for hyperoxia. (MFW/UMS)

655.
FRUCTUS, X.
Bilan de deux ans d'experimentation animale (primate) realisee a la COMEX de mai 1969 a septembre 1971.
[Report on two years of animal experimentation (primates) carried out at the COMEX from May, 1969, to September, 1971].
Marseille, France. CNEXO/COMEX, Rep. on Contract 69/89 and 71/296. 18p. 1971.

Results and conclusions concerning the High Pressure Nervous Syndrome in primates, based on 32 experiments with baboons (Papio papio) are summarized and discussed. The existence of the High Pressure Nervous Syndrome in primates has been demonstrated. In addition, there exists a "safe zone" to 600m in spite of rapid pressurization, and to greater depths (not yet determined) using a new method of slow pressurization. The authors are developing a safe decompression table for confined animals. The influence of an increase of PIO_2 on the appearance and evolution of the High Pressure Nervous Syndrome has been demonstrated. Thresholds of appearance of various anomalies (tremor, EEG signs, seizures, death) as functions of depths and pressurization rates are being determined. Hydrogen-oxygen breathing mixtures have been found to be safe for periods of several hours. EEG studies on nitrogen narcosis have been carried out using baboons at depths too great for man. Further research on the limits of the "safe zone" in which several species of primates are in no danger, and on the physiopathology and pathogeny of the High Pressure Nervous Syndrome is recommended. (MEMH/UMS)

656.
FRUCTUS, X. and P. Fructus.
Programme de recherches sur l'utilisation de divers melanges gazeux pour les plongees tres profondes.
[Research program on using various gaseous mixtures for very deep dives].
Marseille, France, Hyperbaric Exp. Cent., with Wrightsville Marine Biomed. Lab., Wilmington, N. Carolina. 1968.

The Pre-Hydra, Physalie, and Hydra I experiments of 1968 are described. During the preliminary dives, unexpected EEG anomalies, tremors, and a decrement in mental performance occurred. When compression was more rapid, symptoms were exacerbated. The "no joint juice syndrome" was also present, becoming more acute at bottom during physical activity, and lessening during ascent. Vertigo, vomiting, stiffness, and knee pain were present during decompression. The deepest of these dives was 335 m. The Physalie dives — four in all — were also marked by tremors, motor impairment, somnolence and EEG anomalies. In the observations of Dr. A. Gosset regarding somnolence and the cerebellar syndrome (dysmetry), it is noted that the former was more pronounced in one diver, and the latter in the other. Drs. R. Naquet and S. Dimov made observations on the EEG anomalies — theta activity, and the transformation of a curve of wakefulness to one of sleep. In Physalie III, a depth of 365 m was reached, at which point it was decided to terminate the experiment in the interests of safety. In Physalie IV, a slower compression modified the hpns. These dives were considered to be successful in the development of compression and decompression schedules, and in the increased understanding of the stresses involved in very deep dives. Also, and probably most important, they made possible the detailed investigation of hpns. It was found to be controllable to 310m, more pronounced but not acute at 335m, and rapidly intensifying beyond that depth. The use of breathing mixtures other than oxygen-helium, and saturation at an intermediate level to allow for adaptation, could make it possible to achieve 400m with safety. Operation Hydra was directed toward the investigation of oxygen-hydrogen as a breathing mixture. Due to the fire danger, this dive was conducted in the open sea, using a turret. The equipment, including clothing, is described. The dive was aborted at 252 m, due largely to failure of equipment. The heated suits were not satisfactory, and the CO_2 level became too high. The divers suffered from cold and from shortness of breath. In an appendix, a fuller discussion of the hpns is given. (MFW/BSCP)

657.
FRUCTUS, X., C. Agarate, J.P. Charpy, A. Gosset, R. Naquet and J.C. Rostain.
Postponing the high pressure nervous syndrome.
In: Abstracts of the Twenty-fifth congress of Physiological Sciences Satellite Symposium. Recent progress in fundamental physiology of diving, Marseille, France, July 1971, p.54-56. (Proceedings unpublished)

Abstract only: The authors describe the manifestations of the high pressure nervous syndrome, first observed in 1968: tremor, kinetic disorders, lowered vigilance and EEG anomalies. In a dive made in November 1970 (Physalie V) a simulated depth of 1706 feet was reached with minimal hpns manifestations. A new compression curve, based on the theory of gradients of saturation, was used. The authors feel without doubt that hpns is aggravated by rapid compression, and that a method that allows for osmotic dysbarism will postpone the onset of hpns, and also reduce the degree of the symptoms. (MFW/BSCP)

658.
FRUCTUS, X. and C. Agarate.
The high pressure nervous syndrome.
Med. Sport 24:272-278;Nov. 1971.

The High Pressure Nervous Syndrome is characterized in man, by tremors, motor troubles, dizziness and EEG changes appearing around 1100 feet in the case of a fast pressurization (2 metres/minute). It was observed by the authors as well as by Bennett during the Royal Navy simulated 1500 ft dive. It is most certainly enhanced by a fast pressurization which causes it to appear sooner and delayed by long stops at intermediary depths. Nevertheless, it seems it can be overcome down to 1300 feet, but it must appear at greater depths despite the care taken for adapting the divers to the very great depths. (English summary)

659.
FRUCTUS, X.
Down below the great depths.
In: Fructus, X., Ed. Third international conference on hyperbaric and underwater physiology, p.13-22, Paris, Doin, 1972.

It is stated that divers to 850 feet no longer pose physiological problems. Beyond that depth, dives are referred to as "very deep dives" and certain definite problems still exist, both in the nervous disorders that occur during descent and at depth, and in the danger of decompression accidents upon ascent. The Physalie dives of 1968 are described, with emphasis upon compression and decompression schedules and manifestations of the high pressure nervous syndrome (hpns). The symptoms of static tremor, kinetic tremor, dysmetry and theta waves are tabulated for Physalie V in 1970, which went to 1700 feet. As a result of these experiments, the author concludes that the major factor is high pressure under helium-oxygen, aggravated by rapid compression. Symptoms can be reduced by regulation of the compression rate. The author believes that hpns does not present an insurmountable obstacle at depths up to 2,000 feet, and that beyond these depths, respiratory problems would be the limiting factor with or without hpns. (See also Fructus, X. et al., Bull. Medsubhyp. 9:2-6;Mar. 1973) (MFW/UMS)

660.
FRUCTUS, X.
100 heures a 500 metres.
[100 hours at 500 meters].
Med. Sport 46(3):175-178; 1972.

This is a brief account of the COMEX simulated dive which began on February 21, 1972, with a summary of previous dives from 1968 on. The designation of this experiment is Sagittaire II. As a result of data gathered during this series of dives, the author concludes that, at the present state of the art of saturation diving techniques, the depth limit for safe diving and working is 500 meters. New techniques of compression and control of environmental parameters have made it possible for trained and selected divers to function effectively at 400 meters. The hpns symptoms which appeared at the 300-350 meter level became accentuated at 500 meters, and stabilized after 40 hours at this depth. The divers were kept at this depth for 60 more hours. The syndrome was not notably ameliorated until 40 hours later, during ascent, at the 300-meter level. (MFW/BSCP)

661.
FRUCTUS, X.
Physalie VI:610 metres. Nouvelle performance mondiale de plongee profonde en caisson realisee a Marseille, au Centre Experimental Hyperbare de la COMEX, du 16-5 au 2-6-1972.
[Physalie VI:610 meters. New world record in deep chamber diving achieved at Marseille, at the Hyperbaric Experimental Center of COMEX, from May 5 to June 2, 1972].
Med. Sport 46(3):180-182; 1972.

From May 16th to June 2nd, a very deep dive has been carried out in the Hyperbaric Research Center (COMEX — Marseilles). Two divers: Patrice Chemin, aged 24, world recordman at 1706 feet, and Robert Gauret, aged 30, who has already performed a 17 hours saturation dive at 1640 feet, reached the record depth of 610 meters (2001 ft). The overcoming of physiological problems and operational techniques enabled the subjects to remain at this depth for 80 minutes. The data collected will allow us to improve our knowledge of the physiological reactions of man at great depth and to draw a more precise definition of the High Pressure Nervous Syndrome. (English summary).

662.
FRUCTUS, X., ed.
Third international conference on hyperbaric and underwater physiology.
Paris, Doin, 1972.

This conference covered a wide range of subjects in the area of underwater physiology and technology. Specific papers will be found under the following author entries: Appaix, A. and F. Demard; Bornmann, R.C.; Brauer, R.W., M.R. Jordan and R.O. Way; Broussolle, B., E. Bensimon, A. Michaud and C. Vegezzi; Brue, F., J.L. Morcelet, P. Revelat and P. Burtin; Buhlmann, A.A., W.H. Ziegler and J. Muller; Canty, J.M., E.H. Lanphier and R.A. Morin; Chouteau, J.; Christ, M.; Cockett, A.T.K., S.M. Pauley and A.P. Roberts; Conti, V. and F. Sicardi; Ehm, O.F. and A. Piechotta; Fructus, X.; Hempleman, H.V.; Joanny, P. and J. Corriol (two); L'Huillier, J.R., C. Jacquemin and P. Varene; Miller, J.N., O.D. Wangensteen and E.H. Lanphier; Miller, K.W., W.E.M. Paton and E.B. Smith; Muren, A. and K. Wulff; Radomski, M.W.; Rawlins, J.S.P.; Ricci, G.C.; Rostain, J.C. and R. Nacquet; Schaefer, K.E.; Sem-Jacobsen and O.B. Styri (two); Smit, P.J.; Uhlig, G. and G. Haux; Varene, P., C. Jacquemin and J. L'Huillier. (MFW/UMS)

663.
FRUCTUS, X. and J.P. Charpy.
Etude psychometrique de 2 sujet lors d'une plongee fictive jusqu'a 52.42 ATA.
[Psychometric study of two subjects during a simulated dive to 52.42 ATA].
Bull. Medsubhyp 7:3-12;Oct. 1972.

Performance measures carried out during the Physalie V dive to 520m are described. Both sensory-motor tests and mental tests were given. The results are interpreted as follows: First, the hpn syndrome was much less acute than that observed in earlier dives at 400m; this fact is attributed to the compression curve, which was effectively scheduled to postpone the appearance of the syndrome; (the compression schedule is not given). Second, the psychometric tests make it possible to evaluate the real importance of the hpns manifestations. In the manual dexterity tests, the divers showed a 20% diminution of performance at 350m and 420m respectively. However, increase in tremor at 450m and 520m respectively was not reflected in further decline. The effect of hpns on motor coordination was the most apparent, but not necessarily the most important, effect. In the visual choice reaction time tests, performance was more affected than in manual dexterity tests; this suggests that sensory function is involved. Performance degradation in visual choice reaction time tests seems related to the lowering of vigilance indicated by the results of the odd-even test. The lowering of vigilance is always more pronounced in one subject than in the other, and may be a question of intellectual process. The difference of these results might be due to two factors: (1) the less intelligent subject will demonstrate more fragile intellectual processes; (2) the indigenous differences between subjects might result in a difference in motivation and attitude, as these subjects clearly indicated. Relationships, pointed out elsewhere in the literature, between the EEG anomalies and modification of performance must be confirmed and defined before it can be determined whether they would clarify this problem. More findings on a larger number of subjects will help clarify the significance of the degradation in mental performance that was observed in one of the subjects. (MFW/BSCP)

664.
FRUCTUS, X., C. Agarate and J.C. Rostain.
Reflexions sur la courbe de compression des plongees tres profondes.
[Thoughts on the compression curves of very deep dives].
Bull. Medsubhyp 9:2-6 plus illus. Mar. 1973.

The role of the compression schedule upon the HPNS symptoms is studied according to the results obtained during the numerous deep dives carried out at COMEX's hyperbaric research center these last years. It appears that successive improvements of the compression method have permitted the postponement of the appearance of the HPNS and the completion of a 2000-ft dive. Nevertheless, from 1300 feet these symptoms are still present, although attenuated, and further studies of the phenomenon must be under taken. (English abstract)

665.
FRUCTUS, X., R. Lescure and R. Sciarli.
Considerations ethiques dans la recherche hyperbare.
[Ethical considerations in hyperbaric research].
In: Hesser, C.M. and D. Linnarsson, eds. Proceedings of the first annual scientific meeting of the European Undersea Biomedical Society, Stockholm, 13-15 June 1973. Forsvarsmedicin 9:369-372;July 1973.

Hyperbaric research must be constantly based on moral will: a will which will manifest itself by the application of the following principals: a lead to the development of a useful, efficacious, and reliable hyperbaric medicine; to demand of the aquanaut in an experimental situation only that which he can give, without ever putting in danger his health or his life; to demand, on the other hand, the maximum from technology, exacting from the equipment that its constant progress toward perfection contribute to the increase of the security as much as of the efficacy of man in the hyperbaric environment; to concern itself with the long term pathology of professional divers, in order better to prevent or to reduce it. (Authors' conclusion translated by MFW/UMS)

666.
FRYE, J.
Life underseas — with a goal.
Sea Frontiers 19:345-350;Nov./Dec. 1973.

La Chapula is a 50-ft submersible barge, or mobile habitat. For the past year, it has submerged once a month and stayed submerged, with its crew of four scientist-divers and one engineer-diver for two weeks. It is the tool of the Puerto Rico International Undersea Laboratory (PRINUL), the purpose of which is to carry on the work pioneered by Tektite I and II on a continuing basis. It is believed to be the only portable habitat that operates continuously, being towed from spot to spot as the need arises. The breathing mixture used is 9/91 oxygen-nitrogen; after the two-week saturation exposure, decompression takes 18 hours. Pollution studies, fish life studies, coral reef ecology, are among the fields of investigation. Subcom communication equipment is used and 85% of the messages sent from habitat to diver 180 yards away are received. La Chalupa was built by Perry Oceanographics, Inc. Water beds are used for extra ballast. There are three 42-inch viewing ports. Electronic monitoring equipment with sonar follows the divers throughout a 1,000-ft working radius. (MFW/SCD)

667.
FUGITT, R.B. and R.W. Uhrich.
Underwater stereoscopic television and display realism.
U.S. Nav. Undersea Cent., Rep. NUC-TP-358, 37p. July 1973.

Conventional closed-circuit underwater television systems lack display realism, making remote manipulation and positioning difficult. Stereoscopic and head-coupled television systems were developed to provide three-dimensional position and orientation information. Tests show the time required to perform remote positioning and manipulative tasks is reduced when such systems are used. Comparison tests using a single-camera stereoscopic television system and the same system operated in a nonstereoscopic mode showed the average time required to perform a simple precise positioning task was reduced by 24 percent. The average position error was reduced by 60 percent when the stereoscopic system was used. (GRA)

668.
FUGITT, R.B.
Small remotely-manned vehicles.
In: Ocean 73. 1973 IEEE international conference on engineering in the ocean environment, p.260-264. IEEE publication 73-CHO-7740-OCC.

Small, remotely-manned tethered vehicles have been developed for undersea inspection, surveilance, implantment, and recovery. For many applications such vehicles offer several advantages over diver systems or general purpose submersibles. Some of these are: safety, unlimited endurance, low initial and operating cost, portability, ease of operation and availability of information to control personnel. Some features of the vehicle "Snoopy" are closed circuit television, automatic depth control utilizing a variable buoyancy chamber, proportional joystick thruster control, a variable torque grabber, and a compass. "SCAT," a somewhat larger vehicle with greater work capability employs a head-following stereoscopic television and sonar system, automatic depth or altitude control, proportional joystick thruster control, and a two function grabber. A version of Snoopy which is being designed and constructed for deeper operation incorporates a streamlined fiberglass hull and utilizes a single coaxial cable for power and data transmission. (Author's abstract)

669.
FUNK, C.J.
Predicted system performance of improved underwater light sources.
In: Ocean 73. 1973 IEEE international conference on engineering in the ocean environment, p.7-17. IEEE publication 73 CHO 774-0 OCC.

The system performance of the two improved underwater light sources which have been recently developed at the Naval Undersea Center and other advanced light sources is predicted by computer simulation. System performance is evaluated as a function of source-receiver separation, receiver sensitivity, and the angular extent of the beam pattern of the source in representative samples of coastal and deep ocean waters. A figure of merit is calculated for each combination of light source and television camera to provide a convenient reference for comparing the power limitations of the different systems. In addition, signal to backscatter ratios are calculated to provide data on the backscatter limitations of the different systems. (Author's abstract)

670.
FURGANG, F.A.
Carbon monoxide intoxication presenting as air embolism in a diver: a case report.
Aerosp. Med. 43:785-786;July 1972.

A scuba diver suffered loss of consciousness immediately following a rapid ascent. After a five-hour delay, treatment for air embolism was begun in a hyperbaric chamber. A history of antecedent symptoms and strange behavior led to a strong suspicion of carbon monoxide intoxication; this was later confirmed. The problem of a contaminated breathing medium as a contributory factor in diving accidents is discussed. Routine testing of the gas used by diving casualties is suggested. (Author's abstract)

671.
FUST, H.D., K.G. Muller, H. Oser and S. Ruff.
Development of decompression tables for short term 100-200 meter dives.
In: Hesser, C.M. and D. Linnarsson eds. Proceedings of the first annual scientific meeting of the European Undersea Biomedical Society, Stockholm, 13-15 June 1973. Forsvarsmedicin 9:502-506;July 1973.

[An M-value is the maximum value of the partial pressure of dissolved inert gas which can be tolerated in specific compartments of the human body and will permit the diver safely to ascend to the next stop.] The main features of these tables, based on Workman's M-values, were a rather fast initial decompression with overtensions up to 35 m and a slow decompression in the range of depths between 20-0 m. The analysis of the gas tensions at 130 m/60 min-dives showed the following: Some compartments had been exposed to medium overtensions during the first steps; later on the overtensions became negative. During unsuccessful dives they became positive again in the range of depths between 15-0 m. This was correlated with the occurrence of bends. A possible explanation is the formation of a silent bubble produced in the beginning of the decompression which grows to a critical size at 15-0 m. By a slower decompression in this range these positive gas tensions can be avoided, and thus the bends could be circumvented. Problems occurred in using this method to depths beyond 130 m. At a 150 m/30 min-dive bends appeared three hours after decompression; a recompression to 162 m had to be applied. An analysis of the gas tensions indicates a too long exposure to overtensions during the first steps, the effect of which could not be counterbalanced by any treatment at lower depths. Indications were that a decompression schedule no longer can be constructed alone by controlling the values of the gas tensions in the compartments by M-values. The history of a compartment and especially the duration of exposure to overtensions become important. On the basis of these ideas new decompression schedules in the range of 150 - 200 m are proposed. (Authors' abstract)

672.
GABIBOV, V.M. and E.Z. Emirbekov.
Aktivnost' fermentov azotistogo obmena v mozge krys posle deistviya kisloroda pod posyshennym davleniem.
[Activity of nitrogen metabolising enzymes in rat brain in the presence of hyperbaric oxygen].
Ukr. Biokhim. Zh. 45(5):577-580; 1973.

The activity of glutamine synthetase, glutaminase, glutamate decarboxylase, and GABA (γ-aminobutyric acid) aspartate- and alanine-amino-transferases was studied in the rat brain during hyperoxic convulsions and at different times (1, 5, 10, 15, 25, 40, 60 days), after O_2 effect at a pressure of 4 or 6 atm. Hyperbaric O_2 evokes an increased activity of glutaminase and aspartate-, alanine-, GABA-, pyruvate-, and GABA-α-ketoglutarate transaminases and a decreased activity of glutamine synthetase, glutamate decarboxylase and GABA-PAA (oxaloacetic acid) transaminase of the rat brain. At different times after the O_2 effect there are changes in the activity of these enzymes; 40-60 days later the initial level of enzyme activity is restored. (DT) (© BA)

673.
GACAD, G. and D. Massaro.
Hyperoxia: Influence on lung mechanics and protein synthesis.
J. Clin. Invest. 52(3):559-565; 1973.

The time course of the influence of in vivo hyperoxia was studied on lung mechanics and protein synthesis. After 24 hr of exposure to greater than 98% O_2 at one atm there were no alterations in descending pressure-volume curves (air or saline) of lungs excised from O_2-exposed rats compared to control rats. After 48 hr of hyperoxia there was a decrease in lung compliance. To study protein synthesis, as indicated by L-[U-^{14}C] leucine incorporation into protein, lung slices were incubated with L-[U-^{14}C] leucine and surface-active material then obtained by ultracentrifugation of lung homogenates. Radioactivity was measured in total protein and in protein in the surface-active fraction. There were no alterations in incorporation after 12 hr of hyperoxia. After 24 hr of hyperoxia there were significant decreases ($P < 0.05$) in L-[U-^{14}C] leucine incorporation into total protein and into protein of the surface-active fraction. After 48 hr of hyperoxia incorporation into protein of the surface-active fraction wa decreased to a greater extent than incorporation into total protein, $63 \pm 4\%$ and $75 \pm 5\%$, respectively, ($P < 0.025$). Hyperoxia produces a major decrease in protein synthesis, including synthesis of protein in a surface-active fraction, before the onset of any detectable changes in the static compliance of excised lungs. (© BA)

674.
GAIT, D.J. and K.W. Miller.
Novel approach to improved submarine escape performance.
Aerosp. Med. 44:645-648;June 1973.

Conventional compressed air based submarine escape techniques have been developed to the extent where only new approaches will yield a significant increase in performance. The novel approach suggested here is to substitute for nitrogen in the breathing mixture an inert gas which saturates the body tissue more slowly, thus increasing the pressure of gas required to achieve a critical tissue concentration in a given time. Calculations on the rate of uptake of a number of inert gases in men indicate that carbon tetrafluoride is a suitable gas for this purpose. This prediction is tested experimentally by determining the incidence of decompression sickness in mice after short exposures to either nitrogen-oxygen or carbon tetrafluoride-oxygen mixtures. The experiments indicate that substitution of carbon tetrafluoride for nitrogen might increase the depth from which submarine escape may be achieved with a given technique by between 50% and 100%. (Authors' abstract)

675.
GALAKTIONOV, L.G.
Sanitarno-prosvetitel'naya rabotana na podroknykh v more.
[Health education on board submarines at sea].
Voennomed. Zh (5):70-72;May 1971.

One of the most important tasks of the submarine physician, besides treating medical emergencies, is the teaching of the crew simple facts of preventive medicine in underwater conditions. The author outlines two basic forms of medical training for the submarine crew, formal and informal. The formal training consists of planned lectures and courses for the entire crew, teaching them in simple language, the basic physiological concepts of various aspects of underwater life. The informal teaching will be generally unplanned and consists of discussions with small groups or even individuals, answering questions etc. The officer may anonymously post a medical question he does not care to discuss in public. The answer posted by the physician can then be read by all crew members. The most important topics to be discussed by the physician are: metabolic and other physiological changes affecting the organism during underwater stay, the vital importance of regular physical exercise, well planned diet, hygiene of food handling, rational utilization of a limited water supply etc. The author also stresses the importance of stocking the ship library with popular medical educational reading material and the showing of films of similar content. (OLC/SCD)

676.
GALPIN, S.
Achievable performance of acoustic imaging systems.
In: IEEE international conference on engineering in the ocean environment, Panama City, Florida, September 1970. Digest of technical papers, p.79-81. Published by the conference.

Image information content, sonar equations for different target types, and achievable range-resolution performance envelopes are presented. Potential for improved performance and versatility through nonlinear techniques is explored. Illustrations from experiments are provided. (Eng. Ind.)

677.
GANDY, W.F. and F.P. Wittmann, III.
Cruise report #46 FRV Oregon II: July 23-Aug. 9, 1973.
Nat. Oceanic Atmosph. Admin., Nat. Mar. Fisheries Serv. 1973.

The test concept was essentially to deploy an underwater acoustic image device and an optical imaging device over identical targets. Using the optical imagery as a standard, the acoustical image could then be analyzed for resolution, sensitivity and other operational characteristics. The acoustical imagery was acquired using a Side Scan High Resolution Hydroacoustic System developed by Gould, Inc., Advanced Technology Group, Cleveland, Ohio, for the Naval Coastal Systems Laboratory at Panama City, Florida. A detailed technical description is not available because of the system's security classification. System output was monitored on a scope and recorded on strip charts for further analysis. The optical imagery was acquired by means of an underwater photography sled developed by NMFS, and designated RUFAS (Remote Underwater Fishery Assessment System). The system consists of a 35 mm pulsed camera, a closed-circuit television, camera lights, and the necessary control systems to maintain proper altitude and attitude from the ocean floor. The CCTV was monitored, and when an object was spotted the 35 mm camera was activated to photograph the object. A precision Navigation System (RAYDIST) was installed aboard the OREGON II at Pascagoula. The purpose of this system was to obtain precise navigational fix loxations when an obstruction was located. The system also provided an accurate means for maintaining a given track line. The system accuracy is $\pm$ 15.2 meters. (Authors)

678.
GAUDIANO, A.V.
Deep water demands new diving technology.
Offshore 33:39, 40, 42;July 1973.

The author, an official of Taylor Diving and Salvage Co., Inc., describes a typical saturation diving system such as is used by the company: "The control house, placed over the saturation chamber, contains gas console, gas mixer, power distribution, instrumentation and environmental control. The environmental machinery is in a separate room." The saturation chamber consists of two separate chambers, one for active work and the other for decompression. A personnel transfer capsule can mate to either chamber. This transfer capsule has its own life support system, and can also be used in emergency rescue, and in transporting divers from one system to another or to shore. The article is illustrated with diagrams of an underwater saturation diving system and of the basic piping system of a closed circuit free flow underwater breathing system. There is also a table demonstrating gas use and its cost in open, semi-closed and closed breathing apparatus. At 300 feet, for instance, an open circuit system uses one hundred times the gas that a closed circuit system uses. The system illustrated and described here is the first of its kind in commercial use, and is expected to be of prime importance in future deep diving and undertakings. (MFW/BSCP)

679.
GAZEY, B.K.
Visibility and resolution in turbid waters.
Underwater Sci. Technol. J. 2:105-115;June 1970.

In this paper some optical properties of the sea are discussed, particularly those relating to scatterer size and concentration. The effects of scattering particles on the visibility of submerged objects and the inherent resolution limit imposed by the medium are discussed. This has necessitated the use of a scattering theory which unlike most scattering theories in general use, takes account of multiple scatter. This was found necessary in view of the fact that in any real underwater viewing situation the scatterer concentration is sufficiently high that higher order scatter is almost certain to occur. In principle it is possible to predict the inherent resolution limit imposed by the turbidity of the medium itself provided accurate data is available regarding particle size, refractive index and concentration. Unfortunately these parameters vary considerably even within so-called well-defined water mass classifications; consequently each application will have to be treated individually, using scattering functions measured in situ. The experimental work has shown that simple optical systems have no better resolution capabilities than many existing sonar equipments. They are certainly likely to be inferior in range performance and even the use of more sophisticated range-gated laser TV or image dissection techniques (although increasing the useful range of optical imaging by perhaps as much as an order of magnitude) is unlikely to change this situation. (Author's conclusions)

680.
GEE, G.K.
Educational programs for studying man's reactions in water.
In: Applications of marine technology to human needs. Preprints. 8th annual conference and exposition, Marine Technology Society, September, 1972, Washington, D.C., p.173-201. Published by the Society, 1972.

"Man in a Water Evironment" is a pilot undergraduate program [at Corning Community College] designed to introduce students to the principles of underwater physiology as a basis for understanding human body reactions and adaptability in water. The program provides a student the opportunity to explore his capability, limitation and compatibility in the hydrospace for living, useful work and safe recreational activities. The program structure and some experimentations are described. The program serves students in marine biology, oceanography, marine technology and engineering, physical education, environmental medicine, recreation and safety programs. (Author's abstract)

681.
GELFAND, R. and C.J. Lambertsen.
A re-breathing technique for measurement of stable-state CO_2 reactivity.
In: Aerospace Medical Association. 1972 annual scientific meeting, Bal Harbour, Florida, May 1972. Preprints, p.176-177. Published by the Association.

The widely used re-breathing method which produces a linear increase (ramp) in $PACO_2$ for measurement of CO_2 reactivity was investigated. . . The entire experiment lasted 40 minutes, as follows. The subject pre-breathed the test mixture for 10 minutes while the re-breathing system was flushed with the same gas. The subject then was connected to the re-breathing system and breathed CO_2-free gas for 10 minutes (inspired air passing through the CO_2 absorber). The CO_2 absorber was then bypassed and the inhaled CO_2 rose approximately 12mm Hg above the control level during the final 20 minutes of the experiment. Measurements were made at ambient pressures of 0, 100, 200, 300 and 400 feet of sea water (fsw) breathing N_2/O_2, at 0, 400, 700, 900 and 1200 fsw breathing crude Ne/O_2, and at 0, 400, and 900 fsw breathing He/O_2 mixtures. Under these conditions the system was effectively functional for study of respiratory reactivity. (Authors)

682.
GELFAND, R. and C.J. Lambertsen.
Dynamic respiratory response to abrupt change of inspired CO_2 at normal and high PO_2.
J. Appl. Physiol. 35(6):903-913; 1973.

Breath-by-breath measurements of the respiratory tidal volume, frequency, and minute volume transients which resulted when 6% CO_2 was abruptly added to and subsequently abruptly removed from inspired gas were obtained in 14 experiments on a single intensively studied human subject. Analysis of these measurements established that it is possible to identify and quantitatively characterize the dynamic response characteristics of two central nervous system respiratory receptor components in addition to that of peripheral chemoreceptors. The same three components of respiratory response to CO_2 were found in studies on three additional men. The intensively studied subject showed reproducible dynamic response characteristics. At natural levels of alveolar PO_2, his peripheral chemoreceptor contribution to overall respiratory stimulation by CO_2 was small (12%), its onset lag was short (6 sec), and its rate of development was rapid (time constant — 5 sec). O_2 breathing reduced the magnitude of this most rapid component of respiratory control. The CNS-related components both had an extended onset lag (20 sec), with widely differing response rates (T = 10 and 89 sec) and equal contributions to overall respiratory stimulation (44% each). Oxygen breathing also reduced the magnitude of the rapidly responding central component. The response rate of even the slowest CNS-related component implies a perfusion rate for these receptors approximately the same as CNS gray matter; this is inconsistent with a superficial medullary location for such receptors. (Authors' abstract)

683.
GELLER, M., D.E. Altman and G.J. Barstow.
Performance data on cadmium and zinc metal vapor arc lamps as efficient light sources for deep ocean waters.
In: Ocean 73. 1973 IEEE international conference on engineering in the ocean environment, p.18-23. IEEE publication 73 CHO 774-0 OCC.

The optical attenuation characteristics of deep ocean waters show a broad minimum between 460 nm and 510 nm. Optical sources for underwater applications should emit in this ocean window to minimize the required optical power. To fulfill this need for an efficient source, a new pair of arc lamps were developed: zinc-xenon and cadmium-xenon. Performance and engineering data on this type of short-arc lamp with various electrode spacings are presented in terms of spectral-emission curves, line widths, electrical characteristics, and conversion efficiencies. Lamp blackening due to the tungsten-water cycle as a limitation to lamp life is discussed. Sample lifetime data indicate lifetimes in excess of 200 hours are realizable. (Authors' abstract)

684.
GENIN, A.M., M.A. Tikhonov, V.B. Malkin, V.A. Glazkova, Ye.P. Grishin, N.T. Drozdova, Ye.V. Logionova, L.A. Lushina, N.A. Roshchina and V.I. Solov'yev.
[Physiological criteria of manifestations of early toxic normobaric hyperoxia].
Izvest. Akad. Nauk SSSR (Ser. Biol.) 3:380-391;May/June 1973.

A study was conducted (1) on the dynamics of the functional state of the human body during prolonged respiration of pure oxygen under normal barometric pressure; (2) on the selection of the most adequate physiological tests, which characterize the initial toxic signs of hyperoxia; and (3) on the determination of safe time limits of hyperoxia exposure. A series of 79 experiments with 49 healthy male subjects aged 18-23 studied the influence of normobaric hyperoxia (PO_2:720-740 mmHg). These tests lasted from 4-24 hours and studied a number of physiological functions. A description is presented for the developmental dynamics of the symptomocomplex for the toxic manifestations of hyperoxia, changes in the condition of neuropsychic efficiency, the systemic and regional hemodynamic indices, the activity of some lymphocyte enzymes, phagocyte neutrophile activity, and indices of the acid-alkali blood equilibrium. It was shown that the appearance and the dynamics of functional lung deficiencies most adequately characterize the vital capacity and forced vital capacity changes, elasticity, resistance, and diffusional capacity of the lungs. It was found that the development of pathological reaction most probably occurs following 14-16 hours of breathing pure oxygen at normal atmospheric pressure. Possible pathophysiological mechanisms of these reactions are discussed. (S&T Alert)

685.
GIERTSEN, J.C.
Scubadykkerulykker. En diskusjon av 8 fatale tilfelle.
[Fatal scuba diving accidents. A discussion of 8 fatal cases].
T. Norsk. Laegeforen. 12:924-928;May 1972.

No English summary available.

686.
GILARDI, R.C.
Saturation diving gas logistics.
In: The working diver, 1972. Symposium proceedings, February 1972, Columbus, Ohio, p.9-22. Washington, D.C., Marine Technology Society, 1972.

The smooth conduct of saturation diving depends on the availability of substantial quantities of industrial gases in pure and mixed form. Handling and delivery methods may differ from those customary for short duration dives. Gas logistics are discussed in two parts: first, equipment and methods for supplying the gas at the diving scene; and second, techniques for conserving gas to keep the total requirements and costs at manageable levels. (Author's abstract)

687.
GILARDI, R.C.
Production of diving gases.
In: Battelle Columbus Laboratories. Proceedings, 1973 divers' gas purity symposium, November 27-28, 1973, p.VII-1-VII-14. U.S. Navy Supervisor Diving, Nav. Ships Syst. Comm., Rep 2-73, 1973.

Production methods for the gases currently used in diving — oxygen, nitrogen, helium, hydrogen, and neon — are discussed with emphasis on methods of determining purity and the typical purities of these products. Techniques for in-plant and on-site preparation of mixtures and their analysis are cited. Reference is made to extension of gas supplies by recovery and repurification. The conclusion is reached that industry can respond to the total requirements of the diving community with gases as well as broad range of specialized services and hardware. (Author's abstract)

688.
GILBERT, D.E.
Development of electronic technology for deep ocean applications.
UnderSea Technol. 14:24-26;Mar. 1973.

Pressure tolerant electronic (PTE) technology in this article relates to the operation of electronic assemblies immersed in a chemically inert dielectric liquid when these assemblies are submitted to, and experience, ambient hydrostatic pressures of the ocean depths. There are three approaches to the operation — electronic components in a high hydrostatic environment can be: (1) enclosed in hard shells and maintained at normal atmospheric pressure; (2) enclosed in soft shells with a pressure-compensating liquid; or (3) free flooded in the environment. The value and feasibility of the second approach for PTE systems has been documented. This article discusses the rationale, approach, state of the art, and future trends in PTE technology of the second approach — components enclosed in soft shells with a pressure-compensating liquid. (Author)

689.
GILBERT, P.W. and C. Gilbert.
Sharks and shark deterrents.
Underwater J. 5:69-79;Apr. 1973.

After discussing the physical characteristics of the shark, the author mentions the establishment in 1958 of the American Institute of Biological Sciences Shark Research Panel, the purpose of which was to stimulate and coordinate shark research. One of the activities of the panel was to evaluate anti-shark measures, another to set up a shark attack file. The file indicates that about 100 shark attacks occur yearly throughout the world, about half of which are fatal. It has been demonstrated both in Australia and in Florida that sharks can be attracted by low-frequency sound and thus drawn away from an area. An early attempt to combat sharks was the setting of nets parallel to the beach in Sydney, Australia, in 1937. Sharks were captured in the nets, in ever increasing numbers, until at the present time, the shark hazard is practically eliminated. The same method was used successfully in South Africa. During World War II research led to the development of the chemical "shark chaser" which was dissolved in water soluble wax. It was effective against most, but not all, species; it is not effective against sharks that are in a "feeding frenzy". To protect the individual survivor at sea, the Shark Screen is effective. It is a bag with inflatable collars. The submerged part is dark in color, which renders it unattractive to sharks. Various types of electronic barriers are described. Billies, spear guns, and bang sticks are used by swimmers with varying success. The gas gun which inflates a shark by means of a 16 g CO_2 cartridge is at present considered very effective (See McKenney, J. Skin Diver 21:28, 30; Feb. 1972). Another device under development is a piece of buoyant wood that can be attached to a shark, upsetting its hydrostatic balance. Some research has been undertaken to train dolphins to ward off sharks, but was not successful in the case of the bull shark. (MFW/BSCP)

690.
GILL, J.S.
The ARL processor for helium speech.
In: Diving applications in marine research. Proceedings of a seminar, National Institute of Oceanography, Godalming, Surrey, U.K., December 1971, p.127-132. Published by the Institute, 1972.

This paper describes the development of a time-domain processor which restores the intelligibility of speech produced in oxy-helium. . . . Signals from the transducer are filtered by a 12 kHz low-pass filter and then pass through an adustable shaping network to the larynx detector and analogue-to-digital convertor. This adjustable network can provide up to 20 dB lift in the upper part of the spectrum to enhance the unvoiced sounds. The larynx pulse detector selects the most intense 2.5 millisecond-long section of each larynx period.These sections are encoded at 30 kilosamples/sec into 8-bit PCM and read sequentially into shift-register stores. During unvoiced sounds the monostable fires almost continuously and most of the speech is stored. Read shift pulses are applied to the 3 banks of storage which are not currently being written and these signals are interleaved and decoded at four times the read shift rate. The signals from the digital-to-analogue convertor are passed through a 4 kHz low-pass filter which averages the samples from the three stores and removes the unwanted products of the sampling process. The variable frequency oscillator which controls the overall expansion ratio is adjustable over the range 120-40 kHz to provide any ratio which may be required within the range 1:1 to 3:1. This model operated successfully throughout the record-breaking dive to 1500 feet, made by John Bevan and Peter Sharphouse of the RNSS at RNPL Alverstoke during March 1970. The processed speech was at all times highly intelligible. (Author)

691.
GILL, J.S.
The Admiralty Research Laboratory processor for helium speech.
In: Sergeant, R.L. and T. Murry, eds. Processing helium speech: proceedings of a Navy-sponsored workshop, August 1971, U.S. Nav. Submar. Med. Res. Lab., Rep. NSMRL 708, p.34-38. May 22, 1972.

The basis of the method which has been developed at the Admiralty Research Laboratory is to write sections of the speech in a temporary store and then to read them at a lower rate. During voiced sounds these sections are taken from the most intense part of each larynx period and the remainder is rejected. During unvoiced sounds the sections are taken less regularly and are more closely spaced. The frequency compression resulting from the lower replay rate is inversely proportional to the time expansion. The section length must be less than the shortest larynx period, otherwise the larynx periodicity will be destroyed, but it must be sufficiently long to ensure that the first formant of the helium speech is adequately defined. In this application a length of 2.5 milliseconds was chosen to allow operation at larynx frequencies up to 400 Hz. The expanded sections overlap whenever the product of section length and expansion ratio exceeds the larynx period. Four temporary stores are used and at any time one is being written whilst the remainder are being read. This enables the expansion ratio to be varied over the range 1:1 to 3:1, whilst retaining all of the sampled sections. Operation at larger expansion ratios would call for an increase in the number of temporary stores in order to maintain the whole of the 2.5 millisecond sections. . . . This model operated successfully throughout the record-breaking dive to 1500 feet, made by John Bevan and Peter Sharphouse of the RNSS at RNPL, Alverstoke, during March 1970. The processed speech was at all times highly intelligible. (Author)

692.
GILLEN, H.W.
Decompression sickness and its therapy.
Skin Diver 21:8, 10, 13;Apr. 1972.

It is stated that in five cases recently reported in the non-medical literature, the key problems of inadequate treatment of decompression injuries are illustrated: lack of recognition of the extent of the illness by the diver, the supervisor, and the physician. Most important is the physician's failure to recognize the inadequacy of the initial treatment. (See Mullinix, J.M., Skin Diver 20:47-48;Aug. 1971). There is a lack of post doctoral clinical education programs (only one is currently in existence). Increased availability of recompression chambers will help, but not to any great extent until better understanding of the problems is disseminated throughout the diving community. In spite of the efforts of the Committee on Man's Underwater Activities of the Marine Technology Society, of the Undersea Medical Society, and of some of the leading training associations (NAVI, YMCA, PADI, and the British Sub-Aqua Club) to promote diving safety, diving injury recognition, and decompression sickness therapy, there has been little improvement. In conclusion, the author states "The individual's concern for himself is the secret with the development of enough personal recognition of the hazard of a decompression injury to eliminate the ridicule associated with symptoms and cause the prompt recognition of the injury. (MFW/BSCP)

693.
GILLEN, H.W.
Undersea medicine: osteogenic necrosis.
Aerosp. Med. 43:466-467;Apr. 1972.

This is a plea for a centralized national registry of data collection on the subject of osteogenic necrosis (or aseptic bone necrosis). This should include data on "diving experience, radiographic studies, life habits and health characteristics of a large number of exposed persons over many years." Interview and questionnaire techniques must be developed. The collection of data must be on an involuntary basis as a requirement of employment. It is emphasized that the cause of bone necrosis is not known, and there is no therapy in existence at present by which lesions may be reversed. A national registry of data on bone necrosis would reveal collateral significance of data now isolated and dispersed, and might lead to the identification of other safety and health problems. It is estimated that 5,000 persons are regularly employed in commercial diving and caisson work and many others are irregularly so employed. Because a large number of these workers are peripatetic, reliable data are not available under any program now in existence. A national registry must be developed under the Occupational Safety and Health Act of 1970, with the help of the Occupational Safety and Health Administration of the Department of Labor. (MFW/BSCP)

694.
GILLEN, H.W.
International standards designed for offshore operations. I. Diving submersibles.
In: Marine industries: problems and opportunities. Proceedings of the ninth annual conference of the Marine Technology Society, p.623-632. Washington, D.C., Marine Technology Society, 1973.

There are no internationally accepted standards for the design of, or operational characteristics of diving equipment or submersibles. There is not even a mutual understanding of the emergency signals that would be useful except those of the International Rules of the Road. Thread dimensions, pipe and fitting sizes, color coding, equipment maintenace schedules and inspection are as varied as are their national sources. The protection of the man and his operation underwater, whether diving or in a submersible, is required for safe and economically useful offshore activities. The international availability of interchangeable equipment and supplies is now based on specific supply lines rather than on a logical arrangement of international standards. Useful occupational safety and health programs require reliable equipment that is well maintained and widely dispersed. The same programs require excellent supply lines with proven efficacy delivering pre-tested material on schedule. Offshore operations widely scattered need significant logistic support. Material and supplies of uncertain origin or reliability hazard the lives of the personnel and the success of the operation. However, reliable logistic support is best based on pretested equipment and supplies, and advance planning for procurement, when test methods and performance characteristics are accepted and established by the users. This will require prior consensus agreement by the users and multiple regulatory agencies of specific standards, of specific test methods, and of specific re-inspection/maintenance programs. (From author's abstract)

695.
GILLEN, H.W. and R.W. Brauer.
Human toxicologic limits in hyperbaric environments.
In: Battelle Columbus Laboratories. Proceedings, 1973 divers' gas purity symposium, November 27-28, 1973, p.VIII-1-VIII-12. U.S. Navy Supervisor Diving, Nav. Ships Syst. Comm., Rep 2-73, 1973.

Contaminants can arise from the system itself (from solvents, materials, glues, oil, etc.) or from the human (carbon monoxide and methane). Some affect the lung, others pass through the lung into the blood. Recycling of breathing gas will often increase contaminants, such as microbiologic pollution. Cost of toxicological studies, both in time and money, has been a deterrent. HPNS studies are mentioned as instances of attempts to separate effects of compression and compression rate from those of gas. Fluid breathing techniques have made possible animal experiments to distinguish between these effects. Saturation diving because of length of exposure, poses new problems. Toxicological control studies under these conditions have not been made. The possibility of toxicological effects delayed for years, like malignancy from radium, or dysbaric osteonecrosis from exposure to a hyperbaric environment is noted. Without analytic data, and cumulative clinical data, no criteria for toxicology or permissible contaminants in hyperbaric environments can be determined. The problem of tissue sampling, i.e., which type of tissue constitutes an effective test for which contaminant, must be solved. (MFW/UMS)

696.
GIOLAS, T.G., J.R. Duffy, R.J. Duffy, H.S. Cooker and R.L. Sergeant.
Equivalency of sentence intelligibility lists for audiological assessment of naval personnel and navy voice communication systems.
U.S. Nav. Submar. Med. Res. Lab., Rep. NSMRL 759, 9p. Sept. 14, 1973.

The problem was to determine the equivalence of ten Central Institute of the Deaf (CID) sentence intelligibility lists and relate that information to the equivalence of corresponding revisions by the Naval Submarine Medical Research Laboratory (R-CID) of the ten CID Lists. It was found that: (1) Two five-list combinations of the CID Lists yielded equivalent scores. (2) Seven R-CID Lists yielded equivalent scores. (3) The mean scores for eight R-CID Lists were significantly lower than scores obtained with the corresponding CID Lists. (4) Both the CID and the R-CID sets of Lists contain a sufficient number of equivalent lists to render them useful in Navy research and clinical settings. (5) The R-CID lists have an advantage of more equivalent lists and greater sensitivity to frequency distortion. Sentence intelligibility lists can be used to provide oto-audiologists additional evaluation of various hearing problems incurred by Naval personnel. Also, the lists can be used by communications engineers involved in determining figure-of-merit for Navy systems, such as in the case of message sending from hyperbaric or underwater environments which create distortions in speech. (Authors' summary)

697.
GIORDANO, A.R.D., P.G. Tuteur, G.S. Longobardo and N.S. Cherniak.
The effect of increased metabolic rate and denervation on CO_2 storage in muscle.
Resp. Physiol. 18:309-327;Sept. 1973.

The full capacity of muscle to store CO_2 is reached only gradually in the face of disturbances to CO_2 balance. To determine whether this behavior of muscle CO_2 storage capacity is in part caused by the uneven distribution of perfusion within muscle, CO_2 storage was determined before and after an increase in muscle metabolic rate and in innervated and denervated muscle. CO_2 storage was serially measured during disturbed CO_2 balance caused by apneic oxygenation or by artificially ventilating paralyzed dogs with gas mixtures enriched with CO_2. Intravenous dinitrophenol doubled muscle metabolic rate and increased its CO_2 dissociation slope from 1.06 to 1.8 ml/kg/mm Hg PCO_2; while muscle denervation increased the slope from 0.92 to 1.30. Because both types of experiments could have increased CO_2 storage capacity by improving CO_2 diffusion across muscle cell membranes as well as by evening perfusion in muscle, a mathematical model was used to distinguish the relative importance of the two possible effects. The changes in muscle CO_2 storage capacity observed experimentally were best explained by changes in the distribution of the blood flow within muscle tissue. Assumed alterations in the ability of CO_2 to diffuse between extra and intracellular fluid had a relatively small effect on CO_2 storage capacity. The improvement in immediate CO_2 storage capacity observed with vasodilation and increased metabolic rate would tend to stabilize extracellular pH when muscle activity is increased during exercise. (Authors' abstract)

698.
GIORDANO, T., H.B. Rothman and H. Hollien.
Helium speech unscramblers — A critical review of the state of the art.
Gainesville, Fla., Univ. Fla., Commun. Sci. Lab., Rep. CSL/ONR 45, 29p. Aug. 1, 1972.

The development of saturation diving has enabled man to work in the sea at great depths and for long periods of time. This advance has resulted, in part, as a consequence of the substitution of helium for nitrogen in breathing gas mixtures. However, the utilization of HeO_2 breathing mixtures at high ambient pressures has caused problems in speech communication; in turn, electronic aids have been developed to improve diver communication. These helium speech unscramblers attempt to process variously the grossly unintelligible speech resulting from the effects of helium-oxygen breathing mixtures and ambient pressure, and to reconstruct such signals in order to provide adequate voice communication. This report presents a discussion of the effects of HeO_2/P on speech and then describes some of the techniques used to "unscramble" the distorted speech. Included among the techniques are: 1) frequency subtraction, 2) tape recorder playback, 3) vocoder approaches, 4) digital coding and 5) convolution processing. In addition, a generalized evaluation of these approaches is included. (DCD abstract)

699.
GLAUSER, S.C. and E.M. Glauser.
Hyperbaric oxygen therapy: Size of infarct determines therapeutic efficacy.
Ann. Intern. Med. 78(1):77-80; 1973.

Reports of the efficiency of hyperbaric O_2 therapy for thrombotic and embolic states [in humans] differ. An analysis of the volume of tissue necrotized as a function of the radius of tissue originally supplied with O_2 by the occluded vessel was made. The volume of necrosis increases rapidly as the cube of the original radius. The volume of tissue saved by breathing 100% O_2 at 3 atm increases more slowly, as the square of the original radius. Thus, the percent of tissue saved varies according to the reciprocal of the original radius; any phenomena that produce multiple small necrotic areas will respond more favorably to hyperbaric O_2 therapy than any phenomena that produce one large volume of necrosis. (© BA)

700.
GLAZKOVA, V.A. and I.N. Chernyakov.
Vliyanie povyshennogo partsial'nogo davleniya kisloroda na kislotno-shchelochnoe sostoyanie krovi.
[Effect of an increased partial oxygen pressure on the acid-base equilibrium of the blood].
Kosm. Biol. Med. 7(5):68-73; 1973.

The acid-base equilibrium was studied in animals [rats] and humans by the method of Astrup-Siggaard-Andersen. Change in the acid-base equilibrium was shown to depend on PO_2 [oxygen tension] in the breathing air and the time of hyperoxia. The correlation of the acid-base equilibrium with morphologic changes in the lung tissue induced by hyperoxia suggests that morphologic changes may occur and develop in the absence of visible X-ray shifts. (© BA)

701.
GLOVER, J.N., D.H. Kerem, J.A. Kylstra and H.A. Saltzman.
Effects of hyperoxia upon physiologic dead space in normal adults.
J. Clin. Invest. 52(6):33a-34a; 1973.

Abstract only. Entire item quoted: Systematic capillary blood flow is known to decrease on exposure to abnormally high partial pressures of oxygen. A similar response of the pulmonary capillary bed might cause an increase in the physiological dead space. This in turn, might cause alveolar hypoventilation in patients with a decreased ventilatory reserve. The physiological dead space (VD) was measured in 22 normal adults with inspired pressures of oxygen (PIO_2) ranging from 0.4 to 1.53 atmospheres absolute (Ata), at fractional concentrations of oxygen (FIO_2) ranging from 0.21 to 0.81. Gas volumes were determind by spirometry, fractional concentrations of oxygen and carbon dioxide in respired gas were determined by gas chromatography, and partial pressures of oxygen and carbon dioxide in arterial blood were determined electro-chemically. When compared to results obtained at 0.21 Ata of oxygen, values for the physiological dead space (VD) increased from 137.3 ± 44.7 (mean $\pm$ standard deviation in milliliters BTPS) to 158 ± 44.2 at 0.4 Ata of oxygen, from 110.6 ± 27.4 to 140.6 ± 44.8 at 0.5 Ata of O_2 from 143.1 ± 49.0 to 166.4 ± 55.7 at 0.8 Ata of oxygen, and from 110.4 ± 23.7 to 140.0 ± 27.0 ml BTPS at 1.53 of oxygen. Responses were variable, however, and approached statistical significance only at the highest PIO_2 administered ($P < 0.08$ at 1.53 Ata PIO_2). These findings of an increased VD, although not conclusive, suggest a change in the balance between ventilation and perfusion caused by hyperoxia.

702.
GOETERS, K.-M.
Horen unter Wasser: Absolute Reizschwellen und Richtungswahrnehmung.
[Underwater hearing: absolute thresholds and sound localisation].
Meerestechnik 3:191-197;Oct. 1972.

The article deals first with the theoretical foundations of underwater hearing, and the effects of the acoustical characteristics of water on hearing are described. Experiments on the subject are then reviewed. Two aspects of underwater hearing of special interest are discussed. Stimulus transmission: it can be taken as proved that underwater sound is received only by bone conduction. Sound localisation: theory and first experimental results lead to the conclusion that, in water, man can locate the direction of sound at low and at very high tonal frequencies of the audio range, but this ability probably vanishes in the middle range of frequencies. (English abstract)

703.
GOLDEN, F. St. C.
Accidental hypothermia.
In: Cold/wet survival symposium. J. Roy. Nav. Med. Serv. 58:196-206;Winter 1972.

Immersion in cold water produces rapid falls in deep body temperature accompanied by minor alterations in blood pH and electrolytes. The treatment consists of rapid reversal of the body temperature by immersion in a hot bath at 41°C. Generally speaking it is unnecessary and unwise to try and correct the biochemical disturbances. If necessary, then it should not be undertaken until the rewarming is well established. Accidental hypothermia produced in stiuations which involve high muscle energy expenditure over a period of time is usually accompanied by moderate to severe biochemical changes which may require correction, but again only when rewarming is well established. In this instance rewarming should be slow. Attempts at resuscitation must be made even in those apparently dead. (Author's conclusions)

704.
GOLDEN, F. St. C.
Cold water immersion.
In: Cold/wet survival symposium. J. Roy. Nav. Med. Serv. 58:195;Winter 1972.

This is a summary of a brief talk on the rewarming of hypothermia casualties. After the individual is removed from the cold water, an "after drop" always occurs. In most cases, this drop reached its lowest point eight to 12 minutes after immersion in a hot water bath. Every effort must be made to reduce the afterdrop during the rescue phase. (MFW/UMS)

705.
GOLDEN, F.St.C.
Death after rescue from immersion in cold water.
J. Roy. Nav. Med. Serv. 59:5-7;Spring 1973.

It has been suggested that in many cases, death after rescue from immersion in cold water is due to cardiac failure. An account is given of such a case in which the patient was being electrocardiographically monitored at the time of death. Two survivors of a sailing accident died shortly after arriving at hospital, and their deaths were ascribed to drowning. The author believes that treatment for hypothermia might have reversed ventricular fibrillation, which was the terminal event, and which was very possibly brought on by cold. The author cautions that, since ventricular fibrillation is likely to occur during the post-immersion period, it is important to handle the patient very carefully so as to avoid irritating the cold-sensitized myocardium. (MFW/UMS)

706.
GOODEN, B.A.
Effect of face immersion on body temperature and tail blood flow in the rat.
Comp. Biochem. Physiol. (A) 40(3):659-668; 1971.

Changes in tail blood flow, rectal, colonic and tail temperature produced by simulated diving were measured in anesthetised rats, and the temperature changes were compared with those produced by arresting tail flow with a tourniquet. "Diving" produced a rapid fall in tail blood flow from 30 to 40 ml/100 ml per min to zero within 15-30 sec. Tail temperature fell at the same rate whether tail flow was halted by "diving" or tourniquet. Rectal, and some times colonic, temperature fell during "diving"; both rose with tail tourniquet. Colonic temperature fell below pre-procedure level when tail temperature and flow recovered after "diving". Metabolic depression induced by "diving" is suggested. (Author's abstract)

707.
GOODEN, B.A.
Drowning and the diving reflex in man.
Med. J. Aust. 2:583-587;Sept. 9, 1972.

Five hundred and twenty-two people drowned in Australia in the year 1970, and the majority of these deaths were accidental. Children aged from 0 to 9 years had the highest incidence of accidental drowning for any ten-year age group, and one-year-old infants had the highest incidence for any particular year. Knowledge of the physiological adjustments that can occur during submersion is of particular relevance to the survival and resuscitation of the near-drowned. Recent research has shown that submersion of human subjects evokes a reflex cardiovascular response qualitatively similar to that observed in diving mammals, and evidence is accumulating that this diving reflex may act as an oxygen-conserving device in man. (Author's abstract)

708.
GOODEN, B.A.
The tadpole tail as a model for decompression studies.
Aust. J. Exp. Biol. Med. Sci. 51(1):109-112; 1973.

The tail of the tadpole of *Litoria ewingi* (Anura, Hylidae) was used to visualize directly the growth and reabsorption of gas bubbles in living tissue following decompression. Intravascular bubbles were observed to move along the vascular arcades of the transparent tail fins after rapid decompression from 600 lb/in^2. Some blood vessels became so distended with gas that they ruptured at intervals along their length and the bubbles extended into the extravascular tissue. This preparation provides a useful model for studies on the effects of rapid decompression. (© BA)

709.
GOODHILL, V.
Sudden deafness and round window rupture.
Laryngoscope 81:1462-1474; 1972.

[The author puts forward] the concept of labyrinthine window ruptures as a possible explanation for profound, sudden, cochlear deafness associated with exertion. Such membrane ruptures may occur anywhere in the labyrinth with both acoustic and/or vestibular system sequelae. Both explosive and implosive routes may be hypothecated. Combinations of the two routes are not impossible. Such ruptures undoubtedly may heal spontaneously with varying degrees of hearing restoration. The observations in three cases [one of whom was a man who suffered sudden hearing loss after a scuba dive] indicate that, in addition to intracochlear membrane ruptures, there may well occur explosive ruptures resulting in oval window or round window persistent perilymphatic fistulas, perhaps related to an unusual cochlear aqueduct patency. Where there is a distinct exertion history, and where spontaneous improvement is not observed at bed rest, exploratory tympanotomy and careful search for an oval window or round window rupture may be indicated. A persistent perilymphatic fistula may be present and may lend itself to repair if covered with a compatible tissue graft, such as perichondrium. (Author)

710.
GOODHILL, V.
Inner ear barotrauma.
Arch. Otolaryngol. 95:588; 1972.

In this letter to the editor, cases of inner ear barotrauma involving persistent sensorineural hearing loss, reported by Freeman and Edmonds, are discussed briefly. The original authors had suggested the effect of pressure changes on the staples as a possible mechanism involved. The present author suggests, in addition, an implosive force on the round window membrane. Prevention probably consists of more careful consideration of nasal and naso-pharyngeal factors in selection of divers, as well as more emphasis on predive check-ups. Treatment should consist, for the first 48 hours, of absolute bed rest with head elevated. If no improvement is noted, an exploratory tympanotomy, to determine whether or not round window rupture has occurred, is indicated. If rupture is evident, the fistula should be plugged with a membrane autograft. (MFW/SCD)

711.
GOODMAN, M.W. and T.E. Berghage.
The multivariate aspects of depth narcosis.
In: Abstracts of the Twenty-fifth Congress of Physiological Sciences Satellite Symposium. Recent progress in fundamental physiology of diving. Marseille, France, July 1971, p.45. (Proceedings unpublished)

Abstract only. Entire item quoted: If depth narcosis is defined in terms of decrements in human performance, the phenomenon becomes highly complex. Historically, studies of depth narcosis have concentrated on one or two factors, with the main emphasis being given to the partial pressure of various inert gases. This study differs from those of the past in that simultaneous measurements were taken on eight experimental variables. These variables were analysed using an analysis of variance and were combined into a linear model to evaluate the relative contribution of the significant variables. Using this approach the experimenters were able to account for 90% of the variance in the dependent performance variable (two choice reaction times). The interactions between several of the variables were statistically significant and contributed to the prediction of diver performance.

712.
GORDON, A. and M.R. Knittel.
Underwater multiple scattering of light for system designers. Part I. An exponential multiple-scattering model. Part II. Evaluation of the exponential multiple-scattering model.
U.S. Nav. Undersea Cent., Rep. NUC-TP-371, 101p. Nov. 1973.
(AD-771, 357/1GA)

An iterative method is presented which yields an exponential model for underwater multiple scattering in the forward direction. An easily evaluated effective attenuation coefficient is derived which allows rapid prediction of flux through an aperture and on-axis irradiance. Extensive comparison with experimental and Monte Carlo results indicate that our simple approximate expressions retain predictive value out to seven to ten attenuation lengths. (Author) (GRA)

713.
GORMAN, R.R., J.P. Jordan, J.B. Simmons II and D.P. Clarkson.
Biochemical adaptation in rat liver in response to marginal oxygen toxicity.
Biochem. J. 125:439-447; 1971.

Hepatic glucose 6-phosphate dehydrogenase activity was increased in rats exposed to 5lb/in^2 (equivalent to 27,000 ft) 100% O_2 when compared with control animals in a 14.7 lb/in^2 (sea level) air environment. Glyceraldehyde 3-phosphate dehydrogenase, isocitrate dehydrogenase, and succinate dehydrogenase were not affected by the 5 lb/in^2, 100% environment. Animals exposed to the hyperoxic environment consumed food, expired CO_2 and gained weight at the same rate as normoxic control animals. Additionally, blood glucose and liver glycogen concentrations were unchanged in the hyperoxic animals. The only readily apparent physiological difference in the hyperoxic animals was a decreased haematocrit. The increase in glucose 6-phosphate dehydrogenase was eliminated by the injection of actinomycin D or cycloheximide. Expiration of $^{14}CO_2$ from [1-^{14}C] glucose was approximately the same in hyperoxic and normoxic rats. However, $^{14}CO_2$ expiration from [6-^{14}C] glucose was markedly decreased in the animals exposed to the hyperoxic environment. Calculations of the relative importance of the pentose phosphate pathway versus the tricarboxylic acid cycle pulus glycolysis indicated that the livers from animals in the 5lb/in^2, 100% O_2 environment metabolized twice as much carbohydrate by way of the pentose phosphate pathway as did those from the sea-level air control animals. In livers of rats exposed to 5lb/in^2, 100% O_2 the concentrations of pyruvate, citrate and 2-oxoglutarate were increased, that of isocitrate was slightly elevated whereas the concentrations of succinate, fumarate and malate were decreased. An inactivation of both tricarboxylic acid cycle lipoate-containing dehydrogenases, pyruvate and 2-oxoglutarate, under hyperoxic conditions is proposed. The adaptive significance of the induction of glucose 6-phosphate dehydrogenase and the resultant production of NADPH under hyperoxic conditions is discussed. (Authors' abstract)

714.
GORTNER, D.A., A.A. Messier, E. Heyder and K.E. Schaefer.
The effects of elevated atmospheric CO_2 on acid-base balance and red-cell electrolytes of FBM submarine crew members.
U.S. Nav. Submar. Med. Cent., Rep. NSMRL 692; 6p. Dec. 6, 1971.

Blood from twelve volunteers serving on a submarine and breathing elevated levels of CO_2 was analyzed for electrolyte, pH, and PCO_2 levels in the plasma and in red-cell hemolysates. The method for measuring pH and PCO_2 in frozen samples entails certain difficulties due to loss of CO_2 during storage. Empirically determined correction factors were used for pH and PCO_2. After seven days of exposure to the submarine atmosphere, red cell pH was found to be satistically significantly lower than control values while plasma pH showed only a tendency to decrease; plasma chloride was decreased and red cell chloride increased. These findings were considered as evidence suggesting existence of a mild respiratory acidosis. After forty-two days of exposure plasma chloride was still significantly reduced and red-cell chloride slightly elevated. Moreover, red-cell sodium was increased and red-cell potassium decreased, while pH values of plasma and red cells did not differ significantly from control levels. The electrolyte shifts observed after forty-two days have been interpreted as evidence suggestive of an existing acidosis. (Authors' abstract)

715.
GOSOVIC, S.
Nasa zapazanja o linickom toku, incidenciji i iskustva u lijecenju barotraumatske plinske embolije.
[Personal observation of the clinical course, incidence and experiences in the treatment of barotraumatic gas embolism].
Vojnosanit. Pregl. 28:439-443;Sept. 1971.

No English abstract available.

716.
GOSOVIC, S.
Medicinski aspekti ronjenja u suvremenoj armiji.
[Medical aspects of diving in the modern army].
Vojnosanit. Pregl. 30:3-7;Jan./Feb. 1973.

The author outlines the role of deepsea diving in military medicine. Submarine crews shoud receive special training for combat in wartime and underwater research in peacetime. A specially trained medical officer should be attached to every submarine crew his tasks are discussed in detail. Physicians trained for submarine and diving medicine must be well acquainted with all aspects of underwater physiology. The main task of the medical unit is the selection of capable submarine crew members, screened by aptitude tests, their training for prolonged underwater stay and safe use of their equipment. Deepsea divers also have to be taught special underwater safety measures and behavior during survival and rescue operations. Submarine physicians and crew members should be familiar with the health hazards of deepwater operations as well as with preventive measures against, and treatment of diseases occurring during submarine expeditions. The most frequent diseases affecting divers are decompression sickness, so-called oxygen epilepsy, caused by oxygen toxicity and inert gas narcosis. The author describes various therapeutic measures, such as oxygen inhalation therapy, hyperbaric oxygenation, and therapeutic recompression. Special rescue units should be trained for assisting divers to surface from disabled submarines submerged at the bottom of the sea. The author lists various institutions in charge of submarine and diving medicine and research. Among them are: the Kafedra Spetsifisiologii in the USSR, the US Navy Experimental Diving Unit, and the Naval Submarine Medical Research Laboratory in the USA, the Royal Naval Physiological Laboratory in England, and the Institut za Pomorsku Medicinu in Yugoslavia. He emphasizes the importance of the role of submarine and diving medicine in the Yugoslav army and points out, how its safety and performance could be further developed and improved. (OLC/SCD)

717.
GOTTLIEB, S.F.
Effect of hyperbaric oxygen on microorganisms.
Ann. Rev. Microbiol. 50:111-152; 1971.

There are grounds for enthusiasm among microbiologists advocating the use of O_2 as a research and clinical tool. That it may be toxic to microorganisms in vitro and in vivo is established, but the molecular mechanisms are not understood. Microbial responsiveness to high O_2 tensions may be a useful character for differentiating microbial species. Studies on microbial O_2 toxicity may promote understanding of O_2 toxicity in higher life forms as well as provide information contributing to understanding convulsive states. Data on SH compounds in protecting microbes against O_2 toxicity suggest that protozoa may be more profitable to study than bacteria since SH-stabilizing agents, e.g., cysteine, glutathione, or 2,3-mercaptopropanol, are not protective in bacterial systems but do protect protozoa and mammals. Work is needed on in vivo and in vitro model systems based on pure cultures, also on models involving mixed infections. Gnotobiotic animals may be useful in these studies. More study is needed on the effects of O_2, alone and in combination with drugs, on model diseases involving drug-sensitive and resistant pathogens. Zobell's finding that pressure may enhance the bactericidal effects of O_2 raises an interesting possibility. Would increased inert gas pressure enhance the toxic effects of O_2 in vivo and thus become a therapeutic technique? — ignoring, for the present, problems of decompression. What are the conjoint effects of O_2, pressure, and antimicrobial agents? Elucidation of interrelationships between O_2 and the structure-activity relationships of drugs should help delineate drug structures requisite for synergism. Knowledge gained from nutritional or other analytical studies may pinpoint O_2-sensitive enzyme systems, thereby opening a rational approach to new chemotherapeutic agents; it may then be possible to substitute such new drugs for O_2, thus retaining its synergistic action without having to use expensive, cumbersome, and manpower-, time-, and space-consuming gadgetry. (From author's concluding remarks)

718.
GOTTLIEB, S.F. and L.K. Austin.
Effects of inorganic ions on altering central nervous system responses of mice to oxygen under high pressure.
Fed. Proc. 32(3,pt.1):430;Mar. 1973.

Abstract only. Entire item quoted: The principal objective of these investigations was to gain insight into the cellular mechanism(s) of oxygen toxicity. Male Swiss mice were treated acutely or chronically with different concentrations of sodium, lithium, chloride, bromide, iodide, and sulfate ions prior to exposure to increased oxygen tensions. Lithium and bromide ions increased the preconvulsive latency of mice exposed to 5 ATA oxygen. Bromide appeared to exert a greater protective effect than lithium. Independent protective effects of lithium and bromide were neither additive nor synergistic in prolonging preconvulsive latency periods. Lung weight-body weight ratios of mice, exposed to increased oxygen tensions for a constant time period, were markedly increased compared to corresponding 1 and 5 ATA air controls. Lung weight-body weight ratios did not differ significantly among ion-treated animals exposed to increased oxygen tensions.

719.
GOULD, V.E., R. Tosco, R.F. Wheelis, N.S. Gould and Y. Kapanci.
Oxygen pneumonitis in man. Ultrastructural observations on the development of alveolar lesions.
Lab. Invest. 26(5):499-408; 1972.

Lung samples obtained post mortem from 15 patients with oxygen pneumonitis (respirator-lung syndrome) were studied ultrastructurally. Exposure periods ranged from 14 hours to 30 days; oxygen concentrations oscillated between 40 and 110 per cent while total pressure never exceeded 760 mm Hg. All of these patients were known to be free of preexisting pulmonary disease. The earliest changes involved the membranous pneumocytes and endothelial cells eventually leading to widespread sloughing. Granular pneumocytes were also damaged; the septa showed early edema. In five cases, endothelian sloughing was followed by fibrin thrombi formation. After approximately 4 to 7 days of exposure the denuded basal laminae were covered on their epithelial aspect by hyaline membranes. After one week of exposure there was conspicuous reepithelialization of the alveoli by granular pneumocytes. During the above periods of exposure, septal edema persisted. Beyond approximately ten days, there was a considerable septal cell proliferation with deposition of interstitial collagen, elastin, and microfibrils. (Authors' abstract)

720.
GOULD, W.M. and J.W. Burnett.
Effects of 'Chrysaora quinquecirrha' (sea nettle) toxin on sodium transport across frog skin.
Annapolis, Md., Md. Fish Wildlife Admin., Rep. NOAA-72091917, 4p. May 25, 1971.
(COM 72-11233)
(Also published in J. Invest. Dermatol. 57(4):266-268; 1971)

Sea nettle toxin was found to increase the short-circuit current across isolated frog skin. The effect was blocked by hyperimmune serum but not by calcium chloride. In vitro guinea pig kidney (Na+K)ATPase was unaffected by the toxin. The rise in short-circuit current was mimicked by vasopressin but tissue levels of 3'5' cyclic AMP were not found to be elevated over controls. (Author) (GRA)

721.
GRANDPIERRE, R., G. Neverre, J. Rozier and P. Henry.
Etude comparee chez deux primates (Macacus nemestrinus et Papio papio) de la crise comitiale hyperoxique et de sa prevention.
[A comparatie study of hyperoxaemic convulsions and their prevention in two primates, Macacus nemestrinus and Papio papio].
J. Physiol. (Paris) 63:547-550;June/July 1971.

The photosensitivity of the two primates has been used as a means of studying hyperbaric convulsions. Sensitivity to hyperbaric oxygen appears similar in both. However, the preventive effect of Diazepam and of two of its derivatives (R0.05.4023, R0.05.4200) is more definite in the macaque than in the baboon. (English summary)

722.
GRAVE, G.D., C. Kennedy and L. Sokoloff.
Impairment of growth and development of the rat brain by hyperoxia at atmospheric pressure.
J. Neurochem. 19:187-194;Jan. 1972.

The continuous exposure of newborn rats to 70-80 per cent oxygen at atmospheric pressure throughout the first nine days of life significantly inhibited the growth of the brain which normally occurs during this period of life. The accumulations of DNA, RNA, total protein, and proteolipid protein which accompany brain growth during this period were all approximately proportionately depressed by the oxygen-enriched atmosphere. RNA/DNA and protein/DNA ratios were unaffected. The increase in brain mass in the first week of life reflects mainly cell proliferation and since the decreased DNA accumulation occurred with no changes in RNA/DNA and protein/DNA ratios, we conclude that the effect of oxygen was to inhibit cellular division. We estimate that the oxygen exposure caused an approximately 7 per cent deficit in the cell population of the brain. These results indicate that the use of elevated concentrations of oxygen may have serious deleterious effects on the growth and development of the brain. (Authors' abstract)

723.
GRAVER, D.
How to get somewhere in diving.
Skin Diver 22:84-85, 88;July 1972.

The author discusses various ways of moving through the water that will reduce fatigue by making use of different sets of muscles. Most divers use the flutter kick exclusively, and not always correctly. The kick should be done with the knee nearly straight on the down stroke, and locked on the return. It should be as wide as possible. Swimming on the back is an easy method of achieving a wide kick, and is less tiring. With two divers, they can alternate face down and face up positions, so that one can maintain proper directional course. Swimming on the side using the scissors kick is another alternative. A good rest kick is the frog kick, used while swimming on the back. Another method that uses the ankles only, is to lie face down, rotate ankles to the outside so that the fins are perpendicular to the surface, then pull them together and glide. Leg cramps can be caused by fins that are too large and stiff; offset fins are better than straight-bladed fins. Problems of streamlining and of reducing weight are also briefly discussed. (MFW/BSCP)

724.
GRAVES, D.J., J. Idicula, C.J. Lambertsen and J.A. Quinn.
Bubble formation in physical and biological systems: a manifestation of counter-diffusion in composite media.
Science 179:582-584;Feb. 9, 1973.

The counterdiffusion of gases across a composite layer can lead to supersaturation and development of bubbles within the layer. A physicochemical model has been derived to predict the extent of such supersaturation; experiments with inert liquid layers confirm predictions. These findings explain the evolution of cutaneous lesions observed in man during simulated deep-sea dives and the cutaneous lesions and intravascular bubbles experimentally induced in pigs by exchanging certain inert gases across the skin. The phenomena associated with counterdiffusion have widespread physical and biological implications. (Authors' abstract)

725.
GRAVES, D.J., J. Idicula, C.J. Lambertsen and J.A. Quinn.
Bubble formation resulting from counterdiffusion supersaturation: a possible explanation for isobaric inert gas "urticaria" and vertigo.
Phys. Med. Biol. 18:256-264;Mar. 1973.

In recent simulated diving experiments, subjects have experienced intense itching, confluent maculopapular skin lesions and a severe vestibular derangement with vertigo and nystagmus. These effects have been observed when a gas mixture containing nitrogen or neon was being breathed while a second inert gas, helium, was present in the surrounding environment. Attempts to explain this phenomenon led to a study of counterdiffusion through two-layer composites. When the two layers differ in their relative permeabilities to the two diffusing species, and when the layers are arranged in the proper sequence in a counterdiffusion system, a steady-state supersaturation will result within the two layers. Bubble formation in an oil-water system and continual flow of gas into an intermembrane space in a two-membrane system were demonstrated experimentally: both effects were predicted from diffusion theory. In addition to providing a possible explanation for the itching phenomenon and vestibular derangement, the theory has a wide range of applications to physical and biological processes. (Authors' abstract)

726.
GRAY, S.P., J.E.W. Morris and C.J. Brooks.
Renal handling of calcium magnesium, inorganic phosphate and hydrogen ions during prolonged exposure to elevated carbon dioxide concentrations.
Clin. Sci. Mol. Med. 45:751-764; 1973.

Fifteen healthy young men were exposed to an atmosphere of 0.7% CO_2 in air for 7 weeks. For 1 week before and during the exposure to CO_2, serum calcium, magnesium and inorganic phosphate (P_i) levels were measured at intervals, together with 24 h urinary excretion of these three components, and net urinary acid excretion. The urinary excretion of Ca^{2+}, Mg^{2+} and P_i fell during exposure to CO_2, whereas the serum levels of these components increased. Serum levels of calcium were inversely correlated with urinary Ca^{2+} excretion both in control conditions and during exposure to CO_2. An increase in urinary acid excretion in the third to fourth week of exposure to CO_2 was associated with an increase in the urinary excretion of Ca^{2+}, but not of Mg^{2+}. It is suggested that there is a difference from the normal in the renal handling of H^+ and Ca^{2+} ions during exposure to CO_2 which may lead to a retention of Ca^{2+} in the tissues. (Authors' summary)

727.
GREEN, G.C.
Automatic shut-off protection for pressure chambers and diving systems in case of abnormal fluid flow or line rupture.
In: The working diver, 1972. Symposium proceedings, February 1972, Columbus, Ohio, p.85-92. Washington, D.C., Marine Technology Society, 1972.

This report describes the automatic shut-off valves as a basic safety device for hyperbaric pressure chambers. In addition to presenting the basic mechanical operation of these valves, a description of an investigation undertaken at NCSL, Panama City, Florida, to evaluate the performance and operating characteristics of these automatic shut-off valves is summarized. These unique valves provide safety to personnel, systems and property by isolating a failure much the same way an electrical circuit breaker protects its system by shutting off when the current flow rate through it exceeds the maximum desired. They are presently being used in sophisticated diving equipment such as the Navy's Mark II Deep Diving System and will be installed in the Navy's OSF (Ocean Simulation Facility). In the design considerations of hyperbaric chambers, these valves play an integral role. Because of their ability to instantaneously shut off in the event of an excessive flow rate through them, these valves are used in hyperbaric chambers to preserve the pressure integrity within the chambers. They thus prevent inadvertent depressurization of the divers inside in the event of a serious downstream leak or downstream pipe rupture. (Author's abstract)

728.
GREENBAUM, L.J., Jr. and D.E. Evans.
Inert gas narcosis in unanesthetized cats.
In: Abstracts of the Twenty-fifth Congress of Physiological Sciences Satellite Symposium. Recent progress in fundamental physiology of diving. Marseille, France, July 1971. p.45-46. (Proceedings unpublished).

Abstract only. Entire item quoted: Evoked potentials in the lateral geniculate nucleus and visual cortex and excitability cycles of cortical dendrites were used to study neuronal excitability in cats (encephale isole) exposed to 200 psig and breathing the following gas mixtures: oxgen-nitrogen, oxygen-helium, oxygen-argon, and oxygen-neon. With cats breathing an oxygen-helium atmosphere (PO_2 200 and PHe 10129), neuronal excitability was unaltered. When neon, nitrogen or argon was substituted for helium CNS depression was equivalent to 10, 15 and 21 percent respectively. Elevating the PO_2 to 1980, with a concimitant decrease of the inert partial pressure to 7920, increased the severity of narcosis during the oxygen-neon, oxygen-nitrogen and oxygen-argon breathing but not during the oxygen-helium breathing. The increase in narcosis was reversed during hyperventilation. It is suggested that the increased oxygen potentiates the narcosis indirectly by interfering with the buffering capacity of the RBC with a resultant increase in tissue carbon dioxide. This increased narcosis may be due to the combined effect of the inert gas plus the carbon dioxide.

729.
GREENBAUM, L.J., Jr., L.G. Dickens, D.L. Jackson and D.E. Evans.
Toxicologic and physiologic effects of bromotrifluromethane in hyperbaric atmospheres.
Toxicol. Appl. Pharmacol. 21(1):1-11; 1972.

[Bromotrifluoromethane has been successfully employed as a fire extinguishant in hypobaric, normobaric and hyperbaric atmospheres when the O_2 tension exceeded 150 mm Hg (O_2 equivalent for air at atmospheric pressure). Recent physiologic and toxicologic studies with bromotrifluoromethane at sea level pressure has demonstrated some cardiac irregularities and decrement in performance.] ECG's evoked visual potentials and blood gases were recorded in cats breathing bromotrifluoromethane at 165 ft of seawater (73 psig). The cats breathed the bromotrifluoromethane (228 mm Hg) in air for 5 min. Heart rates were not significantly altered, but the QRS intervals were increased from a control value of 0.05 to 0.06 sec. The increase in QRS interval was associated with frequent nodal beats. Respiratory rate and the $PaCO_2$ increased. Small reductions in the amplitude and increased latency of the lateral geniculate response were recorded. In cats sacrificed immediately after exposure, electron microscopic examination of the lungs demonstrated minimal engorgement of alveolar capillaries and small numbers of acute inflammatory cells. The alveolar basement membrane was thickened with vacuolation of alveolar capillary endothelium and alveolar epithelium. No morphologic changes were seen in cats sacrificed 5 days after exposure. (JFL) (© BA)

730.
GREENE, H.L., D.H. Jefferson and C.E. Mengel.
Effect of hyperoxia on red blood cell (RBC), 2,3-diphosphoglycerate (2,3-DPG).
J. Lab. Clin. Med. 78:841;Nov. 1971.

Abstract only. Entire item quoted: Previous studies showed that RBC 2,3-DPG was increased by hypoxia. The present studies were undertaken to explore the effect of in vivo and in vitro hyperoxia on RBC 2,3-DPG. Chow-fed mice exposed to 100% O_2 at 60 p.s.i.a. for 30 min (OHP) had lower, 2,3-DPG (21.1 $\pm$ 1.9 uM per gram of hemoglobin) than control mice (31.1 $\pm$ 3.0) (P 0.001). A linear relationship was shown between the level of hyperoxia and the decrease of 2,3-DPG. The slope of this curve was different (P 0.05) from the slope expressing the relation between hypoxia and the rise of 2,3-DPG. The recovery curves of 2,3-DPG were also different, T1/2 13 hrs return time from the increase due to hypoxia and 30 min for the decrease due to hyperoxia. Tocopherol-deficient mice had lower control values of 2,3-DPG (26.0 $\pm$ 1.7) than chow-fed controls (31.3 $\pm$ 3) (P 0.01) and even lower levels (21.5 $\pm$ 2.3) after OHP (P 0.01). RBCs of tocopherol-deficient mice (known to accumulate H_2O_2 in excess) also formed lipid peroxides during OHP (19.1 muM per milliliter of RBC) in contrast to before OHP (0) and chow-fed mice exposed to OHP (0). RBCs exposed in vitro to diffused H_2O_2 had lower, 2,3-DPG (20.5 $\pm$ 1.83) in contrast to control values (25.8 $\pm$ 2.13) (P 0.001). These data demonstrate an in vivo suppression of 2,3-DPG by hyperoxia. They are consistent with the hypothesis that the decrease is mediated by H_2O_2 accumulation, and that the control mechanisms for change of 2,3-DPG are different for hypoxia and hyperoxia.

731.
GREGORY, E.M. and I. Fridovich.
Oxygen toxicity and the superoxide dismutase.
J. Bacteriol. 114:1193-1197;June 1973.

Oxygen caused an increase in the amount of superoxide dismutase in Escherichia coli B but not in Bacillus subtilis. E. coli B cells, induced by growth under 100% O_2, were much more resistant to the lethal effects of 20 atm of O_2 than were cells which contained the low uninduced level of this enzyme. In contrast, B. subtilis, which could not respond to O_2 by increasing its content of superoxide dismutase, remained equally sensitive to hyperbaric O_2 whether grown under 100% O_2 or aerobically. The catalase in these organisms exhibited a reciprocal response to oxygen. Thus, the catalase of E. coli B was not induced by O_2, whereas that of B. subtilis was so induced. These results are consistent with the view that superoxide dismutase is an important component of the defenses of these organisms against the toxicity of oxygen, whereas their catalases are of secondary importance in this respect. The ability of streptonigrin to generate O_2^-, by a cycle of reduction followed by spontaneous reoxidation, has been verified in vitro. It is further observed that E. coli B which contain the high induced level of superoxide dismutase were more resistant to the lethality of this antibiotic, in the presence of oxygen, than were E. coli B which contained the low uninduced level of this enzyme. This difference between induced and uninduced cells was eliminated by the removal of O_2. These results are consistent with the proposal that the enhanced lethality of streptonigrin under aerobic conditions may relate to its in vivo generation of O_2^- by a cycle of reduction and spontaneous reoxidation. In toto, these observations lend support to the hypothesis that O_2^- is an important agent of oxygen toxicity and that superoxide dismutase functions to blunt the threat posed by this reactive radical. (Authors' abstract)

732.
GRIFFITHS, P.D.
An exposure to risk registry for compressed air workers.
Trans. Soc. Occup. Med. 21:123-125;Oct. 1971.

A central Registry of compressed air workers was established in Newcastle-upon-Tyne in 1964. Data collected form the Tyne Tunnel project in 1948 and subsequent compresssed-air operations were stored and assessed. The data included etiology, sequelae, osteonecrosis, and more recently, diving hazards. In assessing exposure to risk the intensity of the hazard and the duration of exposure are the chief considerations. Data on approximately 10,000 individuals are held. Radiological data are collected on a voluntary basis, and therefore are incomplete. Of the 1660 men who have been radiologically examined, 330 show positive signs of osteonecrosis. Data show that the longer the exposures and the higher the pressure the more likely is the occurrence of osteonecrosis, although cases have been known to occur after a single exposure. Since divers seem to suffer much less frequently from osteonecrosis than do compressed air workers, it is thought that probably the durations of exposure is more important than the degree of pressure. It may be necessary to shorten the work shift, but at present the line of experimentation is in the lengthening of the decompression period. (MFW/BSCP)

733.
GROTE, W., and W.D. Wagner.
Fehlbildungen bei Kaninchen nach hyperbarer Oxygenation.
[Malformation in rabbits following hyperbaric oxygenation].
Klin. Wochenschr. 51:248-250;Mar. 1973.

At the 9th day of gestation pregnant rabbits were exposed to an oxygen pressure of 1.5 or 2.0 ata (absolute atmospheres) for five hours. The mother rabbits were killed on the 29th day of pregnancy. The foetuses were removed and the uteri studied for resorptions. After macroscopic inspection, skeleton preparations were made and inspected for malformations. The results were compared with untreated controls. Hyperbaric oxygen resulted in increased resorption rate and number of malformations. (English summary)

734.
GROUEFF, S.
L'homme et la mer.
[Man and the sea].
Paris, Larousse Paris-Match, 1973. 395p.

This book is splendidly produced, with the superb illustrations and design that are associated with Larousse. The author has ranged over the field of the science of the sea in 34 chapters with reasonable accuracy, but with some romantic overtones. Historically, it begins with Matthew Fontaine Maury. All of the glamour is here — Beebe, Piccard, Cousteau, submarine habitats, and Mohole. More serious and penetrating activities are not neglected, however. A beautiful book for the curious layman. Written in French. (Sea Frontiers)

735.
GUENARD, H., H. Viellefond, J. Timbal, J. L'Huillier and P. Varene.
Les echanges gazeux de l'homme au repos, en hyperbarie, dans une atmosphere He O_2.
[Gas exchange in man at rest in a hyperbaric helium-oxygen environment].
J. Physiol. (Paris) 65 (Suppl.):240A;Oct. 1972.

Abstract only. Four subjects were exposed to pressures of from 1.5 to 31 ATA. Various respiratory parameters (oxygen consumption, carbon dioxide elimination, alveolar ventilation, mean ventilatory debt, respiratory frequency, and dead space) were measured. Before two measurement periods the breathing gas was cooled. Most parameters did not vary significantly with pressure. Variations in oxygen consumption seemed to coincide with cutaneous heat loss.

Augmentation of carbon dioxide elimination, as measured at the cutaneous surface, occurred in direct ratio to the increase in pressure. This augmentation remains difficult to explain. Alveolar carbon dioxide partial pressure also increased slightly. These experiments confirm previous findings, published in the literature, regarding respiratory function under pressure. (MFW/BSCP)

736.
GUENARD, H., J. Timbal, P. Varene and H. Vieillefond.
La deperdition thermique par convection respiratoire en plongee profonde.
[Heat loss by respiratory convection in deep diving].
In: Hesser, C.M. and D. Linnarsson eds. Proceedings of the first annual scientific meeting of the European Undersea Biomedical Society, Stockholm, 13-15 June 1973. Forsvarsmedicin 9:475-480;July 1973.

It appears, from the findings of these experiments, that heat loss by respiratory convection can be estimated, provided ventilation, pressure, and the temperature of the inspired gases of a given breathing mixture are known. The nature of the breathing can have a modifying effect on the specific heat, but not, it seems, on the relation between the temperature of the inspired and expired gas. This relation appears to be independent of ventilation, but dependent upon the hygrometry of the inspired gas. (Authors' conclusions translated by MFW/UMS)

737.
GUILLERM, R., R. Badre and G. Masurel.
Influence de divers parametres sur le taux d'accidents de decompression lors de sequences de compression-decompression rapides chez le lapin.
[Influence of various parameters on the rate of decompression accidents during sequences of rapid compression-decompression in the rabbit].
Bull. Medsubhyp 7:13-14;Oct. 1972.

The rescue of a submarine crew requires passage through an airlock where they are compressed to the ambient pressure. They are then carried to the surface by the buoyancy of a special garment. It is decompression accidents which limit the depth at which rescue is possible. In this connection, experiments have been made with rabbits to learn the importance of various parameters involved in rapid compression-decompression sequences. Experiments with various rates of compression and decompression at various depths led to the following conclusion: air, hyperoxygenated at 40%, and speed of ascent checked during the terminal phase, made it possible to extend the depth limit in the case of the rabbit to between 300 m and 400 m. (MFW/BSCP)

738.
GUILLERM, R., J. Chouteau, J. Hee and J.C. LePechon.
Etude de la pression partielle d'oxygene arterielle chez le lapin lors de la respiration de melanges normoxiques en hyperbarie (O_2N, O_2A, O_2Ne, O_2He).
[Study of oxygen partial pressure in the rabbit while breathing normoxic breathing mixtures in a hyperbaric environment (O_2N, O_2A, O_2Ne, O_2He)].
Bull. Medsubhyp 8:34-37;Nov. 1972.

The authors have attempted to confirm the hypoxic origin of the motor dysfunction observed by Chouteau with his goats, when they reached a certain pressure breathing a normoxic gas mixture. Nitrogen, argon, neon and helium were used as diluents. The experimental animals, rabbits, were submitted to various pressures up to 91 ATA. They were anesthetized, and a probe was injected into the left carotid artery. The only outward sign of behavioral reaction to the experiment was wakefulness under helium at 46 to 51 ATA. The authors concluded from their findings that, while there is undoubtedly a pressure beyond which a normal PaO_2 cannot be maintained while using a normoxic mixture, the resulting hypoxia is not entirely due to pressure, because hypoxia was evident at different pressures with different gases. Density is apparently an important factor, and other properties of the gases are probably involved. Findings agree to some extent with the conclusions arrived at in the goat experiment, except that the hypoxia recorded by the instruments manifested itself at higher pressures and seemed insufficient to account for the disorders observed in the goats. However, if one attributes arterial hypoxia to a disturbance of the alveolo-capillary diffusion caused by elevated inert gas pressure, it is logical to assume that this phenomenon might be amplified at the hemato-encephalic barrier or at the cellular level. Hypoxia in the nervous tissue would thus reach a degree that could explain the behavioral disorders. It is necessary, however, to ascertain whether the arterial hypoxia actually results from a modification of the alveolo-capillary diffusion or ventilation perfusion relationships. (MFW/BSCP)

739.
GUILLERM, R., G. Masurel, M. Monjaret, H. David and B. Schmidlin.
La detection des bulles intravasculaires par ultrasons chez le mini porc apres exposition hyperbare. Role filtrant de poumon.
[Detection of intravascular bubbles by ultrasound in the minipig after hyperbaric exposure. Filtering role of the lung].
Bull. Medsubhyp 10:50-53;Dec. 1973.

A perivascular ultrasonic transducer implanted in minipigs on pulmonary and aorta arteries, combined with special treatment of specific signal of bubbles and use of integrators, allowed a semi-quantitation of apparent bubble flow after hyperbaric exposure. When apparent bubble flow is low, pulmonary filtration is complete; when it reaches a critical value, bubbles flow in systemic circulation. (English abstract)

740.
GUILLERM, R., G. Masurel and J.L. Monjaret.
Detection ultrasonore par effet Doppler des bulles intravasculaires lors de la decompression apres exposition hyperbare du porc.
[Ultrasonic detection by Doppler effect of intravascular bubbles during decompression after hyperbaric exposure of the pig].
Bull. Medsubhyp 10:19-27;Dec. 1973.

A perivascular ultrasonic transducer implanted on pulmonary artery in the pig revealed presence of many bubbles (Doppler effect) after hyperbaric exposure. It appears that bubbles may be present in circulation after conventional intervention dives without giving rise to any symptom of decompression sickness. Special signal treatment allowed easy graphic recording of specific appearance of bubbles, giving objective endpoint when assessing decompression procedure. (English abstract)

741.
GULYAR, S.O., M. Kiklevich, S.O. Pevnii and S.S. Sirota.
Study of some indices of the higher nervous activity of men subjected to underwater environment for many hours.
Fiziol Zh. (USSR) 18:744-750;Dec. 1972.
(Translation JPRS 58484)

The report studies the neurological effect on men subjected to an underwater environment for many hours, and concludes (1) Aquanauts' mental capacity for work, attention, muscle strength and endurance, and speed of sensomotor reactions do not change after 20-30 min. in a water environment. (2) After three hours of physical work under water the ability to perform mental work and the speed of information processing decreased and aquanauts experienced difficulties in counting. Along with the decrease of hand muscle strength, endurance, and the speed of the sensomotor reactions, the frequency of the repeated motions also decreased. The time orientation also worsened. (3) A definite worsening of mental and physical activity, together with time orientation, was observed in aquanauts that spent 26 and 38 hours under water in a state of relative hypodynamics. (4) Basic factors which change the higher nervous activity of aquanauts during a long-term stay under water were spatial stress, sensory isolation, and changes in the thermal balance of the human organism. (Authors' conclusions)

742.
GUNDERSON, E.E.K., R.H. Rahe and R.J. Arthur.
Prediction of performance in stressful underwater demolition training.
J. Appl. Psychol. 56(5):530-432; 1972.

The relevance of selected biographical, physical fitness, and health status measures for success in Underwater Demolition Team training was investigated. A combination of five variables, including a Cornell Medical Index subscale, yielded highly significant cross-validity coefficients with training success. Physical fitness tests were the most important predictors of training success, but prediction also could be enhanced by assessing physical and emotional health status with questionnaire methods. (Authors' abstract)

743.
GUYATT, A.R., C.J. Yu, B. Lutherer and A.B. Otis.
Studies of alveolar-mixed venous CO_2 and O_2 gradients in the rebreathing dog lung.
Resp. Physiol. 17(2):178-194; 1973.

Measurements were made of PCO_2 [CO_2 tension] and PO_2 [O_2 tension] in alveolar gas of dog lungs rebreathing in situ and in the pulmonary arterial blood. The PCO_2 in alveolar gas was almost always higher than that of the blood under a variety of experimental conditions. The PO_2 was also usually higher in alveolar gas than in blood but less consistently than in the case of CO_2. The magnitude of the observed gradients showed no consistent relationship to duration of experiment or rate of blood flow through the lung. Respiratory acidosis increased the CO_2 gradient but reduced that for O_2. Inhibition of blood carbonic anhydrase enhanced the CO_2 gradient. When normalized with respect to plasma bicarbonate concentration, the CO_2 gradient is inversely related to plasma pH. No definitive explanation is offered for these observations. (© BA)

744.
HAAS, G.F. and A.V. Boccabella.
The effect of hyperbaric oxygen on the adult rat testis.
Anatom. Rec. 169:330-331; 1971.

Various tissues from the urogenital systems of rats exposed to 100% oxygen at 3 ATA for six hours, followed by two hours standard decompression time, showed no significant change in weight. Histological examination of testes revealed spermatogenesis and normal-appearing Leydig cells. Also, reproductive organs did not differ histologically from those of controls. Sperm was plentiful and motile. These findings agree with some previous findings and disagree with others regarding the effect of hyperbaric oxygen on the reproductive system. (MFW/UMS)

745.
HAAS, G.F. and E. Hirschberg.
The effect of repetitive hyperbaric oxygen exposures on the adult rat testis.
Fed.Proc. 31:296;Mar./Apr. 1972.

Abstract only. Entire item quoted: As a result of a previous study of the effects of hyperbaric oxygen on adult male rat reproduction and development (Haas, *Anat Rec.* 169:330-331, 1971) the effects of repeated exposures on rat reproductive and endocrine organs were examined. Seven week old Wistar rats received 6 hours exposure to 3 Atmosphere Absolute 100% oxygen, followed by 2 hours decompression. This was repeated 3 times at 12 day intervals. Rats were autopsied at several time intervals during the 48 day period following the first exposure. Gravimetric and histologic evaluation of the reproductive and endocrine organs showed no differences between exposed and unexposed animals. Epididymal suspensions indicated that sperm number and motility were similar in both groups. In addition, a fertility study was carried out by selecting 2 males from each autopsy group and allowing several opportunities to mate with normal females for a two day period before autopsy. Average number of male and female offspring per litter as well as average pup weights were comparable between the control and experimental groups. It is concluded that neither morphologic nor functional defects in the reproductive or endocrine systems occur under the conditions of hyperbaric exposure used in this study. However, the mortality rate of animals exposed to two or more hyperbaric stays was significantly increased, 7 out of 12 animals failing to survive due to lung damage.

746.
HABERER, K., K. Ellebrecht and G. Walther.
Tier experimentelle Untersuchungen uber die Schutzuirkung des Sauerstoffe bei der Druckfallkrankheit.
[Animal experiments on the protective effect of oxygen in decompression sickness].
Beitr. Gerichtl. Med. 29:303-311; 1972.

Experiments were made to find out if there would be a protective effect of pure oxygen breathing in regard to decompression sickness. Guinea pigs were subjected to the following conditions: (1) 3.5 ata air three hours (12 animals); (2) 3.5 ata oxygen three hours (12 animals); (3) 1.0 ata air three hours (10 animals); (4) 1.0 ata oxygen three hours (10 animals). Following rapid decompression (three minutes) group one showed numerous intravascular and intracardial gas bubbles. In some cases the lungs were macroscopically overinflated. Histologic examination showed overinflated areas, atelectasis, ruptured alveolar walls and hemorrhage in the alveoli. In group two some hemorrhage could be seen. Widespread atelectasis, thickened alveolar walls, interstitial edema and subpleural congestion were common. These are typical signs of oxygen poisoning. The animals of group three and four in some cases showed small atelectatic areas. The existence of atelectatic areas in animals of all groups is normal in guinea pigs. Pathologic changes in heart and kidney as a result of rapid decompression could not be demonstrated. The investigation has shown that the typical pathologic changes in blood and lung following rapid decompression are far less severe after oxygen breathing. (English summary)

747.
HACKNEY, J.D.
Effects of oxygen on cell renewal in the mouse lung.
In: Abstracts of BuMed-ONR sponsored Navywide workshop in high pressure biomedical research, U.S. Naval Submarine Base, Groton, Conn., May 1971, p.6. Published by the Naval Submarine Medical Research Laboratory, 1971.

Abstract only. Entire item quoted: The purpose of this study was to determine the effects of continuous exposure to 60 and 80% oxygen on cell renewal in the pulmonary alveoli of mice. In a previous study it had been shown that continuous exposure to 100% oxygen decreased the number of cells preparing to divide from 20.6/1000 alveolar cells to 7.4/1000 alveolar cells after 24 hours' exposure; further decrease occurred with continued exposure up to 96 hours. (Aerosp. Med. 40:1365; 1969). In the present study the authors exosed groups of mice to either 40, 60 or 80% oxygen for up to nine days. At various intervals during this time mice were removed from the chamber and one hour before sacrifice the diving cells labeled with tritiated thymidine. Using autoradiographic technique the number of labeled cells in the alveoli was determined (labeling index). All these groups of animals responded about the same to exposure to oxygen. After four days' continuous exposure to either 40, 60 or 80% oxygen there was little change in the labeling index. However from 5 through 9 days' exposure there was an increase in the number of cells preparing to divide. This increase in labeled cells was due to more endothelial cells preparing to divide. There were no changes in the labeling indexes of Type 2 alveolar cells and alveolar macrophages. These preliminary studies show that after 4 to 5 days' continuous exposure to elevated concentrations of oxygen the number of endothelial cells preparing to divide is increased.

748.
HAGEMAN, W.E., D.G. Wentling and T.P. Pruss.
Interaction of vasoactive agents and micro-emboli on the pulmonary circulation.
Eur. J. Pharmacol. 22:275-303;June 1973.

Micro-embolization of the perfused lobe of the dog lung with diatomaceous earth increased pulmonary perfusion pressure. I.v. administered aminophyline, cyproheptadine and methysergide reduced this effect. Infusions of serotonin, bufotenine and d-amphetamine enhanced the elevation of perfusion pressure produced by diatomaceous earth. Other known pulmonary vasoconstrictors such as 1-norepinephrine, angiotensin II and histamine were without effect. These data indicate that the increase in perfusion pressure elicited by micro-embolization was due to pulmonary vasoconstriction and not to the physical presence of the microemboli. Serotonin release is the mechanism implicated in the elevation of pulmonary vascular resistance induced by micro-emboli. Evidence is also presented to indicate that d-amphetamine produced its enhancement by releasing serotonin within the pulmonary circulation. (Authors' abstract)

749.
HAIGH, K.R.
Propulsion of submersibles.
Underwater J. 5:53-61;Apr. 1973.

The author contends that speed and long-term endurance are not important factors in the design of research submersibles, since in the long run the endurance of the crew will be the decisive factor. With few exceptions, present-day submersibles are powered by electrohydraulic propulsive systems. Habitability problems are acute in small submersibles. The larger submersibles, such as Ben Franklin and Aluminaut might benefit from more power. The use of an inexpensive diesel engine is considered, and rejected because of corrosion problems as well as back pressure and noise levels. Table I gives the advantages and disadvantages of various types of propulsion. Table II gives the battery type of 33 submersibles in current use or in the design stage. Lead acid is by far the most common type. Drawings show submersibles representative of various shapes and sizes, both from the standpoint of habitability and propulsion and manoeuvering configurations. Table III shows speed time endurance, and distance endurance, of lead acid, silver zinc and silver cadmium batteries. Fuel cell batteries are discussed. They are most advantageous as to both weight and volume. The author believes that "the system which shows the most promise for manned civilian submersibles is the hydrogen oxygen combination using cryogenically stored reactants." In his conclusion, he states that "for the deep ocean, electric propulsion is the only current practical proposition. Its nearest rival would appear to be the Stirling engine which is still in the experimental stage. On the continental shelf thermal systems have a limited application where noise and large size can be tolerated." (MFW/BSCP)

750.
HAIGH, K.R.
Submersibles in Europe: offshore oil will be biggest market.
Offshore Services 6:36-37, 49-50;June 1973.

Activity in the development of submersibles in Europe is currently increasing unlike that in the United States, which appears to be, at least temporarily, on the wane. A table lists submersibles, either constructed in Europe, constructed in Canada from UK specifications, built in the United States from UK specifications, or built in the United States and chartered by the U.K. The types include bathyscaphes, manned untethered, manned wet systems, manned towed systems, unmanned untethered systems, unmanned towed systems, unmanned seafloor crawlers, and unmanned tethered systems. Countries of origin include the UK, France, Switzerland, West Germany, the USSR, the Netherlands and Finland. Few are devoted to scientific research, and these are mostly simple, unsophisticated systems of the towed or tethered types. Military use is restricted to recovery and rescue, and in this field the United States has led with the DSRV. The laying and surveying of cable is an important function of several types of submersibles. The author believes that the greatest demand for submersibles in Europe will be in the pipeline burying field, in pre-route survey, inspection during lay and burial, routine inspection and damage and repair inspection. (MFW/SCD)

751.
HAIMSON, N.
A suggested modification in treatment of apparent drowning of scuba divers.
Med. J. Aust. (1):83;Jan. 13, 1973.

In cases where bloody froth is present, due to alveolar damage from sudden surfacing, resuscitation is impossible. It is suggested that the victim be placed head down on a hard surface with jaw extended so as to clear the airway. In the case of cardiac arrest, the supine position is maintained, so that closed heart massage can be applied. Lung compression thus brought about will produce tidal air flow sufficient to clear the airways of froth. Cardiac massage must be continued while the victim is removed to a treatment center where the indicated therapy is administered. In cases where there is a heart beat, the diver is placed head down in a prone position, and a compression form of resuscitation, such as the Schaeffer method, is applied. (MFW/UMS)

752.
HAINES, G.
Instrumentation gains wider applications.
Meerestechnik 4:A18-A20;Oct. 1973.

[The need for a comprehensive seawater testing facility] and designing instrumentation for use in the hostile environment presented by the sea, whether shipborne or underwater, has led to the development of equipment that can do the job for which it was intended, but which can also find applications in other hostile environments. One of the most important developments in proving this instrumentation has been the setting up of a test ground for underwater trials and system evaluation in Scotland, where depths of over 500 ft (152 m) are available close inshore — this facility is thought to be unique in Europe and is typical of the lengths to which British scientists are going to perfect such instrumentation. (Author)

753.
HALL, D.A.
Mark II diving system.
In: Professional diving symposium, New Orleans, Nov. 1972. Mar. Technol. Soc. J. 7:10-12; Mar./Apr. 1973.

The Mark II Mode 0 deep dive system has recently been operationally evaluated and assimilated by Submarine Development Group One. It is a dual complex saturation diving system permanently installed on the surface support ship IX-501, Elk River. This system was originally utilized as the elevator for the Sea Lab III project. A 13-month operational evaluation of the complex has recently been completed. This evaluation included open sea dives as deep as 1,010 feet. The major units of this system include the deck decompression chamber (inner and outer lock; transfer trunk; medical lock), personnel transport chamber, the main control console, life support console and strength/power/communications winch. The Deep Diving System is used in six modes of operation which require different types of control action. The six modes of operation are: (a) saturation dive using mixed gas (normal), (b) hydrostatic dive, (c) air dive, (d) routine diver support, (e) submarine rescue, and (f) decompression. (Author)

754.
HALL, P.
The miniature pig as a model for the study of decompression.
In: Aerospace Medical Association. 1972 annual scientific meeting, Bal Harbour, Florida, May 1972. Preprints. p.221-222. Published by the Association.

Diving for work or sport is increasing rapidly in the mountains of the western U.S. In the central Rocky Mountain region the only readily available decompression tables are the U.S. Navy *sea-level* tables and a theoretical table which uses a Boyle's Law factor to convert depths at altitude to "equivalent" depths below sea-level. This table is set out so that for any depth at any altitude up to 10,000 ft. one can enter the U.S. Navy tables at the calculated equivalent *deeper* depth and decompress for the indicated times at the calculated *shallower* stops. The concept of a proportionality factor which would enable the diver at altitude to use established sea-level decompression tables is very attractive. This simple application of Boyle's Law might seem to be the obvious first approach, but the resulting theoretical table has not been rigorously checked. The author did preliminary testing on the miniature pig, chosen as a model because of its many physiological similarities to man. There is a growing need to develop a set of acceptable air decompression tables for altitude divers. In view of the hazards of decompression at altitude, the miniature pig should be a useful tool in the development of such tables. (Author)

755.
HALL, R.M. and F.R. Margolin.
Oxygen alveolpathy in adults.
Clin. Radiol. 23(1):11-17; 1972.

Ample clinical and experimental evidence indicates that prolonged exposure to high concentrations or partial pressures of O_2 may provide an exudative alveolar reaction progressing to interstitial pulmonary fibrosis. Initially this process appears roentgenographically as diffuse alveolar infiltrate. With progression to the proliferative phase of the disease, a more linear and nodular pattern is observed. No characteristic roentgen features allow specific diagnosis. Emphasis is placed upon the inclusion of O_2 alveolopathy in the differential diagnosis of widespread pulmonary infiltrates in patients who receive respirator therapy. Six examples of this condition in adults are reported. (© BA)

756.
HALLANGER, L.W. and A.M. Parisi.
The buoyancy transport vehicle — concept evaluation.
In: Applications of marine technology to human needs. Preprints, 8th annual conference and exposition, Marine Technology Society September 1972 Washington, D.C. p.655-668. Published by the Society 1972.

The potential utility of the Buoyancy Transport Vehicle as a tool for diver construction work was evaluated. The test program included determination of baseline vehicle performance data plus load handling and load placement capabilities. Basic vehicle characteristics are: maximum operating depth of 850 feet, payload capacity of 1800 pounds. Specific tests investigated vehicle ballasting, speed, maneuverability, and load handling capabilities. Surface support and maintenance requirements were also considered. Test results indicate the Buoyancy Transport Vehicle concept is valid for use in jobs such as construction or salvage where the diver must move multi-thousand-pound loads and precisely position them on the bottom. Concept limitations include visibility requirements, endurance and topside support requirements. (Authors' abstract)

757.
HALLENBECK, J.M., A.A. Bove, R.B. Moquin and D.H. Elliott.
Accelerated coagulation of whole blood and cell-free plasma by bubbling in vitro.
Aerosp. Med. 44:712-714;July 1973.

Bubbles with agitation cause a greater acceleration of the coagulation of whole blood than either agitation alone or contact with glass, whereas bubbles with agitation accelerate the coagulation of cell-five plasma more than agitation alone but less than by contact with glass. Thus bubbles have a capacity to accelerate some hematological reactions through their action on the cellular elements of blood and by the activation of a plasma factor, presumably Hageman. (Authors' abstract)

758.
HALLENBECK, J.M., A.A. Bove and D.H. Elliott.
The bubble as a non mechanical trigger in decompression sickness.
In: Ackles, K.N. ed. Blood-bubble interaction in decompression sickness. Proceedings of an international symposium held at Defence and Civil Institute of Environmental Medicine, Downsview, Ontario, Canada, p.129-139. Published by the Institute, December 1973. (DCIEM Conference Proceedings 73-CP-960)

In studying spinal cord lesions from decompression sickness, the authors sought a mechanism other than arterial embolism; evidence was accumulated supporting venous obstruction. Bubble surface activity can result in protein denaturation, enzyme activation, formation of fat emboli, increased blood viscosity, platelet aggregation, coagulation, and release of vasoactive amines, all of which are factors contributing to decompression sickness. The ultimate effect of these complex and numerous events depends upon the extent of bubble medication. If this is slight, the process can be reversed by elimination of gas, bubble resorption, and inhibiting enzyme activity. In more severe cases a limb bend could occur. In most extreme cases, the process could move to the lung. This organ can deal with moderate dose rates of bubbles and the products of bubble surface activity, but when these limits are exceeded, the cumulative effect on pulmonary vessels is both mechanical and reactive. Experiments with anesthetized dogs demonstrated a series of derangements which led from cardiopulmonary dysfunction to CNS damage by routing bubble-laden venous blood into the epidural vertebral venous system (EVVS). Various manifestations of experimentally produced cord lesions in dogs are described. The authors believe that obstruction of the EVVS, plus rheological disturbances, are sufficient to cause CNS damage without the presence of arterial emboli. (MFW/UMS)

759.
HALSEY, M.J. and E.I. Eger II.
Fluid shifts associated with gas-induced osmosis.
Science 179:1139-1140;Mar. 16, 1973.

It has been proposed that equilibration of nitrous oxide with blood plasma increases osmotic pressure and thereby causes hemodilution. However, calculations show that the 250-torr osmotic gradient produced by 0.7 atmosphere of nitrous oxide dissolved in blood plasma (separated from the other body fluids by a membrane permeable only to water) would be eliminated by a water shift which would dilute the plasma by only 4 percent. Permeability of the membrane to nitrous oxide would further reduce the shift. In vivo measurements confirmed the smallness of any osmotically induced shifts by demonstrating no significant transient changes in hematocrit value when 0.7 atmosphere of nitrous oxide was added to or removed from an inhaled anesthetic mixture in man. These results cast doubt on the suggestions that gas-induced osmosis is an important factor in dysbarism or in clinical anesthesia. (Authors' abstract)

760.
HAMILTON, R.W., Jr. and T.D. Langley.
Exercise in high pressure of neon, helium and nitrogen.
Physiologist 14(3):157; 1971.

Abstract only. Entire item quoted: Deep sea diving at pressures beyond about 7 atm. is usually done using helium as the inert gas. We are investigating the use of crude neon (c. 75% Ne, 25% He) to avoid the excessive heat loss and speech distortion of He. We exposed subjects to pressures of 7, 10, and 13 atm in a dry pressure chamber using either He, N_2 or crude Ne and 10% O_2, and to 16 and 19 atm with Ne and He and 7% O_2. Following 15 minutes of performance testing, divers rode a bicycle ergometer for 10 min. at 140 watts. Breath-by-breath end-expiratory CO_2 was drawn by a nasal catheter into an infrared detector modified for pressure; there were no other restrictions to breathing. Heart rate showed slight increases over control in the pressure experiments, increasing somewhat more at the higher pressures. Respiration rate tended to be less at pressure than control, and was relatively higher in He than the other gases. CO_2 rose at first with exercise while at depth in all cases, returning toward normal with He but leveling off at 8-12 mm Hg above normal with Ne and N_2. No evidence of neon narcosis was seen, but narcosis was quite severe with nitrogen forcing the diver to stop work after 3 min. in the 400 ft/dive. We see no reason why crude neon should not be safe and effective for diving to depths up to 500 ft.

761.
HAMILTON, R.W., Jr. and T.D. Langley.
Comparative physiological properties of nitrogen, helium and neon: A preliminary report. Presented at the annual symposium of the Undersea Medical Society, Houston, 4p. April 1971.

The purpose of this experiment was to test the possibilities of neon as a diving gas. The gas used was crude neon, which is 75% neon and 25% helium. The advantages of neon over helium are that it causes less voice distortion and cooling and also it may have some advantages during decompression. The disadvantages are its greater density and viscosity and its higher cost. These preliminary experiments indicate that crude neon is acceptable at least to depths of 400 feet. (MFW/BSCP)

762.
HAMILTON, R.W., Jr., H.R. Schreiner, M.R. Powell and G.F. Doebbler.
Two approaches to the study of decompression sickness.
In: Abstracts of BuMed-ONR sponsored Navywide workshop in high pressure biomedical research, U.S. Submarine Base, Groton, Conn., May 1971, p.24 Published by the Naval Submarine Medical Research Laboratory, 1971.

Abstract only. Entire item quoted: The study of decompression sickness was approached along two lines: detection of bubbles by the use of ultrasound, and correlating the degree of decompression damage with the rise of certain serum enzymes. The ultrasonic technique involves passing a beam through the tissue under study and measuring attenuation of the signal following decompression. Signals of 5.7 MHz transmitted through the foot of anesthetized rats held for one hour at 6 atmospheres and then decompressed were found to decrease by 10 to 16 db shortly after decompression. Signal strength returned on recompression. A similar profile, but with a short exposure resulted in no attenuation. Bubbles were found in all rats which showed signal attenuation. When the probes were placed across one thigh of similarly decompressed rats and the other thigh examined optically it was found that signal attenuation usually preceded the appearance of visible bubbles. In attempting to correlate exposure time, bubble formation and signs of decompression sickness in unanesthetized rats, it was found that although bubbles and exposure time are correlated the extent of decompression damage is not so easy to predict and is not necessarily related to the extent of visible bubble formation. The time course of signal attenuation parallels that for development of signs of decompression sickness. In a number of controlled and intentionally inadequate decompressions of miniature pigs it has been found that signs of decompression sickness can be recognized by observation of the animals as they walk on a treadmill. Serum lactic dehydrogenase and creatine phosphokinase were followed at appropriate times following decompressions of varying severity and both were found to rise substantially in those animals not properly decompressed, and to a degree which correlated with both severity of symptoms and inadequacy of decompression. Seven lipid constituents similarly followed showed no relation to decompression conditions.

763.
HAMILTON, R.W., Jr. and T.D. Langley.
Neon as a diving gas: Performance compared with nitrogen and helium at 7, 10, and 13 atmospheres.
In: Abstracts of the Twenty-fifth Congress of Physiological Sciences Satellite Symposium. Recent progress in fundamental physiology of diving. Marseille, France, July 1971, p.43-44. (Proceedings unpublished)

Abstract only. Excerpts quoted: These experiments were designed to explore the use of crude neon as a diving gas, as a replacement for helium. Crude neon is a mixture of about 75% neon, 25% helium and can be obtained from properly equipped air distillation plants, at a price roughly comparable to helium. The authors conducted dives to 7, 10 and 13 atm. abs., all with 10% oxygen. Helium, crude neon and nitrogen were used as the inert gases. Appropriate physiological and performance tests were chosen to fit the 30 minute "bottom time" and were conducted in an identical way on all dives. Tests included simple reaction time, manual tapping, simple auditory vigilance, complex auditory vigilance, arithmetic, manual dexterity and two 2-min. determinations of static intention tremor. When normalized and plotted as decrement from control values, results of all these tests were remarkably similar. When plotted against increasing ambient pressure all tests showed a striking decrement as pressure increased when nitrogen was being breathed but in no case is there a clear and distinct difference between results for helium and neon, and decrement while using these gases was minimal. Throughout the dive evoked brain responses were induced by auditory calibrated beeps (rather than clicks). The decrease in amplitude of the evoked potentials as measured by the N_1-P_2 interval followed a pattern similar to that of the performance tests. . . . Decompressions from neon dives were uneventful while "pain only" limb bends, routinely treated, were encountered in 300 feet dives using nitrogen and helium. Although subjects were able to appreciate subjectively the added density of the neon mixtures they did not find them objectionable in any other ways. These experiences and the data strongly support the contention that crude neon can be used as a substitute for helium in diving to moderate depths.

764.
HAMILTON, R.W., Jr.
Comparative narcotic effects in performance tests of nitrous oxide and hyperbaric nitrogen.
Fed. Proc. 32(3,Pt.2):682;Mar. 1973.

Abstract only. Entire item quoted: The anesthetic properties of nitrous oxide allow this gas to be used in light doses as a model for the study of the nitrogen narcosis encountered in diving. We evaluated this model on two subjects by determining dose-response curves. A 25-minute package of cognitive psychomotor and sensory tests was repeated while subjects breathed several normoxic (0.2 atm) mixtures by mask. Five nitrous oxide doses ranged from zero to 0.5 atm. Five nitrogen mixtures (in He) were all breathed at a total pressure of 13.1 atmospheres; doses were from zero to 12.9 atm. In most cases test scores conformed to the upper part of and S-shaped dose-response curve for both gases. Slopes were eye drawn along the steep part of each curve, and the slopes were compared. For psychomotor tests (e.g. tracking) nitrous oxide is about 40 times as potent as nitrogen, but for cognitive tests (e.g. arithmetic) it may be less, about 30 times. Brauer and Way (JAP 29:23, 1970) found a ratio of 25.3 for righting reflex in mice.

765.
HAMILTON, R.W., Jr., D.J. Kenyon, H.R. Schreiner and P.O. Edel.
Computation and testing of no-stop decompression procedures for use from saturation in a nitrogen-oxygen habitat.
In: Aerospace Medical Association. 1973 annual scientific meeting, Las Vegas, Nevada, May 1973. Preprints, p.239-240. Published by the Association, 1973.

This is a report on NOAA OPS I and II, first in a new series of operational experiments whose purpose it is to develop and refine decompression procedures for working from a shallow undersea habitat. The program can be described in four phases: (a) to search out, review and analyze available relevant data on decompression with nitrogen as the inert gas, (b) to use this data base for computing a set of tables describing depth-time limits for no-stop (e.g. "no decompression") excursions from various habitat depths (both ascending and descending), (c) to verify these tables, and (d) to evaluate health and performance aspects of these environmental exposures. Throughout the entire experiment extensive physiological, psychological, biophysical and biochemical surveillance was carried out in cooperation with the U.S. Naval Submarine Medical Research Laboratory. Ultrasonic methods applied to seek evidence of bubble formation, both Doppler and through-pass techniques being tried. Performance tests and evoked brain responses were used to follow the course and degree of adaptation to nitrogen narcosis of the divers. (5) Mass spectrometric analysis was used to study the rate of nitrogen washout from the diver's lungs. Ecological, dental, immunological and microbiological parameters were monitored throughout the program, as well as biochemical factors in blood, urine and saliva. Psychological surveillance was also maintained. There seems to be a definite adaptation to narcosis in divers saturated at 90 and 120 fsw, less in those saturated at 60 and 30 fsw. From 90 and 120 fsw, their performance at 200 and 250 fsw showed little decrement from control levels, but at 300 fsw there was still a substantial effect of nitrogen narcosis. (Authors)

766.
HAMILTON, R.W., Jr., D.J. Kenyon, M. Freitag and H.R. Schreiner.
NOAA OPS I and II: Formulation of excursion procedures for shallow undersea habitats.
Tarrytown, N.Y., Union Carbide Tech. Cent., Environ. Physiol. Lab., Rep. UCRI 731, 179p. July 31, 1973.

This is a report on operational experiments whose purpose it is to develop and refine procedures for working from a shallow habitat. The program was (1) to construct a matrix of ascent-limiting M-values based on several hundred diversified dive logs, (2) to compute no-stop excursion limits for various times and depths, (both ascending and descending), and (3) to verify the resulting tables. [An M-value is the maximum value of the partial pressure of dissolved inert gas which can be tolerated in specific compartments of the human body and will permit the diver safely to ascend 10 ft to the next stop]. The authors devised an efficient method for extracting and utilizing data from previous dives, using a combination of computer and manual methods. Tables were computed using the new matrix and the decompression model which in this case comprises 11 gas loading compartments; the longest limiting half-time used was 480 minutes. Three subjects in tow 14-day dry chamber experiments tested this matrix in twice-daily excursions from normoxic saturation at 30, 60, 90 and 120 fsw, and ascents ranged from 30 to 65 fsw above the habitat depth; excursion times ranged from 8 minutes to 6 hours. Air was breathed on excursions. Results show that this approach produced highly successful tables on the first attempt. Extensive physiological experimentation and medical surveillance was conducted in cooperation with researchers from the U.S. Naval Submarine Medical Research Laboratory. Among the findings was the demonstration that habituation at 90 fsw provides relief from narcosis when subjects are subsequently exposed to 250 fsw of air. (Authors' abstract)

767.
HAMILTON, R.W., Jr.
Current status of the formulation of criteria and standards for commercial diving.
Pressure Med. Physiol. 2(Spec. Insert 4):3;Sept./Oct. 1973.

The Occupational Safety and Health Act (OSHA), passed in 1970, is supposed to establish safety criteria for workers in stressful environments, including commercial divers. Objections to the adoption of the U.S. Navy Diving Manual, by divers and contractors, made it necessary to establish standards for industrial diving. The American National

Standards Institute (ANSI) and The Marine Technology Society's Committee on Man's Underwater Activities (MU/WA) had been attempting to establish such standards under the leadership of Dr. H.W. Gillen. Criteria for decompression and other medical problems had not been sought. Efforts are now being made in this area, by Dr. E. Beckman at Texas A & M, to be reviewed by the NAS/NRC Committee on Underwater Physiology and Medicine under Dr. H. Rahn, and coordinated with criteria set up by the Committee on Salvage and Diving, under Capt. W. Searle. Public hearings will probably be held by OSHA before these combined results will be designated as law. Limited funds are at present delaying completions of the project. (MFW/BSCP)

768.
HAMILTON, R.W., Jr.
Breathing mixtures.
Tarrytown, N.Y.: Ocean Systems, Inc., Res. Devel. Lab., Rep. CRL-T-750, 87p. Dec. 29, 1973.

This report is concerned with the elements involved in the choice of breathing mixtures for diving. . . . The ideal choice of gas is a compromise of several factors. These factors — oxygen toxicity, metabolism, inert gas narcosis, HPNS, density, voice, thermal properties, decompression, fire safety, cost and logistics — are covered by topic. . . . Current diving modes require the selection of optimal breathing mixtures for each of several operational situations. These include scuba, closed and semi-closed breathing rigs, hose-supplied gas, and the atmosphere of both submersible and deck chambers; in addition to the equipment used, the particular diving situation affects the choice of gas. Physiologic factors also are involved; these include duration of exposure, temperature, work load and whether the diver is immersed in a gas or breathing it by mask. . . . [This report was prepared for inclusion in a handbook on underwater bioengineering which is being produced by the Science Communication Division of The George Washington University Medical Center, scheduled for publication in early 1975 by Plenum Publishing Corp]. (from author's introduction).

769.
HAMMER, J.G. and H.S. Zwibel.
Comparative solutions for the response of restrained, rigid-body underwater structures to acoustic shock.
U.S. Nav. Civil Eng. Lab., Tech. Note N-1141, 73p. Jan. 1971.

This study seeks better understanding of the general problem of predicting the response of fixed underwater structures to a shock wave propagating through the water. Two idealized structures are considered: an elastically-restrained rigid sphere and an elastically-restrained rigid cylinder. The shock is assumed to be an exponentially-deacying pressure pulse in an acoustic fluid. Solutions to the exact equations are obtained analytically for the spherical structure and by Bellman's numerical inversion procedure for both structures. Previously obtained solutions for the restrained cylindrical structure, simplified by the curves are given for both structural types over a range of parameters. The effects of drag are discussed. (Authors' abstract)

770.
HAMMOND, R.E. and T.K. Akers.
The effect of sympathetic releasing and blocking agents on the pulmonary system during high pressure oxygen toxicity.
In: Aerospace Medical Association. 1973 annual scientific meeting, Las Vegas Nevada, May 1973. Preprints, p.147-148. Published by the Association, 1973.

Evidence has been presented to indicate that OHP may possibly produce a physical change in the membrane of the effector cell, thus preventing a normal interaction between the adrenergic neurotransmitter and the receptor. . . [The data presented here] indicate that alpha-adrenergic blockade may be of definite value in ameliorating the pulmonary effects of OHP. Further investigation will be necessary before it is certain whether the resultant protection is afforded primarily through the activity of the respiratory bronchioles, through the pulmonary vasculature or partially through extraneous factors such as systemic arterial pressure. The prevention or production of pulmonary edema was in no case directly attributable to a drug effect but rather to damage in pulmonary capillary beds caused by OHP. The development or absence of pulmonary edema is dependent on the hemodynamics of the damaged capillary bed. Therefore, drugs which modify the activity of the autonomic nervous system exert some degree of control over the hemodynamic state of the pulmonary capillary beds. (Authors)

771.
HANNA, J.M. and S.K. Hong.
Critical water temperature and effective insulation in scuba divers in Hawaii.
J. Appl. Physiol. 33:770-773;Dec. 1972.

Thirteen regular scuba divers from Honolulu, Hawaii, were compared with fifteen control subjects in a water immersion test as developed by Rennie et al. (in: Physiology of Breath Hold Diving and the Ama of Japan). Water temperature ranged from 28 to 33°C. Subjects were immersed for three hr or until the onset of shivering; trials were repeated each day until the minimum temperature which could be tolerated for three hours with no visible shivering was determined. This was called critical water temperature (CWT). Divers tended toward a lower CWT at any level of subcutaneous fat thickness, but there were no apparent differences in maximal tissue insulation (I_{max}) that has been reported in other studies. The responses of ten subjects of Japanese ancestry and ten of European ancestry were examined separately. There were no great differences in response between ethnic groups. (Authors' abstract)

772.
HANSEN, M. and J. Madsen.
Effect of oxygen breathing on local blood flow in human adipose tissue.
Scand. J. Clin. Lab. Invest. 30(1):43-48; 1972.

The effect of O_2 breathing at 1 atm on the blood flow of abdominal subcutaneous adipose tissue in man was investigated using the ^{133}Xe washout method. Adipose tissue perfusion was about 25% lower during O_2 breathing than when breathing air. This was the case whether the breathing medium was changed from air to O_2 or from O_2 to air. (© BA)

773.
HANSEN, M. and J. Madsen.
Changes in crural blood flow caused by oxygen breathing at 1 atmosphere.
Acta Physiol. Scand. 87(1):12A; 1973.

Abstract only. Entire item quoted: Change of breathing medium from air to oxygen at 1 atm causes an 11 per cent reduction in calf (Reich et al. 1970) and forearm blood flow (Bird and Telfer 1966) of resting men examined by pelthysmography. Bird and Telfer noticed that the reduction in blood flow persisted for some time after cessation of oxygen administration. Similar observations were made on dog hind limbs. No figures were given for the duration of this "after-effect". The present experiments were carried out to examine the blood flow changes in a calf segment at the beginning and at the end of a 20 min period of oxygen breathing. One experiment was made on each of 9 healthy male volunteers. The subject laid immobile on his back with the calf placed in a water plethysmograph 20 cm above the level of the couch. The arrangement and use of the plethysmograph were essentially as described by Hansen and Madsen (1972). Most readings were taken with 1-2 min intervals. For each 5 min period the average value was used for further calculations. The average flow rate during air breathing before the oxygen period was 1.9 ml . 100 ml^{-1} min^{-1} (S.D. 0.46). Calf blood flow was reduced during oxygen breathing. For each experiment the change was calculated as a fraction of the initial blood flow. The average reduction was -6 per cent in the 0-5 min period of oxygen breathing ($0.1 > P > 0.05$) and reached its maximum value of -12 per cent (S.E. 2.6) in the 5-10 min period ($P < 0.002$). Upon cessation of oxygen breathing the flow increased. This increase became significant in the 5-10 min period after breathing gas change ($P < 0.001$). In the 0-5 min post-oxygen period the flow rate averaged 97 per cent (S.E. 4.2) of the pre-oxygen control flow, in the 5-10 min period 106 per cent (S.E. 2.9). The average values were statistically indistinguishable from the pre-oxygen control values both in the 0-5 and in the 5-10 min periods after resumption of air breathing ($P > 0.05$).

774.
HANSON, R. deG.
Decompression sickness in civilian divers.
J. Roy. Nav. Med. Serv. 59:77-80;Summer 1973.

Most cases resulted from repetitive dives. In general, recompression therapy sufficed. One case is described in detail. Neurological symptoms occurred 15 minutes after two 15-minute dives to 130 feet, and developed over the next two days, consisting of back pain, leg pain, a headache, difficulties in urinating, and some cutaneous anesthesia. Treatment was not initiated until 84 hours after onset of symptoms. Initial recompression to 60 feet cured bladder problems and numbness. After nine days in hospital, the pain subsided (treatment not specified). This survey shows that only a small proportion of divers practicing repetitive diving of short duration suffer from decompression sickness. It is concluded that the Royal Navy decompression tables are too conservative. There is a brief discussion of the calculation of tables, and a comparison of Royal Navy tables and U.S. Navy tables. The desirability of educating divers into decompressing on their last dives is noted. (MFW/UMS)

775.
HARDENBERGH, E., R.G. Buckles, J.A. Miles, Jr., P.W. Schilling and J.B. Eckenhoff.
Cardiovascular changes in anesthetized dogs at 3 and 5 atmospheres absolute pressure.
Aerosp. Med. 44:1231-1235;Nov. 1973.

Cardiovascular changes in anesthetized (chloralose) dogs were studied during exposure to three hyperbaric environments: 3 atmospheres absolute (ata) breathing air; 3 ata oxygen; and 5 ata air. Breathing air at 3 ata appeared to have little effect on physiologic parameters, but breathing oxygen at 3 ata depressed the heart rate and diminished the iliac blood flow (Doppler flow meter) in most of the animals, with little apparent effect on the mean arterial blood pressure (brachial artery). Breathing air at 5 ata, however, increased the blood pressure in all animals and diminished iliac flow and heart rate. These observations are in agreement with other reports. They indicate that physiological changes effected by changes in the gaseous environment, as well as the physical characteristics of the gases breathed, can be contributing factors to the development of oxygen poisoning and bubble formation. (Authors' abstract)

776.
HAREL, D., N. Conforti and S. Lavy.
Influence of deafferentation of the medial basal hypothalamus on the sensitivity of the brain to hyperbaric oxygen.
Aerosp. Med. 44:1223-1226;Nov. 1973.

The electrical activity of the brain in rats after complete deafferentation of the medial basal hypothalamus and in normal controls was examined under hyperbaric oxygen of 6 atmospheres absolute (ata). Continuous electroencephalographic recording was obtained from chronically implanted electrodes. The pattern of background activity was not altered by the procedure. The first paroxysmal electrical discharge was considered to be the first sign of cerebral oxygen toxicity. The pattern of this discharge and the time of onset of first electrical seizures were not altered by the complete deafferentation of the medial basal hypothalamus. The literature dealing with the influence of the medial basal hypothalamus on adenohypophysis and target glands is cited. The lack of response to hyperbaric oxygenation of animals with hypothalamic islands supports our previous observation that adrenalectomy and hypophysectomy do not alter sensitivity of rat brain to oxygen poisoning if first electrical discharge is used as a criterion of oxygen toxicity. (Authors' abstract)

777.
HARICHAUX, P., J. Davidovits, M. Freville, C. Tavernier and J. Lienard.
Asymetrie des transferts gazeux dans un modele experimental et anisotrope de menbrane biologique.
[Asymmetrical gaseous exchanges in an experimental and anisotropic model of a biological membrane].
C.R. Soc. Biol. 165(4):866-870; 1971.

By using a special device and by continuous measurement, the variations of PO_2 [O_2 tension] and PCO_2 exchanges between two sections separated by a synthetic polyamide anisotropic membrane were studied. The gaseous exchanges varied according to the direction of transfer through this membrane which had two different permeability coefficients depending on the face studied. Anisotropy varied with certain physico-chemical factors (membrane thickness, hydration level and the polyamide concentration). (© BA)

778.
HARRIS, E.A.
Accurate analysis of carbon dioxide in oxygen-nitrogen mixtures by infra-red absorption.
Biomed. Eng. 8:66-69;Feb. 1973.

Although infra-red analysers are used widely for the analysis of carbon dioxide in expired air, the accuracy of such instruments is usually less than that obtained by chemical analysis. This paper describes a study of the characteristics of an URASM infra-red CO_2 analyser, with a view to increasing its accuracy. Means are described by which corrections can be made successively for non-linearity of output, and for the dependence of infra-red absorption upon the O_2 and N_2 concentrations of the gas sample. With these corrections the instrument has an accuracy comparable with that of standard chemical analysis. (Author's abstract)

779.
HARRIS, J.A., Jr.
Properties of materials in high pressure hydrogen at room and elevated temperatures.
West Palm Beach, Fla., Pratt Whitney Aircraft, Res. Develop. Cent., Ann. Rep. 2 (NASA-CR-123929), 66p. June 1972.
(N72-32145)

Experimental efforts in this program for this period. Mechanical property tests of wrought and cast nickel-base alloys and one wrought cobalt-base alloy were conducted in 34.5 MN/sq m (500-psig) helium and hydrogen or hydrogen mixtures. Comparison of test results was made to determine degradation of properties due to the hydrogen environments. All testing was conducted on solid specimens exposed to external gaseous pressure. Specific mechanical properties determined and the testing methods used are summarized. (Author) (STAR)

780.
HARRIS, J.D. and P.G. Lacroix.
Audiometric survey on USS Tigrone (AGSS-419) underway during seven days of active sonar operations.
U.S. Nav. Submar. Med. Cent., Mem. Rep. NSMRL 71-3, 11p. May 3, 1971.

Results of a sound level survey undertaken by NUSC/NLON (Naval Underwater Systems Center, New London Laboratory) in January of 1971 disclosed pressure levels (SPLS) aboard USS TIGRONE (AGSS-419) which are considered unacceptable, as a result of high-intensity active sonar operations. Audiometry was undertaken while underway on a representative cross-section of the crew who lived and worked in those spaces considered unacceptable. Audiometric results showed that losses were in general within normal limits. This is not surprising when it is considered that the highest SPL was little more than 100 dB and the attenuation afforded by ear defenders was near 30 dB. Therefore, maximum level at the protected crew member's ear was about 70 dB, which is well within acceptable limits. Specifically, only 8 readings out of 88 showed a loss of greater than 5 dB, only one was greater than 10 dB (15dB) and these losses were counterbalanced by 11 variations of greater than 5 dB in the other direction. Whether future operations of longer duration with more intense SPLs and modified repetition rates would adversely affect hearing, and/or health is still an open question. Changes in environmental conditions aboard USS TIGRONE (AGSS-419) are being watched carefully. (Authors' abstract)

781.
HARRIS, J.D. and R.E. Croteau.
Field evaluation of the effects on hearing and general habitability of own-ship echo-ranging during a submarine patrol.
U.S. Nav. Submar. Med. Cent. and Nav. Underwater Systems Cent., Joint Mem. Rep. NSMRL 71-5, 13p. May 28, 1971.

On a six-day cruise of USS BERGHALL (SSN-667), engaged in active echo-ranging the hearing of personnel and general habitability of the ship were assessed by personnel from Naval Underwater Systems Center, New London Laboratory (NUSC/NLON), and Naval Submarine Medical Research Laboratory (NSMRL). Pulse levels up to 97.8 dB were measured in CPO quarters, and 86-91 dB in the 37-man forward compartment. No temporary hearing changes were found after three hours or less of recovery, and no evidence of deterioration of habitability of living/sleeping quarters was reported by the human factors observer who was aboard. It is concluded that the several hours of own-ship sonar pulses had only a transient effect on hearing and that the levels of 86-91 dB in living/sleeping quarters for this duration are within the range of habitability for healthy, well-motivated young men. (Authors' abstract)

782.
HARRIS, J.D.
The ear and hearing in aquatic and dysbaric environments.
U.S. Nav. Submar. Med. Res. Lab., Rep. NSMRL 746, 47p., May 29, 1973.

A non-quantitative theory of human hearing is sketched for the case of the head immersed in water, based upon what is known of hearing in air and hearing by bone conduction. A consideration is given of four routes by which acoustic waterborne energy is transmitted to the fluids of the inner ear. Quantitative data are presented from recent studies of the thresholds of underwater auditory acuity, and of the relations between airborne and waterborne thresholds. Sound levels possibly hazardous to free swimmers are suggested and the intelligibility of speech passed through water is discussed. Studies on the ability of the human to localize sounds under water are discussed. The acute otorhinological problems of the outer, middle, and inner ear are discussed in both aquatic and dysbaric environments. A bibliography of 250 items is presented which constitutes a valuable reference tool. (Author's abstract)

783.
HARRISON, G.A.
Ultrastructural changes in rat lung during long-term exposure to oxygen.
Exp. Med. Surg. 29:96-107; 1971.

The pathogenesis of oxygen toxicity in the lung of rats was studied by electromicroscopy. Rats, exposed to 100% oxygen at 1 atmosphere in constant environment capsules, were sacrificed at weekly intervals and the lung prepared for ultrastructural study. The first response was a widespread perivascular, interstitial, and intracellular edema. Mitochondria, pinocytotic vesicles and ER cisternae were swollen and the cytoplasm was loosely packed.Edema occurred first in the capillary endothelium, but was quickly followed by changes in the organelles of the alveolar epithelium and other cell types. At this time, the basement membrane became thickened and invaded by fibers. The endothelial cell showed breaks and then was destroyed leaving the basement membrane exposed to the capillary contents. The basement membrane next shredded leaving only a narrow vesiculated strand of epithelial cytoplasma which eventually ruptured. Complete destruction of the alveolo-capillary wall allowed adjacent alveoli to become contiguous. With prolonged exposure, these animals showed emphysema and this destruction of the blood-air barrier, described below, may very possibly be a factor contributing to the pathogenesis of this condition. As the length of exposure increases so, too, does the amount and complexity of the alveolar exudate. After long exposure (4-5 weeks) some of the red blood cells show signs of altered hemoglobin or partial hemolysis. Previous studies of 100% oxygen at 1 atmosphere have been of short duration. In this study, young animals were used and provided a model for long-term chronic exposure to this atmosphere. (Author's summary)

784.
HARRISON, G.A., C. Turnbill and S. Black.
Effects of oxygen on tracheal mucosa.
J. Cell. Biol. 59(2,Pt.2):135a; 1973.

Abstract only. Entire item quoted: Oxygen at high pressure damages the lung considerably and ultrastructural studies reveal damage to and destruction of the alveolo-capillary wall, alveolar exudate, interstitial edema and intracellular edema in the form of swollen or rarified cytoplasm, cytoplasmic blebs and swollen organelles. Bronchioles also exhibit blebbing, sloughing and cellular proliferation. Tracheal mucosa is also affected by oxygen exposure. To study the effects, groups of 12 Sprague-Dawley rats were exposed to 100% oxygen at one atmosphere for periods of 24, 36,

48, 72 or 96 hours. Following sacrifice, the tracheae were removed, and prepared by Critical Point Drying for study in a scanning electron microscope (SEM). Parts of the tracheae were also prepared by routine methods for transmission microscopy (TEM). At 24 hours of exposure some of the microvilli had changed in size and length. After 48 hours exposure, the non-ciliated cells had rounded up, the microvilli were disappearing and some of the mucus coating remained. This coating was even more extensive after 72 and 96 hours. After the tissue preparation processing used, this coating is removed from normal trachea. The fact that it remains suggests a change in composition. At this same time (72 and 96 hours), the microvilli have almost completely disappeared. Ciliated cells are shed and many of the cilia are altered in appearance. In oxygen exposure, the normal muco-ciliary clearance is interfered with in two ways. First, the mucus is altered in composition and second, the cilia are blocked mechanically by cellular swelling of non-ciliated cells or cellular blebbing of the ciliated cells. Good correlation was provided of ultrastructural changes between the SEM and the TEM.

785.
HARRISON, J.A.B.
Aseptic bone necrosis in naval clearance divers.
Proc. Roy. Soc. Med. 64:1276-1278;Dec. 1971.

The author gives the final results of a survey of naval divers undertaken to "establish the presence and assess the incidence" of osteonecrosis; interim findings had been previously published (Elliott, D.H. and J.A.B. Harrison. J. Roy. Nav. Med. Serv. 56:140-161; 1970). Over the period of 1967-1971, of 383 divers, the final results were 356 negative 9 doubtful, and 19 positive. It is noted that during this period, three cases moved from negative to doubtful, one from negative to positive, and one from doubtful to positive. Most of the lesions detected are shaft lesions; most of them preceded symptoms. (MFW/BSCP)

786.
HARRISON, J.A.B.
Aseptic bone necrosis in divers.
Brit. J. Radiol. 45:393. May 1972.

Abstract only. Entire item quoted: The lesions of aseptic bone necrosis which occur in divers were described. The differential diagnosis of aseptic bone necrosis was discussed. A summary of the techniques used and a classification of the lesions and their distribution in a three-year X-ray survey of a sample of 383 naval clearance divers were given. The classification of lesions is now accepted on an international basis. Only the shoulders, hips and knees were X-rayed as a compromise between a complete examination and limitation of radiation exposure. The correlation of lesions to diving experience and the occurrence of decompression sickness was discussed and the subsequent development of the lesions and their progression in the sample X-rayed were reviewed. The incidence of aseptic bone necrosis in the naval sample at the conclusion of the three-year survey was 4.2 per cent. No lesions had so far been detected in a control sample of naval personnel in an age rank distribution equivalent to the divers' sample who had not been exposed to pressure changes. The progress and present results of other surveys of divers were briefly reviewed.

787.
HARRISON, J.R.
Some aspects of medicine in nuclear submarines.
Trans. Soc. Occup. Med. 22:15-18;Jan. 1972.

The medical officer of a British nuclear submarine, in addition to his duties as a physician, has responsibility for the health and safety of the crew. He must run a full radiological protection program, and must also supervise the atmosphere control program. The atmosphere is continuously monitored for H_2, O_2, N_2, F_{12}, CO and CO_2 by gas chromatography. Hydrocarbon contaminants are monitored on charcoal cartridges, and aerosol contaminants by high velocity samplers, and results are analyzed by the Admiralty Materials Laboratory. There are also emergency monitoring facilities (draeger) and special portable instruments for oxygen, hydrogen, and monoethanolamine. An electrolyser is used to produce O_2; scrubbers employing monoethanolamine are used to remove CO_2; H_2, CO, and some hydrocarbons are burned. Dust and aerosol are conrolled by the banning of woolen clothing and other dusty substances such as talcum powder, and the use of polyurethane filters on exhausts; invisible particles are controlled by electrostatic precipitators. The environment must be constantly monitored for temperature and humidity. Airborne bacteria are monitored. Upper respiratory tract infections are particularly prevalent during the first two weeks of a patrol. Hearing conservation is a problem in certain working areas, and ear defenders are used. The effects of occupational stresses on health and performance are an important consideration. Recreational programs, such as films and internal radio broadcasting, competitive games, weekly 50-word telegrams from home, keep morale high. Epidemiological studies carried out incude (1) Effects of CO_2 on acid-base balance; (2) effects of CO_2 on calcium and magnesium metabolism; (3) carboxyhaemoglobin levels in submarines; (4) transfer of bacteria and phage typing; (5) effects of prolonged watchkeeping on circadian rhythms. (MFW/UMS)

788.
HARRISON, R.J. and S.H. Ridgway.
Telemetry in experimental and trained dives by seals.
J. Anat. 111:491;Apr. 1972.

Abstract only. Entire item quoted: Radiotelemetry devices have been implanted in the hypodermis of the back and neck of 12- to 18-month-old grey seals (Halichoerus grypus). The package had electrodes extending across the thorax. The ECG could be broadcast continuously over a period of several months: a magnetic switch incorporated in the transmitter turned the transmitter on and off. This made it possible to carry out prolonged experiments on ECG characteristics and changes in cardiac rhythm in relation to respiratory rhythm on land, during sleep and during diving in unrestrained seals and to compare them with findings in restrained seals. The seals were trained to submerge on command signalled by an underwater light. When the light was turned off and a whistle sounded as a bridging stimulus a fish was delivered by an underwater feeder. Thus the seals could be instructed to make voluntary dives of periods of submersion up to 8 minutes and recordings were made before, during and after the dive. It is contended that there is a maximum dive response as judged by bradycardial characteristics during restrained dives. Forced dives were made with the seal in a small cage. Out of water respiratory rate is 2-12 per minute, heart rate is 120-150 beats per minute but falls to 40-70 during the regularly occurring breath holds. Asleep out of water respiratory rate is 8-15 and heart rate is 140-170. Resting in water respiratory rate is 3-5, heart rate is 110-170 but falls to 33-48 on breath holds. Trained-dive heart rate fals to 20-40 and in forced dives to as slow as 10-40. The onset of the bradycardia is immediate in all types of dive but each seal displays certain individual characteristics in its dive response.

789.
HARRISON, R.J., S.H. Ridgway and P.L. Joyce.
Telemetry of heart rate in diving seals.
Nature 237:280;Aug. 4, 1972.

Radiotelemetry devices were implanted in the hypodermis of the back and neck of seals that had been trained to dive on command. Other seals were forcibly submerged in a tank. Heart rate changes were monitored in both groups. The bradycardial response was found to be stronger (heart rate 10-40 beats per minute) in the forced dives than in the trained dives (20-40 beats per minute, but with a continual fluctuation). (MFW/BSCP)

790.
HARVEY, C.
Naval submarine medical research laboratory conducts shallow saturation dive using compressed air.
Pressure Med. Physiol. 2:2;Sept./Oct. 1973.

A 30-day simulated shallow saturation dive was begun on 1 October at the Naval Submarine Medical Research Laboratory at New London. The project, of which this is the first dive, is designated as SHAD (Shallow Habitat Air Dives). Excursion dives will be made at pressures equivalent to 5 and 235 fsw. Extensive monitoring of the divers was carried out. EEG patterns and visually evoked brain responses were studied. Pulmonary function, respiration rate, ECG and gas analysis were monitored. Blood gas analysis was made. All aspects of vision were measured to determine any possible effects of elevated oxygen partial pressure. At the time of the writing of this account, the dive was not completed, and the findings had not been made. (MFW/SCD)

791.
HASEGAWA, H., M. Sato and H. Tsuruta.
A biochemical study of divers.
Ind. Health 9(3):113-136; 1971.

A strong diver is one who is not susceptible to decompression sickness and a weak one is the converse. Old and fat people are not suitable for diving work. Decompression sickness might be avoidable if the divers could be classified into the two groups by some scientific methods. Twenty divers and ten normal people were examined biochemically and the results were compared with a self-rating by the divers themselves into strong and weak. Total cholesterol content in the blood of the divers was in the normal range, although that of weak divers were larger than the strong. Free cholesterol content in the blood of divers was about 1/3 of that of normal people. Ester cholesterol of weak divers was larger than strong one. The velocity of N_2 gas uptake by the blood of the weak was larger than the strong. O_2 affinity of the Hb molecule of most divers examined showed a marked raise. Most divers examined had a low pH and high CO_2 tension of the venous blood. (JK) (© BA)

792.
HASEGAWA, T.
Coding scheme for underwater digital data transmission.
IEEE international conference on engineering in the ocean environment, Panama City, Florida, September 1970. Digest of technical papers. p.60-62. Published by the conference.

Considerations on the probability of applying Fibonacci code to underwater data transmission, on its synchronization problems (digit, word and frame synchronization) and on its error detecting or correcting ability are presented and discussed. (Eng. Index)

793.
HAUX, G.
Draeger Duocom: a completely new concept of a portable two-man chamber.
Tauchtechnik Inf. 8:29-35;Mar. 1972.

There is a gap between the man-sized stationary chambers for several men which are available only in a few central bases and large diver support vessels, and the one-man chambers which are sometimes available in large numbers. Until now, a small two-man chamber has not been available which would either permit local pressure treatment of a diver with medical assistance, or transportation for transfer to a large chamber under the *same* conditions, i.e. medical assistance even during transportation. This gap is closed by the Draeger Duocom. A system is introduced in which the function alone was determining for the design, without regard to conventional ideas. This is manifested externally in the completely new shape. But new approaches were used down to small details and these approaches might one day set guidelines for the construction of pressure chambers. (Author's summary)

794.
HAUX, G.
Die Unterwasserstationein Stutzpunkt im Meer.
[The underwater-station — a base in the sea].
Meerestechnik 3:233-235;Dec. 1972.

Since 1962 — the year of inception of the first underwater laboratory — there have been more than 50 underwater stations put into operation around the world. According to available information, there are about another 15-20 installations either under construction or in the planning stage. A certain proportion of these installations, on the other hand, were not put into successful operation, or after their first mission they were either scrapped or shut down. Only a few installations were repeatedly used or are in permanent use. With these facts in mind, the author poses the question regarding the future for underwater stations — not forgetting their use in German sea areas. (English summary)

795.
HAWKINS, I.K.
Helium effect on cardiac mitochondria of mice.
Aerosp. Med. 43:775-777;July 1972.

Twenty male A/Jax mice, 50 $\pm$ 5 days old at the onset, were exposed for 90 days at ambient pressure to the effect of substituting helium for nitrogen in respired air. Control animals were held under identical conditions, but their respiratory gas supply contained no helium. All animals were randomly divided into four equal groups. Each group was housed in a separate cage which was placed inside an individual environmental chamber. Electron micrographs of cardiac muscle from the helium treated animals showed varying degrees of diffuse disruption of the internal mitochondrial membranes and cristae. The mitochondrial disruptions were seen predominantely in mitochondria adjacent to the transverse sarcotubular apparatus. (Author's abstract)

796.
HAWKINS, I.K.
Helium effect on skeletal muscle of mice.
Aerosp. Med. 44:374-378;Apr. 1973.

Twenty male A/Jax mice, 50$\pm$5 days old at the onset, were exposed for 90 days at ambient pressure to the effect of substituting helium for nitrogen in respired air. Control animals were held under identical conditions, but their respiratory gas supply contained no helium. All animals were randomly divided into four equal groups. Each group was housed in a separate cage which was placed inside an individual environmental chamber. Photomicrographs of skeletal muscle from the helium-treated animals showed diffuse myopathic lesions of some of the skeletal muscle fibers. Additional indications of muscle tissue degradation were present. (Author's abstract)

797.
HAWKINS, T.L., A.B. Quist and T.C. King.
Open sea evaluation of the Bio Marine CCC-1000 General Electric MK 10 MOD 5, and Westinghouse CCM-1 closed circuit, mixed gas, underwater breathing apparatus.
U.S. Navy Exp. Diving Unit, Rep NEDU-9-72, 79p. Aug. 1972.

The Bio Marine CCR-1000, General Electric MK 10 MOD 5, and Westinghouse CCM-1 closed circuit, mixed gas, underwater breathing apparatus' were jointly evaluated in open sea test operations sponsored by the Navy Experimental Diving Unit during the period 9 March through 13 June 1972 at the Naval Station, Roosevelt Roads, Puerto Rico and at the Naval Amphibious Base, Little Creek, Norfolk, Virginia. Earlier objective and subjective tests were accomplished with the individual SCUBA's and are discussed in the following NAVXDIVINGU reports:
a. Report No. 3-72: BIO MARINE CCR-1000, Mixed Gas, Closed Circuit, Underwater Breathing Apparatus
b. Report No. 6-72: GENERAL ELECTRIC MK 10 MOD 5, Mixed Gas, Closed Circuit, Underwater Breathing Apparatus
c. Report No. 7-72: WESTINGHOUSE CCM-1, Mixed Gas, Closed Circuit, Underwater Breathing Apparatus
General results of these tests concluded that each of the three SCUBAs were satisfactory for employment by Naval Inshore Warfare Forces. The series of tests discussed herein represents a culmination of comparative tests to determine and select a breathing apparatus which could subsequently replace operational scubas now being utilized by U.S. Navy Underwater Demolition and Sea-land-air (SEAL) Teams. The scope of the open sea testing included long distance shallow water swims, deep dives to depths of 160 feet and Swimmer Delivery Vehicle (SDV) operations of six hours in duration. Test results indicated that all of the units tested meet or exceed a six hour operational canister and

gas life requirement. However, some limitations were noted in areas of human engineering, and in compatibility with existing equipments which impose some limitations upon each of the units tested. (Authors' abstract)

798.
HAWKINS, T.L. and T.C. King.
Evaluation of the prototype General Electric model 1500 sensor controlled, closed circuit, mixed gas, underwater breathing apparatus.
U.S. Navy Exp. Diving Unit, Rep NEDU 11-73, 32p. + append. Nov. 1973.

The GE MOD 1500 MBA (General Electric Model 1500 Underwater Breathing Apparatus) is a prototype, closed circuit, mixed gas, diving apparatus independently developed by the General Electric Corporation in response to established operating requirements of Naval Inshore Warfare tactical swimmers. The design goal was to have the UBA meet and/or exceed a desired six hour gas and CO_2 absorbent life support cycle. This project was conducted to determine that the prototype units could meet the design goals and to determine equipment operational capabilities and limitations with respect to general areas of: Operational performance, compatability to existing fleet equipment, reliability (such as could be determined), maintainability and human engineering considerations. A total of 197 hours 48 minutes bottom time was logged in the conduct of these tests. . . . General results of the tests indicate that the prototype equipment is potentially satisfactory for employment by Naval Inshore Warfare Forces. However, several failures were encountered with the equipment which were considered critical in nature, primarily in the electronic design, and should be corrected prior to any further test or procurement action by the Navy. Two separate, but similar prototype units were tested, both having the same inherent functional characteristics. Physical construction of the individual units was varied through "modification update", and differing operational characteristics were noted. For test and reporting purposes, the nomenclature assigned to the equipment was MOD 1500 ALFA and MOD BRAVO. (From authors' abstract)

799.
HAWLEY, S.A.
Electrophoretic separation of conformational states of α-chymotrypsinogen A at high pressures.
Biochim. Biophys. Acta 317(2):236-239; 1973.

When reversible denaturation of chymotrypsinogen is produced at elevated pressures and low temperatures, the transition occurs very slowly. Electrophoretic separation of the transition mixture at high pressures revals the presence of 2 distinct molecular species. This evidence, in conjunction with previously reported spectroscopic data, suggests that a simple 2-state model provides a useful description of the transition phenomena at high pressures. (© BA)

800.
HAYE, E.F.
Underwater imagery by mapping sonar.
In: 1973 Offshore Technology Conference, April/May 1973, Houston, Texas. Preprints, Vol. II, p.265-274. Published by the conference.

This is a discussion of an instrument capable of sea floor mapping with sound waves in a similar fashion to which side looking radar maps the land with radio waves from an airplane. The instrument used is a long range side scan sonar, one developed specifically for geologic mapping of the sea bottom. This particular instrument was developed by Institut Francais du Petrole; the French governmental petroleum research company. It is capable of producing imagery as far as 1/2 mile on each side of a fish towed behind a ship. . . . It is 13 ft long and weighs 2000 lb. In it are mounted transducers that emit sound and receive the echoes from the ocean floor. One pulse is emitted each second. The frequency used is 37-1/2 kilocycles, well out of the range of petroleum seismic sources. Because a much higher frequency is used, the instrument is compatible with marine seismic techniques. The fish can be towed at speeds of up to 10 knots, although the slower speeds of seismic operations are more ideal. . . Sound is emitted in a vertical beam that is 1-1/2 degrees wide on each side of the fish. The vertical sweep can be adjusted from 10 to 30 degrees. In addition to being able to adjust the sweep angle, the look angle of the sweep can also be pointed downward or more horizontally to compensate for changes in water depths. This particular instrument is unique among sonars in that its range is 750 m, or approximately 1/2 mile. (Author)

801.
HAYNES, H.H. and L.F. Kahn.
Behavior of 66-inch concrete spheres under short and long-term hydrostatic loading.
U.S. Nav. Civil Eng. Lab., Rep. NCEL-TR-774, 93p. Sept. 1972.
(AD 748 584)

Fourteen unreinforced concrete and mortar spheres, 66 inches in outside diameter (OD) and 4.125 inches in wall thickness, were subjected to simulated deep-ocean loading conditions. The average short-term implosion pressure for wet concrete spheres was 2,350 psi and for the dry-concrete spheres was 2,810 psi; the average uniaxial compressive strength of the concrete was respectively 7,810 psi and 9,190 psi. Under long-term loading, the concrete spheres failed by static fatigue where the relation between level of sustained pressure and time to implosion was similar to that known for concrete under uniaxial loading. Wet-concrete spheres under seawater pressure as high as 1,670 psi showed an average D'Arcy's permeability coefficient, K sub c, of 10 to the minus 12 power ft/sec; this K sub c value was also similar to that known for concrete under freshwater pressure as high as 400 psi. Design guides were developed to predict the short- and long-term implosion pressures and permeability rates of concrete spheres. (Author) (GRA)

802.
HAYNES, H.H.
Submerged concrete structures.
In: 1973 Offshore Technology Conference, April/May 1973, Houston, Texas. Preprints, Vol. II, p.599-604. Published by the conference.

An overview of the existing technology for submerged, pressure resistant, concrete structures is presented for the offshore engineer. Empirical equations allow predictions of the implosion strength of spherical and cylindrical structures. Other design aspects related to submerged concrete structures such as penetrations, reinforcement, permeability and compressive strength, are also discussed. . . [It is concluded that] the effect of properly designed hull penetrations and conventional steel reinforcement on the strength of concrete structures is negligible. Ocean tests on submerged structures have shown that the permeability of concrete to seawater is not a problem. Sufficient technology exists today for employing concrete for submerged pressure-resistant structures within the depth range of 1000 ft; within the near future, further testing and experience will permit concrete structures to operate at 3000 ft. (Author)

803.
HAYWARD, J.S., M. Collis and J.D. Eckerson.
Thermographic evaluation of relative heat loss areas of man during cold water immersion.
Aerosp. Med. 44:708-711;July 1973.

Infrared thermography was used to provide illustrations of the regional difference of temperature of the surface of the human body before and after immersion in water of 7.5°C for 15 min. Thermal gradients over the surface are increased by cold water immersion, with areas such as the lateral thorax, upper-chest, and groin having the highest temperatures. It is predicted that heat loss in the water would be greatest from such areas and that these findings would be useful in the design of thermally-protective lifejackets and for advice on body posture in the water to minimize heat loss. Swimming activity increased the amount of the body surface having higher relative temperatures, thereby increasing overall heat loss. (Authors' abstract)

804.
HAYWARD, T.
Royal Navy developing saturation diving system for conshelf depths.
Hydrospace 5:22-23;Apr. 1972.

The Royal Navy will use saturation diving techniques to extend its capability to continental shelf depths. Instead of a seated habitat, they will use a surface-supported diving system consisting of two deck decompression chambers, a submersible decompression chamber, and a personnel transfer capsule. Under certain conditions, a lock-out submersible will probably be used. Details of the complex are at present classified information. The ultimate goal is to carry out tasks to depths of 1200 feet. New decompression tables are being evaluated at the Deep Trials Unit, at Alverstoke. (MFW/BSCP)

805.
HAZARD, H.R.
Air pollution and the diver.
In: Battelle Columbus Laboratories. Proceedings, 1973 divers' gas purity symposium, November 27-28, 1973, p.X-1-X-10. U.S. Navy Supervisor Diving, Nav. Ships Syst. Comm., Rep 2-73, 1973.

At the present time, the author knows of no experimental data relating the concentrations of air pollutants in the atmosphere to the concentrations reaching a diver being supplied with compressed air, nor of data on the effects of various pollutants under hyperbaric pressures. In view of current concern with the effects of air pollutants on the general population and upon industrial workers, some research on the potential problems for divers appears warranted. A review of the variation of pollutant concentrations in various cities in the United States shows that air quality is satisfactory everywhere most of the time, but that dangerously high pollutant levels can build up occasionally in any city. Large masses of polluted air can move well out to sea with little dilution under some conditions, consequently affecting off-shore diving operations. Thus, if air pollution proves to be a significant factor affecting divers, the need to monitor air quality and, perhaps, to purify the air supplied to divers should be considered. (Author's conclusion)

806.
HEAVERS, B.A., A.A. Messier, R. Montanti and K.E. Schaefer.
CO_2 effects on acid-base balance in air saturation dives.
U.S. Nav. Submar. Med. Res. Lab., Rep. NSMRL 742, 15p. Apr. 11, 1973.

Blood gas tensions, pH, plasma chloride, sodium and potassium, blood urea, ammonia, and amino acid nitrogen were measured in mature Sprague-Dawley rats at various intervals during and after exposure to pressures equivalent to depth at 50 feet and 60 ft. lasting for 60 and 35 days, respectively. In both experiments, a consistent decrease in pH to values of about 7.30 and a rise in CO_2 tensions to 55-60 mm Hg in the arterial blood were found. Plasma bicarbonate was elevated 5-7 mEq and chloride correspondingly decreased. Plasma potassium was consistently increased in both experiments. These findings indicate the existence of a pronounced respiratory acidosis during the saturation dives to 50 and 60 feet. There is no evidence in the literature which would indicate that, elevated pressures of nitrogen or oxygen, per se; in the ranges observed in these experiments could cause significant acid-base alterations. It must, therefore, be concluded that the increased ambient CO_2 levels in conjunction with the effects of increased oxygen and nitrogen is responsible for the observed changes. When compared with data obtained in rats during acute and chronic hypercapnia, the observed $PaCO_2$, pH, and bicarbonate values correspond to the range of values obtained by exposure to 3% and 5% CO_2. (Authors' abstract)

807.
HECKLY, R.J.
Studies of infections occurring under deep submergence saturated conditions at the Naval Biomedical Research Laboratory.
In: Abstracts of BuMed-ONR sponsored Navywide workshop in high pressure biomedical research, U.S. Submarine Base, Groton, Conn., May 1971, p.15 Published by the Naval Submarine Medical Research Laboratory, 1971.

Abstract only. Entire item quoted: A test chamber system suitable for infecting animals via the respiratory route while under deep submergence hyperbaric pressure conditions has been designed and fabricated. The objectives in design of the hyperbaric system were to provide a controlled environment system with a large central chamber into which small particle size aerosols could be generated and held, and several separate vessels for holding small animals. The system arrangement permits exposure of the animals to the test aerosols and subsequent animal holding for extended periods under maintained pressure conditions. The system has been tested with high helium (97%) gases at 1,000 lb/in^2 and found to leak less than 1% per day. Food and water may be added through air locks and cylinder oxygen is added as required to maintain a partial pressure of 0.2 atmosphere. Oxygen concentration is monitored periodically with a paramagnetic oxygen meter. Carbon dioxide and trace gases are removed with a Baralyme tower and charcoal filter and relative humidity is controlled by recirculating the gas mixture through a chilled surface condenser. Waste is flushed out through air locks. Mice have been held in the system for four weeks without apparent ill effects but infectivity tests have not yet been initiated. Preliminary tests with microbial aerosols indicate that aerosols can be generated by conventional techniques. The concentration of particles can be determined in sites by right angle light scatter measurements and samples of the aerosols can be taken for separate assay of viability and infectivity.

808.
HEIMBECKER, R.O., G. Lemire, I. Koven, K. Richards and W.R. Drucker.
The role of gas embolism in decompression sickness.
Bibl. Anat. 11:488-494; 1973.

Fifty (17%) of animals died of decompression sickness during rapid decompression, and all showed large gas emboli, producing marked embolic obstruction, through all parts of the vascular tree. The remaining animals (83%) survived the severe insult of rapid decompression. There was a marked reduction of tissue perfusion with capillary slowing and statis; intravascular hemoconcentration and red cell agglutination, tissue edema, variable arterial and arteriolar constriction, reaching a peak about 50 min after decompression, and then slowly improving over the next hour. Intravascular gas embolism was rarely observed. Body fluid changes in 13 dogs were followed during compression and decompression, by Cr^{51}, I^{125}, and S^{35}. The latter showing mean increase of ECF volume of 16%, probably due to an increase of interstitial fluid volume. Rapid recompression dramatically improves tissue perfusion but may be incomplete therapy. Measures which would enhance tissue perfusion require further study. The immediate restoration and maintenance of plasma volume with albumin or other plasma expanders may be an important adjunct. Standard decompression tables could be significantly altered by these further therapeutic measures. (Authors' summary)

809.
HEIMBECKER, R.O., I. Koven and K. Richards.
The role of gas embolism in decompression sickness.
In: Ackles, K.N. ed. Blood bubble interaction in decompression sickness. Proceedings of an international symposium held at Defence and Civil Institute of environmental Medicine, Downsview, Ontario, Canada, p.218-226. Published by the Institute, December 1973. (DCIEM Conference Proceedings 73-CP-960).

Fifty (17%) animals died of decompression sickness during rapid decompression, and all showed large gas emboli, producing marked embolic obstruction, through all parts of the vascular tree, but occurring subsequent to a period of red cell agglutination, capillary slowing and stasis. The remaining animals (83%) survived the severe insult of rapid decompression. There was a marked reduction of tissue perfusion with capillary slowing and stasis; intravascular hemoconcentration and red cell agglutination, tissue edema, variable arterial and arteriolar constriction, reaching a peak about 50 min. after decompression, and then slowly improving over the next hour. Intravascular gas embolism was scanty, and late. Body fluid changes in 13 dogs were followed during compression and decompression, by Cr^{51}, I^{125}, and S^{35}. The latter showed mean increase of ECF volume of 16% probably due to an increase of interstitial fluid volume, thus confirming our microscopic observations.Rapid recompression dramatically improved tissue perfusion but may be incomplete therapy. Measures which would enhance tissue perfusion require further study. The immediate restoration and maintenance of plasma volume with albumin or other plasma expanders may be an important adjunct. Standard decompression tables could be significantly altered by these further therapeutic measures. (Authors' summary)

810.
HEISTAD, D.D. and F.M. Abboud.
Response of muscular and cutaneous vessels to stimulation of chemoreceptors by hypoxia and hypercapnic acidosis.
Fed. Proc. 31:392;Mar./Apr. 1972.

Abstract only. Entire item quoted: Stimulation of chemoreceptors by nicotine or cyanide causes constriction in muscular vessels and dilatation in cutaneous vessels (Circ. Res. 27:259, 1970). Experiments were done to determine whether these differential responses are also seen during stimulation of carotid chemoreceptors by hypoxic and hypercapnic blood. Anesthetized dogs were paralyzed and ventilated artificially. The left common carotid artery was perfused, internal carotid artery ligated, and external carotid outflow was returned to the external jugular vein through a Starling resistor to maintain carotid pressure constant. The isolated gracilis muscle and hindpaw were perfused at constant flow, so that changes in perfusion pressure (PP) reflected changes in resistance. Chemoreceptors were stimulated by bubbling nitrogen with CO_2 through the blood perfusing the common carotid, so that PO_2 was increased to 73 ± 5 mm Hg, and pH decreased to 7.13 ± 0.05. Stimulation of carotid chemoreceptors increased muscle PP ($+55 \pm 12$ mm Hg) and decreased paw PP (-10 ± 3 mm Hg). Responses to hypoxia without hypercapnia were less pronounced. Denervation of carotid chemoreceptors abolished the responses. This study indicates that stimulation of carotid chemoreceptors by hypoxia and hypercapnic acidosis causes opposite responses in muscular and cutaneous vascular beds.

811.
HEITKAMP, D.H., R.P. Gruber and M.D. Waters.
Microfiber glass discs, a new support for skin organ cultures.
U.S. Army, Edgewood Arsenal, Rep. EA-TR-4765, 11p. June 1973.
(AD 763 167)

A model system was developed for studies of the direct effects of high pressure oxygen on skin growth and viability. The data demonstrate the feasibility of the system in studies of the effects of hyperoxygenation by exhibiting the toxicity of 100% oxygen under the conditions employed. (Author) (GRA)

812.
HELD, K., L. Symon and N.W.C. Dorsch.
Untersuchungen zue Autoregulation des Hirnkreislaufs. I. Akute druckinduzierte Xunderungen des zerebralen GefaBwiderstandes in Normo- and Hyperkapnie.
[Studies on the atuoregulation of cerebrovascular circulation. I. Acute pressure-induced changes of the cerebral vascular resistance in normo- and hypercapnia].
Z Kardiol. 62:59-74;Jan. 1973.

Pressure induced rapid changes of cerebral blood flow are measures (A) in dogs on the arterial inflow, and (B) in baboons at the venous outflow. The evaluation of the results in "instant" i.-p.-diagrams (A) simulates an increase of cerebral vascular resistance (CVR), which is really caused by an altered pressure/flow relation at the artery, but does not reflect changes of peripheral resistance. In the vascular area of the middle cerebral artery (B) pressure induced changes of CVR beginning after less than one sec. result in an autoregulation within 60-90 seconds. Whereas ischemia abolishes cerebral autoregulation, it is maintained in hypercapnia. The results are discussed as evidence of myogenic vascular reactions, which are "paralyzed" in ischemia. The findings support the suggestion of different mechanisms for the CO_2-reactivity and the autoregulation of cerebral blood flow. (English summary)

813.
HELMREICH, R.
Stress, self-esteem and attitudes.
Austin, Tex., Univ. Tex., Dept. Psychol., Tech. Rep. 12, 24p. Nov. 1970.

The arguments set forth in this paper represent an attempt to tie together several disparate approaches to the study of attitude change. The central assumption is that psychologically stressful situations threaten an individual's self-esteem. This assumption and those derivative from it are based primarily on circumstantial evidence. Although the line of reasoning followed may turn out to be either partly or wholly erroneous, such speculations would still have a desirable outcome if they provoked research aimed specifically at clarifying interactions between stress, arousal, self-esteem and attitude change. Primary emphasis should be placed on isolating relationships between stress and self-esteem. More direct tests of self-esteem-communicator credibility interactions under differing levels of stress should also be performed. Additionally, the effects of nonspecific arousal on communicator credibility need to be assessed. A comprehensive examination of stress and attitude change will involve a program of both field and laboratory studies. Laboratory experimental studies are needed because controlled manipulations which give precise information on causal relationships are essential for the development of theoretical models. But in many areas, particularly the study of stress effects, laboratory research can provide only limited data. In the case of stress, for example, ethical and practical considerations make it impossible to investigate the effects of really severe stress or of prolonged stress (that is, no laboratory manipulation could approximate the levels or duration of stress found in many natural situations such as combat). The investigator concerned with testing the generality and validity of laboratory derived theoretical formulations will be forced into naturalistic research using ongoing social situations. (Author)

814.
HELMREICH, R.
Characteristics of the aquanauts.
In: Miller, J.W., J.G. Van Derwalker, and R.A. Waller, eds. Tektite 2: Scientists-in-the-sea, p.VIII-28-29. Washington, D.C., U.S. Department of the Interior, August 1971.

The aquanauts, as a group, formed a highly qualified and educated population. There were, however, large individual differences in experience and in personality characteristics. In this section, descriptive statistics from the Aquanaut Background Questionnaire and other pre-dive measures are presented to provide an indication of the characteristics of the research group and to show the range of variation present. . . The Allport-Vernon-Lindzey Study of Values (Allport, Vernon and Lindzey, 1960) is a widely used test which measures the relative strength of six major value areas (theoretical, economic, aesthetic, social, political, and religious). . . . the profiles for Tektite scientists and Sea Lab II civilian aquanauts as well as Mt. Everest explorers are almost identical. Scientists undertaking hazardous but professionally rewarding tasks seem to have a similar constellation of values characterized by high theoretical and aesthetic values, low religious values, and average social, economic, and political concerns. Although teams do not differ significantly on background variables, recorded events during childhood and youth are significantly related to individual performance and adjustment underwater. These are discussed. (Author)

815.
HELMREICH, R.
Conclusions and recommendations.
In: Miller, J.W., J.G. Van Derwalker, and R.A. Waller, eds. Tektite 2: Scientists-in-the-sea, p.VIII-59-VIII-62. Washington, D.C., U.S. Department of the Interior, August 1971.

The author summarizes the findings of the behavior and performance aspects of the Tektite 2 experiment. First, it was proven that both male and female aquanauts could adapt successfully to the habitat environment, and could perform even more effectively than under more normal conditions. It is recommended that in programs that are primarily operational, performance standards should be externally imposed. Teams led by a scientist-aquanaut achieved more than those led by engineer-aquanauts. The greater the interrelation between the scientists and the engineers, the more effective the performance. Time spent in sleeping and in leisure were negatively related to performance; however, gregariousness was positively related to performance. The two-way video line seemed effective in reducing feelings of isolation and remoteness from supervisory personnel. Stability of behavior was greater in the long than in the short missions. The Life History Questionnaire has proven to be a most effective predictive instrument. (MFW/BSCP)

816.
HELMREICH, R.
Patterns of aquanaut behavior.
In: Miller, J.W., J.G. Van Derwalker, and R.A. Waller, eds. Tektite 2: Scientists-in-the-sea, p.VIII-30-VIII-45. Washington, D.C., U.S. Department of the Interior, August 1971.

This section describes overall patterns of behavior shown by the ten teams of aquanauts. These data focus on the general patterns of observed behavior in the habitat and also on group differences in behavior across missions. The data are presented in several ways: (1) all ten missions are contrasted using percentage of total mission time spent on each activity as the basis for comparison. In these analyses, missions of different lengths as well as the female and international missions are treated equally; (2) missions of different durations are compared; (3) the reactions of the female crew are related to those of other crews; and (4) relations between scientists and engineers are discussed. (Author)

817.
HELMREICH, R., J. Wilhelm and R. Bakeman.
Prediction of in-habitat behavior.
In: Miller, J.W., J.G. Van Derwalker and R.A. Waller, eds. Tektite 2: Scientists-in-the-sea, p.VIII-30-VIII-59, Washington, D.C., U.S. Department of the Interior, August 1971.

The author discusses the "effectiveness of pre-mission predictive variables in accounting for the actual behavior recorded" during the various missions of Tektite 2. The availability of "continuous, objective, behavioral criteria" makes Tektite 2 a particularly valuable source for the evaluation of predictive measures of performance and adjustment. The principal predictive tool used was the Life History Questionnaire (LHQ), which covered the first 18 years of life. In this discussion, the LHQ variables are related to the criterion of total marine science achievement during the mission. In a very general analysis of the data, it is concluded that members of small families, from small towns, of lower social status, with little religious background or education, and with good academic performance in the elementary grades, tend to become the most effective marine scientists. It was found that first-borns out-performed later-borns, in contrast to findings in Sea Lab. This is explained by the fact that stress was much greater in Sea Lab; where stress is not a factor, first- and only-borns tend to out perform later-borns. Poor health in childhood, followed by heightened physical activity in the teenage years is a characteristic of the top performers. The results of the observations made with the aquanauts, and those made with a very different group of U.S. Navy enlisted men show that certain variables relate to performance in the same degree. It is concluded that the LHQ is a most effective predictive test, applicable both to research into the antecedents of behavior and into selection of candidates for specialized roles. (MFW/BSCP)

818.
HELMREICH, R.
The Tektite 2 human behavior program.
In: Miller, J.W., J.G. Van Derwalker and R.A. Waller, eds. Tektite 2: Scientists-in-the-sea, p.VIII-15-VIII-18, Washington, D.C., U.S. Department of the Interior, August 1971.

The objectives of this program were to study and assess the psychological dynamics of small groups under stress in a hazardous environment. The program was designed to obtain information applicable to crew selection, concepts, and command structure. The data were collected utilizing closed circuit television and open microphones. The results were recorded directly on computer cards. The findings indicated that the techniques used and the criteria applied should provide valuable information with respect to the selection of crews for future under sea and space missions. (Author's abstract)

819.
HELMREICH, R., R. Bakeman and L. Scherwitz.
The behavior observation program Navy-Makai dive.
Austin, Tex., Univ. Tex., Dept. Psychol., Rep. TR-19, 9p. Mar. 1972.
(AD 758 080)

Technical problems prevented the acquisition of sufficient data for a statistical analysis of in-habitat behavior and its relationship to performance. The methodology employed seems highly flexible and easily adaptable to a number of settings and uses. It is recommended that observational programs be continued in subsequent saturation missions and that consideration be given to applying the methodology to other habitability and performance evaluations. (GRA)

820.
HELMREICH, R. and R. Bakeman.
The life history questionnaire as a predictor of performance in Navy diver training.
J. Appl. Psychol. 57:148-153;Apr. 1973.

A new demographic instrument, the Life History Questionnaire (LHQ) is described. The LHQ elicits demographic data longitudinally providing a question-by-year matrix of responses. Variables derived from the LHQ both for prediction and as a research tool is discussed. (Authors' abstract)

821.
HEMMINGS, C.C.
Diving in relation to fish behaviour studies.
In: Diving applications in marine research. Proceedings of a seminar, National Institute of Oceanography, Godalming, Surrey, U.K., December 1971, p.48-67. Published by the Institute. 1972.

The use of diving methods in most branches of science, including the behavioural sciences is only one of a number of available techniques. Because underwater endurance is usually limited by air supply, decompression, water temperature or a combination of all three, the actual time spent under water is short in relation to that spent in pre-dive preparation or subsequent analysis of results. It is therefore essential so to plan and organize this limited time under water as to produce the maximum possible yield of useful information. In studies of fish behaviour, diving is used in two ways. The first is making of simple observations of fish behaviour in the natural environment. These may lead on either to laboratory experiments designed to investigate alternative possible explanations of observed behaviour, or to the second use of diving, in which the setting up or conducting of experiments goes on under water. This paper provides brief examples of ways in which diving has been used in fish behaviour research, and a more detailed description of the investigation of fish behaviour in relation to one type of fishing gear. [It is noted in closing that the use of closed circuit breathing apparatus, which eliminates the bubbles that alarm the fish and interfere with their normal behavior, has made the role of the diver in these studies more important. It has also made much more stringent demands on the degree of knowledge and experience required of divers operating in this area of investigation]. (Author)

822.
HEMPLEMAN, H.V.
Human problems of open sea diving.
In: Diving applications in marine research. Proceedings of a seminar, National Institute of Oceanography, Godalming, Surrey, U.K., December 1971, p.119-126. Published by the Institute. 1972.

The author discusses gas that may be substituted for nitrogen at depths at which nitrogen is narcotic. Neon has been proven by experiments to be non-narcotic at depths up to 1200 fsw, but is prohibitively expensive. Hydrogen presents a possibility, but its explosive quality has prevented (at this time of writing) much experimentation. Helium has been the gas most used. The two main variables are the oxygen and carbon dioxide partial pressures. It has been found difficult to design monitoring apparatus that will be reliable under high pressure. [A tragic example is the Johnson-Sea Link failure]. Heat loss and communication problems with helium mixtures are discussed. Depth limits, decompression schedules, and compression rates are discussed in a general way, with the observation that slow compression seems to be the answer to some of the problems involved in diving to great (1500 ft) depths. During the discussion considerable attention is given to the problem of heat loss, and the death occurring during preparation for Sea Lab III is attributed partly to the fact that the diver had not sufficiently rewarmed before making a second deep dive. The techniques of heating breathing mixtures, and of heating suits are briefly discussed. The electrically heated suit is considered here to be the best solution. (MFW/SCD)

823.
HEMPLEMAN, H.V.
The site of origin of gaseous emboli produced by decompression from raised pressures of air and other gases.
In: Fructus, X., ed. Third international conference on hyperbaric and underwater physiology, p.160-162. Paris, Doin, 1972.

Dead female Wistar rats were compressed at 50 psi/min and decompressed at a rate of 15 psi/min, and the main blood vessels then examined for bubbles. In two sets of experiments, animals were compressed to 100 psig on air for periods of 1, 3, 4 and 5½ hours, and on helium for periods of 1 hour, ½ hour, 15 minutes and 8 minutes. One striking result was the absence of bubbles in the pulmonary vein at all times; another was the fact that when few bubbles were present on the whole, they were always present in the aortic arch, the thoracic aorta, and the abdominal aorta; a third was the presence of bubbles in the helium experiments even at 8 minute exposure, and their absence in hour-long exposures in air. The author discusses these findings and speculates upon their relationship to bubble formation in live animals. He states that it is important to establish "whether the bronchial circulation is the most susceptible body situation for bubble formation." (MFW/UMS)

824.
HENDERSON, J.V. and E.H. Lanphier.
The effects of 7.8 ATA air on the intracellular action potential of the frog sartorius muscle.
In: Aerospace Medical Association. 1973 annual scientific meeting, Las Vegas, Nevada, May 1973. Preprints, p.271-272. Published by the Association, 1973.

Neurological effects seen in high pressure environments may be ultimately attributable to alteration of membrane function in excitable cells. Techniques of intracellular electro-physiology allow direct assessment of membrane function and permit investigation of pressure effects at the cellular level. The action of increased air pressures on the resting and action potentials was studied in frog muscle fibers. Because of expected interactions of pressure and temperature, electrical activity was observed as a function of both variables. . . . This preliminary investigation has shown the feasibility of using microelectrode techniques for electrophysiological studies at increased pressures. Also, significant changes in excitable membrane function have been demonstrated at moderate pressures. It must be noted, however, that this study has not distinguished between possible effects of pressure per se, effects of elevated partial pressures of nitrogen or oxygen, or effects that might arise from combinations of these factors. (Authors)

825.
HENDERSON, N.C., R.J. Eiber, S.C. Ford, W.I. Griffith and D.W. Strauch.
Evaluation of new aluminum gas cylinders for use with the swimmer delivery vehicle.
Columbus, Ohio, Battelle Lab., Final rep. on contract N00014-70-C-0072, 68p. July 1973.
(AD 767 328/8 GA)

A program was conducted to determine the basic performance characteristics for a limited number of new aluminum gas cylinders for use with the Swimmer Delivery Vehicle. This research consisted of five major tasks: virgin burst experiments, cyclic fatigue experiments, computer analysis of existing alternate design configuration, extended time low temperature creep experiments, and buoyancy experiments. It was concluded that the (specified) operating pressure was significantly higher relative to the observed cylinder burst pressures when compared to the operating pressure to burst pressure ratios normally encountered in diving gas cylinders. It was recommended, therefore, that the operating pressure be reduced to 1500 psig. It was further recommended that the cylinders be inspected for cracks every six months or 100 cycles due to the localized high stresses discovered in the end cap. (Authors) (GRA)

826.
HENKENER, J.A. and D.E. Adkins.
An approach to the design of shipboard breathing gas systems.
In: The working diver, 1972. Symposium proceedings, February 1972, Columbus, Ohio, p.23-51. Washington, D.C., Marine Technology Society, 1972.

This paper describes a six-step approach to the design of shipboard breathing gas systems. [The steps are: (1) review ship's diving mission requirements; (2) establish maximum diving operations; (3) calculate storage volume and flow; (4) lay out gas distribution system; (5) calculate line sizes; (6) select gas and air flasks, compressors and mixing components.] It is intended as a guideline for design engineers to use in creating an adequate gas system capable of supporting the required diving operations. The information should also be useful to operational planners in establishing gas volume and flow requirements for various operating conditions. (Authors' abstract modified by MFW/BSCP)

827.
HENNESSY, T.R.
The equivalent bulk-diffusion model of the pneumatic decompression computer.
Med. Biol. Eng. 11:135-137;Mar. 1973.

It is shown that the pneumatic-decompression computer is essentially an analogue of the bulk-diffusion equation into a rectangular slab of tissue. The empirical parameters of the instrument have been used to match the nearest equivalent diffusion time scale which appears longer than that determined by Hempleman (1969) and Hills (1969). The equivalent diffusion coefficient is a linear function of the pressure with consequent faster gas uptake than elimination on a dive. (Author's abstract)

828.
HENRY, F.C.
Hyperbaric problems as they relate to divers.
Trans. Amer. Acad. Ophthalmol. Otolaryngol. 75:1322-1332;Nov./Dec. 1971.

The author reaches the following conclusions: Nitrogen bubbles always form during decompression with certain time and depth quotients; proper decompression eliminates most bubbles, but subclinical bubbles persist for as long as 24 hours. They start out small, and increase in size as they move with the flow of blood. The pulmonary vasculature is capable of absorbing a large number of bubbles, thus preventing them from reaching the heart. Recompression does not completely eliminate bubbles. The sheep is a satisfactory experimental animal. In recent experiments with sheep, the U.S. Navy decompression tables proved inadequate. Data and tables derived from sheep experiments should be more than safe for man. Bubbles do not occur in arterial circulation until extreme conditions are reached. Debubbling after saturation requires 24 hours. Exercise and massage may eliminate bubbles formed in tissue. Oxygen inhalation can cut decompression time in half, by preventing further intake of nitrogen during decompression; also, by some mechanism not yet understood, it aids in elimination of bubbles. (Author's conclusions abbreviated by MFW/BSCP)

829.
HENRY, F.C.
Physical examination of scuba divers.
Northwest Med. 72:133-138;Mar. 1973.

The author lists in Table 1 the physiological problems encountered during descent, those encountered at depth, and those encountered on ascent. In Table 2 are listed contraindications: obesity, cardiovascular disease, ENT disorders, marked visual abnormalities, genito-urinary disease, disqualifying dental problems, disabling skin disorder, marked musculo-skeletal abnormalities, chronic systemic disease (diabetes, chronic gastro intestinal disorders, etc.), respiratory disease, drug or alcohol addiction. A candidate over 40 requires special evaluation. The following laboratory tests are recommended: chest X-ray (essential); glucose tolerance test when indicated; EEG and ECG when indicated; oxygen tolerance test (60 feet for ½ hour on O_2 in a chamber) if diver is to make deep dives or pure oxygen dives. (MFW/UMS)

830.
HERRERO ALDAMA, P.
El EEG de las hipoxias hipoxicas e hiperoxicas en medicina de aviacion y subacuatica.
[The EEG of the hypoxic and hyperoxic hypoxias in aviation and submarine medicine].
Arch. Neurobiol. (Madrid) 36:31-46;Jan./Feb. 1973.

In this review of the literature, the hypoxia of pilots is classified in four categories: (1) due to a diminution of the O_2 content or of its partial pressure (anoxic or hypoxic hypoxia); (2) due to a defect in the mechanism of transport (anemic); (3) due to diminution in the velocity of transport (stagnation); and (4) due to inability of the tissues to utilize the oxygen brought to them (histotoxic). Hyperoxic anoxia is incuded in this category. The central nervous system (CNS) symptomatology of acute hypoxic hypoxia is discussed as are alterations in physiopathology revealed by animal experimentation at high altitudes. After discussing high altitude hypoxia, the authors deal with problems of deep diving (365 meters). Theories are mentioned to explain the effects (including death) resulting from hyperoxia. The relation of oxygen tension to the bioelectric activity of the cerebral cortex is given consideration. Hyperventilation produces a diminution of CO_2, or hypocapnia, which is known to be an important factor in the development of slow waves in the EEG. In hypoxic states the EEG has registered synchronization and activation of the alpha waves, subdelta waves in the vertex, delta waves with sensorial block, predominantly frontal of the slow waves, with recuperation of the human subjects upon resumption of breathing normal air. Hyperbaric chamber studies are cited as regards EEG reactions. Recent studies employing evoked potentials have revealed a reduction of the N_1, P_2 component of the auditory evoked response of the cat and also of man under hyperbaric conditions. This is interpreted as being due to an action on the polysynaptic system of the cortical mantle and elsewhere. Animal experiments on the effects of different O_2 mixtures on electrical activity of different parts of the CNS (cauddal nucleus, intralaminar nucleus of the thalamus; cortex and subcortex of the thalamus, mesencephalon and pontine structures) under hyperbaric conditions are discussed. It is concluded that the genesis of certain changes observed in EEG tracings under hyperbaric conditions might be considered a functional disturbance of biochemical nature, without constant origin, but in which the subcortical structures appear to have an important role. (ART/SCD)

831.
HERRON, J.M., H.A. Saltzman,B.A. Hills and J.A. Kylstra.
Differences between inspired and expired minute volumes of nitrogen in man.
J. Appl. Physiol. 35:546-551;Oct. 1973.

To test the reported production of nitrogen gas (N_2) by man, the differences between inspired and expired N_2 volumes were measured; each N_2 volume was calculated as the product of total gas volume, determined by spirometry, and the volume fraction (FN_2), determined by gas chromatography. During exposure to 79% helium and 21% oxygen, the maximal computed error of $\dot{V}N_2$ was reduced to approximately 2.0 ml min^{-1} STPD at rest as a consequence of lowering the FIN_2 to 0.0015, in comparison to an error of 100 ml min^{-1} STPD when breathing air. Measurements were obtained before and after the ingestion of 36 g protein, while the subjects were resting (n = 27) or performing work (n = 16). As anticipated, $\dot{V}EN_2$ was initially greater than $\dot{V}IN_2$, as a result of washout of body nitrogen stores. The initial range for $\dot{V}EN_2$ - $\dot{V}IN_2$ was -0.1 to 4.4 ml min^{-1} STPD at rest and -2.8 to 7.7 ml min^{-1} STPD during work. Values for $\dot{V}EN_2$ - $\dot{V}IN_2$ were clearly less during the latter portion of each exposure (0.23-0.87 ml min^{-1} STPD after 12 hr), and were not discernibly affected by the ingestion of protein. These findings indicate that metabolic production of N_2 gas by man, if present, is less than the error of conventional experimental techniques. (Authors' abstract)

832.
HERVEY, G.R.
The physiology of cold/wet survival.
In: Cold/wet survival symposium. J. Roy. Nav. Med. Serv. 58:161-170;Winter 1972.

The physiology and effectiveness of the body's thermoregulatory mechanisms are studied. The working of the control system is discussed and its effects demonstrated. The general effect of this thermoregulation on the likelihood of survival is considered, together with the principles of treatment for those suffering from immersion or exposure. (Author's abstract)

833.
HESSER, C.M. and D. Linnarsson.
First annual scientific meeting of the European Undersea Biomedical Society.
Forsvarsmedicin 9:235-529;July 1973.

The meeting consisted of the following sessions: (1) Current Swedish activities in diving research. (2) Oxgyen, hydrogen and inert gases. (3) Ventilation, circulation and gas exchange. (4) Workshop on ethical considerations in hyperbaric research. (5) Workshop on labyrinth disturbances in diving. (6) Performance, heat exchange. (7) Hydrostatic pressure, inert gas exchange and decompression. Specific papers will be found under the following author entries: Adolfson, J.A., L. Fagraeus and C.M. Hesser; Adolfson, J.A. and C. Lindemark; Ardashnikova, L.I. and G.N. Evstropova; Bachrach, A.J. and P.B. Bennett; Balldin, U.I.; Balouet, G., L. Barthelemy, J. Chouteau, J. Corriol, E. Girin, J. LeChuiton, A. Michaud and J. Parc; Balouet, G., L. Barthelemy and A. Belaud; Barnard, E.E.P. and R. de G. Hanson; Barnard, E.E.P., R. de G. Hanson, B.J. Reid and J. Williams; Bennett, P.B. and D.G. Blenkarn; Bennett, P.B. and J.A. Kylstra; Bonnet, M., J. Chouteau, M. Hugon, C. Imbert and J.P. Roll; Broussolle, B., F. Brue, A. Chaumont, R. Hyacinthe, D. Monget and B. Pineau; Broussolle, B., R. Hyacinthe, G. Mainart, J.F. Stoltz and F. Streiff; Buhlmann, A.A.; Burgess, D.W. and A.N. Dossett; Charpy, J.P., J.P. Deyts and P. Wide; Coles, R.R.A.; Conti, V. and R. Sciarli; Conti, V. and G. Segui; Cox, P.T.; Dahlback, G.O. and C.E.G. Lundgren; Demard, F.; Deroanne, R., J. Dujardin, M. Lamy, R. Marechal, J.M. Petit and F. Pirnay; Edmonds, C.; Eklund, B., L. Kaijser and A. Melcher; Fagraeus, L., J. Haggendal and D. Linnarsson; Fagraeus, L. and D. Linnarsson; Fagraeus, L. and D. Linnarsson; Fant, G.; Farmer, J.C., Jr. and W.G. Thomas; Fructus, X., R. Lescure and R. Sciarli; Fust, H.D., K.G. Muller, H. Oser and S. Ruff; Guenard, H., J. Timbal, P. Varene and H. Vieillefond; Issaakjan, L.A., G.V. Troshikin and A.G. Zhironkin; Kirkness, C.M. and A.G. MacDonald; Krol, J.P.; Kurenkov, H.; Lang, J. and I. Rozsahegyi; LeMaire, C., H. Monod and J.C. Rostain; Lundgren, C.; Miller, J.N. and M. Winsborough; Muren, A.; Obrist, W.D., H.A. Saltzman, I.A. Sulg, L.W. Thompson and R.E. Townsend; Rockert, H.; Rostain, J.C.; Thornstedt, H.; Tjernstrom, O. It should be noted that in each case the authors are listed alphabetically rather than by seniority. (MFW/BSCP)

834.
HESTER, R.
Provisional medical statistics for personnel attached to nuclear powered submarines: FY 66-69.
U.S. Nav. Submar. Med. Cent., Rep. NSMRL 674, 56p. 1971.

A statistical summary of admissions to the sick list and deaths among personnel attached to nuclear powered submarines during fiscal years 1966-69 inclusive is reported. Data were obtained by search of Navy Bureau of Medicine and Surgery ADP tape files; and in view of the file search procedure certain admissions to the sick list, notably admissions to non-naval medical facilities, are missing. Compared to Navy and Marine Corps service-wide experience for corresponding years the hospitalization rates for the submariners were very low; and in general preliminary findings were negative. Possible implications of these data with respect to prolonged exposure to the nuclear powered submarine environment upon crew health are explored. (© BA)

835.
HEYDER, E.
Studies of calcium and inorganic phosphorus levels in plasma and erythrocytes during acute and chronic hypercapnia.
U.S. Nav. Submar. Med. Cent., Rep. NSMRL 702, 29p. Feb. 29, 1972.

To ascertain the effects of acute and chronic hypercapnia on blood levels of calcium and inorganic phosphorus, guinea pigs were exposed to 1%, 3% and 15% CO_2 for various periods up to seven days. Plasma and erythrocyte calcium and inorganic phosphorus and serum ionized calcium were determined. Blood from submariners on FBM patrol, exposed up to 1% CO_2 for three weeks and followed by one week recovery, was analyzed for plasma electrolytes and erythrocyte calcium. The serum ionized calcium of guinea pigs during acute exposure to each concentration of CO_2 shows a pH dependent inverse relationship of a 4.5-5% change per 0.1 unit pH change. During chronic hypercapnia, elevation of total plasma calcium and depression of inorganic phosphorus in those animals exposed to 3% and 15% CO_2 would suggest increased parathyroid function. In those guinea pigs exposed to 1% CO_2, a depressed total plasma calcium in the presence of increased serum ionized calcium is interpreted as suggesting a possible functional hypoparathyroidism. In the guinea pigs, increases in erythrocyte calcium and inorganic phosphorus and plasma inorganic phosphorus accompanied by a decrease in total plasma calcium, during the acute phase of respiratory acidosis, are interpreted as pH dependent inhibition of active transport and/or increase in membrane permeability. In the submariners exposed to up to 1% CO_2, both total plasma calcium and inorganic phosphorus tended to decrease although the changes did not become significant. Erythrocyte calcium, however, increased gradually and became significant after three weeks' exposure. This finding suggests inhibition of active transport and/or increase in red cell permeability to calcium. After one week recovery in air, the erythrocyte calcium had returned to control levels. (Author's abstract)

836.
HEYDER, E. and D.V. Tappan.
Mineral and electrolyte responses following severe decompression stress.
U.S. Nav. Submar. Med. Res. Lab., Rep. NSMRL 743, 8p. plus append. May 3, 1973.

Blood and urinary minerals and electrolytes, and urinary hydroxyproline from adult male rats were measured for periods up to five days following compression and severe decompression, (neither explosive, resulting in 100% mortality, nor "completely safe", giving no symptoms). During the first hour after acute decompression stress, serum ionized calcium and inorganic phosphorous increased and sodium decreased. Within one day, ionized calcium, as well as total calcium, decreased and continued to do so throughout the three-day post-dive study period. Serum sodium returned to control levels by the third day whereas inorganic phosphorus, which had returned toward control levels during post-dive days one and two, experienced a second rise at the end of three days. No significant changes occurred in serum potassium or chloride. Total urinary excretion of sodium, potassium, calcium, phosphorus and hydroxyproline became depressed below control values one day following severe decompression. This period was followed by a general rebound effect by the third day post-dive. By the fifth day, calcium and hydroxyproline again fell while sodium excretion continued to increase. The one-hour-serum and one-day-urinary mineral and electrolyte changes resulting from severe decompression are interpreted as adrenal cortical responses to the dysbaric stress and reflect a post-stress hemoconcentration. The subsequent mineral and electrolyte changes away from control values seem to represent rebound effects resulting from the interaction of recurring hemoconcentration episodes and the tendency of metabolic processes to move toward an equilibrium. These findings reinforce observations that several days are required for the re-establishment of homeostasis following decompression stress. (Authors' abstract)

837.
HEYDER, E. and D.V. Tappan.
Excretion of minerals and nitrogen metabolites following exosure to increased air pressures (2 or 7 ATA).
U.S. Nav. Submar. Med. Res. Lab., Rep. NSMRL 765, 9p. Oct. 10, 1973.

Urinary minerals, electrolytes, nitrogen metabolites, and steroids were measured in Navy divers following exposure to air at 2 and 7 ATA for 45 minutes. Total urinary excretion of osmoles, sodium, potassium, calcium, phosphorus, urea nitrogen, uric acid, creatinine, keto- and ketogenic steroids were depressed below control values during the first day following exposure to either 2 or 7 ATA. The mineral and electrolyte changes are related to reduction in urine volume, which may result from an anti-diuretic hormone (ADH) mediated response to a hypovolemia induced by dysbaric stress. Although a general rebound effect began to occur by the second post-dive day, a continued depression of uric acid, creatinine, and ketosteroids throughout four days of observation suggests a prolonged period of recovery from diving. Increasing excretion of hydroxyproline for several days by those men exposed to 7 ATA, implies a latent response in the metabolism of cartilage and bone to this stress. (Author's abstract)

838.
HIGH, W.L.
Submersibles for marine biological research.
Seattle, Wash., Nat. Mar. Fish. Serv., NOAA-71100713, 5p. 1971.
(COM 72 10929)
(Also published in Proceedings of the IEEE Engineering in the Ocean Environment conference, 1971, p.37-40)

Submersibles provide a direct means of studying the living ocean resources. Basic submersible types include bathyscaphs, bathyspheres, tethered propelled subs and selfcontained subs. Biological scientists require a submersible that is stable, can pinpoint and maintain its position, has variable speed with long endurance and provide excellent viewing and data monitoring systems. Few existing subs meet these needs. Subs can be used to monitor resources not available to other sampling gear, observe relationships of animals to their environment, and determine characteristics of conventional sampling gear. Sophisticated support vessels and diver lockout features will improve the versatility of new generation submersibles. (Author) (GRA)

839.
HIGH, W.L., I.E. Ellis, W.W. Schroeder and G. Loverich.
Evaluation of the undersea habitats — Tektite II, Hydro-Lab, and Edalhab — for scientific saturation diving programs.
Helgolander Wiss. Meeresunters 24(1-4):16-44; 1973.

The assessment of three undersea habitats — Tektite, Hydro-Lab and Edalhab — is based primarily upon the experience of the authors during a total of 62 man-days under saturation diving conditions while conducting biological research programs. A number of desirable and undesirable features were found in each habitat system; none of the individual systems included all of the desirable features. The paper discusses advantages and disadvantages of various features of the habitats including work and living areas, support equipment and techniques, operations and safety. The authors offer their experiences and suggestions to contribute to improvement of habitats and undersea diving operations. (Authors' summary)

840.
HILDEBRAND, C.E. and E.C. Pollard.
Hydrostatic pressure effects on protein synthesis.
Biophys. J. 12:1235-1250; 1972.

The effect of high hydrostatic pressure on several phases of cell-free protein synthesis have been examined. The initial rate of polyuridylic acid (poly U)-directed synthesis of polyphenylalanine showed an apparent increase at 100 atm, above which the synthetic rate was reduced sharply with increased pressure up to 640 atm where 95% inhibition was observed. The magnitude of the inhibition of polyphenylalanine synthesis with increased pressure depended strongly on the magnesium salt concentration in the reaction system. Misreading of the poly U message, as measured by insertion of leucine in place of phenylalanine, dropped rapidly with increased pressure from 1 to 350 atm. above which the amount of misreading increased. Enzymatic activation of transfer RNAs (tRNAs) was reduced by increased pressure in the range 100-640 atm, where the rate of tRNA aminoacylation was 80% inhibition. Both nonenzymatic attachment of phenylalanyl-tRNA (phe-tRNA) to the poly U-ribosome complex and stability of the phe-tRNA-poly U-ribosome complex were decreased at high pressures (100-900 atm). The results of the action of pressure on the various phases of cell-free protein synthesis suggest that the major pressure-sensitive element in the protein synthetic machinery is the ribosome. (Authors' abstract)

841.
HILL, G.B. and S. Osterhout.
Experimental effects of hyperbaric oxygen on selected clostridial species. I and II.
J. Infect. Dis. 125:17-35;Jan. 1972.

The in-vitro effect of hyperbaric oxygen (HBO) on clostridia was investigated for evaluation of HBO therapy for clostridial infection. Log-phase bacteria in solid medium or broth were exposed to various pressures of O_2 (usually 3 atmospheres absolute pressure); bacterial inactivation was quantitated by anaerobic incubation and viable counts. Hyperbaric oxygen was bactericidal for Clostridium perfringens. Clostridium novyi, Clostridium histolyticum, and Clostridium tetani were similarly sensitive to O_2, but Clostridium bifermentans and Clostridium septicum were more resistant. Spore suspensions of C. perfringens, C. histolyticum, and C. bifermentans were resistant to 18 hr of O_2 at 3 atmospheres absolute pressure. Whole blood partially blocked the inactivation of C. perfringens in HBO. The basis for this protection was the enzymatic destruction of H_2O_2 by catalase. Other clostridia were not protected to the same extent by catalase, suggesting that they might be more sensitive to H_2O_2 or to other inactivating effects of HBO. (Authors' abstract)

842.
HILL, G.B.
Hyperbaric oxygen exposures at 3 and 4 atmospheres absolute pressure for experimental gas gangrene: succinate protection against oxygen toxicity.
Antimicrob. Agents Chemother. 2:384-389;Nov. 1972.

The concurrent effect of succinate administration to protect against oxygen toxicity and of hyperbaric oxygen (HBO) exposures to treat model gas gangrene in mice was tested to determine whether succinate would interfere with the therapeutic efficacy of HBO. HBO (seven 90-min exposures) at 3 atmospheres absolute pressure (ATA) had been shown to reduce significantly the mortality of mice injected with Clostridium perfringens suspended in 10 ug of adrenalin. When succinate was tested with this system, mortality of HBO-exposed infected animals was again significantly reduced (79% control mortality versus 17% HBO-exposed mortality), indicating that succinate does not interfere with the action of HBO. Exposures to 4 ATA of O_2 were evaluated in the same model clostridial infection with succinate used to prevent oxygen toxicity. Five 30-min exposures at 4 ATA reduced the mortality of infected animals (62% control versus 6% HBO-exposed mortality). Intraperitoneal succinate injections (10 mmoles/kg) were given 20 to 25 min prior to four of the seven 3-ATA exposures and before three of the five 4-ATA exposures. The intermittent succinate injections gave significant protection against the development of oxygen toxicity in infected and noninfected mice at both O_2 pressures. These studies support the potential clinical use of succinate or other oxygen-protective agents (i) to shorten HBO exposure times by using higher pressures to deliver the necessary O_2 dose, (ii) to increase the O_2 dose for difficult clinical situations by using maximal exposures at 4 ATA or more prolonged exposures at 2 or 3 ATA, and (iii) to continue HBO exposures in patients who require treatment but develop symptoms of oxygen toxicity. (Author's abstract)

843.
HILL, P.M.
Hyperventilation, breath holding and alveolar oxygen tensions at the breaking point.
Resp. Physiol. 19:201-209;Nov. 1973.

The influence of hyperventilation on subsequent breath holding was investigated in eight male subjects. Breath holding was performed after normal breathing and after 8, 16 and 24 vital capacity breaths taken at a rate of 24 per minute both at 1 ATA and during simulated "dives" produced by rapid compression and decompression to and from 2 ATA in a dry pressure chamber. Measurements were made of expired volume during hyperventilation; inspired and expired volumes of the breath held; PAO_2 and $PACO_2$ at the beginning and end of breath holding; and the duration of breath holding. Each of these measurements produced a wide scatter of results. The PAO_2 at the breaking point fell as hyperventilation increased but the extent of the fall was unpredictable. In one subject, hyperventilation produced dangerous hypoxia without significantly increasing the duration of apnoea. The results suggest that it is not possible to determine a "safe" level of hyperventilation that will permit a breath-hold diver to increase the duration of his dive without risking loss of consciousness from cerebral hypoxia. (Author's abstract)

844.
HILL, T.A.
The hyperbaric toxicity of sulfur dioxide.
In: Abstracts of BuMed-ONR sponsored Navywide research in high pressure biomedical research, U.S. Submarine Base, Groton, Conn., May 1971. p.44. Published by the Naval Submarine Medical Research Laboratories, 1971.

Abstract only. Entire item quoted: Although much work has been done on the toxicity of "inert" or noble gases under hyperbaric conditions, there is little information on the in vivo effect of toxic gases under pressure. Previous studies with CO, an asphyxiant, have indicated that there is no difference in toxicity at 1 and 8 atm absolute (ata). In the present study, male Sprague-Dawley derived rats were exposed for four hours to SO_2 at 1 and 8 ata to evaluate the pressure-related response to an irritant gas. Oxygen partial pressure was automatically controlled at 160 ± 10 mmHg, and chamber temperature was regulated to provide a nonstressful thermal environment. Carbon dioxide and humidity were controlled by a constant purge of the chamber with the exposure mixture. There was no significant difference between the four hour L050 expressed as mg/m^3 at 1 and 8 ata. These data support the hypothesis that within the range of pressures studies a constant mass concentration of toxic contaminant elicits a response independent of the total environmental pressure, provided partial pressure of oxygen is maintained constant throughout the pressure range.

845.
HILLS, B.A.
Studies underlying the computation of diving tables.
In: Abstracts of BuMed-ONR sponsored Navywide research in high pressure biomedical research, U.S. Submarine Base, Groton, Conn., May 1971, p.39. Published by the Naval Submarine Medical Research Laboratories, 1971.

Abstract only. Entire item quoted: The author's work is primarily concerned with the fundamental aspects of decompression sickness which can be conveniently classified into several vital issues underlying the computation of diving tables. The most important concerns the separation of the gas phase from solution during an asymptomatic decompression. Recent success has been obtained using inductometric methods to detect finely-dispersed extra-vascular gas as a change in electrical conductance monitored without electrodes and the associated interfacial problems. Indirect methods for elucidating the physical state of the tissue during decompression include a quantitative study of 'surface excursion' diving and surface decompression. These results cast further doubts upon the popular assumption of a critical degree of super-saturation in tissue as conventionally expressed by a decompression ration. The work has also indicated a means of selecting type I or type II bends as the marginal symptoms induced by 'titrating' decompression time, so providing a convenient model for studying the treatment of C.N.S. symptoms. Studies directed at the mechanism for aspetic bone necrosis in divers have included measurements of intramedullary pressure and direct estimations of bone blood flow during all phases of hyperbaric exposure. It has been shown that sealed bones are effective osmometers and that nitrogen can induce osmosis across articular cartilage — a fact which may explain hyperbaric arthralgia. So far, it would appear that the compression is as likely to cause bone lesions as the decompression. An intensive study of gas-induced osmosis has revealed that it is active *in vivo* and can correlate the narcotic potency of many inert gases. Preliminary trials indicate that it may also play a role in oxygen toxicity — particularly in lung. Separate ventilation of the two lungs of the same animal with normoxic mixtures of N_2 versus N_2O have shown a relative hydration of the lung acting as a source for the more soluble gas.

846.
HILLS, B.A.
The driving force for inert gas elimination during decompression.
In: Abstracts of the Twenty-fifth Congress of Physiological Sciences Satellite Symposium. Recent progress in fundamental physiology of diving, Marseille, France, July 1971. p.60-62. (Proceedings unpublished)

Abstract only. Excerpt quoted: An overall review of the experimental evidence leaves little doubt that the gas phase is present during a conventional asymptomatic decompression, the relevant physical condition being one of phase equilibration in at least one fully-nucleated micro-region rather than supersaturation. This raises the question of what driving force there can be for the elimination of inert gas from such "equilibrated" zones. Analyses of subcutaneous gas pockets and total tension in rigid cavities suggest that O_2 and CO_2 remain at essentially normal venous values, PVO_2 and $PVCO_2$ respectively, in gas separated from solution in tissue. A simple pressure balance can then be applied to derive the driving force (Δp) for inert gas elimination from that separated gas in a man breathing a mixture of inert fraction x at an absolute pressure P as: $\Delta p = (1\text{-}x)P - PVO_2 - PVCO_2 - PW + \delta$ where PW is body water vapour pressure and δ is a small "mechanical" term to allow for elastic deformation of tissue and any surface tension effects. The above expression implies a greater driving force at greater pressure (P) and hence an overall redistribution of decompression time towards deeper stops than employed in conventional Naval tables.

847.
HILLS, B.A.
Chemical engineering principles in medicine and biology.
Br. Chem. Eng. 16:700-703;Aug. 1971.

Engineering principles underly the function of many organs — a realization which is just starting to be appreciated by the more progressive universities and research institutes. In this respect the chemical engineers are late starters yet, in the end, their contribution could be far greater than that of their colleagues. . . Each tissue is effectively a fixed-bed reactor in which the gross distribution of reagents and the collection of products is effected by the circulation. The blood controls the supply of solutes necessary for the interstitial fluid to provide the environment ideal for the well-being of the cells to which metabolism is confined. This process can take a great many biochemical pathways with innumerable reagents, products and intermediates, but molecular oxygen is invariably necessary and carbon dioxide produced. Thus the gas transport aspect is termed 'tissue respiration' and can be studied in excised sections severed from their blood supply and exposed to gaseous oxygen. . . It has proved most rewarding to regard these sections as heterogeneous reactors in which the biochemist's data refer only to the medium within the cells. A chemical engineering analysis of this type in which allowance is made for the purely physical processes such as diffusion in each phase, has provided a better correlation of experimental data and provided a simply physical explanation for an effect which biologists have termed 'active transport of oxygen' . . . Reactor models can also be used to determine transient distribution of inert gases in tissue following change in the partial pressure of that gas in the breathing mixture. . . The reactor model can thus be used to estimate both the steady-state assimilation of oxygen by tissue as well as the transient accumulation of inert gas upon compression of an individual. Thus the total gas tension distribution throughout the tissue can be calculated and hence the imminence of cavitation occurring during decompression. This has led the writer to propose a method of decompressing divers and caisson workers totally unlike that published in standard Naval tables based effectively upon the simple stirred-tank concept in which only inert gases are considered relevant. The 'reactor' model has produced tables which have enabled total decompression times to be reduced by as much as 35% when tested upon goats using the type of equipment shown. (Author)

848.
HILLS, B.A.
Clinical implications of gas-induced osmosis.
Arch. Int. Med. 129:356-362;Feb. 1972.

A review of the evidence for believing that gas concentration gradients can induce water movement in vivo shows that this could be a significant physiological parameter in many tissues, depending upon the magnitude of the gas-osmotic pressures. Estimation of these has suggested two experiments whose results show (1) that reflexion coefficients for gases may be appreciably higher than determined previously, (2) that water flow rates are high, and (3) that the list of semipermeable tissues should include articular cartilage. The clinical implications of gas-induced osmosis are then discussed with particular reference to gaseous anesthesia, hyperbaric arthralgia, gouty arthritis, aseptic bone necrosis, hyperbaric urticaria, pulmonary edema, and the edematous separation of tissue boundaries in general. (Author's abstract)

849.
HILLS, B.A.
Peak osmotic water displacement induced by gases in tissue.
Phys. Med. Biol. 17:277-287;Mar. 1972.

An analysis has been undertaken of the osmotic displacement of water in tissue induced by a transient gas concentration gradient. This is applied to the particular cases of (a) switching the inspired inert gas at constant pressure, as in anaesthetics, and (b) a diver or caisson worker undergoing compression to his working pressure while breathing a mixture of constant composition. The derived time courses for transient water displacement are then discussed in connection with several possible manifestations of gas-induced osmosis, such as inert gas narcosis and hyperbaric arthralgia, and shown to be compatible with many of their clinical features. (Author's abstract)

850.
HILLS, B.A. and R.S. Straley.
Aseptic osteonecrosis: a study of tibial blood flow under various environmental conditions.
Aerosp. Med. 43:724-728;July 1972.

The direction of change of blood flow in the tibiae of five large rabbits and nine mongrel dogs has been monitored at various stages of exposure to compressed air and to various breathing mixtures at normal atmospheric pressure. The results show a definite increase in flow 4-7 mins after compression to 4 ATA in air and upon exposure to normoxic nitrous oxide. These effects are essentially reversed upon return to air at normal atmospheric pressure or upon exposure to pure oxygen, while I.V. alcohol can cause appreciable variations in either direction. The duration and extent of ischemia observed were not considered sufficient to initiate the aseptic necrosis of bone commonly found in compressed-air workers and alcoholics. Discussion of this disease indicates that it may not be a symptom of decompression sickness, as generally assumed, and may even be induced by the compression phase of an exposure to compressed air. (Authors' abstract)

851.
HILLS, B.A.
Gas-induced osmosis in the lung.
J. Appl. Physiol. 33:126-129;July 1972.

A preferential retention of water, and even fluid expulsion, has been demonstrated in lungs ventilated with a normoxic mixture of nitrous oxide compared with contralateral controls separately ventilated with air under otherwise identical conditions. This is considered a manifestation of gas-induced osmosis. The probable magnitude of such osmotic pressures is calculated and discussed as a possible factor influencing homeostasis. (Author's abstract)

852.
HILLS, B.A.
Neurologic oxygen toxicity: effects of switch of inert gas and change of pressure.
Aerosp. Med. 43:716-723;July 1972.

A switch from N_2O to N_2 as the inert gas inspired at the same absolute pressure and inspired PO_2 was found to induce convulsions in 21 rats in appreciably less time than taken using either inert gas alone. A switch from N_2 to N_2O had the opposite effect. Decompression upon an N_2O:O_2 mixture was found to induce particularly violent convulsions. It was found that full developed seizures could be stopped for several minutes by further rapid compression on pure O_2. These findings constitute five basic tests whose results are compatible with the concept that spontaneous nervous activity can be increased by cellular dilution induced osmotically by gases. This approach has been extended to show how fluid shifts can be caused by steady-state gas concentration gradients induced by hyperoxia. This is shown to offer a simple physical contributing mechanism consistent with the basic features of neurologic oxygen toxicity. (Author's abstract)

853.
HILLS, B.A.
Chemical facilitation of thermal conduction in physiological systems.
Science 182:823-825;Nov. 23, 1973.

Experimental evidence supports the concept that solutes capable of reversible chemical reaction can passively facilitate thermal conduction within their solutions. Myoglobin and bicarbonate are suggested as energy carriers in muscle, having the combined capacity for conveying all waste metabolic heat produced under normal physiological conditions. The concept is extended to convective heat transfer in vivo; this implicates hemoglobin. . . for instance, in hyperoxia, to the extent that when Hb in venous blood is saturated with O_2 there can be no chemical removal of heat from tissue by blood. Heat can then accumulate in a tissue, such as the brain, which is not readily able to increase its perfusion rate. Hence it is interesting that neurological oxygen toxicity becomes manifest at about the point of venous saturation of hemoglobin and that it is particularly sensitive to temperature — a man with fever readily convulses in hyperbaric oxygen. (Author)

854.
HILPERT, P., R. Bahr, H. Junger and W. Rosendahl.
CO Diffusionskapazitat, Compliance und Lungenvolumina nach hyperbarer O_2-Atmung (3 ata uber 3 Std) bei Lungengesunden.
[CO diffusion capacity, compliance and lung volumes after hyperbaric oxygenation].
Pneumonologie 149:75-81; 1973.

The effect of oxygen toxicity on the lung was studied in six normal subjects who breathed oxygen at a pressure of 2050 mm Hg in a pressure chamber for 3 hours. There were no significant changes in vital capacity, maximal breathing capacity, dynamic compliance, maximal transpulmonary pressure gradients and single-breath CO-diffusion capacity. All subjects had signs of general malaise and fatigue. Visual impairment, substernal distress and coughing was seen only occasionally in some subjects. (English abstract)

855.
HIRSCH, A.E. and A.K. Ommaya.
Lethal effects on man of underwater detonation of a firecracker.
AGARD Conf. Proc. 88:15-1 - 15-5; 1971.

A firecracker exploded in contact with the skin within six inches of the skull base in a young man while he was swimming underwater. The resultant severe head injury and death appeared to be directly related to this underwater explosion. Reconstruction of the mechanics of this injury indicate that when the head is subjected to impact energies between 440 and 1800 in-lb and impact impulse between 1.8 and 3.5 lb.sec., both skull fracture and brain injury can occur. (Authors' abstract)

856.
HITTLEMAN, R.L.
Remote vehicle has human reactions.
Hydrospace 4:42-44;Apr. 1971.

The Dillingham Corporation, working with the Naval Underwater Research and Development Center, has developed a remote controlled, miniature, unmanned submersible, in which the operator's head motion and direction is coupled to that of the vehicle and its TV camera. Thus is demonstrated the "feasibility of directing underwater systems using acoustic and visual sensors which acquire information in the same manner as does the human mechanism." The camera and sensors are contained in a 20-inch plastic sphere. Tests of the vehicle indicated that such a coupling can contribute a valuable new technique. It was shown that the operator could follow the movements of a diver who was taking evasive action. (MFW/BSCP)

857.
HITTLEMAN, R.L. and W. Forman.
Anthropomorphic vehicle system.
In: Duntley, S.Q., J.L. Lones, and H.S. Weisbrod, eds. Proceedings of the society of photo-optical instrumentation engineers. Underwater photo-optical instrumentation applications. March 1971, Honolulu, p.73-76. Published by the Society, 1972.

The efficient performance of any task in the hostile underwater environment requires that due care be exercised in the design of the man-machine interface to take full advantage of the enormous potential available in the human mechanism. In particular, it was believed that significant benefits could be realized if the human brain was introduced as an integrally functioning element of an underwater remote controlled vehicle system. (Authors' introduction)

858.
HLASTALA, M.P. and J. Butler.
Transient state diffusion of diethyl ether in subcutaneous tissue.
Physiologist 16:343;Aug. 1973.

Abstract only. Entire item quoted: The initial transient state of growth or decay of a decompression sickness bubble is very important since it involves a major change in bubble volume. Gas flux is heavily dependent on the diffusion characteristics of surrounding tissue. Transient state diffusion of an inert gas was measured in the subcutaneous tissue of rats. An existing subcutaneous gas pocket was surgically opened exposing the inner surface with the perfusion intact and a rigid, transparent chamber was mounted on the exposed surface. The chamber could be completely flushed with gaseous diethyl ether in four seconds. The uptake of gas by tissue was measured as a change in chamber pressure using an attached pressure transducer. The uptake rate could be accurately predicted using a mathematical model in which the tissue if perfused by an infinite number of infinitesimally small capillaries. This technique allowed measurement of the rate of gas flux across the gas tissue interface during both the initial transient state — the build-up of a diffusion gradient in the tissue — and the later steady state. The transient state was relatively independent of tissue perfusion and allowed measurement of the diffusivity of diethyl ether which was .000752 $\pm$ .000058 cm^2/min (mean + SEM) at a mean temperature of 38.4°C. This phase was over in 5 to 10 minutes depending on the perfusion. The steady state was strongly dependent on tissue perfusion which varied between experiments.

859.
HLASTALA, M.P. and L.E. Farhi.
Absorption of gas bubbles in flowing blood.
J. Appl. Physiol. 35:311-316;Sept. 1973.

Resorption of N_2 bubbles (radius 500-2,500 μ) was measured in vitro in moving streams of saline, red cells suspended in saline, plasma, or whole blood. The absolute volume of the bubble was determined every 4 min by a compression technique. The diffusion characteristics are described in terms of the mass transfer coefficient which decreased from 0.0059 to 0.0022 cm/sec as the viscosity of the perfusing liquid increased from 1 to 8 centistokes. The results are also interpreted in terms of generalized parameters which allow comparison of these results to those of other investigators using different systems. For a bubble in blood, the mass transfer characteristics are similar to heat and mass transfer from solid spheres to moving liquid. (Authors' abstract)

860.
HOBSON, E. and E.H. Chave.
Hawaiian reef animals.
University Press of Hawaii, 1972. 135p.

People in ancient Hawaii lived in harmony with the sea. Hawaiian folklore is filled with the names of sea creatures, their legendary and true habits, and with the taboos and rituals surrounding them. Today, burdened by the growing complexity of modern life in the Islands, few people have retained this familiarity with the sea, even though the near-shore reefs still abound with life. For those who want to know more about Hawaii's reef life, this book depicts the fishes and other reef animals. Eighty-seven full-color, full-page photographs are integrated with a text that combines natural history with legends and folklore. The photographs show the animals in their natural settings, just as a person swimming and diving in Islands waters would see them. This book covers the majority of the fishes and the more prominent invertebrates — the corals, crabs, sea urchins, and mollusks. It also gives accurate taxonomic information for the animals in terms easily understood by the layman. Snorklers and divers will find this book to be a valuable guide and reference. Among the material presented is cautionary advice on approaching and handling sea creatures that might be harmful to man. Finally, this book will be a welcome addition to the library of anyone interested in tropical marine life. (Publisher)

861.
HOCHACHKA, P.W., D.E. Schneider and T.W. Moon.
The adaptation of enzymes to pressure. I. A Comparison of trout liver fructose diphosphatase with the homologous enzyme from an off-shore benthic fish.
Amer. Zool. 11:479-490; 1971.

At low temperature (3°C), in the absence of substrate and cofactor, trout fructose diphosphatase (FDPase) is inactivated by exposures to relatively low pressures. FDP and Mg^{2+} protect against this inactivation; hence, maximum catalysis at pH 7.5 is pressure insensitive, while at more alkaline pH, it is markedly accelerated by pressure. The volume change of activation (ΔV^*) at saturating FDP and Mg^{2+} concentrations is about -40 cm^3/mole. The apparent K_m for FDP and the K_a for Mg^{2+} are markedly increased by pressure. At low FDP or Mg^{2+} levels these kinetic properties outweigh ΔV^* in determining the reaction rate; hence, under these conditions, pressure retards catalysis. Similarly, the K_i for AMP is notably pressure sensitive. Comparable effects of pressure on the kinetic constants for liver FDPase from benthic Coryphaenoides are much less pronounced, suggesting that in these off-shore species enzyme substrate, enzyme-cofactor, and enzyme-modulator interactions have been tailored through evolution for pressure independent catalytic function. (Authors' abstract)

862.
HOCHACHKA, P.W.
Enzyme mechanisms in temperature and pressure adaptation of off-shore benthic organisms: the basic problem.
Amer. Zool. 11:425-435; 1971.

The degree of participation of any given enzyme reaction in metabolism is not determined by energy-volume relationships, but rather by enzyme affinities for key regulatory ligands. In temperature adaptation, enzyme-substrate affinities often decrease as thermal kinetic energy increases, thus compensating for temperature-induced changes in reaction velocity at low substrate concentrations. Since the effects of pressure are not unidirectional (some enzymes are accelerated; some are unaffected; some are decelerated), a more functional solution in pressure adaptation is to elaborate enzymes whose affinities for key metabolites are pressure independent. In consequence, at physiological substrate concentrations, the pressure sensitivities of catalysis and control of catalysis are probably held at a minimum. (Author's abstract)

863.
HOCHACHKA, P.W., H.W. Behrisch, and F. Marcus.
Pressure effects on catalysis and control of catalysis by liver fructose diphosphatase from an off-shore benthic fish.
Amer. Zool. 11:437-449; 1971.

At low temperature (2°C) in the absence of FDP and Mg^{2+}, the enzyme fructose disphosphatase (FDPase) extracted from the liver of an off-shore benthic Coryphaenoides species, is inactivated by exposures to relatively low pressures. The substrate, FDP and the cofactor, Mg^{2+}, protect against this inactivation, so that catalysis per se is not retarded by pressure. In contrast, at alkaline pH, pressure dramatically accelerates the catalytic rate when FDP and Mg^{2+} are saturating. The volume change of activation (ΔV^{*}) for Coryphaenoides FDPase under these conditions is about -40 cm^3/mole. At low concentrations of FDP and saturating concentrations of cofactor, the reaction rate at alkaline pH is pressure-independent. Similarly, at low concentrations of Mg^{2+} but saturating concentration of FDP, the reaction rate is pressure-independent. The K_m for FDP does not change measurably with pressure, while the K_a for Mg^{2+} concentrations, it is evident that the reaction rate is determined by the kinetic characteristics of the enzyme and not by its energy-volume relationships, a situation which would appear to be of functional and selective significance to an organism living under constantly high hydrostatic pressure. AMP is potent specific inhibitor of Coryphaenoides FDPase. The K_i for AMP is essentially pressure-independent both at neutral and alkaline pH, suggesting that efficiency of AMP control of this enzyme is comparable at all pressures likely to be encountered in nature. (Authors' abstract)

864.
HOCHACHKA, P.W., T.W. Moon and T. Mustafa.
The adaptation of enzymes to pressure in abyssal and midwater fishes.
In: The effect of pressure on organisms. Symposia of the Society for Experimental Biology, No. 26, p.175-195. London, Cambridge University Press, 1972.

Two enzyme systems, liver fructose diphosphatase (FDPase) which is pressure-activated, and muscle pyruvate kinase (PK) which is inhibited by pressure, are compared in detail with the homologous enzymes extracted from tissues of the rainbow trout, Salmo gairdnerii. . . For each enzyme, specific steric and mechanistic requirements of the reaction per se place tight restrictions upon those characteristics which are adaptable and those which are inviolate. These mechanistic parameters will determine the degree to which the inherent pressure sensitivity of the enzyme-catalysed reaction can be reduced. The large reduction in the volume change of activation of the PK and FDPase reactions from midwater organisms probably approaches such a lower limit for these reactions, and beyond this limit evolution cannot go. But whereas the evolutionary process cannot contradict or negate the basic energy-volume relationships, it can largely circumvent them, and this indeed seems to be the basic 'ground rule' for natural selection. Thus, it is not the volume change of activation or the activation energy, but it is enzyme-substrate, enzyme-cofactor, enzyme-modulator affinities which are most carefully tailored during pressure adaptation of enzymes. By dramatically reducing the pressure sensitivities of these enzyme-ligand interactions, uncontrollable effects of pressure on in vivo enzyme functions are prevented inboth midwater and abyssal organisms. (Authors)

865.
HOCHACHKA, P.W.
Multiple end products of anaerobiosis in diving vertebrates.
Physiologist 16:343;Aug. 1973.

Abstract only. Entire item quoted: When oxygen availability to working muscle in diving animals is limited by peripheral vasoconstriction, the muscle ferments carbohydrate and amino acids simultaneously, in effect coupling two additional energy-yielding reactions to those of glycolysis. Multiple anaerobic end products accumulate as a result. Succinate is the chief end product of anaerobic amino acid catabolism, alanine is a minor end product, while pyruvate and lactate are produced by glycolysis. During recovery following diving, increased blood concentrations of all four metabolites can be readilly measured in the green sea turtle, the harbor seal, the sea lion, and the porpoise.

866.
HOCHWALD, G.M., C. Malhan and J. Brown.
Effect of hypercapnia on CSF turnover and blood-CSF barrier to protein.
Arch. Neurol. 28:150-155;Mar. 1973.

Formation of cerebrospinal fluid (CSF) and transfer of albumin from blood to CSF was measured during steady state ventricular perfusion. In both normal and experimentally induced hypercephalic cats elevation of arterial carbon dioxide pressure (PCO_2) by 10% carbon dioxide (CO_2) inhalation resulted in a decrease in absorption of CSF by approximately 50%. Under these conditions, there was no increase in CSF formation. The pH, PCO_2 and their changes in perfusate and CSF were similar and reflected those measured in blood. Hypercapnia caused more than an 11-fold increase in the influx of albumin into the perfusate of normal cats only. This effect was rapid and to a large extent reversible when the 10% CO_2 was removed from the breathing gas. The failure to detect a similar increase in permeability of the blood-CSF barrier to protein in hydrocephalic cats was attributed to the pathological changes in the choroid plexus due to the kaolin. (Authors' abstract)

867.
HOCTOR, F.
Break the silent gap — the Hellephone.
Skin Diver 22:32-33;Dec. 1972.

The Hellephone promises to give a new dimension to safety, training and time saving in both commercial and sport scuba diving. It has been checked out in all the situations mentioned above, in depths of 200 feet and at distances of a quarter mile and greater. The Hellephone is a complete communications system, although it can be purchased in units and expanded as needed. The underwater portions for diver-to-diver work include a power unit which straps to the air tank, a microphone encased in a standard U.S. Divers mask, and a small receiver to slip inside the hood just behind the ear. Wireless like a two-way radio, but using sound waves rather than radio waves for transmission, the Hellephone provides clear voice communication underwater for distances up to one-quarter mile. With it, divers can talk to other divers and to their surface ship over a two-way swimmer unit that weighs less than four pounds topside or eight ounces submerged, and operates for 50 hours on eight "AA" penlight batteries. Operation is automatic the moment the Hellephone is submerged, and a single "press-to-talk" switch is all the diver needs to concern himself with when using the device underwater. Automatic gain control keeps hearing volume the same at any distance. The system operates at a frequency of 42 kHz, using amplitude modulation (AM). The topside unit of the Hellephone can be used from ship to dock to communicate with working divers, or poolside as a training aid, and also combines transmit and receive functions. It operates for 400 hours from a single 12-volt lantern battery. For communicating topside, there's a surface transceiver in a compact, rugged case with just one switch to operate. It is especially designed to facilitate instruction, coordination of underwater activities and salvage, and to increase all-around diver safety. Completely sealed, the Hellephone weighs only eight pounds. Although it is a new product, the Hellephone has been proven a valuable diver communication aid in an unusual variety of research, commercial and recreational projects. (Author)

868.
HODGSON, R.T. and D.R. Caldwell.
Application of Fourier techniques to underwater image transmission: a test of the linear-invariant hypothesis.
J. Opt. Soc. Amer. 62:1434-1438;Dec. 1972.

The modulation transfer functions of some aqueous solutions were calculated in two ways: (a) by measuring the sine-wave response through observation of the contrast transmittance of a resolution grating, and (b) by computing the Fourier transform of the image of a line source. For linear-invariant systems, to which Fourier techniques are applicable, both schemes will yield the same result. In the experiments, significant differences were found, caused by small temperature fluctuations in the solutions. The indiscriminate application of Fourier techniques to image transmission in natural bodies of water is questioned. (Authors' abstract)

869.
HODY, G.L., J.J. Kacirk and A.A. Pilmanis.
Direct "in situ" measurement of thermal insulation quality underwater.
In: Ocean 73. 1973 IEEE international conference on engineering in the ocean environment, p.133-136. IEEE publication 73 CHO 7740 OCC.

Thermal insulation is one of the most critical components involved in life support in a large number of operations undersea. The degree to which thermal insulation is effective in blocking the flow of heat depends both upon its properties and also upon the environment. For example, the common closed cell wet-suit material compresses and loses efficiency as a function of pressure at depth. The factors involved in thermal protection of divers are very difficult to evaluate in theory or in the lab, thus a method of "in situ" measurement was developed. The method is based upon direct measurement of the heat flow through the thermal insulation by the use of thermoelectric heat flow transducers applied in series with the principal heat flow path. The temperature difference (Δ t) between the outer surface of the insulating layer and the skin is also determined and the thermal resistance is then computed as the ratio of Δt/heat flow. Typical resistance units, readily convertible to "Clo", are $^{o}C \times watt^{-1} \times meter^{-2}$. The feasibility of the method was tested at moderate depths in Catalina waters, with wetsuited divers, using open circuit SCUBA and "hooka" breathing systems. The instruments proved reliable. The thermal resistance, an indication of the functional quality of the wet suits, was measured for several suit configurations. Regional differences within a single suit as well as surface-averaged data for the whole suit were obtained. These data are reported as thermal resistance given as a function of location on the suit. The method would be equally applicable to the walls of habitats, or personnel transfer capsules, heated or passively insulated. The development of better thermal barriers for personnel protection undersea should be aided by this direct measurement method. (Authors' abstract)

870.
HOFF, D.G., W.H. Cline, Jr., J.D. Dexter and C.E. Mengel.
CNS epinephrine tone, a possible etiology for the threshold in susceptibility to oxygen toxicity seizures.
Aerosp. Med. 43:1194-1199;Nov. 1972.

The nature of the earlier defined circadian rhythm in susceptibility to Oxygen at High Pressure (OHP) seizure was explored by proposing CNS epinephrine as a possible candidate for a chemical which sets a receptor tone in the CNS, and thus perhaps the threshold of susceptibility to seizure. Albino, Sprague-Dawley rats (200-400 gm.) were divided into eight groups, which were defined by 2 criteria: (1) the time of day of decapitation (A=0130-0230 hrs, B=0730-0830 hrs., C=1330-1430 hrs., D=1930-2030 hrs.) and (2) whether the animal was on a regular or reversed sleep wake cycle. Immediately upon decapitation the brain was removed and areas of cerebral cortex, hypothalamus and brainstem were dissected out over ice. Epinephrine and norepinephrine determinations using a modified automated trihydroxy-indole fluorometric method were then performed on each area. The results showed a daily rhythm of epinephrine in the hypothalamus and brainstem resembling the susceptibility of the regular cycled animals to OHP seizure which could also be reversed by sleep-wake reversal of the animals. (Authors' abstract)

871.
HOFFERT, J.R., D.A. Baeyens and P.O. Fromm.
The resistance of teleost ocular tissues to oxygen toxicity.
Invest. Opthalmol. 12:858-861;Nov. 1973.

White grunts were used in this experiment. Homogenate of liver tissue demonstrated marked inhibition of cellular oxygen consumption after 5 atm. of pure oxygen for one hour at room temperature. Ocular tissues, with the exception of the retina after a six hour exposure, did not demonstrate oxygen toxicity. The cornea and lens tissues showed increases in oxygen consumption under hyperbaric oxygen, indicating resistance to oxygen toxicity. The authors hypothesize that a protective agent from either the retina or the pseudo-branch (also demonstrated to be resistant to oxygen toxicity) enters the ocular fluids and is thus carried to the vicinity of the cornea and the lens. (MFW/UMS)

872.
HOGBERG, T. and U. Soderberg.
Effects of high ambient pressure on resistance to anoxia in mice.
Acta Anaesthesiol. Scand. 17:159-162; 1973.

The resistance of mice to asphyxiation in pure nitrogen at 5 ata, after equilibration with a high pressure atmosphere (4.2% O_2 in N_2, 5 ata; "normal" Po_2) producing a nitrogen anaesthesia, has been compared to the resistance of mice exposed to pure nitrogen at 1 ata after atmospheric air breathing. The anoxic resistance was increased by 58% by the nitrogen anaesthesia. (Authors' abstract)

873.
HOGG, W., J. Brunton, M. Kryger, R. Brown and P.T. Macklem.
Gas diffusion across collateral channels.
J. Appl. Physiol. 33(5):568-575; 1972.

Various indexes of ventilation distribution were studied before and after airways were occluded by beads insufflated into bronchi of excised lobes. In the dog, this delayed the multiple-breath N_2 washout and increased the slope of the alveolar plateau of the single-breath N_2 curve. A five-minute breath hold was required for the slope to return to normal. The distribution of inspired gas to alveoli via collateral channels is reduced, and gas diffusion occurs slowly across collateral channels. Single-breath inflations with He:SF_6 mixtures with sampling of gas during expiration revealed the initial gas in control lobes to be SF_6 enriched and later gas He enriched, indicating that a small degree of incomplete diffusion mixing normally exists. After obstruction, the initial gas was He enriched and later samples SF_6 enriched, although absolute concentrations of both gases fell throughout expiration. Breath holding reversed both effects. Gas sampled from a catheter wedged in the airway of an otherwise normal lobe was consistently SF_6 enriched. These results are attributed to separation of He and SF_6 due to Taylor diffusion within the tracheobronchial tree, allowing the denser gas to penetrate more deeply into the lung. (© BA)

874.
HOKE, B.
Respiratory heat loss from breathing cold gas at high pressure.
In: Abstracts of BuMed-ONR sponsored Navywide research in high pressure biomedical research, U.S. Submarine Base, Groton, Conn., May 1971. p.45. Published by the Naval Submarine Medical Research Laboratories, 1971.

Abstract only. Entire item quoted: Respiratory heat loss (RHL) was measured in two men while breathing cold oxyhelium at the surface, at 200, 400, 600, 800 and 1,000 feet of sea water in a warm, dry chamber. Four exercise levels were used to vary the respiratory minute volume (RMV). RHL is directly related to inspired gas temperature, RMV, and depth. At 800 feet, one subject demonstrated excessive heat loss in spite of exercise, and the other subject experienced acute respiratory difficulty from excessive secretions. Nine other subjects were studied at 850 feet with moderate exercise while breathing cold gas and the data show that when RHL exceeds about 350 watts the diver will be in danger, sooner or later depending on individual characteristics, because of excessive heat loss.

875.
HOLLAND, C.R.
A life support instrumentation consideration for hyperbaric facilities.
In: Ocean 73. 1973 IEEE international conference on engineering in the ocean environment, p.126-128. IEEE publication 73 CHO 774-0 OCC.

The creation of special atmospheres for exploration of inner and outer space raises questions relating to control levels and methods for safety and success. This paper discusses the "solution" employed in the design and construction of the Ocean Simulation Facility in Panama City, Florida. Because all compounds are not life critical, the problem is simplified by defininig two instrumentation categories. Category one involves continuous measurement of constituents vital to short term physiological well being. Category two involves infrequent detection and identification of constituents which may have a long term physiological effect. The instrumentation provided adequately determines the level of any constituent, but the follow-on control is rudimentary. (Author's abstract)

876.
HOLLAND, J.A., W.G. Wolfe and J.A. Kylstra.
Helium: Absence of antiarrhythmic effect in anesthetized dogs.
J. Thorac. Cardiovasc. Surg. 66:478-480;Sept. 1973.

In this study, 22 healthy dogs, anesthetized with pentobarbital and ventilated mechanically, were evaluated for cardiac arrhythmias. Blood flow in the left circumflex coronary artery was interrupted by ligation and transection. The incidence of cardiac arrhythmias during two hours after ligation while the animals breathed either 75% helium and 25% oxygen, or else 75% nitrogen and 25% oxygen was not significantly different. These results are at variance with similar recent studies on the antiarrhythmic effects of helium in anesthetized dogs. (Authors' summary)

877.
HOLLAND, J.A., W.E. Davis, W.G. Wolfe and J.A. Kylstra.
Evaluation of clotting factors during hyperbaric exposure.
In: Ackles, K.N. ed. Blood bubble interaction in decompression sickness. Proceedings of an international symposium held at Defence and Civil Institute of Environmental Mecicine, Downsview, Ontario, Canada, p.238-246. Published by the Institute. December 1973. (DCIEM Conference Proceedings 73-CP-960)

It had been thought that the presence of bubbles in blood samples during decompression might produce artifacts that would confuse coagulation testing. A dialysis unit was developed to eliminate dissolved gas from the blood. Slowly decompressed blood samples, both dialized and non-dialized were tested, as were rapidly decompressed blood samples. The study indicates that dialysis of blood samples is not necessary for accurate hematologic evaluation. Reliable results were obtained from non-dialized as well as from dialized blood. (MFW/UMS)

878.
HOLLIEN, H.
Studies of diver communication and retrieval.
In: Miller, J.W., J.G. Van Derwalker and R.A. Waller, eds. Tektite 2: Scientists-in-the-sea p.X-1-X-10. Washington, D.C. U.S. Department of the Interior, August 1971.

The author discusses first the intelligibility of diver-to-surface communication systems as a function of distance. A small version of the Diver Communication Research System (DICORS) was designed for the Tektite 2 studies. The DICORS was floated at 15 feet in 30 feet of water, and hydrophones were placed at 50, 250, 500, 1000, 2000 and 4000 feet from the diver/talker. The systems studied were the Raytheon Yack-Yack, the Bendix Watercom, the Scuba-com, the Aquasonics 420, the ERUS-2-3A, the Sub-Com prototype and the PQC-2. The last four are amplitude modulated systems and require special receiving equipment. The results of these evaluations are not given. Another group of tests involved sound localization. It is rather inconclusively indicated that trained divers are capable of a certain degree of sound localization, and that there is little difference between results in salt water and in fresh water. In the diver recall studies it was tentatively concluded that the type of explosive sounds now generally employed are only minimally affective. In the tests of diver performance as affected by the use of communication systems, it appeared that performance was better without than with communication systems. Extensive diver training is required in order to make use of the existing systems, which in themselves are much in need of improvement. (MFW/BSCP)

879.
HOLLIEN, H., H. Rothman and S. Feinstein.
Annual summary report.
Gainesville, Fla., Univ. Fla., Commun. Sci. Lab., Rep. CSL/ONR 48, 13p. July 1, 1972.

This report summarizes the work accomplished during the contractual year, June 1971-May 1972. Studies completed were: 1) Diver-to-surface communication (near field and over distance); 2) Diver-to-diver communication; 3) Speech modification in helium at 300 feet; 4) Off-line evaluation of the RELA unscrambler; 5) Underwater microphone evaluation; 6) Diver auditory acuity; 7) Minimum audible angle of Scuba divers. Studies nearing completion: 1) Speech intelligibility in neon at depths of 300-680 feet; 2) Speech feedback (divers underwater hear their own speech immediately after their utterances and attempt modification for better intelligibility). (DCD abstract)

880.
HOLLIEN, H. and S. Feinstein.
The conribution of the external auditory meatus to human underwater auditory sensitivity.
Gainesville, Fla., Univ. Fla., Commun. Sci. Lab., Rep. CSL/ONR 40, 12p. July 1, 1972.

Support for, and a refinement of, the hypothesis that divers hear primarily by bone conduction was provided by Hollien and Brandt. (Journal of Acoustical Society of America, 46, 384-387, 1969). To further test this hypothesis, the thresholds of seven submerged listeners were obtained (at frequencies of 0.25, 0.50, 1.0, 4.0 and 8.; kHz) under three different conditions: 1) while they wore a full 3/16" wet suit with no hood, 2) while wearing a full 3/16" wet suit with a 3/16" hood and 3) while wearing a full 3/16" wet suit and hood with 1/4" rubber tubes passing through the hood to the external auditory meatuses. There were no significant differences between the conditions involving the use of a hood but thresholds were significantly lower in the middle and high frequencies for the no-hood condition. These findings provide further support for the hypothesis that underwater sound energy is transduced by bone conduction rather than by the normal middle ear linkage. (DCD abstract)

881.
HOLLIEN, H. and H.B. Rothman.
Evaluation of helium speech unscramblers under controlled conditions.
Gainesville, Fla., Univ. Fla., Commun. Sci. Lab., Rep. CSL/ONR 46, 17p. July 1, 1972.

Man's attempts to probe and utilize "inner space" have to a large degree, been hampered by inadequate voice communication. One of the specific sources of speech degradation is the use of helium as an inert breathing gas in the deep diving situation. In turn, electronic devices have been developed which are designed to improve speech intelligibility distorted by the effects of high ambient pressures and HeO_2 breathing mixtures. In order to evaluate the effectiveness of these HeO_2 "unscramblers" the Communication Sciences Laboratory at the University of Florida has undertaken a four-part project: (1) to evaluate available unscramblers on-line; (2) to test them off-line; (3) to develop a standardized off-line test for the evaluation of all types of unscramblers; and (4) to establish guidelines for the development of optimum equipment of this type. This report provides the results of two evaluations of a number of unscramblers available to our laboratory and the U.S. Navy. The first evaluation was conducted "on line" during the training of SeaLab III aquanauts at EDU; it was followed by an off-line (bench) test. Also described is a test consisting of 57 word lists that have been developed for standardized off-line evaluations of electronic aids to speech communication in HeO_2/P environments. Briefly, the on-line evaluation showed that the NASL unscrambler in combination with the Roanwell microphone provided greatest intelligibility; a later off-line test revealed the IRPI unit to be superior. The first use of the off-line test indicates that it is a valid method for evaluating helium speech unscramblers. (DCD abstract)

882.
HOLLIEN, H., S.H. Feinstein, H.B. Rothman and P. Hollien.
The auditory sensitivity of divers at high pressures.
Gainesville, Fla., Univ. Fla. Commun. Sci. Lab., Rep. CSL/ONR 50, 17p. Feb. 1, 1973.

A theory that divers hear primarily by bone conduction has been proposed by Hollien and Brandt (JASA, 1967, 42:966-971, and JASA, 1969, 46:384-387). This hypothesis is based on 1) theoretical postulations, 2) the results of studies of hearing sensitivity conducted under high ambient pressure (up to 105 feet), 3) investigations of underwater auditory acuity and 4) the authors' own research program in these areas. The present status of this theory will be reviewed, as will the past theoretical concepts and data from reported experiments. Further, our research program will be discussed — including a review of the methodologies utilized. These experiments have focused on auditory sensitivity in the hyperbaric situation and in water as a function of basic response, depth, contents of the external ear and contents of the middle ear. Data from a new experiment also will be reported. Specifically, in a further test of the hypothesis, the thresholds of seven submerged listeners were obtained (at frequencies of 0.25, 0.50, 1.0, 4.0 and 8.0 kHz) under three different conditions: 1) when wearing a full 3/16" wet suit with no hood, 2) when wearing a full 3/16" wet suit with a 3/16" hood, and 3) when wearing a full 3/16" wet suit and hood with 1/4" rubber tubes passing through the hood to the meatuses. There were no significant differences between the second two conditions but thresholds were significantly better for condition one. These findings provide further support for the hypothesis that underwater sound energy is transduced to the cochlea by bone conduction rather than by normal external and middle ear linkage. Implications of this theory relative to divers' auditory functioning underwater are discussed. (DCD abstract)

883.
HOLLIEN, H., H.B. Rothman, S.H. Feinstein and P. Hollien.
The speech characteristics of divers in HeO_2 breathing mixtures at high pressures.
Gainesville, Fla., Univ. Fla., Commun. Sci. Lab., Rep. CSL/ONR 49; 10p. Feb. 1, 1973.

The development of saturation diving has enabled man to work in the sea for long periods of time — and at great depths. This situation has created problems in speech communication due to the effects of breathing HeO_2 gas mixtures at high ambient pressures. This paper will describe a program of empirical research (conducted at depths ranging from 250 to 825 feet) used to investigate the effects of HeO_2/P on speech. Specifically, a series of experiments will be described that relate the distorting effects of the HeO_2/P environment to: 1) intelligibility levels, 2) phonemic confusions, 3) non-linearity of vowel formant shifts, 4) speech adaptation over time, and 5) speech modification techniques to improve intelligibility. We have found that breathing HeO_2 under high ambient pressures reduces speech intelligibility by approximately 50% for every 200 feet of depth. A method for analyzing listeners' phonemic confusions of consonants has been developed which enables us to compare the relative intelligibility of each phoneme with other phonemes in the utterance or with the same phoneme in various other situations. A linear vowel formant shift occurs due to the introduction of helium to the vocal system; a non-linear vowel formant shift occurs in the lower formant frequencies because of cavity wall vibration and pressure. Our research demonstrates that the intelligibility of a diver's speech under HeO_2/P conditions improves over time, i.e., even unsystematic speaker adaptation to the environment occurs as a function of the length of time the diver remains in HeO_2/P. Finally, we have found that divers can *systematically* manipulate their speech characteristics in order to be more intelligible in the HeO_2/P milieu. Implications of these research results to theory and to the improvement of divers' speech communication in the HeO_2 environment are discussed. (DCD abstract)

884.
HOLLIEN, H., C.L. Thompson and B. Cannon.
Speech intelligibility as a function of ambient pressure and HeO_2 atmosphere.
Aerosp. Med. 44:249-253;Mar. 1973.

Speech intelligibility was obtained on Navy divers at sea level (in air) and at 200, 450 and 600 feet in helium-oxygen breathing mixtures. Subjects were personnel in training for DSSP's Sealab 3 at the Experimental Diving Unit, Washington Navy Yard. A total of 46 diver/talkers were studied; 28 at 0 and 200 feet, 22 at 0 and 450 feet, and nine at 0 and 600 feet. A reasonably nonreverberant recording environment was provided by an enclosure fabricated from mattresses available in the chamber's sleeping compartment. Listeners were 11-15 University of Florida students trained for tasks of this nature. The combined effects of HeO_2 mixtures and high ambient pressures were extremely detrimental to speech intelligibility which was reduced by approximately 50% for each increase of 200 feet of depth. It was also found that intelligibility level rankings at the surface do not predict similar rankings at depth. (Author's abstract)

885.
HOLLIEN, H.
Underwater sound localization in humans.
J. Acoust. Soc. Amer. 53:1288-1295;May 1973.

Theory and some empirical evidence would predict that humans should exhibit little ability to localize sounds underwater; however, other observations seemed to contradict this position. In order to provide relevant data on the issue, a pilot study was conducted; its results suggested that man can localize sounds underwater — at least to some degree. Accordingly, a major experiment was carried out utilizing 17 divers who were free to move their heads but not their bodies, in an underwater localization task. In order to allow precision in the experiment, a Diver Auditory Localization System (DALS) was developed; its design is based on previous structures employed in underwater communication research and consists of an open polyvinyl choloride (VPC) framework to which five 3-m arms and other equipment are attached. The five arms allow placement — at ear level — of underwater projectors at angles (to the diver) of 0°, 45°, 90°, 270°, and 315°. Subjects respond to four different signals — 250-, 1000-, and 6000-Hz sinusoids and thermal noise — at 110 dB SPL (re 0.0002 dyn/cm^2); this level is approximately 40 dB re underwater hearing thresholds. Responses to stimuli were accomplished by means of a specially constructed five-position underwater switch coupled to an IBM key punch at the surface. The obtained scores were substantially above chance and demonstrate that humans are capable of at least some sound localization underwater. (Author's abstract)

886.
HOLM, B. and S.C. Sorensen.
The role of the carotid body in the diving reflex in the duck.
Respiration Physiol. 15:302-309;July 1972.

The role of the carotid body in the development of bradycardia during diving was examined in the duck. In six ducks studied between two and seven days after denervation of the carotid body with nicotine and cyanide in anesthetized and unanesthetized spontaneously breathing animals caused hyperpnea and tachycardia, but the cardioaccelerator response was delayed relative to the ventilatory response. Stimulation of the carotid body with nicotine in anesthetized and artificially ventilated animals which were paralyzed with curare, did not affect the heart rate. Stimulation of the carotid body with nicotine in artificially ventilated and in non-ventilated unanesthetized animals caused bradycardia during submersion in water. We suggest that the afferent input elicited by immersion of the head in water by facilitation or disinhibition opens a reflex pathway which mediates a decrease in heart rate upon chemoreceptor stimulation by hypoxia. (Authors' abstract)

887.
HOLMQUIST, C.O.
The Navy and the challenge of deep diving.
Nav. Res. Rev. 25:1-13;Mar. 1972.

The author recounts the history of diving as it has been practised in the U.S. Navy over the past 50 years. One of the earliest problems was nitrogen narcosis, which led to the use of helium as a breathing gas. The necessity of lengthy decompressions for short times led to saturation diving, in which divers can remain at depth for days or weeks without necessitating a longer decompression time. Experimentation in saturation diving started with Genesis I a simulated dive under the direction of Capt. George Bond at the Submarine Medical Research Laboratory in New London, and continued through Sea Lab I and II under the Office of Naval Research. Other experiments have taken divers to 850 ft in the open sea, and it is planned to go to 1000 feet. Techniques for both habitat saturation divers and short-term divers at these depths are being developed, so that the ability to explore the continental shelf will be attained. The underwater tasks undertaken by the Navy include rescue, salvage, reconnaissance, repair, construction and engineering as well as undersea warfare. Physiological research into the problems of decompression sickness, inert gas narcosis, gas density and viscosity, and thermal balance is being undertaken. If these problems are solved, the final barrier will be the direct effects of hydrostatic pressure. It is possible that some effects now ascribed to nitrogen narcosis and to carbon dioxide, could actually be the result of hydrostatic pressure. Possible bone-muscle effects of hydrostatic pressure must be investigated. Still in the early experimental stage is fluid breathing. If this can be made practicable, the problem of decompression sickness and inert gas narcosis would be circumvented, since no inert gas would dissolve in the blood and tissues of a diver with fluid-filled lungs and depth limits would be imposed only by the cellular effects of hydrostatic pressure. Work on artificial gills, which could enable man to obtain oxygen by diffusion from water, is underway, and one such gill has already been patented. Technological problems in life support of the diver are chiefly concerned with development of more accurate devices for providing a safe breathing mixture and the improvement of closed-circuit breathing apparatus. Currently, the Mark 10 apparatus extends the diving time to six hours at any depth of the continental shelf. The greater the depth attained, the more acute becomes the problem of heat loss; here, the crucial need is to develop a compact energy source. Technological problems in functional support consist chiefly in the development of tools that will compensate for the weightlessness of the diver, and inert waterproofing and pressure requirements. Communication, navigation, sonar and propulsion equipment also come in this category. Current developments in self-sustaining ocean floor habitats will constitute a great step forward in underwater capability. Brief mention is made in conclusion of the psychological pressures to be encountered, about which little is yet really known. (MFW/BSCP)

888.
HOLNESS, D.E. and M.W. Radomski.
Uptake of a metabolically inert amino acid by brain tissue during high pressure oxygen exposure.
Experientia 28:1277;Nov. 15, 1972.

It is known that gamma-aminobutyric acid (GABA) protects against convulsions induced by hyperbaric convulsions, but it has not been possible to prove that the brain GABA levels have actually been raised, thereby indicating that hyperbaric oxygen has some effect on the blood-brain barrier. Investigations were made into the absorption of the inert amino acid alpha-aminoisobutyric acid (AIB) into the brain from the blood. Male Wistar rats were used. Results indicate that this absorption depends upon serum concentration and is not increased by hyperbaric oxygen. The functional integrity of the blood-brain barrier was apparently unaltered by hyperbaric oxygen. It is suggested that the protective action of GABA might not be due to its accelerated transport into the brain. (MFW/BSCP)

889.
HONG, S.K., Y.C. Lin, D.A. Lally, B.J.B. Yim, N. Kominami, P.W. Hong and T.O. Moore.
Alveolar gas exchanges and cardiovascular functions during breath holding with air.
J. Appl. Physiol. 30:540-547;Apr. 1971.

Nine male subjects capable of breath holding (BH) for times from two to four minutes were employed in the investigations. The residual volume of each subject was measured by the nitrogen-dilution method of Rahn, et al. (1949), and the resting oxygen consumption was determined by using a 13-liter Collins recording spirometer. During 4 min BH the lung supplied 700 ml of oxygen into the blood while it gained only 160 ml of carbon dioxide from the blood, indicating a significant retention of carbon dioxide in the blood and tissues. Mixed venous oxygen pressure and content approached arterial blood values toward the end of BH. (Aerosp. Med.)

890.
HONG, S.K., Y.C. Lin, D.A. Lally and T.O. Moore.
Alveolar gas exchanges and cardiovascular functions during breath holding with air.
In: Abstracts of the Twenty-fifth Congress of Physiological Sciences Satellite Symposium. Recent progress in fundamental physiology of diving. Marseille, France, July 1971. p.16-17. (Proceedings unpublished)

Abstract only. Entire item quoted: This investigation was undertaken to study, during a prolonged breath-holding (BH) with air, (1) changes in the alveolar gas pressures and the time course of alveolar O_2 and CO_2 exchange, (2) changes in arterial blood gas pressures and contents, (3) changes in the cardiac output, and (4) changes in the arterial, right atrial and esophageal pressures. Nine male subjects (5 divers and 4 nondivers, average age of 30 years) were employed. A. Alveolar Gas Exchange: In general, PAO_2 fell continuously but at a diminishing rate during 4 min BH, whereas $PACO_2$ increased rapidly during the first 20-30 sec. after which they increased very slightly. The terminal PAO_2 and $PACO_2$ were 30 and 56 mm Hg, respectively. During BH, the rate of O_2 removal from the lungs was considerably greater than that of the addition of CO_2 to the lungs. The overall R during BH was approximately 0.2. By the end of the maximal BH beginning with TLC, the total amount of O_2 removed from the lungs was equivalent to 70% of VO_2. About 80% of total CO_2 produced are retained in the blood and other tissues by the end of 4 min. BH. B. Blood Gas Composition: PaO_2 was approximately 10 mmHg lower than $PACO_2$ throughout the entire BH period. $PaCO_2$ also became consistently lower than $PACO_2$ after 60 sec of BH. The maximum $(A\text{-}a)CO_2$ gradient was as high as 5 mmHg. Arterial pH declined continuously during BH, with the lowest level of 7.29 at 4 min BH. CaO_2 decreased slowly during the first 2 min after which it decreased at a faster rate. $P\bar{V}O_2$ and $C\bar{V}O_2$ did not change appreciably until 2 min of BH after which they began to fall. At 4 min $P\bar{V}O_2$ and $C\bar{V}O_2$ became almost equal to those of arterial blood. $P\bar{V}CO_2$ became almost equal to $PaCO_2$ at 30 sec of BH although it became slightly lower than $PaCO_2$ during the rest of BH period. $C\bar{V}CO_2$ became equal to $CaCO_2$ after 90 sec of BH. As a result, mixed venous pH became higher than arterial pH. C. Cardiac Output. The cardiac output, as measured by Cardiogreen-dilution method, tended to increase during BH ($p > 0.05$). On the other hand, the heart rate tended to decrease while the stroke volume tended to increase during BH ($p > 0.05$). Both the central blood volume (estimated by the flow times the mean transit time) and the peripheral resistance also tended to increase somewhat. D. Blood Pressure and Intraesophageal Pressure: In general, the arterial blood pressure increased only slightly during the first minute after which it increased progressively toward the end of BH. On the average, the systolic pressure increased to a greater extent than the diastolic pressure, causing a progressive increase in the pulse pressure during the later phase of BH. The right atrial pressure increased instantly with the onset of BH to approximately 10 mmHg and maintained this level throughout the entire BH period. The intraesophageal pressure increased in the same manner as the right atrial pressure at the beginning of BH and gradually decreased to zero at 140 sec. The heart rate decreased to approximately 15% within 20 sec of BH and more or less maintained this level during the rest of the BH period. In other words, this bradycardia developed in the absence of any significant change in arterial blood pressure. The blood lactate level began to increase linearly after 2 min of BH. Moreover, there was a further increase in blood lactate at 20 sec after BH.

891.
HONG, S.K.
Pattern of cold adaptation in women divers of Korea (ama).
Fed. Proc. 32:1614-1622;May 1973.

Pattern of cold adaptation in ama who daily dive in water of 27-28°C in summer and 10°C in winter has been systematically studied from 1959 to 1969. The total extra heat loss for diving work is estimated to be 1,000 kcal/day throughout the year. The following adaptive phenomena to cold are found in Korean ama as compared with non-divig Korean women: (1) a consistent, reversible increase in basal metabolic rate of ama in winter (i.e. metabolic adaptation), which seems to be associated with increased utilization of thyroid hormone; (2) a very small (but significant) increase in VO_2 in response to exogenous norepinephrine in winter; (3) a lower critical water temperature at a comparable subcutaneous fat thickness throughout the year (i.e. insulative-hypothermic adaptation); (4) a significantly greater maximal thermal insulation at a comparable subcutaneous fat thickness throughout the year; (5) a lower heat flux from the limb coupled with a higher blood flow throughout the year during whole-body immersion in water of critical temperature; suggesting a more efficient countercurrent heat exchange system in the limb; and (6) a lower finger skin temperature and blood flow in winter during hand immersion in 6°C water (i.e. vascular adaptation). These results indicate that the basic pattern of cold adaptation in man is qualitatively similar to that observed in women divers of Korea (ama). (Author's abstract)

892.
HONG, S.K., T.O. Moore, D.A. Lally and J.F. Morlock.
Heart rate response to apneic face immersion in hyperbaric heliox environment.
J. Appl. Physiol. 34:770-774;June 1973.

Bradycardial responses to simple breath holding (BH) and apneic face immersion (FI) in 30°C water were studied in five divers in 4.0, 6.6, and 12.5 Ata heliox environments and in 1 Ata air. Maximal percent reduction in heart rate (ΔHRmax) during apnea at 1 Ata averaged 5.3 and 15% during BH and 30°C FI, respectively. As ambient pressure increased, ΔHRmax increased to 22% (BH) and 37% (30°C FI) at 12.5 Ata. During both BH and FI, ΔHRmax was greater at 6.6 and 12.5 Ata than in 1 Ata air (< 0.05). ΔHRmax was correlated with ambient pressure in the FI series ($r = 0.485$, $P < 0.01$). ΔHRmax during 30°C FI in 4.0, 6.6, and 12.5 Ata heliox were equivalent to those in 1 Ata during FI in 12.5, 10, and 6°C water, respectively. In addition, eight male subjects performed BH and FI experiments after breathing 75% He-25% O_2 at 1 Ata for 15 min. In the lower heart rate (HR) group (mean resting HR $\simeq$ 60 min^{-1}, 4 subj), Δ HRmax during BH and FI were generally potentiated. Resting HU was unchanged. In the higher HR group (mean resting HR $\simeq$ 80 min^{-1}, 4 subj), resting HR was lower during He-O_2 breathing while Δ HRmax in BH and FI tended to be attenuated. Breathing 75% Ar-25% O_2 did not alter resting HR or Δ HRmax in the lower HR group. These results are discussed in terms of 1) altered behavior of thermal receptors and 2) possible suppression of the sympathetic system by He. (Authors' abstract)

893.
HORNE, T.
Diuresis in the rat, induced by hyperbaric oxygen.
In: Wada, J. and I. Takashi, eds. Proceedings of the fourth international congress of hyperbaric medicine, Sapporo, Japan, Sept. 1969, p.161-163. Baltimore, Williams and Wilkins, 1970.

In this experiment, as in earlier ones, it was observed that the volume of urine under hyperbaric conditions increased threefold, on an average. Potassium, calcium and phosphate were excreted proportionately to the urine volume, but sodium and chloride amounts increased 11 and 12 times, and magnesium increased seven times. (MFW/BSCP)

894.
HORVATH, F. and I. Rozsahegyi.
Chronische caisson-osteoarthropathie in der Gelenkpfanne des Schulterblattes.
[Chronic caisson osteoarthropathy in the glenoid cavity of the clavicle].
Fortschr. Geb. Roentgenstr. Nuklearmed 117:733-734;Dec. 1972.

A case of chronic osteoarthropathy of the right shoulder blade in a 48-year old diver and caisson worker is reported. X-ray photographs of the shoulder show a widespread uneven subchondral and cranial sclerosis which extends to a lesser degree to the upper joint surface of the humerus. The joint itself was not compromised, and the patient, although complaining of pain in the right hand, arm and shoulder, had good mobility in the joint. The authors have noted only four cases of shoulder blade arthropathy among the 150 cases of caisson arthropathies which they have examined. (MEMH/SCD)

895.
HORVATH, F. and T. Vizkelety.
Experimentelle Untersuchungen der osteoartikularen Manifestation fer Caisson-Krankheit. [Experimental studies on osteocaricular manifestations of caisson disease]. Arch. Orthop. Unfall-Chir. 75:28-42; 1973.

Based on their experimental investigations the authors are of the opinion that in cases of identical decompression time the bone and joint changes of caisson disease develop according to the degree of pressure and according to the number of repetitions. As the epiphyseal circulation is quickly damaged necrotic areas develop in the articular cartilage, in the growth plate and in the metaphysis. In cases of severe lesion large necrotic areas form also in the region of the main nutrient artery. The marrow cavity has the appearance of a cellular reaction following ischaemic necrosis. The necrosis and the reparative processes are balanced in cases of slight circulatory disturbances. No signs of regeneration in the diaphysis and insignificant regeneration in the epiphysis are characteristic of severe defects of the blood supply. Radiological bone changes were especially typical of groups in which the decompression treatment was performed with the critical 2-2.5 atm pressure. Authors found a subchondral and a solitary circumscribed cystic lesion, both of them situated in the distal femoral epiphysis. A further case was observed with a radiological picture of the femur resembling myeloma multiplex. The distal femoral metaphysis of rabbits of the group treated with one atm pressure presented very slight, partly sclerotic, partly porotic structural changes. (English summary)

896.
HORVATH, F. and I. Rozsahegyi.
Bedeutung der Tomographic fur die Diagnose der chronischen Caisson-Osteoarthropathie. [Importance of tomography for the diagnosis of chronic caisson osteoarthropathy]. Forschr. Geb. Roentgenstr. Nuklearmed. 119(5):610-618; 1973.

Radiographic symptoms of bone manifestations of caisson sickness in 123 caisson workers are reviewed. Most common localizations were the proximal humeral epiphysis and metaphysis and the caput and collum femoris; bone changes were also noted in the scapula, acetabulum, and in the ends of the tibia and femur forming the knee. Radiographic symptoms include osteosclerosis, isolated or multiple geode formations, and isolated or multiple cystic formations of various sizes. These symptoms are discussed in detail and illustrated by a series of photographs. The author recommends the routine use of tomography in the diagnosis and ongoing evaluation of caisson osteoarthropathy. (MEMH/UMS)

897.
HOULIHAN, R.T., M.D. Altschule, Z.L. Hegedus and M.H. Cross.
Rheomelanin accumulation in the blood and lungs, and hemolysis in rats poisoned by hyperbaric oxygen.
In: Wada, J. and I. Takashi, eds. Proceedings of the fourth international congress on hyperbaric medicine, Sapporo, Japan, Sept. 1969, p.61-66. Baltimore, Williams, and Wilkins, 1970.

Adrenochrome and adrenolutin have been implicated in a number of neurological disorders, and have been shown to induce hemolysis; all of these phenomena resemble some of those caused by oxygen toxicity. Hence, the production of these compounds may explain the toxicological response seen during increased oxygen tension. The unstable nature of these compounds in biological media points not only to their high reactivity, but also to the problems involved in determining their presence. This report shows that substances similar to adrenochrome derivatives are present in the plasma and lungs of animals subjected to increased oxygen pressures. . . The destruction of red cells is owing either directly to the accumulation of aminochrome derivatives or else to the loss of some inhibiting factor in plasma that is protective to red blood cells. The data presented here favors the idea that increased aminochrome production explains how increased oxygen tension leads to disturbances in metabolism, to convulsions, and to the loss of red cell mass found during exposure to high concentrations of oxygen. (Authors)

898.
HOULIHAN, R.T. and B. LaLone.
In vitro epinephrine oxidation during exposure to hyperbaric oxygen.
In: Aerospace Medical Association. 1971 annual scientific meeting. Houston, Texas, April 1971. Preprints, p.64-65. Published by the Association, 1971.

The purpose of this experiment was to ascertain the effect of hyperbaric oxygen on epinephrine oxidation. Sprague-Dawley rats were bilaterally adrenalectomized. Some were treated with aldosterone, some with hydrocortisone, before being placed in the hyperbaric chamber. Some were adrenalectomized and not treated, and some were kept intact. After compression to five atmospheres for about one hour, the rats were removed and decapitated; the trunk blood was collected in heparinized tubes, then centrifuged. The plasma was incubated with epinephrine. Separation of the aminochromes adrenochrome, epinephrine and adrenolutine produced during the incubation of the four different sets of plasma is shown in a diagram. Lowest concentration of the aminochromes occurred in the aldosterone treated blood; the highest was in blood from the intact rat and in that of the adrenalectomized, hydrocortisone-treated animals. The adrenalectomized non-treated animal was partially protected from oxygen toxicity. Results indicated that adrenalectomized, aldosterone-treated animals were protected not only from oxygen toxicity, but also from the endogenous oxidation of epinephrine. It appears that manifestations of oxygen toxicity are produced by the metabolites of epinephrine intoxication. (MFW/BSCP)

899.
HOULIHAN, R.T.
Untitled.
In: Abstracts of BuMed-ONR sponsored Navywide workshop in high presure biomedical research, U.S .Submarine Base, Groton, Conn., May 1971. p.11. Published by the Naval Submarine Medical Research Laboratory, 1971.

Abstract only. Entire item quoted: It has been reported recently that the endocrine state of an animal clearly affects its response to oxygen toxicity but it is not known whether hormones directly after effects of oxygen at the cellular level. The author previously noted that an adrenocortical hormone production increase correlates very well with the symptom of oxygen toxicity. He also notes that the convulsions associated with oxygen toxicity are accompanied by a large sympathoadrenomedullary discharge. It had been shown that removal of either the adrenal cortex or medulla affords some protection to the toxicity of oxygen. An association between both these glands and oxygen toxicity could be in an increased metabolism of epinephrine via the indole pathway with the increased circulation adrenal steroids during exposure to hyperbaric oxygen. In the present study the authors report the proposed indole pathway of epinephrine metabolism. A modification of Hornings gas liquid chromatographic (GLC) separation of bioamines is usable in separating adrenochrome and adrenolutine from biological fluid. The data presented demonstrates the GLC spectra, high resolution mass spectroscopy of these compounds. These data are compared in adrenalectomized and steroid treated rats. They show a consistent correlation between an increased aminochrome production and symptoms of oxygen toxicity.

900.
HOULIHAN, R.T. and J.R. Downs.
Parotid gland response following exposure to oxygen at high pressure.
Physiologist 15:174;Aug. 1972.

Abstract only. Entire item quoted: During recent years, evidence has accumulated substantiating an increased epinephrine oxidase activity as one factor in acute oxygen toxicity. The earlier controversy regarding this enzyme led to questions of its in vivo activity and to indications that it was in highest concentration in the parotid gland. It was, therefore, considered necessary to examine the parotid gland, both in terms of its histology and possible changes in epinephrine oxidase following exposure to oxygen at high pressure (OHP). For this study, 200 gm. male Sprague-Dawley rats were used. These animals were adapted to the laboratory regimen of a 12 hour photoperiod with food and water ad libitum for two weeks. The animals were exposed to OHP at 60 PSIG for 45 minutes, by which time all of the animals had exhibited severe convulsions. The animals were slowly decompressed, the parotid glands removed and fixed in formalin or homogenized in normal saline giving a 10% homogenate. The fixed glands were sectioned and stained with hematoxalin and eosin for examination. One ml alequates of the homogenate were incubated with and without 5 mg. L-epinephrine for 30 minutes. One hundred ul of the incubate was chromatographed to separate the formed indoles which were then quantitated with GLC. The results of this study indicate the parotid gland is maximally stimulated by exposure to OHP. The tubule cells show significant lysis of the zymogen granules. The acinar cells are swollen. The nucleus is displaced and exhibits considerably hyperchromia. Measurements of epinephrine oxidase activity differ from the plasma enzyme. It is more reactive and produces less products of epinephrine with a preponderance of adrenochrome.

901.
HOULIHAN, R.T.
The effects of oxygen at high pressure on catecholamine metabolism.
Pontiac, Mich., Mich. Coll. Osteopath. Med., Rep. 301, 7p. Dec. 31, 1972.

In previous reports on contract (N00014-70-A0159-0001), consideration was given to renal function blood flow, adrenocortical, and sympathoadrenomedullary activity during the progression of oxygen toxicity. These studies led to proposing the involvement of epinephrine oxidation and indole production during acute oxygen poisoning. At the termination of this contract, cyclic oxidation of epinephrine has been verified. Adrenalectomy, which protects animals from oxygen toxicity, inhibits indole production. Enzyme activity is significantly increased during exposure to high pressure oxygen. There are species differences with respect to lung changes following seizures induced by hyperbaric oxygen. (Author's abstract)

902.
HOW, J. and G. Chan.
Management of delayed cases of decompression sickness — 3 case reports.
Singapore Med. J. 14(4):532-535;Dec. 1973.

Decompression sickness may give rise to a variety of symptoms and signs. Paralysis or paresis is the common presenting complaint because the victims, usually fishermen divers, ignore "minor" signs and symptoms. Three cases of decompression sickness were treated by therapeutic recompression using hyperbaric oxygen in September/October 1972 at the SAF Diving Centre. Only one session of therapeutic recompression lasting 285 minutes was carried out on each patient because of satisfactory results. The patho-physiology and symptomatology of decompression sickness and the rationale of using hyperbaric oxygentation in therapy are discussed. (Authors' synopsis)

903.
HOWE, G.R.
Untitled.
In: Abstracts of BuMed-ONR sponsored Navywide workshop in high pressure biomedical research, U.S. Naval Submarine Base, Groton, Conn., May 1971 p.10. Published by the Naval Submarine Medical Research Laboratory, 1971.

Abstract only. Entire item quoted: Experiments have been designed to test the effects of hyperbaric compression upon reproduction in laboratory rodents. Current methods have been developed so that only two experimental variables exist, namely, total level of compression and compression interval. Initial studies with male and female rats showed that short term continuous (96 hrs) or intermittent (5 hrs daily for 5 days) compression at 4-10 atmospheres had little effect on overall reproduction. Vaginal cycle length, however, was significantly decreased following increasing compression intervals. Such data suggested a relationship between level and/or duration of compression and reproductive capacity. Subsequent studies have subjected groups of mice (10 females and 3 males) to continuous compression at 3-6 atmospheres for varying intervals of 5 to 15 days. Total compression at 3 or 4 atmospheres for five days had no effect upon conception rate when compared to controls in the animal colony room or the pressure chamber at room atmospheres for 15 days resulted in lowered conception rates of 50 and 10 per cent respectively. These few existing conceptions did take place under the hyperbaric conditions. The conception failure was not irreversible in that normal conception rates were obtained in all females when they were exposed to males three weeks following termination of their hyperbaric exposure. Future studies will attempt to reveal the specific level(s) of total compression and/or compression interval that is deleterious to reproductive capacity. In turn, studies will then be conducted to isolate the specific mechanisms involved with impaired fertility so that preventive measures may be applied to future hyperbaric programs.

904.
HOWE, G.R.
Hyperbarism and reproduction: II. The conception rate of mice under different hyperbaric conditions.
Aerosp. Med. 44:5-7;Jan. 1973.

The exposure of sexually mature mice to compression at 3, 4, and 6 atmospheres for 5 consecutive days did not alter conception rate. In contrast, there was an inverse relationship between conception rate and hyperbaric duration greater than 5 days at all three levels of compression. The reproductive dysfunction was reversible within 3 weeks post hyperbaric termination. Litter size was not influenced by any of the experimental treatments. A histological examination of the gonads and adrenals did not reveal evidence of endocrine pathology from chronic hyperbarism. The degree of alteration in reproductive capacity was related to both level and duration of compression. (Author's abstract)

905.
HUANG, N.C. and G. Funk.
Inelastic buckling of a deep spherical shell subject to external pressure.
Notre Dame, Ind., Notre Dame Univ., Coll. Eng., Rep. UND-73-7, 69p. July 1973.
(AD 764 085)

The report is concerned with the investigation of the inelastic buckling of a deep spherical shell subject to a uniformly distributed external pressure. The geometry of the shell is considered to be axisymmetrical while the shell thickness may vary as a function of the polar angle. The edge of the shell is supported elastically. The material of the shell is assumed to satisfy the generalized Ramberg-Osgood stress-strain relations and a power law of steady creep. The analysis is based on Sanders' nonlinear theory of thin shells expressed in an incremental form and Hill's theory of inelastic bifurcation. Computations are carried out by a numerical iterative procedure associated with a finite difference method. Solutions are sought for both the axisymmetrical inelastic buckling and the asymmetrical bifurcation. (Authors) (GRA)

906.
HUBER, G.L., S.L. Porter, S.W. Burley, F.M. La Force and R.J. Mason.
The effect of oxygen toxicity on the inactivation of bacteria by the lung.
Chest 61(Suppl.):66S;Feb. 1972.

The effect of prolonged oxygen administration on host defense mechanism in the lung was evaluated by comparing the intrapulmonary inactivation of gram positive and gram negative bacteria. . . . Prolonged administration of 100 percent oxygen (PO_2.700 mmHg) resulted in progressive impairment of antibacterial defenses proportional to the duration of oxygen exposure. . . These studies demonstrate that excess oxygen is toxic to the pulmonary alveolar macrophages and to their antibacterial function in a dose-dependent relationship and provide a pathophysiologic basis for the pulmonary infection frequently associated with prolonged oxygen administration. (Authors)

907.
HUBER, G.L., C. O'Connell and M. Laforce.
The role of pulmonary surfactant in the bactericidal activity of alveolar macrophages during oxygen toxicity.
J. Clin. Invest. 52(6):422; 1973.

Abstract only. Entire item quoted: Although the alveolar macrophage (AM) is the key cell in antibacterial defenses in the lung, the bactericidal role of pulmonary surfactant is controversial. Prolonged exposure to 100% oxygen resulted in progressive depression in vivo of the intrapulmonary inactivation of an aerosolized challenge of radiolabeled (^{32}P) Staphylococcus aureus. Oxygen exposure also induced progressive increases in alveolar surface tension forces (quantified by pressure-volume relationships and correlation of alveolar bubble stability indices with ultrastructural morphometry) and decreases in surface activity and phospholipid phosphorus recoverable by brancho-pulmonary lavage. However, AM from control and oxygen-toxic rats were comparable in number, viability, and phagocytic uptake to staphylococci in vitro. Bacterial precoating with an acellular surfactant fraction (SF), recovered by centrifugation of lavage fluid (40,000 g), was required for intracellular killing by AM when evaluated in vitro with lysostaphin, in spite of the presence of excess strain-specificity antibody and fresh complement. SF by itself had no bactericidal activity. Incorporation of SF from control animals provided equivalent bactericidal activity for both control and oxygen-toxic AM, whereas incorporation of SF from oxygen-toxic animals resulted in no intracellular killing by either control or oxygen-toxic AM. In vivo adaptive tolerance to oxygen toxicity, induced by intermittent exposure to oxygen and characterized morphometrically by proliferation of granular pneumocytes (cellular origin or surfactant), attenuated the impairment in bactericidal activity and in recoverable surfactant. These experiments imply that bacterial coating with normal SF stimulates bactericidal activity of both control and oxygen-toxic AM and that the depressed bactericidal activity in the oxygen-toxic lung is secondary to alterations in SF rather than to a direct impairment in the AM.

908.
HUETER, T.F.
Twenty years in underwater acoustics: generation and reception.
Seattle, Wash., Honeywell Inc., Marine Systems Center, Rep. 2306, 21p. May 1971. (AD 756 063).
(Also published in J. Acoust. Soc. Amer., 51(3,Pt.2):1025-1040; 1972)

Development in the art of transducer design and array configuration has been spurred on mainly by two motivating forces: (1) Extensive research in underwater propagation has established the advantages of increasingly lower frequencies for long-range detection and localization of targets and noise sources. (2) The advent of new piezoelectric and structural materials and solid-state electronic devices has led to substantial improvements in transducer performance with regard to sensitivity, power output, and depth of submersion. Theory has kept abreast with these developments, particularly in handling large arrays with their mutual impedance problems, in pointing to digital multibeamforming techniques, and in revealing the significance of waveform design to detection performance. A few new concepts were born and have won acceptance during this period. These include: the generation of sound by hydroacoustic means, the employment of compliant metal tubes for acoustic focusing and reflection, the exploitation of structural flexing modes for sound radiation, and the use of free-flooded cavity structures as deep submergence sources. (Author) (GRA)

909.
HUGHES, D.M.
The real meaning of safety regulation to the diver, customer and contractor.
In: Professional diving safety. Second annual symposium, New Orleans, 1971. Mar. Technol. Soc. J. 6(34-40;Jan./Feb. 1972.

This is an informal discussion of some of the provisions of the American National Standards Institutes Z-135 Diving Procedures section; which had not been completed in final form at the time of this presentation. The author points out the lack of licensing procedure, which would adequately ensure a diver's qualification. Requirements at present tend to emphasize safety of equipment and procedures; personnel qualification standards require only proof of certain basic experience. Various provisions of the standards are discussed, including the requirement that responsibility for the safety of an operation be fixed on a designated individual, that a diving bell be used in all dives below 200 feet, that a stand-by diver be used in all dives requiring decompression, and in shallow water under unusually hazardous conditions. It is noted that too few specifications as to record-keeping are included. The advisability of quick-release weight belts is questioned; it is felt that they should be prohibited under certain conditions. Other requirements discussed include that of a double-lock decompression chamber below 130 feet; the provision that "for air dives deeper than 130 feet the diver must use equipment with a reserve air supply capable of life support for a minimum of five minutes at his working depth. This system must function independently of surface control or surface reserve supply"; requirements concerning open-bottom and pressure-capability diving bells. The question is raised as to real necessity of diving bells at 200 feet, and is left unanswered. (MFW/BSCP)

910.
HUGHES, D.M.
The evolution of commercial diving bells.
Oceanol. Int. 7:30-32;Mar. 1972.

The author refers to the diving bell, for the purpose of this article, as SWC (submersible work chamber). Modern SWCs differ from the old diving bell in that, as well as providing a refuge and a source of breathing gas, they provide a means of returning the divers to the surface under pressure, so that they can decompress on the surface. The two-compartment SWCs developed recently by American companies — Ocean Systems, Divcon and Avco, are discussed briefly.The purpose of two separate compartments is to permit supervisory personnel to stay at atmospheric pressure in the upper compartment, while the divers can operate out of the lower compartment at ambient pressure. These have proved cumbersome and costly to maintain, and the trend now is toward the single-compartment SWC. Breathing gas can be supplied by umbilicals from the surface or by the storage cylinders mounted on the SWC. They are all equipped with releasable ballast, so they can be made positively buoyant when necessary. Methods of giving SWCs a certain degree of horizontal mobility — towing, diving along tracks — are briefly discussed. Lock-out submersibles are a completely mobile form of SWC. Perry Shelf Diver and Deep Diver are cited as examples. The more complicated mobile habitat is being developed but is not yet in use. The aspect of SWC design and technology which needs the most improvement at present is the launch and recovery system. (MFW/BSCP)

911.
HUGHES, D.M.
Many factors affect deepwater dives.
Offshore 33:57-64;Aug. 1973.

The author points out the advantage of bounce diving as opposed to saturation diving in industry, because of the much shorter decompression time required. Most working dives can be completed within half an hour, and almost all tasks could be accomplished in two half-hour dives. However, it is emphasized that, due to a lack of firm data and adequate field research, a saturation decompression is required whenever a diver has been at 300-400 feet for more than one hour, or at 400-600 feet for more than half an hour, even though the diver has obviously not become saturated in this time. In diving deeper than 600 feet, hpns becomes a problem. Since the only way to avoid hpns at present is to compress slowly, a diver going to 1000 feet in order to do an hour's work would require 25 hours of compression time and ten days of decompression time. The central problem of deep diving in the near future is the development of a conventional, or bounce, diving system that has a saturation capability. Problems of human factors, atmosphere control, and support of the diver on the bottom are discussed. Much work needs to be done to meet these requirements. (MFW/UMS)

912.
HUGON, M., J. Chouteau, J.P. Roll, M. Bonnet and G. Imbert.
A study of spinal reflexes in baboons during saturation exposures to 16 and 21 ATA of $N_2 + O_2$.
In: Abstracts of the Twenty-fifth Congress of Physiological Sciences Satellite Symposium. Recent progress in fundamental physiology of diving. Marseille, France, July 1971, p.40-41. (Proceedings unpublished)

Abstract only. Entire item quoted: A study of the effects of hyperbaric normoxic oxygen-nitrogen atmosphere was performed on two Papio papio, pressures ranging from 1 to 21 ATA. The animals show their activity slowing with increasing depth, giving way to prostration at -160 m. During this diminishing activity, cardiac frequency and rate of respiration are also decreasing. The electrophysiological phenomenon in nerves and muscles are maintained without any obvious change in excitability or conductivity of nerves, or synaptic transmission during the whole experiment. The monosynaptic Hoffmann reflexes are small or null at depth, but the tendon reflexes (jerk) evoked in the same muscle (soleus) are increased by the same time. Latency and duration of these reflexes are constant during the dive. The cutaneous polysynaptic flexion reflexes are facilitated as obvious through their shorter latency or higher amplitude and longer duration. Apparently peripheral neuromuscular physiology is unimpaired. Spinal physiology displays only minor changes in this case. Apparently the main behavioural troubles could be due to some supra spinal dysfunction; possibly hypoxia is responsible in this dysfunction.

913.
HUNSINGER, R.
Repetitive dive calculator.
Skin Diver 20:48-49;July 1971.

NAUI Instructor Ralph Maruscak, who holds a degree in physics and is currently doing post graduate work in Ocean Engineering at the University of Southern California, has created an ingenious method of performing a repetitive dive calculation. He has rearranged the U.S. Navy Repetitive Dive Tables eliminating the need for any repetitive group designation for a no decompression dive and reduced the time required for a calculation to a fraction of the previous computation. These calculations, which are copy-righted and therefore cannot be reproduced, are available on a plastic card for the dive scene or a 30X40 inch chart for classroom presentation. It's a must for every diver who makes more than one dive a day. (Author's abstract)

914.
HUREVICH, M.I., N.V. Ilchevich, A.G. Kartseva, V.V. Bratus and E.A. Dykhin.
Pro fizichnoi roboti pid vodoyu na sertsevo-sudinnu sistemu lyudini.
[Effect of underwater physical activity on the cardiovascular system in man].
Fiziol. Zh. 18(606-613;Sept./Oct. 1972.

Ten amateur deepsea scuba divers, aged between 18-20 years, participated in this experiment. Cardiovascular function was tested at rest, with and without the diving gear. The data obtained served as control for the observations during immersion and underwater work. The following hemodynamic measurements were taken: systemic arterial pressure (measured by ocillagraphy), heart contraction rate (ECG), pulse rate, minute volume of blood (rheography), general and peripheral vascular resistance, the working index of the left ventricle, duration of the cardiac cycle and electric systole during expulsion. Immediately after submersion of the aqualung type 2 to the depth of 5-10 m the arterial pressure of the divers was found to be elevated, the pulse rate and blood minute volume (cardiac output) decreased, the total peripheral resistance increased. It was concluded that performance of underwater physical activity and exertion causes increased cardiac arterial pressure, decreased pulse rate, increased peripheral vascular resistance. A complex study of the character of these hemodynamic changes revealed a series of compensatory interrelationships between the various hemodynamic data. Further detailed studies are needed for the better understanding of the compensatory and adaptational reactions of the human cardiovascular system in order to develop an optimal underwater regime for deepsea diving. (OLC/SCD)

915.
HURLOCK, R. and A.H. Malin.
Case report: underwater contact lens correction.
Amer. J.Optom. 50:653-655;Aug. 1973.

This is a report of an underwater contact lens fitting procedure, a survey of the literature and an evaluation of the method. One of the major visual limitations imposed upon the diver in underwater activities is the constriction of the visual field due to the obstruction of the various masks in common use. . . . The method was to first fit what would have been an optimal fenestrated scleral lens, i.e. no blanching of the conjunctival blood vessels at the edges, centering on the lens in extreme rotation of the eye, and using sodium flourescein, ample clearance at the limbus and past it, apical clearance and a moveable air bubble. Although this case was successful, the method has not had widespread use for the following reasons: 1. The individual diver's conjunctival reaction to the water. 2. The need for a different breathing habit using a double-hose breathing regulator in order to avoid bubbling exhaust air across the eyes and eyelashes. 3. The expense compared to the diver's mask. 4. The additional effort and care required to place and remove the lens as compared to a face mask. The advantages are:1. The wide field and range. 2. The stability of the lenses in turbulent water. 3. The absence of mask squeeze while descending and ease in clearing the ears by being able to pinch the nose directly. 4. The freedom from fogging of the lenses. (Authors)

916.
HUSS, J.H.
Medical aspects of skin and scuba diving.
J. Sch. Health 42:238-242;Apr. 1972.

The problems encountered on descent include mechanical injuries known as "squeeze", which are brought about by the inequality of pressure between the air-containing spaces of the body, such as the inner ear, paranasal sinuses and the lungs, and the fluids and tissues of the body. These forms of squeeze usually heal spontaneously. Another form of squeeze can result from an air pocket under a faulty filling, inlay or cap of a tooth. In these cases, replacement is necessary. Thoracic squeeze, which occurs most often in skin divers diving too deeply, can be fatal. The problems encountered at depth include nitrogen narcosis, oxygen toxicity, and carbon dioxide poisoning. Hyperventilation by a skin diver can result in shallow water black-out caused by hypocapnia; this can cause drowning. Toxic properties in the breathing mixture, such as carbon monoxide from exhaust gases or oil vapors from compressors, are other hazards. The chief problem encountered on ascent is decompression sickness, caused by nitrogen bubbles in body tissues and fluids. The chief preventive measures are limitation on depth and bottom time and careful observation of decompression tables. Treatment is recompression. It is noted that methods of detection of bubbles before they reach the size to produce symptoms are being developed. These techniques include flowmeters and sonic detectors. The most common cause of fatal injury in sport divers is air embolism. This occurs when air enters the blood stream because of lung rupture; the bubbles usually enter the circulation of the brain. Symptoms occur within seconds of surfacing and include bloody, frothy sputum, confusion, deterioration in vision and in balance, paralysis, convulsions, and unconsciousness. In the case of the scuba diver, the appearance of bloody, frothy sputum should be assumed to be an indication of air embolism. In the case of a skin diver, it is probably due to thoracic squeeze. Either air embolism or decompression sickness must be assumed for an unconscious diver and recompression should be instituted as soon as possible. The importance of medical examinations of prospective divers is emphasized. The following areas are crucial: (1) heart disease; (2) respiratory disease; (3) chronic middle ear infection or tympanic membrane rupture; (4) diabetes mellitus; (5) chronic gastrointestinal disorders; (6) chronic musculo-skeletal disorders; (7) neuropsychiatric problems. (MFW/BSCP)

917.
HWANG, K.C.
A transient performance method for CO_2 removal with regenerable adsorbents.
Los Angeles, Cal, Airsearch Mfg. Co., Rep. 72-8786, NASA-CR-112098, 241p. Oct. 1972.
(N 73-10173)

A computer program is described which can be used to predict the transient performance of vacuum-desorbed sorbent beds for CO_2 or water removal, and composite beds of two sorbents for simultaneous humidity control and CO_2 removal. The program was written primarily for silica gel and molecular sieve inorganic sorbents, but can be used for a variety of adsorbent materials. Part 2 of this report describes a computer program which can be used to predict performance for multiple-bed CO_2 removal sorbent systems. This program is an expanded version of the composite sorbent bed program described in Part 1. (Author) (STAR)

918.
HYACINTHE, R. and B. Broussolle.
Etude de la mecanique ventilatoire au cours d'une plongee fictive a 51 ATA en helium-oxygene. [Study of the ventilatory mechanics during a simulated dive at 51 ATA with helium-oxygen]. Bull. Medsubhyp 8:4-6;Nov. 1972.

The respiratory function of two experienced divers was studied during a simulated helium-oxygen dive to 51 ATA, both as regards gas exchange and ventilatory mechanics. Dynamic lung compliance did not change. Expiratory resistance increased by 1.75. The isovolume pressure-flow curve reached a plateau at 41 ATA. At 51 ATA, the maximal expiratory flow at 75% of vital capacity decreased 62%, and the maximum voluntary ventilation decreased 58%. Oxygen and carbon dioxide partial pressures remained normal. The maximal voluntary debit was higher than the expiratory debit. The authors conclude that the limit of the ventilatory capacity at work probably occurs at about 61 ATA. (MFW/BSCP)

919.
HYACINTHE, R., B. Broussolle and D. Desbruyeres.
Affinite de l'hemoglobine pour l'oxygene chez l'homme en milieu hyperbare (31 ATA). [The affinity of hemoglobin for oxygen in man at 31 ATA]. Bull. Medsubhyp 10:44-46;Dec. 1973.

The affinity of hemoglobin for oxygen was studied in three divers during a simulated saturation dive at 31 ATA. The blood was withdrawn inside of the chamber, analysis was made outside. At 31 ATA, the oxygen affinity of hemoglobin increased (the P_{50} decreased from 28 mm Hg at sea level in air to 18 mm Hg). This change appeared after a period of 48 h; it was reversed during decompression. This increased affinity of hemoglobin for oxygen improves the alveolar uptake, but it may cause a cellular hypoxia as is suggested by the release of creatine phosphokinase after muscular exercise in cold water. (English abstract)

920.
HYACINTHE, R., B. Broussolle and F. Brue.
Affinite de l'hemoglobin pour l'oxygene en hyperoxie chronique chez le rat. [Affinity of hemoglobin for oxygen in chronic hyperoxia in rats]. J.Physiol. (Paris) 67:198A-199A; 1973.

Abstract only: Rats were exposed to pure normobaric oxygen for 48 hours, then to air for 5 hours, then again to oxygen. Blood samples were taken on the 5th, 10th and 20th day for measurements of (1) hemoglobin-oxygen affinity, measured by the P_{50} obtained by tonometry at 37°C and a pH = 7.40; and (2) erythrocyte 2,3-DPG concentration, plasma lactic acid, and hemoglobin level. P_{50} decreases constantly with exposure time from 34.2 mmHg to 29.4 mmHg. 2,3-DPG concentration, which is at 8.5 moles/ml in control animals, is maintained on the 5th day, and then falls to 5.9 moles/ml erythrocytes the 20th day; the molar 2,3-DPG/hemoglobin ratio, 1.53 for controls, falls to 1.05 the 20th day. Lactic acid increases to a maximum the 10th day. Increased affinity of hemoglobin for oxygen is clear in normobaric hyperoxia. It should be verified in more moderate, hyperbaric hyperoxia. (Transl. MEMH/UMS)

921.
IDICULA, J.
Perplexing case of maxillary sinus barotrauma. Aerosp. Med. 43:891-892;Aug. 1972.

Most cases of sinus barotrauma occur as the ambient pressure rises either while diving or while descending in an aircraft. It is reported in the literature that maxillary sinus barotrauma can cause neural symptoms (though rare) due to pressure on the infraorbital nerve which has its course through the infraorbital on the roof of the maxillary sinus. In the case presented here the barotrauma occurred while the subject was being decompressed from a 680-foot dive. This is possible, but rare, and is due to a pressure buildup inside the sinus due to blockage of the ostium by a ball-valve mechanism. The other interesting feature was the occurrrence of numbness in the distribution of the infraorbital nerve which was especially perplexing because the subject was decompressing after treatment for a knee bend. However, differentiation from neural decompression sickness was possible on recompression due to the sudden disappearance of symptoms with a hissing sound in the nose. Post-dive X-rays of the sinuses showed protrusion of the mucous membrane suggestive of chronic sinusitis. (Author's abstract)

922.
IHA, R.Y.
Portsmouth Naval Shipyard chamber modifications — 1971. U.S. Navy Exp. Diving Unit, Rep. NEDU-1-72, 12p. Jan. 1972.

Extensive modifications to the Navy Experimental Diving Unit Hyperbaric Facility were performed by the Portsmouth, New Hampshire Naval Shipyard during 1971. This report describes and documents the modifications which consist of installing penetrators, modifying hatch seals, magnetic particle testing welds and repair welding performed on the pressure hull. (Author's abstract)

923.
IMBERT, G., J. Chouteau, C. Roman and J. Corriol.
Somatovegetative and EEG dysfunction in goats during saturation exposure to high pressure (111 ATA).
In: Abstracts of the Twenty-fifth Congress of Physiological Sciences Satellite Symposium. Recent progress in fundamental physiology of diving. Marseille, France, July 1971, p.42. (Proceedings unpublished)

Abstract only. Entire item quoted: Chronically implanted electrodes allowed in ten goats continuous recordings of EEG, EKG, and EMG from postural muscles, diaphragm and gastric wall (reticulum). First trials were designed to definite patterns associated with classical stresses encountered during hyperbaric exposures (nitrogen narcosis, hypoxia, hyperoxia). In further experiments two subjects were compressed respectively to 111 and 91 ATA, where death occurred after severe hypoxia crises. Vegetative dysfunctions including arrests of gastric motility and flattening of circadian rhythms were observed long before the behavioural and irreversible EEG disturbances.

924.
INAMDAR, A.R., M. Wittner and R.M. Rosenbaum.
Control of rate-limiting enzymes in tryptophan metabolism during pulmonary O_2 toxicity.
J. Appl. Physiol. 33:234-237;Aug. 1972.

Exposure of rats to 100% oxygen at normal atmospheric pressure for 48-55 hr resulted in two- to threefold increases over control values of tryptophan pyrrolase activity in rat liver but had no effect on enzyme activity up to 24 hr of exposure. A slight increase in enzyme activity was observed in experimentally produced O_2-tolerant rats. Increased levels of tryptophan pyrrolase in intact animals under oxygen toxicity was presumably due to de novo synthesis of enzyme protein. Pyrrolase activity did not increase over air control values in adrenalectomized rats exposed to 100% oxygen for 55 hr but treatment of such animals with hydrocortisone increased enzyme activity in O_2-exposed animals, suggesting adrenocortical hormones are necessary for the induction of enzyme rather than a direct O_2 effect. Hepatic tryptophan hydroxylase activity remained unchanged in both O_2-toxic and O_2-tolerant rats at equivalent exposures to oxygen. (Authors' abstract)

925.
INGMANSON, D.C. and W.J. Wallace.
Oceanology: An Introduction.
Belmont, California. Wadsworth Publishing Co. Inc., 1973, 325p.

Although a beginner's text in oceanology it has a great deal of interest to the marine biologist and the diver. For the marine biologist the chapters on: Diversity of Marine Life; The Marine Environment: and the Contaminated Ocean. The Diversity of Marine Life is extensive in its coverage, profusely illustrated and easily read. For the underwater person the chapters on Motion of the Waters, The Contaminated Ocean, and Man and Technology are particularly appropriate. The entire text is beautifully styled with over 400 drawings and photographs, and with quotations and poetry at the beginning of each chapter. A detailed outline also precedes each chapter and a list of further reading follows each chapter. (CWS/UMS)

926.
INGVAR, D.V., J. Adolfson and C. Lindemark.
Cerebral air embolism during training of submarine personnel in free escape: an electroencephalographic study.
Aerosp. Med. 44:627-635;June 1973.

It is concluded that the incidence of lung rupture and/or air embolism (proven or suspected) during free ascent is about 3.5 per cent with the present careful observation technique. About one-half of the cases suffering from this complication may develop general or focal neurological symptoms as well as EEG disturbances, which, however, in the cases observed in the main series were transient. It is concluded that EEG recordings are valuable in the diagnosis and in the follow-up of cases in which air embolism has taken place. An EEG record taken before the beginning of the diving training was also found helpful to evaluate subsequent EEG abnormalities caused by air embolism. As a screening method for submarine personnel EEG has, however, been found to be of less value than current general medical procedures. (From authors' abstract)

927.
INNES, G.S.
Introduction to physical and chemical hazards.
In: Innes, G.S. ed. The production and hazards of a hyperbaric oxygen environment. Proceedings of a symposium held at University College, London, Jan. 1968, p.53-56. Oxford, Pergamon Press, 1970.

Mechanicals hazards are listed as underdesigning, bad handling and irradiation damage. Chemical hazards are listed as lack of oxygen, pocketing of carbon dioxide (these are unlikely to occur under routine procedures) and toxic chemicals from components (these should be designed especially to withstand high pressures and changing pressures). One of the chief dangers is fire or flash. Causes can be chemical ignition (such as the ignition of grease in a regulator); static spark; electrical breakdown; cable parting spark; (it is emphasized that the metal parts should be solidly bonded together and earthed); hot circuit; mechanical spark (abrasion). (MFW/BSCP)

928.
INNES, G.S. ed.
The production and hazards of a hyperbaric oxygen environment. Proceedings of a symposium held at University College, London, January 1968.
Oxford, Pergamon Press, 1970. 121p.

With this rapid expansion in the use of hyperbaric environments, the U.K. Liaison Committee felt that a Symposium was needed which would collate the available information. The papers given and which are reproduced in this book cover not only the advantages of hyperbaric treatment, the risks and their prevention, but also the underlying principles involved in the clinical application of hyperbaric oxygen. [Specific papers will be found under the following author entries: Brennand, R.; Denison, D.M.; Innes, G.S.; Ledingham, I. McA.; Purser, P.; Reeks, T.; Van Den Brenk, H.A.S.] (Author)

929.
INSTITUTE OF ELECTRICAL AND ELECTRONICS ENGINEERS.
IEEE international conference on engineering in the ocean environment, Panama City, Florida, September 1970. Digest of technical papers.
Published by the conference, 1970.

Most of the papers read at this conference were of a highly technological nature. Those that might have some bearing on man-oriented underwater activity will be found under the following author entries: Arndt, W.R.; Ballard, A.S.; Bares, W.A.; Chey, Y.H.; Flaherty, R.J., J.F. Tobin and E.H. Jones; Fulton, D., J. Irgon, J. Joye, R. Baccaglini and K. Rogers; Galpin, S.; Hasegawa, R.; Kies, J.A., R.L. Sanford and D.R. Mulville; Lee, J.V.; Lesster, L.E. and J.C. Frye; London, A.J.; Nielsen, T.W. and F.R. O'Brien; Pfeiffer, R.E.; Siegel, M. and R.W.P. King. (MFW/BSCP)

930.
INSTITUTE OF ELECTRICAL AND ELECTRONICS ENGINEERS.
1970 IEEE international conference on engineering in the ocean environment, Panama City, Florida, 21 September. Digest of tutorial papers.
New York, Lewis Winner, 1970.

The papers published in this Digest that might bear relation to man-oriented underwater activities will be found under the following author entries: Fischer, K.H.; Porter, R.B. and R.H. Banks; Vail, E.G. (MFW/BSCP)

931.
INSTITUTE OF ELECTRICAL AND ELECTRONIC ENGINEERS.
Ocean 73. 1973 IEEE international conference on engineering in the ocean environment.
IEEE publication 73 CHO 774-0 OCC. 623p. 1973.

The three session of this conference which were most directly related to the problems of man underwater were Session II-A: Underwater imaging and viewing; Session IV-B: Buoys and submersibles; Session III-A: Diving and life support systems. Specific papers will be found under the following author entries: Burrows, D.W. and J.F. Hadwin; Burt, J.F., Jr. and A.J. Dietrich; Fugitt, R.B.; Funk, C.J.; Geller, M., D.E. Altman and G.J. Barstow; Hody, G.L., J.J. Kacirk and A.A. Pilmanis; Holland, C.R.; Jacobson, J.O., D.P. Haugen and M.N. Hogman; Kashiwagi, H. and Suzuki; Mine, H., T. Hasegawa, K. Ohno and H. Kawai; Moritz, W.E.; Nakatsui, M., J. Suzuki, T. Takasugi and R. Tanaka; Sakurai, K., H. Kashiwagi, M. Kasamatsu, T. Sato and Y. Suzuki; Rolle, A.L.; Uhrich, R.W.; Waltz, A.R.; Watanabe, S. and T. Homma; Berju, K.K., E.L. Daniels and E.M. Strohlein. Strohlein. (MFW/UMS)

932.
INWOOD, M.J.
Experimental evidence in support of hypothesis that intravascular bubbles activate the hemostatic process.
In: Ackles, K.N. ed. Blood bubble interaction in decompression sickness. Proceedings of an international symposium held at Defence and Civil Institute of Environmental Medicine, Downsview, Ontario, Canada, p.171-200. Published by the Institute, December 1973. (DCIEM Conference Proceedings 73-CP-960) (Author's conclusions)

After experimental decompression sickness studies using rats, followed by experimental protective use of drugs, it was concluded that the mechanisms that implicate the hemostatic system during pathogenesis of decompression sickness occur in three stages. The first is platelet consumption, which probably begins as soon as the gas bubble enters the vessel. Thrombocytopenia occurs when platelets can no longer be released, and the platelet count will probably not return to normal for several days. Second, with increasing bubble load, the blood coagulation mechanism is activated; increase in coagulability is in direct ratio to the number of bubbles present. Third, when the circulation is severely hampered by acidosis, hypoxia, and gross microcirculatory perfusion defects, consumption of intrinsic coagulation factors and increased activation of the fibrinolytic system occur. This stage can be called disseminated intravascular coagulation (DIC), and reflects a general breakdown of protective mechanisms. The role of drugs in decompression sickness is both prophylactic and therapeutic. An agent active against platelet adhesiveness, such as the dipyridamole analogues, combined with potential danger of hemorrhage. As a therapeutic agent, PF-68 appears to be preferable to some others, in correction of the perfusion defect. Heparin may be required, but its use is fraught with many complications. (MFW/UMS)

933.
ISHERWOOD, D.M., D.R. Isherwood and W. Annan.
Factors affecting the precision and accuracy of PO_2 measurements using the Clark electrode.
Clin. Chim. Acta 42(2):295-301; 1972.

The results of a laboratory quality control survey for oxygen tension estimation were given. The scheme was based on the interchange between laboratories of human blood specimens arriving for routine analysis, of partially equilibrated blood samples, and of O_2-N_2 gas mixtures. The analytical results of these samples were used to detect and quantitate errors in the measurement of PO_2. A major cause of both systematic and random errors in the PO_2 results was the technique of sampling standards for calibration of the electrode. Different methods for calibrating the O_2 electrode were compared by analyzing standard O_2-N_2 gas mixtures. Atmospheric air was a reliable standard, and O_2-N_2 gas mixtures provided a convenient and accurate means of assessing the prevision and accuracy of routine PO_2 measurements. (© BA)

934.
ISHIKAWA, S. and M.S. Segal.
Re-appraisal of helium-oxygen therapy on patients with chronic lung disease.
Ann. Allergy 31:536-542;Nov. 1973.

The authors investigates the use of helium-oxygen mixtures on patients with chronic obstructive lung disease, in order to assess the respiratory gas exchange which accompanied the use of these breathing mixtures. It was found that clinically stable patients were able to maintain oxygen and carbon dioxide partial pressures through the use of this mixture, and in two cases, the oxygen partial pressure increased and the carbon dioxide partial pressure decreased. These findings may be of some interest to the diving community, because of the prevalence of the use of helium-oxygen. (MFW/UMS)

935.
ISHIZUKA, R., K. Miyakawa, T. Maekawa, B. Imamura, T. Akashi, N. Tanaka, Y. Kasai, H.C. Jockin and W.F. Bernhard.
Pulmonary surface characteristics in oxygen toxicity.
In: Wada, J. and I. Takashi, eds. Proceedings of the fourth international congress on hyperbaric medicine, Sapporo, Japan, Sept. 1969, p.16-21. Baltimore, Williams and Wilkins, 1970.

Group 1 showed the longest survival time. Nevertheless, pulmonary damage was remarkable in relation to surface characteristics. Pulmonary oxygen toxicity was suspicious of main cause of death. Group 2 which underwent controlled respiration showed the moderate compliance reduction. However, since 20% of the material were induced on pulmonary edema at their critical stage, much attention should be paid on surfactant damage when continuous mechanical respiration is applied. Group 3 showed the highest depression of surface activity among OHP groups. Pulmonary oxygen toxicity was also considered as in Group 1. Group 4 and Group 5 died in fairly short hours after oxygen exposure. There were remarkable symptoms of disturbance in central nervous system which was suspicious of a fatal cause of death in oxygen toxicity. However, pulmonary surface characteristics are generally within normal limits. (Authors' summary)

936.
ISHIZUKA, R., K. Miyakawa, T. Maekawa, K. Tajima, T. Nagao, I. Onodera, T. Sato and Y. Kasai.
The role of protective agents against oxygen toxicity; influence on the SH enzymes and correlated metabolic components.
In: Wada, J. and I. Takashi, eds. Proceedings of the fourth international congress on hyperbaric medicine, Sapporo, Japan, Sept. 1969, p.49-54. Baltimore, Williams and Wilkins, 1970.

Single shot of the so-called protective agents against oxygen toxicity failed to get any significant effect to prolong the survival time of materials at 1 ATA oxygen. Blood chemistry revealed no significant difference among them. Gross and microscopic findings of the main viscera revealed typical pulmonary edema. Histochemical study in the brain, kidney and liver proved marked reduction of succinic dehydrogenase activity regardless of drug preparations. (Authors' summary)

937.
ISSAAKJAN, L.A., G.V. Troshikhin and A.G. Zhironkin.
The influence of increased atmospheric pressure on oxygen availability in muscle tissue of rats.
In: Hesser, C.M. and D. Linnarsson, eds. Proceedings of the first annual sicentific meeting of the European Undersea Biomedical Society, Stockholm, 13-15 June 1973. Forsvarsmedicin 9:357-359;July 1973.

Wistar rats were exposed to various pressures of helium and nitrogen breathing mixtures. Oxygen partial pressure was maintained at 0.21 ATA. The oxygen availability (O_2a) in the m. quadriceps femoris was measured. In He-O_2 mixtures, at 20 and 40 kgp/cm^2 pressure, and 28°C temperature, O_2a in the muscle decreased 20 and 40% as compared with air at atmospheric pressure; rectal temperatures decreased by 2.7 and 3.2°C respectively. When the He-O_2 mixture was raised to 3°C, O_2a decrease did not occur. Neither did it occur when N_2-O_2 was used at a pressure of 6 kgp/cm^2 and 26°C. A rise of pressure of 20 kgp/cm^2 resulted in 20% lowering of O_2a. In the case of He-O_2, it could be due to density effects on respiration, to anesthetic action of nitrogen, or to decrease of blood flow. (MFW/UMS)

938.
JACEY, M.J. and K.E. Schaefer.
The effects of chronic hypercapnia on blood phosphofructokinase activity and the adenine nucleotide system.
Resp. Physiol. 16:267-272;Oct. 1972.

Phosphofructokinase activity and adenine nucleotide levels were determined in blood of guinea pigs exposed to 15% CO_2 in 21% O_2, balance N_2, for varying periods of time up to one week. Acute exposure produced a decrease in enzyme activity while the chronic phase increased activity without attainment of control values. These alterations in blood phosphofructokinase activity strikingly paralleled the biphasic changes in blood pH during acute and chronic hypercapnia. These findings demonstrate that blood phosphofructokinase activity is capable of responding to in vivo fluctuations in blood pH. Arterial ATP, ADP, and AMP concentrations and the energy change were virtually unchanged during both phases indicating that hypercapnia is characterized by conservation of high-energy phosphates. (Authors' abstract)

939.
JACEY, M.J., D.V. Tappan and K.R. Ritzler.
Hematologic responses to severe decompression stress.
In: Aerospace Medical Association. 1973 annual scientific meeting, Las Vegas, Nevada, May 1973. Preprints, p.198-199. Published by the Association, 1973.

A study was undertaken to investigate and identify potential hemotological alterations during a period of recovery from dysbaric stress. Mature male rats of the Sprague-Dawley strain were pressurized and decompressed according to a schedule previously determined by us to give a proper degree of survival. . . . The data demonstrate an apparent recovery from hypovolemia associated with severe dysbaric stress which may be followed by the development of microcytic, hypochromic anemia-like condition with an accompanying hemoconcentration. Acute decompression stress also caused a transient leucopenia due to a reduction in lymphocytes. A neutrophilia which was both relative and absolute accompanied the lymphopenia. All white cell parameters returned to control values at one day and remained at these levels for the duration of the observation period. (Authors)

940.
JACEY, M.J., D.V. Tappan and K.R. Ritzler.
Hematologic responses to severe decompression stress.
U.S. Nav. Submar. Med. Res. Lab., Rep. NSMRL 744, 12p. May 3, 1973.

Red and white blood cell parameters were measured in the blood of mature Sprague-Dawley rats at various times up to three days following compression and severe decompression. Acute decompression stress (one-hour post-surfacing) produced an increase in red cell count, hematocrit and hemoglobin, without concomitant alterations in red cell indices. This was taken as evidence of hemoconcentration. The normalization of red cell parameters by one day post-decompression was indicative of a spontaneous resolution of the acute hypovolemia. During the late phase of the observation period (day two), red cell counts again rose without changes in hematocrit and hemoglobin levels. At day three, red cell counts further increased with accompanying hematocrit elevation but without alteration in hemoglobin. During this period (days two and three) mean corpuscular volume and mean corpuscular hemoglobin declined. Parallel decreases in these indices are indicative of microcytic hypochromic morphology and may be caused by the time-related hypertonic plasma. At no time was evidence of retibulocytosis or decrease in red cell counts, hemoglobin or hematocrit levels noted. The increase in hematocrit and red cell count at the end of the experiment suggests another episode of hemoconcentration. These data demonstrate, then, that an apparent recovery from severe dysbaric stress may be followed by the development of a microcytic hypochromic condition, with an accompanying hemoconcentration. Acute decompression stress caused a transient lymphocytic leucopenia together with a concomitant neutrophilia which was both relative and absolute. All white blood cell parameters returned to control values at one day post-decompression and remained at these levels for the duration of the observation period. The acute leucocytic changes following exposure to severe decompression fit the classical concept of adrenal cortical responses to stress. (Authors' abstract)

941.
JACEY, M.J., D.V. Tappan and J.J. Wojtowicz.
A compression-decompression schedule for producing dysbaric stress in mature rats.
U.S. Nav. Submar. Med. Res. Lab., Rep NSMRL 749, 7p. Aug. 8, 1973.

A need arose to develop a compression-decompression table that would insure a proper degree of severe decompression stress in rats. Severe decompression stress has been defined as that stress which is neither safe, allowing complete

(100%) survival, nor excessively hazardous (explosive) resulting in a 90-100% death rate within one hour post-surfacing. By these criteria, then, a 66% survival rate documents severe decompression. This report details a schedule with 72 minutes of chamber time which will routinely produce severe decompression stress in rats. This schedule was employed as a model for a study of the effects of decompression accidents which may be encountered by human divers. (Authors' abstract)

942.
JACOBSON, J.O., D.P. Haugen and M.N. Hogman.
Ultrasonic detection of bloodstream emboli.
In: Ocean 73. 1973 IEEE international conference on engineering in the ocean environment, p.141-147. IEEE publication 73 CHO 7740 OCC.

Quantitative assessment of decompression-induced emboli in the blood flow may provide important information relating to physiological changes associated with decompression. A CW transmitter-receiver unit and a chest-mounted transducer probe have been developed for non-invasive ultrasonic monitoring of pulmonary blood flow using Doppler shift techniques. Preliminary spectral analysis of signals obtained during simulated dives in a hyperbaric test facility indicates that the spectrum of abnormal emboli signals is significantly different from that of normal blood flow. A preliminary theory explaining the observed spectra is offered. (Authors' abstract)

943.
JACOBSON, M.J. and L.A. Stallworth.
Sound transmission in an isospeed ocean channel with depth-dependent current.
Troy, N.Y., Rensselaer Polytech. Inst., Dept. Math., Rep. RP1-Math-98, 17p. Aug. 6, 1971. (AD 750,974)
(Also published in J. Acoust. Soc. Amer. 51(5, Pt. 2):1738-1750; 1972.

A constant sound-speed (isospeed) channel with horizontal boundaries and a current of constant direction and linear depth-dependent magnitude is considered. Ray paths are closely approximated by connected circular helical arcs. Expressions for the travel time and spreading loss of individual arrivals are found when necessary and sufficient conditions for the ray paths to be plane are satisfied. For a bottom-mounted source and receiver, it is shown that a current gradient can significantly affect the ray geometry, travel time, and spreading loss of each arrival. The total field for a 33-kmX40-m channel is calculated. It is found that small changes in the current gradient can produce large variations in the amplitude and phase of the field including the amplitude fade-phase offset phenomenon. (Authors) (GRA)

944.
JACQUEMIN, C., P. Varene and J. L'Huillier.
Aspects respiratoires de l'environnement thermique hyperbare.
[Respiratory aspects of the hyperbaric thermal environment].
J. Physiol. (Paris) 63:293-295;May 1971.

The authors attempt to develop a predictive equation of the specific heat of a ventilated gas as a function of the environment and of the activity of the subject. The experimental side of this study comprised an attempt to measure $T_{ex} - T_{in}$ (where T_{ex} = temperature of exhaled gas and T_{in} = temperature of inhaled gas) by means of thermocouples temporarily lodged in the esophagus. Experiments were carried out at 1 and 5 Ata, at rest, in normal and hypernea induced by the inhalation of dry gaseous mixtures. No correlation was found between T_{ex} and ventilation, but T_{ex} appeared to be a function of the first degree of T_{in}, as shown in Figure 1 (p. 294). The study of esophagal temperatures also enabled the authors to describe exactly the mechanisms of this thermal exchange: they conclude that, in man at least, the pulmonary thermal exchanger is controlled by the gas-exchange regulatory system, not by the thermo-regulatory system. A constant alveolar temperature is maintained by means of heat exchanges between the inhaled gases and the surrounding tissues of the respiratory tract. (MEMH/BSCP)

945.
JAMES, J.E.A. and M. DeB. Daly.
Some mechanisms involved in the cardiovascular adaptations to diving.
In: The effect of pressure on organisms. Symposia of the Society for Experimental Biology, No. 26, p.313-341. Cambridge, University Press, 1972.

The authors discuss the following cardiovascular adaptations which occur in diving mammals such as seals and whales: cardiac output, arterial blood pressure, and regional vascular resistance. They then discuss some of the mechanisms which might be related to these adaptations: changes in intrathoracic pressure, trigeminal nerve reflexes, vagus nerve reflexes from upper respiratory tract, asphyxia, role of arterial chemoreceptors, reflexes from the thorax, pulmonary vagal reflex, central "irradiation," role of arterial baroreceptors, and other possible mechanisms. In conclusion, they emphasize "the role played by integrative mechanisms of the automatic nervous system," in these cardiovascular responses, noting at the same time that understanding of which cardio-respiratory inputs to the CNS are concerned is still very incomplete. (MFW/SCD)

946.
JASKUNAS, S.R., E.J. Stork, and B. Richardson.
Effects of a hyperoxic environment on erythropoietin production.
Aerosp. Med. 44:1112-1116;Oct. 1973.

Experiments were performed to clarify the mechanisms by which hyperoxia suppresses erythropoiesis. Increased plasma erythropoietin levels induced in rats by phlebotomy or phenylhydrazine were suppressed by a hyperoxic environment. The stimulation of erythropoiesis by testosterone propionate, presumably resulting from increased production of erythropoietin, was also suppressed by hyperoxia. No effect on the activity of erythropoietin was found. The results suggest that decreased levels of circulating erythropoietin can be attributed to decreased production rather than increased clearance or reduction in the activity of erythropoietin. (Authors' abstract)

947.
JASTRZEBSKI, J., M. Slomkowski, R. Michalowska and E. Kostrezewska.
Zachowanie sie adhezji krwinek plytkowych pod wplywem wzrostu cisnienia czastkowego tlenu (P_aO_2) w krwi tetniczej.
[The behavior of blood platelet adhesiveness under the effect of increased oxygen tension (PO_2) in arterial blood].
Acta Haematol. Pol. 2:355-337;Oct./Dec. 1971.

Experiments have been performed on the effect of increased oxygen pressure on platelet adhesiveness. It was found that with increased partial pressure there is a decreasing tendency in platelet adhesiveness. The observed variations are statistically significant and there is a negative correlation between the increase in the pressure of molecular oxygen and the adhesiveness of platelets (the greater the PO_2 the smaller the adhesiveness). This may partially explain the occurrence of hemorrhagic complications in the course of protracted hyperoxygenation. Tests were performed on 8 subjects, 3 males, 5 females, aged 17-29. No surgery was performed. Blood was drawn from the radial artery twice: once during breathing of atmospheric air; and then after 5-10 min of breathing of pure oxygen. Differences in partial pressure are highly significant. No changes were observed in the acid-base equilibrium. It has been noted in past studies that iron and copper compounds in blood participate in oxygen transport. The excess of oxygen in blood platelets disturbs the hemostatic activity of blood platelets. Studies are also being conducted on the relationship between blood platelets and Factor III. (OLC/SCD)

948.
JEGOU, A.
Deep diving and cold water — some practical results.
In: The working diver, 1972, Symposium proceedings, February 1972, Columbus, Ohio, p.127-143; Washington, D.C., Marine Technology Society, 1972.

Foundation COMEX, a new Canadian Company, was chosen by Tenneco Oil and Minerals, Ltd., to furnish diving assistance during Tenneco's 1971 summer operations off the coast of Labrador (Canada) with the drilling vessel Typhoon belonging to the Storm Drilling Co. Despite very adverse conditions, including a water depth of 570 ft. a bottom water temperature of 30°F., bottom currents up to one knot, and danger of icebergs, all required underwater operations were successfully carried out. The deep diving equipment had to permit saturation diving (at least very long decompression) and back-to-back bounce dives, and it had to be usable without guidelines in case of necessity. Last, but not least, it had to suit available space. The personnel were carefully selected and trained for the job. Before the beginning of operations, all divers were tested in wet and dry pressure chambers in Marseilles, France, simulating 660 ft., of depth in water at 28°F. The decompression procedures specially computed are quick and safe for optimum utilization. The key factor in making this a successful performance was the utilization of a new type of individual diving rig by the divers. The equipment was developed basically for a saturation dive at 840 ft and it has been improved during a series of tests under the conditions mentioned above (660 ft. and 28°F). The divers have worked in water for 70 minutes, though this is not a limit. The special individual equipment consists of (a) a constant-volume dry suit; (b) an electrically heated undergarment with a low voltage supply controlled by the diver; (c) an electric gas heater maintaining a constant gas-inhalation temperature. (Author's abstract)

949.
JENKINS, J.F.
Analysis of hydrophone support structure after 52-1/2 months exposure at a depth of 5270 feet in the Barking Sands Test range, Kauai, Hawaii.
U.S. Nav. Civil Eng. Lab., Rep. NCEL-TN-1267, 15p. Mar. 1973.
(AD 759 674)

The condition of the support structure for hydrophone 4-7 of the Barking Sands Test Range, Kauai, Hawaii, was analyzed after 52-1/2 months of exposure to seawater at a depth of 5270 feet. The types and severity of corrosion on the various structural components are described and analyzed. A prediction of the additional lifetime to be expected from similar structures at this location is made. Recommendations for extending the useful lifetimes of similar structures at this site are made. (Author) (GRA)

950.
JENKINS, W.T.
A summary of diving techniques used in polar regions.
U.S. Nav. Coastal Syst. Lab., Preliminary Rep. under ONR Res. Proj. RF 51-523-101, 100p. July 1973.

The contents of this manual are as follows: Chapter 1 — Introduction: Purpose and scope, Background, The environment, Thermal protection; Chapter 2 — Logistics: General, Ground transportation, Air transportation, Surface Effect Vehicles (SEV's); Chapter 3 — Equipment: Exposure suits, Regulators, Dive support; Chapter 4 — Operational: Dive plan, Water entry/exit, Navigation, Emergency procedures; Chapter 5 — Biomedical: Physiological stress, Types of cold injury, Prevention of cold injury, Selection of personnel, Psychological stress. The report concludes with an extensive bibliography and a glossary. (MFW/BSCP) [This report has since been supplemented by "A guide to polar diving" prepared by the same author for Office of Naval Research and published in September, 1974].

951.
JENNINGS, C.
Inflatable diving suit.
Skin Diver 20:40-42; 66-67;Apr. 1971.

The Unisuit, manufactured by A.B. Aqua Sport in Sweden, comes in two models: the Super, for extra heavy duty, and the Explorer, for normal diving conditions. The former has an extra nylon lining; both are made of 1/4 inch neoprene. They can be worn with heavy underwear in cold conditions and light underwear in warmer temperatures. A layer of air is kept next to the skin. The suit can be inflated and deflated easily by pressing an air intake button to inflate and an exhaust button to deflate. There is a zipper that passes from the chest between the legs and up between the shoulder blades in the back. It is of a special design that is waterproof and pressure-proof. The suit is very flexible, even when inflated. In performing underwater tasks, a diver can lift as much as he can hold with one hand, by utilizing the buoyancy of the suit. The chief advantage of the Unisuit, however, is the thermal comfort that it furnishes. (MFW/SCD)

952.
JENSEN, C.B., S.J. Brumleve and B. De Boer.
An electronystagmographic study of post-rotatory nystagmus duration, number of beats, and frequency in 10 atmospheres absolute helium and oxygen and during decompression.
Physiologist 16:353;Aug. 1973.

Abstract only. Entire item quoted: Adult, male guinea pigs weighing 700 gm ($\pm$ 100 gm) were chronically implanted with periorbital, silver, disc electrodes for the purpose of recording electronystagmus. Each was individually restrained in a plexiglas restraining cage, secured to a turntable, and placed in a hyperbaric chamber for subsequent experimentation. Vestibular nystagmus was induced by rapidly stopping the turntable following ten rotations at 40 rpm. Post-rotary electronystagmograms were recorded by a polygraph, and all eye movements were monitored on an oscilloscope. Nystagmus duration, number of eye beats, and frequency were manually determined from the polygraph recordings. Post-rotary nystagmus samples were recorded in room air, 1 atmosphere absolute (ata) helium and oxygen (He-O_2), 10 ata He-O_2, and at four stages (7.7 ata, 5.0 ata, 3.5 ata, and 1.0 ata) during six different decompression rates (0.4, 0.06, 0.08, 0.10, 0.12, and 0.15 ata/min). Slight changes in post-rotatory nystagmus duration, number of beats, and frequency were observed in each of the test environments. The greatest post-rotatory nystagmus variations occurred during decompression, and the fastest decompression rates provided the most significant alterations. Spontaneous nystagmus was present during rapid decompression, and the possibility of its serving as a warning of impending decompression trauma was evaluated.

953.
JERRETT, S.A.
Seizures, H_2O_2 formation, and lipid peroxides in brain during exposure to oxygen under high pressure.
In: Aerospace Medical Association. 1972 annual scientific meeting, Bal Harbour, Florida, May 1972. Preprints, p.127-128. Published by the Association.

The purpose of this study was to determine if H_2O_2 occurs in brain during OHP and if it has any relation to lipid peroxidation and seizures and to study any morphologic alterations that acute OHP exposure causes in brain. Mice of equal age and weight were divided into two groups; one was fed chow and the other a tocopherol deficient diet. One-half of the chow fed mice were then given tocopherol intraperitoneally (i.p.) prior to study. All the tocopherol deficient and 50% of the chow fed mice seizured whereas none of the tocopherol supplemented ones did. The brain H_2O_2 of the tocopherol deficient mice at room air was higher (34 u) than that in chow fed mice (27 u) at the .01 level of significance. Chow fed mice exposed to OHP, however, demonstrated brain H_2O_2 levels of 41 u vs the 34 u for tocopherol deficient animals at room air ($P < .025$). Tocopherol deficient mice under OHP demonstrated the greatest elevation of H_2O_2 (71 u) which was significantly elevated ($P < .005$) above all other groups. The tocopherol supplemented mice were seen to have the lowest level of H_2O_2 of all groups ($P < .025$). (Author)

954.
JERRETT, S.A., D. Jefferson and C.E. Mengel.
Seizures, H_2O_2 formation and lipid peroxides in brain during exposure to oxygen under high pressure.
Aerosp. Med. 44:40-44;Jan. 1973.

Mice and rats of varying tocopherol status were exposed to oxygen under high pressure (OHP). Brain levels of lipid peroxide and H_2O_2 were measured and the animals monitored for clinical seizure activity. H_2O_2 levels were highest in OHP exposed tocopherol-deficient animals. Brain levels of lipid peroxide paralleled H_2O_2 formation. Seizures occurred in 100% of tocopherol-deficient, 50% of chow-fed, and 0% of tocopherol-supplemented mice. Tocopherol-deficient rats exposed to OHP and compared with controls showed elevation of lipid peroxides at 5 minutes; H_2O_2 was elevated at 15 minutes. At these times, there was no clinical evidence of seizures. Tocopherol-deficient mice exposed to acute OHP showed no CNS lesions under light microscopy or ultrastructure analysis. The data are consistent with the hypothesis that CNS oxygen toxicity is caused by peroxidation of membrane lipid. The role of H_2O_2 and lipid peroxide as enzyme toxins is discussed. (Authors' abstract)

955.
JOANNY, P., J. Corriol, J. Calcet and F. Giannellini.
Oxygene hyperbare: taux de malonaldehyde dans le plasma, les hematies et le tissu cerebral du Rat.
[Hyperbaric oxygen: malonaldehyde levels in the plasma, erythrocytes and cerebral tissue in rats].
C.R. Soc. Biol. (Paris) 165:1341-1346; 1971.

Malonaldehyde levels of rat plasma, red blood cells and cerebral tissue were studied in an attempt to determine the possible relationship between cerebral hyperexcitability under hyperbaric oxygen and lipid peroxydation. Twenty-eight male and female Wistar rats were exposed to 100% O_2 in small caissons. The pressure of 4.6 Ata was reached in ten minutes, and maintained for 3 hours. CO_2 given off by the animals was eliminated by soda lime and a constant flow of gas. A plexiglass window permitted constant observation. For the analysis of results, the rats are divided into three groups: (a) unexposed animals; (b) exposed animals which did not suffer convulsions; and (c) exposed animals which presented convulsions. A significantly higher malonaldehyde level was found in the cerebral tissues of groups b and c than in group a; further, the difference in malonaldehyde levels between groups b and c were significant. For the erythrocytes, the difference between the control group and the exposed rats was not considered significant, but a very significant difference was found between groups b and c. For the plasma, there was no significant difference between groups b and c, but a significant difference was noted between the exposed rats and those of the control group. (Specific details of results are given in the Table, p. 1345.) It is speculated that a critical level of lipidic peroxydation may be a determinant of the convulsive crises noted under hyperbaria; research on this and related topics should be encouraged. (MEMH/BSCP)

956.
JOANNY, P. and J. Corriol.
Cytotoxicite nerveuse de l'oxygene hyperbare.
[Nerve cell toxicity of hyperbaric oxygen].
In: Fructus, X., ed. Third international conference on hyperbaric and underwater physiology, p.205. Paris, Doin, 1972.

The authors studied the elimination of $^{14}CO_2$, the consumption of glucose and glycolytic activity of sections of the cerebral cortex and cardiac tissue of the rat, as well as of isolated retinas of oxen. Results showed a significant increase in glycolysis in nerve tissue in proportion to the oxygen partial pressure and the duration of the exposure; the increase was slight in the cardiac tissue. The findings suggest that under hyperbaric oxygen, when the cellular structure is kept intact, the route of Embden-Meyeroff cannot be considered as a limiting metabolic factor. (MFW/UMS)

957.
JOANNY, P. and J. Corriol.
Etude sur des coupes de tissus cerebral de mammifere des effets de l'oxygene hyperbare sur divers parametres metaboliques et la repartition ionique.
[Study of the effects of hyperbaric oxygen on various metabolic parameters and ionic distribution in slices of cerebral tissue].
In: Fructus, X., Ed. Third international conference on hyperbaric and underwater physiology, p.203-204, Paris, Doin, 1972.

The authors attempted to link functional modifications of the nervous tissue to cytotoxicity of hyperbaric oxygen, manifesting itself particularly at the level of certain parameters of oxydative metabolism, and of the apparent intracellular ionic distribution. Although specific mechanisms of oxygen toxicity remain to be demonstrated, it has been shown in these experiments with rats and guinea pigs that peroxides may play an important role in its genesis. The inactivation of thioenzymes, structural alterations of lipoproteins involved in the transfer of energy, or of electrons, can modify considerably the permeability of the mitochondrial membrane or of the external membrane. (MFW/UMS)

958.
JOANNY, P., J. Calcet, J. Corriol and F. Giannellini.
Peroxidation des lipides cerebraux et crises convulsives hyperoxiques.
[Peroxidation of cerebral lipids and convulsive hyperoxic seizures].
J. Physiol. (Paris) 67:199A; 1973.

Abstract only: In order to examine the possible role of lipid peroxidation in the determination of disturbances noted under hyperbaric oxygen, we used for the first time a method of specific ultra-microanalysis of the peroxide groups of the cerebral poly-unsaturated fatty acids. Groups of 2 rats were subjected to a PO_2 of 4.6 ATA in the same caisson. The brains were separately analysed as soon as convulsive seizures appeared in one animal. The levels of peroxidation were found to increase significantly in the following order: normoxic rats: 0.64 x 10^{-8} at O_2g-1; hyperbaric rats without convulsions: 0.87 x 10^{-8}; rats presenting convulsions: 1.62 x 10^{-8}. In addition, comparative analysis of cerebral malonaldehyde (an end product of peroxide cleavage) in the same two latter classes confirms these results. In vitro, more intense peroxidation of cerebral tissue, which can be related to PO_2 and exposure time, is observed. Pre-exposure to hyperbaric oxygen in vivo is accompanied by a significant rise in this peroxidation in vitro. We may conclude from this study that elective peroxidation of cerebral lipids is a concomitant of the appearance of hyperbaric disturbances. (transl. MEMH)

959.
JOHNSON, P.C., T.B. Driscoll, W.C. Alexander and C.J. Lambertsen.
Body fluid volume changes during a 14-day continuous exposure to 5.2% O_2 in N_2 at pressure equivalent to 100 fsw (4 ata).
Aerosp. Med. 44(7, Sec. II):860-863;July 1973.

Blood volume, intracellular volume, and extravascular-extracellular water volume were measured in six subjects before, during and after exposure for 14 days to a hyperbaric (4 ata) atmosphere containing 94.8% nitrogen and 5.2% oxygen (natural PO_2). These studies showed a significant decrease in red cell mass during (-25%) and following (-16%) the exposure, associated with a decrease ^{51}Cr red cell survival but no significant change in iron kinetics. Plasma volume decreased 19% during the period in the chamber. Most of the plasma volume decrease was caused by a water loss from the plasma space rather than a protein loss. The interstitial space increased 17% and the intracellular water volume decreased 13% during the hyperbaric exposure. The losses in extravascular fluid volume were partially reversed during the early post-exposure period. (Authors' abstract)

960.
JOHNSON, S., L. Harris, D. Malik, D. O'Connell, G. Simmons, E. Finder, F.M. LaForce and G.L. Huber.
Recovery of lung injury and host antibacterial defenses following experimental oxygen toxicity.
Clin. Res. 20:888;Dec. 1972.

Abstract only. Entire item quoted: Pulmonary infection is a frequent complication of oxygen therapy. Our previous studies have demonstrated a dose-dependent impairment in pulmonary alveolar macrophage antibacterial defenses following prolonged exposure to 100% oxygen. The rate of recovery of this impairment is ambient air after exposure to oxygen is not known. Following exposures to 100% oxygen of 24, 48, 72, or 96 hours oxygen-treated mice recovered in ambient air for variable durations and were then challenged with an aerosol of radiolabeled (32p) Staphylococcus aureus. Intrapulmonary bacterial inactivation was evaluated by quantifying bacterial viability and radiotracer activity in homogenized lungs of each animal six hours after challenge with the aerosolized bacteria. Controls inactivated 90.8 ± 1.6% of the organisms. With exposure to 100% oxygen, bacterial inactivation was depressed to 79.3 ± 2.4% at 24 and 69.7 ± 3.5% at 48 hours. Intrapulmonary bacterial replication exceeded bacterial inactivation at 72 and 96 hours exposure to oxygen. In all studies, a period of recovery in ambient air equal to the duration of exposure to 100% oxygen was required for bacterial inactivation to return to normal (24, 48, 72 and 96 hours recovery following 24, 48, 72, and 96 hours exposure). These studies help define the duration of increased risk to infection following a finite exposure to 100% oxygen and provide some understanding of the recovery process in the oxygen toxicity.

961.
JOHNSON, W.P., D. Jefferson and C.E. Mengel.
In vivo production of H_2O_2 in RECs of mice exposed to oxygen under high pressure.
In: Aerospace Medical Association. 1971 annual scientific meeting. Houston, Texas, April 1971. Preprints, p.48-49. Published by the Association, 1971.

Tocopherol deficient mice were exposed to OHP and RBC catalase determinations were carried out to determine whether or not H_2O_2 was generated in vivo. The results demonstrated that tocopherol deficient mice form H_2O_2 at atmospheric conditions and that this process is greatly accelerated upon exposure to OHP. (Authors' summary)

962.
JOHNSON, W.P., D. Jefferson and C.E. Mengel.
In vivo formation of H_2O_2 in red cells during exposure to hyperoxia.
J. Clin. Invest. 51:2211-2213;Aug. 1972.

Chow-fed and tocopherol-deficient mice were given aminotriazole (AT) exposed to 100% O_2 at 60 pounds per square inch absolute for 1 hr (OHP), and red blood cells were assayed for catalase activity and lipid peroxide levels. A decrease of catalase activity (CA) in the presence of AT can be taken as evidence of excess formation or accumulation of H_2O_2. No differences of CA were observed among chow-fed mice, with or without AT and/or OHP. Tocopherol-deficient mice with AT had lower CA (0.174 ± 0.040) than chow-fed mice with AT (0.225 ± 0.028) $P < 0.01$. Tocopherol-deficient mice with AT exposed to OHP had even lower CA, $.0137 \pm 0.024$, $P < 0.01$. The data are consistent with the hypothesis that H_2O_2 is formed or accumulated in excess in red cells of tocopherol-deficient mice, an effect that is enhanced in the presence of hyperoxia. They imply that tocopherol plays a role in the detoxification of H_2O_2. (Authors' abstract)

963.
JOHNSON, W.P., D. Jefferson and C.E. Mengel.
In vivo hemolysis due to hyperoxia: role of H_2O_2 accumulation.
Aerosp. Med. 43:943-945;Sept. 1972.

Chow fed and tocopherol deficient mice were given aminotriazole (AT), exposed to 100% O_2 for one hour (OHP) and red blood cells were assayed for catalase activity and lipid peroxide levels. A decrease of catalase activity (CA) in the presence of AT can be taken as evidence of excess formation or accumulation of H_2O_2. No differences of CA were observed among chow fed mice, with or without AT and/or OHP. Tocopherol deficient mice with AT had lower CA ($.174 \pm 0.040$) than chow fed mice with AT (0.225 ± 0.028) $P < 0.01$. Tocopherol deficient mice with AT exposed to OHP had even lower CA $.137 \pm 0.24$, $P < 0.01$. The data are consistent with the hypothesis that H_2O_2 is formed or accumulated in excess in red cells of tocopherol deficient mice, an effect that is enhanced in the presence of hyperoxia. They imply that tocopherol plays a role in the detoxification of H_2O_2, and that the excessive formation of H_2O_2 is responsible for the observed features of oxygen toxicity. The data support the contention that tocopherol may be considered a protective agent against oxygen toxicity. (Authors' abstract)

964.
JOLY, R.
Les problemes d'aptitude a la plongee en scaphandre dans la Marine Nationale.
[Scuba diver aptitude problems in the French Navy].
Med. Sport 46(3):164-169; 1972.

The author believes that diving accidents result from the lack of knowledge of the fundamental rules of diving safety, and of the basic physiological or physiopathological concepts on which they are founded, and also from inadequate methods of selection, both from the medical and psychological points of view. The five classes of divers in the French Navy are: (1) "ordinary" divers who dive occasionally, in open-circuit compressed air apparatus, to 30-40 meters; (2) mine-clearing divers, who go to 60-70 meters on open circuit compressed air apparatus, and occasionally use semi-closed high-oxygen mixtures at lesser depths, and carry out tasks in cold, turbid water; (3) combat swimmers, who are qualified to carry out numerous tasks, and who operate on closed-circuit pure-oxygen equipment, at depths shallow enough to preclude the dangers of oxygen toxicity; (4) hard hat divers, experienced divers with additional qualifications enabling them to work long hours under difficult conditions, to depths of 60 meters, on air; (5) itervention divers, selected from the most experienced mine-clearing divers, who go to depths greater than 200 meters, on experimental and test dives, on binary or ternary helium breathing mixtures. The medical examinations given to all candidates are briefly described: The respiratory system, the cardiovascular system and the nervous system, must show no abnormalities; other examinations include: hematological and urinological; dental (removable dentures are contraindicating); vision (requirements are not high); otolaryngological (these are of the utmost importance, and any chronic disorders of the passages are definite contraindications); while acute conditions are temporary contraindications. Three essential tests are (1) audiogram, (2) vestibular function, (3) tube permeability. Specific tests of cardiovascular function are described. For the depth divers, psychological tests are important. Life history questionnaires are valuable. Personality tests to determine social attitudes, and personal interviews directed especially toward motivation are important. Stability, maturity, judgment, flexibility of intelligence, and sharpness of memory and attention, plus a high degree of sociability, are necessary qualifications. It is indicative that in the 19-year age group, 75% were eliminated, while in the 23-year age group only 12% were eliminated. Motivation is fundamentally important; it must stem from a genuine ambition accompanied by a healthy self-criticism, and not from a neurotic wish to be a hero. (MFW/BSCP)

965.
JOLY, R.
Recherches experimentales et indications therapeutiques de l'oxygene hyperbare.
[Experimental research and therapeutic indications of hyperbaric oxygen].
Rev. Tuberc. (Paris) 36:85-102;Jan./Feb. 1972.

The authors give a table of admissible durations of exposure to certain pressures from the point of view of avoidance of oxygen toxicity: 7 meters-7 hours, 8 meters-3 hours, 10 meters-50 minutes, 20 meters-30 minutes, 25 meters-10 minutes. The various types of toxicity are described: acute, sub-acute, chronic, and cytological. Certain preventive agents for acute toxicity are discussed, and the authors state that barbiturates, novacaine, serotonine, sodium hydroxybutyrate, THAM, vitamin B6 and potassium succinate have a protective effect. Current therapeutic uses of hyperbaric oxygen are discussed, among which is the treatment of decompression sickness; it is noted that the use of pure oxygen in recompression therapy speeds up the process of resorption of nitrogen bubbles. The other uses of hyperbaric oxygen therapy has no relevance for this bibliography. (MFW/BSCP)

966.
JONES, D.R.
Anaerobiosis and the oxygen debt in an anuran amphibian, Rana Esculenta (L.).
J. Comp. Physiol. 77(4):356-382; 1972.

Artificially ventilated curarized frogs consumed 23% less O_2 than animals breathing naturally but their respiratory quotient was significantly increased. Artificial ventilation maintained arterial oxygen tension at normal levels but arterial CO_2 tension fell significantly. When 90% of the Hb was combined with CO, O_2 consumption was reduced by 40% and the respiratory quotient was increased. During apnea both normal animals and those exposed to CO showed reductions in O_2 uptake of about 45%. Heart rate also declined by 20-40%. During apnea respiratory quotient of both groups of animals was significantly elevated. In normal animals arterial and venous O_2 tensions fell during apnea, arterial tensions to 20% of the ventilation value and venous O_2 tensions fell during apnea, arterial tensions to 20% of the ventilation value and venous oxygen tensions to a slightly higher value. Arterial O_2 content fell from 9.6 to 3 volumes per 100 ml. Arterial CO_2 tensions and contents increased during the apnea and arterial pH fell. When ventilation was restored frogs consumed about 109-130 μ 1 more oxygen in the 1st 10 min than in comparable periods before the apnea. Animals with 90% of the hemoglobin combined with CO showed only a gradual return to the preapneic level of O_2 consumption. Heart rate, respiratory quotient and blood gas tensions returned to preapneic levels within 30 min of the resumption of artificial ventilation. The excess O_2 consumed during the 1st 10 min was equal to the amount of O_2 calculated to have been removed from the O_2 store of the blood during apnea. The blood has a function in maintaining O_2 metabolism in both ventilated and apneic frogs. Oxygen stores, including that of the blood, make little contribution to O_2 metabolism during apnea and appear to be replenished immediately lung ventilation is restored. (© BA)

967.
JONES, D.R. and G.F. Holeton.
Cardiac output of ducks during diving.
Comp. Biochem. Physiol. (A) 41:639-645;Mar. 1972.

Blood flow in one pulmonary artery has been measured, using an electromagnetic flowmeter, in lightly restrained ducks before, during and after submergence. This method gave values for cardiac output at rest (control) of 393.9 ± 53.8 ml/min ($\pm$ S.E.M.) and stroke volume of 2.2 ± 0.33 ml. Stroke volume increased slightly but not significantly during diving and after 2 min submergence cardiac output was 25.9 ± 5.4 per cent of control and heart rate 21.1 ± 2.1 per cent of control. Heart rate and cardiac output increased sharply on emergence and after 10 sec were 136.7 ± 12.2 and $141.\pm7.8$ per cent of control values respectively. The present results confirm that the intense bradycardia that occurs during diving is accompanied by a reduction in cardiac output of the same order of magnitude as the fall in heart rate. (Authors' abstract)

968.
JONES, D.R., H.D. Fisher, S. McTaggart and N.H. West.
Heart rate during breath-holding and diving in the unrestrained harbor seal (Phoca vitulina richardi).
Can. J. Zool. 51:671-680;July 1973.

Heart rate and breathing movements have been monitored in three unrestrained harbor seals. On voluntary submergence heart rate fell markedly in all seals, and after 2-3 s submergence stabilized at about 40-50% of the predive level. Heart rate increased before the animals broke surface at the end of the dive and, when breathing began again, a postdive tachycardia was observed. Two of the three seals frequently showed anticipation of the dive as judged from their heart-rate response. Heart-rate during feeding dives was generally more variable; in fact one seal exhibited no bradycardia in 20% of its feeding dives, although another seal showed a significantly greater bradycardia than was seen in routine dives. When breathing rate was low (less than five breaths min^{-1}) respiratory variations in the heart rate occurred, although the onset of bradycardia was much more rapid during diving than during breath-holding. Because of the flexibility of the response it is concluded that the generation of diving bradycardia in the seal is a complex phenomenon which, aside from any responses set in train by peripheral receptors, must also involve some form of associative learning. (Authors' abstract)

969.
JONES, D.R.
Systemic arterial baroreceptors in ducks and the consequences of their denervation on some cardiovascular responses to diving.
J. Physiol. (London) 234:499-518;Nov. 1973.

In the duck systemic arterial baroreceptors which cause bradycardia in response to induced hypertension are located in the walls of the ascending aorta, innervated by the depressor nerves. The location of the baroreceptors was confirmed both histologically and by recording activity from the depressor nerve. Stimulation of the central cut end of a depressor nerve caused transient bradycardia and a fall in blood pressure which was maintained throughout the period of stimulation. Cardiovascular adjustments to submergence of 2 min duration were monitored in intact, sham-operated and denervated ducks. The sham-operated and denervated ducks were used in the experiments some 20-50 days post-operation. The denervations were checked at post-mortem. In the first series of experiments on young ducks mean arterial pressure during a 2 min dive fell by 30% in intact, 17.5% in sham-operated, and 48% in denervated ducks. In all ducks heart rate was reduced by 84-85%. In a second series of experiments on older ducks sciatic artery blood flow was also recorded and mean arterial blood pressure fell by 9.2% in intact and by 53% in denervated animals, although there were no significant differences in heart rate during the 2 min dives. In normal animals sciatic vascular resistance increased after 2 min submergence by 7.86 $\pm$ 1.7 times, whereas in denervated ducks it increased by only 2.32 $\pm$ 0.5 times. The role of systemic arterial baroreceptors in generation of the cardiovascular responses to submergence in ducks is discussed in terms of the input supplied by the baroreceptors to the central nervous system. (Author's summary)

970.
JONES, J.C.
Oxygen toxicity.
Rocky Mountain Med. J. 69:49-52;July 1972.

The purpose of this paper is to remind all of us that we must take a modern and careful look at oxygen. It is only within the past few years that we have recognized the potential for danger to the patient from oxygen. Once we looked upon oxygen almost as a panacea, but this is possible no longer. We must view it as a drug, just as we do digoxin. As with an anesthetic agent, most anesthesiologists feel that one ought to give just enough, and no more. So it is with oxygen. In order to give oxygen properly, it must be monitored, and the facilities to do so are available. The toxic effects of oxygen are a function of time and concentration, in addition to the patient's individual susceptibility, and when blood gas analyses show oxygen to be needed no longer, it should be stopped. (Author's summary)

971.
JORDAN, J.P.
Metabolic effects of artificial environments.
Fort Collins, Col., Col. State Univ., Rep. NASA-CR-62079, 40p. Oct. 31, 1971.
(N72-21041)

The mechanisms by which inert gases influence metabolism were investigated from several viewpoints. Groups of rats were exposed at the thermal neutral temperature of the respective mixtures, to normoxic (PAO_2= 100 mmhg) environments with argon, helium or nitrogen as the diluent at a total pressure of one atmosphere. The possible influence of diluent gases on oxygen transport to the cell was examined with hypoxic (PAO_2 = 70 mmHg) mixtures of the same diluent gases. Metabolic measurements included food, water, and oxygen consumption, CO_2 production, hematocrit and the rate $C_{14}O_2$ of expiration subsequent to intraperitoneal injection of acetate-1-C_{14} or glucose UL-C_{14}. Argon-exposed animals showed a consistently decreased metabolic rate while, on the other hand, helium-exposed rats did not significantly alter metabolic rate relative to nitrogen. Certain indices, including acetate and glucose utilization, suggested that helium attenuated the imposed hypoxia at the cellular level while argon facilitated it as compared with nitrogen. These results suggest that metabolic influence of helium is largely thermal in nature while argon has a significant direct metabolic effect and that diluent gases may selectively influence oxygen availability to the interior of the cell. (Author) (STAR)

972.
JORDAN, J.P., L.J. Huston, J.B. Simmons, II, D.P. Clarkson, W.W. Martz and C.L. Schatte.
An environmental chamber system for prolonged metabolic studies on small animals.
Space Life Sci. 4(3/4):424-433; 1973.

Measurement of metabolic adaptation to marginally stressful environments requires both precise regulation of a variety of atmospheric factors for extended periods of time and the capacity to employ sensitive parameters in an undisturbed subject. A metabolic chamber system which can simultaneously maintain groups of small animals in two completely separate closed environments having different pressures, temperatures and gas compositions for an indefinite period is described. O_2 consumption, CO_2 production, food and water consumption and animal activity cycles can be continuously monitored and quantified 24 h per day while the animals are in an unrestrained state. Each chamber can be serviced and the animals handled, injected and sacrificed without subjecting them to barometric stress. Several unique electrical and mechanical components allow semi-automated data collection on a continuous basis for indefinite periods of time. (© BA)

973.
JOSEPHSON, S., E. Berglund, T.C. McAslan, M. Mina and P. Herzog.
Lung machines and respiratory gas exchange during pulmonary air embolization in the dog.
Scand. J. Clin Lab. Invest. 32(3):265-270; 1973.

Lung mechanics and blood gases were studied in 7 open-chest dogs and 1 whose chest was intact. Balloon occlusion of 1 pulmonary artery iduced inconsistent changes except for a 3-13% decrease in compliance. After air embolization, on the other hand, pulmonary compliance fell on an average 30%, pulmonary airflow resistance increased 19%, arterial O_2 pressure decreased markedly, and mean pulmonary arterial pressure doubled. The fall in compliance and the rise of PA pressure were not significantly correlated. Compliance and arterial O_2 values were restored, at least temporarily by hyperinflation of the lungs. The changes in pulmonary ventilatory mechanics and arterial blood gases acutely after embolization are probably caused by constriction in peripheral bronchioles. (© BA)

974.
JOYCE, J.W. and R.L. Woods.
A fleuric gas-concentration sensor for diver breathing gases.
In: Battelle Columbus Laboratories. Proceedings, 1973 divers' gas purity symposium, November 27-28, 1973, p.XIV-1-XIV-14. U.S. Navy Supervisor Diving, Nav. Ships Syst. Comm., Rep 2-73, 1973.

This paper describes a passive flueric resistor bridge that is capable of sensing the concentration of carbon dioxide (CO_2) or oxygen (O_2) in a helium nitrogen environment. The resolution of the sensor is about 0.0005 atm of CO_2 in helium-nitrogen at a total pressure of 50 atm, which makes the device useful for diver breathing gas applications. Analytical and experimental results are presented. (Authors' abstract)

975.
JOZSA, L., O. Szekely and A. Reffy.
Pulmonary changes caused by hyperbaric oxygenation.
Magy. Traumatol. Orthrop. 15:53-64; 1972.

Experimental animals have been placed by the authors for 7 hours into overpression (3 atmospheres) oxygen and the ultrastructural pulmonary changes — due to the inspiration of hyperbaric oxygen — have been examined. It has been found that the developing pulmonary changes are partly due to the oxygen intoxication (vacuolization of the alveolar epithelial cells, degeneration and casting off of the mitochondria, interstitial edema, swelling and detachment of the capillary endothelium, narrowing of the capillaries). These changes may develop even at the inspiration of oxygen of 1 atm. In the authors' opinion, the lesions of the superficial membrane of the pulmonary alveoli (thinning, splitting up, vacuolization, casting off) —, as well as the increased secretion in the adenocytes of the bronchioles are due to the overpression treatment. The authors presume that the pulmonary changes due to the hyperbaric oxygen treatment impair — after their development — the respiratory metabolism of the lung and the blood's oxygenation. (English summary)

976.
JUGEL, M.K.
An analysis of civil diving in the United States and the implications of the results on diver training.
In: Marine industries: problems and opportunities. Proceedings of the ninth annual conference of the Marine Technology Society, p.279-288. Washington, D.C. Marine Technology Society, 1973.

A special analysis [of non-military diving] was started approximately a year ago by the MUS&T Program with the assistance of the Technical Analysis Division of the National Bureau of Standards. The analysis covered commercial diving, scientific/educational institutional diving, non-military governmental diving, and recreational diving. From the resulting information, various conclusions can be reached on training. In commercial diving, the information indicates there should be careful counseling of individuals considering training for a career in the field because of supply and demand, earnings, and characteristics of the field. In the scientific/educational institutional field, there is considerable use of diving by faculty and students in marine science and engineering programs at institutions with curricula in marine sciences and related fields. Non-military governmental organizations were found to rely heavily on recreational diver training organizations for initial training. The largest number are associated with a police or fire department and while jurisdictions with large teams generally make provision for continued training, the majority of the divers are not believed to have this opportunity. With regard to recreational diving, it appears that recent changes in training are both improving safety and reducing the number of individuals who "dropout" after completing training. (From author's abstract)

977.
KAISER, D., P. Eckert, O.H. Gauer and H. Linkenbach.
Circulation and water balance during immersion in a water bath.
Arch. Ges. Physiol. 278(52):52-53; 1963.
(Translation: Silver Spring, Md., Techtran Corp., NASA-TT-F-14834, Mar. 1973)
(N73-19124)

Immersion of the human body in a temperature-controlled bath leads to a three-fold increase in water diuresis, mainly at the expense of the blood plasma. (Authors) (GRA)

978.
KAISER, R.J. and D.W. Klopp.
Hyperbaric air and corneal vascularization.
Ann. Ophthalmol. 5:44-47;Jan. 1973.

Hypoxia is one of the factors postulated as promoting vascularization of the cornea; however, previous experiments designed to increase tissue oxygen for short or intermittent periods have had no effect in retarding neovascularization. The present study utilizes rabbit exposure to hyperbaric air for continuous periods of up to two weeks to increase tisue oxygen, and demonstrates no effect on the neovascularization caused by sodium hydroxide burns of the cornea. This confirms previous experimental results and tends to rule out inadequate time periods or intermittency of exposure as factors in previous negative results. (Authors' abstract)

979.
KANABIS, W.G.
Signal fluctuations in shallow water: BIFI 48-hr tests.
U.S. Nav. Underwater Syst. Cent., Rep. NUSC TR 4441, 63p. May 10, 1973.
(AD 763 360)

Short- and long-term fluctuation studies were made in the 37-kyd Block Island-Fishers Island (BIFI) Shallow Water Acoustic Range at a frequency of 1700 Hz. It is shown in this report that time smear analysis may be used to predict the extent of short-term signal fluctuation by taking into account the energy content of the 'front' and the 'tail' of the received signal. This method is then applied to an actual received signal with good results. Long-term fluctuation, such as that caused by tide is considered in terms of normal mode theory and the results of the time smear analysis are used to provide an estimate of the relative strengths of the modes. When applied to the BIFI range, the estimate predicts that tidal effects will cause negligible fluctuations in the received signal because of the absence of other than the fundamental modes — a prediction that has been verified by experiment. At shorter ranges, interactions of several modes cause relatively large fluctuations in the signal as water depth changes during the tidal cycle. Measurements of frequency smear over the BIFI range are also described. The non-uniformity of the smearing of energy into the side-bands that is apparent in the measurements is explained. (Author) (GRA)

980.
KANAI, N., T. Hayakawa and H. Mogami.
Blood flow changes in carotid and vertebral arteries by hyperbaric oxygenation.
Neurology (Minneapolis) 33:159-163;Feb. 1973.

The effect of hyperbaric oxygentation on blood flows in the common, internal and external carotid and the vertebral arteries were investigated with the use of transcutaneous ultrasonic blood rheography in 14 subjects who had no cardiac and pulmonary disorders. Oxygen inhalation at 2 ATA resulted in marked reductions of blood flows in the common, internal and external carotid arteries, but the blood flow in the vertebral artery was little changed or showed a tendency to increase rather than decrease. The significance of the difference between blood flow changes in the carotid and vertebral arteries by oxygen inhalation at high atmospheric pressure are briefly discussed in relation to clinical results of hyperbaric oxygen therapy for head injury and cerebrovascular diseases. (Authors' summary)

981.
KANEVSKAYA, E.B., A.B. Zimin and P.V. Matekin.
O dykhanii poikilotermnykh zhivotnhkh v gelio-kislorodnoi atmosfere.
[Respiration of poikilothermic animals in a helium-oxygen atmosphere].
Kosm. Biol. Med. 7(6):17-19; 1973.

By the Warburg manometric method, the O_2 consumption by larval Chironomus plumosus L. in the air and a He-O_2 atmosphere was studied. The use of He in place of N did not affect the gas exchange of *Chironomus* larvae. This may be accounted for by a low temperature gradient between poikilothermic animals and the surrounding environment. (JJB) (© BA)

982.
KAPANCI, Y. and R. Tosco.
Oxygen pneumonitis in man. Light- and electron-microscopic morphometric studies.
Chest 62:162-169;Aug. 1972.

Morphometric analysis of the lungs of six patients given 60 percent to 100 percent oxygen for 14 hours to 13 days revealed a considerable increase in air-blood barrier thickness. This was essentially due to an increase in interstitial tissue; epithelial hyperplasia was less prominent. Other morphometric findings included a decrease in alveolar and capillary surface densities, and in capillary volume. Endothelial volume was greatly reduced, arguing in favor of pronounced endothelial cell injury. These morphometric findings were qualitatively similar to those for monkeys exposed to prolonged hyperoxia. The functional implications of these findings are discussed, and it is postulated, on the basis of morphometric data, that the diffusion capacity of the air-blood barrier should be highly reduced in patients given 60 percent to 100 percent oxygen for periods longer than three days. (Authors' abstract)

983.
KAPLAN, E. Ya., V.I. Shubin and I.M. Epshtein.
Vliyanie antioksidantov na skorost' deoksigenatsii krovi zhivotnhykh, posvergavshikhsya vozdeistviyu izmenennoi gazovoi sredy.
[Effect of anti-oxidants on the rate of blood deoxygenation of animals exposed to changed atmospheres].
Kosm. Biol. Med. 7(1):9-14; 1973.

By polarographic coulombmetry the effects of hypoxia and hyperoxia on the rate of blood deoxygenation and the influence of antioxidants (mexamine) were studied on mice. The rate of blood deoxygenation increased in response to i.p. injections of antioxidants under the normal, hypoxic and hyperoxic conditions. The preparations affected the blood directly, penetrating through the red blood cell membranes. The mechanism of action of antioxidants on the dissociation of hydroxyHb is probably related to their capacity to vary hydrogen ion concentration in the plasma and within red blood cells. (JJC) (© BA)

984.
KAPLANSKY, A.S., G.N. Durnova and V.V. Portugalov.
Techenie infektsionnogo protsessa i funktsional' naya aktivnost makrofagov v legkikh u myshei, nakhodivshikhsya v srede s povyshennym coderzhaniem kisloroda.
[The course of the infection process and functional activity of alveolar macrophages in mice exposed to a hyperoxic atmosphere].
Kosm. Biol. Med. 7:6-9; July/Aug. 1973.

The effect of a hyperoxic atmosphere (PO_2 304 mm Hg) on the course of the infection process in the lungs of mice infected intranasally by Klebsiella pneumonia on the 10th experimental day was studied. The infected animals developed interstitial pneumonia which was not fatal. The pathological process in the lungs of the infected mice developed similarly in experimental and control mice from both the qualitative and quantitative point of view. No pathological changes were found in the lungs of noninfected animals sacrificed on the 20th experimental day. The phagocytic activity of alveolar macrophages of experimental mice remained unchanged whereas activity of succinate dehydrogenase and NAD-dependent and NAD-independent α-glycerophosphate dehydrogenase in the macrophage cytoplasm decreased significantly. No changes in the activity of $NADH_2$, $NADPH_2$, malate and lactate dehydrogenases were found. No alternations were noted in the content of lipids and PAS-stained substances. It is suggested that an assessment of the succinated dehydrogenase activity in alveolar macrophages can be used as a test to measure the toxic effect of oxygen. (English summary)

985.
KAPPLER, J.R. and C.B. May.
A space maintainability experiment aboard the Ben Franklin submersible during the 30-day Gulf Stream drift mission.
Presented at American Institute of Aeronautics and Astronautics, Man's role in space conference, Coco Beach, Fla., Mar. 1972, paper 72-232, 15p.

In the summer of 1969, a deep submersible drifted for 30 days below the surface of the Gulf Stream, while operated by a six man crew. The main purpose of the mission was oceanographic research. The crew's activities and completely self-contained environment resembled those of a space station such as Skylab. Because of these similarities aspects of on-board vehicle maintenance during the actual conduct of a scientific mission were investigated. The maintainability study was accomplished in six distinct phases. Two useful plots of manpower distribution were developed. A maintenance action summary is presented in a table. (GR) (IAA)

986.
KASHIWAGI, H. and Y. Suzuki.
Laser beam behavior in the sea water.
In: Ocean 73. 1973 IEEE international conference on engineering in the ocean environment, p.35-38. IEEE publication 73 CHO774-0 OCC.

Behaviors of laser beams propagating through the sea water were measured, which are a beam profile and an attenuation characteristic. The maximum distance detecting a laser beam was obtained by using a photon counter to 26.5 attenuation length. The propagation experiment was conducted at Sakaide Bay in Seto inland sea. A new towtype α meter was constructed to measure a cluster of optical and oceanic parameters which are required on applying laser beams to the marine electronics. (Authors' abstract)

987.
KASKEL, D. and J. Neumann.
Investigations on the influence of CO_2 and O_2 partial pressure upon the intraocular pressure in rabbits.
Ophthalmic Res. 2(3/4):211-216; 1971.

Investigation on the influence of different respiratory gases on intraocular pressure (IOP) were made with 15 rabbits under Somnifen narcosis. During a 10-min. period of exposure to the test gases, IOP and blood pressure were recorded every min. Inhalation of 7% CO_2 induced a marked increase of IOP, blood pressure remaining constant. With 15% CO_2 the decrease of blood pressure was more marked than that of IOP. One hundred percent had no influence on IOP and blood pressure. (© BA)

988.
KATS, B.G., B.A. Kheifets-Tetel'baum and E.E. Rozov.
Ispol'zovanie dekompressionn'ykh kamer dlya lechebnoi kompressii i oksigenobaroterapii. [The use of decompression chambers in therapeutic compression and oxygen barotherapy]. Voennomed. Zh. (7):67-69;July 1971.

Therapeutic hyperbaric oxygenation is used mainly in the treatment and prevention of specific divers' diseases, but also in treatment of other conditions. The treatment consists of repeated exposure to 1.2-2 atm pressure in the chamber for periods ranging from 45 to 75 min. In postoperative gas embolism this was found to be the only successful treatment since it helped to dissolve the gases causing embolism. In the authors' experience with hemorrhagic and traumatic shock oxygen barotherapy helped to prevent the formation of gangrene and promoted collateral circulation. The authors consider oxygen barotherapy as being at the present time the only effective method in the treatment of gas embolism of various origins, even in extremely severe cases. It is also effective in some hypoxic conditions. Other therapeutic uses of hyperbaric oxygen, not related to the subject area of this bibliography, are discussed. (OLC/BSCP)

989.
KATSURA, R. and K. Sato.
[The effects of high pressure on the activity level of the central nervous system]. J. Anthropol. Soc. Nippon 80(1):78; 1972.

Abstract only: The authors studied the effects of high pressure on the activity of the central nervous system in an animal experiment. Chronic electrodes were implanted in the cerebral cortex of rabbits kept individually in cages without anesthesia or restraint. As indicators of central nervous system activities, N_1 and P_2 amplitudes of evoked potentials and recovery curves from the dual stimulation were derived. An 85 db click sound was used as a stimulus and the evoked potential was computed by adding the potentials reactive to the stimulus. It was noted that the amplitudes of N_1 and P_2 of auditory evoked potentials decreased with an increase of ambient pressure and returned to normal when the pressure was reduced. It was observed that at 4 atm., the central nervous system activity level was reduced. The recovery curves were derived by computing the percentage of the N_1 and P_2 amplitudes 6 hours, 12 hours, and 24 hours, respectively, following the hyperbaric exposure. Five series of experiments have been conducted up to now but no conclusion has been reached from these studies. (OLS/UMS)

990.
KAWASHIRO, T.
[Physiological aspects of pulmonary function tests — application of inert gases in pulmonary function tests. (1) The alveolar gas exchange with different solubility and diffusion coefficients]. Jap. J. Thorac. Dis. 10:535-536;Oct. 1972.

For more practical quantification of uneven distribution of pulmonary gases in ventilation and perfusion, compartmental analysis was performed. In the compartments M and N, blood volume was expressed as Qm, and Qn and ventilation volume as Vm and Vn respectively. Admixture of gas X in the arterial blood was expressed as: PmxQm + PnxQn = PaxQ. Similar formulation could be drawn for gases Y and Z. Kx expressed solubility of the gas X corrected by coefficients for pressure and temperature. Fick's formula for gas X in compartment M was: PmxVm = KxFvxQm - KxpaxQm. With the use of three gases in both compartment M and N, there were six Fick's formulas at this point. Further, Qm + Qn = Q relationship was added to these and, altogether ten equations were derived. Ten unknowns — partial gas pressure, blood volume, and ventilation volume in each compartment — were expressed in the ratios to partial pressure of each gas in venous admixture, overall blood flow volume and overall ventilation volume. Further, by adding overall ventilation and blood volume values, ventilation-perfusion ratio and blood and ventilation volumes in each compartment were derived. Theoretically, the relationship among arterial blood, venous admixture blood and indicator gas X in the inspired air is expressed in: CVx = Cax + Ve/Q Fex. Values derived in experiments using dogs were applied to this formula and found valid. Thus, if only two of three data on arterial blood, venous admixture blood and inspired air are given, the third may be calculated. In the clinical application of the above mentioned method, the need for drawing of venous admixture blood is eliminated by analyzing the arterial blood and inspired air only, without sacrificing the accuracy of the test. (OLC/SCD)

991.
KAWASHIRO, T.
[Experimental studies on the tissue gas exchange]. Jap. J. Thorac. Dis. 11:195-200;Apr. 1973.

Gas pockets were formed by injection of air into the dorsal subcutaneous tissue of rats. . . By measuring gas tensions in the pockets and the overall O_2 consumption of rats breathing gas mixtures of varied O_2 tensions, it is possible to get information on the O_2 tension difference between the pocket and the blood perfusing the pocket-tissue. Data of this experiment lead to the following conclusions: (1) O_2 tensions in the pockets went down and CO_2 tensions tended to elevate as the days went by after preparation of the gas pockets. (2) A granulomatous tissue layer proliferated on the inner surface of the pocket and this layer grew thicker as the days went by after initial air injection. (3) When applying the subcutaneous gas pockets to the physiological study, it seemed reasonable to use the pockets only formed on the same day. (4) The overall O_2 consumption of rats breathing pure O_2 under 1 ATA was 3.27 ml. 100 g

B.W.$^{-1}$ min^{-1} in average. There was no statistically significant difference between the O_2 consumption of rats breathing pure O_2 under 2 ATA. (5) The difference between O_2 tension in the pocket and that in the blood perfusing the surrounding tissue of the pocket was greater under higher inspired O_2 tension than under lower inspired O_2 tension. (From English abstract)

992.
KAZAKOV, A.I., G.I. Meleshko and Yu. V. Pepelyayev.
Dynamics of the content of carbon monoxide in an atmosphere regenerated by chlorella.
Space Biol. Med. 6(2):18-22;May 18, 1972.
(JPRS 56030)

This paper presents experimental results indicating that carbon monoxide can be accumulated in the enclosed environment of a Chlorella reactor in a "man-Chlorella" system and remain at a relatively constant level. The stabilized level of the carbon monoxide content in an enclosed atmosphere may vary. It is likely to be associated with the photosynthetic activity of Chlorella cells, which as was shown previously, may absorb carbon monoxide from the atmosphere. (Authors' abstract)

993.
KAZEMI, H., N.S. Shore, V.E. Shih and D.C. Shannon.
Brain organic buffers in respiratory acidosis and alkalosis.
J. Appl. Physiol. 34:478-482;Apr. 1973.

To determine the role of organic buffers in brain and cerebrospinal fluid (CSF) during respiratory acidosis and alkalosis, changes in glutamic acid, glutamine, and ammonia concentrations were measured in brain, cisternal CSF, and arterial blood before and after six hr of hypercapnia and hypocapnia in anesthetized dogs. During respiratory alkalosis there were no significant alterations in brain, CSF, or arterial glutamic acid, glutamine, or ammonia concentrations. Thus reduced brain CO_2 buffering and decreased CSF bicarbonate observed in respiratory alkalosis are not related to these substances. After six hours of respiratory acidosis brain glutamic acid decreased 23.0 mg/100 ml or 1.6 mEq/kg. CSF and blood glutamic acid remained unchanged. Brain glutamine increased 18.6 mg/100 ml or 1.3 mEq/kg and CSF and blood glutamine showed parallel increases. Ammonia concentration increased from 1,027 to 1,604 μg/100 g brain tissue in respiratory acidosis concomitant with increases in CSF ammonia content. The fall in brain glutamic acid concentration and increase in ammonia content can account for part of the increased brain CO_2 buffering capacity and secondarily for elevated CSF bicarbonate in respiratory acidosis. The mechanism responsible for the fall in brain glutamic acid in respiratory acidosis may be similar to that in kidney tissue described in metabolic acidosis. (Authors' abstract)

994.
KEATINGE, W.R.
Cold immersion and swimming.
In: Cold/wet survival symposium. J. Roy. Nav. Med. Serv. 58:171-176;Winter, 1972.

Experiments to indicate the effects on survival after immersion in water of such factors as subcutaneous fat, exercise and clothing are described. The causes of sudden death in water are discussed and advice is given on action to be taken to preserve life after immersion. (Author's abstract)

995.
KEBKALO, V.I. and V.P. Ponomarev.
Lung ventilation and gas exchange of a man breathing different gas mixtures while swimming under water.
Fiziol. Zh. SSSR 57:1802-1807;Dec. 1971.
(Translation NASA-TT-F-14,260, May 1972)

Eight healthy men, 19 to 26 years of age, were trained in aqualung swimming from a distance of 500 meters at maximum speed and at a depth of about 2 meters. For breathing they used air and normoxic mixtures of argon and helium. The respiratory minute volume, oxygen consumption and carbon dioxide discharge increased when shifting to breathing of a less dense mixture. At the peak work load, the resistance to breathing increased in direct relation to the density of the mixture. The respiratory minute volume increased, in inverse proportion to the mixture density. The consumption of oxygen and the discharge of carbon dioxide while breathing air and the argon-oxygen mixture were practically the same, and during breathing of the helium-oxygen mixture they increased significantly. (Authors) (STAR)

996.
KEELE, B.B., Jr. and S. Schanberg.
The distribution of superoxide dismutase in tissues of normal rats and rats exposed to hyperbaric oxygen.
Ala. J. Med. Sci. 9:434-435;Oct. 1972.

Superoxide radicals (O_2) are known to be produced both in vivo and in vitro. It is also known that hyperbaric oxygen can increase the oxygen tension with tissues and therefore increase the level of the superoxide radical. Young rats were exposed to both normal and hyperbaric conditions and the levels of the enzyme superoxide dismutase were measured. Superoxide dismutase activity was observed in lung, adrenal glands, and all portions of the brain of both normal rats and rats exposed to hyperbaric oxygen. No differences were observed in the enzyme levels between the two groups of animals. (Authors' abstract)

997.
KEIDEL, W.N., L. Gluck, M.V. Kulovhich and M.J. Westberg.
Effect of prolonged oxygen exposure on pulmonary surfactant.
Pediatr. Res. 7:429/201; 1973.

Abstract only. Entire item quoted: Pathogen free rats exposed to 90% O_2 at one atmosphere for 75 hours had no respiratory distress until day 3 of exposure. Shown below, lungs of study rats were 2.3 x heavier than controls with significant increase in total lipid of lung tissue and alveolar wash (AW). Phospholipids (PL) comprised 69% of AW lipids in control rats and 34.5% of O_2-exposed rats. Significant changes occurred in composition of AW PL but lung tissue PL were relatively unchanged. Prolonged O_2 exposure produced major changes in lipid composition of pulmonary surfactant. Further study is needed to determine if these changes are produced by disordered lipid metabolism and/or pulmonary edema and cell death.

	Body Wt (gm)	Lung Wt (gm)	AW Lipids (mg)	Tissue Lipids (mg)	
Study	286.5 ± 14.9	3.7 ± 0.6	4.8 ± 1.2	77.4 ± 7.5	
Control	292.0 ± 6.0	1.6 ± .3	1.9 ± .5	47.9 ± 3.7	
	AW PL (mg)	% Lec	% Sph	%PDME	% PE
Study	1.6 ± .5	59 ± 14	7 ± 5	21 ± 5	13 ± 6
Control	1.4 ± .2	93 ± 4	6 ± 5	tr	tr
	Tissue PL (mg)	% Lec	% Sph	%PDME	% PE
Study	59.5 ± 11.8	65 ± 4	11 ± 3	tr	23 ± 6
Control	33.2 ± 3.6	49 ± 4	23 ± 3	tr	38 ± 5

998.
KELLAND, N.C.
The diver as a geophysical tool.
Hydrospce 3:31-35;Dec. 1970.

Because of the difficulties associated with underwater time limitation, cold, poor visibility — the information given by the diver can be (a) unrepresentative, (b) inadequate, (c) inaccurate, and (d) expensive. When divers are used in conjunction with marine geophysical tools, however, some of these limitations can be avoided. The author discusses several of these tools and their uses. Among those discussed are boomers and pingers for seismic profiling, and side scan sonar which is used in conjunction with seismic profiling equipment. The diver is most useful when his role is that of correlating the geophysical data acquired by the forementioned two tools. The author gives specific examples of underwater work projects in which the work of the divers is optimized by being planned on the basis of the results of geophysical surveys. (MFW/BSCP)

999.
KELLAND, N.C.
Diver support of offshore geological surveys.
In: Diving applications in marine research. Proceedings of a seminar, National Institute of Oceanography, Godalming, Surrey, U.K., December 1971. p.88-118. Published by the Institute. 1972.

The diver trained geologist or geophysicist is able to assist in overcoming some of the limitations and problems mentioned above. The author's geological diving experience has been drawn from university projects, commercial offshore operations, and investigation work with a government research unit. The dives have covered a wide range of applications which can be divided into four types: (a) Geological sampling and observation dives; (b) Equipment evaluation and monitoring dives; (c) Underwater navigation and positioning dives; (d) Panic dives [to deal with emergencies such as propellers fouled by cables, or lost or damaged equipment]. As an example, over the past two years, the Unit of Coastal Sedimentation (UCS) diving team has carried out 112 man dives composed of 24 geological sampling and observation dives, 53 equipment evaluation and monitoring dives, 25 underwater navigation and positioning dives and 10 panic dives. (Author)

1000.
KELLY, D.L., K.R.L. Lassiter, A. Vongsvivut and J.M. Smith.
Effects of hyperbaric oxygenation and tissue oxygen studies in experimental paraplegia.
J. Neurosurg. 36:425-529;Apr. 1972.

This study demonstrates that the tissue PO_2 of the normal spinal cord of dogs can be modified by ventilating the animals with oxygen and carbogen. Following trauma to the cord, the tissue PO_2 responded only to hyperbaric oxygen. A series of animals rendered paraplegic and treated with oxygen recovered to a greater degree than those in an untreated control group. (Authors' abstract)

1001.
KENMURE, A.C.F., W.R. Murdoch, I. Hutton and A.J.V. Cameron.
Hemodynamic effects of oxygen at 1 and 2 Ata pressure in healthy subjects.
J. Appl. Physiol. 32:245-251;Feb. 1972.

Hemodynamic measurements were made in 20 healthy men at rest while breathing air at 1 Ata and 100% oxygen at 1 and 2 Ata pressure for successive periods of 45 min. Inhalation of oxygen at 2 Ata caused a statistically significant 10% fall in cardiac index which was brought about mostly by a fall in heart rate. There was a 15% increase in systemic vascular resistance, an 80% decrease in left ventricular work, and a statistically insignificant 3% rise in mean arterial pressure. Similar but less pronounced effects occurred with inhalation of pure O_2 at 1 Ata. (Authors' abstract)

1002.
KENNEDY, J.L.
Sub developed for hostile waters.
Oil Gas J. 71:51-55;June 4, 1973.

Sub Sea Oil Services of Milan has designed a work submersible, the Phoenix 66, which has an operating range of up to 400 miles, maximum power of 540-625 hp, and a depth capability of 1200 feet. It will accommodate a crew of seven for seven days, at one atmosphere or ambient pressure, as well as the decompression stages in between. It could operate in hostile conditions (sea force 8). Manipulators are controlled from within. It can hover, and is equipped for long-range underwater navigation. A transfer system can move the occupants from living to working quarters in whatever environment is desirable. Divers can also lock out. An earlier submarine habitat, Capshell, is also described. This is a working habitat which enables divers to work dry in a one-atmosphere environment. The chamber was developed in Italy, and used in Borneo by Brunei Shell Petroleum. (MFW/UMS)

1003.
KENNEDY, R.S.
A bibliography of the role of the vestibular apparatus under water and pressure: content-oriented and annotated.
U.S. Nav. Med. Res. Inst. Rep. 1 on M4306.03.5000BAK9, 119p. Aug. 10, 1972.

This report contains about 965 references dealing with the role of the vestibular apparatus in compressed air work. The sources for this bibliography include the diving medicine reference works as well as the literature dealing with vestibular functions. In addition, there are many items in the bibliography which would not typically be seen when consulting the standard reference works in diving medicine or vestibular physiology. These include obscure references and/or translations of articles not previously translated. The references are sorted by subject matter into six categories: Category I. Vestibular Symptomatology as a Sign of Decompression Sickness (Compression Effects: Isobaric?); Category II. Clinical Investigation of Vestibular Symptomatology; Category III. Tests of Positive Function of Vestibular Apparatus; Category IV. Perceptual Illusions Occasioned by the Environment SOme of Which May be of Vestibular Origin; Category V. The Use of the Vestibular System as an Inertial Guidance System; and Category VI. Auditory Studies Which Have Relevance for Understanding Vestibular Function Underwater. The major category is Category I (293 references). Most of the citations are annotated and many are cross-referenced between and within categories. It is felt that the role of the vestibular system in compressed air work is presently underestimated. This bibliography calls attention to the incidence of vestibular involvement in compressed air work and provides reference to the background material essential for understanding and future study of vestibular problems. (Author's abstract)

1004.
KENNEDY, R.S.
The role of the vestibular apparatus under water and high pressure.
U.S. Nav. Med. Res. Inst., Rep. 3, 34p. Mar. 1973.
(AD 761 616)

The report briefly reviews literature relating to vestibular functions in underwater medicine, and introduces a more complete reference list, 'A bibliography of the role of the vestibular apparatus under water and pressure: content-oriented and annotated.' The author states that the role of the vestibular system in compressed air work is presently underestimated. This review and the broader bibliography call attention to the incidence of vestibular involvement in compressed air work and provides reference to the background material essential for understanding and future study of vestibular problems. (Author) (GRA)

1005.
KENNY, J.E.
Business of diving.
Houston, Texas, Gulf Publishing Co., 1972, 302p.

The main text is written to be understood by an intelligent reader with little exposure to diving. The content is designed to provide a knowledge of human physiological characteristics that permit reentry into the ocean, a brief summary of man's past attempts to reenter, an overview of the latest diving equipment and systems, a review of diving activity in all major segments of the field, and an analysis of diving as a business, both from the inside looking out and the business as a customer. For those with a previous knowledge of diving, each section relating to technology contains a supplement with in-depth discussion of the latest developments and theory. Appendices are located at the end of the section. They should be considered a must for the experienced, and optional for those who do not require that degree of technical assistance. (Author's preface)

1006.
KEPTYA, E.B. and E.A. Mukhin.
Vliyanie etirona na techenie kislorodnogo otravleniya i soderzhanie askorbinovoi kisloty v tkanyakh.
[Effect of etiron on the course of oxygen poisoning and an ascorbic acid content in tissues].
Kdravookhr 15(5):31-33; 1972.

In this study 138 rats were used, 130 of which were exposed 50 min to hyperbaric O_2. Etiron (ethylisothiuronium bromide), 20 mg/kg, was given intra-abdominally, 10-15 min before rats were placed into the chamber. Etiron demonstrated pronounced protection: only 11-14% of the rats suffered from severe poisoning, while in the unprotected group 75% had severe signs of O_2 poisoning with asphyxia. This effect was explained by etiron's beneficial influence on ascorbic acid metabolism in vital organs. (MDS) (© BA)

1007.
KEREM, D., R. Elsner and J. Wright.
Anaerobic metabolism in the brain of the harbor seal during late stages of a maximum dive.
Fed. Proc. 30:484; 1971.

Abstract only. Entire item quoted: Young, unanesthetized, restrained harbor seals Phoca vitulina were subjected to a simulated maximum dive by submerging their heads until the appearance of high voltage slow waves on the electroencephalogram. Arterial and cerebral venous blood samples were drawn simultaneously before and during EEG slowing. Catheters were placed high in the arterial tree through either brachial or femoral arteries and were advanced in the intravertebral vein to the level of C-1. This vein lies above the dura of the spinal cord and is the major drainage of the seal's brain. Independent measurements of blood flow in the intravertebral vein suggest that brain blood flow remained substantially unchanged during the dives. During the last five minutes of the dives, which averaged 17 minutes, cerebral oxygen extraction, $(a\text{-}v)O_2$, diminished and cerebral lactate production, (v-a)L, increased. At EEG slowing PaO_2 and PvO_2 were 10 and 1-3 torr, respectively, and were consistent over a wide range of pH and PCO_2 values. The results indicate that during advanced asphyxial hypoxia the seal's brain can tolerate a fall in oxygen consumption and derives part of its energy anaerobically before EEG signs of functional disturbance. Such metabolic changes have not been demonstrated in terrestrial mammals, probably because of their low tolerance to asphyxia.

1008.
KEREM, D., G. Kooyman, J.P. Schroeder, J.J. Wright and C.M. Drabek.
Hyperbaric oxygen-induced seizure in a marine mammal, the seal.
Amer. J. Physiol. 222:1322-1325;May 1972.

A female yearling northern elephant seal, Mirounga angustirostris, and a female yearling harbor seal, Phoca vitulina, were subjected to breathing oxygen at a pressure of 4.5 ATA in the restrained unanesthetized state inside a wet pressure chamber. The elephant seal showed first signs of central nervous system poisoning after ten min. of a 15-min. compression period. A full-fledged convulsive seizure ensued shortly after decompression. The harbor seal was compressed for 20 min. The first apparent toxic symptoms occurred after 9 min. They increased gradually and were completely relieved by decompression. Recovery of both animals was complete. Compared to other mammals these species seem especially vulnerable to acute oxygen toxicity, possibly on account of their breathing pattern. (Authors' abstract)

1009.
KESTIN, J., S.T. Ro and W.A. Wakeham.
Viscosity of the binary gaseous mixture, neon-krypton.
Providence, R.I., Brown Univ., Div. Eng., Rep. AROD-8117:8-E.
(AD 748 787)
(Also published in J. Chem Phys. 56:4086-4091;Apr. 15, 1972)

The paper presents new relative measurements of the viscosity of binary mixtures of neon and krypton and repeated determinations of the viscosity of the pure gases neon, krypton and argon. The experiments were performed using an oscillating disk viscometer; the measurements were made at atmospheric pressure and in the nominal temperature range 25-70°C. Tables of consistent values of the thermal conductivity of the mixture as well as of the pure gases are given. The binary diffusion coefficient for the mixture has also been computed. (Authors) (GRA)

1010.
KHAN, M.A., I. Alkalay, S. Suetsugu and M. Stein.
Acute changes in lung mechanics following pulmonary emboli of various gases in dogs.
J. Appl. Physiol. 33:774-777;Dec. 1972.

Air emboli produces elevations in total lung flow resistance and decreases in dynamic lung compliance and arterial oxygen tension similar to changes produced by autologous thromboemboli. These effects were blocked by heparin, by rendering the animal thrombocytopenic, and infusions of a serotonin antagonist. The mechanism of airway constriction appeared to be related to thrombin-induced serotonin release from platelets. Emboli of pure CO_2 produced no changes in lung mechanics probably due to the rapid solubility of the gas and/or a bronchodilator effect. High concentrations of CO_2 in inspired gas also prevented airway constriction in animals embolized with air. Emboli of nitrogen and oxygen produced airway constriction while helium, neon, argon, and xenon failed to produce significant alterations in lung mechanics. (Authors' abstract)

1011.
KHAN, M.Y.
Compressed air illness.
J. Indian Med. Ass. 58:95-96;Feb. 1, 1972.

A case history is described. An experienced diver worked at 3.94 atmospheres for one hour and surfaced without making the recommended stop of ten minutes at ten feet. Decompression sickness symptoms in the right elbow appeared after one-half hour and he was put back into the water for lack of a recompression chamber. His pain disappeared, and he was brought back at 2 ft/3 min to 70 feet, 2 ft/5 min to 35 feet, and 2 ft/8 min to the surface. He appeared well except for the effects of extreme cold. There was no recurrence of symptoms. (MFW/BSCP)

1012.
KHEIFETS-TETELBAUM, B.A. and E.E. Rozov.
Izmenenie rentgenograficheskoi kartiny pridatochnykh pazukh nosa u vodolazov v protsesse professional/noi deyatel'nosti.
[Changes in the X-ray picture of the accessory sinuses of the nose in divers during their occupational activities].
Gig Tr. Prof. Zabol. 16(7):49-51; 1972.

From roentgen pictures of the accessory sinuses of 72 divers, the various changes in the nasal passages of 7(14.5%) were determined. The number of divers with noted changes of the accessory sinuses increased 4 times (25.4%) after 2-4 yr of work. The changes were apparently of a physiological character and related to a reciprocative reaction of the mucous membrane under favorable occupational conditions. (MDS) (© BA)

1013.
KHEIFETS-TETELBAUM, B.A. and E.E. Rozov.
Izmenenie rentgenograficheskoi kartiny pridatochnykh pazukh nosa u vodolazov v protsesse professional'noi deyatel'nosti.
[Changes in the x-ray image of the paranasal sinuses occurring in the course of professional activities in divers].
Gig. Tr. Prof. Zabol. 16:49-51;July 1972.

This is a comparative study of changes detected in the x-ray image of the paranasal sinuses in a group of 72 professional deepsea divers and 40 control subjects. The controls were working with the divers, regularly accompanying without taking part in the actual diving. Both groups were examined at the beginning of their professional careers and again after 2-4 years of continued work. Radiological changes, found significantly more often in the divers, consisted mainly of lowered pneumatization of the paranasal sinuses and thickening of the mucous membranes. Divers are exposed to high atmospheric pressure, elevated partial pressure of oxygen, nitrogen and helium, low ambient temperature and low temperature of breathing mixtures. The mucous membrane of the upper respiratory tract undergoes morphological, but non-pathological changes. Since none of the divers exhibiting these changes had any subjective symptoms, the authors believe that these changes indicate an adaptive reaction of the mucous membrane to continued exposure to the underwater environment. (OLC/UMS)

1014.
KHEIFETS-TETELBAUM, B.A. and E.E. Rozov.
[The use of oxygen in the decompression and remedial recompression of divers].
Voennomed. Zh. (12):52-54;Dec. 1970.
Def. Res. Inform. Cent., Orpington, U.K., DRIC-Trans-3095, 9p. Apr. 1973.
(AD 760 743) (N73-26069/7)

Prevention of decompression sickness requires strict control of the oxygen part of the decompression regime by the doctor, following underwater submersion. In cases where decompression sickness occurs, the application of oxygen in the stage when pressure is reduced during remedial recompression is a very promising technique. The increase in the rate of desaturation of the organism from inert gases, governed by the inhaling of pure oxygen, offers the opportunity to use less protracted regimes and makes it possible to increase the time of subjection to maximal remedial pressure; this improves conditions for the dispersion of gas bubbles in the organism of the patient. (GRA)

1015.
KIES, J.A., R.J. Sanford and D.R. Mulville.
Reliability and safety aspects of glass as a deep ocean structure.
IEEE International conference on engineering in the ocean environment, Panama City, Florida, September 1970. Digest of technical papers, p.203-205. Published by the conference.

Accurate predictions of the probability of a failure originating at an internal flaw are made based on an assumed Weibull distribution of strengths. This analysis includes the effects of size and dissimilarities between the strength distributions of test specimens and the actual structure. (Eng. Index)

1016.
KIESOW, L.A., J.W. Bless and J.B. Shelton.
Oxygen dissociation in human erythrocytes: its response to hyperbaric environments.
Science 177:1236-1238;Mar. 23, 1973.

There are at least three different ways by which hyperbaric nitrogen could cause the observed effects on the oxygen dissociation in erythrocytes. The effect could be the result of the hydrostatic pressure associated with the use of hyperbaric nitrogen; it could be the result of molecular nitrogen gas itself; or it could be the result of a trace contaminant in the nitrogen gas, although it was of the highest purity available. Figure 1c shows that hyperbaric helium also produces shifts in the RBC oxygen dissociation curve to lower oxygen partial pressures. However, the increase in the affinity of hemoglobin for oxygen caused by 100 atm of helium gas is quantitatively smaller than the increase produced by an identical pressure of nitrogen. Therefore, it would appear that hydrostatic pressure itself is at least not the only cause of the increased oxygen affinity, if indeed it is a cause at all. Hyperbaric gases themselves seem to interfere with functions of the hemoglobin molecule to an extent that depends on their concentration and on their chemical nature. (Authors)

1017.
KIM, J. and C.E. Zobell.
Agarase, amylase, cellulase, and chitinase activity at deep-sea pressures.
J. Oceanogr. Soc. Jap. 28(4):131-137; 1972.

An agarase produced by a marine bacterium, a bacterial amylase, a fungal cellulase and an actinomycetal chitinase were examined for their stability and hydrolytic activity at hydrostatic pressures existing in the deep sea. All 4 enzymes were from barophobic organisms which fail to grow at pressures exceeding 400-500 atm, but some observations were made on the hydrolase activity of barophilic bacteria grown at 500-1150 atm. Although differing in the rates at which they catalyzed the hydrolysis of agar, starch, cellulose and chitin respectively, all 4 enzymes were active at deep-sea pressures and temperatures. These glycoside hydrolases were much more baroduric than most oxidoreductases, transferases and ligases (synthetases) which were investigated. The chitinase and α-amylase were about as stable at 1000 atm as at 1 atm. Cellulase was also baroduric and active at 1000 atm at pH 4.2, its pH optimum at 1 atm. The pressure tolerance of cellulase was much less at higher pH values characteristic of normal sea water, i.e., near pH 8.2. The activity of agarase (synthesized at 1 atm) was retarded by increased pressure, due largely to the inactivation of this enzyme system. Barophilic bacteria, isolated from the deep sea, synthesize agarases which are active at 1000 atm as indicated by the hydrolysis of agar. (© BA)

1018.
KIMZEY, J.H.
Fire extinguishment in hypobaric and hyperbaric environments.
In: Conference on materials for improved fire safety, Houston, Tex., Manned Spacecraft Center, 1970; p.163-169. Washington, D.C. National Aeronautics & Space Administration, 1971. (NASA-SP-5096)
(N 72-16429)

Work that has been performed to provide information on the effects of various fire extinguishing agents in special atmospheres is discussed. Data used in the development of both equipment and techniques for manned spacecraft and related equipment are discussed. The equipment includes a hypobaric chamber suitable for low pressure use and a hyperbaric chamber for high pressure operation. The effectiveness of agents in weightless environment is also discussed. (Author) (STAR)

1019.
KINDWALL, E.P.
First aid for pressure related accidents.
Skin Diver 22:60-61;Sept. 1972.

The two most common diving accidents are air embolism and decompression sickness. The first usually manifests itself within a minute or two of surfacing. It results from over distension of the lungs during ascent which forces air into vital organs. Symptoms may include unconsciousness, convulsions, paralysis, and bleeding from the mouth. The patient should be placed with his feet elevated, kept warm, and transported to a recompression chamber as quickly as possible. The appearance of decompression sickness symptoms may be delayed for as long as 24 hours, but usually occurs within a few hours, and more gradually than those of air embolism. Ninety per cent of all cases have pain, usually in a limb; 25 per cent of cases of neurologic symptoms such as numbness, paralysis, vertigo, visual disorders. Respiratory symptoms, or "chokes", appear in only 2 percent of cases. In attempting to differentiate between air embolism and decompression, it is helpful to remember that the latter occurs only after dives to 33 feet or more and then only when bottom time has been sufficient for nitrogen absorption. Paralysis due to decompression sickness is usually of the lower half of the body, while in air embolism it is usually one half of the length of the body. Speed of transportation is most essential. Oxygen should be administered during transportation. Air embolism should be recompressed to 165 feet. In cases of very ill patients, it is preferable to administer inadequate recompression than to delay several hours until adequate recompression can be reached. In cases of decompression sickness, the Navy's low pressure oxygen tables (V and VI) are preferable to air tables. Recompression in the water is not recommended. (MFW/BSCP)

1020.
KINDWALL, E.P.
Treatment of decompression sickness.
Hyperbaric Med. Newsletter 9:1-3;Jan./Feb. 1973.

The author discusses the theory of recompression therapy for decompression sickness, and the development of the use of oxygen breathing. The disadvantage of oxygen breathing is that it cannot be used at depths of more than 66 feet, and the time period must be kept within the latent period for oxygen toxicity. However, it has been proven effective despite these disadvantages, reducing greatly the percentage of failures both for initial recompressions and for Type 2 cases. The author attributes this efficacy to the hypothesis that more surface area in the bubbles, due to less recompression facilitates nitrogen diffusion, while at the same time tissues are adequately oxygenated despite incomplete circulation. Tables for use in case of blow-ups from various depths are discussed. From a depth greater than 165 feet, that developed by Dr. H.V. Hempleman should be used; it may be shortened by oxygen breathing at the shallow end. The use of low molecular weight Dextran 6 recommended in all cases in which symptoms persist for two hours or longer; it should be given at once in severe cases. Steroid therapy is useful in cases presenting CNS symptoms. Repetition of hyperbaric oxygen on the second day is helpful, if symptoms have not completely disappeared. Heparin is effective in cases of shock, as is also digitalis. The importance of examination for neurologic symptoms before initiating treatment is stressed. An extremely conservative approach should be maintained under all circumstances. (MFW/BSCP)

1021.
KINDWALL, E.P.
Corrections and additions regarding article on treatment of decompression sickness — Last issue.
Hyperbaric Med. Newsletter p.4:Mar./Apr. 1973.

Referring to an article written for the previous issue of Hyperbaric Medicine Newsletter the author apologizes for entitling the table for use in cases where the depth is greater than 165 fsw, compiled by Dr. Hempleman, "Long British Air Table," since the preferred mixture is helium-oxygen. The use of air with this table might narcotize both the patient and the tender, thus seriously confusing the procedure. Peter Edel has recently compiled a treatment table for use after blow-up from a depth greater than 165 feet. The purpose was to provide a table which off-shore personnel could use in an emergency. It is based on the assumptions of a maximum bottom time of 120 minutes and a depth of 200 fsw, with a breathing mixture of 85-15 helium-oxygen. Two tables are given, one to be used with helium oxygen and one to be used when only air is available. In the first the diver is switched to air at 110 fsw. The air table takes 57-1/2 hours (maximum), starting at 300 fsw, which is the depth limit; the helium-oxygen tables take 36-1/2 hours. It is emphasized that these tables are theoretical and have never been put to use. (MFW/BSCP)

1022.
KINDWALL, E.P.
Divers' asceptic bone necrosis.
In: Professional diving symposium, New Orleans, Nov. 1972. Mar. Technol. Soc. J. 7:36-38; Mar./Apr. 1973.

Aseptic or avascular necrosis is a disease which can affect anyone working under increased ambient pressures, in excess of 38 feet of sea water, who does not follow sound decompression procedures. It is too early to say with certainty what the incidence of this disease will be in those people using present saturation diving techniques, but it has appeared on the Gulf Coast in saturation divers. The shoulders and hips are most often affected. It is difficult to correlate the incidence of bone necrosis with the number of times a man has decompression sickness. Treatment consists of placing the joint at rest in the early stages or performing surgery if actual destruction of the joint has taken place. Pre-employment and yearly x-rays are becoming prevalent among diving companies to prevent liability and minimize the destruction caused by the disease should it occur. (Author's abstract)

1023.
KINDWALL, E.P.
Treatment of air embolism.
Hyperbaric Med. Newsletter, p.1-2;May/June 1973.

The author describes the development of the treatment of air embolism. Previous to the middle 60's, because of CNS involvement, it was treated by recompression using U.S. Navy tables III or IV., which meant 20 to 38 hours of decompression after recompression to 165 fsw. Captain Charles Waite, USN, carried out a series of experiments with dogs, in which it was indicated that decompression on the standard U.S. Navy tables for 10 min at 170 feet was adequate. It must be noted that the head-down Trendelenburg position is advisable. If symptoms do not disappear after 30 min at 165 fsw, the patient may be kept at that pressure for up to two hours, then decompressed on the U.S. Navy Exceptional Exposure Air Tables at 60 feet, where the low pressure oxygen table is then used. A case is described in which the patient suffered from a dense right hemianopsia which failed to respond to recompression; at the beginning of the oxygen table at 60 feet, improvement was noticeable, and recovery was complete by the completion of decompression. Helium-oxygen is recommended as the breathing mixture to be used during treatment. If a 6 ATA chamber is not available, effective treatment may be carried out in a 2 or 3 ATA chamber, using pure oxygen. Steroids should be used liberally starting with 19 mg I.V., at arrival at the 30-ft stop; 4 m.g. can be injected intramuscularly every six hours thereafter, for as long as 72 hours. The author recommends Decadron. (MFW/SCD)

1024.
KINDWALL, E.P.
Massive surgical air embolism treated with brief recompression to six atmospheres followed by hyperbaric oxygen.
Aerosp. Med. 44:663-666;June 1973.

A case of massive air embolism stemming from open-heart surgery is described. Twenty-two minutes elapsed before cardio-pulmonary bypass could be reestablished. The patient reached the hyperbaric chamber 3 hr 17 min after embolization occurred. Only a brief 9 min stay at 6 ata was used, followed by treatment with low-pressure oxygen requiring a total chamber stay of 5 hr 13 min. The patient was discharged from the hospital with only minimal neurologic residuae. The practical advantages of this brief treatment schedule versus the standard 38 hr table are discussed. Pre-embolic heparinization probably played a major role in survival. The author feels that initial brief exposure to 6 ata followed by hyperbaric oxygen is superior in the treatment of air embolism to the longer 38 hr schedule. (Author's abstract)

1025.
KINDWALL, E.P.
Comparison of hematologic data in tunnel workers working in free air, at 38 pounds and those suffering from decompression sickness.
In: Ackles, K.N. ed. Blood bubble interaction in decompression sickness. Proceedings of an international symposium held at Defence and Civil Institute of Environmental Medicine, Downsview, Ontario, Canada, p.247-257. Published by the Institute, December 1973. (DCIEM Conference Proceedings 73-CP-960)

Data derived from blood samples taken from compressed air workers in Milwaukee are presented. Blood samples were taken from the compressed air workers at the beginning of their shifts, but after several days of compressed air work. These samples, compared with blood from fresh air workers, showed: no significant difference in hematocrit or red cell count; a significant increase in mean corpuscular hemoglobin; an important increase in erythrocyte sedimentation rate; no significant difference in hemoglobin and white cell counts. Platelet counts were not reliable because of faulty methodology. There was no significant difference in creatinine phosphokinase. In cases of bends, the white cells rose, the hematocrit declined, and the creatinine phosphokinase rose. It is noted that most of what is known about bubbles in relation to decompression sickness has to do with bubbles in the blood, because blood is easily available for study. The author suggests that something is happening in the tissue, perhaps related to ionic bonds, on an ultra-micro scale, but possessing great force, that actually triggers decompression sickness. (MFW/UMS)

1026.
KINLOUGH-RATHBONE, R.L.
The physiology of blood platelets.
In: Ackles, K.N. ed. Blood-bubble interaction in decompression sickness. Proceedings of an international symposium held at Defence and Civil Institute of Environmental Medicine, Downsview, Ontario, Canada, p.19-30. Published by the Institute, December 1973. (DCIEM Conference Proceedings 73-CP-960)

The structure and function of platelets are described and well illustrated with drawings, electromicrographs and diagrams. The principal role of platelets is concerned with the response of blood to injury. They have the ability to aggregate, to release their constituents, to adhere to surfaces, to phagocytose particulate material, and to participate in blood coagulation. Platelet function can be altered by non-steroidal anti-inflammatory compounds, by pyrimo-pyrimidine drugs, and by anticoagulants. In the first group, aspirin has been found beneficial in the treatment of decompression sickness. Other drugs that have been found useful are aminophyline, caffeine, theophylline, papaverine, dextrans and heparin. The protective effects of these drugs are probably not entirely due to their interference with platelet function. (MFW/UMS)

1027.
KINNEY, J.A.S., C.L. McKay, A. Mensch and S.M. Luria.
The visual evoked cortical response as a measure of stress in Naval environments: methodology and analysis (2) Rapid Flash rates.
U.S. Nav. Submar. Med. Cent., Rep. NSMRL 681, 15p. Oct. 6, 1971.

[The problem was] to evaluate the use of rapid flash rates as a technique for obtaining visual evoked responses (VERs) from the human cortex. With this method, the rate of presentation is purposely too rapid for a single evoked response to be completed before the next flash occurs. [It was found that] the technique results in VERs which are easy to quantify and interpret statistically. Furthermore, these VERs appear to be composed of elements of the complete, evoked response and of an additional rhythmical response superimposed upon it. The method evaluated in this report plus those described in the previous paper, SMRL #669, together afford an excellent technique for assessing the VER. All were evolved in order that the VER can be used to measure man's response to typical Naval problems, such as the hyperbaric or narcotic conditions imposed on a diver. (Authors' summary)

1028.
KINNEY, J.A.S., C.L. McKay and S.M. Luria.
Visual evoked responses for divers breathing various gases at depth to 1200 feet.
U.S. Nav. Submar. Med. Cent., Rep. NSMRL 705, 12p. Mar. 23, 1972.

Visual evoked responses were recorded from men subjected to hyperbaric conditions simulating 400, 700, 900, and 1200 feet of seawater in a saturation dive conducted at the Institute for Environmental Medicine, University of Pennsylvania, Philadelphia, Pa. Various breathing mixtures were used. At any given depth the VERs were the same for helium-oxygen and neon-oxygen but were sizeably reduced with nitrogen-oxygen, both in amplitude and in regularity. The possibility of an overall loss in VER amplitude with depth deserves further study since one subject did show such a decrement while the other did not. (Authors' abstract)

1029.
KINNEY, J.A.S., S.M. Luria, S.H. Ferris and H.M. Paulson.
Optical and visual tests on the navy prototype hard hat diving system.
U.S. Nav. Submar. Med. Res. Lab., Rep. NSMRL 731, 18p. Dec. 12, 1972.

The Navy prototype surface-supported, hard-hat system was subjected to a battery of tests to assess both its optical quality and its characteristics for visual performance. Optical tests were performed in the laboratory; visual measures were made on divers wearing the full suit in clear, well-lighted water. For comparative purposes, the same tests were performed with two other diving systems: the Mark 5 hard-hat system, which is the current hard-hat system, and normal SCUBA gear. Visual performance in the prototype suit was generally as good as, or better than in the Mark 5 or SCUBA equipment, but it was felt that the optical quality could be improved. (Authors' abstract)

1030.
KINNEY, J.A.S., S.M. Luria and M.S. Strauss.
Measures of evoked responses and EEGs during shallow saturation diving.
U.S. Nav. Submar. Med. Res. Lab., Rep. NSMRL 761, 28p. Sept. 14, 1973.

Visual evoked responses (VERs) and electroencephalograms (EEGs) were recorded during the course of a long-term, shallow, nitrogen/oxygen saturation dive. Measures were made during excursion dives and at the saturation level prior to and following each excursion. Comparison with a control series, in which bounce dives were made from the surface, revealed that some adaptive changes took place in the VER; complete adaptation however, did not occur. Reduction in frequency and amplitude of alpha, in the EEG, also was found during the course of the saturation period. (Authors' abstract)

1031.
KIPP, J.E. and R.G. Nevins.
Performance and life support in altered environments.
Manhattan, Kan., Kan. State Univ., Inst. Environ. Res., Rep. AFOSR-TR-72-2464, 50p. Oct. 31, 1972.
(AD 754 216)

Multidisciplinary studies of performance and life support in altered environments have been carried out. A summary of these investigations, including goals, personnel, and bibliographical data, is provided. Final phase progress reports as well as an over view of the results of this study when viewed as a single integrated study are also included. (Authors)

1032.
KIRK, B., S. Marks and R.L. Sergeant.
Variability among ten talkers of word intelligibility in noise.
U.S. Nav. Submar. Med. Cent., Rep. NSMRL 693, 13p. Jan. 12, 1972.

In an effort to determine what acoustic differences render one voice more intelligible than others, especially in the presence of noise, or reverberation, or when breathing helium gas mixtures, experiments were conducted using ten young adult talkers. The work of numerous other researchers who have worked with this problem is also reviewed and discussed (32 refs.) It is concluded that it may not be good practice to depend upon a single voice in assessing the performance of a communication system. Even when each of ten talkers with dialect-free speech were equated for acoustic intensity, when speaking at a comfortable level, one talker yielded performance of 75.5% words correct, another only 47.5%. It would be necessary to take the average intelligibility of any five of these talkers in order to properly assess a communication system. (Authors' abstract)

1033.
KIRKNESS, C.M. and A.G. MacDonald.
Effect of helium pressure on the narcotic potency of nitrogen in dividing cells.
In: Hesser, C.M. and D. Linnarsson eds. Proceedings of the first annual scientific meeting of the European Undersea Biomedical Society, Stockholm, 13-15 June 1973. Forsvarsmedicin 9:310-313;July 1973.

Inhibition of cell division in Tetrahymenaphyriformis was inhibited by 60 atm N_2: this was revised by the addition of 40 atm He, and cell division was nearly normal at 100 atm total pressure. The combination of 30 atm N_2 and 70 atm He, however, caused severe inhibition. Thus, a sub-effective dose of N_2 is potentiated by pressure, while an effective dose is antagonized by pressure. The practical application of these findings lies in the possibility that a low partial pressure of nitrogen used to offset the hyperexcitability effects of pressure during a dive might have a deleterious effect on growing tissue. (MFW/UMS)

1034.
KISLYAKOV, Yu. Ya.
Effect of PO_2 and PCO_2 of the arterial blood on the tension of these gases in the blood and brain tissue (mathematical modelling).
Biophysics 18(1):98-104; 1973.
(Transl. of Biofizika 18(1):98-104; 1973.)

On the basis of the idea of Krogh on a tissue cylinder as an averaged functional unit reflecting the processes of metabolism, a mathematical model of gas exchange in the brain is devised. In constructing the model the authors used the actual relations between the concentrations of O_2 and CO_2 in the blood and their partial pressures. Comparison of the results of modelling with experimental findings enabled them to choose the mean dimensions of the tissue cylinder (external radius $R = 30\mu$, length $1 + 640\mu$). The model was used to run a quantitative investigation in static conditions of the dependence of the O_2 and CO_2 tensions in the blood and brain tissue on the levels of PO_2 and PCO_2 in the arterial blood. The results obtained are used to interpret physiological experiments. (Author's abstract)

1035.
KIWULL, P., W. Wiemer and H. Schone.
The role of the carotid chemoreceptors in the CO_2-hyperpnea and hyperoxia.
Pfluegers Arch. 336:171-186; 1972.

In anesthetized rabbits rebreathing oxygen or inhaling constant mixtures of CO_2 and O_2 the influence of inactivation of the carotid sinus nerves by section or temporary cold blocking on the respiratory response to increased $PACO_2$ was investigated. In some of the experiments the vagi were intact, in others they were cut. Even during respiration of pure oxygen, in part of the animals blocking of the sinus nerves caused a slight diminution of ventilation which was significant only in the vagotomized preparation (average decrease by 11.4%). However, the diminishing effect of the blockade did not increase, but rather decreased, with increasing $PACO_2$. Similarly, section of the sinus nerves did not cause a significant shift or decrease of slope of the $PACO_2$ response curve. Evidently in the rabbit carotid chemoreceptors do not contribute essentially to the steady-state hyperpnea caused by hypercapnia under hyperoxic conditions. (Authors' abstract)

1036.
KLEPSER, W.F., Jr. and A. Morales, Jr.
A study of the impact of SSN688 class submarine design on a generalized advanced casualty ship control training device.
Groton, Conn., Gen. Dynamics Corp., Elect. Boat Div., Rep. NAVTRAEQUIPC-71-C-0200-1, 65p. June 1973.
(AD 764 086)

The study (1) evaluates the feasibility of providing advanced casualty ship control training for SSN688 class submarine crews, (2) determines what modifications to the detailed functional characteristics of the proposed device must be made to incorporate SSN 688 class advanced casualty training capabilities, and (3) determines the impact of such a device on the Navy's existing submerged ship control training programs. Recommendations were made concerning the implementation of an integrated, generalized training program and the development of the proposed device to support that program (Authors' abstract modified by GRA)

1037.
KLIMA, O.
Technological interrelationships between aerospace and hydrospace.
J. Hydronautics 4(3):126-128; 1970.

There are, of course, some areas of specific technology transfer: computers, solid-state electronics and microcircuitry, power generation, heat transfer, and communications are among the most obvious. And while there are dissimilarities in applying some of these technologies, depending on whether your interest is aerospace or hydrospace, there is sufficient commonality in terms of skills and knowledge required to make the prospects for closer relationships real and rewarding. Benefits emerging from these relationships already are evident. Certainly, more will follow, especially once the hydrospace community succeeds in acquiring a nationally accepted goal. Even in this, the fields share a certain commonality. As with the skeptics in aerospace of a few years ago, many people today feel that probing the sea to depths of several miles involves insurmountable obstacles. These same people, however, quickly accepted men flying at 18,000 mph in orbit for periods of several weeks. Yet a hard engineering evaluation of the obstacles in the deep submergence undertakings to date shows them to be no more difficult than those involved in space flight. (Author's conclusions)

1038.
KLINTSEVICH, G.N.
Etiologiya i profilaktika porazheniya kholodom na flote.
[Etiology and prevention of cold exposure in naval personnel].
Voennomed. Zh. (8):58-59;Aug. 1971.

There are two main causes of freezing: the lowering of the environmental temperature and the presence of factors reducing the body's local or general resistance to cold. Exposure to cold is a frequently occurring danger to naval personnel and deepsea divers. At the depth of 30-40 m the water temperature sinks to or below 4°C. Exposure to such temperatures for more than an hour can be extremely dangerous. In divers it may cause common cold, prohibiting further underwater activity, as well as decompression sickness by inhibiting the dissolution of blood gases. The author lists various measures for the prevention of freezing. He points out the importance of systematic intensive physical training of divers and naval personnel, as well as education in self preservation and mutual assistance, especially in cases of shipwreck. (OLC/BSCP)

1039.
KNOX, C.
Acoustic-optical imaging as a means of detecting bubble formation during decompression.
In: Abstracts of BuMed-ONR sponsored Navywide workshop in high pressure biomedical research, U.S. Submarine Base, Groton, Conn., May 1971, p.23. Published by the Naval Submarine Medical Research Laboratory, 1971.

Abstract only. Entire item quoted: The acoustic-optical imaging process utilizes Bragg diffraction of light by a beam of sound to produce an optical image of an acoustically irradiated object. Inasmuch as many materials which are quite opague to light are, to varying degrees, transparent to certain acoustic frequencies, the technique offers the possibility of visually examining the internal structure of optically opaque bodies. The imaging of internal features is made possible by the fact that different materials and structures often have different acoustic characteristics, thus causing the sound to be reflected, scattered, absorbed and diffracted. These factors cause perturbations in the acoustic wavefronts which are transformed in the light-sound interaction into a visual image, in real time, which may be observed by eye, photographed by a camera, or processed by other conventional optical methods. Acoustic-optical imaging in being applied to the detection of decompression bubbles in vivo. Investigations have included both analytical and experimental studies of the physical parameters (resolution, signal-to-noise ratios, power levels, etc.) which affect the feasibility of the application. Preliminary work has been done with hamsters.

1040.
KOBULIYA, N.S., L.E. Gedymin, F.R. Chernyakhovsky and O.P. Arkhipova.
Izuchenie pronitsaemosti gisto-gematicheskikh bar'erov pri razlichnykh rezhimakh giper barich eskoi oksigenatsii v eksperimente.
[Permeability of histo-haematic barriers in different regimes of hyperbaric oxygenation].
Eksp. Khir. Anest. 17:31-33; 1972.

The permeability of the histo-haematic barrier was studied experimentally on 70 guinea pigs subjected to 100% oxygen in therapeutic (1-2.2 up to 3 ata) and toxic (4-5 ata) regimes of hyperbaric oxygenation during 1-4 hours. Histology and radioactive indication (with streptomycin-S^{35} in the dose of 20,000 units per kg and with the activity of 14.2 microcuries in 1 ml) were used to assess various levels of permeability of the histo-haematic barriers of the lungs, liver, kidneys, spleen, myocardium and brain at the above regimes of hyperbaric oxygenation. Toxic regimes were accompanied by a universal increase of permeability of the vascular walls conditioned by structural lesions of the histo-haematic barriers. With therapeutic regimes vascular permeability rose only in the spleen, liver and kidneys, i.e. in the organs with an increasing functional activity under conditions of hyperbaric oxygenation and was not accompanied by changes in histostructure of the main elements of the histo-haematic barrier. (English summary)

1041.
KOCH, G.H. and R.Y. Nishi.
Decompression procedures for caisson work — a review of various techniques.
Downsview, Ontario, Def. Div. Inst. Environ. Med., Def. Res. Board, Rep. DCIEM 905, 24p. Nov. 1972.

Many different procedures are in effect for decompression after exposure to pressure in caisson work although they differ little in their basic concepts. The main principle is to prevent decompression sickness and aseptic bone necrosis in workers while affording rapid (and therefore economical) decompressions. In order to determine which of the new and highly favoured procedures is the most safe and economical, an analysis was carried out comparing the Ontario, Washington State, and British "Blackpool" caisson decompression procedures, and the U.S. Navy and Royal Navy diving decompression procedures with the DCIEM Kidd-Stubbs decompression model. The conclusions reached are that the Ontario procedure is safe provided the second shift is eliminated for exposures to pressures greater than 14 psig, and that the Washington State and British "Blackpool" procedures become increasingly unsafe as the exposures become longer over all the pressure ranges up to 50 psig. It is noted that these "unsafe" exposures have not generally been used in practice. Recommendations for caisson decompression are suggested. (Authors' abstract)

1042.
KOCHERGA, D.A. and T.L. Zhigailo.
Vpliv giperkapnii na elektrichni rozryadi bul'barnikh, dikhal'nikh neironiv ta neiromotornikh odinits' dikhal'nikh m'yaziv.
[Effect of hypercapnia on electrical discharges of bulbar respiratory neurons and neuromotor units of respiratory muscles].
Fiziol. Zh. 18:636-643;Sept./Oct. 1972.

Changes in impulse activity of different populations of bulbar respiratory neurons and neuromotor units of respiratory muscles during respiration of animals in the gas mixture containing 6% of CO_2 in the air were investigated in experiments on cats under nembutal-chloralose narcosis. It is shown that at the level of the bulbar respiratory center, the intensification of the respiration is brought on by an increase of inspiratory and expiratory neurons. At the level of an efferent link — respiratory muscles — intensification is due mainly to the activation of previously inactive neuromotor units and also partly to a slight increase in the frequency discharge of the functioning neuromotor units. A comparison of reactions of bulbar respiratory neurons and neuromotor units of respiratory muscles with hypercapnia results in a conclusion that an increase in neuron discharge frequency is a necessary condition for bringing new functional units into activity. (From English summary)

1043.
KOEHLER, G.J. and S.F. Gottlieb.
Effects of increased tensions of O_2, N_2, and He on the activity of a Na-K-Mg ATPase of rat intestine.
Aerosp. Med. 43:269-273;Mar. 1972.

The Na-K-Mg ATPase from rat intestine was found to be a pressure-sensitive enzyme. O_2, 15 psia and in the range of 90-135 psia, inhibits ATPase activity. In the range of 150-240 psia, O_2 enhances ATPase activity. Substrate protection did not account for failure of O_2 to exert marked inhibition. Nitrogen, in the range of 15-105 psia, does not inhibit ATPase activity. In the range of 30-80 psia, N_2 activates the enzyme. A progressive increase in degree of inhibition of ATPase occurs in the range of 120-285 psia. At PN_2 greater than 285 psia activation of ATPase activity occurs. Effects of He on ATPase activity are qualitatively similar to that of N_2. Quantitative differences between He and N_2 were observed in the ranges of 15-90 psia and 105-260 psia. At the lower pressure range, He exerted a more marked stimulatory effect than N_2; and at the higher pressure range, the increase of ATPase inhibition as a function of pressure was steeper with He than N_2. (Authors' abstract)

1044.
KOLGANOV, M.S., G.A. Povarnitsyn and G.V. Yakemenko.
Printsipy naznacheniya resursa klinicheskoi ekspluatatsii odiomestnykh lechebnykh barokamer.
[Principles of testing equipment for clinical utilization of individual decompression chambers].
Med. Tekh. 2:36;Mar./Apr. 1973.

The authors describe the methods for testing the durability of the material used for the dome-shaped glass-like covering of individual (single unit) decompression chambers for submarines. Mathematical calculations, based on static and dynamic hydraulic tests, will determine the resistance and durability of the material best suited for the dome. When in operation, it will be exposed to the varying pressures and temperatures of oxygen from the inside and water from the outside. After serial testing of various materials, a decompression chamber prototype should be designed, constructed and tested and uniform guidelines established for the manufacturing of each type of decompression chamber. Recently a specific type of single-unit decompression chamber, called "hyperbaric bed," has been tested. For its dome-shaped covering polymethylmethacrylate (organic glass) has been used. During testing it has been established that after 5000 hours of use its resistance will be considerably lowered. Deterioration of the plastic material constitutes a more than tenfold loss of durability. The authors supply several mathematical tables for the illustration of the hydraulic tests. They conclude that during clinical use for any individual decompression chamber periodic hydraulic testings are imperative, the frequency of check-ups depending on the use of the equipment. Parts of the chamber, when found defective and beyond repair, should be discarded and replaced. (OLC/SCD)

1045.
KOMORDIN, I.P.
O lechebnoi rekonipressii pri barotravme legkikh.
[Therapeutic recompression in pulmonary barotrauma].
Voennomed. Zh. (2):69-71;Feb. 1972.

The author criticizes an earlier communication by D.M. Verin (Voennomed. Zh. 10:68-69; 1969) in which two cases of successful treatment of barotrauma of the lungs in divers were reported. The author of the present paper points out that, in spite of the successful outcome of Verin's cases, there were two basic deficiencies to this treatment: organizational and medical. The organizational deficiency lay in the lack of an immediately available recompression chamber. Medical examination was also unduly delayed. The author points out several medical errors in the chosen therapeutic method: namely the sudden exposure of the patients to 10 atm pressure in the recompression chamber; the recommended safe pressure is 7 atm. The second error was the repeated exposure of one of the patients to 10 atm pressure when he showed "insufficient improvement of the neurological status." The second exposure was not indicated since the so-called neurological symptoms may have been caused by hypoxia of the nervous tissues and should have been treated with oxygen inhalation therapy. The only indication for repeated recompression therapy would be recurrence of barotrauma, which in the opinion of the author, practically never occurs. The author strongly disapproves of D.M. Verin's recommendation for military physicians to use repeated recompression in the treatment of barotrauma of the lungs when the first treatment results in insufficient improvement. Repeated recompression in these cases is not only contraindicated but may be extremely hazardous to the patient. The physician should use his own judgment in the choice of treatment of each individual patient. (OLC/BSCP)

1046.
KOMORDIN, I.P.
Nekotorye osobennosti men'erovskogo sindroma u vodolazov glubokovodnikov.
[Some aspects of Meniere's syndrome in deep sea divers].
Voennomed. Zh. (5):66-67;May 1973.

Meniere's syndrome in deepsea divers has two main forms: one results from the formation of gaseous bubbles in the endolymph; the other presents itself in the form of gas embolism of the labyrinthine blood vessels. The latter can be relieved by prompt therapeutic decompression. The author studied eight cases, each one occurring in deepsea divers emerging from 40-50 m depth, exposed to more than 150 m atm pressure, while breathing an air-helium mixture. Symptoms were: vertigo, nausea, vomiting, hearing and orientation disorders. Skin rash, joint and muscle pain, often found in decompression sickness, were absent. Successful treatment consisted of prolonged therapeutic decompression, initiated immediately. Since individual predisposition to Meniere's syndrome seems to be a main factor, careful testing and selection of divers is of primary importance. Fatigue and stress also may contribute to susceptibility. A balanced regimen of work and rest for divers, in order to avoid fatigue during deepsea expeditions is desirable. (OLC/UMS)

1047.
KOOYMAN, G.L.
Deep diving behaviour and effects of pressure in reptiles, birds, and mammals.
In: The effect of pressure on organisms. Symposia of the Society for Experimental Biology, No. 26, p.295-311. Cambridge, University Press, 1972.

In summary, the several aspects of deep diving which are discussed in this paper are: (1) Some species of reptiles, birds, and mammals dive to considerable depths. (2) The deep diving behaviour of only a few species has been studied in detail. In these, depth change rates can be very rapid and the most prolonged dives are not necessarily the deepest. (3) Pressure differentials are avoided in gas cavities either by exceptional flexibility of the structure surrounding the cavity, i.e. thorax, or by blood vessels expanding and acting as a space filler, i.e. middle ear. (4) Relative to body weight, the diving gas volume — the source of inert gas — is largest in penguins and smallest in seals. (5) Calculations show that even in seals blood N_2 tension could reach dangerous levels if all the gas were absorbed. (6) Measured blood N_2 tensions reach higher levels in sea turtles and penguins than they do in seals. (7) Avoidance of elevated blood N_2 tensions in most diving mammals is probably achieved by displacement of most of the gas into the rigid, nonabsorptive upper airways. Avoidance of, or tolerance to, high blood N_2 tensions in sea turtles and birds is obscure. (Author)

1048.
KOOYMAN, G.L. and W.B. Campbell.
Heart rates in freely diving Weddell seals, Leptonychotes weddelli.
Comp. Biochem. Physiol. (A)43:31-36;Sept. 1972.

Heart rates of seals were recorded during four activity levels) while they were sleeping in ice holes, before, during and after dives. Resting heart rates averaged 64/min during eupnea and 34/min during apnea. Rates before and after dives averaged 85/min. Rates during dives up to 5-min duration averaged 36/min. Rates during the first 45 sec of dives longer than 5 min were as low as 16/min. There appears to be an inverse relationship between heart rate and length of the dive. This relationship as well as other observed behavioral events that seem to correlated with heart rate indicate that the seals anticipate the nature of the dive. (Authors' abstract)

1049.
KOOYMAN, G.L., J.P. Schroeder, D.M. Denison, D.D. Hammond, J.J. Wright and W.P. Bergman.
Blood nitrogen tensions of seals during simulated deep dives.
Amer. J. Physiol. 223:1016-1020;Nov. 1972.

Three species of seal were subjected to a total of 65 simulated deep dives equivalent to depths ranging from 30 to 272 m (4-28.2 atm absolute (ATA)) in a hydraulic pressure chamber. Lung volume and arterial and venous N_2 tension were measured during these dives. Mean lung volume at the beginning of the dive was 20.4 ml x kg^{-1} in elephant seals and 22.6 ml x kg^{-1} in harbor seals. Lung volume was not determined in the Weddell seal. Soon after maximum pressure was achieved, arterial N_2 tension, which had risen at least 2-5 ATA, declined. It was always lower than theoretically possible considering the ambient pressure. Venous N_2 tension lagged behind arterial tension, and although it was low at the beginning of the compression period, it rose to about 2 ATA in elephant seals and as high as 5 ATA in harbor seals. Based on the lung volume and low arterial N_2 tensions, it was concluded that seals experience absorption collapse of the lung alveoli during time at depth and that this event is probably hastened by some degree of compression collapse during descent. In some instances with harbor seals N_2 tensions were high enough to be of possible concern with regard to N_2 narcosis and decompression sickness. (Authors' abstract)

1050.
KOOYMAN, G.L., D.H. Kerem, W.B. Campbell and J.J. Wright.
Pulmonary gas exchange in freely diving Weddell seals, Leptonychotes weddelli.
Resp. Physiol. 17:283-290; 1973.

Composition of end-tidal samples collected from the first expiration after resting apneusis and weight was 425 kg. Also determined was respiratory exchange ratio (R) and oxygen consumption ($\dot{V}O_2$). After an average resting apneusis of 4.5 min the end-tidal O_2 tension (PAO_2) averaged 59 mm Hg and CO_2 tension ($PACO_2$) averaged 50 mm Hg. After deep dives of an average submersion of 11.5 min the PAO_2=70mm Hg and $PACO_2$=27mm Hg. The exploratory dives, which ranged from 25-47 min, averaged PAO_2=40 mm Hg and $PACO_2$=36 mm Hg. It is concluded that the marked difference in the end-tidal composition of the deep dives is a result of hyperventilation preparatory for the dive and subsequent lung collapse and little gas exchange during the dive. Resting R was 0.69, but after dives R was highly variable. It began low and usually rose above 1.0 and subsequently fell to near 0.70. Mean resting VO_2 was 309 ml x kg^{-1} x hr^{-1} whereas $\dot{V}O_2$ after dives was initially as high as 2.4 L x kg^{-1} x hr^{-1} but fell precipitously during the ventilation period. Mean overall $\dot{V}O_2$ which included both the ventilation and the submersion period was 254 ml x kg^{-1} x hr^{-1}. The reasons for diving $\dot{V}O_2$ being lower than resting $\dot{V}O_2$ are discussed and it is concluded that the cost of diving is not great. (Authors' abstract)

1051.
KORCHANOV, L.S., V.A. Belov and N.D. Popov.
Dinamika pokazatelei tromboelactogramm pri giperbaricheskoi oksigenatsii v eksperimente.
[Dynamics of thromboelastographic indices in experimental hyperbaric oxygenation].
Voennomed. Zh. (7):51-54;July 1972.

The authors studied the changes in the thromboelastographic indices under the effect of hyperbaric oxygenation. In a series of experiments on rabbits they observed an increased coagulability of the blood. Several other authors have noted the rising of blood coagulation indices in patients treated with hyperbaric oxygenation for traumatic shock or acute arterial occlusion. In the present study a group of 28 rabbits were exposed to 1, 2 and 3 atm. pressure of oxygen respectively, during 1-2 hrs. Animals exposed to 3 atm. for 2 hrs. did not survive the toxic effect of O_2. The authors submit a detailed mathematical explanation in addition to a chart demonstrating the changes occurring in the thromboelastogram under hyperbaric oxygenation. With the increase of the pressure and exposure time some of the thromboelastographic constants are increased, a few remain unchanged. Hypercoagulation of the blood under increased oxygen pressure was the most significant finding. The authors, in agreement with other investigators, found that hyperoxia has a stimulating effect on the liver and the hypercoagulation indices observed are in accordance with the heightened activity of the functional processes of the liver. The authors recommend that patients undergoing hyperbaric oxygen therapy be kept under constant supervision, and, should hypercoagulation occur, treated with anticoagulant drugs. (OLC/BSCP)

1052.
KOROSTOVTSEVA, N.V., V.I. Baev, G.A. Valeeva and S.A. Bratseva.
Soderzhanie anniaka i glyutamina v golovnom mozge krys pri okhlazhdenii, giperka pnii i gipolsii.
[Amount of ammonia and glutamine in the rat brain during hypercapnia and hypoxia].
Fiziol. Sh. SSSR 59:713-717;May 1973.

The single and repeated effects of hypercapnia, hypoxia, and cooling on changes in the ammonium hydrate and the blutamine contents in the brain and the cerebellum, were studied in adult white male rats. The single impact resulted in a sharp alteration of nitrogen metabolism, and repeated impacts led to adaptive changes in the structures under study. (English summary)

1053.
KORZ, R., F. Fischer and C. Behn.
[Renin-angiotensin system in simulated hypervolemia induced by immersion].
Klin. Wochenschr. 47(23):1263-1268; 1967.
(Translation NASA-TT-F-14885, April 1973)
(N73-22036)

The relationship between plasma renin activity, sodium and potassium excretion, and plasma volume was studied during a control period and after immersion in neutral-temperature water (34-34.5°C) for six hours. Plasma renin activity decreased by 28% and the Na/K ratio increased, possibly reflecting decreased aldosterone secretion. Plasma volume decreased by 14%; no inverse relationship to plasma renin activity is found. The early natriuretic effect of immersion is concluded to be independent of aldosterone secretion. The early increase in tubular sodium load is considered to cause the decreased renin activity, inducing a reduction in aldosterone secretion, in turn responsible for altered electrolyte excretion after prolonged immersion. (AUTHOR((STAR)

1054.
KOSKI, W.S. and K.M. Wilson.
Untitled
In: Abstracts of BuMed-ONR sponsored Navywide workshop in high pressure biomedical research, U.S. Submarine Base, Groton, Conn., May 1971, p.22. Published by the Naval Submarine Medical Research Laboratory, 1971.

Abstract only: A miniature apparatus suitable for biological and physico-chemical studies at pressures up to 200 atm is described. A study was made of "the effect of iso-narcotic pressures of inert gases and some standard anesthetics on the cholinesterase system of sub-cellular particle derived from rat brain". Apparent activation of the enzyme occurred; the significance of this in relation to the effects of inert gases is discussed. A current investigation attempts to rank anesthetic agents and inert gas in the order of their narcotic potency; brine shrimp and amphipods are being used. Studies are being started on "the interaction of rare gases and anesthetics on spin labelled model membranes using ESR techniques." Finally, calculations on the interaction of a rare gas with a portion of a model membrane have been started. (MFW/BSCP)

1055.
KOSKI, W.S., J.J. Kaufman and K.M. Wilson.
Physiochemical aspects of the action of general anaesthetics.
Nature 242:65-66;Mar. 2, 1973.

The authors cite the theory that narcosis results from the occupation of a critical fraction of space in the membrane by an anesthetic agent, and is due to physical rather than chemical action of the molecule. They examine here the "Correlation between anesthetic potency of molecules and the van der Waals α constant." Temperature dependence and the antagonism of pressure in anesthesia are noted. It is concluded that "The correlation of log of anesthetic pressure against $\sqrt{\alpha}$ has a sound Thermodynamic basis and may express a general principle of narcosis by chemically inert materials." (MFW/UMS)

1056.
KOTTIK, P.
Bionik — gezeigt am Beispiel beweglicher Unterwassersysteme.
[Bionics — shown on the example of mobile hydrospace systems].
Meerestechnik 4:59-64;Apr. 1973.

Bionics, the new science between biology and engineering was born out of our time and its great problems. By exact analysis of biological systems, their construction and the way they work, we are able to construct new technical systems which are working better and specially are corresponding with their surrounding ecological systems. Mobile hydrospace systems are a good example to show the basics of bionics as they have all parts biology and engineering use to build up their systems [sic]. [The following examples are illustrated]: (1) Comparison between technical forms of pressure bodies and biological systems of pressure bodies. (2) An underwater vehicle, built in France, in which the crew fitted with diving suits is transported to the point of operation inside the flooded vehicle, is adjusted to a biological model. (3) Design for a cyclic ventilation system based on principles of bionics. Semipermeable membranes or permanently porous artificial materials (plastics) can be used, for instance, for oxygen admission and carbon dioxide exhaustion. (4) An "artificial dolphin-skin" has been developed in accordance with bionic discoveries which may be used as the outside element of underwater vehicles. (5) Design for mechanical and chemical transforming elements for energy transmission. (Author)

1057.
KOVALENKO, Ye. A.
[Questions on the theory of gas dynamics in the organism].
Fiziol. Zh. (2):315-324;Feb. 1973.

The article examines present concepts concerning the manner in which O_2 and CO_2 enter and leave the organism. Two oppositely directed and constantly functioning fluctuations of partial pressures of O_2 and CO_2 are considered as a general schematic of gas dynamics in the tissues, blood, lungs, and atmosphere. A hypothesis is advanced concerning the existence, in the organism, of a unique, dynamically changing topography of PO_2 and PCO_2 levels in various organs and tissues. The problem is examined from the viewpoint of analysis of diffusion of the gases and the convective transfer of the O_2 and CO_2 molecules. Models of various diffusion fields of oxygen in the tissues are analyzed in detail and shown in two detailed diagrams. For the first time, particular attention is paid to convective means of oxygen transfer in the tissues with flexible means of extra- and intracellular fluid. The question of changes in the penetrability of cell membranes for oxygen is raised. The author proposes a new version of the model of oxygen supply to the tissues which incorporates both the opposed bloodflow of K. Diemer (Naturwissenshaften 50:617; 1963) but also a random arrangement of capillaries, even at angles to each other, which substantially more accurately reflects the actual situation and explains the averaging of PO_2 levels actually recorded in various portions of dog brain tissues. (S & T alert).

1058.
KOWAL, J.P.
Cold and the diver.
Sea Frontiers 16:42-47; 1970.

The author discusses the investigations carried on by Dr. Hugh M. Bowen, made in a flooded rock quarry in Rhode Island using a movable platform which tested divers at 65°F and 45°F. Touch sensitivity, gross manual dexterity and hand and eye coordination, mental and memory function, and group assembly capability were tested on dry land and at both water temperatures. The water effect, noticeable at 65°F consisted of simple motor impairment, due to instability, neutral buoyancy, water resistance and lowered sensory functions. The cold effect, which occurs at temperatures lower than 55°F in a normal wet suit during a 30-min. dive, consists of marked lessening of touch sensitivity, finger dexterity and grip strength, and impairment of mental and memory function. The more complex the task, the greater the deterioration. The degree of impairment varies greatly among individuals. An attempt will be made to determine what factors contribute to this variation. Provided the diver is protected against narcosis, cold is the single greatest deterrent to performance. Heated suits as they present exist relieve the cold stress but are so cumbersome that they greatly impair motor function. (MFW/BSCP)

1059.
KOZLOV, A.N.
Ultrasonic Doppler cardiography in a medical monitoring system.
Space Biol. Med. 6(2):68-73;May 18, 1972.
(JPRS 56030)

Due to its high information content, stability and comfortable conditions for signal monitoring, ultrasonic Doppler cardiography seems to be promising when used in medical evaluations of enclosed men. Use of narrow-band filters, threshold limitations, and selection of the proper site for fixation of sensors make it possible to isolate a single complex from the ultrasonic Doppler cardiographic signal during every cardiac cycle for determining the heart rate in the medical monitoring system. (Author's abstract)

1060.
KREKELER, H., W. Liese and G. Von Nieding.
Effect of increased pressure and ambient gas compositions on alveolar-arterial O_2 pressure gradient.
In: Abstracts of the Twenty-fifth Congress of Physiological Sciences Satellite Symposium. Recent progress in fundamental physiology of diving, Marseille, France, July 1971, p.68. (Proceedings unpublished)

Abstract only. Entire item quoted: The alveolar-arterial oxygen pressure differences were determined during breathing of 20.9% oxygen in different inert gases and at different pressures. A second series of experiments was done, in which the O_2 partial pressure was kept constant at 0.2 ata. (1) At normal atmospheric pressure and at constant inspiratory PO_2 the arterial PO_2 fell from an average of 89.7 Torr at a N_2-O_2-mixture to 83.1 Torr at a He-O_2-mixture and 79.1 Torr respectively at a Ar-O_2-mixture. The AaD-O_2 rose from 8.7 Torr at N_2-O_2 to 15.3 Torr at He-O_2 and 16.3 Torr respectively at Ar-O_2. (2) Similar differences in arterial PO_2 were found between N_2 and He at rising pressures up to 6 ata and corresponding increase of inspired PO_2. The AaD-O_2 rose from 54.0 Torr to 65.0 at 2 ata, from 64 to 91 at 3 ata, from 131 to 186 at 4 ata and from 92 to 123 Torr at 5 ata respectively. (3) At a constant inspiratory PO_2 and increasing nitrogen pressure up to 4.8 ata the arterial pO_2 rose slightly or remained unchanged, but decreased significantly when nitrogen was replaced by helium. The AaD-O_2 rose from 7.1 Torr at N_2-O_2 to 22.6 Torr at He-O_2 at a pressure of 4.8 ata.

1061.
KREKELER, H., K. Muysers, W. Liese and G. von Nieding.
The influence of inert gases on the alveolar and arterial PO_2 and PCO_2.
Scand, J. Resp. Dis. (Suppl.)77:57; 1971.

Abstract only. Entire item quoted: The alveolar-arterial oxygen pressure difference was determined during breathing of 20.9% O_2 in different inert gases. At a constant inspiratory PO_2 the arterial PO_2 fell from an average of 89.0 torr (ten subjects) at a N_2-O_2 mixture to 83.1 torr at a He-O_2-mixture and 79.1 torr at a Ar-O_2-mixture. The A-a PO_2 rose from 8.7 torr at N_2-O_2, to 15.3 torr at He-O_2 and 16.3 torr at Ar-O_2-mixture. When the inspiratory O_2 pressure was kept constant at 0.2 ata and the nitrogen pressure was increased up to 5.8 ata there was no significant change in the arterial O_2-pressure. A significant decrease of arterial PO_2 was found when nitrogen was replaced by He. Corresponding differences in arterial PO_2 were found breathing 20.9% oxygen in N_2 or He at increased pressures up to 6 ata. The pronounced depressing effect of He and Ar mixtures on arterial PO_2 was also observed in patients with chronic bronchitis breathing He-O_2 or Ar-O_2 mixtures at ambient pressure.

1062.
KREKELER, H., G. Von Nieding, W. Liese and K. Muysers.
Sauerstoffpartialdruck im arteriellen Blut und im Capillarblut des hyperaemisierten Ohrlaeppchens in Norm-, Hyper- und Hypoxie.
[O_2-partial pressure in the arterial blood and in the blood of the hyperemisized ear lobe in norm-, hyper- and hypoxia].
Pneumonologie 146(1):34-44; 1971.

In 11 healthy subjects the O_2 partial pressure in the blood of the arteria brachialis and in the "arterialized" blood of the hyperemisized ear lobe was compared in norm-, hyper- and hypoxia. In norm- and hypoxia there was good congruence between PaO_2 (arterial O_2 tension) and Pcap (ear) O_2 (capillary O_2 tension). In hyperoxia Pcap (ear) O_2 was systematically lower than PaO_2. The mean differences between arterial and capillary blood were, when breathing a 15% O_2-N_2 mixture 0.4 torr; 20.9%, 0.5 torr; 30.0%, 5.7 torr; 40%, 6.9 torr; 50%, 16.0 torr; 70%, 11.9 torr; 85%, 106 torr; and 100%, 23.9 torr. (© BA)

1063.
KREKELER, H., G. von Nieding, K. Muysers, P. Cabarrou and D. Fust.
Washout of inert gases following hyperbaric exposure.
Aerosp. Med. 44:505-507;May 1973.

After hyperbaric exposure we determined the elimination of helium and argon by the lungs. In two different experiments in a compression chamber all subjects breathed for four hours at 1.8 ata a mixture of 0.2 ata oxygen and either 1.6 ata helium or 1.6 ata argon. Fifteen minutes after leaving the compression chamber the determination of the helium and argon partial pressures in the sampled alveolar gas by means of a mass spectrometer was started. At this moment the alveolar partial pressure for helium as well as for argon was less than seven torr. The subsequent washout for both gases was multiexponential. Eight hours later — in some cases even 24 hours later — the alveolar partial pressure of helium was still significantly increased (5.7×10^3 torr) in comparison with the ambient partial pressure of helium (3.5×10^3 torr). After the same time the elevation of argon was more distinct, it ranged from 7 to 21×10^1 torr above the ambient level (6.63 torr). The calculated desaturation half-time of helium for the slowest compartment ranged from 159 to 241 min. with a mean of 204 min. The desaturation half-time of argon for the slowest compartment amounted frm 610 to 672 min with a mean of 652 min. The amount of gas eliminated between 15 min and 8 hours after leaving the compression chamber was 1500 ml to 1800 ml STPD for helium and 2400 ml to 3200 ml STPD for argon. There was no clear correlation between these amounts and either body height or weight. The measured time constants of the slowest compartments for the washout of both helium and argon are greater than those given in literature. This leads to the conclusion that either the perfusion of the slowly eliminating tissues is less than formerly assumed or that other processes are the limiting factors for the washout. (Authors' abstract)

1064.
KRISHNAMURTI, S., M. Akhtar and N.R. Krishnan.
Myocardial infarction in patients undergoing hyperbaric oxygen therapy.
Indian Heart J. 25:107-110;Apr. 1973.

Two patients of peripheral arterial disease developed myocardial infarction while being treated with hyperbaric oxygen at 2½ absolute atmospheres daily as a therapeutic procedure. The episodes occurred after 22 and 24 exposures and 10 hours and 15 hours respectively, after the last exposure. The first patient, aged 37 years, died suddenly without any premonitory symptom of ischaemic heart disease and post-mortem revealed evidences of a fresh as well as an old myocardial infarction. The second, aged 29 years, had severe epigastric and retrosternal pain and was diagnosed on ECG as a case of acute myocardial infarction, involving the anterior wall. He was treated with bed rest, analgesics and anti-coagulants and made an uneventful recovery. Hyperbaric oxygen is reported not to cause hypercoagulability, leading to thromboembolism. In fact, it is used as an adjunct to the treatment of acute myocardial infarction. In these two cases the exact relationship between hyperbaric oxygen therapy and myocardial infarction is not immediately apparent. (Authors' abstract)

1065.
KRISS, A. Ye., ed.
Zhiznenyye Protssessy i Gidrostaticheskoye Davleniye.
[Vital processes and hydrostatic pressure].
Moscow, Izd-vo Nauka, Moscow, 1973. 271pp.

The monograph surveys foreign and Soviet research on the biological action of high hydrostatic pressure on proteins, nucleic acids, enzymes, plant, animal and human viruses, microorganisms and multi-celled organisms. Much original material by the author and his co-workers is also included, especially on the physiology of microorganism metabolism. Some relatively recent trends in this field are discussed, such as comparative research on the metabolism of microbes capable of multiplying under both normal and increased pressure. (S & T Alert)

1066.
KRITZ, A.C. and G.E. Miller.
Underwater display legibility as a function of water turbidity, display illumination color and brightness.
U.S. Nav. Electron. Lab. Cent., T.N. NELC 2074, 26p. July 14, 1972.
Unpublished report.

The legibility of an electrical meter was measured in four different water turbidities (bay, lake, tap, and distilled), using three illumination colors (white, green, and red) and three levels of illumination (0.02, 0.05, and 0.08 ft-lamberts). Mean response times are significantly reduced as brightness increases ($p < .001$) but errors tend to increase. There is a significant tendency for response times to increase as turbidity increases but errors tend to decrease. Turbidity and color interact significantly ($p < .05$). Green illumination results in the shortest latencies in bay and distilled water and the longest latencies in lake and tap water. White display illumination is suggested for underwater display systems since reading response time is as fast as any color, produces fewer errors, and requires less power to produce equal intensities than any other color investigated in all water conditions. A display brightness of 0.02 ft-lamberts is adequate for display legibility. Increases to 0.05 and 0.08 ft-lamberts result in shorter latencies but increased errors. (Authors' abstract)

1067.
KROHN, J.
Untersuchungen zum Problem: GFK-Propeller fuer U-Botte.
[Investigation on the problem of glass fiber reinforced plastic propellers for submarines].
Hamburg, W. Germany, Schiffbau-Versuchsanstalt, Rep. BMVG-FBWT-73-8, 28p. 1973.

The hydrodynamic behavior of glass fiber reinforced submarine propellers was compared with that of bronze propellers. The chord lengths were calculated for different thicknesses of blade sections based on the hydrodynamic conditions and geometric data of an existing bronze type. The expected bending stresses were calculated. For these blade sections with different dimensions, the behavior with respect to cavitation and efficiency were considered. The results of the investigations show that the hydrodynamic behavior of a glass fiber reinforced propeller is not worse than that of a bronze propeller. (ESRO) (GRA)

1068.
KROL, J.P.
An electronic measurement system for the assessment of mental load in the submarine environment.
In: Hesser, C.M. and D. Linnarsson eds. Proceedings of the first annual scientific meeting of the European Undersea Biomedical Society, Stockholm, 13-15 June 1973. Forsvarsmedicin 9:443-446;July 1973.

The purpose of this paper was to determine the feasibility of using a binary choice task in a submarine environment, in order to measure fluctuations in performance. Navy frogmen were tested in danger free and in stressful conditions. The task was self-paced, that is, the next stimulus was not presented until the previous response had been made. The subjects had to respond to aural or visual binary stimuli by pressing keys or pedals. Performance was registered at the surface. It was found that on an average choice making capacity was reduced by 25% under the more stressful, or dangerous, conditions. The subjects belonged to two groups, rated by their instructors as better and lesser divers. Group performance reflected the ratings. There was little individual difference. In the case of one novice diver, who had demonstrated normal responses before submersion, a completely chaotic performance was registered after entering the underwater habitat. (MFW/UMS)

1069.
KRUGER, P.
Mit dem Tauchboot zur Korallenernte.
[To coral harvest with the submarine].
Meerestechniik 4:12-14;Feb. 1973.

A Lubeck firm has developed a series of 12 commercial-industrial submarines called TOURS (Tourist, Observation, and Underwater Research Submersible). The equipment, operation and use of the TOURS 66 is described here. The submarine, 7.8 m long and 3.8 m wide, takes a two-man crew, and can reach depths of 300 m. The craft is towed to the work site and is always accompanied by a supply boat. For harvesting coral, the submarine has hydraulically operated manipulators and a freight net, in addition to the usual light, sonar, ventilation, and communications equipment. (MEMH/SCD)

1070.
KUEHN, L.A. and D.M.C Sweeney.
Canadian diving data: a computerized decompression data bank.
Comput. Biomed. Res. 6:266-280; 1973.

The study of decompression sickness is of major concern at various hyperbaric laboratories throughout the world. Although many data pertinent to decompression exist in various laboratories, few are circulated in any consistent format in the open literature. The development of an adequate decompression model that is suitable not only for shallow-depth short-time excursions but also for deep lengthy exposures requires the application of computer techniques and storage facilities. This computer methodology will make possible an efficient review of all pertinent data which in turn will lead to a better appreciation and elucidation of the important physiological parameters relevant to decompression sickness. Such an approach has proven successful in the collation and analysis of medical statistics. This report describes the development and use of such a computerized system to store, collate, and evaluate an extensive body of decompression information collected at the Defence and Civil Institute of Environmental Medicine (DCIEM). The system is known as Canadian Diving Data and is referred to by the acronym CANDID. . . The merits of this computerized data bank on decompression appear to be: (1) Evaluation of the success of pneumatic analogue decompression computers in providing safe decompression profiles that are efficient in terms of time and life-support facilities. The quantitative measure of success is the "bends" incidence at various depths and times of hyperbaric exposure. (2) Evaluation of current theories of safe decompression models or techniques such as the USN and RN diving tables. (3) Correlation of various parameters of hyperbaric exposure (such as time of dive, date of dive, earlier incidences of decompression sickness, etc.) with the bends incidence at various depths and exposure times in an attempt to elucidate predisposing trends or factors in the etiology of decompression sickness. Extensions of the CANDID system have been prepared and are in the planning stage. These include: (1) Incorporation of all diving information in Canada into CANDID in an acceptable format for analysis by the CANDID system. It is hoped that diving information from European and American laboratories will also become part of the data bank. The deposition of such information into CANDID would entitle the donor to access to and analysis of all the data in the system. (2) Incorporation of the biomedical characteristics and medical histories of all divers in the data bank into the CANDID system. This information could then be searched for any predisposition of these personnel toward decompression sickness. (Authors)

1071.
KUNZ, A.L.
Dynamics of alveolar CO_2 control.
In: Abstracts of BuMed-ONR sponsored Navywide workshop in high pressure biomedical research. U.S. Naval Submarine Base, Groton, Conn., May 1971, p.3. Published by the Naval Submarine Medical Research Laboratory, 1971.

Abstract only. Entire item quoted: It has been suggested that rate changes in CO_2 concentration may be important to respiratory control. The chicken prepared for unidirectional artificial respiration is convenient for studying rate change effects since dead space and washout volume are minimized. The chicken is awake, upright, and intact. Air forced into the trachea passes sequentially through the lungs, air sacs and prosthetic ports to the outside. Air flow is kept constant at 5 l/min (9 x normal); its CO_2 concentration is varied by an electropneumatic transducer and monitored by an LB-1 CO_2 analyzer. Ventilatory movements are measured with a whole body plethysmograph. Step function CO_2 inputs produce a gradual crescendo of ventilation (15 sec. time constant) and no overshoot. Sinusoidal oscillation of CO_2 about a mean of 4% appeared to produce the same ventilation as 4% CO_2 without oscillations. However, in spite of this apparent lack of derivative control, oscillations of CO_2 do effect ventilation. It has been found that with careful selection of the frequency and phase of the CO_2 oscillation the chicken can be entrained to breathe synchronously with each CO_2 oscillation. Once locked onto the oscillation the frequency can be carried over a range of about two octaves. In the externally closed-loop studied, the Co_2 is computerized to follow the algorithm: $\% \ CO_2(t) = \int [\dot{Q} - \dot{V}_{I\ (t\ -\ T)}]dt$, where $\dot{Q}$ is the analog of the rate of CO_2 production, V_I is inspirationary ventilation and T is the time delay. This closed-loop preparation comes to a steady state CO_2 level. If the CO_2 is momentarily disturbed to a higher or lower value it returns to the same steady state level. This steady state value is dependent upon $\dot{Q}$. There is a range of $\dot{Q}$s over which a large change in $\dot{Q}$ produces only a very small (but demonstrable) change in steady state mean CO_2. This demonstrable change in % CO_2 indicates the presence of load error and rules out the possibility of integral control.

1072.
KURENKOV, G.I. and B.O. Yakhontoe.
Potreblenie kisloroda pri napryaxhemmoi myshechnoi rabote v usloviyakh povyshennogo atmosfernogo davleniya.
[Oxygen requirement in intense muscular work under high atmospheric pressure].
Fiziol. Zh. SSSR 42(12):1812-1816; 1971.

Under 5 atm. pressure with a work load gradually increased from 900 to 1050 kgm/min a linear increase in O_2 requirement was observed. The respiratory frequency decreased, while depth of respiration increased. Airway resistance and the intensity of respiratory muscle activity increased depending on the density of the inhaled gas mixture. The second series was undertaken to study the extent of O_2 requirement under 5 atm. pressure during standard work load of 900 kgm/min. The average O_2 requirement under high pressure was found to increase by 67%, the aerobic component of energy metabolism by 51.1% and the anaerobic by 137.7%. Under high atmospheric pressure standard work performance requires a higher energy level because of the intensification of the respiratory activity. Increased O_2 deficit causes increased O_2 requirement and consumption. The authors suggest that one way of lowering the energy metabolism, while increasing physical working capacity under high atmospheric pressure seems to be the use of light density gas mixtures (helium-air or helium-O_2). Also, muscular work needs to be classified according to various degrees of intensity of the physical load. (OLC/UMS)

1073.
KURENKOV, G.I.
Muscular work in man under hyperbaric pressure.
In: Hesser, C.M. and D. Linnarsson eds. Proceedings of the first annual scientific meeting of the European Undersea Biomedical Society, Stockholm, 13-15 June 1973. Forsvarsmedicin 9:332-336;July 1973.

Professional divers engaged in muscular activity were observed during saturation exposures of 7-14 days, in an O_2-N_2 environment at 5 ATA, and underwater at 60 meters. Muscular activity in these environments is accompanied by increased oxygen consumption, oxygen deficit, CO_2 retention, pH increase, respiratory acidosis increase, and heightened cardiac activity. It is stated that the increase in oxygen debt is due to an increase in the lactate fraction. Arrhythmia was observed in two subjects. Results indicate a breakdown of the cardiac and hormonal regulatory systems. Urinary excretion of steroids increased in both environments, but much more greatly under water than in the dry chamber. Combination of these factors may reduce capacity for adaptation, thus leading to the development of respiratory and cardiac disorders. (MFW/UMS)

1074.
KUSTOV, V.V., L.T. Poddubnaia and V.I. Mikhailov.
K voprosu o toksichnosti vydykhaemogo vozdukha.
[Problem of the toxicity of expired air].
In: Chernigovskii, V.N. ed. Problems of cosmic biology, p.196-198. Moscow, Izdatel'stov Nauka, 1971.

Male albino mice were placed in an atmosphere consisting of air expired by humans. In order to distinguish effects attributable only to the elevated carbon dioxide content, some animals were subjected to a control run involving a higher concentration of this gas as the only deviation from normal air. It is shown that a number of gaseous toxic products present in air expired by humans induce neurohumoral changes which stimulate some inhibitory reactions in the central nervous system. (Aerosp. Med.)

1075.
KUTZLEB, R.E.
Current activity in deep ocean search and recovery.
In: Applications of marine technology to human needs. Preprints, 8th annual conference and exposition, Marine Technology Society, Sept. 1972. Washington, D.C. p.507-517. Published by the Society, 1972.

All phases of search and recovery — call out, survey, mobilization of resources, operations and demobilization — are discussed. Special search techniques include various sensor and other systems. Those discussed here are portable and therefore capable of quick response. Deep diving, requiring special breathing mixtures and decompression is not used in search activities except when (1) no other techniques are available or effective; (2) the target position is closely defined; (3) temperature and current conditions are favorable. (4) visibility is from 10 to 30 feet. It is noted that the diver is a most valuable asset in helping to prevent damage to the object while it is being salvaged. In many cases, classification prior to recovery is accomplished by television and/or video-tape record, so that the diver can be familiar with the situation at the outset. (MFW/SCD)

1076.
KYLSTRA, J.A.
Static recoil and maximum expiratory flow from saline and fluorocarbon filled lungs.
In: Abstracts of BuMed-ONR sponsored Navywide workshop in high pressure biomedical research, U.S. Naval Submarine Base, Groton, Conn., May, 1971. p.2. Published by the Naval Submarine Medical Research Laboratory, 1971.

Abstract only. Entire item quoted: Pseudo-static pressure-volume curves of FC-80 fluorocarbon and air filled dogs lungs reveal approximately equal hysteresis. Deflation isovolume pressure of air filled lungs > FC-80 filled lungs > saline filled lungs. In excised dog lungs, at transpulmonary pressures from 10 to 50 cm H_2O:

$$\int_{FRC + 250}^{FRC + 650} \frac{\dot{V}(air)}{\dot{V}(saline)} = 39.8 \pm 6.1$$

In spite of the fact that FC-80 is approximately twice as dense and viscous as saline:

$$\int_{FRC + 250}^{FRC + 650} \frac{\dot{V}\ (air)}{\dot{V}\ (FC\text{-}80)} = 31.6 \pm 4.6$$

These results indicate that FC-80 does not abolish surface tension at the alveolar interface and suggest that the alveolar lining layer is a surfactant micelle with polar groups facing the alveolar lumen.

In a healthy 40 year old man (left lung):

$$\int_{FRC + 330}^{FRC + 830} \frac{\dot{V}_{max}\ (air)}{\dot{V}_{max}\ (saline)} = 38$$

Ventilation at a rate of 6 l/min or more should be feasible in saline or fluorocarbon breathing divers if time allotted for inspiration and expiration are proportioned optimally. Since the solubility of CO_2 in FC-80 is 1.6 times greater than air at 37C, it seems likely that the effective alveolar ventilation of a mechanically assisted FC-80 breathing diver would suffice for critical operations at great depths.

1077.
KYLSTRA, J.A. and W.H. Schoenfisch.
Alveolar surface tension in fluorocarbon-filled lungs.
J. Appl. Physiol. 33:32-35;July 1972.

The quasi-static pressure-volume relationship of excised dogs' lungs filled with air and subsequently with FC-80 fluorocarbon liquid and of lungs first filled with air and then with 0.9% NaCI in water was determined by volume displacement plethysmography. At comparable lung volumes, the static recoil pressure of air-filled lungs > FC-80-filled lungs > saline-filled lungs. It is concluded that alveolar surface tension is not abolished in a fluorocarbon-filled lung. (Authors' abstract)

1078.
KYLSTRA, J.A., W.H. Schoenfisch, J.M. Herron and G.D. Blenkarn.
Gas exchange in saline-filled lungs of man.
J. Appl. Physiol. 35:136-142;July 1973.

During volume controlled lung lavage in a patient with alveolar proteinosis and a healthy volunteer, the PO_2 and PCO_2 of end-tidal liquid remained virtually unchanged as the time between the beginning of infusion to the end of drainage of a tidal volume increased from less than 30 to more than 200 sec while the arterial and mixed venous PO_2 and PCO_2 remained essentially the same. It is concluded that diffusive gas tension equilibrium between alveolar capillary blood and alveolar contents was established within 30 sec in these saline-filled human lungs. (Authors' abstract)

1079.
LAAN, J.
Devices for making underwater work safer.
Sea Grant 70's 3:2;May 1973.

Ali Sevieg and Amr Baz of the University of Wisconsin Sea Grant Program, have been working on depth, decompression and orientation control devices. The orientation control device consists of a movable weight which can be manipulated by the diver, so that he can operate at the most effective angle for the task at hand. Depth control devices use pressure sensors and enable the diver to control his rate of ascent and descent. The decompression device controls decompression automatically and is designed to work with the depth controller. The devices are designed for ease of removal. They have been tested in a swimming pool, and will be further tested while at the same time physiological monitoring goes on. (MFW/BSCP)

1080.
LaCERDA, J.
Embolism disaster averted.
Skin Diver 21:22-25;Mar. 1972.

This is an account of an occurrence of air embolism that lodged in the spine of an experienced diver making a routine slow ascent because of a leaking mask. At ten feet, she stopped and took a deep breath to blow into her mask to clear it, and may have drifted upward a foot or two while holding her breath. Her legs and arms felt swollen and weak, and she was taken home where she soon became unable to walk. She phoned for help, was taken to the Perry plant where she was placed in a demonstration chamber. Recompression and decompression lasted 41 hours. A diving companion, a doctor, went into the chamber with her and attended her during the treatment, measuring intake and output, forcing fluids orally and intravenously, and sending out blood for tests. Navy Decompression Table IV was used, and authorities were consulted by long distance phone. (Dr. David Youngblood in New Orleans and Dr. Joseph MacInnis in Toronto). Intermittent oxygen breathing was used during ascent. Three days later, a three-hour hyperbaric oxygen treatment was administered. The patient is still on crutches, is undergoing intensive neurotherapy, suffers from numbness and tremor, but is expected to make a full recovery eventually. (MFW/BSCP)

1081.
LACKNER, F., M. Baum, H. Benzer and J. Neumark.
Die Moglichkeiten erweiterten Monitorings atemphysiologischer Parameter in der hyperbaren Kammer.
[Possible methods for fuller monitoring of respiratory parameters in hyperbaric chambers].
Pneumonologie 149:97-106; 1973.

A small hyperbaric chamber (Vickers) was modified in order to facilitate amplified monitoring. ECG, basal temperature, central venous and arterial blood gases, blood pressure pneumotachygraphy and ventilation pressure were monitored in a cerebral trauma case. With rising pressure in O_2 atmosphere rises in venous PO_2 and in arterial PCO_2 were observed. When the patient was ventilated with a fluid-logic ventilator there was a higher rise in arterial PCO_2 and in venous PO_2, as hyperbaric atmosphere was gained. The pneumotachygraphic registration and the ventilation pressure showed that the fluid-logic ventilator can not comply with requirements in critical situations and especially when used as an assistor. The interpretation of these findings is discussed in the light of current knowledge in this field. Uncontrolled use of the fluid-logic ventilator is deprecated and the modification of the Vickers chamber is recommended for monitoring in selected cases. (English abstract)

1082.
LAI, Y.L., B.A. Attebery and E.B. Brown, Jr.
Intracellular adjustments of skeletal muscle, heart, and brain to prolonged hypercapnia.
Resp. Physiol. 19:115-122;Nov. 1973.

The in vivo apparent CO_2 buffer values ($\Delta HCO_3^-/\Delta$ pH) of extracellular fluid, skeletal muscle, cardiac muscle, and brain were determined on tissues from rats that had breathed 10% CO_2 for periods of 1 to 24 hr. The patterns of early changes in pH and HCO_3^- in extracellular fluid, skeletal muscle, and brain were similar. There was a rapid fall in pH to its lowest value at 1 hr followed by an increase over the next few hours. These pH changes reflected an increasing HCO_3^- concentration in these 3 tissues over the first few hours. By contrast the intracellular pH of cardiac tissue decreased very slowly over the first 4 hr, reflecting a rapid rise in HCO_3^- during the first hour of CO_2 breathing. When these data are expressed as apparent CO_2 buffer values; extracellular fluid, skeletal muscle, and brain increased while cardiac tissue decreased over the 4 hr of CO_2 breathing. Although nephrectomy altered the pattern of HCO_3^- increase in extracellular fluid and skeletal muscle, it did not alter the order of relative buffering in the 4 tissues studied. (Authors' abstract)

1083.
LAI, Y.L., B.A. Atterberry and E.B. Brown, Jr.
Mechanisms of cardiac muscle adjustment to hypercapnia.
Resp. Physiol. 19:123-129;Nov. 1973.

It has been previously demonstrated both in dogs and in rats that cardiac tissue has an ability to buffer CO_2 far greater than that of skeletal muscle in vivo under conditions of hypercapnia. This increased CO_2 buffering by cardiac tissue may be due to one of three factors. 1) A larger inherent noncarbonic buffer content. 2) An enhanced ability to form noncarbonic buffer during hypercapnia. 3) An enhanced exchange of bicarbonate and/or hydrogen ions between intracellular and extracellular fluid in response to hypercapnia. The in vitro CO_2 buffer values of homogenates of cardiac and skeletal muscle were compared and skeletal muscle had the higher in vitro CO_2 buffer value. This eliminated factor number 1. Rats were exposed for 2 hr to 10% CO_2 before the tissues were obtained for in vitro CO_2 buffer value determination, and there was no significant difference between CO_2 buffer values of tissues from hypercapnic and normocapnic animals. This eliminated factor number 2. By elimination these data suggest that the mechanism responsible for the high in vivo CO_2 buffer value of cardiac tissue is an enhancement of the mechanism(s) responsible for the transfer of bicarbonate into, or hydrogen ions out of, cardiac intracellular fluid. (Authors' abstract)

1084.
LAI, Y.L., E.D. Martin, B.A. Attebery and E.B. Brown, Jr.
Mechanisms of extracellular pH adjustments in hypercapnia.
Resp. Physiol. 19:107-114;Nov. 1973.

An estimate was made of the relative contributions of 1) chemical buffering and distribution, 2) exchange between extracellular fluid and other body compartments, and 3) renal compensation, to the pH adjustment of extracellular fluid in rats breathing 10% CO_2 for periods of 15 min to 21 days. At the end of one hour 33% of the increase in extracellular bicarbonate was attributed to chemical buffering, 22% to exchange with other body compartments, and 45% to renal compensation. After 48 hr the contributions were 8%, 12%, and 80%, respectively, and after 21 days the values were 7%, 11%, and 82%. The overall response expressed as "%pH adjustment" (Siesjo, 1971) increased from 8% at 15 min to 72% at 21 days with most of the adjustment taking place in the first 48 hr. (Authors' abstract)

1085.
LAMBERT, R.J.W.
The nuclear submarine environment.
Proc. Roy. Soc. Med. 65:795-796;Sept. 1972.

The author discusses briefly the environmental problems of the nuclear submarine, such as the presence of toxic gases, the ready exchange of bodily flora, the absence of ultraviolet light, and climate control. The four ways of meeting the situation are summed up as follows: (1) accept the risk and do nothing; (2) correct the environmental factors, even though the cost in terms of money, space and power might make this impracticable; (3) intensify selection requirements with emphasis on specific susceptibilities; (4) consider protective routines, either in diet or in prophylactic drugs, to correct the imbalances of the environment. (MFW/BSCP)

1086.
LAMBERTSEN, C.J.
Integrated studies of respiratory gas effects.
In: Abstracts of BuMed-ONR sponsored Navywide research in high pressure biomedical research, U.S. Submarine Base, Groton, Conn., May 1971, p.37. Published by the Naval Submarine Medical Research Laboratories, 1971.

Abstract only. Excerpt quoted: The areas of physiological activities, have included oxygen effects upon respiration, pulmonary and ophthalmological oxygen toxicity, inert gas narcosis by nitrogen and nitrous oxide, pulmonary and respiratory function at extreme gas density, and decompression optimization. Special attention has been given to the design and establishment of an "International Decompression Data Bank", for the selection, storage and dissemination of decompression data of exceptional quality. A series of sustained exposures to inert gas-oxygen mixtures at increased pressure has provided the means of applying the methods of acute studies to the investigation of physiological adaptions during chronic, multiday exposure to high gas density and narcosis. Studies thus far have included (a) a 48 hour open sea exposure of two men to a depth of 432 feet; (b) participation in a two day laboratory chamber exposure of two men to a pressure equivalent to 650 feet of sea water; (c) laboratory and open sea studies of four men exposed for 60 days to a pressure of 42 feet of sea water; (d) laboratory chamber studies of six men exposed for 14 days to nitrogen-oxygen atmosphere at a pressure equivalent to 100 feet of sea water. Present high pressure chamber studies involve separate investigation of hydrostatic narcotic and gas density effects through use of nitrogen, neon and helium at increased ambient pressure.

1087.
LAMBERTSEN, C.J.
Chronic nitrogen exposure study.
In: Miller, J.W., J.G. Van Derwalker and R.A. Waller, eds. Tektite 2: Scientists-in-the-sea, p.IX-25-IX-35. Washington, D.C. Department of the Interior, August 1971.

The objectives were: 1. To study the increased respiratory airway resistance produced by the four-fold increase in density of respired gas. At rest and in exercise this airway resistance should lead to an increase in work of breathing and, at some elevated ambient pressure, to a decrement in alveolar ventilation at work and even at rest. Such decrement, by interfering with uptake of oxygen from the lungs by the blood and elimination of carbon dioxide from the blood and lungs, should lead to hypoxia, elevation of arterial carbon dioxide tension, and decrease in motor and intellectual performance. 2. To study the narcotic influences of nitrogen. 3. To appraise the influence of ambient pressure and increased nitrogen partial pressure upon blood cellular constituents, body fluid volumes, and blood chemical composition. . . . There appear to be no gross performance-limiting influences of the increased atmospheric density, pressure, and nitrogen partial pressure. The primary cautions are as follows: The narcotic influence of nitrogen is expressed to different degrees in different individuals. The highly motivated, skilled, and intelligent subjects used in the laboratory study had, for physical, mental and physiological functions, such reserve and compensatory ability that their performance was superior even in the narcotic atmosphere. Other individuals are obviously more affected and would be endangered by exposure to severe physical stress in diving or by a requirement for use of fine judgment or a high order of technical skill. The dangers for such individuals would lie largely in work in the water outside the habitat. (Author)

1088.
LAMBERTSEN, C.J.
Carbon dioxide tolerance and toxicity.
Philadelphia, Pa., Univ. Pa. Med. Cent., Inst. Environ. Med., 76p., Oct. 1971.

Carbon dioxide is a normal body constituent, continually produced by oxidative metabolism. Its hydration leads to formation of hydrogen ions and the establishment of a bicarbonate buffer system in blood and other vital body fluids. In its numerous normal roles in body function, carbon dioxide is a key chemical messenger substance in the linking of respiration, general circulation and local vascular response to the demands of metabolism both at rest and in exercise. In its normal, active role as an agent in the respiratory, circulatory and renal control systems, intrinsically produced carbon dioxide is not a toxin. It is an essential factor in the determination of the normal acid-base balance required for enzymatic reaction. *Inhaled* carbon dioxide produces the same physiological effects as does carbon dioxide produced metabolically. These effects appear to result from the acidosis induced by carbon dioxide reaction with water, rather than by the CO_2 molecule itself. Toxic effects of CO_2 do occur when such high concentrations of CO_2 are inhaled that severe and disruptive cellular acidosis occurs. This acidosis and its effects are alleviated by lowering the inhaled concentration of CO_2. Adaptation to moderate inspired concentrations of carbon dioxide (to three and four percent) occurs in normal men who can tolerate continuous inhalation of three percent inspired CO_2 for at least one month and four percent inspired CO_2 for over a week. Because the effects produced by low and moderate concentrations of carbon dioxide be increased from 0.5 to 2.0 percent in inspired air. This level has not been shown to induce decrement in performance or in normal physical activity. (Author's abstract)

1089.
LAMBERTSEN, C.J. and H. Bardin.
Decompression from acute and chronic exposure to high nitrogen pressure.
Aerosp. Med. 44(7, Sec.II):834-836;July 1973.

Exposure of men to a nitrogen-oxygen mixture at 4 ata ambient pressure for 14 days required that decompression schedules be devised for the saturation exposure of the subjects, for the nonsaturation acute exposures of the subjects, and for acute exposures of investigators and support personnel. The schedules developed for the 100-ft, 14-day chamber study were to serve as the decompression schedules for the planned 100 ft. open-sea phase of Project Tektite II. That phase was not carried out. (Authors' abstract)

1090.
LAMBERTSEN, C.J. and W.B. Wright.
Multiday exposure of men to high nitrogen pressure and increased airway resistance at natural expired oxygen tension: a 14-day exposure to 5.2% O_2 in N_2 at 4.0 atmospheres absolute pressure.
Aerosp. Med. 44(7, Sec.II)826-833;July 1973.

[The study, conducted in June-July 1970, concerned] factors limiting the tolerance or adaptation of man to increased atmospheric pressure. These have included: The degree of impairment of respiratory control and pulmonary gas exchange by the combined effects of increased work of respiration and the narcosis produced by nitrogen; The alterations of mechanical and other pulmonary functions in response to acute and sustained exposure to increased resistance to breathing; The rate of successful adaptation to the stresses upon pulmonary function and respiratory control and the rate of deterioration of these functions at rest and in work where adaptation is not successful; The degree of decrement in specific aspects of mental performance induced by the inert gas narcotic, nitrogen, and the pattern of adaptation or failure of these functions when the narcotic exposure is continued; The influence of nitrogen upon formation and destruction of cellular constituents of blood; The patterns of chemical, endocrine, and metabolic adjustment to the prolonged, high pressure exposure. . . . A conclusion of this study is that normal, intelligent, highly motivated young individuals in excellent physical condition can carry out strenuous physical or meticulous intellectual tasks for extended periods of time in a high-pressure nitrogen atmosphere. . . . An equally important conclusion relating this study to previous, acute investigations of high nitrogen pressure is that individuals less well endowed in physical capacity, competitive drive, intellectual capacity or pulmonary reserve can be expected to show gross detrimental and possible incapacitating effects of exposure to the same environment. [The introductory section is followed by individual articles concerning specific aspects of the experiment, such as decompression, pulmonary function, respiration and gas exchange, hematological, biochemical and immunological studies, body fluid volume changes and nitrogen narcosis]. (Authors)

1091.
LAMBERTSEN, C.J., R. Gelfand, M.J. Lever, G. Bodammer, N. Takano, T.A. Reed, J.G. Dickson and P.T. Watson.
Respiration and gas exchange during a 14-day continuous exposure to 5.2% O_2 in N_2 at pressure equivalent to 100 fsw (4 ata).
Aerosp. Med. 44(7, Sec.II):844-849;July 1973.

Exposure to the narcotic influences of high nitrogen pressure, the interference with carbon dioxide elimination at high respiratory gas density, and the mechanical influences of increased work of breathing all may conceivably alter the normal patterns of respiratory control. Study of these possible influences of acute and sustained exposure to a nitrogen-oxygen breathing medium at 4 ata ambient pressure produced no deleterious effects related to respiratory control at rest or in exercise. A slight diminution of respiratory response to carbon dioxide was observed but was probably more related to density of the respiratory gas than to narcotic influences of the respired nitrogen. In exercise, in spite of elevated respiratory resistance, competent performance of vigorous work was practical without gross deficiencies in respiratory gas exchange. (Authors' abstract)

1092.
LAMMERANT, J. and I. Becsei.
Response of the coronary circulation to hyperoxia in the anaesthetized intact dog infused with adenosine.
Arch. Int. Pharmacodyn. 200:309-319; 1972.

In closed-chest anaesthetized dogs, the mean coronary resistance was lowered close to one-fourth of normal value by infusing adenosine into the right atrium. While the infusion was maintained, a significant decrease in myocardial blood flow and increase in coronary resistance were observed when ventilating the animals with pure oxygen at ambient pressure. Despite the occurrence of coronary constriction, the myocardial blood flow remained considerably higher than normal. The coronary venous oxygen tension reached values similar to that reported for exposures to oxygen at 3 atmospheres absolute pressure without adenosine infusion. (Authors' abstract)

1093.
LAMY, M.L. and M.M. Hanquet.
Modern aspects of treatment of decompression sickness.
Acta Anaesthesiol. Belg. 3:215-229;Oct. 1973.

Treatment of decompression accidents no longer consists in just recompressing the patient. The physiopathology of these accidents, if not yet completely explained, affords better understanding of the importance of oxygen during recompression and of the drug therapy. If the bubbles of inert gas represent the primary aetiologic agent, they involve an important series of progressive deteriorations in the tissues; the result is a new pathological state, decompression sickness, with its neurovegetative, humoral, cardiovascular and respiratory disorders. Modern treatment consists principally in oxygen recompression at minimal pressure (no more than 4 ATA) and in drug therapy for decompression sickness. This treatment is best made in intensive care units. Pulmonary overpressure warrants the same kind of treatment but it should be started with greater speed still. A penumothorax may necessitate punctures or surgical draining. If the patient is situated at a distance of less than two hundred kilometres from a well-equipped treatment centre the best procedure would be to convey him by ambulance under normobaric oxygen and with an intravenous perfusion of low molecular weight dextran. Transportation chambers can be dangerous and should only be used with much circumspection and care. At the moment, two therapeutical possibilities of decompression accidents exist in Belgium: the multiplace chamber of the Naval Force in Ostend and the monoplace Draeger chambers devised for hyperbaric oxygen therapy in resuscitation centres. (Authors' summary)

1094.
LANDSBERG, P.G.
Carbon dioxide changes in hyperventilation and breath-hold diving.
South African Med. J. 46:777;June 19, 1972.

Abstract only. Entire item quoted: Breath-hold dives to a depth of 10 m in fresh water at 1,640 m above sea-level, at atmospheric pressure (Pb) mmHg, were performed by 5 male divers. The water pressure at 10 m at this altitude is approximately 1.83 ATA (1,368 mmHg.). Peripheral venous blood from the right antecubital vein was analysed for combined CO_2 content ($^cCO_2$) by the Van Slyke method, and expressed in $^cCO_2$ vol% and cross-checked in $^2CO_2$ mEq/L. The CO_2 content of peripheral venous blood is lowered by hyperventilation and increased by repeated breath-hold diving. Individual divers had different rates of CO_2 elimination from blood to alveolar air. CO_2 elimination is also not the same in any one diver from day to day. It is postulated that the effects of hyperventilation are unpredictable in different divers under the same diving conditions. This may have contributed to the deaths of several divers in South Africa.

1095.
LANDSBERG, P.G.
Bradycardia during human diving.
Presented at Science Week, 1972, University of Witwatersrand, South Africa, July 1972.

Abstract only. Entire item quoted: During the hyperventilation-breath-hold-dive cycle in man, several cardiac arrhythmias occur, of which bradycardia is the most consistent, and is thought to be part of an atavistic "diving reflex" which conserves oxygen within the organism. The physiological mechanism is not fully understood. The carbon dioxide content of the peripheral venous blood is correlated with the extreme bradycardial response found in prolonged apneic diving. Extreme bradycardia during diving may cause unconsciousness and drowning. The bradycardial response under different conditions of apnea and diving is compared, and the various electrocardiographic arrhythmias are tabulated. Diving bradycardia is compared to fetal bradycardia recorded during labour.

1096.
LANE, C.
Literature review of the effects of helium on the mechanics of respiration, with clinical correlations.
U.S. Nav. Submar. Med. Res. Lab., Rep. NSMRL 741, 8p. Mar. 5, 1973.

A review of the pertinent literature [through 1970] relating to the physiology of ventilatory dynamics using helium-oxygen breathing mixtures is presented together with conclusions regarding the indications and contraindications for their use in clinical medicine. A review of relevant studies in diving medicine is included because of the clarification which these investigations lend to problems of pulmonary ventilation. The bibliography is representative but not all-inclusive. (Author's abstract)

1097.
LANG, J. and I. Rozsahegyi.
Damage to the vestibular function of caisson workers.
In: Hesser, C.M. and D. Linnarsson eds. Proceedings of the first annual scientific meeting of the European Undersea Biomedical Society, Stockholm, 13-15 June 1973. Forsvarsmedicin 9:423-427;July 1973.

Vestibular function of 400 compressed air workers engaged in the construction of the metro in Budapest was examined; the eighth cranial nerve was markedly sensitive to decompression accident — the cochlear branch more so than vestibular. Previous cranial trauma appears to predispose to decompression sickness; particularly to the vestibular nerve. Damage to the vestibular nerve can occur without symptoms of decompression sickness. Otoneurological examination is an important part of any medical fitness examination for compressed air work. Any disorder involving the eighth cranial nerve should be considered disqualifying. (MFW/UMS)

1098.
LANGLEY, T.D. and R.W. Hamilton, Jr.
Comparison of helium versus crude neon as inert gas components.
In: Abstracts of BuMed-ONR sponsored Navywide workshop in high pressure biomedical research, U.S. Submarine Base, Groton, Conn., May 1971, p.31. Published by the Naval Submarine Medical Research Laboratory, 1971.

Abstract only. Excerpts quoted: The authors conducted a series of two-man dry chamber "dives" centered around the use of crude neon (72-87% neon, with the balance helium) and compression at 100 ft/min. These dives comprise a matrix of three gases — helium, nitrogen, and crude neon, all with 10% oxygen in 30 min. exposures to depths of 200, 300 and 400 fsw. Auditory evoked brain responses and the on-going EEG and ECG were monitored continually on both divers during rests of postural tremor on the outstretched arm, manual tapping, arithmetic, simple reaction time, alpha blocking, simple auditory vigilance, relatively complex auditory vigilance and nut-and-bolt assembly. In general the performance tests showed no measurable differences between helium and crude neon as inert components. Most tests showed a decrement when the inert gas was nitrogen. Of particular interest was the 400 ft. nitrogen dive, an exposure to nearly 12 atmospheres of nitrogen, the equivalent to 460 feet of air and one of the most extreme nitrogen exposures on record. Computer averaging of the evoked responses and statistical treatment of other results are in progress.

1099.
LANGLEY, T.D.
Neurophysiological investigations of inert gas effects on the central nervous system.
Tarrytown, N.Y., Ocean Systems Inc., Final report on N00014-69-C-0405, 10p. Apr. 25, 1973. (AD 766,298/4)

The chief factors studied were the effects of ultra-high pressures, rapid compression, and inert gas narcosis. Following experiments with squirrel monkeys, experiments with human subjects, using helium-oxygen breathing mixtures, demonstrated that compression at 100 fsw/min to 800 fsw, then a 22-minute stop, followed by compression to 1,000 fsw at 50 fsw/min was feasible with experienced divers if the environment was properly controlled. In subsequent 1,200 fsw saturation experiments carried out at the Institute for Environmental Medicine of the University of Pennsylvania, a new technique referred to as somatic evoked brain response measurement was introduced. Constant-current electrical stimuli of the median nerve at the wrist were recorded by means of scalp electrodes located over the primary cortical projection area for the hand. With increasing pressure, the somatic responses increased, indicating drowsiness. Mental and psychomotor tests were employed, in which no distinction could be made between neon and helium in their effects on performance. In two two-week saturation dives conducted jointly with the Naval Submarine Medical Research Laboratory, divers made excursion dives of 10 minutes to five hours to 300 fsw and upward to the surface from saturations at various depths, the greatest of which was 120 fsw. Measurements made by means of somatic evoked brain responses, as well as performance tests, indicated that deep excursions after saturation induced less narcosis than similar excursions from sea level, thus demonstrating adaptation to narcosis following residence in a habitat containing a nitrogen breathing mixture. (MFW/BSCP)

1100.
LANGLEY, T.D. and R.W. Hamilton, Jr.
Somatic evoked brain responses as indicators of adaptation to nitrogen narcosis.
In: Aerospace Medical Association. 1973 annual scientific meeting, Las Vegas, Nevada, May 1973. Preprints, p.265-266. Published by the Association, 1973.

The authors tested the hypothesis of adaptation to nitrogen narcosis, and also the "rebound effect" from nitrogen narcosis when relatively rapid decompression is used. It has been found that narcosis during a bounce dive will be less after a saturation dive than at other times. There is less narcosis during excursion dives from saturation when the excursion dives take place a few days into the saturation period rather than at the beginning. Also, during a long excursion dive, narcosis decreases toward the end of the period. The "rebound effect" occurs immediately after decompression from short bounce dives from sea level, and immediately after decompression from excursions from habitat level. Two of the subjects showed steady adaptation as evinced by progressive decrements in the evoked response during the course of a two-week saturation dive (simulated). Other subjects showed less consistent changes. Bounce dives before and after saturation were made to test the "rebound" hypothesis. The recordings made after the bounce dives before saturation showed a much greater degree of rebound than those made following bounce dives which took place ten days after saturation. (MFW/BSCP)

1101.
LANGLEY, T.D. and J.B. MacInnis.
Vestibular function: equilibrium and balance.
Tarrytown, N.Y., Ocean Systems, Inc., Res. Devel. Lab., Rep. CRL-T-749, 74p. Dec. 29, 1973.

The vestibular sense is of major importance in diving, particularly when visibility is poor. Dysfunction, indicated primarily by vertigo, nausea and vomiting is a life threatening emergency when the diver is in the water; with bell-diving it is incapacitating but not life-threatening when an assistant is available to perform essential functions. Vertigo may be a prime cause of accidents with shallow water scuba diving. With deep diving (greater than 300 fsw) for both research and operational purposes, vestibular dysfunction is increasing as the number of deep dives increases and as greater depths are reached. At sea, remoteness and unfamiliarity with diagnosis and treatment have complicated many cases. Permanent damage to the vestibular system is a serious hindrance to a diver's occupation; partial and complete recoveries from vestibular problems have occurred, permitting these divers to resume normal activities. There is a need for a world-wide review of vestibular dysfunction in Navy, commercial and institutional deep diving so that relevant elements of the diagnosis, treatment and prevention can be clarified. [This report was prepared for inclusion in a handbook on underwater bioengineering which is being produced by The Science Communication Division of The George Washington University Medical Center, scheduled for publication in 1975 by Plenum Publishing Corp.]. (Authors' summary)

1102.
LANPHIER, E.H.
Untitled.
In: Abstracts of BuMed-ONR sponsored Navywide research in high pressure biomedical research, U.S. Submarine Base, Groton, Conn., May 1971, p.36. Published by the Naval Submarine Medical Research Laboratories, 1971.

Abstract only. Entire item quoted: A major portion of effort in the High Pressure Laboratory has been focused upon plans, preparations, and developmental work for the large new 170 atm chamber. This is expected to be installed and in use later in 1971. The chamber and its adjuncts will include a number of departures from usual practice. If successful in use, these will be of considerable interest to other laboratories. Recent research in the more usual sense includes continued study of the respiratory effects of gas density. Interest is directed not only at ventilatory aspects but toward diffusion in denser media. A recently-instituted study concerns cardiovascular effects of compression and will include intracellular electrode measurements in myocardial tissue. In addition to pressure facilities, the new Laboratory of Environmental Physiology will provide capability for studies in submergence, altitude, heat, cold, high-G and exertion under various conditions. Research in several other areas of the Department relates to high pressure problems in various ways.

1103.
LANPHIER, E.H.
Human respiration under increased pressures.
In: The effect of pressure on organisms. Symposia of the Society for Experimental Biology, No. 26, p.379-394. Cambridge, University Press, 1972.

Increased pressure influences human respiration primarily through the effects of increased gas density. With air and other relatively dense gases, diving encroaches upon the reserve of ventilatory capacity at any depth, and the capacity for physical exertion is progressively reduced beyond a certain depth even with optimal breathing apparatus. The use of $He\text{-}O_2$ mixtures restores much of this capacity and markedly increases the depth of useful activity. However, the full extent of this benefit is not yet precisely known. Additional benefits with hydrogen may be very great, but predictions are even less confident at this time than those for helium. Present thinking suggests that ventilatory limitations will become consequential only at pressures greatly beyond those yet reached by man. A potentially more serious problem is presented by the 'Chouteau effect', which very possibly represents impaired diffusion of oxygen in dense gas. Use of hydrogen-oxygen breathing mixtures cannot be expected to enhance diffusion greatly, but it may decrease diffusion deadspace through increased 'disturbance mixing' and should permit more effective compensation. Hydrogen appears to be an acceptable component of gas mixtures for deep diving and man's ultimate depth as a useful diver may depend upon possible respiratory benefits of its use. (Author's summary)

1104.
LANSCHE, J.M.
Deaths during skin and scuba diving in California in 1970.
Calif. Med. 116:18-22;June 1972.

The diving deaths in California during 1970 totaled 33. Of these, 23 were due to drowning, five to air embolism, and one each to decompression sickness and hemopneumothorax. More deaths occurred in the 41-45 year age group than in any other. The following statistics are tabulated: Incidence of drowning; activity being engaged in at time of death by drowning; location of death by drowning (type of body of water); causes of death in diving; incidence by age and sex; expired time and depth of recovery of bodies; incidence as related to experience; systems failure groupings — (equipment, judgment, training, rescue operation). In the latter case, training failure was the most frequent type of system failure. The difficulty of reaching definite conclusions in this type of investigation is emphasized. The importance of good physical condition and thorough training becomes obvious. Seventeen of the accidents in which data were available, could probably have been avoided by better endurance, use of the buddy system, experience with equipment, use of distress signals, buddy breathing, and knowledge of decompression sickness. (MFW/BSCP)

1105.
LARKIN, E.C., W.T. Williams and F. Ulvedal.
Human hematologic responses to 4 hr of isobaric hyperoxic exposure (100% oxygen at 760 mm Hg).
J. Appl. Physiol. 34:417-421;Apr. 1973.

Four males breathed 100% oxygen at 760 mm Hg via face mask for 4 hr. Prior to the exposure, during the exposure and after the exposure at various intervals the following measurements were obtained: hematocrit, hemoglobin, red blood cell (RBC) count, reticulocyte count, serum bilirubin, plasma hemoglobin, red cell osmotic fragility, red cell population density distribution, red blood cell glutathione (GSH), red blood cell glutathione stabilities, white blood cell count with differebutal count, and platelet count. During exposure, there was progressive increase in red blood cell osmotic fragility and decrease in mean red blood cell density. Hyperoxia also resulted in a plasma hemoglobin rise and abnormal RBC GSH stabilities. Abnormal RBC osmotic fragilities, RBC population density distributions, and plasma hemoglobin levels persisted after exposure. A small population of red cells was lysed. Another population of red cells appeared to have persistent abnormalities following isobaric hyperoxic insult. (Authors' abstract)

1106.
LaROCCA, J.J.
Federal regulation of diving.
In: Professional diving safety. Second annual symposium, New Orleans, Nov. 1971. Mar. Technol. Soc. J. 6:32-33;Jan./Feb. 1972.

The author, who is with the Occupational Safety and Health Administration of the Department of Labor, reports on the progress of the development of the American National Standards Institute's Z-135 standard for diving operations. The problems of industry-government communications are touched upon, and it is suggested that a training program be set up for field compliance officers to enable them better to understand the operational situations they will be called on to evaluate. In addition to the ANSI Z-135 further standards may have to be developed under section 6(b) of the Occupational Safety and Health Act. Many standards now operative under the OSHA also apply to the diving industry, in such areas as occupational health, hazardous materials, compressed gas equipment, etc. (MFW/BSCP)

1107.
LARSON, C.R., D. Sutton, E.M. Taylor and J.D. Burns.
Visual evoked potential changes in hyperbaric atmospheres.
Tempe, Ariz., Ariz. State Univ., Tech. Rep. 71-02, October 1, 1971.

The VEP in chloralose-anesthetized cats decreased in amplitude as a function of increasing pressure. This was true for compression with PO_2 = 200 or 1,000 mm Hg. Maintained pressure while changing PO_2 from 200 to 1,000 mm Hg or from 1,000 to 200 had little effect. If PO_2 — 1,000 mm Hg had been used in a session, variability in VEP measurements was extremely high, i.e., the VEP amplitude dropped to zero at 100 FSW for some cats, while other cats showed little effect at 500 FSW. Limited information on decompression indicates the VEP may be recovered from its depressed state at 500 FSW by slow decompression. Rapid decompression results in the VEP remaining depressed or being reduced in amplitude even further. The VEP was not a reliable index for determining decompression stops. (Authors' summary)

1108.
LAURENT, P. and J.-D. Rouzeau.
Afferent neural activity from pseudobranch of teleosts: Effects of PO_2, pH, osmotic pressure and Na^+ ions.
Resp. Physiol. 14(3):307-331; 1972.

Morphological study of the pseudobranch of teleosts has established the presence of a rich, sensory innervation composed of several types of receptors which are associated with the "true" pseudobranch, the existence of a sensitivity to chemical factors in the plasma was studied. Analysis of the electric activity in the pseudobranchial nerve revealed 2 types of impulses. Abrupt changes in hydrostatic pressure resulted in a burst of large amplitude impulses. For similar types of impulses, increase in the concentration of Na^+ ions in the perfusing solutions brought about an average increment frequency of more than 3%½/meq L^{-1}. The frequency of small amplitude impulses is influenced mainly by the PO_2 and osmotic pressure. The average increment of frequency is greater than 1%/torr below $PO_2 = 100$ torr and more 2% mOsm. [osmotic pressure equivalents] below 269 mOsm L^{-1}. There are at least three types of receptors found, which is in good agreement with the morphological findings. It follows that the function of the pseudobranch, still unknown, might concern ion and ventilatory regulation mechanisms. (© BA)

1109.
LAUVESTAD, V.R.
Acoustic scattering by objects whose shapes permit separation of variables.
La Spezia, Italy, Saclant ASW Res. Cent., Rep. SACLANTCEN-TM-180, 33p. Sept. 1, 1972. (AD 750,754)

Descriptions of the field scattered by finite objects in the presence of a radiating acoustic source are among the investigations fundamental to antisubmarine warfare, but progress from idealised tractable models to more realistic 'target' shapes is a slow business of great theoretical difficulty, leaving aside the complications introduced by the properties of the medium. In this paper a selective reivew of existing treatments is first briefly and critically made. Then, because of the insight that generalisations may give, a general treatment is formulated of the acoustic scattering problem that includes the whole class of cases in which the Helmoltz's equation separates and partial wave analysis is applicable. Care is taken to indicate the practical shortcomings of the class of solutions that this exact treatment provides. Possible means by which some of these shortcomings might be overcome are indicated. (Author) (GRA)

1110.
LAVERNE, A.A., D.J. DiMaio and A.J. Fernandez.
Occupational, accidental, explorational carbon dioxide inhalation poisonings, and prevention.
Behav. Neuropsychiat. 4:33-48;Feb.-Sept. 1973.

Pathological and toxicological findings related to CO_2 inhalation deaths of the therapeutic and non-therapeutic variety are described. CO_2 has long been used experimentally and therapeutically in medicine for one hundred years in concentrations of 5 to 80% in oxygen mixtures. It has been so used in acute and chronic debilitating diseases in all age groups. Submarine personnel exposed to CO_2 levels reaching 3 to 15% in the ambient air for several weeks developed chronic fatigue and non-specific pathological reversible syndromes. In the two recent minisub deaths similar chronic CO_2 exhalation buildup caused toxic CO_2 levels for a period of hours causing death. [The medical examiner's report of the Johnson Sea-Link disaster is included in the article. The extreme cold suffered by the divers who later died of CO_2 poisoning is given as the reason that they were unable to attempt to leave the submarine and come to the surface]. One acute accidental CO_2 inhalation poisoning is also reported. To establish CO_2 as the cause of death, in any type of CO_2 inhalation poisoning, autopsy findings must show petechial hemorrhages and anoxic vascular changes. Valuable scientific data is now provided to supplement the body of knowledge that has been compiled in therapeutic CO_2 inhalation over the past forty years. It appears that CO_2 inhalation, whether therapeutic or non-therapeutic, can be as safe or as dangerous as the conditions created in each specific situation. The knowledge of control and prevention of side-effects in the therapeutic area of CO_2 research can be applied to the occupational fields of endeavor such as submarine and space exploration, which may prevent irreversible side-effects, as has occurred in the minisub and other CO_2 poisonings. (Authors' abstract)

1111.
LAVY, S., H. Shoham and D. Harel.
Sensitivity of the brain to repeated exposures of hyperbaric oxygen.
Aerosp. Med. 44:254-255;Mar. 1973.

A preliminary study investigating the susceptibility of rats to repetitive daily exposures to HOP was carried out. When the first electrical discharge is used as an early sign of oxygen toxicity, the latency of its appearance remains unchanged and it can be assumed that the animals suffered no permanent brain damage. This finding does not support the previous reports that repetitive exposures increase susceptibility to oxygen poisoning. (Authors' abstract)

1112.
LAWSON, W.H., Jr.
Effects of drugs, hypoxia and ventilatory maneuvers on lung diffusion for CO in man.
J. Appl. Physiol. 32:788-794;June 1972.

We measured the effect of hypoxia, hyperventilation, epinephrine, or isoproterenol infusion, and the release of a Valsalva maneuver on pulmonary diffusing capacity for CO (D_{CO}) and pulmonary capillary blood flow ($\dot{Q}c$) in normal subjects breath holding at total lung capacity both seated and supine. D_{CO} and $\dot{Q}c$ increased significantly in all five tests, mean of 116 and 153% of control ($P < 0.001$). "Control" and test D_{CO} for hypoxia were measured at similar low alveolar PO_2 so that the rate of reaction of CO with erythrocytes in the pulmonary capillaries (Θ_{CO}) would be similar. $\dot{Q}c$ varied with the duration of hypoxia, ten seconds in control and five to ten minutes in test measurements. The increase in D_{CO} per unit increase in $\dot{Q}c$ in a given subject was similar for all tests and is similar to that observed during exercise by others. The possible exception is hypoxia which may have a larger $\Delta D_{CO}/\Delta \dot{Q}c$. Perhaps the transmural vascular pressure responsible for opening capillaries in the lung correlates with $\dot{Q}c$ in these widely varying conditions. (Author's abstract)

1113.
LEACH, C.S., W.C. Alexander, C.L. Fischer, C.J. Lambertsen and P.C. Johnson.
Endocrine studies during a 14-day continuous exposure to 5.2% O_2 in N_2 at pressure equivalent to 100 fsw (4 ata).
Aerosp. Med. 44(7, Sec.II):855-859;July 1973.

Vigorous activity as experimental subjects and technicians — during multiday exposure of normal men to the increased nitrogen partial pressure, and increased density of respired gas — was accompanied by changes in endocrine hormone concentrations in blood and urine. Measurements in blood included insulin, tri-iodothyronine, thyroxine, angiotensin, and cortisol. Unexplained decreases in thryoid hormone concentrations occurred, while insulin and angiotensin I concentrations in plasma increased and cortisol concentrations were not systematically changed. Measurements in urine showed increase in norepinephrine and cortisol excretion during the exposure, with a decrease in antidiuretic hormone excretion and no change in aldosterone excretion. These changes were accompanied by a diuresis that persisted from the second day until the end of the exposure period. (Authors' abstract)

1114.
LEDINGHAM, I. McA.
Clinical applications of hyperbaric oxygen in a large air-compressed pressure vessel.
In: Innes, G.S. ed. The production and hazards of a hyperbaric oxygen environment. Proceedings of a symposium held at University College, London, January 1968, p.29-37. London, Pergamon Press, 1970.

Among the clinical applications of hyperbaric oxygen, the author lists decompression sickness. It is noted that the use of compressed air or oxygen in these cases is "based upon the fact that the size of a gas bubble in a blood vessel or in the tissues will diminish in proportion to an increase in the gaseous pressure around it." It is further noted that the use of hyperbaric oxygen, as compared to hyperbaric air, has the advantage of reducing the pressure requirement, thus reducing the risks to the chamber personnel while not appreciably altering the efficiency of the treatment. (MFW/BSCP)

1115.
LEDINGHAM, I.McA. and J.K. Davidson.
Hazards in hyperbaric medicine.
In: Wada, J. and I. Takashi, eds. Proceedings of the fourth international congress of hyperbaric medicine, Sapporo, Japan, Sept. 1969, p.527-530, Baltimore, Williams and Wilkins, 1970.

There has rightly been concern amongst hospital personnel and those responsible for their safety that the dangers of a hyperbaric environment might be too high a price to pay for any therapeutic benefit to be gained. These data at present support the claim that, while there is no room for complacency, pressures of air in the range 1-3 ATA are relatively safe for use in a specialised medical hyperbaric environment. It remains entirely conjectural as to whether the modifications added to the conventional decompression programmes, such as the breathing of oxygen and the introduction of extra stops during decompression, have had any bearing on these findings. (Authors' discussion)

1116.
LEE, J.V.
Underwater acoustic interferometer.
IEEE international conference on engineering in the ocean environment, Panama City, Florida, September 1970. Digest of technical papers, p.63-65. Published by the conference.

Measurements have been made showing the limitations a seawater medium imposes on the resolving power of underwater acoustic equipment. An interferometer was designed that is capable of measuring the "visibility" of the interference fringes in the far field of an acoustic radiator. Phase and amplitude fluctuations of the divided acoustic wavefront are analyzed utilizing correlation techniques. (Eng. Index)

1117.
LEE, K.J.V.
Underwater submersible navigation.
Meerestechnik 3:122-128;June 1972.

Subsurface navigation has long been used by naval submarines, which normally employ sophisticated inertial systems, but various reasons, including cost and weight, preclude their use for commercial purposes. This article deals with the navigation of submersibles. To satisfy the wide variety of their applications, several types of submersible have been made for use in many parts of the world. Tethered and untethered free-swimming versions and the tethered bottom crawler are considered here. Their navigation can be achieved either by a surface-referenced or a sea-bed-referenced system, supplemented by certain basic instrumentation. (Author's abstract)

1118.
LEE, S.H.
[Studies on the energy metabolism and respiratory functions in Korean UDT divers].
Yonsei J. Med. Sci. 5(1):197-208; 1972.

Among the various lung volumes measured, residual volume and functional residual capacity were significantly smaller in the UDT (underwater demolition team) compared to that of controls. Breath holding time of the UDT (122.3 sec) was significantly longer than that of controls (76.6 sec). Both the maximal inspiratory and expiratory pressure at different lung volumes were significantly higher in the UDT than that of controls. Ventilatory response to a 5% CO_2 breathing mixture, among other cardiopulmonary responses, was significantly diminished in the UDT compared to the controls. The daily energy expenditure was higher in winter than in summer, i.e. 5036 cal/day and 4378 cal/day, respectively. This difference was attributed to a larger heat loss during dives in winter. The results of breath holding time and ventilatory response to CO_2 in the UDT are comparable to those of other reports, suggesting that there was a decrease of sensitivity of the respiratory center to CO_2. However, the maximal inspiratory pressure at each lung volume was distinctly higher in Korean ama (female skin divers) [see Song, S.H. et al., J. Appl. Physiol. 18:466-470;May 1963] and Japanese ama [see Kobayasi S. et al., Acta Med. Biol. (Niigata):249-260;Mar. 1971], whereas both the maximal inspiratory and expiratory pressures were higher in the UDT. This may be because the ama engage in negative pressure breathing during skin diving, while the UDT members are engaged in positive pressure breathing during scuba dives. Results indicate that the UDT members who practice a mixed type of dive also develop adaptive changes to the aquatic environment. (BCT) (© BA)

1119.
LEE, W.H., Jr.
Physical and biologic sequelae of blood-gas interfacial reaction.
In: Ackles, K.N. ed. Blood bubble interaction in decompression sickness. Proceedings of an international symposium held at Defence and Civil Institute of Environmental Medicine, Downsview, Ontario, Canada, p.227-232. Published by the Institute, December 1973. (DCIEM Conference Proceedings 73-CP-960)

A distinct similarity exists between the pathophysiology of decompression sickness and the problems arising from gas-blood interface in the pump oxygenators used during heart surgery. Numerous pathophysiologic events have been observed following the protein denaturation which occurs in exposures to such interface while using oxygenators. It would be logical, therefore, to investigate denaturation of proteins occurring during post-dive decompression. Other subjects worthy of investigation are: changes in blood rheology, alterations in immunologic surveillance, alterations in vascular permeability, alterations in the enzymatic function of blood proteins, and the possible presence of denatured protein in the lymph effluent from tissue containing decompression-related bubbles. (MFW/UMS)

1120.
LEEK, J.H. and R.L. Riess.
Traumatic sudden deafness.
Minn. Med. 56:608-610;July 1973.

The authors describe a case of a scuba diver who suffered significant hearing loss after diving to 43 ft. On reaching this depth, severe pain in the left ear forced him to ascend a few feet; the same pain recurred on repetitions of the descent. When the diver surfaced he became aware of hearing loss, pressure, fullness and tinnitus in the left ear. At first the condition was diagnosed as middle ear barotrauma which would spontaneously heal. On the fourteenth day, tympanotomy revealed a small rupture in the round window membrane. When this was repaired with a plug of fat from the ear lobe, hearing was restored to normal. The authors caution against assuming that round window membrane rupture is always the cause of sudden deafness; the circumstances under which it is likely to be the case are a popping sensation immediately preceding hearing loss and lack of vestibular symptoms. Emergency action is advised against, since such cases have been known to heal spontaneously after as long as 18 days. (MFW/SCD)

1121.
LE FAN, J.H. and R. Helmreich.
Methodology.
In: Miller, J.W., J.G. Van Derwalker and R.A. Waller, eds. Tektite 2. Scientist-in-the-sea, p.VIII-18-VIII-26. Washington, D.C., U.S. Department of the Interior, August 1971.

Data collection was conducted in four ways: (1) pre-mission testing; (2) continuous observation of in-habitat behavior; (3) self-report questionnaires filled out daily by aquanauts during their dive; and (4) structured debriefing of aquanauts immediately after decompression. . . The bulk of the research effort was directed at collecting complete quantitative data on personal and interpersonal activities during the total stay underwater. The variables observed can be used to form criterion variables or factors for the prediction of behavior and can also be used for analyses of trends in behavior over time and the study of interrelations of discrete behaviors. The pre- and post-dive measures provide variables to correlate with the objective data available on each aquanaut's reactions to the undersea environment. (Authors)

1122.
LEFEVRE, P. and G. Federspil.
Effets d'un exercice musculaire continu (nage forcee) sur le metabolisme du tissu adipeux du rat.
[The effects of continuous muscular exercise (forced swimming) on adipose tissue metabolism in rats].
Arch. Int. Physiol. Biochim. 79(3):565-572; 1971.

In rats, forced swimming in tepid water is accompanied by a stimulation of true lipolysis at the level of the adipose tissue and a considerable reduction in the process of fatty acid reesterification by the adipocyte. This decrease is quantitatively important in the mechanisms assuring fatty acid mobilization in this type of exercise. Two endocrine variations were recorded during the experiment: an increase in the plasma corticosterone level and a significant decrease in the blood insulin level. (SLR) (© BA)

1123.
LE GUENEDAL, J.Y. and Baret.
Activites enzymatiques seriques et autres parametres biochimiques sanguins et urinaries au cours d'une plongee fictive a saturation en melange helium-oxygene a 31 ATA (equivalent a 300 metres) avec long sejour a la pression maxima.
[Serum enzyme activity and other blood and urine biochemistry parameters during a simulated saturation dive to 31 ATA (equivalent to 300 metres) using a helium-oxygen mixture, with a prolonged stay at the maximum pressure].
Cent. Etud. Rech. Biophysiol. Appl. Mar., Rep. CERB 73-15, 22p. 1973.

Serum enzyme measurements show: 1) that no cellular lesion is observed during this deep dive, neither during the phases of pressure variation, nor during the long stage at the maximum pressure; 2) that a slight change in cellular permeability may exist, and would explain the few slight rises in [the cellular enzymes] SGOT and LDH observed by these and by other authors; 3) that cellular hypoxia may exist, during adaptation to the maximum pressure, at the time of muscular exercise and is probably related to the increased affinity of hemoglobin for oxygen which has been shown elsewhere; 4) the discovery of a correlation between decompression accidents and a marked rise in serum alkaline phosphatases will lead us toward the study of isoenzymes in the near future. (Authors' conclusions, transl. by MEMH/UMS)

1124.
LE GUENEDAL, J.Y., B. Broussole, H. Burnet and F. Mantoux.
Les proteins solubles du lavage endobronchial du rat sous oxygene.
[Soluble proteins of the endobronchial lavage of the rat under oxygen].
Cent. Etud. Rech. Biophysiol. Appl. Mar., Rep. CERB 73-05, 10p. 1973.

Rats were exposed to oxygen for five or ten days, then three endobronchial lavages were made and centrifuged to eliminate the cellular elements. Findings led to the following conclusions: the protein content of the alveoli increases in proportion to the duration of the oxygen exposure. Phospholipids increased fourfold, while proteins increased fifteenfold. The protein rate reflects to a large extent the intensity of endamatous process. Two possible hypotheses are presented: (1) An optimum phospholipid-protein relationship is destroyed by pulmonary edema; (2) the proteins in excess are degraded proteins. These investigations do not permit firm conclusions, but open perspectives of research on the role of proteins in the functional study of pulmonary surfactant (MFW/SCD)

1125.
LE GUENEDAL, J.Y., B. Broussolle and C. LaJeune.
Les enzymes seriques au cours d'une plongee fictive a 300 metres, comportant un long sejour au fond.
[Serum enzymes during a simulated dive to 300 meters with a long stay at bottom].
Bull. Medsubhyp 10:47-49;Dec. 1973.

The serum enzymes: SGOT, SGPT, SLDH, SCPK, total PAL and PAL inhibited by L. phenylalanine (intestinal origin) were studied in three divers (DIG, FOU, GAU) during a simulated dive at 31 ATA with a PIO_2 = 0.30 bar. The groups of measures were done: at sea level, after 4 days at 1.5 ATA, two groups at 21 ATA separated by 48 hours, three groups at 31 ATA (48 h, 6th and 12th days), two groups during decompression (19.7 ATA and 6.5 ATA) and 48 hours after return to the surface. SGPT level did not change. SGOT and SLDH increased slightly at the beginning of the dive and 48 hours after return to the surface. SGPK increased from 30 UI/L to 125 UI/L for FOU and DIG 24 hours after exercise in cold water. GAU had only 44 UI/L but his exercise was done 72 hours before measurement. PAL did not change except for FOU during decompression. At 21 ATA this diver presented severe knee bends. The measures show: no real cellular lesion during a deep dive, but there may exist a slight change of the cellular permeability; the possibility of a slight muscular hypoxia after light exercise at depth; the evidence of a correlation between decompression sickness and an increased level of PAL with a participation of PAL inhibited by L. phenylalanine. (English abstract)

1126.
LEITNER, L.-M.
Sensibilite des recepteurs pulmonaires d'etirement du chat et du lapin aux variations de tension de CO_2.
[Sensibility of the cat and rabbit pulmonary stretch receptors to changes in CO_2 partial pressure].
C.R. Acad. Sci. (Paris) (Serie D) 275:1151-1153;Sept. 11, 1972.

The sensitivity of the pulmonary stretch receptors to weak hypercapnia were studied in anesthetized cats and rabbits. In half of the cases, hypercapnia brings on a weak diminution (less than 10%) of the discharge frequency of the vagal fibres innervating the receptors. This lowering seems insufficient to modify the intensity of the Breuer-Hering reflex. (Author's abstract translated by MFW/SCD)

1127.
LEITNER, L.-M., M. Roumy and P. Remy.
Role du reflexe de Breuer-Hering dans la regulation du regime respiratoire du lapin et du chat anesthesies au cours de l'hypercapnie hyperoxique progressive.
[Role of the Breuer-Hering reflex in the regulation of respiration in the anesthetized rabbit and cat during progressive hyperoxic hypercapnia].
C.R. Acad. Sci. (D) (Paris) 276:2701-2704;May 9, 1973.

The Breuer-Hering reflex has an important role in the respiratory function of the anesthetized rabbit and cat submitted, under hyperoxia, to progressively increasing hypercapnia. This role is much more important in the rabbit than in the cat. In animals that have been bilaterally vagotomized, other reflex mechanisms must intervene at more elevated thresholds in order to maintain respiratory function. (Authors' abstract translated by MFW/SCD)

1128.
LEMAIRE, C. and H. Monod.
Capacite de travail statique et electromyographie en hyperbarie et hyperoxie.
[Static work capacity and electromyography in a hyperbaric environment and in hyperoxia].
Bull. Medsubhyp 8:22-25;Nov. 1972.
(Also published in Maroc Med. 568:306-308;May 1973)

The authors chose to test the fatigability of muscles used in static rather than dynamic work in a hyperbaric environment. Static work is defined as that which calls into play a small number of muscles which require a low expenditure of energy. Thus, the findings are not confused by the hampering effects of respiratory limitations and possible joint pain that might accompany dynamic work. The tests consisted of holding various weights, with the forearm extended perpendicular to the upper arm, for as long as possible, with five to eight minute rests between each test. Electromyographs of the brachial biceps were recorded. As a result of these tests, the authors conclude that work capacity of the muscle is retained at 300 meters, in a hyperbaric chamber. However, work capacity in water will be diminished by the resistance of the liquid medium, which absorbs some of the strength. (MFW/BSCP)

1129.
LEMAIRE, C., J.C. Rostain and M. Bergonzi.
Frequences cardiaques au repos et pendant le travail musculaire au cours d'une saturation a 500 metres (50.68 ata) en hyperoxie moderee (Sagittaire II).
[Heart rate at rest and exercise during a saturation dive at 500 meters (50.68 ATA) in moderate hyperoxia (Sagittaire II)].
Bull. Medsubhyp 9:7-12;Mar. 1973.

Heart rate was recorded at rest every four hours on the two divers of "Sagittaire II". It shows a moderate increase during compression and stay at 500 metres. A relative increase during static and dynamic work is noted. It is greater for one of the two subjects and may be related to a higher fatigability than at surface level. Roles of helium and pressure are discussed. (English summary)

1130.
LeMAIRE, C., Mond and J.C. Rostain.
Frequence cardiaque en hyperbarie (51 et 62 ATA).
[Heart rate in a hyperbaric environment (51 and 62 ATA)].
In: Hesser, C.M. and D. Linnarsson, eds. Proceedings of the first annual scientific meeting of the European Undersea Biomedical Society, Stockholm, 13-15 June 1973. Forsvarsmedicin 9:346-351;July 1973.

During the whole of two very deep dry chamber dives (to 500 and 610 metre) under oxy-helium mixture (.4 ATA PIO_2), measurements at rest were obtained every four hours during the day and every hour during sleep. Exercise was performed by the two humans every day and heart rate was then continuously monitored. Results show an increase of rate at rest around 350 metres reaching higher values than the control ones (obtained during predive at 10 metres.) During decompression, a slow decrease is noted for all the subjects. During static exercise, the known increase is observed, and is independent of depth and stay at depth. During muscular work on bicycle ergometer at 140 and 100 Watts, heart rate is slower than at the surface level even at 565 metres, and cardiac cost is unchanged. Oxygen, pressure, temperature and inert gases combine to explain bradycardia at depth. The variations observed may be related to the increased pressure or to a specific effect of helium. (From authors' abstract)

1131.
LEMAIRE, C.
Excitabilite de la fibre nerveuse en hyperbarie.
[Excitability of nerve fibre in hyperbaric environment].
Marseille, France, Univ. Provence, Cent. St-Jerome, and COMEX, 20p. Sept. 1973.

The possible activation of single motor axons with threshold stimuli applied to the median nerve at the elbow has been described by Bergmans (1970). With electromyographic recordings from the thenar eminence, it is possible to follow the recovery of the excitability of the nerve fibre in response to supraliminal stimulation. The recovery of the excitability was studied with three subjects, first at the laboratory of Faculte des Sciences St-Jerome (I ATA air), then in hyperbaric oxy-helium atmosphere at 1.8 ATA and 31 ATA during a saturation dive carried out at the Hyperbaric Research Centre of COMEX. The recovery of the excitability was not modified during our whole experiment. Neither helium, high pressure, nor stay at great depths had effects on excitability. The muscular responses were not modified. So we can conclude that nerve and muscle fibres were not altered, neither in excitability nor in conduction velocity. This means that ion-permeability of the membrane keeps in normal range during the whole saturation dive. (English abstract)

1132.
LENFANT, C.
NIH Program as to underwater problems.
In: United States-Japan conference on natural resources development. Proceedings of the first joint meeting of the U.S.-Japan panel on diving and technology, Tokyo, p.116-120. Japan, Ministry of Agriculture and Forestry, 1972.

The goals of this program are (1) to promote research in underwater physiology; (2) to focus particularly on human adaptation to immersion, and (3) to improve equipment and techniques. Specific areas that have been investigated so far include (1) cardiorespiratory response to immersion, (2) exercise capacity during immersion, (3) effect of breathing mixtures on cardiorespiratory function, and (4) behavioral and psychological factors. Liquid breathing has also been studied. Diving reflexes in marine mammals are the adaption of marine life to high hydrostatic pressure and to hypoxia have been studied. These programs are carried out both by large hyperbaric facilities, and under small research grants. (MFW/UMS)

1133.
LENNARD, D.E., A.J.H. Joseph and M.B.F. Ranken.
U.K. industry's research requirements in diving technology and underwater engineering.
London, CIRIA Underwater Engineering Group, 1971, 111p.

The authors describe over 70 research projects in this field, and classify them as long- or short-term and as top, intermediate or low priority. In the section on diving, some of the long-term projects mentioned are: improved diving capability (compilation of helium-oxygen decompression tables, physiological research, and development of saturation diving techniques) and research into aids to diver vision. Some of the short-term projects are improved semi-closed circuit breathing apparatus, suits, masks, communication systems, power tools, work techniques, and the developments of a new type of container for divers' breathing mixture called Vehicle Escape System Air (VESA). Of top priority are improved diving capability, communication systems, a manual on underwater work techniques, power tools, aids to diver vision and better underwater welding equipment. In the section on navigation, the theoretical study and development of hardware for submersibles and divers is considered long-term and of intermediate priority. (MFW/BSCP)

1134.
LENNOX, T.J. Jr., M.H. Peterson, J.A. Smith and R.E. Groover.
Marine corrosion studies: the effects of dissimilar metal couples and toxicants from antifouling paints on the corrosion of 5086 and 6061 aluminum alloys and their response to cathodic protection.
U.S. Nav. Res. Lab., Rep. NRL-MR-2444, 86p. May 1972.
(AD 746 099)

Aluminum alloy 5086-H32 when not coupled to dissimilar metals was observed to be corrosion resistant in seawater or in the Potomac River at Washington, D.C. Severe corrosion occurred in seawater however when coupled to any of the following dissimilar metals: copper nickel, 10%; yellow brass; 304 stainless steel; or mild steel. This galvanic corrosion could not be completely prevented by cathodic protection. A magnesium anode also caused severe corrosion of the aluminum in sea water. Aluminum alloy 6061-T6 was severely corroded when continuously immersed in quiescent seawater or in the Potomac River. In seawater corrosion caused by the cuprous oxide toxicant was not as severe as that observed on uncoated and unprotected 6061-T6 aluminum, but in the Potomac River the depth of corrosion was significantly increased by the cuprous oxide antifouling coating. (Authors) (GRA)

1135.
LEONARD, R.G. and P.G. Morken.
Development of end-closure systems for undersea concrete pressure resistant cylindrical hulls. San Francisco, Cal., Bechtel Corp., Rep. NCEL-CR-72.017, 119p. May 1972. (AD 747 217)

The purpose of this study was to develop end-closure systems for undersea concrete pressure resistant hulls. These end-closures must seal and lock concrete cylinders ranging from 20 to 60 feet in diameter. They must be removable permitting full access when the cylinders are located on the ocean floor in 1000 feet of water and when the cylinders are located on land. The study considers end-closure configuration including geometry and material, actuation or handling methods and sealing and locking alternates. Areas requiring additional research and development are identified. (Authors) (GRA)

1136.
LEONG, J.K.L., W.W. Schultz, E. Zebovitz and N.A. Schlamm.
System for studying uninfected and virus-infected cell cultures in hyperbaric chambers. Appl. Microbiol. 26:258-263;Sept. 1973.

Equipment and techniques previously used to investigate the effect of hyperbaric gases on bacteria were modified to permit comparable investigations with uninfected and virus-infected tissue cell cultures. This report describes the modified equipment and related methodology. Use of the system is illustrated with findings on the effect of oxygen-helium mixtures at 68 atm on cell physiology and virus growth in two cell types. Our results suggested that, under those experimental conditions, several synthetic processes in chick fibroblast monolayers are inhibited but that Sindbis virus growth in the cells is increased. Growth of Japanese encephalitis virus in procine kidney cells was found to be unaffected by oxygen-helium gas at partial pressures of oxygen between 0 and 700 mm Hg, but morphological alterations in the cells occurred at low and high pO_2 levels. (Authors' abstract)

1137.
LEONOV, A.N. and V.A. Barsukov.
Nekotorye osobennosti metabolizma v miokarde pri ostrom defitsite krovi v usloviyakh giperbaricheskoi oksigenatsii.
[Some characteristics of metabolism in the myocardium during acute blood deficit under conditions of hyperbaric oxygenation].
Kardiologiya 11(5):140-142; 1971.

Hyperbaric oxygenation of white rats at 2 atm for 40 min prevented suppression of cell respiration, increased the number of SH-groups and decreased the free radical content observed in the myocardium in the moribund state. A moribund condition did not develop in the majority of rats after bloodletting and hyperbaric oxygenation, although the degree and duration of the posthemorrhagic anemization was the same as that in untreated animals. (NLG) (© BA)

1138.
LePAGE, A. and P. Wide.
Deep diving from a dynamically positioned drill ship.
In: 1973 Offshore Technology Conference, April/May 1973, Houston, Texas. Preprints, Vol. I, p.528-531. Published by the conference.

The use of dynamic positioning of the drill ships raises the demands on diving systems on board. Such problems as increasing diving depths are, to a great extent, already solved or are on the verge of being solved from the physiological point of view. The 1972, 2001-ft dive at the hyperbaric facility of COMEX, Marseille, shows the human capacity. From the technical point of view, however, the dynamic positioning leads to problems until now unknown in the use of deep diving systems such as guiding and positioning the bell between the surface and the work site, handling without guidelines, supply of gas and power, safety aspects, etc. Principally and practically, these problems have been solved and the first diving systems are already working from dynamically positioned drill ships, such as the Pelican from which in Dec. 1972, about 50 dives had been carried out. . . The experiences of the first diving systems aboard dynamically positioned vessels show that a conventional diving bell connected to the surface vessel by a heavy umbilical cable is not the ultimate system since it does not take full advantage of the freedom in positioning that the surface vessel gives. Probably the future solution will be a small submarine with diver lock-out capability, connected to the surface vessel only by a small, high voltage power cable. The submarine could be connected to the decompression chambers to permit long saturation dives necessary for very deep diving operations. In fact, a submarine of this type has already been built and has operated for one year. It is the Comex Marco submarine.It is a small submarine of seven tons displacement, capable of carrying three divers with lockout capacity down to 200 m and a maximum working and observation depth of 300 m. [What is termed "a diving bell" is apparently a personnel transfer capsule]. (Authors)

1139.
LESCURE, R.
Bibliographie medicale de la plongee et de l'hyperbarie. Volume VII.
[Medical bibliography on diving and the hyperbaric environment. Volume VII].
Marseille, France, Societe Francaise de Medicine Subaquatique et Hyperbare, 1973.

The citations listed in this bibliography are divided into six categories: (1) Respiration, breathing gas, and energy metabolism; (2) Pressure and decompression; (3) Diving, sport medicine and diving, swimming, pools; (4) Drowning and resuscitation; (5) Naval, aeronautic, and space medicine; (6) Marine biology, oceanography, fish, and shellfish. The material is drawn chiefly from the period 1970-1972. Many of the references have a general application and are only peripherally concerned with underwater physiology or the hyperbaric environment. The volume lists members of the Society, lists other similar societies throughout the world, as well as doctors throughout the world that are engaged in underwater research. (MFW/UMS)

1140.
LESSTER, L.E. and J.C. Fye.
Electrical integrity on DEEPSTAR 20,000.
IEEE international conference on engineering in the ocean environment, Panama City, Florida, September 1970. Digest of technical papers, p.193-195. Published by the conference.

DEEPSTAR 20,000 is a battery powered submersible vehicle with 20,000 ft depth and 16 hr dive endurance capability. This paper describes briefly the overall electrical system of the DEEPSTAR 20,000 as background, and shows some of the steps taken to ensure safe operation particularly in the area of insulation. (Eng. Index)

1141.
LETICH, M.J.
New priorities in ocean engineering.
In: Marine industries: problems and opportunities. Proceedings of the ninth annual conference of the Marine Technology Society, p.491-497. Washington, D.C., Marine Technology Society, 1973.

This paper deals chiefly with the engineering problems of designing large tankers and barges. A final section entitled "Underwater ocean engineering structures" mentions the "Guide for the classification of underwater vessels and related systems," which will include new sections on the following: (1) Lock-in lock-out submersibles; (2) Tethered submersibles; (3) Submersible vehicles; (4) Small submarines; (5) Stationary underwater vessels; (6) Support ships; (7) Diving systems; (8) Launch and recovery gear; (9) Equipment including requirements on anchors and chains, lines and umbilical cords. It is a revised version of the "Guide for the classification of manned submersibles," published by the American Bureau of Shipping. The submersible VOL 1 is described. It is a 32-foot lock-out submersible that is carried aboard a surface ship. The submersible mates to a decompression system aboard the surface ship, then takes on new divers and resubmerges. The sub can operate at 1200 ft. carry a payload of 2,000 lbs, and travel at 5 knots. The Lockheed one-atmosphere work capsule which can be attached over a wellhead is also briefly described. (MFW/UMS)

1142.
LEUENBERGER, P., U. Karmann and D.R. Held.
Does chronic hypercapnia entail an adaptive improvement of extra-cellular space buffering against acute PCO_2 changes?
Eur. J. Clin. Invest. 3:295-298; 1973.

Schwartz and coworkers have shown recently that chronic hypercapnia entails a marked decrease of the $d(H+)/dPCO_2$ ratio plasma, in response to acute PCO_2 changes in vivo. They have interpreted this finding as an indication of improved CO_2 buffering performance by the extracellular space, mediated by an unidentified mechanism. This hypothesis is reviewed in the light of a theoretical treatment of CO_2-titration regarding extracellular space as an isolated buffered solution. — It is concluded here that renal compensation during chronic hypercapnia without changes in the buffering properties can account for much if not all of the observed effect through the quantitative relationships governing CO_2 equilibrium. Reasons for the use of Van Slyke's "buffer value" rather than the $d(H+)/dPCO_2$ ratio as an analytical parameter of extracellular CO_2-buffering performance are presented by reference to the general theory of titration. (Authors' abstract)

1143.
LEVISON, H. and R.M. Cherniak.
Interdependence between mechanical resistances to breathing and the ventilatory response to hypercapnia and hypoxia.
Clin. Res. 19:803; 1971.

Abstract only. Entire item quoted: Mechanical factors may play a major role in limiting the ventilatory response to inhaled carbon dioxide. It has been suggested that when the work of breathing is increased in normal subjects, they tolerate hypercapnia rather than expend the effort required to increase the ventilation and keep the arterial carbon dioxide tension at a normal level. To determine whether this situation is also applicable to hypoxic conditions we studied the effects of added work on the ventilatory response to hypoxia and compared them to the effects of added work on the ventilatory response to carbon dioxide. The ventilatory response to hypercapnia was lowered by increased work of breathing due to high non-elastic resistance but not by an increase due to high elastic resistance. In contrast, the ventilatory response to hypoxia was not influenced by an increased work of breathing due to either high elastic or non-elastic resistance. The data suggest that when the work required to overcome non-elastic resistance is increased, the body may tolerate hypercapnia rather than work harder, but would rather work harder than tolerate more hypoxia.

1144.
LEVITT, M.D. and D.G. Levitt.
Use of inert gases to study the interaction of blood flow and diffusion during passive absorption from the gastrointestinal tract of the rat.
J. Clin. Invest. 52:1852-1862;Aug. 1973.

Measurement of the relative absorption rates of inert gases (H_2, He, CH_4, SF_6, and ^{133}Xe) was used to investigate the interaction between diffusion and blood flow during passive absorption from the stomach, small bowel, and colon of the rat. If uptake is blood flow limited, the gases should be absorbed in proportion to their solubilities in blood, but if diffusion limited, uptake should be proportional to the diffusion rate of the gases in mucosal tissues. The observed absorption data were fitted to a series of models of interaction between perfusion and diffusion. A simple model accurately predicted the absorption rates of the gases from all segments of the bowel. In this model, gas is absorbed into two distinct blood flows: one which flows in proximity to the lumen and completely equilibrates with the lumen, and a second which is sufficiently rapid and distant from the lumen that its gas uptake is entirely diffusion limited. The fraction of the total absorption attributable to the equilibrating flow can be readily calculated and equalled 93%, 77%, and 33% for the small bowel, colon, and stomach, respectively. Thus, the rate of passive absorption of gases from the small bowel is limited almost entirely by the blood flow to the mucosa, and absorption from the stomach is largely limited by the diffusion rate of the gases. The flow which equilibrates with the lumen can be quantitated, and this flow may provide a useful measure of "effective" mucosal blood flow. (Authors' abstract)

1145.
LEWIS, J.W.
Design of a controlled depth, submerged barge and tug system for Arctic marine transportation.
In: 1973 Offshore Technology Conference, April/May 1973, Houston, Texas. Preprints, Vol. I, p.743-756. Published by the conference.

This paper describes the feasibility design of an Arctic marine, crude oil transportation system. The system consists of a depth controlled, submerged barge towed by a powerful, surface ice-breaking tug. The design of the tug, barge, towing system, and control systems are described. Because the cargo is carried below the icewater surface, the system is capable of achieving advance speeds through a given ice field which are greater than an equivalently powered conventional surface system. This feature when combined with total system costs, can give the system an economically competitive edge over alternative marine systems. The paper concludes that the system is technically feasible and that with a suitable development program, an operational system could be realized with present day technology. (Author's abstract)

1146.
LEWIS, W.F., R.J. Lee and B.M. Hoffert.
The quality of breathable air utilized by Canadian Forces scuba clubs.
In: Battelle Columbus Laboratories. Proceedings, 1973 divers' gas purity symposium, November 27-28, 1973, p.XVII-1-XVII-8. U.S. Navy Supervisor Diving, Nav. Ships Syst. Comm., Rep 2-73, 1973.

The quality of breathable air utilized by Canadian Forces' SCUBA clubs was investigated. Samples of compressed air were collected from each of twenty-two clubs and analyzed for oxygen, moisture and trace contaminants using standard Defence and Civil Institute of Environmental Medicine's analytical techniques. Results were compared to the limits specified in Canadian Forces Regulations. One sample contained a dangerous amount of carbon monoxide. All but two samples showed excessive amounts of water vapour. A regular quality assurance programme to monitor and regulate gas purity was recommended. (Authors' abstract)

1147.
L'HUILLIER, J.R., C. Jacquemin and P. Varene.
La dissipation de chaleur par convection respiratoire en plongee.
[Heat loss due to respiratory convection in diving].
In: Fructus, X., ed. Third international conference on hyperbaric and underwater physiology, p.137-144. Paris, Doin, 1972.

The factors governing thermal exchange in the respiratory tract are discussed, and mathematical models of these phenomena are proposed. In addition to the ambient atmospheric temperature, atmospheric pressure and composition and ventilatory volumes play a role in determining respiratory heat loss. (MEMH/UMS)

1148.
LIBERATORE, G.L., E.J. Dyckman, J.A. Montemarano and M.L. Cohn.
Antislime coatings. Part II. Preconditioning value of slime for barnacle attachment.
Nav. Ship. Res. Devel. Cent., Rep. NSRDC-28-233, NSRDC-3597, 28p. Aug. 1972.
(AD 750 122)

Investigations of the relationship between barnacle attachment and the presence of a primary slime film on submerged surfaces has been completed. Using laboratory-reared barnacle cyprids in a statistical settlement survey, it has been determined that the number of barnacle cyprids settling on a slimed surface consistently exceeds by a factor of ten the number that settle on a cleaned control surface. Data describing the slime factor as a naturally occurring surface-preconditioning agent affecting the settlement of other sessile organisms are evaluated. (Author) (GRA)

1149.
LIESE, W., R. Schibli, H. Gehring and A.A. Buhlmann.
Decompression after air dives in mountain lakes.
Abstract submitted to first annual scientific meeting of the European Undersea Biomedical Society, Stockholm, 13-15 June 1973. (Paper not published).

Abstract only. It is stated that the major factor in decompression sickness is the ratio of nitrogen pressure in the tissue to ambient pressure. Therefore, for the same depth and duration at a lower ambient pressure, i.e., at high altitude, longer decompression times are necessary. One hundred and six chamber dives, and 108 actual dives, were made under conditions of simulated altitude of 3000 meters and real altitude of 1250 meters respectively. Decompression was calculated by the usual method, but allowing for lower surface pressure, without altering the nitrogen half-time spectrum of 5-640 minutes nor the oversaturation factors. Both the real and simulated dives in these experiments can be classified as repetitive dives. These experiments, which were carried out without decompression sickness symptoms, form the basis for decompression tables for diving at altitude, including rules for repetitive dives. (MFW/UMS)

1150.
LIFFICK, G.L. and S.A. Black.
Power sources for underwater hydraulic tools.
In: The working diver, 1972. Symposium proceedings, February 1972, Columbus, Ohio. p.215-238. Washington, D.C., Marine Technology Society, 1972.

The Naval Civil Engineering Laboratory is developing hydraulic power sources for underwater hydraulic tools. Diesel-hydraulic and electro-hydraulic power sources have been successfully developed and evaluated. The operational testing was conducted with divers utilizing hydraulic tools to work underwater. The criteria for selecting a particular hydraulic circuit and the components for an underwater hydraulic power source are different from those used for designing a surface hydraulic power source. For example, a hydraulic pump's tolerance for salt water and reliability are generally more important than the pump's volumetric efficiency. Pressure and flow gages must be able to withstand severe mechanical vibration, hydraulic fluid shock, and salt spray corrosion. Hydraulic hose expansion under pressure must be minimized but not at the expense of excessive weight. Hydraulic hose couplings should be easy to couple and uncouple but should not separate when dragged over the side of a boat. Hydraulic fluid must provide adequate lubricity, have a low viscosity in cold water. Appraisal of the relative merits of different hydraulic circuits and components is based on experience gained during NCEL's power source evaluation program. Final component selection, however, is dependent on the user's particular requirements. (Authors' abstract)

1151.
LIFFICK, G.L. and F.B. Barrett.
Hydraulic tools and equipment for underwater salvage.
U.S. Nav. Civil Eng. Lab., Rep. NCEL-TN-1229, 38p. July 1972.
(AD 748 585)

Commercially available hydraulic pumps, rigging, load handling and cutting equipment have been evaluated to determine characteristic diver performance and mechanical suitability for underwater operation. Manually operated hydraulic pumps were modified and pumped against a load cell to determine reasonable levels of diver exertion. Tests have shown that divers can be utilized as prime movers for small jobs and that some conventional surface hydraulic equipment can be used underwater for reasonable periods of time with a minimum of additional maintenance. Surface hydraulic equipment suitable for underwater operation includes manual pumps, rams, cylinders and several cutters. (Authors) (GRA)

1152.
LIGHTFOOT, N.F.
Chronic carbon monoxide exposure.
Proc. Roy. Soc. Med. 65:798-799;Sept. 1972.

In submarines, carbon monoxide is introduced primarily by smoking. Improvements in carbon monoxide removal techniques have reduced the levels to 25 parts/10^6 and even down to 8-10 parts/10^6. The relationship between ambient carbon monoxide and carboxyhemoglobin levels (in non-smokers) can be expressed by the following equation: COHb % = 0.16 x ambient CO parts/10^6. The current permissible carbon monoxide level is 25 parts/10^6, which can result in a 5% carboxyhemoglobin level in non-smokers. Some detrimental effects have been reported at this level. At the level of 8-10 parts/10^6, the carboxyhemoglobin level in non-smokers is only 1.6%, which is well within the safety limits. The level in smokers can go up to 18% in the case of heavy smokers. (MFW/BSCP)

1153.
LILJA, B.
Regional lung function and central hemodynamics during hypoxia, hyperoxia, and breath-holding.
Scand. J. Clin. Lab. Invest. 30(1):11-15; 1972.

In thirteen healthy men, pulmonary blood flow distribution (PBFD) pulmonary artery pressure (PAP) and cardiac output ($\dot{Q}$) were measured during 10% and 100% O_2 breathing and after maximal breath-holding preceded by breathing air and 100% O_2. The PAP and $\dot{Q}$ increased and the PBFD became more even during 10% O_2 breathing and after maximal breath-holding during air breathing. There were no significant changes in the $\dot{Q}$ and PBFD during 100% O_2 breathing nor after prolonged breath-holding during 100% O_2. During the latter experiment PAP increased somewhat. (© BA)

1154.
LIN, Y.C.
Autonomic nervous control on the cardiovascular responses of unanesthetized rat during diving.
Fed. Proc. 31:368;Mar./Apr. 1972.

Abstract only. Entire item quoted: The diving effect was produced by submerging the head of unanesthetized rats confined in a wire mesh cone for 15 sec. The relative importance of the autonomic nervous controls on the cardiovascular system was studied by means of differential blockades of autonomic nervous activity. The responses to diving (mean ± SE, 6 rats/group) of heart rate (A, bpm) and mean arterial blood pressure (B, mm Hg) were summarized as follows:

	Control (Saline)	Atropine (1 mg/Kg)	Propranolol (8 mg/Kg)	Reserpine (5 mg/Kg)
A. Predive	399 ± 12	464 ± 8	297 ± 9	209 ± 11
Dive	143 ± 6	418 ± 17	133 ± 23	103 ± 8
B. Predive	118 ± 2	123 ± 2	140 ± 11	105 ± 5
Dive	136 ± 5	168 ± 3	169 ± 11	77 ± 4

It is calculated, according to Walsh (Amer. J. Physiol. 217:1139, 1969) from the above results that vagal tone increased 326% while sympathetic tone decreased 45% during diving from predive values. Catecholamine depletion eliminated vasoconstrictor responses during diving, while bradycardia was present. Since β adrenergic receptor blockade did not affect vasoconstrictor responses, it is concluded that α adrenergic receptors and neurotransmitter availability are responsible for hypertension during diving. Increased vagal tone and decreased sympathetic tone are responsible for diving bradycardia.

1155.
LIN, Y.C.
Depression effect of respiring helium-oxygen (80-20%) on the heart rate in the unanesthetized male normotensive and spontaneously hypertensive rats.
Physiologist 16:377;Aug. 1973.

Abstract only. Entire item quoted: Until recently, He gas has been considered devoid of cardiovascular actions. However, over the past 3 years, there have been reports that breathing He-O_2 mixture induces a protection against the arrhythmic effect of coronary ligation in dogs. It is of interest to see whether He affects the heart rate in the intact animal. The comparison of the heart rates under the two breathing gas mixtures was based on iso-aerobic requirements. The oxygen consumption ($\dot{V}O_2$) was varied by altering the ambient temperature (T_a), and was measured with a ventilated chamber and an oxygen analyzer. The T_a was varied from 10-35°C and 25-35°C for breathing air and He, respectively. The heart rate was obtained by direct wiring through an air-tight entry port to the animal chamber which was submerged in water for temperature control. The results are summarized in the following table, where X is $\dot{V}O_2$ in ml/min/kg, and Y is heart rate in beat/min:

	Normotensive (Sprague-Dawley)	Hypertensive (Okamoto)
air	Y = 5.4X + 191 (n=40, r=.6304)	Y = 3.8X + 210 (n=26, r=.7558)
He-O_2	Y = 5.0X + 161 (n=16, r=.7537)	Y = 3.4X + 115 (n=22, r=.6331)

The heart rate was lower in the rats breathing He than rats breathing air at all $\dot{V}O_2$ as indicated by similar regression coefficients with distinct intercepts. The effect of He breathing was similar in both normotensive and hypertensive rats. However, the sensitivity of the heart rate changes in response to the changes in $\dot{V}O_2$ was lower in the spontaneously hypertensive rats than that of the normotensive rats as indicated by lesser slopes of the regression lines.

1156.
LINDEROTH, L.S., Jr.
Duke University's hyperbaric chamber.
In: Professional diving symposium, New Orleans, Nov. 1972. Mar. Technol. Soc. J. 7:53-57; Mar./Apr. 1973.

The paper describes the facilities of the F.G. Hall Laboratory for Environmental Research and the pertinent instrumentation and medical facilities to support research projects in simulated diving environments to depths up to 1000 feet for human subjects and deeper for animal experiments. It continues with illustrations and descriptions of three important deep dive projects; a 1000-foot dive, made in December 1968, to study the capability of a diver to do useful work at this depth and the physiological behavior of his body functions; a 600-foot dive to study the effect on the diver of working in cold water; and a 300-foot dive to study the effect of gas density on the respiratory functions of the diver. The paper also describes some animal experiments on rapid decompression schedules. In conclusion a brief review of comparable European research centers is given. (Author's abstract)

1157.
LINDQVIST, J.
Present and future work in underwater communications at the speech transmission laboratory in Stockholm.
In: Sergeant, R.L. and T. Murry, eds. Processing helium speech: proceedings of a Navy-sponsored workshop, August 1971, U.S. Nav. Submar. Med. Res. Lab., Rep. NSMRL 708, p.22-25. May 22, 1972.

The author discusses the effect of pressure on speech, and gives a diagram showing formant frequency as a function of the air pressure. He then describes investigations carried out in the Swedish Navy's pressure tank in Stockholm, regarding the effects of helium; these are the increase of the velocity of sound and the shifting upward of the resonant frequencies of the vocal tract. Pressure and helium distortions can be corrected by an unscrambler. Distortions caused by breathing mask can only be minimized by the use of a microphone which has a frequency response at least up to 8 kHz. A piezoelectric microphone which could be used either as a contact microphone or in the mask was developed by the author and his colleagues. For helium speech correction, a frequency correction with +12dB/oct up to %kHz, and +6dB/oct up to 8kHz will give the best result. (MFW/BSCP)

1158.
LINN, W.S. and J.D. Hackney.
Nitrogen and helium "closing volumes": simultaneous measurement and reproducibility.
J. Appl. Physiol. 34:396-399;Mar. 1973.

A system has been developed for measuring "closing volumes" simultaneously by the nitrogen-dilution technique and by a modification of the inert-bolus-distribution method using a bolus of helium and a critical-orifice analyzer. Nine subjects, seated erect, were tested repeatedly with this equipment in an investigation of variability and possible errors in the measurement. Measured "closing volumes" in normal non-smokers were highly reproducible (standard deviations less than two percent of vital capacity), were similar when measured simultaneously by nitrogen and helium inspiration, and were comparable to published normal values. Variability was greater in smokers and exsmokers. Variations with time (period of hours or days), volume history, recent smoking, different observers, and variations in the test procedure were investigated. None of these variables was found to have any significant effect on measured "closing volume." (Authors' abstract)

1159.
LIPTON, B., A. Toth and J.H. Jacobson II.
The hyperbaric chamber and pulmonary oxygen toxicity: A clinical and pathologic study.
Mt. Sinai J. Med. 40:7-19;Jan./Feb. 1973.

This study is a retrospective survey of patients sent to the hyperbaric chamber of the Mount Sinai Hospital, New York City, in severe respiratory failure. Of thirty patients only eight survived, five probably because of the use of intermittent hyperbaroxia. One patient was treated by means of extracorporeal oxygenation with a membrane oxygenator for 36 hours. Postmortem examination of his lungs indicated that oxygen toxicity had already progressed to the irreversible proliferative phase. Thirteen postmortem examinations in patients who had had prolonged oxygen therapy revealed toxic pulmonary lesions described as exudative, intermediate and proliferative. The use of corticosteroids may prevent the development of the proliferative phase. The etiology and prevention of pulmonary oxygen toxicity is discussed. Extracorporeal blood oxygenation by means of venovenous bypass and a disposable membrane oxygenator may be used to treat acute respiratory failure in patients where there is insufficient functioning lung tissue to support life or where pulmonary oxygen toxicity has been superimposed on the original disease process. (Authors' summary)

1160.
LONDON, A.J.
FMEA. Reliability tool and management aid on scuba.
In: IEEE international conference on engineering in the ocean environment, Panama City, Florida, September 1970. Digest of technical papers, p.198-199. Published by the conference.

Failure modes and effects analysis (FMEA) is used for evaluating the reliability and safety aspects of a life support system. (Eng. Ind.)

1161.
LONES, J.J. and J.D. Stachiw.
Deep submergence windows for optical systems.
In: Duntley, S.Q., J.J. Lones and H.S. Weisbrod, eds. Proceedings of the society of photo optical instrumentation engineers. Underwater photo optical instrumentation applications, March 1971, Honolulu, p.77-83, Published by the Society, 1972.

Spherical shell sector windows have been found to have a higher structural efficiency under hydrostatic loading than conical frustums of same thickness to diameter ratio. Although acrylic plastic windows of spherical shell sector shape have been found to be ideal for panoramic windows in continental shelf depths, glass or glass ceramic will have to be utilized for abyssal depths. Some exploratory tests with glass windows of spherical shell sector shape have shown considerable promise for such application. (Authors' abstract).

1162.
LONG, R.W. and N.E. Smith.
Hot water: an economical approach to increased diver performance and safety in the offshore oil industry.
In: 1972 Offshore Technology Conference, May 1-3, Houston, Texas. Preprints. Vol. I, p.521-532. Published by the conference. 1972.

Since the beginning of diving, cold has been one of the limiting factors to man's performance in the sea. An economical approach to solving this problem was introduced utilizing hot water to replace the heat normally lost by the diver to the cold water. Since its introduction in 1965, several improvements have been made to insure efficient diver performance in the offshore oil industry. This system has supported divers in the open sea for periods in excess of eight hours, and in depths down to 850 feet. This approach increases the diver's performance when properly applied and makes an everyday reality of what was once considered technically and economically impossible. [The use of hot water in heating suits, bells, chambers and breathing gas is discussed]. (Authors' abstract)

1163.
LONG, R.W.
Hot water diving — state of the art.
In: The working diver, 1972. Symposium proceedings, Feb. 1972, Columbus, Ohio, p.239-250. Washington, D.C., Marine Technology Society, 1972.

The use of hot water as a heat transfer vehicle has experienced an ever widening acceptance for heating other equipment and facilities as well as divers. Presented here is a brief on hot water theory; a description of present day equipment being used in the field is discussed, both military and civilian. Various types of power sources are discussed. Both closed loop and open circuit systems are presented together with combinations utilizing both approaches. Methods of utilizing the approach for bell chamber heating and facilities are reviewed. Formats are presented for the engineer to establish his needs and analyze trade-off to assist him in making his equipment selections. Hot water has proven itself to be a safe, highly reliable and economical approach to solving some of the problems experienced when diving in extreme and arduous conditions. (Author's abstract)

1164.
LOOMIS, J.L., W.C. Nicholas, L. Barlett, P. Carroll and E.R. Buskirk.
Flow control valve for expired gas collection from scuba-equipped swimmers.
J. Appl. Physiol. 32:869-871;June 1972.

Measurement of pulmonary ventilation and oxygen consumption of scuba-equipped swimmers by continuous collection of discrete expired air samples above the water surface has proved to be impossible with existing equipment. Scuba regulators are actuated by the pressure difference from within the breathing hose to that of the surrounding water. If a swimmer's exhalation hose is vented to the water surface the scuba regulator will "free flow" continuously. A flow control valve was developed which prevented free flow and facilitated the necessary measurements. Comparative ventilation and oxygen consumption measurements were first made while the subjects worked on a bicycle ergometer. It was found that the flow control valve, if used with a Collins triple-J valve, and a double-hose scuba regulator, yielded essentially the same pulmonary ventilation and oxygen consumption as was conventionally measured during high work loads with a Collins triple-J valve and mouthpiece. Successful collections of expired air were also made during underwater swimming at high work loads. Ventilation and oxygen consumptions were lower during fin-kicking in water as compared with riding a bicycle at equivalent relative work loads. Development of the flow control valve should facilitate studies of mobile scuba-equipped swimmers at heavy work loads in which an assessment of ventilation and energy expenditure is required. (Authors' abstract)

1165.
LUNDGREN, C.E.G. and H.C. Ornhagen.
Oxygen consumption in liquid breathing mice.
Aerosp. Med. 43:831-835;Aug. 1972.

Oxygen consumption was measured in mice spontaneously breathing fluorocarbon liquid oxygenated at different pressures. Body temperature was varied from 16°C and upwards and oxygenation pressures ranged from 1.0 atm to 7.8 atm. Intraperitoneal buffer (THAM) injections did not appreciably influence survival time which was usually too short for oxygen consumption measurements at temperatures above 34°C. It was found that up to a body temperature of about 22°C the oxygen uptake was not influenced by the oxygenation pressure. Above this temperature the oxygen pressure had to be increased to yield a maximal oxygen uptake about 3.5 atm of oxygen pressure apparently being adequate at all body temperature levels. Oxygen uptake increased with body temperature in a seemingly curvilinear fashion reaching (by extrapolation) about 2.8 ml O_2 x g^{-1} x h^{-1} at 37°C as compared to 1.6 ml O_2 x 6^{-1} x h^{-1} in oxygen breathing Nembutal anesthetized mice. The difference was presumably to a great extent due to the heavier work of breathing imposed on the liquid breathing animals. (Authors' abstract)

1166.
LUNDGREN, C.E.G.
On alternobaric vertigo: epidemiologic aspects.
In: Hesser, C.M. and D. Linnarsson, eds. Proceedings of the first annual scientific meeting of the European Undersea Biomedical Society, Stockholm, 13-15 June 1973. Forsvarsmedicin 9:406-409;July 1973.

Alternobaric Vertigo (AV) has been recognized as a reaction to inadequate pressure equilibration in the middle ear in connection with changes in environmental pressure. It can occur in divers, caisson workers and fliers who are exposed to such pressure changes, but it may also be provoked in some individuals by auto-inflation of the middle ear. In both diving and flying AV occurs most frequently in connection with ascent, and it appears to be related to overpressure in the middle ear. (Author)

1167.
LUNDSGAARD, J. and H. Degn.
Digital regulation of gas flow rates and composition of gas mixtures.
IEEE Trans. Biomed. Eng. 20:384-387;Sept. 1973.

A digital principle is described which permits a linear regulation of gas flow rate. The regulator unit consists of a set of on-off valves connected to parallel flow resistors. The conductivities of the resistors are 1,2,4,8...,n and combinations of the resistors give the flow rates 1,2,3,4...,2^n-1. Thus a stepwise regulation with a unit step of less than 1 percent of the maximal flow rate can be obtained by a set of 7 valves and resistors. By using two-way valves and complementing with a second gas, binary mixtures of controlled composition (molar fraction) are produced. An apparatus is described which utilizes the above principle for mixing oxygen and nitrogen. The flow resistors are made of plastic tubing, and magnetic valves are used to permit electric control. The limitations of the applicability of tubular resistors due to nonlinear phenomena are discussed. (Authors' abstract)

1168.
LURIA, S.M.
Effect of limited peripheral cues on stereoacuity.
Psychon. Sci. 24:195-196; 1971.

The purpose of this experiment was to learn whether the introduction of peripheral stimuli into a "Ganzfeld" situation will improve stereoacuity. The "Ganzfeld" situation is defined as "an attempt to produce a featureless field of view around the test apparatus by having the observer look through a small circular aperture in a white hemisphere which afforded him a view only of a white screen with a rectangular window through which the [stereoacuity measuring apparatus] was visible." When magazine photographs were hung on the outer limits of the screen, thus introducing peripheral stimuli, stereoacuity was markedly improved. (MFW/BSCP)

1169.
LURIA, S.M.
Review of recent underwater and chamber research conducted in the vision branch.
In: Abstracts of BuMed-ONR sponsored Navywide research in high pressure biomedical research. U.S. Submarine Base, Groton, Conn., May 1971, p.54. Published by the Naval Submarine Medical Research Laboratories, 1971.

Abstract only. Entire item quoted: Vision underwater is affected by a wide variety of physical, physiological and psychological factors. Light waves, the physical basis of vision, are greatly and selectively attenuated by the watery environment, dispersed by suspended impurities, and refracted in passing from the water into air. Studies have been carried out of the effects of these phenomena (1) on the visibility of colors and paints underwater and the ability of divers to identify colors in various bodies of water; (2) on resolution and stereoscopic acuity and means of improving acuity in the water; (3) on the ability of divers to estimate both size and distance in water of varying turbidity. Attempts have also been made to specify the factors effecting perception of size and distance, and to devise procedures and training methods for improving such judgments; (4) a closely related problem is that of hand-eye coordination. This has been studied in the water, and various procedures for improving the speed of learning to coordinate hand-eye movements are being evaluated. In addition to these physical variables, which affect the stimulus for vision, there are a wide variety of factors under water which may affect the diver himself or his visual system. These include of course, the increased pressure and the unusual breathing mixtures. A recently completed study investigated the effect of various pressure-levels and susceptibility to nitrogen narcosis on visual evoked potentials and the perception of the staircase illusion. Finally, both confinement in sealed capsules and the necessity of breathing through a facemask raise questions of the effects of carbon monoxide and other atmospheric pollutants. A study has recently been completed testing the effects particularly of low levels of carbon monoxide on a wide variety of visual processes. These latter studies confirm the sensitivity of the visual system as an indicator of physiological stress.

1170.
LURIA, S.M. and J.A.S. Kinney.
Peripheral stimuli and stereoacuity under water.
Percept. Psychophysics 11:437-440; 1972.

A variety of attempts were made to improve stereoacuity under water by providing limited additional peripheral stimulation. It was concluded that acuity is most improved when the peripheral stimuli are at the same distance from the O as the target. As the peripheral stimuli are moved closer to the O than the target, their beneficial effects are decreased, and beyond a certain point, their presence degrades acuity. This effect seems to be enhanced by increasing turbidity of the water, which decreases the contrast of the distant target relative to that of the nearby peripheral stimuli. These and previous findings implicate several distinct processes in the degradation of stereoacuity in the water. (Authors' abstract)

1171.
LURIA, S.M.
Vision with chromatic filters.
Amer. J. Optom. 49(101):818-829; 1972.

Detection and resolution thresholds for blue and yellow targets against blue, green, and yellow backgrounds were measured while wearing yellow and blue filters. Yellow filters improved thresholds for yellow targets against blue backgrounds. Their effectiveness decreased (i) as the wavelength of the background increased, (ii) as the size of the target decreased, and (iii) with the age of the observer. The blue filters were generally ineffective. The results are for the most part explained on the basis of changes in target contrast brought about by the filters. The effectiveness of yellow facemasks for divers under certain conditions is discussed. (Author's abstract)

1172.
LURIA, S.M. and J.A.S. Kinney.
Accommodation and stereoacuity.
U.S. Nav. Submar. Med. Res. Lab., Rep. NSMRL 711, 12p. June 5, 1972.

[The problem was] to determine the causes of the marked decline in stereoacuity under water with a view toward remedial action. [It was found that] the major cause of the degradation of stereoacuity in water of even the greatest clarity is the increase in accommodation. This is brought about by two factors: (1) the production of a virtual image of the target at 3/4 its physical distance by the refraction of the light rays passing through the water-air interface of the face mask, and (2) the presence of higher contrast peripheral stimuli closer to the diver than the primary target. These results lead to the conclusion that at least part of the reduction in stereoacuity in the water can be reversed through the use of a face mask with compensating lenses which increase the apparent distance of the target. (Authors' summary)

1173.
LURIA, S.M., C.L. McKay and S.H. Ferris.
Handedness and adaptation to distortions of size and distance under water.
U.S. Nav. Submar. Med. Res. Lab., Rep. NSMRL 724, 12p. Aug. 28, 1972.
(Also published in J. Exp. Psychol. 100:263-269;Oct. 1973)

Both before and after 15 minutes of adaptation under water, 20 right-handed and 20 left-handed or ambidextrous subjects made size matches to standard rectangles and were tested for hand-eye coordination. Nearly all showed a reduction in the amount of distortion to position after adaptation with no significant differences as a function of handedness. In other respects, however, the two groups showed great dissimilarities. The results for the right-handers were consonant with previous reports of a negative correlation between magnitudes of adaptation to size and distance, but this was not true for the left-handers. The effect of previous diving experience also differed for the two groups. Finally, the left-handers consistently showed increased distortion in the perception of size after adaptation, but the right-handers did not. Thus, only the left-handers showed true counteradaptation (increased distortion after adaptation) but only the right-handers showed negative correlations between two modalities of adaptation. Misinterpretation of the word "counteradaptation" is cautioned against. (Authors' abstract)

1174.
LURIA, S.M. and C.L. McKay.
Effect of low levels of carbon monoxide on visual processes: a preliminary study.
U.S. Nav. Submar. Med. Res. Lab., Rep. NSMRL 727, 14p. Sept. 5, 1972.

[The problem was] to determine which of several different visual processes is most sensitive to low levels of carbon monoxide toxicity. [It was found that] night-vision sensitivity, reaction-time, and evoked cortical potentials often appeared to show a decrement after 90 minutes of exposure followed by improvement after 3 hours of exposure. No reliable changes were found in several other tests, such as field of view, stereoacuity, and the appearance of the retina. These results indicate that exposure to 200 ppm CO for three hours produces slight effects on visual performance and only the most sensitive of the visual processes are affected. These results are relevant to the question of tolerable levels of atmospheric CO contamination and which visual process can be used as the most sensitive test of CO toxicity. (Authors' summary)

1175.
LURIA, S.M., S.H. Ferris, C.L. McKay, J.A.S. Kinney and H.M. Paulson.
Vision through various scuba facemasks.
U.S. Nav. Submar. Med. Res. Lab., Rep. NSMRL 734, 15p. Dec. 15, 1972.

The visual performance of divers was compared utilizing five commercial facemasks. [Masks tested were (1) a standard oval mask, (2) a kidney-shaped mask, (3) a wrap-around wide-field mask, (4) a goggle-type mask, and (5) a mask with a lens system to compensate for underwater distortion]. Measurements were made of visual fields, visual acuity, stereoacuity, hand-eye coordination, accuracy of distance estimates, and accuracy of size estimates at both near and far distances. In addition, the optical properties of the masks were measured and the susceptibility of each mask to fogging was tested. There were significant differences between the masks for every visual process tested. Some masks were superior for one purpose, and inferior for another purpose. For example, the compensating mask improved size and distance estimates and hand-eye coordination but degraded acuity and stereoacuity. In every test, the results for the goggles fell bewteen those for the compensating mask and those for the other three masks. The results were not explained on the basis of susceptibility to fogging. (Authors' abstract)

1176.
LURIA, S.M. and J.A.S. Kinney.
Accommodation and stereoacuity.
Percept. Psychophysics 13:76-80; 1973.

Stereoacuity and resolution acuity were measured (1) through apertures set at various distances from 0 and (2) through plus lenses producing an accommodative error for the target equal to that produced by the presence of the apertures. Stereoacuity was degraded by the apertures but not by the lenses, whereas resolution acuity was degraded by the lenses but not by the apertures. Although stereoacuity progressively declined with decreasing target distance, it did not change significantly if accommodation remained constant. The decline of stereoacuity in the water is attributed to increased accommodation resulting from different sources and to a "Ganzfeld" effect of the typical underwater scene. (Authors' abstract)

1177.
LUSHCHITSKIF, M.A., O.B. Porembskii and M.V. Grinev.
O vozmozhnykh metodakh obezbolivaniya pri khrurgicheskikh operatsi yakh na podrodnykh lodkakh.
[Methods of anesthesia suitable for surgery on board submarines].
Voennomed. Zh. (5):68-71;May 1972.

Military physicians assigned to submarines during long expeditions may be confronted with surgical emergencies caused by injuries or acute abdominal complications. As the most frequently occurring diseases, the authors list acute appendicitis, perforated peptic ulcer and injuries to the extremities and abdominal organs. The best possible anesthetic method for surgery performed on board submarines is local anesthesia with premedication. However, in some complicated cases, when local anesthesia is insufficient, it may be combined with intravenous alcohol-thiopental anesthesia. A morphine-scopolamine mixture is used as pre-anesthetic medication. The authors conclude that neuroleptanalgesia may be considered as best method of the future but needs further testing. They also recommend further studies on anesthetic equipment especially suited for use in sealed underwater environment. (OLC/BSCP)

1178.
LUTHER, G.
UWL "Helgoland" — an underwater laboratory for rough sea conditions.
Helgolander Wiss. Meeresunters. 24:45-53; 1973.

The Helgolander underwater laboratory, or habitat, was designed to be used in rough North Sea waters. It consists primarily of a horizontal cylinder ballasted to a negative buoyancy of 16T. Emergency supplies make independence of the surface possible for 10 days. Communications consist of one TV system and two radio systems. Because of rough weather conditions, there is a decompression chamber within the habitat. Energy, compressed breathing mixtures, and water are supplied from a floating buoy that is controlled by the crew of the habitat. Other supplies are brought in containers without diver assistance. Extra breathing gas, and also nitrogen, are stored on the sea floor. (MFW/UMS)

1179.
LUXA, J. and V. Dolezal.
The effect of hyperbaric air and hyperbaric oxygen on the thyroid hormone-binding proteins and on the excretion of the metabolites of the catecholamines.
Acta. Univ. Palacki Olomuc Fac. Med. 65:304; 1973.

Abstract only. Entire item quoted: The group of ten sitting volunteers was examined in the hyperbaric chamber in 3 ata. The men breathed the air or the oxygen for 10 or 120 minutes. The blood and the urine samples were collected before, during and after the experiments for the determination of the thyroid hormone-binding proteins (T_4BG and T_3BG) and 3-methoxy-4-hydroxy-mandelic and 3-methoxy-4-hydroxy-penylacetic acids (VMA and HVA). The rates of T_4BC and T_3BG were determined using thyroid hormones labelled J 134 ("in vitro") and paper electrophoresis with the agar-agar impregnation, VMA and HVA using two dimensional paper chromatography. We found that T_4BG significantly descended in pressure of air in 60 minutes, while T_3BG did not change. The excretion of VMA and HVA show the same trend. During the 120 minutes exposition of O_2 T_4BG and T_3BG sank significantly, while VMA significantly rises. It seems, that the blood thyroidal hormones increase, together with the TBG decrease, is in relation with the duration of the oxygen pressure breathing. The VMA rising is related to the degree of the stress.

1180.
LYTHGOE, J.N.
Vision.
In: Woods, J.D. and J.N. Lythgoe, eds. Underwater science: An introduction to experiments by divers, p.103-139. London, Oxford University Press, 1971.

In his introduction, the author states that "No problem in underwater vision can be solved without regard both to the physiology of the eye and to the optical properties of the water; the two phases of the problem can be separated but they cannot be divorced." The aspects of underwater vision dealt with in this comprehensive review are: light under water, the color of water and the attenuation of light, the radiance of the water background and the distribution and polarization of light, the reduction of contrast, the eye and the face plate, the eye and vision, dark adaptation in dark water, brightness contrast and visual range, polarized light and vision, colored face plates, spectra sensitivity, and visual range, color recognition, conspicuous colors, and liminal color differences. The many illustrations include the following: a diagram of visually important optical events occuring as light penetrates water; down welling irradiance at various depths in clear water; relationship between the planes of natural underwater polarization and the sun's altitude; various devices for measuring visibility parameters; the spectral sensitivity of the eye to different wave-lengths at low light intensities; the relationship between the threshold for contrast perception, the brightness of the background and the angle subtended by target at the eye; the brightness contrast and visual range; the visible range of 16 15 x 20 cm mat-painted gray targets; the spectral reflectance of yellow and red fins of fish, and also of yellow, orange and red perspex targets. (MFW/BSCP)

1181.
LYWOOD, D.W. and D.B. Jennings.
An environmental chamber for studying chronic hypercapnia in dogs.
J. Appl. Physiol. 33(6):831-834; 1972.

An inexpensive chamber for studying the effects of chronic hypercapnia in large dogs was described. The system utilized the CO_2 production of the dog supplemented with CO_2 from a tank to provide an elevated chamber CO_2 concentration. A system for removing CO_2 from the chamber ($CO_2 < 0.5\%$) for control studies was also described. During a study of chronic hypercapnia in dogs over periods of fourteen days, the chamber had the following performance characteristics: mean PO_2 was generally between 146 and 142 mmHg; mean temperature varied between 19.6 and 21.9°C; the mean daily drift of the CO_2 system from the set 5% varied between 0 and 0.12% CO_2; and the mean average deviation of the relative humidity from set (30, 35, and 40%) was between 1.7 and 3.4%. (© BA)

1182.
MACEDO, I.C. and W-J Yang.
Acoustic effects on gas bubbles in the flows of viscous fluids and whole blood.
J. Acoust. Sc. Amer. 53:1327-1335;May 1973.

Gas-bubble behavior in a liquid flowing inside a circular tube subjected to an acoustic pressure field is studied analytically and experimentally. Consideration is given to both viscous fluids and whole blood, with the effects of acoustic radiation and viscosity taken into account. Slug flow and laminar parabolic flow cases are treated. Analytical solutions are obtained which predict the trajectory of bubble motion and the location where the bubble can be brought to a standstill on the tube wall by the acoustic force. It is disclosed that the trajectory is strongly dependent upon the acoustic pressure amplitude, flow velocity and liquid viscosity. By either increasing the acoustic pressure amplitude or decreasing the flow velocity or liquid viscosity, the bubble can be brought to a standstill in the first half-wavelength from the tube entrance, at the node or antinode depending upon its size. The theory is in good agreement with experiments performed in water and SEPARAN AP30 polymer solutions. The later fluids resemble whole blood in rheological properties. (Authors' abstract)

1183.
MacINNIS, J.B.
Arctic diving and the problems of performance.
In: The working diver, 1972. Symposium proceedings, February 1972, Columbus, Ohio, p.159-174. Washington, D.C., Marine Technology Society, 1972.

In 1970 and 1971, the author led two expeditions for underwater studies in the Canadian high Arctic. The objectives were to begin focusing on the performance problems of scientists working in this extreme environment and to make preliminary surveys of local marine biology and geology. Sixty-three shallow scuba dives were made during winter and summer conditions in water at a temperature of 28.9F. In order to improve understanding of the problems of performance almost half the dives were carried out by doctorate level scientists attempting meaningful work. At times the ice was six feet thick and air temperatures reached 50 below zero. Standard scuba equipment as well as the General Electric Mk X, the Poseidon Unisuit, and a portable communications station were evaluated. From these two expeditions and others in near-arctic conditions the author has begun to clarify the factors which enhance and degrade shallow diving performance beneath polar seas. (Author's abstract)

1184.
MACKAY, R.S.
Non-invasive cardiac output measurement.
Microvasc. Res. 4:438-452; 1972.

A sound beam in the 2-MHz frequency range can be shown down from the suprasternal notch or across through an intercostal space to look along the lumen of the aortic arch, thus returning a Doppler-shifted frequency which measures instantaneous velocity of flow. Circuits are described for continuously graphing indicated flow distribution, including the direction of flow. The rate of increase of velocity (acceleration) is a measure of myocardial contractility. In combination with a radiographic or ultrasonic determination of aorta diameter, the integrated curve of velocity as a function of time gives stroke volume, with apparently useful accuracy. Possible errors are discussed, and a combination of standard commercial items is described for producing these results. (Author's abstract) [According to personal communication from the author, this technique is useful in circumstances related to underwater medicine. Ed.].

1185.
MACKAY, R.S.
High pressure state simulation studies as an aid to understanding diving problems.
IEEE Trans. Biomed. Eng. 19:140-143;Mar. 1972.

Some of the earliest biological system models used to guide the affairs of man were employed to avoid the "bends" in diving. A brief discussion of decompression sickness, as it can affect tunnel workers, airplane pilots, or divers, is given, along with an analog computer configuration to represent the situation. The configuration itself has proved helpful in aiding engineers to understand some of the mechanisms involved, and the recordings that result seem helpful in supplying to physiologists and divers a feeling for the probable effect of a change in circumstances associated with a proposed dive. The effect of changing a gas mixture or changing the time course of a dive is readily visualized, for example, as are the results of using a continuously variable gas mixture and continuous ascent for minimum decompression time. (Author's abstract)

1186.
MACKAY, R.S.
Study of decompression sickness (bends) using ultrasonic imaging of bubbles.
Presented at Ultrasonics International 1973, London, 27-29 March 1973.

Small bubbles are readily noticed during ultrasonic imaging, which allows study of the bends. This presentation largely consists of a motion picture showing work with George Rubissow, in which diverse structures in animal and human legs are observed by both continuous Doppler and pulsed systems during pressure changes. Using a fast sector scan with combined brightness and deflection display, and a synchronized movie camera, one can observe the pattern of bubbles come and go, especially in vessels and in the vicinity of fat pads. The equipment and methods have some novel aspects, and have allowed decompression by ultrasonic observation alone. (Author's abstract)

1187.
MacKINNON, J.R.
Development of techniques for measuring performance in the undersea environment.
New London, Conn., Conn. Coll., Dept. Psychol., 10p. Apr. 15, 1972.
(AD 748 036)

The overall objective of the project was to develop precise, reliable techniques for monitoring changes in human performance during exposure to unusual environmental conditions. Specifically, this research was designed to provide base-line information on the usefulness of a selected task as an instrument in assessing performance degradation under adverse conditions germane to the diving situation. The task selected for investigation was a modified version of the Stroop Color-Word Interference Test (CWIT). Experiments conducted were designed to determine the efficiency of this test in evaluating the effects of environmental and psychological stress on cognitive functioning. (GRA)

1188.
MacMILLAN, V. and B.K. Siesjo.
The effect of hypercapnia upon the energy metabolism of the brain during arterial hypoxemia.
Scand. J. Clin. Lab. Invest. 30:237-244; 1972.

In order to evaluate whether hypercapnia affects the energy metabolism of the hypoxic brain, lightly anesthetized rats were maintained for 30 min at a PaO_2 of close to 28 mm Hg and a $PaCO_2$ of close to 65 mm Hg, and compared with normocapnic rats maintained either at a normal PaO_2 or at a PaO_2 of close to 28 mm Hg. The results showed that in the hypoxic rats the energy state of the tissue, as evaluated from the energy charge of the adenine nucleotide system, was unaffected by the added hypercapnia. The hypercapnia decreased the accumulation of lactate during hypoxemia and affected the tissue levels of carbohydrate substrates in a direction suggesting decreased metabolic flux. It is concluded that during hypoxemia, and in the absence of ischemia, carbon dioxide protects rather than disrupts the energy metabolism of the brain. (Authors' abstract)

1189.
MacMILLAN, V. and B.K. Siesjo.
The influence of hypocapnia upon intracellular pH and upon some carbohydrate substrates, amino acids and organic phosphates in the brain.
J. Neurochem. 21:1283-1299;Nov. 1973.

In order to evaluate the influence of hypocapnia upon the energy metabolism of the brain, lightly anaesthetized rats were hyperventilated to arterial CO_2 tensions of 26, 15 and 10 mm Hg respectively, with subsequent measurements of intracellular pH and of tissue concentrations of carbohydrate substrates, amino acids and organic phosphates. At $PCO_2 = 26$ there was a moderate increase in the intracellular pH but when the CPO_2 was reduced further to 10 mm Hg the intracellular pH returned to normal, or slightly subnormal, values. The reduction in PCO_2 was accompanied by increased cerebral cortical concentrations of lactate, pyruvate, citrate, α-ketoglutarate, malate and glutamate and by decreased aspartate concentrations. It is concluded that the accumulation of metabolic acids explains the normal value for intracellular pH at very low CO_2 tensions. Previous results obtained in man indicate that there is an increased anaerobic production of lactic acid in the brain in extreme hypocapnia. At comparable CO_2 tensions the present results showed a small fall in phosphocreatine and a small rise in ADP. However, since the ammonia concentrations were normal or decreased and since there was an increase in citrate, the results give no direct support to the hypothesis of an activation of phosphofructokinase. Since the cerebral venous PO_2 was reduced to 20 mm Hg at an arterial CO_2 tension of 10 mm Hg the accumulation of acids was probably secondary to tissue hypoxia. However, since there was no, or only a very small, increase in the calculated cytoplasmic NADH/NAD+ ratio, it appears less likely that acids accumulated due to lack of NAD+. (Authors' abstract)

1190.
MADSEN, J. and E. Jacobsen.
Decompression disease and its treatment.
Ugeskr. Laeg. 134:1157-1160;May 29, 1972.

The treatment of decompression disease has been modified in recent years, the classical recompression treatment being replaced by oxygen breathing under moderate recompression. This regimen has also proved valuable in the treatment of aeroembolism. It has further been shown that hypovolemic shock has a prominent place in the syndrome of decompression and that its treatment is equally important as recompression. Other aspects of the treatment of decompression disease are discussed. (English summary)

1191.
MAESTRACCI, P., J.P. Rigal, W. Amzallag and G. Plante-Longchamp.
Les accidents de la plongee et leur traitement actuel.
[Diving accidents and their current treatment].
Maroc Med. 50:349-361;June 1970.

The author describes the mechanisms, circumstances under which they occur, the clinical symptoms, and the recommended therapy for the most common types of diving accidents. The formation of air embolisms is graphically illustrated. Both the American and the French therapeutic tables are given, as is a therapeutic decompression schedule of 44 hours duration. Another table shows the recommended schedules for various types and degrees of accidents. Another illustration shows the effect of heightened pressure on the tension of a bubble. In the authors' conclusion, it is stated that the most serious diving accidents are pulmonary barotrauma and air embolism. Their pathogenesis, although widely known, is not entirely understood. Treatment should consist of recompression in a multiplace chamber, followed by a very carefully regulated decompression. If there is injury to the central nervous system, medical treatment of the microcirculation must accompany this therapy. If all of these methods can be utilized (and this necessitates major equipment and a numerous and well-trained staff) the results can be considered excellent, taking into consideration the alarming clinical condition of most of these patients upon arrival. (MFW/BSCP)

1192.
MAISON, J.R. and J.D. Stachiw.
Acrylic pressure hull for Johnson-Sea-Link submersible.
Presented at the American Society of Mechanical Engineering meeting, Washington, D.C., November 28-December 2, 1971.

The design, fabrication technique, and test data developed by the Navy for the 600-ft-operational depth NEMO acrylic-plastic (a-p) submersible were extrapolated at a minimum cost to an a-p capsule with 1000-ft-operational depth for the Smithsonian Institution's Johnson-Sea-Link (JSL) submersible. Being able to use existing data from the NEMO a-p hull program for man-rating a-p capsule with greater operational depth than NEMO's is an important milestone in the development of a-p capsules for submersibles. The paper summarizes the guidelines used in extrapolating the NEMO data to the JSL and the data validation by experimental means. (Authors' abstract)

1193.
MAKAROVA, V.G.
K. voprosy o perekrestnoi adaptatsii organizma k giperboksii i gipoksii v ontogeneze.
[Cross adaptation of the organism to hyperoxia and hypoxia in ontogenesis].
Pathol. Fiziol. Eksp. Ter. 17:50-54;Mar./Apr. 1973.

It was revealed in experiments on young (3-4 weeks), adult (9 months) and old (24 months) rats that adaptive changes in metabolism to high altitude hypoxia were more pronounced in the young animals. Prolonged training of the animals under oxygen pressure of 1 to 1.5 atmospheres reduced the toxic effect of high oxygen pressure (3.5 atmospheres). Training to hypoxia does not produce cross adaptation to high altitude hypoxia; anaerobic changes in tissue metabolism were more pronounced than in intact rats placed under hypoxic conditions. (English summary)

1194.
MAKOVKINA, T.V.
Dinamika izmeneniya vesa i vesovye indeksy vnutrennykh organov u belykh myshei v zavisimosti ot sostava gazovoi sredy i pitaniya.
[Changes in body weight and visceral weight indices of white mice in relation to the composition of the atmosphere and diet].
Kosm. Biol. Med. 7(4):30-34; 1973.

The effect of inert gases on the visceral weight indices and water content and body weights of white mice was studied with respect to various diets. Visceral weight indices showed no significant changes under the influence of the gas composition. The body weight and visceral weight indices depended mainly on the diets. In a helium-oxygen atmosphere body weight decreased significantly on the 5th and 10th experimental days. The effect of exposure to an argon-oxygen or nitrogen-oxygen atmosphere was less pronounced. The visceral water content was not affected either by the atmosphere or the diets. (ML) (© BA)

1195.
MANGHNANI, M.H., A. Quattrochi and J.F. Ferraro.
Pressure and temperature studies of glass spectra; infrared spectra or several glasses at high pressures; infrared absorption spectra of sodium silicate glasses at high pressures.
Phys. Chem. Glasses 13:116-121; 1972.
(Also published in J. Appl. Phys. 43:4595-4599; 1972)
(AD 753,323)

Interrelated studies of the pressure and temperature dependence of elastic and infrared vibrational properties of silicate glasses are reported in three published papers. In the first paper, a study of six Na20-Ti-Si02 glasses containing 20 or 25 mol % Ti02, is presented. In the second paper, the infrared absorption characteristics of alpha-quartz, fused silica, and Pyrex and Vycor (Corning Glass Works) glasses are compared at ambient and high pressures to 58.5 Kbar. Gruneisen parameters were calculated. A similar study of twelve Na20-Si02 glasses of varying composition (10 to 45% Na20), reported in the third paper, shows that the pressure dependences of all the infrared absorption frequencies studied are positive. (GRA)

1196.
MANO, Y. and I. Nashimoto.
Diving data recorder (DDR).
In: United States-Japan conference on natural resources development. Proceedings of the first joint meeting of the U.S.-Japan panel on diving and technology, Tokyo, 1972, p.170-171. Japan, Ministry of Agriculture and Forestry, 1972.

The diving data recorder monitors the physiological condition of the diver. It can operate over a period of four hours, recording diving time, depth, and the ECG of the diver. The data are analyzed by means of a demodulator and an oscillograph. Other data which can be recorded include water temperature and body temperature. The purpose of the instrument is to study the relationship between the underwater environment and the physiological state of the diver, thus making possible the development of more efficient diving techniques. (MFW/UMS from English summary)

1197.
MARGARIA, R., E. Camporesi, P. Aghemo and G. Sassi.
The effect of O_2 breathing on maximal aerobic power.
Pfluegers Arch. 336(3):225-235; 1972.

Time of performance, blood lactic acid concentration (LA) heart rate (HR) and maximal O_2 consumption ($\dot{V}O_2max$) were measured during air and O_2 breathing in 11 subjects performing a supramaximal exercise with an O_2 requirement of 70 to 80 ml/kg.min to exhaustion. The subjects were tested for maximal aerobic power with an indirect method. In one subject the rate of lactic acid increase in blood was also measured. The $\dot{V}O_2max$ measured with both the direct method appeared to be about 8% higher when breathing pure O_2; lactic acid production rate decreased correspondingly. Maximal HR and maximal LA concentration were the same. In submaximal exercise the steady state HR was lower by about 8-9 beats/min when breathing O_2. When breathing O_2 the HR was a linear function of the work load. From experimental data obtained in subjects of different $\dot{V}O_2max$ breathing both air or O_2, the energy equivalent of LA amounted to 47 ml of O_2 or 235 cal/g of LA produced. (© BA)

1198.
MARGOLIS, G., L.R. Mills and A. Naitove.
Augmentation of neurotoxic effects of experimental aortography by the vascular reflexes induced during simulated diving.
J. Neurosurg. 37:332-338;Sept. 1972.

Augmentation of the neurotoxic sequelae of retrograde aortography in the dog is produced by the cardiovascular responses evoked by a simulated diving procedure. This action is explained by profound peripheral vasoconstriction and resultant diversion of aortic outlfow toward the neral vascular bed. These findings are in agreement with previous studies made with the use of Levarternol in conjunction with aortography. The new findings also demonstrate that physiological circulatory reflexes pose the same hazards for arteriography as do pharmacologically induced vasopressor responses. (Authors' abstract)

1199.
MARINE TECHNOLOGY SOCIETY.
Applications of marine technology to human needs. Preprints, 8th annual conference and exposition, September 1972, Washington , D.C.
Washington, D.C., published by the Society, 1972. 782p.

The emphasis of this conference was on engineering. Specific papers related to the subject areas of this bibliography will be found under the following author entires: Camfield, F.E., W.L. Prelan and H. Wang; Gee, G.K.; Hallanger, L.W. and A.M. Parisi; Kutzleb, R.E.; Miller, J.W. and D.C. Beaumariage; Sherwood, W.G.; Walrod, R.A.; Wozniak, J., C.K. Raft and R.W. Alperi. (MFW/BSCP)

1200.
MARKHAM, J.
Navigating Britain's underwater vehicles.
Hydrospace 3:40-43;Aug. 1970.

This article deals with the problems of navigation as they are dealt with in the cases of the Cammell Laird SBV and the Vickers Pisces/Vickers Venturer. In the first instance, the problem was chiefly one of position fixing. The problem is basically the same as that on land — the resolution of azimuth and distance into cartesian coordinates. It was decided to adapt the computer of the Sperry Land Navigator and the Sperry CL 11 Directional gyroscope. In the case of the Vickers Pisces/Vickers Venturer, a navigation system was specially designed and produced by Marcom International Marine Co. It is described as follows: "The surface unit transmits at 24KHz from an omnidirectional transducer mounted at the center of the ship's hull. This pulse is received by the submersible and retransmitted at 48KHz. The returning pulse is received by receiving transducers mounted fore and aft on the support ship. The time taken from transmission to reception gives a measure of the range of the submersible while the time delay between reception at the fore and aft receiving transducers gives the bearing." (MFW/BSCP)

1201.
MARONE, G., S. Cifaldi, A. Scapicchio, L. Bianchi and F. Boccalatte.
Modificazioni elettroencefalografiche, elettrocardiografiche ed ematochimiche nel coniglio sottoposto a 6 ata di ossigeno.
[Electroencephalographic, electrocardiographic and hematochemical changes in the rabbit subjected to 6 atmospheres of oxygen].
Rass. Med. Sper. 19(1):1-12; 1972.

Studies were made of ECG and EEG behavior in relation to changes in O_2 and CO_2, pH and alkaline reserve of arterial and venous blood. EEG alterations, which were evident before 6 atm absolute was reached, were observed first, ECG alterations, proportional to alterations in CNS performance, also became evident. Blood data revealed that the animals were able to tolerate the hyperbaric situation. As soon as the compensatory mechanisms stopped working, the animals died. (CMM) (© BA)

1202.
MARONE, G., A. Colantuoni and S. Cifaldi.
Effetto protettivo dell' α-mercapto-propionil-glicina nella intossicazione acuta la ossigeno iperbarico.
[The protective effect of alpha-mercaptopropionylglycine in acute intoxication from hyperbaric oxygen].
Boll. Soc. Ital. Biol. Sper. 48(23):1062-1064; 1972.

The toxic action of hyperbaric O_2 may be due to the oxidation of sulfhydryl groups in enzymes such as pyruvate oxidase, thus inhibiting the oxidation of cerebral pyruvate. The administration of α -mercaptopropionylglycine (Thiola) in rats does not produce an increase in blood SH concentrations and is realtively less toxic. Thiola yields SH groups gradually during metabolism. Test rats received i.p. injections of Thiola ranging from 200-1600 mg/kg in 5 ml physiologic saline, while controls received saline. Forty min after treatment, the rats were placed in a stainless steel hyperbaric O_2 chamber and, after removal of atmospheric N, were subjected to O_2 at 6 atm for 30 min. At the maximum Thiola dose (1600 mg/kg) all rats survived at the time of decompression while 200 mg/kg produced zero survival. However, 24 h after decompression, all rats on the 1600 mg/kg dose were dead, presumably due to the inherent toxic action of the substance, but at lesser doses survival increased, reaching a maximum at 800 mg/kg, which under the conditions of the experiments seemed to combine maximal protection against hyperbaric O_2 with minimal toxicity. (PHVI) (© BA)

1203.
MARQUET, W.M.
Submerged navigation and submersible instrumentation.
In: Woods Hole, Mass., Woods Hole Oceanog. Inst., Rep. WHO1-72-90, p.4-7, Nov. 30, 1972.

The objective of the submerged navigation development program is to develop and conduct at-sea evaluations of an acoustic navigation system for submersibles and their support ships. The program began in February 1971. The first six months were spent detailing the basic real time system, procuring the major components, building a prototype of the submersible electronics unit, building a prototype of the support ship system. This report covers the period 1 April 1971 through 31 January 1972 during which the system was debugged and tested at sea. (Author)

1204.
MARRIOTT, J.
Submarine rescue methods.
Meerestechnik 3:115-120;June 1972.

All navies have had their share of submarine disasters, and many astonishing escapes from trapped submarines have been made, but so far all of them have been in relatively shallow water. With the advent of the nuclear submarine, capable of diving to hitherto unprecedented depths and of staying submerged and supporting life for much longer periods, a new problem has been posed to the designers of rescue methods. This article examines the current thinking by the British and the Americans on methods of rescue and describes the latest escape equipments now in use or under development. (Author's abstract)

1205.
MARTIN, F.E., J.E. Hudgens and J.W. Wonn.
Manned hyperbaric demonstration of incipient bubble detection using nonlinear ultrasonic propagation.
Annapolis, Westinghouse Electric Corp., Ocean Res. Eng. Cent., Rep. OER-73-16, 45p. May 31, 1973.
(AD 761 222)

A series of hyperbaric chamber dives were planned and executed which had potential for producing bubbles within the human system and yet allowed recompression therapy prior to overt decompression sickness. The test subjects were instrumented with Westinghouse designed ultrasonic transducers and signal processing set-up. Continuous recordings of transducer response before, during and after the dives, were made. These tests further demonstrated that the Westinghouse Nonlinear Ultrasonic Propagation Technique can detect bubbles both within the venous and the capillary system, that it can count and otherwise characterize these bubbles, that it can do so at a power level well below the recommended "safe level," and that it can do so well before diver awareness of symptoms. (Authors) (GRA)

1206.
MARTIN, H.L., R.C. Durant, W.V. Hudak and S. Friess.
Alterations in chemical blockade of cat gastrocnemius-soleus tissues under hyperbaric HE/O_2 atmospheres.
U.S. Nav. Med. Res. Inst., Med. Res. Prog. Rep. 67, 11p. Nov. 29, 1971.
(AD 751,121)
(Also published in Toxicol. Appl. Pharmacol 23:82-90; 1972.)

The blockade responses of gastrocnemius-soleus (G-S) tissues to infusion with the quaternary ester tropine-p-tolyacetate methiodide (T) have been studied in vivo in the cat as a function of the composition and total pressure of the environmental breathing atmosphere. The G-S preparation itself is fully viable and capable of performing sustained isometric work under burst stimuli (40, 100 Hz) to the nerve for periods in excess of 2 hr, at tissue saturation with pressures ranging from 1 absolute atmospheric pressure (ata) (N_2/O_2) to 266 psig (He/O_2). The standard blockade at 1 ata elicited by slow infusion of 01 M ester T amounts to extinction of response tension within 3.8 mm. As the pressure is increased to 100 psig using He/O_2 mixture, the degree of blockade induced by T at reference infusion times is sharply reduced, remains low at a total saturating pressure of 200 psig, and rises somewhat at 266 psig to modest levels that are still well below the blocking efficacy met at atmospheric pressure. Reasons for this striking dependency of blockade potency of a quaternary ester on external pressure are sought in terms of a deformable pore or crevasse model for receptor surfaces in striated muscle systems. (Authors) (GRA)

1207.
MARTIN, J.L. and R.M. Jacobs.
Untitled.
In: Abstracts of BuMed-ONR sponsored Navywide research in high pressure biomedical research, U.S. Submarine Base, Groton, Conn., May 1971, p.50. Published by the Naval Submarine Medical Research Laboratories, 1971.

Abstract only. Entire item quoted: This report discusses results of tests with capillary viscometer designed to be operated at a number of hydrostatic pressures. Also presented are tests conducted with a falling venturi viscometer, which can be operated at hydrostatic pressure to fifty atmospheres. The most important information to be presented is the observed slight increase in apparent viscosity of blood treated with anticoagulants when hydrostatic pressure increases markedly. The two unusual test units designed for this project are discussed briefly, and pictures obtained with the falling venturi unit are presented.

1208.
MARTIN, K.J. and G. Nichols.
Observations on platelet changes in man after simulated diving.
Aerosp. Med. 43:827-830;Aug. 1972.

Five trained divers and ten non-divers volunteered to take part in a simulated dive on compressed air to 30.5 metres (100 feet sea water). The non-divers were divided into two groups, one of which completed the dive and the other, similarly prepared but without their knowledge, were not subjected to pressure while in the chamber, thus providing a negative control group. Platelet levels were estimated daily both before and after the dive. Under the specific conditions of the experiment and with the particular techniques used, both groups subjected to pressure showed a platelet depression maximal on the third post-dive day. This fall was not apparent in the control group, indicating that the depression was a true effect of pressure and not a psychosomatic situation response. The prothrombin consumption index was also recorded and showed no change. (Authors' abstract)

1209.
MARTIN, K.J.
Observations on haematological and biochemical parameters.
In: The Association of Clinical Pathologists: 89th general meeting. Symposium II. Decompression sickness. J. Clin. Pathol. 25:1004-1005;Nov. 1972.

Abstract only. An attempt was made to determine normal levels, in the context of a symptomless hyperbaric exposure, of the following hematological and biochemical parameters: platelets, lipids, enzymes, plasma cortisol, and coagulation factors. The purpose was to differentiate between the true effects of pressure and the psychosomatic response. Immediate effects indicated metabolic changes affecting steroids and free fatty acids. Changes in euglobulin lysis indicated a psychosomatic response. Delayed effects were found in platelets, and various enzymes. Residual effects of previous diving experience may have contributed to some of the enzyme patterns. It was concluded that in a symptom-free hyperbaric exposure some changes occur that are similar to those observed in a post-traumatic situation; these changes may produce short- or long-term effects, in terms of adaptation and of pathology. (MFW/BSCP)

1210.
MARTIN, K.J., S.P. Gray and G. Nichols.
Effect of a short simulated dive on selected blood constituents in man.
Aerosp. Med. 44:516-522;May 1973.
(Also published as Roy. Nav. Physiol. Lab. Rep. 6/72, Aluritike, England 1972)

Nine non-divers and five trained divers agreed to take part in a short simulated dive on compressed air to 30.5 metres. Five of the non-divers were, without their knowledge, not subjected to pressure while in the chamber, thus providing a negative control and enabling a differentiation to be made between the psychosomatic response to the situation and the true effect of pressure. Selected fat, steroid, enzyme, and coagulation factors were estimated daily both before and after the dive. Under the conditions of this experiment the results showed immediate and delayed effects. The immediate response was both metabolic as depicted by changes in the levels of plasma cortisol and unesterified fatty acids and psychosomatic as shown by the pattern of euglobulin lysis activity. Delayed effects were noted in relation to creatin phosphokinase, alkaline phosphatase and aspartate aminotransferase. Residual effects of previous diving experience were apparent. (Authors' abstract)

1211.
MARTIN, K.J.
Current research into the normal dive.
In: Ackles, K.N. ed. Blood-bubble interaction in decompression sickness. Proceedings of an international symposium held at Defence and Civil Institute of Environmental Medicine, Downsview, Ontario, Canada, p.71-103. Published by the Institute, December 1973. (DCIEM Conference Proceedings 73-CP-960)

Studies of numerous blood parameters made during a series of simulated dives at the Royal Naval Physiological Laboratory at Alverstoke are described. The following measurements were made: fibrinogen and FDP count pre- and post-dive; the effect of heparin on various enzyme levels in a goat with a severe spinal bend; clotting time and platelet count pre- and post-dive in human subjects; unesterified fatty acids, plasma cortisol, alkaline phosphotase, aspartate amino-transferase, alkaline phosphatase, glutamic-oxalacetic transaminase, creatine phosphokinase were all measured pre- and post-dive. The results show that during a chamber dive a number of factors are operating at asymptomatic levels, indicating, among other things, a metabolic influence, a psychosomatic response, residual effects of recent diving on enzyme patterns. The author concludes by saying "It is against this type of background of sub-clinical change which reflects a normal base line range of immediate and delayed effects that the changes relevant to decompression sickness are superimposed." (MFW/UMS)

1212.
MARTIN, R.R., N.R. Anthonisen and M. Zutter.
Effect of gas density on respiratory gas exchange in the anesthetized dog.
In: Abstracts of the Twenty-fifth Congress of Physiological Sciences Satellite Symposium. Recent progress in fundamental physiology of diving, Marseille, France, July 1971, p.26. (Proceedings unpublished)

Abstract only. Excerpts quoted: Dogs were studied breathing air, $He\text{-}O_2$ and $SF_6\text{-}O_2$ at one ATA and breathing $N_2\text{-}O_2$ and $SF_6\text{-}O_2$ at four ATA; O_2 diffusivity should be about 25 times faster in He at 1 ATA than in SF_6 at 4 ATA. Inspired O_2 tensions were constant at 0.2 ATA in all experiments. Pulmonary gas exchange was not effected by gas density either at the surface or breathing $O_2\text{-}N_2$ at depth. However, when SF_6 was breathed at 4 ATA, pulmonary gas exchange became more efficient whether judged by alveolar-arterial PO_2 differences, calculated venous admixture, or inspired-arterial PO_2 differences. This was the opposite of what was expected. . . . It is possible that very dense gas improved the ventilation of units with low compliance; the existance of such units is hypothetical, however. Finally, it is possible that inspiring dense gas, by increasing convective mixing of the inspirate with lung gas, reduces pre-existent diffusion dependent gas tension gradients in peripheral lung units.

1213.
MARTIN, R.R., M. Zutter and N.R. Anthonisen.
Pulmonary gas exchange in dogs breathing SF_6 at 4 ATA.
J. Appl. Physiol. 33:86-92;July 1972.

The effects of inspired gas density on alveolar-arterial oxygen tension differences ($(A\text{-}a)DO_2$) and dead space-to-tidal volume ratios (V_D/V_T) were studied in anesthetized artificially ventilated dogs. With an inspired PO_2 of 150 $\pm$ 8 mm Hg dogs breathed He, SF_6 and N_2 at 1 ATA and N_2 and SF_6 at 4 ATA. No changes in gas exchange were noted with changes in inert gas at 1 ATA, nor were there significant differences between gas exchange at 1 ATA and that breathing $O_2\text{-}N_2$ at 4 ATA. However, breathing SF_6 at 4 ATA produced a consistent decrease in $(A\text{-}a)DO_2$ and a small increase in V_D/V_T. The decrease of $(A\text{-}a)DO_2$ appeared to be due to an increased efficiency of pulmonary O_2 exchange. It was not dependent on lung volume or end-expiratory pressure. It was however, diminished by vagotomy. These results were compatible with the presence in the normal dog lung of low $\dot{V}_A/\dot{Q}$ units which were badly ventilated due to low compliance but which had low resistance; the ventilation of such units might have been increased by increased gas density. Alternatively, SF_6 at 4 ATA could have, by improving convective mixing in the airways, eliminated preexistent stratified inhomogeneities of gas tension. (Authors' abstract)

1214.
MASLOVA, M.N., E.V. Ozirskaya and L.V. Reznik.
Izmeneniya v kore bolyshikh polusharii mozga krys pri giperoksii (sopostavlenie funktsional'no-biokhimicheskikh i morfologicheskikh dannykh).
[Changes in the rat brain under hyperoxia (comparison of functional-biochemical and morphological evidence)].
Tsitologiia 15:16-21;Jan. 1973.

The functional, biochemical and ultrastructural changes were followed in the rat central nervous system at the different stages of the acute hyperoxia. The fine structure of the liver cells of the same animals was studied to determine the order of changes beginning at the ultrastructural level. The data obtained showed the hypoxia-induced changes in behaviour reactions, acetylcholinesterase activity in the brain and in the ultrastructure of brain neurons and of liver cells. The changes of the mitochondrial apparatus in these cells were especially noticeable and it is the changes in the liver cells that were more pronounced. The alterations observed are directly correlated with the strength and duration of the influence applied and with the general state of the animals. They have a non-specific character. (English summary)

1215.
MASSARGIN, A.G.
Neirotropnii efekt glibokoi giperkapnii.
[Neurotropic effect of deep hypercapnia].
Fiziol. Zh. 17:695-697;Sept./Oct. 1971.

Changes in the nervous system of rabbits were investigated after a one min exposure to carbon dioxide producing acute hypercapnia. Previously conditioned defensive reflexes were maintained after hypercapnia. The development of hypercapnia is divided into three stages, beginning with a prenarcotic phase during inhalation of carbon dioxide. The subsequent narcotic phase covers a portion of the inhalation period and continues some time after removal of the animal from the carbon dioxide atmosphere. The last stage entails a phase of recovery to normal activity of the organism. (Aerosp. Med.)

1216.
MASSARO, D.
Hyperoxia influence of food deprivation on protein synthesis by lung.
Proc. Soc. Exp. Biol. Med. 143(3):602-603; 1973.

Rats which are deprived of food and exposed for 48 hr either to $>98\%$ O_2 or compressed air lose an equal amount of weight. Under these conditions the incorporation of leucine-^{14}C into protein is less in lung slices from rats exposed to compressed air. (PLW) (© BA)

1217.
MASSARO, D.
Protein synthesis in lung recovery from exposure to hyperoxia.
J. Appl. Physiol. 35:32-34;July 1973.

Previous work has shown that in vivo hyperoxia decreases in vitro protein synthesis by the lung. In the present study I measured the incorporation of leucine-^{14}C into protein by lung slices during the 24 hr of room air breathing immediately following 48 hr exposure to hyperoxia or compressed air. Four hours of breathing room air following 48 hours of hyperoxia is not sufficient for protein biosynthesis to return to control values. Twenty-four hours after return to room air leucine-^{14}C incorporation into total protein is 1.9 times greater in rats previously exposed to hyperoxia than compressed-air-exposed rats and incorporation into protein of the surface-active fraction is 1.5 times greater than in compressed-air-exposed rats. The greatest difference is in the proteins of a midzone nonsurface-active fraction where the protein specific radioactivity is 2.2 times greater in the rats exposed to hyperoxia compared to those exposed to compressed air. These findings suggest that during recovery from hyperoxia the augmentation of the synthesis of nonsecretory protein is greater than that of secretory protein. (Author's abstract)

1218.
MASSARO, G.D. and D. Massaro.
Hyperoxia: A stereologic ultrastructural examination of its influence on cytoplasmic components of the pulmonary granular pneumocyte.
J. Clin. Invest. 52(3):566-570; 1973.

The technique of lineal analysis was used to study the influence of 48 hr of hyperoxia on cytoplasmic organelles of pulmonary granular pneumocytes with particular reference to their lamellar bodies. This study was undertaken because lamellar bodies are considered to be storage granules for pulmonary surfactant and hyperoxia decreased [^{14}C] leucine incorporation into protein of a surface-active lung fraction. For lamellar bodies the percent cytoplasmic volume was 12.8 $\pm$ 1.5 and 8.4 $\pm$ 2.2, the organelle area (μm^2) per organelle was 0.98 $\pm$ 0.13 and 0.62 $\pm$ 0.10 and the organelle volume (μm^3) was 0.35 $\pm$ 0.04 and 0.18 $\pm$ 0.01 for air- and O_2-exposed rats, respectively, ($P =< 0.05$). The surface density of the lamellar body membrane was 7.05 $\pm$ 0.47 and 9.36 $\pm$ 0.96 ($P =< 0.05$) for air- and O_2-exposed rats. There were no differences in lamellar body number per cytoplasmic area or per pneumocyte between air- and O_2-exposed rats. There were no statistical differences in these parameters between mitochondria of air- or O_2-exposed rats. The surface density of the rough endoplasmic reticulum was the same in both groups. Granular pneumocytes of rats exposed to hyperoxia have the same number of lamellar bodies as control rats but the lamellar bodies are smaller. This finding is consistent with the hypothesis that the hyperoxia-induced decrease in protein synthesis by lung represent at least in part a decreased synthesis of the secretory lipoprotein-pulmonary surfactant. (© BA)

1219.
MATSUDA, M., Z. Ito, T. Kaminaga, H. Nakayama and A. Morita.
Toxic effects under high-pressure oxygen atmosphere.
In: Wada, J. and I. Takashi, eds. Proceedings of the fourth international congress on hyperbaric medicine, Sapporo, Japan, Sept. 1969, p.5-9. Baltimore, Williams and Wilkins, 1970.

For developing the air saturation diving technique, 4 healthy subjects, aged 26-31, well trained and experienced divers were exposed in a dry and wet chamber complex or therapeutical chamber for 24 and 72 hours of the bottom time at 100 ft (4 ATA). Before, during and after exposure some physio-psychological examinations were performed. As results the decrease of red blood cells count in peripheral venous blood was discovered and was also found to recover within 4 days. And all of subjects exposed to air complained of paresthesia at the finger tips. Some discussions and also experiments were performed for clarifying the mechanism of those signs and symptoms under estimation of oxygen toxicity. (Authors' summary)

1220.
MATSUDA, M.
Seatopia (undersea habitation experiment) project in Japan.
In: United States-Japan conference on natural resources development. Proceedings of the first joint meeting of the U.S.-Japan panel on diving and technology, Tokyo, 1972, p.88-93. Japan, Ministry of Agriculture and Forestry, 1972.

The Seatopia project consisted of the construction of an undersea habitat, two personnel transfer capsules, three deck decompression chambers, and one support buoy. Construction was completed in March 1971. The habitat measures 10.85 m in length, 4.5 m in width, and 6.525 m in height, and weighs 68 T. Drawings of the habitat and of the support buoy are given. It is planned that four aquanauts will live and work underwater, first at 30 m, then at 60 m, then at 100 m. The purpose of the program is to study the performance of man in the sea, the physiology and psychology of man in a hyperbaric environment, and to evaluate the usefulness of undersea habitats and of saturation diving. A complete schedule of the first experiment, at 30 m., is given. It took place during August 1972. Most of the month was spent in setting up and inspecting the system. The men actually lived in the habitat for only two days. (MFW/UMS)

1221.
MATTHYS, H. and A.A. Buhlman.
Erfahrungen mit der hyperbaren Sauerstoffeinwirkung beim Menschen.
[Experience with hyperbaric oxygenation in man].
Schweiz. Med. Wschr. 100:1313-1316; 1970.

Above normal O_2 pressure may produce tissue damage in the upper respiratory tract, the lungs and the central nervous system. Experience is reported of pressure chamber tests realizing 100% O_2 at pressures of up to 2.5 atm for periods of 20 min to several hours, and O_2/N_2 or O_2/He mixtures at O_2 pressures of 0.55 to 1.0 atm for periods lasting several hours to 7 days. CNS tolerance is independent of the percentage of the inert gas and of the humidity of the mixture. It is lowered by physical effort. The tolerance of the respiratory organs is somewhat increased by a high percentage of inert gas and of humidity. The early symptoms of O_2 damage of the upper respiratory tract and CNS disappear rapidly when O_2 pressure decreases, the radiologic changes in the lung less rapidly. For exposures of several weeks the average O_2 pressure should not be higher than 0.3 atm. (English summary)

1222.
MATTSSON, J.L., J.M. Stinson and C.S. Clark.
Electroencephalographic power-spectral changes coincident with onset of carbon dioxide narcosis in rhesus monkey.
Amer. J. Vet. Res. 33(10):2043-2049; 1972.

Rhesus monkeys were exposed to continually increasing chamber CO_2 concentrations to determine narcotic levels of environmental CO_2 (barometric pressure was 656 mm of Hg; chamber N_2 was replaced by CO_2 at 7.5%, 15% or 30%/hr). Due to the inaccessibility of the monkeys in an environmental control chamber, the criterion for narcosis was loss of all signs of body movement in response to loud noise. Transition from barely responsive to unresponsive occurred at CO_2 concentration of 16.8 $\pm$ 1.6%. The uncertainty of the rellationship of loss of overt response to loud noise and onset of CO_2-induced narcosis led to cortical EEG as a validating method. Examination of EEG power-spectrums as CO_2 increased demonstrated that a close relationship existed between the power loss at the 10-14 Hz. range and loss of consciousness. As narcotic concentrations of CO_2 were approached, 10- to 14-Hz power markedly decreased. When narcotic concentrations were exceeded, further 10-14-Hz power loss was minimal. This distinctive change in EEG power lent strong support to the contention that loss of overt response to loud noise and onset of narcosis were related events, and conversely, that the transition point between degraded consciousness and CO_2 narcosis could be determined by examination of EEG power-spectrums. (© BA)

1223.
MAXWELL, A.E.
Technical progress report, advanced marine technology. 1 August 1971-31 January 1972.
Woods Hole, Mass., Woods Hole Oceanogr. Inst., Rep. WHO1-72-90, 66p. Nov. 30, 1972.

This is a progress report for the period 1 August 1971 - 31 January 1972 on the following projects in Advanced Marine Technology: (a) Submerged Navigation and Submersible Instrumentation (development of precise navigation for a small submersible). (b) Handling and Transfer at Sea (use of energy absorbers in small boat and buoy handling alongside in rough weather;. (c) Bottom Reconnaissance and Detailed Site Survey (use of submersible in geological mapping). (d) Near Bottom Magnetic Studies Using a Deep Submersible. (e) Near Bottom Gravity Studies from a Deep Submersible. (f) A Self-Contained Deep Sea Rock Drill. (g) Development of Equipment for Use in Deep Ocean Biological Research (observation and collection under pressure of benthic biology). [For specific sections see the following author entries: Marquet, W.M.; Uchupi, E. and R.D. Ballard; Phillips, J.D.] (DD abstract)

1224.
MAY, G.
Underwater sound waves, barrier to killer-sharks.
Electron. Dig., p.11-12, 14;Jan./Feb. 1972.

Australia is the center of an attempt to develop a sonic shark repellant. While a sonic shark attractor has been developed, by which sharks can be successfully led away from one area into another, all the repellents that have been tried so far work for some species but not for all. In one experiment, the transmitter of the attracting signal was placed in a narrow coral cave. The sharks reached a stage of frenzy trying to locate the source of the sound, and battered themselves to death in the narrow opening of the cave. It is expected that before long a sonic repellent will be found. The transmitter can be placed in a small enough container to be used as part of a diver's equipment. It is also expected that they will be placed in the fusilage of aircraft that fly over the ocean. (MFW/BSCP)

1225.
MAZZARELLA, M.A.
Effects of dental aerosols on operatory and undersea environments.
In: Abstracts of BuMed-ONR sponsored Navywide workshop in high pressure biomedical research, U.S. Submarine Base, Groton, Conn., May 1971, p.13. Published by the Naval Submarine Medical Research Laboratory, 1971.

Abstract only. Entire item quoted: Recent work in aerobiology has shown that dental procedures disseminate airborne particulate matter of varied concentration, size and composition. The microbes sent airborne by dental procedures were found to remain buoyant for prolonged periods and could be collected and distributed by self-contained, recycling air conditioning systems. This situation could also be true for submarine personnel on prolonged submerged missions or in specialized underwater habitats working for long periods breathing recycled mechanically purified air. The aerobiological equipment used for definition of aerosol characteristics were slit-samplers to scribe upon nutrient agar a time-tracing of the microbial atmospheric burden and Andersen stage-samplers to determine particle size distribution of bacteria. A log was kept noting the time and type of dental procedure performed in order to determine relations between procedure and amount, particle size and extent of aerosol propagated. An environmentally-controlled air hood, a lavatory with 14 sinks, and two smaller submarine lavatories were studied for the reflection of toothbrushing procedures on the microbial burden of enviromental air. Toothbrushing was found to disseminate particles of varied sizes; one group large enough to have ballistic trajectory, the other group (1-3 u) small enough to travel to the alveoli of the lungs in an airborne state. Toothbrushing in the hood disseminated 2,500 bacterial particles per cubic foot of air per minute per subject. In determinations of the microbial burden of Fleet Ballistic Missile (FBM) submarine air, two of the areas with greatest amounts of viable bacterial particles were the lavatories (10 organisms/cubic foot). Subjects brushing teeth in the 14-sink room caused a 200% increase in recovery of bacteria causing a hemolytic reaction in blood agar when short-term sedimentation plates were used. This room of 2,700 cubic feet in size had an hourly fallout of 67.3 viable particles (VP) when unoccupied. This bacterial shower increased significantly to 883.2 VP when filled with subjects brushing teeth and reduced significantly to 77.6 VP 15 minutes after treatment.

1226.
McBRIDE, T.I., J.P. Vance and I. McA. Ledingham.
Changes in myocardial blood flow and oxygen consumption during acute and prolonged exposure to hyperbaric oxygen.
In: Wada, J. and I. Takashi, eds. Proceedings of the fourth international congress of hyperbaric medicine, Sept. 1969, Sapporo, Japan, p.236-238. Baltimore, Williams and Wilkins, 1970.

This study clearly demonstrates the alterations produced by high partial pressures of oxygen in myocardial blood flow and oxygen consumption. Reduction in blood flow to an organ is a well-recognised phenomenon and the myocardial blood vessels are no exception to the general rule. Unpublished data from this laboratory indicates that the vasoconstriction is likely to be due to a direct effect of oxygen on arteriolar smooth muscle. Reduction of oxygen consumption in the intact organism at partial pressure of oxygen about 1,000 mm Hg is unusual although it is known that when the partial pressure of oxygen surrounding cells exceeds 150 mm Hg enzyme inhibition occurs. Haugaard showed that oxygen consumption of rat heart homogenates was impaired during exposure to oxygen at normal pressure. The changes described in the present study may be explained on the basis of physiological adjustment to an altered environment but the possibility of a toxic action of oxygen cannot be excluded. Oxygen is known to be toxic to other organ systems but the possibility of harmful effects on the myocardium has not been extensively investigated. (From authors' discussion)

1227.
McCALLUM, R.I.
Tunnelling in compressed air and bone necrosis.
Trans. Soc. Occup. Med. 22:2-6;Jan. 1972.

The author summarizes the findings of the Medical Research Council Decompression Sickness Panel from 1923 to the time of writing (1972) concerning osteonecrosis in compressed air workers. Knowledge concerning its nature and development has been gained from following the tunnelling operations: (1) The Tyne pedestrian and cycle tunnels (1948-1950); (2) The Dartford tunnel (1963-1969); (3) The Clyde tunnels (1958-63); (4) The Tyne Road tunnel; (5) The Dungeness "B" power station (1966-1968). It has been impossible to ensure that all compressed air workers have pre-exposure and follow-up radiographs. Thus, no epidemiologically satisfactory investigation of osteonecrosis has been possible. The Panel has succeeded, however, in establishing the existence of the problem, in defining diagnostic criteria and in advising on the use of new procedures. A code of practice to raise the medical standards of compressed air work was being considered. (MFW/UMS)

1228.
McCALLUM, R.I.
Pneumoconiosis and caisson disease of bone.
Trans. Soc. Occup. Med. 22:63-68;July 1972.

These two occupational diseases are treated together because of their common dependence upon radiology for detection and management. The problems connected with radiology are discussed, and the work of The Decompression Sickness Panel in England, in the preparation of an album of illustrative lesions (Radiographic appearance of bone lesions in compressed air workers, 1968) is commended. As to radiation dose, it has been established that three routine joint examinations per year are acceptable, provided adequate protective measures are taken. Because of the fact that a lesion does not become radiographically visible until necrosis is too far advanced, other methods of detection, such as bone scans with strontium 85 or fluorine 18 are being studied. (MFW/UMS)

1229.
McCALLUM, R.I.
Aetiology of decompression sickness.
In: The Association of Clinical Pathologists: 89th general meeting. Symposium II. Decompression sickness. J. Clin. Pathol. 25:1004;Nov. 1972.

Abstract only. The author briefly describes type I and type II decompression sickness, and mentions chronic sequelae (osteonecrosis, neurologic complications and vestibular disturbances). No decompression procedures in current use are infallible. The bubble theory of the etiology of decompression sickness is at present being questioned, but no completely satisfactory explanation has been formulated. The author believes that bubbles always occur but that other body changes may be important contributors. It is stated that osteonecrosis occurs in 20% of compressed air workers and divers, and it is noted that it may result from several factors present during compression, decompression, or both. Further observations of human bone tissue are essential to the understanding of this disease. (MFW/BSCP)

1230.
McCARTHY, C., J. Slade, D. O'Connell, G. Simmons, E. Finder, M. LaForce and G.L. Huber.
Comparative resistance to pulmonary inactivation of bacterial species by the lung in oxygen toxicity.
Clin. Res. 20:879;Dec. 1972.

Abstract only. Entire item quoted: The effect of prolonged oxygen administration on host defense mechanisms in the lung was evaluated by comparing the intrapulmonary inactivation of a gram-positive and gram-negative bacterial challenge. Six hours after aerosolization of radiolabeled (^{32}P) Staphylococcus aureus, Proteus mirabilis, or Pseudomonas aeruginosa, bacterial viability and radio-tracer activity in the lungs of approximately 500 mice were quantified. Control animals (PO_2: 120 mm Hg) inactivated 92.9%, 89.5% and 90.1% of the inhaled staphylococci, proteus and pseudomonas, respectively. Prolonged administration of 100% oxygen (PO_2: 700 mm Hg) resulted in progressive impairment of antibacterial defenses proportional to the duration of oxygen exposure in all bacterial species. The initial impairment was linearly dose-dependent following exposure to 100% oxygen, with inactivation values of 78.5% and 69.2% at 24 and 48 hours of exposure for S. aureus, of 78.2% and 66.9% at 24 and 48 hours for P. mirabilis and of 87.6% at 24 hours for P. aeruginosa. Bacterial replication exceeded bacterial inactivation at 72 and 96 hours of oxygen administration with both staphylococci and proteus, and at all points beyond 48 hours with pseudomonas. Thus, host defenses in the lung are impaired in a dose-dependent manner following exposure to 100% oxygen and this impairment appears to be somewhat more severe with gram-negative organisms.

1231.
McCORMICK, J.G., T.L. Higgins, R.M. Clayton and R.W. Brauer.
Auditory and vestibular effects of helium—oxygen hyperbaric chamber dives to convulsion depths.
J. Acoust. Soc. Amer. 51(1, Pt.1):103;Jan. 1972.

Abstract only. Entire item quoted: Compressing at 24 atm/h, guinea pigs were dived in a helium-oxygen environment (0.5 atm oxygen) to a depth where the animals convulsed — 2640 ft (80 atm) to 2970 ft (90 atm). A modified Haldane decompression profile was used (28 h, 11 min from 80 atm, 22 h. 18 min from 90 atm). Post dive auditory function was assessed with cochlear potential measurements. Animals with myringotomies and tubes did not convulse significantly deeper than nontubed animals. One animal exhibited post-dive bends symptoms. This animal also had severe post-dive vestibular disorders and a severe neurosensory hearing loss. All other animals had severe or slight loss of auditory function. Much of this loss was conductive due to ear drum barotrauma. Some loss was probably neurosensory due to barotrauma or some yet undefined cause. The vestibular loss noted was similar to vestibular loss previously observed in four squirrel monkeys after two hydrogen-oxygen dives.

1232.
McCORMICK, J.G., T.L. Higgins, H.S. Daugherty and P.E. Johnson.
Cochlear dysfuncton associated with decompression from 300-ft hyperbaric chamber dives.
J. Acoust. Soc. Amer. 51(1, Pt.1):103;Jan. 1972.

Abstract only. Entire item quoted: J.D. Harris has reported [U.S. Naval Submarine Medical Center, Conn., Rep. 591, 5 Aug. 1969] severe neurosensory hearing loss in Navy divers due to decompression sickness. In an attempt to develop an animal model for this condition with verification of cochlear involvement, guinea pigs were compressed at 1 atm/min to 300 ft in air. Time at 300 ft was held constant at 6 min while decompression schedules were shortened from Navy diving tables. Animals were dived with an open bulla to eliminate barotrauma to the ear drum, and cochlear potentials were measured postdive. The general finding was the onset of auditory loss 10-15 min postdive. Severe loss (40-50 dB) was usually present by at least 1 hr postdive. The loss remained stable 2-5 h postdive, and became more severe 6 h postdive.

1233.
McCORMICK, J.G., T. Philbrick, W. Holland and J.A. Harrill.
Diving induced sensori-neural deafness: prophylactic use of heparin and preliminary histopathology results.
Laryngoscope 43:1483-1501;Sept. 1973.
(Also published in Proceedings of the 76th annual meeting of the American Laryngological, Rhimological and Otological Society, St. Louis, April 1973, p.1-19.)

[It has been] postulated that hypercoagulation, embolic, and thrombotic problems may precipitate sudden deafness by affecting the microcirculation of the inner ear. These syndromes have been found to occur in decompression sickness and deafness and vestibular attacks are known to occur with diving. The authors were able to demonstrate severe cochlear potential losses in guinea pigs with the induction of decompression sickness. The problem was largely prevented by the prophylactic administration of heparin. Preliminary studies of the temporal bones of a guinea pig with a severe post-dive vestibular attack and loss of cochlear potential function showed the presence of hemorrhage in the perilymph of the auditory and vestibular system. The above results are interpreted as evidence that hypercoagulation, embolic and thrombotic problems may precipitate a loss of cochlear dysfunction — most likely in a diving situation and potentially in cases of sudden deafness not related to diving. (Authors' abstract)

1234.
McCORMICK, J.G., T. Philbrick and W. Holland.
The pathophysiology of diving induced sensory neural deafness as elucidated by beneficial prophylactic use of heparin.
In: Ackles, K.N. ed. Blood bubble interaction in decompresion sickness. Proceedings of an international symposium held at Defence and Civil Institute of Environmental Medicine, Downsview, Ontario, Canada, p.272-297. Published by the Institute, December 1973. (DCIEM Conference Proceedings 73-CP-960)

Electrodes were implanted on the round window of the guinea pigs ears, to measure cochlear hearing loss during a 300-foot chamber dive, carried out according to the U.S. Navy tables except for the ommission of the 20-foot and 10-foot decompresion stops. A significant loss of sensitivity occurred, and even persisted 21 hours post-dive, although there was some spontaneous recovery. Measurement of cochlear potential intensity function showed a severe loss of maximum potential, for both 1,000 cycles per second and 10,000 cycles per second, at two hour post-dive. Some spontaneous recovery occurred, followed, by a severe residual loss at 22 hours post-dive. Damage was much less in the heparin-treated (2.5 mg/kg) animals; although there was slight hearing loss. It is noted that in considering bubbles as etiological factors diving-related deafness and vestibular dysfunction, it is also necessary to consider coagulation, thrombic problems and platelet aggregation. (MFW/UMS)

1235.
McCULLOUGH, D.
The great bridge.
New York, Simon and Schuster, 1972. 636p.

This account of the building of the Brooklyn Bridge contains chapters that deal mainly with decompression sickness, which was at that time very little understood. At about the same time, Paul Bert was publishing his research into the etiology of the disorder, but his bubble theory was not universally accepted in the United States. The St. Louis bridge across the Mississippi was constructed just ahead of the Brooklyn Bridge. Fifteen fatalities from decompression occurred. Three are here described at the Brooklyn Bridge. Dr. Andrew Smith was hired as medical advisor. He had little to go on except the data gathered by Dr. Jaminet during the building of the St. Louis bridge. He set up a system of medical fitness examinations and set forth a list of safety regulations. While rejecting Bert's bubble theory, Smith did recognize the combined importance of speed of decompression, degree of pressure, and duration of exposure. He recognized the therapeutic value of recompression, and recommended the construction of a surface pressure chamber, but this recommendation was apparently not followed. (MFW/UMS)

1236.
McELROY, P.T.
Use of a coherent frequency synthesizer in echo-sounder studies of deep scattering layers.
Woods Hole, Mass., Woods Hole Oceanog. Inst., Rep. WHOI-72-30, 12p. May, 1972.
(AD 742 824)

A coherent frequency synthesizer under computer control is used to generate a pulse train which is power amplified and drives a UQN transducer. A pulse train at the two frequencies, 9.5 and 17 kHz, is used to examine the deep scattering layers at 35 degrees 00 min N, 48 degrees 00 min W during the sunset migration. Striking differences in the scattering returns, as displayed on a facsimile recorder, show the utility of this method for increased frequency coverage in studies of deep scattering layers. (Author) (GRA)

1237.
McEVOY, J.D.S., N.L. Jones and E.J.M. Campbell.
Alveolar-arterial PCO_2 difference during rebreathing in patients with chronic hypercapnia.
J. Appl. Physiol. 35:542-545;Oct. 1973.

Six patients in chronic respiratory failure due to chornic obstructive bronchitis rebreathed mixtures of CO_2 in O_2 in order to obtain an equilibrium of CO_2 in the gas passing between the rebreathing bag and lungs. Arterial blood was sampled duirng the maneuver, 5 sec being allowed for the lung-arm circulation time. In 23 comparisons between the PCO_2 of alveolar gas and of arterial blood, the mean gas-blood difference was 0.3 mm Hg ($\pm$SD 1.76 mmHg). It was concluded that there is no significant alveolar-arterial CO_2 difference during rebreathing in patients with chronic hypercapnia. (Authors' abstract)

1238.
McHALE, E.T.
Habitable atmospheres which do not support combustion.
Alexandria, Va., Atlantic Research Corp., Rep. on Contract DAHC 19-71-C-0026, 155p. Mar. 1972.
(AD-741,808)

It is believed that atmospheres can be developed which will not support combustion of ordinary materials such as paper, plastics, solvents, etc., and in which humans will be able to live and function normally for extended periods of time. Such atmospheres would contain relatively small amounts (10-20%) of certain fully-fluorinated agents (CF4, C2F6, or C3F8) added to air. The presence of the agents would not appreciably affect the life support process. The objective of the present study was to evaluate the validity of this concept. The toxicity tests included acute and ten-day inhalation studies on rats and guinea pigs and cardiac sensitization tests on dogs (with CF4). (Author) (GRA)

1239.
McKEE, D.L.
A study of underwater diver tactile sensitivity.
U.S. Nav. Postgrad. Sch., Thesis, 53p. Mar. 1972.
(AD 743,709)

The thesis examines the effects of underwater submersion and prolonged underwater submersion on a diver's tactile sensitivity. The method of constant stimulus is used to determine size discrimination thresholds. The stimuli used are squares of hard acrylic plastic into which holes of varying diameters have been drilled. Four tests were administered to each subject. One test was administered on dry land in the open air and served as the standard. The other three tests were administered underwater at various time intervals. The conclusion drawn from this research is that a diver's tactile sensitivity as measured by his ability to make size discrimination is not affected by underwater submersion or even prolonged underwater submersion of sixty-six minutes. Furthermore, the thresholds of approximately one millimeter, determined in this thesis are consistent with the findings of past research in this field. (Author's abstract)

1240.
McKENNEY, J.
Mako Purus air compressor.
Skin Diver 20:24-25; 80;Jan. 1971.

The article describes a portable air compressor, the Mako Purus, developed by Mako Products in Miami. It can fill a standard tank in 36 minutes. It weighs only seven pounds, measures 12 inches by 18-1/2 inches by 26 inches. Machines are adjusted to vent off when the pressure reached 3,200 psi, but this adjustment can be set lower if desired. The basic compressor is of German manufacture (Bauer). It is driven by Sachs gasoline engine. The type of oil used is most important. Details of maintenance are discussed. Frequent checking inspection, cleaning and oil changing are essential. (MFW/SCD)

1241.
McKENNEY, J.
The Farallon DPV.
Skin Diver 20:24-27;Oct. 1971.

It is noted that the use of a diver propulsion vehicle (DPV) to transport a diver to and from a work site, or on an inspection of underwater installations, will greatly enhance his range and time by preventing fatigue and conserving his air supply, which would be used up much more quickly during the exertion of swimming unaided. The DPV's described here are the Farallon DPV MK-II and MK-III. The latter allows for a wide range of power thrusts, which enables it to increase its duration of operation. At full speed, both have a duration of one hour, but there is available as an extra accessory a battery pack which will double this time. The cylindrical aluminum units, anodized and finished with international orange, carry a 109,000 candle power 12-volt headlamp and a three-bladed 7 1/2 inch propeller made of unbreakable polycarbonate. They weigh 50 pounds in air, and have a one-half pound positive buoyancy in sea water, which is adjustable to two pounds negative. They pull the diver along at about the speed of a strong swimmer. They are guaranteed to 300 feet, but have been used successfully to 512 feet. They are in wide use internationally, both by navies and by professional diving companies. (MFW/BSCP)

1242.
McKENNEY, J.
Aqueon — the underwater swimming machine.
Skin Diver 20:30, 57;Nov. 1971.

The Aqueon consists basically of a tubular aluminum shaft with wooden crosspieces at each end. It is fastened to the diver via leg boards. To propel the machine the swimmer holds his body as straight as possible, arms forward, bends the knees slightly, then briskly straightens them out, thus activating the front blades. In a test made with Navy divers, a 1500 yard swim which took 44 minutes and 30 seconds with fins, took 24 minutes with the Aqueon. It has been demonstrated that actual muscular effort output with Aqueon was one-fifth of what it would be with fins. Depth control is found to be excellent. (MFW/BSCP)

1243.
McKENNEY, J.
The Farallon shark darts.
Skin Diver 21:28, 30;Feb. 1972.

The various models of the shark dart range from a small (12-1/2 inch) version, through medium and large-sized versions, to a repeater version that operates on compressed air. The dart was originally developed by the Naval Undersea Research and Development Center, and further elaborated by Farallon Industries. Because of the small size of the shark brain, it is most difficult to incapacitate the animal by a spear gun. The shark's abdominal cavity contains all his vital organs and when he is hit anywhere in this cavity with a dart, the high pressure gas (1000 psi) demolishes his internal organs, blows his stomach out of his mouth and forces him to the surface. It is emphasized that this is purely a defensive weapon, and is not intended for use in the hunting and killing of sharks for sport. (MFW/BSCP)

1244.
McKENNEY, J.
The ACR Firefly rescue light.
Skin Diver 22:16;July 1972.

The light is 4 3/8 inches by 2 5/8 inches by 1 inch, weighs 7 1/2 ounces, and is pressure tested to 200 feet. It consists of a strobe light with a xenon tube, and a 4.6 V mercury battery. Maintenance consists merely of a freshwater rinse, cleaning the o-ring, and keeping the battery compartment dry. It is useful in rescue situations, and also in cave diving, night diving and wreck diving. It has a visibility of 150 feet underwater, five miles at sea level, and 15 miles from the air. A small styrofoam float will keep it upright on the surface. (MFW/SCD)

1245.
McKENNEY, J.
Cave diving is not for sport divers.
Skin Diver 22:4-5;May 1973.

The author discusses at some length the alarming increase in cave diving fatalities in the Florida springs and the steps that are being taken to combat it. The National Association for Cave Divers has conducted research into accidents, recovered many of the victims, conducted seminars, and compiled a set of safety rules, which are given here, and a list of specialized equipment mandatory for cave diving. They have trained and certified 11 cave diving instructors. The NACD has explored and mapped most of the more popular caves, and have posted warning signs. They have issued several publications which are available at moderate cost from Jack Banbury, Publications Chairman of NACD, Institute of Marine Science, 10 Rickenbacker Causeway, Miami, Fla. 33149. (MFW/BSCP)

1246.
McKENNEY, J.
Up to our snorkels in masks.
Skin Diver 22:18-21;June 1973.

The author covers the masks currently on the market which retail for $10.00 or more. A chart tabulates for each mask its price, basic shape, purge valve size and type, weight in ounces, retaining band material, type of band fastener, type of strap fastener, volume, and special features. Numerous models are illustrated by photographs. In selecting a mask, the author states the most important points to be fit, air-tightness, pliability of the skirt, low volume, tempered and hardened lenses for eye protection in case of breakage. A mask is an exceedingly personal piece of equipment and must be selected with the individual's comfort and special requirements as the chief considerations. (MFW/BSCP)

1247.
McSHERRY, C.K. and H. Gilder.
Pulmonary oxygen toxicity and surfactant.
In: Wada, J. and I. Takashi, eds. Proceedings of the fourth international congress on hyperbaric medicine, Sapporo, Japan, Sept. 1969, p.10-15. Baltimore, Williams and Wilkins, 1970.

The acute exposure of rabbits to increasing concentration of OHP is associated with a progressive decrease in lung surfactant as measured by the incorporation of C^{14} palmitic acid into lung phospholipids. Chronic OHP exposures are also associated with alterations in surfactant but the response is not dose dependent. Surfactant is believed to have an important role in the pathogenesis of pulmonary oxygen toxicity. (Authors' summary)

1248.
McSHERRY, C.K.
The role of surfactant in the etiology of pulmonary oxygen toxicity.
In: Abstracts of BuMed-ONR sponsored Navywide workshop in high pressure biomedical research, U.S. Naval Submarine Base, Groton, Conn., May 1971, p. 7. Published by the Naval Submarine Medical Research Laboratory, 1971.

Abstract only. Entire item quoted: The authors summarize the background data which suggested that the inactivation of surfactant by oxygen was important in the pathogenesis of pulmonary oxygen toxicity. The methods employed for measuring lung surfactant are described including the use of the modified Wilhelmy tonometer, and the biochemical assay of surfactant utilizing the incorporation of ^{14}C-labelled fatty acid into lung phospholipid. Improvements in the latter technique by the application of thin layer chromatography are discussed. In an effort to correlate the extent of lung damage induced by oxygen breathing with the degree of inactivation of surfactant, a dose response curve has been constructed for rabbits exposed to 2 ATA and 3 ATA for 1, 3 and 5 hours. The author has also attempted to correlate surfactant levels with chemical, dietary and hormonal factors known to alter the pulmonary response to oxygen breathing. To date the effect of THAM, dibenzyline, tetraethylammonium chloride, hexamethonium, low fat and vitamin E deficient diets have been studied and will be described. The author concludes the presentation with a plan for studying the synthetic pathways of dipalmitoyl lecithin, the principal surface active substance in the lungs.

1249.
MECKELNBURG, R.L.
To dive or not to dive.
Delaware Med. J. 44:91-92;Mar. 1972.

The author lists the following as absolute contraindications to diving: epilepsy, diabetes, inability to equalize pressure in middle ears and sinuses, alcohol or drug addiction, mental retardation, and unrepaired facial defects. Relative contraindications are: overweight, poor physical condition, high blood pressure, perforated ear drums, sinus problems, claustrophobia, asthma, emphysema, myocardial infarction and cardiac defects, and pregnancy. The conditions in the second group are discussed briefly, and the relative quality of these possible deterrents is emphasized. It becomes a matter chiefly of degree, and of careful analysis of the individual case. (MFW/BSCP)

1250.
MELESHKO, G.I., A.A. Antonyan, A.I. Kazakov and Ye. K. Lepedeva.
Investigation of the effect of increased oxygen concentrations on chlorella metabolism.
Space Biol. Med. 7:60-65;May 15, 1973.
(JPRS 59015)

The intensity of Chlorella photosynthesis is linearly dependent on atmospheric oxygen concentration. In the range of 5-50% O_2 an increase in the oxygen concentration by 10% decreases photosynthesis intensity on the average by 15% of the initial level. An increase in atmospheric oxygen concentration results in an increase in the content of biogenous elements in algal cells. An increase in the nitrogen content in cells was caused by the nonprotein fraction of organic nitrogen, whereas an increase in the quantity of phosphorus in cells occurs at the expense of the acid-soluble fraction of organic phosphorus. (Authors' abstract)

1251.
MELKA, L.A. and J.A. Henkener.
Oil contamination and control in diver's breathing air.
In: Battelle Columbus Laboratories. Proceedings, 1973 divers' gas purity symposium, November 27-28, 1973, p.XIX-1-XIX-24. U.S Navy Supervisor Diving, Nav. Ships Syst. Comm., Rep 2-73, 1973.

The U.S. Navy has been focusing more and more attention on the quality of air that their divers receive from compressed air breathing systems. One of the major contaminate areas and the most difficult to detect and control is oil mist, which is introduced by oil lubricated compressors. Considerable control of oil mist contamination originating from air compressors can be accomplished by proper system design and periodic air sampling and analysis. To properly design a diver's breathing air systems, all elements of the system must be considered in relationship to each other. The insights and information obtained from field inspections at three diving activities are discussed in this report to assist designers and operators in more effectively limiting the oil mist contamination in diving compressed air breathing systems. (Authors' abstract)

1252.
MENGEL, C.E.
The effects of hyperoxia on red cells as related to tocopherol deficiency.
Ann. N.Y. Acad. Sci. 203:163-171;Dec. 1972.

The studies reported herein deal primarily with the damaging effects of hyperoxia on red blood cells and the relationship between susceptibility to these effects and tocopherol status. . . [It was found] that tocopherol-supplemented animals had normal hematocrits before being exposed to hyperoxia and showed no change afterwards. Their cells were also resistent to lysis by hydrogen peroxide. Similar results were obtained in chow-fed animals. In contrast, the red cells of tocopherol-deficient mice showed an increased in vitro lytic sensitivity to hydrogen peroxide and also a marked hemolytic susceptibility to hyperoxia, as illustrated by the fall in hematocrit from 49% to 25%. . . These series of studies have shown that the tocopherol status of animals can be an important determinant of red cell viability under conditions of oxidant stress. It would appear that either environmental or drug induced oxidant stress may result in alterations of red cells as a consequence of tocopherol deficiency. Although the basic mechanisms responsible for this are not entirely clear, it appears that the predominant mechanism in the damage and lysis of red cells in these circumstances is the peroxidation of lipids, with the rupture of unsaturated fatty acid bonds, the loss of integrity of red cell membranes and ultimate osmotic lysis. (Author)

1253.
MESSETER, K. and B.K. Siesjo.
The intracellular pH in the brain in acute and sustained hypercapnia.
Acta Physiol. Scand. 83(2):210-219; 1971.

The regulation of intracellular pH in the brain was studied in rats exposed to about 11% CO_2 for periods of 15 min-72 hours. At the end of each exposure period cisternal cerebrospinal fluid and supratentorial parts of the brain were sampled and analyzed for CO_2 contents. The intracellular HCO_3- concentration was calculated assuming extracellular volumes of 12, 15, and 20%, respectively, and the intracellular pH was derived from the HCO_3- concentration and mean tissue CO_2 tension. Acute hypercapnia (15 min) was associated with an increase in the intracellular HCO_3-concentration of about 6 meq/kg of i.c. water. With an extracellular volume of 15% the corresponding decrease in intracellular pH [pH_i] was from 7.06 to 6.93. When the hypercapnia was upheld there was a further increase in the intracellular HCO_3- concentration of about 5 meq/kg and an increase in pH_i to about 7.03. Most of this regulation of pH_i occurred during the first three hours. An analysis of the regulating mechanisms suggests that physicochemical buffering, metabolic consumption of acids, and transmembrane fluxes of H^+ or HCO_3- each controlled about one-third of the total accumulation of bicarbonate in the cell during hypercapnia. (© BA)

1254.
MESSETER, K., U. Ponten and B.K. Siesjo.
The influence of deep barbiturate anesthesia upon the regulation of extra- and intracellular pH in the rat brain during hypercapnia.
Acta. Physiol. Scand. 85(2):174-182; 1972.

To study the influence of deep barbiturate anesthesia upon the regulation of extra- and intracellular pH in the brain, hypercapnia was induced in rats anesthetized for maximally three hours with either 200-250 mg/kg of phenobarbital, or with 0.6% halothane. There were no differences in the regulation of the CSF [cerebrospinal fluid] pH between the groups studied. Both at 15 min. and at three hours, phenobarbital anesthesia was associated with a less efficient regulation of the intracellular pH. At 15 min the regulation observed came close to that expected on the basis of pure physicochemical buffering. Deep phenobarbital anesthesia, probably due to its effect on metabolism, can interfere with the mechanisms which regulate intracellular pH during hypercapnia. (© BA)

1255.
MESSIER, A.A., E. Heyder and K.E. Schaefer.
Effect of 90-day exposure to 1% CO_2 on acid-base status of blood.
U.S. Nav. Submar. Med. Cent., Rep. SMRL 655, 10p. Mar. 2, 1971.

The problem was to determine whether a prolonged exposure to an equivalent of 1% CO_2 in a simulated space-station environment is similar in its effect on the acid-base status of blood to a prolonged exposure in a Fleet Ballistic Missile (FBM) submarine. The results of this study showed a mild respiratory acidosis during the first three weeks of exposure followed by a return to control values during the fourth to seventh weeks of the experiment. The acid-base and electrolyte shifts during this time period are consistent and comparable with data obtained during FBM patrols of seven to eight weeks' duration. As the exposure extended into the eighth week, a mild secondary respiratory acidosis developed. The development of this secondary acidosis was related to a fluctuation that occurred in the CO_2 level of the space-station simulator resulting from difficulties with the solid amine CO_2 scrubber system. This report will be valuable to those interested in acid-base and electrolyte shifts occurring in long-term, low-level CO_2 exposures in closed environments, such as in undersea habitations or in space stations. (Authors' summary)

1256.
MESSIER, A.A. and K.E. Schaefer.
The Bohr effect in chronic hypercapnia.
U.S. Nav. Submar. Med. Res. Lab., Rep. NSMRL 732, 10p. Dec. 13, 1972.
(A similar paper was published in Resp. Physiol. 19:26-34;Oct. 1973)

Male guinea pigs (Hartley strain, 400-600 grams) were exposed to 15% CO_2, 21% O_2, balance N_2 for varying periods of time up to seven days. The Bohr effect factor, $\Delta \log P_{50}/\Delta pH$, was determined by a CO_2 titration method. Blood pH, PCO_2, standard $[HCO_3^-]$, Base Excess, 2,3-Diphosphoglycerate (DPG), 50% oxyhemoglobin saturation (P_{50}), and other hematological parameters were measured concurrently. The Bohr effect was significantly elevated (+22%) above control during the first three days of exposure and approached the control level by the seventh day of exposure (+5%), although it remained still significantly increased. In this in vivo model, the Bohr effect was correlated with blood pH and PCO_2 levels but not with DPG levels. The effective Bohr effect, which is calculated as the additional O_2 released at 50% oxyhemoglobin saturation when blood is acidified from pH 7.4 to 7.3 was found to be elevated during the periods of uncompensated respiratory acidosis (i.e., 1 hr., 6 hrs., 1 day), indicating facilitation of O_2 delivery to the tissues. If the P_{50} values were calculated for in vivo pH and body temperature, the opposing actions of a direct pH effect on hemoglobin causing an increased Bohr effect and the indirect pH effect changing the DPG concentration via metabolic alterations could be separated. The increased Bohr effect was found to compensate the displacement of the oxygen dissociation curve to the left produced by the fall in DPG concentration. A high correlation of P_{50} to the base excess (-.96) existed during this period. These findings are of interest to personnel concerned with toxicological aspects of increased carbon dioxide exposure as potentially found in Navy submarine and diving environments as well as other hazards which might induce an acidosis such as hyperbaric hyperoxia. The demonstration of an alteration of the Bohr effect factor may be of interest to clinicians who generally use a constant Bohr effect. (Authors' abstract and application)

1257.
MEUNIER, J.-L.
Les accidents auriculaires barotraumatiques chez les plongeurs sous-marins.
[Auricular barotraumatic accidents in underwater divers].
Rev. Laryngol. Otol. Rhinol. 93:586-594;Sept./Oct. 1972.

The author first mentions the widely known clinical and physio-pathological features which characterize baro-trauma to the middle ear, and then emphasizes the possibility of the development of a perceptive deafness caused by barotrauma to the inner ear, during or immediately after diving. He divides these into two types: deafness caused by compression, encountered during the diver's descent, and deafness caused by decompression, which occurs during [or after] surfacing. The clinical features, physio-pathology, and treatment of these two types of deafness are discussed. (English summary)

1258.
MEYER, E.F.
Analysis of underwater acoustic propagation loss math models in current training devices.
U.S. Nav. Training Equip. Cent., Rep. NAVTRAEQUIPCEN-IH-200, 46p. Aug. 1972.
(AD 750,694)

The report analyzes and compares the various simulation designs and math models of underwater acoustic simulation presently being used in current training devices developed by the Naval Training Device Center. The analysis contains model simplifications and their effects on acoustic propagation loss. The results of these models are compared with the results of the ray trace model developed by the Naval Air Development Center. (Author) (GRA)

1259.
MEYRICK, B., J. Miller and L. Reid.
Pulmonary oedema induced by ANTU, or by high or low oxygen concentrations in rat — an electron microscopic study.
Brit. J. Exp. Path. 53:347-358;Aug. 1972.

Pulmonary oedema has been experimentally induced in rats using either an intraperitoneal injection of alpha-naphthyl thiourea (ANTU) or by variation of atmospheric oxygen content. For the first time an electron microscopic study of the development of ANTU-induced lung oedema has been made. At 2 hours blebbing and scalloping of endothelial cells and interstitial oedema were observed, each showing increasing severity with increase of dose-3, 10 and 50 mg/kg doses. By 6 hours in the 50 mg/kg treated animals, epithelial damage was also apparent. No alteration in mean alveolar size or in the distribution of alveolar lining cells was found. The breathing rate of the rats was slowed for the first 3 hours and then increased well above normal levels. Hyperoxic conditions (99-100% O_2 at 1 atm/pressure) produced interstitial oedema by 6 hours, followed at 24 hours by both endothelial and eipithelial damage. Hypoxic conditions (7-10% O_2 at 1 atm/pressure) did not produce these effects. Both hyperoxic and hypoxic conditions were associated with a significant increase in the mean alveolar size, an apparent decrease in number of Type III pneumonocytes and in the macrophages when related to alveolar cell number, while the counts of Types I and II pneumonocytes remained within the normal range. (Authors' summary)

1260.
MICHAELSON, E.D. and B. O'Byrne.
Effects of varying inspired oxygen concentrations (FIO_2) on pulmonary mechanics.
In: Aerospace Medical Association. 1973 annual scientific meeting, Las Vegas, Nevada, May 1973. Preprints, p.40-41. Published by the Association, 1973.

One of the adverse effects of breathing pure oxygen is the occurrence of absorption atelectasis in alveoli distal to areas of temporary obstruction. These occluded areas may be present with certain pulmonary diseases, during anesthesia, or during airway closure which occurs when the lung is exposed to $+G_z$ accelerative forces. Unfortuantely, these are also the circumstances in which a high FIO_2 is desirable, and in which a vicious cycle of increased atelectasis, shunting, and oxygen requirement can occur. It is generally agreed that the presence of atelectasis is reflected by a fall in pulmonary compliance. To the extent that this is true, our data reflect the relationship between FIO_2 and the development of atelectasis. The similar changes in compliance and functional residual capacity (FRC) as a function of FIO_2 suggest that the observed reductions in compliance are directly related to the degree of atelectasis. Although the alveoli have elastic resistance to atelectasis, a positive transpulmonary pressure is required to open them if they are completely collapsed. Intermittent sighing or positive pressure breathing would be expected to minimize the development of collapse during oxygen breathing, although their effectiveness might be limited by the very factors which render the lung prone to absorption atelectasis. It appears that a 70/30 or 60/40 O_2/N_2 mixture would provide a reasonable compromise for minimizing atelectasis during acceleration, general anesthesia, and in certain pulmonary diseases where supplemental oxygen is required. (Authors)

1261.
MICHAUD, A., J. LeChuiton, J. Parc, L. Barthelemy, G. Balouet, E. Girin, J. Corriol and J. Chouteau.
Bilan d'une experimentation animale de plongees aux melanges hydrogene-oxygene.
[Report on an animal experiment in dives with hydrogen-oxygen mixtures].
Toulon, France, Marine Nationale, Groupe d'Etudes et Recherches Sous-marines, Rep. 01/73/GERS, 51p. 18 June 1973.

Oxygen hydrogen breathing mixtures, which would seem to bring about an improvement in ventilatory dynamics and alveolocapillary gas exchange because of their lighter density, give hope of pushing back further the depth limits reached with oxygen-helium mixtures. However, the authors have established the existence of a toxic effect of these mixtures, which seem to occur only after a certain duration of exposure, which differs according to the species of animal used; thus the hope remains that oxygen-hydrogen mixtures can be used under certain conditions and for brief exposures in human diving. Use by man should not be envisaged until definitive conclusions have been reached with animals. (Authors' conclusion translated by MFW/SCD)

1262.
MICHEL, D.
Electronics are important to diving.
Offshore 32:36, 38, 42;Aug. 1972.

In this article the following applications of electronics in diving equipment are discussed: (1) communications, (2) television, and (3) instrumentation. Two underwater telephone systems are the Landry phone and the Helle phone; a phone similar to the former is currently manufactured in the laboratory of the Taylor Diving and Salvage Company. The first moderately successful helium speech unscrambler was Model 702A, produced by Integrated Electronics; this gave 85 per cent intelligibility at 1000 feet. The currently most widely used unscrambler is Helle Engineering's Model WP 10H. This has been 100 percent successful at 600 feet. Wireless communication systems for scuba divers operate on high frequencies (42 KhZ) to avoid interference, since long distance communication between divers is unnecessary. The Helle Model HE10 can be encapsulated into a very small cylinder. Television is discussed as an essential tool in well-head monitoring, search and recovery, inspection and survey, as well as in monitoring divers wherever they happen to be. Video tapes are invaluable as permanent records. Under the heading of "instrumentation," the author discusses saturation diving techniques as employed since 1965 in the oil industry. The system consists of a deck chamber pressurized to bottom in which the workers live for the duration of a particular job, a pressurized diving bell in which they travel to the work area, and some type of work chamber or habitat on the bottom. Instrumentation comes into the picture in the form of atmosphere control: oxygen controller, sensors for temperature and humidity control, carbon dioxide removal, and monitors of oxygen and carbon dioxide levels. Depth and pressure are also recorded electronically. Physiological monitoring of divers is carried out electronically in diving research laboratories, such as that operated by Taylor Diving at Belle Chasse. Another form of electronic instrumentation is test equipment. Taylor Diving, for instance, operates a 1250 square foot laboratory devoted exclusively to electronics. Also, every major diving job employs at least one electronics expert. (MFW/SCD)

1263.
MICHENFELDER, J.D., R.H. Miller and G.A. Gronert.
Evaluation of an ultrasonic device (Doppler) for the diagnosis of venous air embolism.
Anesthesiology 36:164-167;Feb. 1972.

While being operated on in the upright position, 69 patients were monitored with an ultrasonic device (Doppler) to detect venous air embolism. A right atrial catheter had been inserted previously. Air embolism was suspected or confirmed on 29 occasions in 22 patients. Twenty episodes were signaled by change in the Doppler sounds and confirmed by aspirating air bubbles from the atrium; only one patient developed clinical air embolism. Seven episodes suspected because of characteristic Doppler sound changes were not confirmed by aspirating air or by the development of clinical signs. Two episodes were signaled by the onset of a systolic murmur and confirmed by aspirating air from the atrium; neither was accompanied by changes in Doppler sounds. No patient had complications secondary to air embolism. It is concluded that air embolism is common during operations with the patients upright; that serious sequelae can be minimized by early diagnosis and prompt treatment; and that the Doppler device detects air embolism sensitively but imperfectly. (Authors' abstract)

1264.
MILLARD, R.W., K. Johansen and W.K. Milsom.
Radiotelemetry of cardiovascular responses to exercise and diving in penguins.
Comp. Biochem Physiol. (A) 46(2):227-240; 1973.

Cardiovascular adjustments to voluntary exercise and diving were studied in 2 species of penguins (*Pygoscelis papua* and *P. adeliae*) using techniques for telemetry of blood flow, blood pressure and heart rate. Free exercise resulted in a rise in heart rate (from 122-278 beats/min), mean blood pressure (from 92—163 mm Hg) and femoral blood flow (from 24—59 ml/min). This response was little modified when birds were exercised on a treadmill. Arterial O_2 tension (PaO_2) during exercise rose from 70—80 mm Hg while venous O_2 tension (PVO_2) fell from 38 to 28 mm Hg, resulting in increased O_2 utilization. Severe exercise reduced arterial pH from 7.55 to 7.25. In free swimming, heart rate was 227 beats/min, femoral flow 50/min and carotid flow 55 ml/min. During voluntary dives heart rate fell to approximately 1/3rd femoral flow to 1/4th, and carotid flow by 30%. Forced dives differed by causing considerable struggling accompanied by transient changes in heart rate and blood flows. Only minor changes in blood O_2 tensions and pH were observed after free diving. Forced dives of 90-120 sec caused reductions of PaO_2 from 82.4 to 33.5 mm Hg, PVO_2 from 43.5 to 27.5 mm Hg while pH fell from 7.48 to 7.37. Recovery showed a continued but transient decline in pH and PVO_2. At 30 sec pH was 7.27 and PVO_2 25 mm Hg, while PaO_2 rose near control, 71.5 mm Hg. (© BA)

1265.
MILLER, E.F. and A. Graybiel.
Semicircular canals as a primary etiological factor in motion sickness.
Aerosp. Med. 43:1065-1074, Oct. 1972.

Data are presented which support the view that the semi-circular canals of humans can act as the essential factor for the production of motion sickness and the evocation of symptoms characteristic of this malady in the absence of "motion". Quantitative grading of acute symptoms demonstrated that motion sickness can be evoked by stimuli which are adequately provocative and unique for the canals. These results are compared with those of two provocative rotational tests that introduce Coriolis (cross-coupled angular acceleration) forces or generate a rotating linear acceleration vector. Wide interindividual differences but only slight intraindividual differences among the six provocative test conditions are revealed, indicating that individuals usually possess an overall susceptibility to motion which is relatively independent of its type. The pattern of symptoms manifested by the group of ten subjects at the test end point, moderate malaise, is also similar among these tests. The fact that typical symptoms of motion sickness (M IIA endpoint) were produced also by bithermal irrigation of several subjects who represented a wide range of susceptibility adds to the evidence that semicircular canals can act as the primary etiological factor in this malady. (Authors' abstract)

1266.
MILLER, J.D.
The effects of hyperbaric oxygen at 2 and 3 atmospheres absolute and intravenous mannitol on experimentally increased intracranial pressure.
Eur. Neurol. 10(1):1-11; 1973.

Hyperbaric O_2 at 2 atm absolute, which increased arterial PO_2 [O_2 tension] to 1227 mm Hg, caused a 30% reduction in intracranial pressure, which had been artificially increased in anesthetized dogs by cerebral cold injury. The accompanying changes in cerebral venous blood gases were consistent, with a reduction of cerebral blood flow. Hyperbaric O_2 at 3 atm absolute increased arterial PO_2 to 1891 mm Hg, but failed to reduce intracranial pressure. The cerebral venous blood gas measurements suggested that there was no cerebral vasoconstriction. I.v. mannitol solution, administered at the end of the experiments, produced a 37% reduction of intracranial pressure. (© BA)

1267.
MILLER, J.N., O.D. Wangensteen and E.H. Lanphier.
Respiratory limitations to work at depth.
In: Fructus, X., ed. Third international conference on hyperbaric and underwater physiology, p.118-123. Paris, Doin, 1972.

In summary, expiratory flow is limited by the inherent mechanical properties of the lung-airway system, and not by the effort required to expel gas from the lungs. This mechanism is the main factor contributing to the limitation of pulmonary ventilation at depth. Attempting to maintain external work at a depth beyond that at which ventilation is limited results in carbon dioxide retention and consequently, limitation of the work performed itself. It is unlikely that this sequence of mechanisms limits the performance of work done underwater with conventional underwater breathing apparatus. The resistance afforded by commercially available breathing valves is such that although effort-independent expiratory flow may be attainable, perhaps it may not be sustained. In that event the work of breathing through the external applied resistance would then become the limiting factor. (Authors)

1268.
MILLER, J.N. and M. Winsborough.
The effect of increased gas density upon $\dot{V}A/\dot{Q}$ and gas exchange during expiratory flow-limited exercise.
In: Hesser, C.M. and D. Linnarsson eds. Procedings of the first annual scientific meeting of the European Undersea Biomedical Society, Stockholm, 13-15 June 1973. Forsvarsmedicin 9:321-331;July 1973.

The authors compared the effect on gas exchange and $\dot{V}A/\dot{Q}c$ (alveolar ventilation/cardiac output) with subjects breathing air and those breathing SF_6O_2 (a five-fold increase in density). The overall results indicated that the regional distribution of gas exchange was not affected by increased density, and the decrease in $\dot{V}A/\dot{Q}c$ was a function of insufficient pulmonary ventilation. Increased gas turbulence tends to offset regional maldistribution of gas in the blood. Tables, drawings, graphs and diagrams illustrate in detail the various phases of the experiments. (MFW/UMS)

1269.
MILLER, J.W., J.G. Van Derwalker and R.A. Waller.
Tektite 2. Scientists-in-the-sea.
Washington, D.C., U.S. Department of the Interior, August 1971. 618p.

This is a complete report on the Tektite 2 project. Unlike Tektite 1, which was primarily a feasibility study, Tektite 2 had as its main purpose basic scientific programs. A large part of the report deals with the marine science studies, but there are numerous sections which deal with such things as equipment evaluation, habitability, behavior and performance, medical aspects, and communications. Specific sections have been abstracted separately and will be found under the following author entries: Bakeman, R. and R. Helmreich; Beckman, E.L., R.G. Masson and E.M. Smith; Chandeysson, P.L.; Cobet, A.B.; Deutsch, S.; Helmreich, R. (four); Helmreich, R., J. Wilhelm and R. Bakeman; Hollien, H.; Lambertsen, C.J.; LeFan, J.H. and R. Helmreich; Nowlis, D., H.H. Watters and E.C. Wortz; Schmidt, R.J.; Smith, M.C. Jr.; C.S. Huber, G.A. Swaney and C. Stadler; Tanney, J.B., Jr.; Waller, R.A. (three); Watters, H.H.; Wilhelm, J. (MFW/BSCP)

1270.
MILLER, J.W.
Diving technology.
In: United States-Japan conference on natural resources development. Proceedings of the first joint U.S.-Japan panel on diving and technology, Tokyo, 1972, Ministry of Agriculture and Forestry 1972, p.161-169. Japan, Ministry of Agriculture and Forestry, 1972.

The areas of diving technlogy considered of primary importance by the National Oceanic and Atmospheric Administration are: (1) diver communication; (2) diver navigation; (3) bubble detection; (4) closed cycle rebreathers; (5) diver heating; (6) tracing the movement of solid material on the sea floor from a submersible by the neutron activator system and (7) development of undersea laboratories, with emphasis on the laboratory aspect of habitats. The author briefly describes the nature of the work going on in each of these areas, and concludes with a description of a habitat being built in Puerto Rico which NOAA plans to use in some of its research projects. (MFW/UMS)

1271.
MILLER, J.W. and D.C. Beaumariage.
NOAA's manned undersea science and technology program.
In: Applications of marine technology to human needs. Preprints, 8th annual conference and exposition, Marine Technology Society, September 1972 Washington, D.C. p.727-735. Published by the Society, 1972.

This presentation describes the formation of NOAA's Manned Undersea Science and Technology Program. Included is the program philosophy, the major goals, areas of emphasis and a description of field projects accomplished during the first year of operation. These projects range from geological studies on the carbonate platforms of British Honduras, to undersea investigation of the Pacific Walrus under the ice in the Bering Sea. . . . In addition to the marine science programs, a program was initiated to develop vertical excursion limits for divers saturated on nitrogen oxygen breathing mixtures. Such information is necessary, both from a medical safety standpoint and is essential in order to properly locate future ocean floor laboratories so as to permit optimum vertical excursion ranges in steep topographic areas. These excursion ranges are being developed under contract with Union Carbide Corporation using their computer program. Portions of the resulting tables will be validated in the research chamber facility. A civilian diving manual is under development that will address problems of scientific diving as well as working and sport diving. This document will complement Navy manuals and will integrate information contained in many sources, i.e. universities and other organizations concerned with diving. Close liaison is being maintained with the Navy, the National Research Council on Underwater Medicine, commercial diving organizations and those agencies currently having the charge of developing national diving standards. (Authors)

1272.
MILLER, J.W.
PRINUL — Mission #6. April 24-May 4, 1973.
Nat. Ocean. Atmosph. Admin., Manned Undersea Sci. Technol., Unpublished report, 14p. 1973.

Three separate studies are described. The first was concerned with upward vertical excursion diving tables. The second with underwater color visibility, and the third (unsuccessful for technical reasons) dealt with cosmic ray physics. In the first study, chamber dives at Union Carbide's hyperbaric chambers were made first to validate the table, then 23 excursions were made from a submerged habitat, from saturation depth of 95 feet, to various shallower depths, from 66 fsw to 25 fsw. No symptoms of bends were noticed except for a very slight "niggle" on several occasions, always with the same diver. It is emphasized that upward excursions should not be made within 18 hours of downward excursions. In the color visibility studies, the results for the spherical targets were, from best to worst: fluorescent green, white, fluorescent orange, and black. For flat targets, black was the most visible, except for the closest target, in which case oragne was. These differences were probably due to the background color. (MFW/BSCP)

1273.
MILLER, K.W.
Pressure effects on the intact animal.
In: Abstracts of the Twenty-fifth congress of Physiological Sciences Satellite Symposium. Recent progress in fundamental physiology of diving. Marseille, France. July 1971. p.24. (Proceedings unpublished)

Abstract only. Entire item quoted: Many of the signs and symptoms when small animals are exposed to high pressure have also been observed in primates and man. The anticonvulsant properties of the inert gases, when considered in the light of the ability of pressure per se to antagonise anaesthesia in small animals, points the way to the development of gas mixtures which may enable man to penetrate to yet deeper depths.

1274.
MILLER, K.W., W.D.M. Paton and E.B. Smith.
Experiments on animals at ultra high pressures.
In: Fructus, X., ed. Third international conference on hyperbaric and underwater physiology, p.31-34. Paris, Doin, 1972.

Newts anaesthetised with 34 Ata nitrogen at room temperature (20+1°C) showed nearly complete loss of ability to follow the revolving drum, but when the pressure was further increased with helium this ability was almost restored by ensures that narcosis need never prove a limiting problem and also means that narcotic gases may be used in breathing mixtures at very deep depths to combat hyperexcitability. In addition it was noted that above 140 Ata considerable protection against muscle contraction was afforded. Similar exposures to twice the anaesthetic dose of nitrogen, to a single dose of SF_6, and to an aqueous solution of 0.4 mg/mi sodium pentobarbitone showed that pressure restored activity, although in these cases muscle contraction became important before complete restoration of activity. The latter experiment demonstrates that the narcosis is antagonised by pressure per se and not by some interaction with helium. In conclusion the authors speculate on the meaning of this work for man. The reversal of narcosis by pressure will allow high concentrations of narcotic gases to be breathed and this may be beneficial as the work of Brauer demonstrates, in controlling hyperexcitability and convulsions. At a depth of not more than about 4,000 ft. (1,200 m) man will be confronted with a new barrier to his progress to greater depths. Our knowledge of the nature of this barrier is rather incomplete, but the narcotic gases may be of some benefit. Narcotic gases of small molecular size appear to be most beneficial and this fact may be related to recent observations on the antagonistic effect of anaesthetics and pressures on membrane permeability. (Authors)

1275.
MILLER, K.W.
Inert gas narcosis and animals under high pressure.
In: The effects of pressure on organisms. Symposia of the Society for Experimental Biology, No. 26, p.363-377. Cambridge, University Press, 1972.

The author reviews work in the area of high pressure effects (tremor, convulsions, respiratory distress, effect of compression rate on lethal thresholds). The influence of increased gas density was studied; findings indicated that death was related to pressure per se, rather than to respiratory stress due to increased density. Experiments demonstrating the reversal of anesthesia by pressure are discussed, and it is suggested that narcotic gases at partial pressures sufficient to suppress high pressure convulsions might be included in breathing mixtures. The author then discusses the atempt to develop a "semi-quantitative model with predictive value." The model is based on the theory that "anesthesia occurs at constant volume fraction rather than constant mole fraction," and is referred to as the "critical volume model." The model predicts that helium and neon will not be anesthetic, because gas-induced expansion of tissue will be more than offset by pressure. This prediction agrees with observed fact. In the case of hydrogen, the model predicts that gas-induced expansion is approximately balanced by pressure; this is consistent with the observed anesthetic pressure of hydrogen which is higher than predicted by the simple solubility model. It is suggested that the model may possibly be useful in relation to high pressure excitability, which is possibly caused by membrane compression. (MFW/BSCP)

1276.
MILLER, K.W., W.D.M. Paton, E.B. Smith and R.A. Smith.
Physicochemical approaches to the mode of action of general anesthetics.
Anesthesiology 36:339-351;Apr. 1972.

The anesthetic potencies (ED_{50}) of seven gaseous anesthetics have been determined in mice, using a criterion abolition of the righting reflexes by the rolling response, with the following results: C_2F_6 17.7 ATA; SF_6 5.4 ATA; Ar 15.2 ATA; Kr 4.5 ATA; Xe 0.95 ATA; N_2O 1.50 ATA. These results are combined with previous measurements to test the correlations upon which current physical theories of anesthetic action are based. The best correlation is found with the lipid solubility theories, while the hydrate theory receives little support. It is not possible with these data to decide between the two versions of the lipid theory that postulate constant-mole fraction (Meyer-Overton) and constant-volume fraction (Mullis) at equianesthetic doses. The two approaches, however, predict slightly different environments for the anesthetic site. (Authors' abstract)

1277.
MILLER, K.W., W.D.M. Paton, R.A. Smith and E.B. Smith.
The pressure reversal of general anesthesia and the critical volume hypothesis.
Mol. Pharmacol. 9:131-143;Mar. 1973.

The anesthetic potencies (ED_{50}) of four gaseous anesthetics and five liquid anesthetics were first determined in newts, using the abolition of righting reflex measured by the rolling response at 20°. The following results were obtained: N_2O, 0.69 atm; N_2, 21.5 atm; SF_6, 1.82 atm; CF_4, 11.0 atm; $CHCl_3$, 0.89 mM, butanol, 16.7 mM, pentobarbitone sodium, 0.85 mM, halothane, 0.39 mM, ether, 25 mM. The ability of elevated pressures to antagonize the effect of these anesthetics was then studied. For the liquid anesthetics, a graded respone to pressure was observed and the reversibility of the antagonistic effect was demonstrated. Dose-response curves were obtained for the interaction of pressure with the gaseous anesthetics, and, from these, ED_{50} values at various pressures have been interpolated. The data are used to compare the Meyer-Overton and the critical volume hypotheses; the latter not only is consistent with the data but also provides explanations for the antagonistic phenomenon and the lack of anesthetic effect for helium, neon, and hydrogen. The critical volume hypothesis is developed for three solvent model systems, from which estimates of the compressibility of the site of action are made. (Authors' abstract)

1278.
MILLER, W.C., R. Toon, H. Palat and J. Lacroix.
Experimental pulmonary edema following re-expansion of pneumothorax.
Amer. Rev. Resp. Dis. 108(3):664-666; 1973.

The development of acute edema in a lung that is re-expanded after a pneumorthorax was studied in Rhesus monkeys (*Macaca mulatta*). In 12 animals, unilateral pneumothorax with 80-100% collapse of the lung was induced and maintained for 3 days. In 6 of the animals, rapid re-expansion of the lung by applying suction at a pressure of -10 cm Hg produced marked, acute pulmonary edema ipsilaterally within 2 h. Re-expansion of the lung by underwater seal in the other 6 animals did not result in pulmonary edema. In 6 other monkeys, pulmonary edema did not develop when the lung was re-expanded with a pressure of -10 cm Hg within 1 h after the pneumothorax was induced. A large pneumothorax of 3 or more days' duration and the application of a large negative pressure to reexpand the lung were factors predisposing to pulmonary edema. These factors were also commonly present in reported human cases of the syndrome. (© BA)

1279.
MILNE, A.R.
Methods for launch and recovery of sea bottom instrument packages.
Underwater J. 5:213-220;Oct. 1973.

The journey to the sea-bottom of sensors and recorders and the return of recorded information are two essential stages in a successful visit by a self-contained instrument package. Launching procedures, whether free-fall or controlled, will depend on the relationship of sensors to bathymetry. Recovery techniques are basically those of acquiring stored information and range from the use of underwater telemetry to a return of all the hardware. Techniques are described for launching and recovering instrument packages which are applicable to shallow and deep water as well as temperate and frozen seas. (Author's abstract)

1280.
MILNE, P.H.
Seabed surveying by divers.
Underwater J. 5:120-122;June 1973.

Most of the survey work was carried out in relatively shallow water, 0 to 9m, where divers could work all day without risk of decompression. However, it will be noted that the King's Knowe dives average one hour and that of Stava Geo, one hour 20 minutes. The limitation on time was due to the coldness of the water temperatures in Shetland, 11-12°C, in which, after one hour, a wet suit diver was very cold. Divers involved in underwater surveying, especially the table operator and staff man, are often motionless, so good protection against the cold is essential.The author combatted the cold with a dry Unisuit and nylon-fur underwear, using twin $60ft^3$ ($3.3\ m^3$) cylinders encased in a Sceptre backpack. This equipment gave the author effective control of the survey work during which, on one occasion, the diving time approached two hours without discomfort. In addition to providing extra warmth the Unisuit also gave very effective buoyancy control which simplified the lifting and movement of the plane table underwater. (Author)

1281.
MILNER, C.G.
Developments in underwater services and equipment.
Meerestechnik 4:A15-A17;Oct. 1973.

Submersibles are now used in the North Sea for pipeline survey and inspection, cable laying, salvage survey, recovery and sea-bed sampling. For shallow depths and tasks of short duration, lock-out submersibles and divers are used. The one atmosphere armored suit, known as JIM, is another new development. It is stated here that "pioneering work by the Royal Navy in the use of free escape techniques and bottom bounce diving down to depths of 200 meters or more provided much knowledge on physiological aspects and operating procedures which is now feeding across into commercial work." Strongwork Diving Ltd. is utilizing divers in the design of underwater installations and equipment with emphasis on improved operation and maintainability. Another important tool is side-scan sonar, used in pipeline survey, equipment location, bottom search, and navigation. The Sonafix transponder, for position fixing, can give accurate bearing and range data at distances of 2 km at depths of 500 meters. (MFW/SCD)

1282.
MINE, H., T. Hasegawa, K. Ohno and H. Kawai.
An optimal maintenance policy for deep submergence equipment, part 2.
In: Ocean 73. 1973 IEEE international conference on engineering in the ocean environment, p.269-272. IEEE publication 73-CHO-7740-OCC.

This report presents additional results obtained after the presentation of the report entitled, "An Optimal Maintenance Policy for Deep Submergence Equipment," at Ocean 72. In the model of the deep submergence equipment, it is assumed the following assumptions hold: (1) the system deteriorates with time and finally fails to operate; (2) it is impossible either to repair the system or to observe its level of deterioration without bringing it to the surface; (3) even in a badly deteriorated state, the system can perform its function although with a substantial loss; (4) the observation and repair of the system are quite expensive because of assumption (2). The previous paper presented at Ocean 72 deals with an optimal maintenance policy of the system for which the operating duration is assumed to be given and finite, while this report deals with one for infinite operating duration. (Authors' abstract)

1283.
MIREJOVSKY, P. and E. Mirejovska.
Vliv hyperbaroxie na granulacni tkan.
[The influence of hyperbaroxia upon granulation tissue].
Cesk. Patol. 7:1-5;Feb. 1971.

Since hypoxia is regarded as a stimulus of fibroproduction, an attempt was made to estimate the influence of hyperbaroxia upon fibrotisation. For this purpose, granulation tissue surrounding polyethylene sponges implanted in rats was studied. In one experiment, the animals were exposed to hyperbaroxia of 1.5 to 3 ATA for 6 hours daily for 7 days; in another one the animals had been exposed to an increased pressure of 3 ATA for 4 hours daily for 4 weeks prior to the implantation of the sponges. No changes were disclosed in the granulation tissue exposed to 1.5 ATA. Pressures between 2 to 2.5 ATA caused a gradual mitochondrial alteration presenting as spherical transformation or even myelin degeneration, mitochondrial fusion and lysosomal activation, particularly within pericapillary fibroblasts and endothelia. At 3 ATA cytosegresomes were formed and cell necrosis occurred in both experiments. The appearance of the proteosynthetic apparatus of the fibroblasts remained uninfluenced by hyperbaroxia. (English summary)

1284.
MIRON, I.
Response des larves de Perla burmeisteriana Claassen (Plecoptera) aux variations de la pression hydrostatique.
[The response of larvae of Perla burmeisteriana Claassen (Plecoptera) to variations in hydrostatic pressure].
Hydrobiologia 42(2/3):345-354; 1973.

To explain the reactions of larvae of P. burmeisteriana to an ecological change following the impoundment of a man-made lake on River Bistritza (Romania), some experiments on the responses of this species to variations of hydrostatic pressure were undertaken. Experiments were carried out in Lake Bicaz France. Observations were direct, either by diving or by monitoring the situation visually from a submerged laboratory. Sets of 40 specimens were exposed to pressure of 1, 1.5 or 2 atmospheres. Survival time of the larvae decreased as pressure increased. This phenomenon is temperature dependent. Pressure influences gaseous exchange, by altering the rate of elimination of CO_2. This finally leads to hypercapnia. (HJV) (© BA)

1285.
MISSFELDT, S.
Der pathophysiologische mechanismus und die versicherungsmedizinische problematik des badetodes.
[Physiopathological mechanism and health insurance medical problems of the death from drowning].
Lebensversicherungsmedizin 22:6-13;Jan. 1970.

Noting that sudden, apparently inexplicable deaths occur regularly, though infrequently among users of swimming facilities, the author tries to clarify the life-insurance question of "external" or "internal" cause of death. He identifies four possible mechanisms of such deaths: (1) Effects of a water-drop which irritates the mucous membranes of the larynx. (2) Effects of water pressure on an overly-full stomach. (3) Panic. (4) Panic and hyperventilation. The first case, in his opinion, is clearly an "external" cause, requiring settlement of an accidental-death claim; the second is not. In the third and fourth cases, he points out that the panic may be triggered by any one of a number of occurrences, the psychological state of the victim may be seen as a contributory cause, and insurance benefits must be paid. He suggests, however, that since in practice these different mechanisms are not easily distinguished, insurance liability in such cases should be limited. (MEMH/BSCP)

1286.
MISSIRLIU, C.
Questionnaire permettant l'auto-evaluation du candidat plongeur.
[Questionnaire permitting self-evaluation of the diver candidate].
Cinesiologie 49:1-4; 1973.

In this brief article, the author presents a "medical decalogue for the diver candidate: (1) Circulation: valvular anomalies followed by infarct is a certain contraindication; (2) Respiration: asthma or chornic bronchitis are definite contraindications, while former tuberculosis or a healed scar that does not affect the vital capacity could be tolerated; (3) Emotion: overwork, anxiety, over-emotionalism would predispose to panic; (4) Neurological: loss of consciousness, convulsions, loss of balance, even several years previously, would require a very highly specialized and thorough examination; (5) Ears: perforated eardrums, mastoid operations, and chronic sinusitis generally rule out diving, while cases of ears that are particularly sensitive to pressure changes would require examination by a specialist; (6) Eyes: in cases of severe myopia, detachment of the retina is a danger, and conjunctivitis is a danger in pools; (7) Tetany: does the candidate gasp or pant under emotion?; (8) Glands: diabetes or thyroid irregularity would be contraindications; (9) Nutrition: extreme obesity or thinness, and enlarged liver or spleen, would be unfavorable; (10) Hernias: non-operated, even when small, could be affected by exertion and by the effects of pressure. The author notes that he has omitted the necessity of dental care, in case of caries, and consideration of vaccinations in the case of young trainees, as being in the category of generally understood preventive medicine. (MFW/UMS)

1287.
MIYAZAKI, M.
Effect of some respiratory maneuvers on cerebral and peripheral circulation, with special reference to maximum breathing, voluntary hyperventilation and the Valsalva maneuver.
Jap. Circ. J. 37:455-460;May 1973.

Circulatory effects of maximum breathing, voluntary hyperventilation and the Valsalva maneuver on both cerebral and peripheral hemodynamics were examined in four young and four elderly males, by means of an ultrasonic Doppler apparatus. Blood pressure, heart rate, and PO_2, PCO_2 and pH were also recorded. Results were as follows: (1) Maximum breathing: blood flow was increased in both areas, as were blood pressure and heart rate; respiratory alkalosis was recorded. (2) Voluntary hyperventilation: cerebral, but not peripheral, blood flow was decreased; blood pressure and heart rate were not significantly affected, and respiratory alkalosis was observed. (3) Valsalva maneuver: blood flow in both areas was decreased, blood pressure was decreased, heart rate was increased, and respiratory alkalosis was observed. The pathphysiology and clinical significance of each maneuver are discussed. (Author's summary condensed by MFW/UMS)

1288.
MIYOSHI, D.
Data-gathering system for studying underwater light and bioluminescence.
Albuquerque, N. Mex ., Sandia Labs., Rep. SC-DC-714400, 18p. Mar. 1972.
(SC-DC-714400)

A data-gathering system has been developed for studying the properties of underwater light and bioluminescence. The photodetector output is used to generate a count-rate distribution that is characteristic of the light being observed. Proper analysis of this distribution reveals the pressure of bioluminescence and greatly enhances the signal-detection capabilities of the system. Results of sea operations off Santa Barbara California, are presented. (Authors' abstract)

1289.
MOCHIZUKI, M. and S. Takahashi.
Effective breath holding time in the measurement of the pulmonary diffusing capacity by single breath method.
Jap. J. Physiol. 21:241-249;June 1971.

Discussion of the error arising in pulmonary diffusing capacity measurements by the single-breath method when the inspiration time is included in the breath-holding time. A correction factor is developed to eliminate this error in a modified version of this method which relies on the effective inspiration time. A nomogram is designed to facilitate a convenient determination of the effective inspiration time. (Aerosp. Med.)

1290.
MODELL, J.H., E.J. Kuck, B.C. Ruiz and H. Heinitsh.
Effect of intravenous vs. aspirated distilled water on serum electrolytes and blood gas tensions.
J. Appl. Physiol. 32:579-584;May 1972.

This study was designed to separate the effects of water, per se, from those of respiratory obstruction under conditions simulating freshwater drowning and near-drowning in dogs. Forty-five mongrel dogs were divided into five groups and subjected to either (a) a rapid intravenous infusion of distilled water; (b) acute airway obstruction; (c) both; or (d) aspiration of the same quantity of distilled water. In the absence of hypoxia, rapid intravenous infusion of 44 ml/kg of distilled water produced a mild, transient decrease in serum electrolyte concentrations and pH, and a transient increase in pulmonary artery pressure. There were no significant changes in cardiac output, arterial blood pressure, PaO_2, $PaCO_2$, or hemolysis; all of these dogs survived. However, when acute respiratory obstruction was superimposed hypoxemia, hypercarbia, acidosis, hemolysis, hypotension, hyperkalemia, hypochloremia, hyponatremia and a decrease in cardiac output occurred. If untreated, death ensued. If ventilation and oxygenation were supplied within 5 min. of water infusion and airway obstruction, an 80% survival rate was observed. We concluded that acute airway obstruction with persistent hypoxemia and acidosis is the single most important consequence of near-drowning requiring emergency therapy. (Authors' abstract)

1291.
MOELLER, G. and J.R. MacKinnon.
Development of diver performance measurement methods.
In: Abstracts of BuMed-ONR sponsored Navywide workshop in high pressure biomedical research, U.S. Submarine Base, Groton, Conn., May 1971, p.28. Published by the Naval Submarine Medical Research Laboratory, 1971.

Abstract only. Entire item quoted: The aim of work to be reviewed is development of reliable, standardized measures of well-understood behavioral functions for assessment of human performance capabilities in hyperbaric environments. At this time, efforts are concentrated on obtaining a better understanding of some tasks often used in studies of diver integrity under hyperbaric conditions. In addition, attempts to define behavioral analogs of those tasks for primates and to relate performance therein to the complex of biomedical events found under high pressure have been initiated. Implications of NAVSUBMEDRSCHLAB studies of mental arithmetic, the Stroop test, and tracking (simulated vehicle control) for identification of behavior functions tapped by those tasks and for improved experimental control of task performance measurement in hyprbaric studies will be described. The effects of repeated measurement, variation in task characteristics, and tactics of task performance on the stability and sensitivity to stress of task performance are reviewed.

1292.
MOELLER, G. and C.P. Chattin.
Identification of tasks sensitive to hyperbaria with determination of time interval effects on performance.
U.S. Nav. Submar. Med. Res. Lab., Rep. NSMRL 762, 10p. Sept. 14, 1973.

[The problem was] to identify tasks sensitive to the stresses of hyperbaric environments and to determine the effects of variation in the time interval between such exposures upon task performance. [It was found that] an adaptive tracking task proved sensitive to narcotic effects of 7 ATA air, two mental arithmetic tasks did not. With intervals of 5-20 days between exposures at 7 ATA, much larger decrements in tracking performance were found in the first exposure than in the second. Preceding, or intervening, exposures at 2 ATA did not moderate narcotic effects of the "deeper" exposure in any way. The findings suggest that: (1) susceptibility to narcosis during an hyperbaric exposure can be reduced substantially by an orientation exposure only if its profile closely resembles those working exposures to follow; and (2) studies of the depth-performance relationship must provide for measurement of the effect of sequence of exposures when subjects are tested at several depths. (Authors' summary)

1293.
MOKIEVSKII, O.B. et al.
[Some results from, and prospects for the use of underwater habitats in marine research]. Moscow, Nauka, 1973. 146p.

Various authors have contributed chapters on specific Russian underwater habitats, their design and their use, and also on biomedical problems of the underwater and/or hyperbaric environment. Individual chapters listed alphabetically by senior author, are: Ajazova, L.E. et al.: Some oceanographic experiments utilizing the underwater habitat-laboratory "Sprit"; Ajbulatov, N.A.: The research programme for "Chernomor-68"; Ajbulatov, N.A. et al.: Some problems relevant to the organization of scientific research work carried out from the underwater laboratory "Chernomor"; Akhlamov, E.A. et al.: Medical and physiological observations made during the experiment "Jetheander-67"; Akhlamov, E.A. et al.: Underwater research carried out the "Jetheander" club; Barats, Yu.M., et al.: The underwater habitats "Jetheander-66" and "Jetheander 67"; Denesov, N.E.: A discussion of the experience gained in carrying out biological work from the underwater habitat "Chernomor" in 1968 (preliminary report); Gramenitskj, P.N.; Physiological characteristics of decompression phenomena; Korolev, A.B. et al.: Pneumatic underwater habitats and sanctuaries; Korotaev, E.A. et al.: Medical and physiological experiments made during the experiment "Sadko-2"; Kuliev, I.P. et al.: Prospects for the use of underwater habitats and chambers in developing oil deposits: Ponomavev, V.P. et al.: The narcotizing effects of nitrogen and helium at elevated pressures (results obtained from experiments with animals); Shabalin, V.N. et al.: Particular features of the design of underwater habitats and the prospects for their application; Vasikshikov, N.V.: A discussion of the design project for an integrated Black Sea underwater observatory MGU; Zaltsman, G.L.: The condition and ability of a man to work in conditions of increased pressure and optimal compositions of the gas medium; Zaltsman, G.L.: Principle features of the saturation (desaturation) and oversaturation of the body and the principals of calculating decompression regimes for extended residence under pressure; Zhironkin, A.G.: Safe oxygen concentrations in breathing mixtures during prolonged exposure. (MFW/UMS)

1294.
MOLE, G.
Safe electric power for divers.
Hydrospace 4:29-31;June 1971.

Intrinsically-safe electric power supplies for divers and aquanauts should be used wherever possible, because they eliminate completely the risk of a lethal electric shock. The basic principles and practical capabilities of intrinsically-safe systems are surveyed. It is shown that systems working on either the current-limitation principle or on the voltage-limitation principle are practicable. Elimination of the risk to divers and aquanauts is the most urgent problem at present associated with underwater electric power. Once it is realised that intrinsically-safe systems are possible, the benefits of electric power will become fully available to divers and aquanauts. (Author's abstract)

1295.
MONEY, D.F.L. and P.J. Strong.
Underwater diving, oxygen poisoning and vitamin E.
New Zealand Med. J. 75:34-35;Jan. 1972.

In this brief letter to the editor, the authors give a brief history of experimentation into the relationship between vitamin E and oxygen toxicity, going back as far as 1946. The neurological symptoms of oxygen toxicity are described. It is noted that British diets tend to be deficient in vitamin E, and also that while there has been proven to be a direct relationship between vitamin E deficiency and the toxicity of hyperbaric oxygen in animals, premature infants, and astronauts, there has been no reference in the literature to the importance of vitamin E intake to the underwater diver. The authors feel strongly that this oversight should be remedied. (MFW/BSCP)

1296.
MOON, T.W., T. Mustafa and P.W. Hochachka.
The adaptation of enzymes to pressure. II. A comparison of muscle pyruvate kinases from surface and midwater fishes with the homologous enzyme from an off-shore benthic species.
Amer. Zool. 11:491-502; 1972.

Pyruvate kinase (PK) maximum catalytic rate is dramatically decelerated by increasing hydrostatic pressure. In four different species inhabiting different portions of the water column, muscle pyruvate kinase displays (1) a reduction in the volume change of activation (ΔV^*) at high temperatures, (2) a pH independence of ΔV^*, and (3) a general increase in the activation energy at increased pressures. Although shared by the four different pyruvate kinases examined, none of these characteristics is critically involved in the regulation of PK catalysis. In contrast, pressure effects on another set of characteristics, all vitally important to control of PK catalytic function, depend upon the species origin of the enzyme. In the case of the rainbow trout, Salmo gairdneri, high pressure dramatically reduces pyruvate kinase affinities for the two substrates (PEP and ADP), the cationic cofactor (Mg^{2+}), and the negative modulator (ATP). The homologous muscle enzyme from Oligoplites mundus, another surface dewelling species, displays similar responses to pressure. On the other hand, muscle PK affinities for the same key regulatory ligands are much less pressure sensitive in the abyssal rattail fishes (Coryphaenoides sp.) and are essentially pressure independent in a vertically migrating midwater sea bass, Ectreposebastes imus. In these latter two species, PK catalytic rates under probably physiological conditions are determined largely by these kinetic properties rather than by energy-volume parameters. (Authors' abstract)

1297.
MOON, T.W., T. Mustafa and P.W. Hochachka.
Effects of hydrostatic pressure on catalysis by different lactate dehydrogenase isozymes from tissues of an abyssal fish.
Amer. Zool. 11:473-478; 1971.

The predominant lactate dehydrogenases (LDHs) occurring in liver, heart, and muscle of a benthic Coryphaenoides species are electrophoretically distinguishable from each other. Maximum rates of pyruvate reduction catalyzed by heart and muscle LDHs show an optimum pH near neutrality, while liver LDH activity displays an unusual alkaline pH optimum. Pyruvate saturation curves areMicaelis-Menten in form for all three preparations. Maximum catalytic rates and the apparent K_m (pyruvate) are pressure independent for liver and heart LDHs. In the case of muscle LDHs, the maximum catalytic rate is also pressure insensitive, but the K_m is dramatically increased by pressure. These experiments clearly indicate that, at low substrate concentrations, the precise effects of pressure on enzyme-catalyzed reactions depend upon the nature and origin of the catalyst. (Authors' abstract)

1298.
MOORE, T.O., D.A. Lally and S.K. Hong.
Apneic bradycardia in man: effects of temperature and depth of immersion.
In: Abstracts of the Twenty-fifth Congress of Physiological Sciences Satellite Symposium. Recent progress in fundamental physiology of diving. Marseille, France, July 1971, p.10-11. (Proceedings unpublished)

Abstract only. Excerpts quoted: The schools of thought regarding the mechanism's of apneic bradycardia in man have been (1) hemodynamic and mechanical properties of the cardiovascular system, (2) afferent discharge from peripheral receptors, and (3) both neural and mechanical factors modulating basic apneic bradycardia — a multiple factor theory. . . . As a result of these experiments, the author concludes that there is bradycardia due to apnea alone. Face immersion potentiates the bradycardia, maximally in cold water, although face wetting is not essential. During body immersion, low water temperature governs the response, although immersion at depth produces an attenuation unrelated to gas density or PO_2 elevation, but probably the result of increased hydrostatic pressure. The multiple-factor theory appears the more tenable concept.

1299.
MOORE, T.O.
Thermal problems
In: United States-Japan conference on natural resources development. Proceedings of the first joint meeting of the U.S.-Japan panel on diving and technology, Tokyo, 1972, p.130-134. Japan, Ministry of Agriculture and Forestry, 1972.

The dive made in Aegir, in Hawaii, had three main objectives. The first was to document all heat loss, the second to document energy metabolism, and the third to investigate the fluid and salt balance. It is noted that respiratory heat loss in a helium hyperbaric environment is different from that in air at the surface. The harder the diver works, the higher the heat loss. It is concluded that breathing mixtures will have to be heated. There is also a loss of body fluid. Maintenance of fluid and salt balance is an important factor in meeting problems of thermal balance. During the discussion, the question of nutrition and weight loss is brought up. At 500 feet of depth, the divers consumed 6400 calories a day and still lost weight. (MFW/UMS)

1300.
MOORE, T.O., Y.C. Lin, D.A. Lally and S.K. Hong.
Effects of temperature, immersion, and ambient pressure on human apneic bradycardia.
J. Appl. Physiol. 33:36-41;July 1972.

Heart rate (HR) responses to 60 sec breath holds (BH) were recorded during (1) face immersion (FI) with varied water and air temperatures; (2) FI with and without face wetting, (3) whole-body immersion at different temperatures, (4) wet dives to 18.3 m; (5) dry chamber dives to 30.2 m and (5) chamber dives with gases of different percent oxygen. HR decreased during apnea in air, the response was potentiated by FI, and greatest bradycardia appeared with 5C FI. This pattern was similar in 25 and 5 C ambient air, but bradycardia was not different during FI in 5C water whether the face was wetted or protected. Apneic bradycardia during whole-body immersion was similar to FI alone and appeared to be temperature rather than immersion dependent. Wet ocean dives and dry chamber dives indicated an attenuation of bradycardia with depth (wet) with some evidence that elevated oxygen tension was responsible within certain ranges. It was concluded that multiple rather than single factors are responsible for the HR response to apnea. (Authors' abstract)

1301.
MOORE, T.O., R. Elsner, Y.C. Lin, D.A. Lally and S.K. Hong.
Effects of alveolar PO_2 and PCO_2 on apneic bradycardia in man.
J. Appl. Physiol. 34:795-798;June 1973.

Heart rate to 40 sec of apnea was monitored under conditions which would selectively alter alveolar PO_2 and PCO_2 — air or O_2 prebreathing, rest, exercise, and rebreathing maneuvers. Face immersions were also included to potentiate the observed apneic bradycardia. During both rest and exercise, the bradycardial response was potentiated in the presence of low alveolar PO_2, attenuated under conditions of high PAO_2, and appeared to be independent of $PACO_2$ levels. These data support the theory that the "diving" bradycardia in man is also an oxygen-conserving mechanism as has been postulated for diving marine mammals. While PAO_2 levels do not initiate the bradycardia response to apnea, they should be included in the multiple factors which modify the response. (Authors' abstract)

1302.
MORARIU, I.G. and C. Ignatescu.
Le laboratoire submerge L.S.-1.
[The underwater laboratory L.S.-1].
In: CIESM. Rapports et proces-verbaux des reunions, No. 22(4), p.767. Monaco, Commission Internationale pour l'Exploration de la Mer Mediterranee, 1972.

The Romanian underwater habitat L.S.-1 consists of a cylindrical chamber 33 m^3 in size, which rests on four legs. It has observation portholes. At present the habitat is supplied with air and electricity from the surface, but will eventually be independent. Facilities exist for atmosphere control, heat, light, telephone and television communication with the surface; equipment required for the research program is also installed. The habitat will be first tested at a depth of ten meters in an interior lake, then on the continental shelf of the Black Sea. It is expected that greater depths will be attained, and a work program will be developed that will make the resources of the Black Sea available to Romania. (MFW/UMS)

1303.
MORETTI, G. and S. Fontanesi.
Techniche, sistemi e mezzi di immersione profonda. Rassegna panoramica della loro evoluzione.
[Technics systems and means for deep immersion. Panoramic review of their evolution].
Ann. Med. Nav. 74:317-539;Aug. 1969.

Making a review of the most significant events in the diving evolution, from apnea to saturation techniques, from submarine eyes to modern SDC or turrets, and from bathyscaphes to the lock-out submersibles of today, the authors deal with the major physiological and engineering problems related to hyperbarism. Both industrial and military projects involving the continental shelf are emphasized, as well as the relations between diving improvements and submarine escape possibilities. (English summary)

1304.
MORETTI, G., S. Fontanesi and L. Ghittoni.
La narcosi da gas inerti in condizioni di iperbarismo ambientale: rassegna degli aspetti piu salienti della letteratura mondiale.
[Inert gas narcosis in a hyperbaric environment: the world literature].
Ann. Med. Nav. (Roma) 77:173-198;Apr.-June 1972.

An historical review of world research on inert-gas narcosis under hyperbaric conditions is presented. After a brief description of the first observations of behavioral disturbances under hyperbaria and of early explanations, attempts at precise evaluation of the nature and extent of the disturbances are discussed, primarily in terms of N_2-O_2 breathing mixtures. A short discussion of the narcotic effects of other gases follows. Various etiopathogenic theories of narcosis are summarized; pressure, psychological factors, O_2 partial pressure, CO_2, and inert-gas partial pressure have been considered responsible for the syndrome. Scientific support of the last has been accumulating steadily, and the development of this knowledge is discussed. The presumed mechanism of inert-gas narcosis is also outlined.Several suggestions for the prevention of narcosis terminate the article. (MEMH/BSCP)

1305.
MORETTI, G., S. Fontanesi and L. Ghittoni.
La mallattia da decompressione: analisi di una serie di 96 casi trattati nello ambito della marina militare nel triennio 1969-71.
[Decompression sickness: Analysis of a series of 96 cases treated under the auspices of the Italian Navy, 1969-1971].
Ann. Med. Nav. 78:499-522;Oct./Dec. 1973.

The authors summarize a series of 96 cases of decompression sickness with emphasis on evaluating the recompression-decompression therapeutic protocol. Most patients underwent recompression-decompression in accordance with Van der Aue's table; in a few cases, Workman's Table was used. Osteomyoarthralgic symptoms regressed completely under Van der Aue type repressurization therapy, but neuro-sensory symptoms were resolved only about 60% of the time. It is suggested that in cases with cardio-respiratory involvement, as well as in cases with neuro-sensory symptoms, the Workman-Goodman method, using pure oxygen, may be preferable. The authors note also that in "Neuro-sensory" cases in which treatment is instituted within 5-6 hours of the decompression accident, the prognosis for complete cure is greatly improved. (MEMH/UMS)

1306.
MORIN, R.A. and E.H. Lanphier.
Application of a man-rated centrifuge in underwater research.
Med. Sport 24:279-284;Nov. 1971.

Underwater research is one of the most important aspects of the new Laboratory of Environmental Physiology presently under construction at the State University of New York at Buffalo. A unique feature of this new unit will be a ring-shaped submergence basin, 8 ft wide and 8 ft deep (2.43 m) built around the area swept by a man-rated centrifuge. This circular test basin permits a man to swim for long periods of time without having to change direction. The centrifuge motors will operate over a very wide range of precisely controlled or servo-regulated speeds. By connecting a removable platform to the centrifuge capsule we will be able to precede, lead, or tow a swimmer at any pre-set speed or to follow him accurately at any speed he maintains on a moment-to-moment basis. The platform will be able to carry an observer and apparatus, sampling tubes and monitoring leads, and will thus allow us to use the centrifuge instrumentation and, in effect, the entire laboratory for the experiment. Studies of propulsion, drag, and work in currents will be conducted readily. The outer basin wall will have large transparent sections for observation and photography. Parts of the submergence basin can be isolated for specific purposes such as temperature regulation studies. The outer wall will be surrounded by an ample walkway at a level that places the water surface at lab-bench height. The circular walk-way will be continuous, with its outer portion banked to provide a running track for use in exercise studies. This concentric arrangement of facilities provides multiple laboratory capability under one roof at very moderate cost. (Authors' summary)

1307.
MORITA, R.Y. and R.R. Becker.
Hydrostatic pressure effects on proteins.
Corvallis, Ore., Ore. State Univ., Final progress rep. on contract N00014-67-A-0369-0002, 6p. 1972.
(AD 749 342)

A very brief description is given of the effects of hydrostatic pressure on a model protein which, in turn, will permit an insight into the effects of hydrostatic pressure on cellular constituents. The aggregation of polyvalylribonuclease A (PVRNase) has been studied as a model. (GRA)

1308.
MORITZ, W.E.
Physiologic monitoring in hyperbaric environments.
In: Abstracts of BuMed-ONR sponsored Navywide research in high pressure biomedical research, U.S. Submarine Base, Groton, Conn., May 1971. p.49. Published by the Naval Submarine Medical Research Laboratories, 1971.

Abstract only. Entire item quoted: A compact, swimmable package of instrumentation has been developed to allow for the physiologic monitoring of divers in various hyperbaric environments. The parameters to be measured include electrocardiogram, five body temperatures, inspired and expired gas temperatures, inspired gas volume and environmental pressure and temperature. In addition, an expired partial pressure oxygen device is being obtained for inclusion with this system. The analog signals are multiplexed into a single wire for transmission over an umbilical to the surface. Power is provided over the same umbilical. Hyperbaric exposures are being conducted in dry and wet chambers and a 100-ft deep water tank. In addition, the system will be used to monitor divers in the open sea. The data obtained is fed into a small digital computer and stored on magnetic tape for later analysis by the computer. While the system is primarily designed and calibrated for use at depths up to 150 feet with air as a medium, it is felt that it could be modified for use in deep helium environments. A portable underwater ergometer has also been constructed to impose measurable amounts of work on the divers in each of the four environments. The diver sits in the device and moves his legs against a known load over a measured distance. The results expected from these experiments should quantify man's response to the four types of environments mentioned above and provided additional insights into his physiological limits. The system will also be used to evaluate the performance of various thermal protection systems for divers.

1309.
MORITZ, W.E. and R.G. Buckles.
A computer based instrumentation system for use in biomedical research.
In: 25th Annual conference for engineering in medicine and biology, Bal Harbour, Florida, October 1972. Preprints, p.421. Washington, D.C., Alliance for Engineering in Medicine and Biology, 1972.

A complete system of bioinstrumentation is described which uses a minicomputer for real-time analysis and data acquisition. The system can also be used to analyze the data off-line. Examples of some application of the system in hyperbaric physiologic research are given. The system is capable of measuring a wide variety of physical and physiological variables, a partial list of which follows: electrocardiogram, heart rate, arterial and venous blood pressure, core temperature, various tissue temperatures, respiratory gas flow, respiration rate, radioisotope activity level at 5 sites, environmental pressure and temperature and partial pressure of oxygen. Additional parameters can be incorporated into the system as needed. (Authors)

1310.
MORITZ, W.E., P.A. Van Akkeren and R.G. Buckles.
A computer based physiologic monitoring system.
U.S. Nav. Med. Res. Inst., Rep. 1 on M4306.04-1023B, 21p. June 5, 1972.

A versatile data acquisition/analysis system has been built for conducting extensive physiological experiments — particularly those concerned with hyperbaric medicine. It is capable of analyzing up to 16 channels of analog and 5 channels of digital information and storing the data on magnetic tape for later analysis. The system is built around a minicomputer which adds greatly to the optimum utilization of the hardware. Since the Varian 620i is a general purpose digital computer and has been interfaced with a variety of input/output devices it serves as a powerful tool in the acquisition and analysis of vast amounts of data from a wide range of experimental protocols. An initial series of inert gas experiments has been carried out and the results are currently being analyzed with the system. In addition, an extensive program is underway which is concerned with evaluating man's physiologic response to hyperbaric exposures. In this particular program most of the signal conditioning is done in the instrument package on the man, thus bypassing some of the equipment discussed here. Follow-on experiments are planned for the inert gas studies in the near future. A program to evaluate the effectiveness of an electrically heated suit designed to protect divers from cold water stress has recently been completed. The data acquisition system served not only to analyze the data during these tests but also continuously monitored the divers' physiologic condition and provided alarms when various parameters (core temperature, for instance) exceeded preset limits. Since the cost of a system such as has been described in this paper may exceed $100,000, it will not be practical for all types of experiments. If, however, the protocols call for a large number of measurements to be taken continuously over long periods of time (1 hour) and for real time analysis and monitoring of the data, a computer based data acquisition system such as this can prove invaluable. The ability of the investigator to interact with the system during the analysis phase can also be of considerable benefit. (Authors' summary)

1311.
MORITZ, W.E. and H.C. Langsworthy.
Evaluation of Marine Corps battery powered electrically heated diving dress.
U.S. Nav. Med. Res. Inst., Rep. 1 on M4306.02-1015, 19p. June 22, 1972.

In order for Marine Reconnaissance Divers to perform their tasks with safety and efficiency, a supplemental heat source is required. This heat source must be compact in size, lightweight, capable of providing adequate power for the lowest water temperatures a diver will encounter, and be so designed as not to interfere with the diver's mobility. In answer to these needs the Suchy Division of the Reflectronic Corporation developed a battery package which supplies power to an electric diving suit. At the request of the United States Marine Corps a test and evaluation program was conducted to determine if this battery system was capable of providing a diver with a sufficient amount of heat, while motionless, in 1-3°C water for a period of 2 hours at depths less than 100 feet. The battery package is a cylinder 1 foot in diameter and 2 feet in length weighing approximately 41.5 lbs. The cylinder contains 18 40 amp. hour silver zinc cells that are connected in series, each cell being charged to 2 volts. The test and evaluation revealed a number of weaknesses in the battery system during the course of routine handling. These weaknesses are discussed individually in the report. It appears that the battery system will provide adequate supplemental heat for a diver in depths of 10 feet or less with water temperatures from 1.5 to 3.5°C. At deeper depths in similar water temperatures the battery system will not provide sufficient heat for the diver's thermal comfort. (Authors' abstract)

1312.
MORITZ, W.E. and P.A. Van Akkeren.
A 15 channel multiplexed analog data transmission system.
U.S. Nav. Med. Res. Inst., Rep 1 on M4306.04-1023B, 37p. Aug. 30, 1972.

As Navy divers explore greater and greater depths in the sea, the need to monitor their physiological condition becomes increasingly important. A vital part of this monitoring is the data transmission link between the diver and the surface. An inexpensive, highly reliable multichannel data transmission system has been designed and built specifically for this purpose. The system utilizes a pulse-amplitude modulation multiplexing scheme and transmits 15 channels of analog data over 2 conductors. Input voltages may range from +5.0 to -3.5 volts and the frequency response of each channel is 25 Hz with a 4 KHz system clock. This is more than adequate to reproduce electrocardiograms and most other signals of interest. Automatic synchronization is provided. The diver-mounted transmitter occupies approximately 1.5 cubic inches and operates on + 15 volts DC. Power consumption of the transmitter is approximately 500 milliwatts. This may be provided by batteries on the diver or by adding an additional 2 conductors to the umbilical from the surface. The addition of one more wire would allow the monitoring of 15 channels of data from each of two divers operating on the same general area. Integrated circuits have been used extensively throughout the system and result in reduced cost and ease of construction and maintenance. The cost of parts for a dual diver system, including power supplies and hardware is approximately $1,500. (Authors' abstract)

1313.
MORITZ, W.E.
A diver monitoring system for physiologic studies in all hyperbaric environments.
U.S. Nav. Med. Res. Inst., Rep 3 on M4306.04-1023B 22p. Oct. 18, 1972.

A package instrumentation has been assembled that can monitor the following parameters on divers: electrocardiogram, respiratory gas flow, core temperature, up to 8 skin or gas temperatures, environmental temperature and ambient pressure. The signal conditioners are carried on the diver in a stainless steel cylinder capable of operation at 1700 feet of sea water. The output of each signal conditioner is fed to a 15 channel multiplex data handling system for transmission to the surface monitoring station. All sensor inputs, power and the multiplex output are made through underwater connectors to increase the versatality of the system. The unit has been used extensively in wet and dry hyperbaric chambers as well as deep water tanks and the open sea. The data can be displayed on a strip chart recorder or analyzed on a computer based data analysis system. (Author's abstract)

1314.
MORITZ, W.E. and W.H. Mints.
An ergometer for use in all hyperbaric environments.
U.S. Nav. Med. Res. Inst., Rep. 4 on M4306.04-1023B, 13p. Nov. 20, 1972.

An ergometer has been fabricated and tested that can stress divers in both wet and dry environments. The work load is generated by operating foot pedals against linear springs while the subject is seated in the device. A signalling/timing system is described which enables remote personnel to control the rate and duration of each work cycle. Electronic counting circuitry provides direct, real-time measurement of the work done by the diver. The system can easily provide work loads between 250 and 1400 kg-m/min and has been readily accepted by nine subjects engaged in two research programs. It is small enough (0.45 m x 0.85 m x 1.28 m) to fit through most chamber hatches normally used by divers and relatively light weight (22.7 kg). The device has been used in both wet and dry experiments at depths to 150 feet. (Authors' abstract)

1315.
MORITZ, W.E.
A system for studying the physiologic response of divers to hyperbaric environments.
In: Ocean 73. 1973 IEEE international conference on engineering in the ocean environment, p.129-132. IEEE publication 73-CHO-7740-OCC.

A fifteen channel hardwire, multiplexed physiologic monitoring system for use on divers in all environments is described. Parameters include ECG, respiratory gas flow, temperatures, work out-put and ambient pressure. The system may be used in a duel diver mode. The data may be analyzed on a computer based data acquisition system. A specially designed ergometer is described. The data will be useful in assessing man's capabilities and limitations in the sea. Preliminary results indicate that the system described here is useful for monitoring thermal stress on divers as well as general physiologic response to imposed work loads. (Author's abstract)

1316.
MORRIS, J.E.W.
Microbiology of the submarine environment.
Proc. Roy. Soc. Med. 65:799-800;Sept. 1972.

In a survey of airborne bacteria in Royal Navy submarines, results compared favorably with conditions in occupied spaces ashore and in surface ships, as reported in World War II. It is noted, however, that a high proportion (20%) of the bacteria were Gram-negative rods; genera included escherichia, proteus, acinetobacter, enterobacter, alcaligines, and pseudomonas, suggesting the source to be sewage tanks or lavoratories. There is evidently no increase in respiratory and intestinal infections in submarine crews during patrol. Further studies are being undertaken regarding the importance of environmental factors, for example, increased carbon dioxide levels, affecting tissue pH, might favor survival of certain species at the expense of others. (MFW/BSCP)

1317.
MORRISON, J.B. and W.S. Butt.
Effect of underwater breathing apparatus and absolute air pressure on divers ventilatory capacity.
Aerosp. Med. 43:881-888;Aug. 1972.

Maximum voluntary ventilation (MVV) studies were undertaken using three divers. Measurements were made at 1, 2, 4, and 8 atm abs, breathing air in all cases. In addition to measurements under normal conditions, the tests were repeated with the subject partially immersed in water and wearing underwater breathing apparatus. A two-stage open circuit supply system (SABA) of the type used by RN divers was used in the experiments. The relationship obtained of normal MVV to absolute air pressure for the three subjects was in agreement with that established by previous investigators. When breathing from the underwater breathing apparatus, the values of maximum ventilation at each depth was reduced but the form of the relationship was not greatly altered. At 8 atm abs maximum ventilations of over 60 litres/min were achieved. The mean results of three subjects indicate that in general, at any given pressure within the range of 1 to 8 atm abs, when breathing air from an open circuit demand valve of the type used, a diver can expect to achieve between 85% and 95% of his normal maximum voluntary ventilation at that pressure. (Authors' abstract)

1318.
MORRISON, J.B. and I.C. Mayo.
Gas-mixture supply at constant PO_2 for semi-closed circuit breathing apparatus.
Underwater J. 5:23-27;Feb. 1973.

A method of supplying a variable gas mixture to a semi-closed circuit breathing apparatus is designed in such a way that the gas mixture in the counter-lung will have an oxygen partial pressure which is relatively constant and independent of depth. This is achieved by regulating the total gas mixture supply to the set with a constant volume flow measured at the prevailing ambient pressure. The supply of oxygen to the set is at a constant mass flow at all depths. Oxygen is supplied through a constant mass flow jet (commercially available) and oxygen and inert gas is then supplied to the counter-lung via a laminar flow element. The supply of inert gas is regulated to ensure a constant pressure drop across the laminar flow element and hence a constant volume flow of gas mixture. An experimental model of the system has been constructed and tested over the range 1 to 7 atm. The results obtained indicate that the theoretical system described for supplying a gas mixture at constant oxygen partial pressure to semi-closed circuit breathing apparatus can be reproduced in practice. (Authors' abstract)

1319.
MORRISON, J.B.
Oxygen uptake studies of divers when fin swimming with maximum effort at depths of 6-176 feet.
Aerosp. Med. 44:1120-1129;Oct. 1973.

Analytical techniques were developed to measure oxygen uptake of divers breathing from semi-closed circuit underwater breathing apparatus. A series of trials was carried out under pressure in which the oxygen uptake of clearance divers was measured when fin swimming at maximum sustained effort. The divers, breathing an oxygen-nitrogen mixture from CDBA, swam against a trapeze in a wet chamber for periods of 10 mins. at depths of 6 ft., 78 ft. and 176 ft. The mean maximum sustained oxygen consumption was calculated to be 2.6 liters/min NTP, and individual values of up to 3.4 litres/min were recorded. On the basis of the results, some problems regarding the design, safety and efficiency of semi-closed circuit underwater breathing apparatus are discussed. (Author's abstract)

1320.
MORROW, C.T.
The initial speech transducer and its environment.
In: Sergeant, R.L. and T. Murry, eds. Processing helium speech: proceedings of a Navy-sponsored workshop, August 1971, U.S. Nav. Submar Med. Res. Lab., Rep. NSMRL 708, p.18-21. May 22, 1972.

A type of translator is necessary for understanding speech produced in deep submergence helium atmospheres. In combination with this translator, an adequate microphone such as the one used in this investigation is necessary. The microphone discussed in this presentation performs as a gradient microphone to 10 kHz or better in helium. It is insensitive to mask cavity acoustics and it withstands pressurization, decompression and the marine environment. (Author)

1321.
MOSSBACHER, R.R.
Navy's new ocean simulation facility.
In: Professional diving symposium, New Orleans, Nov. 1972. Mar. Technol. Soc. J. 7:58-62; Mar./Apr. 1973.

The author describes the Ocean Simulation Facility under construction at the Naval Coastal Systems Laboratory at Panama City, Florida. Parameters include: pressure to 1000 psi on 2,250 fsw; vacuum to 150,000 feet altitude; temperature (wet chamber; 29°F to 90°F, (dry chambers) 50°F to 110°F; humidity (dry chambers) 50 to 95 percent; salinity (wet chambers) 0 - 40 parts per thousand, with turbidity and light level as needed. Floor plans of the building, showing the location of the large wet chamber and the five smaller dry chambers, plus all the auxiliary areas, are shown. Photographs show the control room and parts of the chamber complex. The facility is expected to be in full operation by late 1960. Its stated mission is "to be the principal Navy research, development, test and evaluation center for the application of science and technology associated with military operations carried out primarily in the coastal region, and to perform investigations in related fields of science and technology." Among these are swimmer/diver support systems; to this end the Navy Experimental Diving Unit will move to Panama City. A large experimental diving facility, with additional chambers is expected to be built starting in 1974. The entire complex will serve government agencies other than the Navy, as well as industrial and educational institutions. (MFW/BSCP)

1322.
MOUNT, T.
The art of safe cave diving.
Skin Diver 20:69-70;Aug. 1971.

The chief dangers of cave diving are "the inability to make free ascents, the danger of becoming lost, running out of air, loss of visibility by stirring up silt, and panic." In order to avoid stirring up silt, the diver must keep off the cave floor by careful use of buoyancy devices — either flotation vest or air bottle. Safety devices such as reels and light systems are discussed. Buddy breathing should be carried out with an octopus rig: (a single hose regulator with two second stages). Three is usually the best number for cave diving. Watch, depth gauge, submersible dive tables and/or decompression meters should be used. Dives of long penetration should require a buddy tank of 20 - 40 cubic feet with its own regulator, as well as an additional air supply tied off for decompression. A good dive plan includes a divemaster, and flexibility to allow for premature termination due to adverse circumstances; maximum depth and penetration should be set, and the capabilities of the least experienced diver should be taken into consideration. Each diver should limit his dive to his own limitations, and not extend himself because of confidence in his buddy. (MFW/BSCP)

1323.
MOURRET, A., C. Agnius-Delord and M.R. Rinaldi.
Effet de l'oxygene hyperbare sur les proprietes radioprotectrices de trois heterocycles azotes et influence de ces substances sur la toxicite de l'oxytene hyperbare.
[Effect of hyperbaric oxygen on the radioprotective properties of 3 nitrogenous compounds and effect of these substances on the toxicity of hyperbaric oxygen].
C.R. Acad. Sci. (D) (Paris) 275:2985-2988;Dec. 1972.

In order to study the effect of oxygen on the radioprotective properties of imidazole, benzimidazole, naphazoline, and cysteamine, mice were injected with one of these substances and placed in a pressurized radiation apparatus; oxygen pressure was maintained at the desired level (1.1, 1.5, 2, or 2.5 atmospheres) for the duration of exposure to radiation. Survival times were noted. A study of the oxygen-protective properties of these compounds was carried out by injecting mice with one of the compounds and then exposing them to high pressures of oxygen (3.5, 4, 5, and 5.8 atmospheres). Survival times were again noted. It was observed that imidazole and benzimidazole tend to increase oxygen toxicity, and are less effective as radio-protectors under hyperbaric oxygen, than are naphazoline and cysteamine. In addition, the observations of other writers on the greater oxygen sensitivity of males of this strain (C_3H/He/Orl) were confirmed. (MEMH/SCD)

1324.
MUENCHEN, K.
Tierexperimentelle dekompressionsversuche in abhaengigkeit vom wasserhaushalt des organismus.
[Decompression experiments with animals as a function of the water balance of the organism].
Bad Godesberg, West Germany, Deutsche Forschungs Und Versuchsanstalt Fuer Luft-und Raumfahrt, Inst. Fuer Flugmedizin. Rep. DLC-FB-71-20, 45p. Ph.D. Thesis. Mar. 1971.
(N73 14075)

The responses of the organism to decompression as a function of water balance were investigated. Experiments were conducted on 842 guinea pigs with diuretic Lasix. There was an increased mortality rate after treatment with different doses of Lasix compared with nontreated animals. The hematocrit increased after treatment with Lasix as well as after high pressure exposure. The results are discussed and an attempt is made to elucidate the factors possible influencing these results. (Author) (GRA)

1325.
MUENKER, G., P. Pedersen and S. Grundmann.
The testing of eustachian tube function in a hyperbaric chamber: Registration by means of a differential manometer.
Arch. Klin. Exp. Ohren-Nasen Kehl-Dopfheilkd. 201(3):249-257; 1972.

The assessment of tubal function in a hyperbaric chamber is usually based on the sensations experienced by the subjects examined. The registration of tympanic-membrane movements during pressure changes in the chamber requires that the pressure in the ear canal, occluded by the recording instrument, is continually equalized to that in the ambient air. A differential manometer is described that, owing to the action of a low-frequency bypass, is only sensitive to quick drum movements, but not to slow changes in ambient air pressure or those due to slowly-occurring displacements of the tympanic membrane. These quick drum movements are indicative of pressure equilibrations between the outside air and that in the middle ear and are caused by a momentary opening of the eustachian tube. This new method facilitates a quantitative determination of eustachian-tube action when equilibrating the differential pressure across the tympanic membrane while the ambient pressure is being altered. In all cases with mobile, intact tympanic membranes, reproducible and objective results were obtained. (© BA)

1326.
MULLINIX, J.M.
Diary of a tragedy.
Skin Diver 20:47-48;Aug. 1971.

This is an account by a diver of her first dive to 180 feet, which resulted in either air embolism or severe decompression sickness with CNS involvement. The cause was apparently the misguided helpfulness of a companion in filling her air jug too full, thus causing her to shoot up 60-80 feet. Another diver was able to dump some of the air and halt her ascent. (The jugs are used in cave and sink diving to regulate buoyancy). Within a few minutes of surfacing, severe chest pain, weakness, and a widespread tingling sensation occurred followed by pain in the neck and elbow. The diver was taken to a nearby hospital where she was X-rayed for air embolism (negative) and then given recompression to 60 feet, with alternate oxygen breathing. Apparently the minimal extent of the therapy was determined by the fact that she was only a minute or two at 180 feet, and the nature of her symptoms was largely ignored. After therapy, tingling persisted, and was followed by paralysis from the waist down. During her stay in the hospital the patient was given physical therapy, but no further recompression. At the time of writing, a few months later, her condition was considerably improved, but not normal. (MFW/BSCP)

1327.
MUNTON, S.V. and J.R. Buck.
Design and certification of submerged systems handling equipment.
In: 1973 Offshore Technology Conference, April/May 1973, Houston, Texas. Preprints, Vol. II, p.163-172. Published by the conference.

This paper presents the basic design criteria and procedures for certification of submerged systems handling equipment. The authors discuss the total design evolution from establishment of design parameters to certification documentation. The philosophy and the need for certification are also discussed. Examples of design and certification of submerged systems for the U.S. Navy are highlighted. The intent of this paper is to present a useful guideline to be used by engineers designing handling equipment for submerged systems. . . . What is stressed in this paper is certification of handling equipment. As it stands now, however, the only civilian submerged system that is required by law to be certified is the pressure chamber. It is evident to anyone familiar with submerged systems that the pressure chamber is only one portion of the total system. Life support and handling equipment are equally as important as the pressure chamber. As such, this equipment should stand the scrutiny of certification. (Author)

1328.
MUREN, A. and K. Wulff.
Carbon dioxide distribution in the divers helmet.
In: Fructus, X., ed. Third international conference on hyperbaric and underwater physiology, p.99-100. Paris, Doin, 1972.

Problems had arisen in deep diving in the Swedish Navy which were attributed to an uneven distribution of carbon dioxide in the helmet, resulting in performance detriment, headache, dizziness, sometimes loss of consciousness. A device was constructed consisting of "an airtight metal cap around the interior part of the exhaust valve, with a passage for the chin button, the opening directed downwards. . . A thick plastic tube about one inch in inner diameter and 25-30 cm. long is connected to the cap. The lower end of the tube, which is perforated, is placed under the breastplate. The exhaust valve takes the air from the lowest part of the compartment, thus lowering the level of CO_2 — contaminated air. It was found that the CO_2 partial pressure was reduced by 30 to 40%, and the divers experienced less narcosis and no headache. (MFW/UMS)

1329.
MUREN, A., J. Sundlof and L. Troell.
Medicina aspekter pa modern kykeriu tieckling.
[Medical aspects of modern developments in diving].
Lakartidningen 70:2491-2496;June 27, 1973.

The rapid developments which have taken place internationally in diving during the last 10 years have been dictated partly by military requirements but also to a large extent by the increased public interest in exploiting the riches of the sea in a practical manner. Man's penetration into the deeps of the sea to depths of several hundred meters and his staying at these depths for weeks and months have meant that a number of new medical problems have come into existence, in addition to the special problems connected with conventional diving, which are still to a large extent unsolved. Sweden has maintained its position in this field well, largely owing to good collaboration between the Navy, civil research establishments and private firms. However, better co-ordination and more effective utilization of the potential resources in the country will be required if Sweden is to be one of the leading nations in the diving sphere also in the future. (English abstract)

1330.
MUREN, A.
Nitrox diving with constant oxygen partial pressure.
In: Hesser, C.M. and D. Linnarsson, Eds. Proceedings of the first annual scientific meeting of the European Undersea Biomedical Society, Stockholm, 13-15 June 1973. Forsvarsmedicin 9:251-252;July 1973.

It was found that increasing inspiratory PO_2 from 0.2 ata to 1.6 ata resulted in a decrease of heart rate from 120 to 103, of respiratory frequency from 14.5 to 12.3, and CO_2 elimination from 1.53 to 1.35 L/min. There was a reduction in minute ventilation from 36 to 30 L/min, and an increase in end tidal PCO_2 from 46 to 51 mm Hg between 0.2 and 0.8 ata O_2, but no further change with increased PO_2. Work seemed lighter while using the high oxygen mixture (nitrox with 40% O_2). Nitrox diving with a constant PO_2 of 1.5 ata for periods of up to three hours appears to be satisfactory, although the possibility of increased CO_2 retention should be kept in mind. (MFW/BSCP)

1331.
MURRAY, T.
Helium speech unscrambler simulations at the speech transmission laboratory.
In: Sergeant, R.L. and T. Murry, eds. Processing helium speech: proceedings of a Navy-sponsored workshop. August 1971. U.S. Nav. Submar. Med. Res. Lab., Rep. NSMRL 708, p.26-28;May 22, 1972.

The author presents diagrams illustrating the effects on speech of a 600-foot helium atmosphere; of the restoration effects of vocoder methods, with both analysis and synthesis filters; of restoration with methods in the frequency domain; restoration with a combined heterodyne and time domain method. With vocoder methods, original formants tended to leak through. In the time domain method, "micro segments of the divers' speech are stretched by the transposition of factor k", which necessitates discarding part of the speech signal. A better correction of the pressure effect is achieved by using a heterodyne method to move the formant frequencies down in parallel before the time domain method is applied. However, in his conclusion the author states that the time domain method without heterodyne seems to give the best intelligibility; a device based on this principle has been designed. (MFW/BSCP)

1332.
MURRY, T. and R.L. Sergeant.
Response variations of three types of microphones pressurized to 19 Ata.
U.S. Nav. Submar. Med. Cent., Rep. NSMRL 690, 11p. Dec. 3, 1971.

The Navy's interest in deep diving has brought on the need to calibrate instruments and test equipment used for such dives. This study presents the result of changes in the frequency response characteristics of three microphones when pressurized to 19 ata in a helium-oxygen gas mixture. A microphone which was previously calibrated under the same conditions using the reciprocity technique (a technique by which no acoustic standard is necessary) provided the standard against which the other microphones were compared. The results suggest that "off-the-shelf" microphones do not maintain their sensitivity and frequency response when subjected to high ambient pressures. It is apparent that specially designed microphones which maintain a flat response under high ambient pressures are necessary in order to accommodate helium speech unscramblers. Of the three microphones observed, the ceramic microphone was most consistent with changes in ambient pressure, and furthermore, it was the only one of the three to return to its pre-dive electrical characteristic. (Authors' abstract)

1333.
MURRY, T.
Hyperbaric chamber noise during a dive to 100 feet.
J. Acoust. Soc. Amer. 51(4,Pt.2):1362-1365; 1972.

Sound-pressure levels of the noise in a diving chamber, pressurized to a depth equal to 100 feet of sea water, were measured. In the first of two dives, measurements were taken during compression and decompression with a piezoelectric microphone oriented so that it was approximately in a horizontal line with the diver's ear and facing away from the vent. In the second dive, the microphone was at the same position in the chamber, but hanging downward at the diver's ear level. The microphone was previously calibrated under pressure using a reciprocity calibration technique. Measurements wre taken with an octave-band noise analyzer located outside the chamber. The noise levels were highest in the frequency range between 300 and 4800 Hz. Hyperbaric noise levels are discussed in relationship to recently proposed damage risk criteria for exposure to noise. (© BA)

1334.
MURRY, T.
The intelligibility of processed helium speech at diving depths greater than 1000 feet.
U.S. Nav. Submar. Med. Cent., Rep. NSMRL 697, 6p. Jan. 17, 1972.

The purpose of this study was to evaluate the intelligibility of a helium speech unscrambler undergoing development by the Admirality Research Laboratory, Teddington, England. Tapes of divers reading sentence lists at three depths in a helium-rich environment were played to five panels of listeners, each containing 15 members. Fifty words within each sentence list were chosen for evaluation. The overall mean intelligibility score for two divers at 1050 and 1500 feet and one diver at 1250 feet was 92.2 percent. The average score at the deepest depth was slightly lower than the average score at 1050 feet. For the limited conditions evaluated, the unscrambler appeared to operate effectively. Additional evaluation under various conditions using standardized intelligibility test material is necessary to determine the overall applicability and effectiveness of this device. (Author's abstract)

1335.
MURRY, T., E.J. Nelson and E.W. Swenson.
Speech intelligibility during exercise at normal and increased atmospheric pressures.
U.S. Nav. Submar. Med. Cent., Rep. NSMRL 700, 6p. Feb. 9, 1972.

The purpose of this study was to assess the effects of work loads at increased atmospheric pressures on speech intelligibility. Six subjects were exposed to depths equivalent to 0, 50, 100 and 150 feet of sea water. At each depth, the subjects recorded one 25 word PB list at each of four work loads 0, 50, 100 and 150 watts. Subjects were exercised on an ergometer and pedalling was maintained at the desired work load by monitoring a preset metronome. Heart rate and respiratory rate were monitored continuously using EKG electrodes and a nasal thermister. The speech signals were recorded with a microphone attached to a headband thus maintaining mouth-to-microphone distance constant. The recordings were played to naive listening panels to obtain speech intelligibility scores. The results indicate that at rest, speech intelligibility decreases by approximately 20 percent from surface to 150 feet. With the addition of a work load, there is an additional drop in intelligibility; however, intelligibility does not continue to decrease as work load increases. (Authors' abstract)

1336.
MURRY, T. and P.G. Lacroix.
Speech discrimination in noise and hearing loss at 3000 hertz.
U.S. Nav. Submar. Med. Res. Lab., Rep. NSMRL 719, 11p. July 11, 1972.

Navy personnel with normal hearing and with hearing losses at 3kHz and above were evaluated on tests of speech discrimination in noise. Two tests were used, one previously designed for use in audiological clinics and one constructed at this laboratory with background noise similar to that found in the enginerooms of nuclear submarines. The results indicate that subjects with hearing losses at 3kHz and above may score as much as 11 per cent but more generally at least five per cent below normal for a speech discrimination task in noise. For the two types of noise used in these tests, there was little or no difference in the general trend of test results. The correlation coefficients obtained between the puretone audiometric findings and the speech discrimination tasks in noise were found to be nonsignificant for the most part. From these results, it appears that hearing loss at 3 kHz reduces one's ability to discriminate speech in noise but this reduction is minor. (Authors' abstract)

1337.
MUSACCHIA, X.J.
Heat and cold acclimation in helium-cold hypothermia in the hamster.
Amer. J. Physiol. 222:495-498;Feb. 1972.

A study was made of the effects of acclimation of hamsters to high, 34-35°C, and low 4-5°C, temperatures for periods up to 6 wk on the induction of hypothermia in hamsters. Hypothermia was achieved by exposing hamsters to a helox mixture of 80% He and 20% O_2 at 0°C. Hypothermic induction to Tb [body temperature] 7°C was most rapid (2-3 hr) in heat-acclimated hamsters and slowest (6-12 hr) in cold-acclimated hamsters. The induction period was intermediate (5-8 hr) in room temperature non-acclimated animals (controls). Survival time in hypothermia was relatable to previous temperature acclimations. Heat-acclimated hamsters lived longest (2-2.5 days), cold-acclimated animals were short lived (12-18 hr), and nonacclimated control animals were intermediate (18-24 hr). The longevity of hypothermia in heat-acclimated hamsters compares favorably with the periods of hibernation experienced by this species. The hypothesis that thermogenesis in cold-acclimated hamsters would accentuate resistance to induction of hypothermia was substantiated. (© BA)

1338.
MUSACCHIA, X.J. and M. Jacobs.
Helium-cold induced hypothermia in the white rat.
Proc. Soc. Exp. Biol. Med. 142(3):734-739; 1973.

Exposure to a helox mixture of 80% He and 20% O_2 and low ambient temperature induces hypothermia in Sprague-Dawley white rats. Hypothermia to body temperatures of about T_{re} (rectal temperature) 14-15°C in the white rat is tolerated for various periods, for example, after four hr 88% survived and after 6 hr 25% survived. Rewarming to normothermic body temperature is achieved by exposure to room temperature, about 21-22°C. Additional sources of external heat moderately enhanced survival after rewarming. There is a direct relationship between body weight and percent survival. Despite the fact that they require a longer period in order to become hypothermic, the heavier animals are better able to survive. Spontaneous rewarming from low body temperatures of T_{re} 13.5-17°C to normothermic body temperatures, T_{re} 37°C, occurred routinely in those animals placed at 16°C ambient temperatures. Survival rates were substantial; 65% of the 60 animals used in the latter experiment survived indefinitely. Spontaneous rewarming is a consequence of the ambient cold room temperature rather than the body temperature (within limits) reached during induction. Comparisons with previously published data concerned with other methods of induction of hypothermia in the white rat indicate that the He cold method described is slightly more efficacious. The white rat is in no manner comparable to the hamster, in terms of depth of body temperature; T_{re} 7°C and lengths of 1-3 days of hypothermia induced by this same method in the hamster. (PGH) (© BA)

1339.
MUSTAFA, T., T.W. Moon and P.W. Hochachka.
Effects of pressure and temperatures on the catalytic and regulatory properties of muscle pyruvate kinase from an off-shore benthic fish.
Amer. Zool. 11:451-466; 1971.

Muscle pyruvate kinase from an abyssal Coryphaenoides species occurs as a single electrophoretic form with an isoelectric point of about pH 6.0. Maximum catalytic rates are dramatically reduced by pressure. For catalysis at 3°C the volume change of activation (ΔV^*) is about 44 cm^3/mole (calculated between 14.7 and 8000 psi). The value of

ΔV^* decreases at higher temperatures but is pH independent. The activation engery for rattail muscle pyruvate kinase at 14.7 psi is about 13 Kcal/mole and doubles at 12,000 psi. Mg^{2+} saturation kinetics involve positive site-site interactions. Hill plots yield n values of about 2.4 and K_a values of about 2 mM (at 3°C), and these constants are pressure independent. The K_m values for ADP increase slightly with pressure. PEP saturation curves are complex; at high PEP concentrations, the n values are about 2-2.5, while at low PEP levels, values for the Hill constant are about 1.0. The Hill constant for PEP is not affected by pressure, but the apparent K_m increases somewhat with pressure. FDP dramatically activates rattail muscle pyruvate kinase (500% activation with 0.1 mM FDP) by (1) reducing the Km_{PEP}, (2) increasing the maximum velocity and (3) overriding negative ATP modulation of the enzyme. The latter control feature is strictly dependent upon pressure and is not observed at low pressure. In the presence of FDP, the K_m for PEP decreases at high pressures, in this way countering the inhibitory effects of pressure. Under low concentrations of substrates, pyruvate kinase activity is probably determined by its kinetic properties and not by energy-volume relationships (Authors' abstract).

1340.
MUYSERS, K. and U. Smidt.
The nitrogen problem. New aspects of nitrogen elimination through the lungs.
In: Abstracts of the Twenty-fifth Congress of Physiological Sciences Satellite Symposium. Recent progress in fundamental physiology of diving. Marseille, France, July 1971, p.65-66. (Proceedings unpublished)

Abstract only. Excerpts quoted: During a typical prolonged expiration argon at first decreases and only very late it increases above the inspiratory level. Nitrogen behaves completely different: its concentration exceeds the inspiratory level at the same instant where the CO_2 concentration rises and the O_2 concentration fails respectively. The N_2 concentration increases further till to the end of expiration. This increase is rather linear with time. This finding indicates that relatively more nitrogen is exhaled than argon. . . . To test whether this represents a nitrogen release by the lungs or not the following measurements were made. (1) We examined 20 healthy subjects, who breathed at first for 10 min room air through a check valve before the expired air was collected for 15 min in neoprene bags. The analysis of collected expired air showed a higher increase of nitrogen than of argon. All subjects showed a nitrogen release at rest between 1.5 and 9.1 ml/min and a mean value of 3.1 ml/min for the female subjects and 5.87 ml/min for the male subjects. During exercise on a bicycle ergometer the nitrogen release increased to a mean value of 8.1 ml/min for the female and 23.1 ml/min for the male subjects. (2) During breathing in a closed system the volume of the system should increase by the amount of eliminated nitrogen, when the oxygen concentration is kept constant and the CO_2 is fully absorbed; or, if the so-called O_2 stabilization is performed by keeping constant the volume of the system, the O_2 concentration should decrease due to replacement by nitrogen. By both ways we calculated for 8 subjects a nitrogen release between 5.6 and 9.1 ml/min. The nitrogen diffusion through the skin cannot account for this nitrogen excretion of the lungs. From the data of Klock, Gurtner and Farhi (1963) one can calculate a skin diffusion of 0.8 ml/min only, which is about 10% of the nitrogen excretion through the lungs.

1341.
MUYSERS, K., U. Smidt, G.v. Nieding, H. Krekler and K.E. Schaefer.
Diffusional and metabolic components of nitrogen elimination through the lungs: effects of pressure.
U.S. Nav. Submar. Med. Res. Lab., Rep. NSMRL 736, 18p. Jan. 16, 1973.

The contributions of cutaneous diffusion of atmospheric nitrogen to pulmonary nitrogen elimination was determined by mass spectrometric analysis. In short term experiments, subjects were enclosed in gas-tight bags containing helium, O_2, N_2 or air while breathing room air. Moreover 24 hr studies of nitrogen elimination were carried out in a pressure chamber in which the ambient gas composition as well as the total pressure was varied. A linear relationship between ambient PN_2 and nitrogen elimination through the lungs was established. At zero PN_2 ambient nitrogen elimination was present after 18 hr and amounted to 0.5 ml/min. This is considered the metabolic component of gaseous nitrogen excretion. Although this amount appears very small, it can account for the frequency found deficit between nitrogen intake (in food) and nitrogen elimination via urine and faeces. Mass spectrometric analysis of ambient and expired air samples collected during three saturation excursion diving experiments showed in all seven subjects cyclic variations in the ratio of expired/inspired nitrogen while the simultaneously measured respiratory quotient remained constant. Whether these delayed nitrogen excretions are due to release of nitrogen from pools in poorly perfused tissues or altered metabolic processes cannot be stated at this time. One example of the development of large differences between expired and inspired nitrogen was found during decompression of a diver following an air dive to 198 feet. Breath-by-breath monitoring with a mass spectrometer demonstrated a sudden increase washout curve while breathing oxygen. This occurred at the same time the diver experienced skin bends. The latter lasted for about one hour and 40 minutes as did the increase in PN_2E/PN_2I. In this case the development of bends appears to be associated with inability to eliminate nitrogen properly. (Authors' abstract)

1342.
MYRBERG, A.A. Jr., S.J. Ha, S. Walewski and J.C. Banbury.
Effectiveness of acoustic signals in attracting epipelagic sharks to an underwater sound source.
Bull. Mar. Sci. 22(4):926-949; 1972.

Three experimental studies were carried out in the field to determine the effectiveness of various acoustic signals in attracting free-ranging silky sharks, Carcharhinus falciformis, into the immediate vicinity of an underwater sound source. These studies were carried out over deep water in the Straits of Florida, USA, miles from the mainland, as well as at a moored buoy in the Tongue of the Ocean, Bahamas. All of the octave bands of noise used in the tests resulted in attraction, with the level of attraction increasing as the frequency spectrum decreased, respectively, from 500-1000 Hz, to 250-500 Hz, to 75-150 Hz and finally to 25-50 Hz. Irregularly pulsed signals were also more attractive than regularly pulsed signals, with the latter increasing in attractiveness as the pulse rate increased from 1, to 5, to 10, and finally to 20 pulses/sec. Additionally, it was established that, at least under certain conditions, sharks can be drawn away from one vessel by transmitting irregularly pulsed, low-frequency signals from another vessel, stationed a few hundred meters distant. Various behavioral actions of individual sharks after approaching a sound source, are described. (© BA)

1343.
MYRICK, J.A.
A rescue system for medical diving emergencies.
In: 1972 Offshore Technology Conference, May 1-3, Houston, Texas. Preprints. Vol I, p.557-561. Published by the conference, 1972.

A plea is made to begin develpopment of an emergency hyperbaric rescue system for this country. One such candidate system proposed here consists of a light-weight portable hyperbaric chamber, a heavy lift, high-speed rescue helicopter and a shore-based medical facility for comprehensive care. The use of the U.S. Coast Guard HH-3F Helicopter is recommended as the transportation vehicle. A chamber of glass-filament-wound composite material weighing around 1000 pounds will provide the necessary hyperbaric environment. A typical rescue mission is described and flight times estimated. (Author's abstract)

1344.
NAGAITSEV, N.G., B.M. Rezvyi, A.I. Kuznetsov and V.V. Polonskii.
Raxvitie gemorragicheskogo sindroma pri legkovodolaznykh spuskakh.
[The development of hemorrhagic syndrome in divers during light diving experiments].
Voennomed. Zh. (11):60-62;Nov. 1971.

Hemorrhages in the skin, mucous membranes and internal organs of the upper part of the body, as well as in the conjunctiva, may occur in divers under the effect of pressure. The authors attribute these hemorrhagic phenomena partly to the fact that the pressure inside the diver's helmet is lowered in relation to the surrounding pressure. The authors observed a group of 21 cases of multiple disseminated hemorrhages in divers during training for light diving expeditions. The experiment consisted of relatively short time (12-18 min) exposure to relatively low (0.9-2.2 atm) partial pressure of oxygen. All divers developed hemorrhagic symptoms, 10 had to be hospitalized, the rest received ambulatory treatment. The hemorrhagic symptoms were accompanied by general fatigue, headache, sweating and cardiac symptoms, as well as a lowered thrombocyte count. Even short time exposure to relatively low oxygen partial pressure contributed to the incidence of hemorrhage in the various tissues and organs of the upper half of the body. The authors theorize that most of the divers taking part in the experiment may have been affected with some latent respiratory infection at the time or prior to the experiment. Such infection would increase the capillary permeability, thereby making the patient susceptible to hemorrhages. Other contributing factors may have been vitamin deficiency and tendency to thrombopenia. The authors conclude that further studies are needed on the effect of compressed oxygen on the vascular wall. It is also possible that in subjects with heightened susceptibility, the hemorrhagic syndrome is the first manifestation of oxygen toxicity. (OLC/BSCP)

1345.
NAKAMOTO, T. and J.W. Bean.
Influence of oxygen at atmospheric and high pressure on the developing tooth germ in rat embryos.
J. Dent. Res. 51(5, Pt.2):1397-1403; 1972.

Repeated exposure of pregnant rats to O_2 at high pressure (65 psi) twice a day for seven days increased the height of the tooth germ and ameloblastic layer of the embryo, but the width and odontoblastic layer were not changed. Exposure of pregnant rats to O_2 at atmospheric pressure stimulated the body growth of the embryo in utero. (© BA)

1346.
NAKAMOTO, T. and J.W. Bean.
Differences in growth pattern of bone and incisor of rats exposed to O_2 atmospheric and high pressure.
Arch. Oral Biol. 17:799-810;May 1972.

Three groups of young rats (age 22 days) were exposed intermittently (49 times), over a period of 44 days, group one to O_2 at atmospheric pressure (OAP), group two to O_2 at high pressure (OHP) (60 psig) and the third to air at atmospheric pressure (AAP) as controls. The average food consumption for the AAP group was 18.85 g, for the OAP 17.55 g and for the OHP 17.07 g. per rat per day. The change in the body weights of each of these groups was followed throughout the experiment which continued 13 days after the last exposures. Bone growth of the maxilla, mandible and femur diaphysis and incisor growth were not altered by the OAP exposures, but were decreased by the OHP exposures; incisor growth, however, was increased. Hardness of the bone (by Tukon Hardness Tester) was increased in the OAP and OHP exposures as compared with that of the AAP, but the hardness of the incisors was not altered. (Authors' summary)

1347.
NAKAMOTO, T. and J.W. Bean.
Growth of the tooth germ in newborn rats exposed to oxygen at atmospheric and high pressure.
J. Dent. Res. 52(3):558-562; 1973.

Newborn rats were exposed intermittently to O_2 at high pressure (93 psig) 15 times for a period of eight days. Growth of the tooth germs was the same as that of the control rats in air at atmospheric pressure, with the exception of the enamel and dentin layers, which grew less. The width of the tooth germ of rats exposed to O_2 at atmospheric pressure increased. (© BA)

1348.
NAKATSUI, M., J. Suzuki, T. Takasugi and R. Tanaka.
Nature of helium-speech and its unscrambling.
In: Ocean 73. 1973 IEEE international conference on engineering in the ocean environment, p.137-140. IEEE publication 73 CHO 7740 OCC.

Present status of voice communication in the deep and/or saturation diving situation is unsatisfactory. The use of helium solves physiological problems, but it creates the problem of "helium-speech," the degradation of speech intelligibility. A number of studies on the helium distortions have been carried out. The helium-speech is recorded under the controlled condition. Various aspects of the analysis and observation are made to clarify the nature of helium-speech and to provide the useful data for designing the helium-speech unscrambler. Two types of unscramblers are developed. Analysis-Synthesis type is an extended version of the conventional formant vocoder and is computer-simulated to study various schemes. After a simulation of the Segmentation, Partial-Rejection and Expansion (SPREX) type to get the optimum condition, a digital hard-ware of the SPREX is built. (Authors' abstract)

1349.
NARAHARA, K.A., F.W. Booth and C.L. Giannetta.
The effect of chronic hypercapnia (4% CO_2) on myocardial contractility in man.
In: Aerospace Medical Association. 1973 annual scientific meeting, Las Vegas, Nevada, May 1973. Preprints, p.151-152. Published by the Association, 1973.

To evaluate hemodynamic changes during chronic hypercapnia, the cardiovascular dynamics of young men were monitored for 2 weeks while the individuals were exposed to 4% CO_2 in a closed environment. The level for cardiac performance as indicated by the maximal oxygen consumption increased during the CO_2 exposure period. However, myocardial contractility decreased and cardiac output appeared to remain unaltered during basal measurements. These observations suggest that significant and possibly progressive alterations in cardiovascular performance may attend chronic exposure to increased levels of CO_2 in the inspired air. (Authors)

1350.
NASHIMOTO, I.
A method of adjusting decompression schedule for repetitive high pressure exposures.
In: Wada, J. and I. Takashi, eds. Proceedings of the fourth international congress of hyperbaric medicine, Sapporo, Japan, Sept. 1969, p.105-108. Baltimore, Williams, and Wilkins, 1970.

The author discusses the problem of accumulated nitrogen in the tissues, when two compressions are undergone within a period (6 to 12 hours) insufficient for the elimination of nitrogen. A nomogram is developed which takes this factor into account. By giving the values of the residual gas pressure coefficient in the decompression table, the time between two successive compressions, and the subsequent working pressure in the nomogram, the adjustment time is obtained. This adjustment time is added to the actual exposure time, thus giving a schedule adequate for successive compressions. (MFW/BSCP)

1351.
NASHIMOTO, I. and Y. Mano.
Experimental decompression sickness.
In: United States-Japan conference on natural resources development. Proceedings of the first, joint meeting of the U.S.-Japan panel on diving and technology, Tokyo, 1972, p.172-182. Japan, Ministry of Agriculture and Forestry, 1972.

Rats, frogs, tadpoles and goldfish were exposed to pressure of 5 to 200 kg/cm^2 then rapidly decompressed. They were then examined macro and micro-scopically. The authors concluded (1) gill-breathing animals can suffer from decompression sickness under air compression, but not under water compression; (2) lowering of body temperature in these animals prevents decompression sickness; (3) anesthetized animals have greater tolerance to decompression; (4) rats are more susceptible to decompression sickness than the other animals. (MFW/UMS from English abstract)

1352.
NASHIMOTO, I. and Y. Mano.
Oxygen decompression — its effectiveness in preventing decompression sickness and shortening decompression time.
In: United States-Japan conference on natural resources development. Proceedings of the first joint meeting of the U.S.-Japan panel on diving and technology, Tokyo, 1972, p.122-129. Japan, Ministry of Agriculture and Forestry, 1972.

The disadvantages of oxygen decompression are: (1) the danger of oxygen toxicity and (2) the increased fire hazard. The latter has been considerably lessened by the development of breathing equipment which discharges expired oxygen directly out of the chamber. In a recent total of 1,417 trials in Japan, 1,381 used oxygen decompression. In the oxygen breathing group, the incidence of decompression sickness was 1.32%, while in the remainder it was 8.93%. For deep and prolonged diving, oxygen decompression should be very useful. (MFW/UMS)

1353.
NASHIMOTO, I. and Y. Baba.
Regulation and decompression schedule for diving works in Japan.
In: United States-Japan conference on natural resources development. Proceedings of the first joint meeting of the U.S.-Japan panel on diving and technology, Tokyo, 1972, p.95-99.1 Japan, Ministry of Agriculture and Forestry, 1972.

The Japanese regulations governing industrial diving and compressed air work are described. There are now in Japan 20,000 licensed divers who have completed the required training, which covers diving operations, apparatus and equipment, air supply, descent and ascent, and pressure-related disorders. Most of the professional divers are fishermen; the remainder are salvage or underwater construction workers. There are two accepted decompression tables: one for compressed air workers who work at 1.0 kg/cm^2 with two shifts a day, and the other for both divers and compressed air workers who work at 1.0 to 9.0 kg/cm^2 or at depths from 10 to 90 m, without limitation on number of exposures. The tables include diving depths, bottom time, decompression stops, residual gas pressure coefficient, required time between exposures, required time after final exposure that a diver or worker must remain at or near the work site so as to be near recompression equipment, and the upper limit of total working time diving one day. A special nomogram has been devised to provide for the dangers of repetitive diving. (MFW/UMS)

1354.
NAZARKIN, V. Ya.
Izmenenie chuvstvutel'nosti zhivotnykh k dekompressionnoi bolezni v khronicheskikh eksperimentakh.
[A change of animal sensitivity to caisson disease in chronic experiments].
Patol. Fiziol. Eksp. Ter. 16:88-89;May/June 1972.

Experiments were carried out on male cats. There was a reduction of their sensitivity to caisson disease on condition of gradual — from experiment to experiment — increase for one to two minutes of the duration of exposure under increased (8 atm) pressure: the time of harmless exposure of the animals under the mentioned pressure increased by one to five minutes. Following 13-minute exposure under the pressure of 8 atm and subsequent three-minute decompression, caisson disease developed in 57 per cent of the experimental cats. (English summary)

1355.
NEFF, T.A. and T.L. Petty.
Tolerance and survival in severe chronic hypercapnia.
Arch. Intern. Med. 129(4):591-596; 1972.

A study was done of 10 patients, mean age 56 yr, with a mean forced expiratory volume in 1 sec (FEV_1), 0.41 1 (range, 0.31-0.67), and mean level of CO_2 in the arterial blood ($PaCO_2$) of 90mm Hg (range, 75-110 mm Hg). This chronic steady state can exist for many mo. :mean survival of 17 mo. after 1st determination of $PaCO_2$ (74 mm Hg) and is well tolerated. Elevated CO_2 does not cause CNS dysfunction with the possible exception of a fine tremor in some patients. Well oxygenated steady state chronic severely hypercapnic patients have the ability to maintain a high plasma bicarbonate level; mean, 45 mEq/l and nearly normal arterial pH; mean, 7.32. The judicious use of corticosteroid and diuretic therapy did not produce a primary metabolic alkalosis. (DTS) (© BA)

1356.
NELLEN, J.R. and E.P. Kindwall.
Aseptic necrosis of bone secondary to occupational exposure to compressed air: roentgenologic findings in 59 cases.
Amer. J. Roentgen. 115:512-524;July 1972.

Aseptic necrosis of bone is not an uncommon disease among workers employed under hyperbaric conditions. Our limited experience with a relatively small number of compressed-air workers has yielded a high incidence of positive roentgenographic findings. Seventy-one per cent of these lesions are juxta-articular and potentially disabling. Asymptomatic individuals may also harbor multiple bone lesions which may eventually be a source of crippling joint disease. Routine roentgenographic examinations of compressed-air workers are advocated both on a pre-employment basis and on a regular annual basis in an attempt to prevent aseptic necrosis and its sequelae. It is imperative that radiologists be trained to recognize the early lesions of aseptic necrosis in the shoulder and hip. Because of the anticipated increased use of compressed air in construction projects, civil engineers and contractors will be calling upon radiologists to make these determinations with increasing frequency. (Authors' summary)

1357.
NEPTUNE, E.M.
Lipdi peroxide formation in rat brain and liver microsomes and influence of PO_2, NADPH, metallo-ions and ascorbate.
In: Abstracts of BuMed-ONR sponsored Navywide workshop in high pressure biomedical research, U.S. Submarine Base, Groton, Conn., May 1971, p.19. Published by the Naval Submarine Medical Research Laboratory, 1971.

Abstract only. Entire item quoted: Recently other workers (J. Biol. Chem. 245:2295, 1970) have explored the enzymatic characteristics of the lipid peroxidizing system of rat liver microsomes and noted a requirement for FE^{3+} but no dependence on PO_2 above 152 mmHg. The authors have found a pronounced requirement for iron but Fe^{2+} leads to a V_{max} at $12x10^{-5}$ M compared to a V_{max} at $12x10^{-2}$ M for FE^{3+}. Their system is stimulated by increasing oxygen tensions up to 3800 mmHg. Increasing stimulation occurred with increased, added NADPH up to the highest concentration tested ($3x10^{-3}$M). The kinetics of malondialdehyde and KI oxidation values are somewhat different from the work cited above. Since their eventual interest is the question of the possible role of lipid peroxides in the etiology of acute oxygen toxicity in the CNS, studies similar to those with liver were conducted with brain microsomes. The reaction in brain is heat stable, requires iron, is enhanced by increased PO_2 and is completely suppressed by added α-tocopherol. These findings indicate the possible merit of re-evaluating lipid peroxides in acute oxygen toxicity.

1358.
NETT, L. and T.I. Petty.
Oxygen toxicity.
Amer. J. Nurs. 73:1556-1558;Sept. 1973.

In summary, oxygen toxicity of the lungs is a real entity. Although the clinical, X-ray, and histologic findings are not specific, a definite lesion and physiological abnormality can be related to excessive oxygenation. The toxicity is primarily due to the oxygen tension within the alveolus. Oxygen toxicity is due to both concentration and duration of excessive oxygenation. At a concentration of 0.4, this oxygen fraction is certainly tolerated for weeks or a few months, but even lower oxygen fractions can produce tissue change following many months or years of oxygen exposure. In clinical practice, we must constantly minimize the risk of oxygen toxicity by using the lowest flow rate or fraction of oxygen that will provide adequate arterial oxygenation and tissue oxygen delivery. (Authors)

1359.
NEVINS, R.G. and J.E. Kipp.
Performance and life support in altered environments.
Manhattan, Kan., Kan. State Univ., Inst. Environ. Res., Rep. AFOSR-TR-1683, 55p. Aug. 1971.
(AD 748 284)

The Interim Project Themis Report deals with research on (1) physiologic rhythmicity in altered environments, (2) human performance changes in altered environments, (3) effects of environment on microbial flora in clothing, (4) systems analysis and optimization studies, (5) individual cooling, (6) thermal physiological effects of localized ventilation, (7) air flow in confined spaces, and (8) comparative psychophysiology in environmental extremes. (Authors) (GRA)

1360.
NEWBURY, H.G.
Analysis of diving bells.
In: Professional diving symposium, New Orleans, Nov. 1972. Mar. Technol. Soc. J. 7:7-9; Mar./Apr. 1973.

The primary functions of the diving bell are considered fourfold: 1. It must be able to transport divers safely between the deck and bottom worksite. This includes protection from the hostilities of the open sea, and operation of an adequate life support system. It also permits the divers to be removed from the water without undergoing the waterstop decompression currently required on deep surface dives. 2. It provides a bottom safety refuge for the working diver. 3. It functions as an observation chamber at one atmosphere pressure for bottom viewing by divers without committing the diver to pressurization. 4. It contains a mating capability to permit the bell divers to transfer under pressure to a deck complex for decompression. [Diving] bells are considered essential in deep diving and together with the deck decompression chambers, control house, handling system and gas supply make up the complete package known as a Bell Diving System. [The major design parameters discussed are pressure rating, configuration, size, hull material, mating system, viewports, manways, and hatches, certification, outfitting, and buoyancy. (Author and MFW/BSCP)

1361.
NEWMAN, A.V. and F. Ingenito.
A normal mode computer program for calculating sound propagation in shallow water with an arbitrary velocity profile.
U.S. Nav. Res. Lab., Rep. NRL-MR-2381, 70p. Jan. 1972.

A computer program has been written in FORTRAN 3400/3600/3800 which solves the Z dependent part of the Helmholtz equation for a two fluid shallow water model by means of a finite difference technique. Sound speed profiles for the model are entered as discrete sets of points. The first fluid is subdivided into N incremental layers to permit the use of the finite difference equations. A linear interpolation is performed between the profile depths at which the incremental layers are defined to give sound speeds for the latter. The boundary conditions for continuity of acoustic pressure and the vertical particle velocity are matched at the interface between the two fluids. The effect on each normal mode amplitude in the first fluid due to an assumed small absorption in the second fluid is found. (Authors) (GRA)

1362.
NICHOLAS, N.C.
The propagation of sound in the deep ocean. A wave formulation.
Silver Spring, Md., Johns Hopkins Univ., Appl. Physics Lab., Rep. APL-TG-1152, 139p. Sept. 1971.
(AD 754 371)

Sound propagation in the deep ocean is not adequately described by the high frequency ray acoustics approximation, and existing wave formulations are limited. A wave solution (valid at low frequencies) is formulated for an idealized representation of the sound speed profile in the deep sound channel. Perturbation theory is applied to the ideal case to form solutions for sound speed profiles found in the ocean. Extensive calculations are made to detail the ideal solutions and to show the validity of the perturbed solutions for some realistic sound speed profiles. (Author) (GRA)

1363.
NICHOLS, C.W., C. Puglia, C. Haytmanek and C.J. Lambertsen.
Ocular effects of hyperbaric oxygen in the squirrel monkey.
Fed. Proc. 31:562;Mar./Apr. 1972.

Abstract only. Entire item quoted: It has been shown that hyperbaric oxygen can produce constriction of the visual field in man and also irreversible changes in the animal retina. Squirrel monkeys were subjected to hyperbaric oxygen at several pressures from 2.5 to 4.0 atmospheres absolute (ATA). Times to onset of gross manifestations of central nervous system (CNS) and pulmonary oxygen toxicity were noted. Fifteen of 19 monkeys exposed to hyperbaric oxygen showed aberrations of pupillary light reflex. The altered pupillary responses varied from mildly reactive to totally unreactive to light stimuli. Pupillary functions gradually returned to normal in all cases over a 24-hour period following return to air at 1 ATA. The ocular fundus of all animals was observed opthalmoscopically before, at the conclusion of, and daily after oxygen exposure. On selected animals, fluorescein angiography was performed. The most striking vascular findings apeared in the choroid although retinal hemorrhages were occasionally seen. All monkeys were killed 7 to 21 days after oxygen exposure and their eyes examined histologically for manifestation of vascular changes, and for residual neuronal damage.

1364.
NICHOLS, C.W., M. Yanoff, D.A. Hall and C.J. Lambertsen.
Histologic alterations produced in the eye by oxygen at high pressure.
Arch. Ophthal. 87:417-421;Apr. 1972.

Groups of albino guinea pigs were exposed to high concentrations of oxygen at several pressures and the eyes of the animals examined for histological changes both immediately and several months following the exposures. Normal animals as well as animals exposed to conditions of anoxia and hyperbaria were also examined. Ocular changes were observed only in the animals exposed to 100% oxygen at 3 and 5 atmospheres absolute. The primary alterations, which were found to be irreversible over the time of observation, included thinning of the corneal endothelium with darkening and condensation of the cytoplasm and pyknosis of the nuclei, and pyknosis and loss of nuclei from the epithelium of the lens. (Authors' abstract)

1365.
NIELSEN, T.W. and F.R. O'Brien.
Two-compartment chamber for long-term animal studies at gaseous pressures up to forty atmospheres.
In: IEEE international conference on engineering in the ocean environment, Panama City, Florida, September 1970. Digest of technical papers, p.230-232. Published by the conference.

A high pressure chamber for long-term animal experimentation is described. A gate valve separates two compartments; each can be held at pressures up to 40 atm. Controlled parameters are — temperature, humidity, and gaseous composition. (Eng. Ind.)

1366.
NIINIKOSKI, J., R. Goldstein, M. Linsey and T.K. Hunt.
Effect of oxygen-induced lung damage on tissue oxygen supply.
Acta Chir. Scand. 139:591-595; 1973.

Pulmonary oxygen toxicity was studied in rabbits by exposing them to pure oxygen at one atmosphere for 2 to 4 days. Tissue oxygen tension was measured periodically by means of a 13 cm Silastic tube implanted subcutaneously in the backs of the rabbits. The tube was perfused continuously with anoxic saline which equilibrated at the PO_2 of the surrounding tissue medium due to the high O_2 permeability of Silastic. The tissue PO_2 was recorded serially during oxygen breathing and after exposure to air. The arterial blood PO_2 was measured simultaneously in ear blood. A dramatic fall in both PaO_2 and tissue PO_2 was observed after 2 days' exposure to oxygen. Between days 2 and 4 a further decrease in PO_2 values occurred. Concurrently with these changes a marked respiratory distress and pulmonary edema developed in the rabbits within the first 3 days of oxygen breathing and half the rabbits died on the fourth day. At autopsy, histologic examination of lungs revealed typical signs of oxygen-induced pulmonary damage. (Authors' abstract)

1367.
NISHI, R.Y.
Ultrasonic detection of bubbles with Doppler flow transducers.
Ultrasonics 10(4):173-179; 1972.

Doppler blood-flow transducers have been used to detect gas bubbles in the circulatory system during hyperbaric decompression. This paper describes briefly the theoretical acoustic scattering properties of bubbles and then describes various experimental procedures used to determine the properties of these flow transducers. The capabilities and limitations of the transducers for the detection of bubbles were investigated by studying the scattering from both solid objects and air bubbles moving through the acoustic field. In vivo experiments indicate that it would be difficult to obtain any correlation between the output of these transducers and bubble size. (© BA)

1368.
NISHI, R.Y.
Calibration procedures for pneumatic analogue decompression computers.
Downsview, Ontario, Canada, Def. Div. Inst. Environ. Med., Def. Res. Board, Rep. DCIEM 918, 30p. Jan. 1973.

The Kidd-Stubbs pneumatic analogue decompression computer is used for the real-time prediction of the safe ascent depth of a diver exposed to pressure. Calibration procedures for the pneumatic section of the computer are described for two types of operational computers, the Mark VIS pneumatic-mechanical computer and the hybrid pneumatic-electronic computer. Experimental calibration data are presented for these computers as well as the tolerance levels of the calibration parameters derived from the theoretical decompression model. (Author's abstract)

1369.
NISHI, R.Y. and L.A. Kuehn.
Digital computation of decompression profiles.
Downsview, Ontario, Canada, Def. Civ. Inst. Environ. Med., Def. Res. Board Rep. DCIEM-884, 28p. Jan. 1973.
(AD 765 704/2)

The Kidd-Stubbs pneumatic analogue decompression computer is used for the real-time prediction of the safe ascent depth following an excursion to depth. The theoretical model which is derived from the decompression computer can be solved using numerical techniques on a digital computer, or can be solved on an analogue computer. This report describes a series of Fortran IV programs which have been written to solve this theoretical model under a variety of conditions. The basic program can be used to calculate the safe ascent depth for a standard dive or for repetitive dives, and if desired, the safe ascent height for flying after diving. Modifications to the basic program are described which permit the use of the model for applications such as the design of pneumatic computers and the analysis of decompression tables. (Author) (GRA)

1370.
NISHI, R.Y. and S.D. Livingstone.
Intravascular changes associated with hyperbaric decompression: theoretical considerations using ultrasound.
Aerosp. Med. 44:179-183;Feb. 1973.

Doppler blood flowmeters have been used to detect intravascular gas bubbles which are considered to be a major cause of decompression sickness. However, observations by various investigators have indicated that other factors such as red cell agglutination, platelet aggregates and coalescence of lipids may be involved in decompression sickness. The possibility of using the Doppler flowmeters to detect such particles in the blood has been investigated theoretically. Experimental results from these devices implanted around the inferior venae cavae of rabbits are presented showing the waveform for bubbles as well as changes which appear in the blood flow waveform during decompression. The latter may indicate aggregation of erythrocytes and/or platelets. (Authors' abstract)

1371.
NISHIDA, K.
The structural behavior of glass pressure hulls.
U.S. Nav. Ship Res. Develop. Cent., Rep. NSRDC-3863, 111p. June 1972.
(AD 746 878)

A report on glass vessels for deep submergence is presented. Emphasis is on the structural response of spherical and hemispherical glass shells under external hydrostatic and cyclic pressure. Results of earlier programs are reviewed. A computerized analysis trading off the variables in the joint problem is presented. Final joint geometries are discussed and data on chemically strengthened glass hemispherical shells with equatorial joint rings under fatigue conditions are presented. The results indicate relatively efficient (W/D = 0.5), small pressure vessels of chemically strengthened glass are practical for unmanned noncritical applications to 20,000 ft. Nine 10-inch diameter chemically strengthened glass hemispherical shells of PPG 1080 glass with overall weight to displacement ratios of 0.5 survived at least 3000 cycles to 20,000 feet. Each hemisphere was then subjected to a proof test to 30,000 feet. (Author) (GRA)

1372.
NODDIN, E.M.
Studies in enlisted submariner motivation I: Some etiological factors related to devolunteering of submarine school candidates.
U.S. Nav. Submar. Med. Cent., Rep. NSMRL 703, 14p. Mar. 2, 1972.

Questionnaire data pertaining to the circumstances surrounding a submarine crewmember's decision to devolunteer were collected from 101 enlisted men following Submarine School graduation. Thirteen classes of motives resulted from a content analysis of these data. The four major motivational categories in descending order of incidence were: Habitability factors, Motivation deficiencies, Maladjustive indices, and Family problems. Habitability factors and motivation deficiencies account for most of the devolunteering of the lower paygrade men assigned to the diesel submarine fleet. In contrast, the higher-rated, nuclear-trained submariners appeared to have devolunteered largely because of problems related to family adjustment, and to a lesser extent, because of the perceived dangers of submarine duty. Across all subgroups within this sample, 25% or more apparently had some type of maladjustive trend associated with and probably causally related to the decision to devolunteer. Several approaches counteractive to the major causes of devolunteering delineated by this study were presented. (Author's abstract)

1373.
NOLTE, H. and K. Von Schnakenburg.
Einflusse der Hyperoxie auf das Zentralnervensystem.
[The influence of hyproxia on the central nervous system].
Pneumonologie 149:87-96; 1973.

Two main types of side effects must be considered in hyperbaric oxygenation: respiratory disturbances or pulmonary changes and central nervous system lesions. The effects on the central nervous system may lead to a tonoclonic seizure. Light- and electron-microscope examination of the brain after experimental hyperbaric oxygen convulsions revealed typical predilection sites for nerve cell alterations which are not identical to localizations of changes caused by other noxious agents. They are regarded as specific changes due to the hyperoxia and their localization in the brain stem correlates to the origin of electrical discharges in hyperbaric oxygen convulsions. Pharmacological investigations on the symptoms of oxygen intoxication revealed the alternating effects between pulmonary and central nervous system changes. (English abstract)

1374.
NOLTE, H. and K. Von Schnakenberg.
Morphologische and pharmakologisch-toxikologische Aspekte der Hyperoxie.
[Morphologic and pharmacologic-toxicologic aspects of hyperoxia].
Int. J. Clin. Pharmacol. 7:340-347;July 1973.

Pulmonary changes due to oxygen at high pressure, known as Smith-effect, develop depending on oxygen partial pressure and length of exposure. They also occur following a generalized tonoclonic convulsion (Paul Bert-effect) brought about by very high oxygen pressure. Histological alterations of nerve cells in the rat brain were found in typical predilection sites after such an oxygen convulsion. The effects of centrally acting drugs on the lung changes occurring simultaneously with oxygen convulsions demonstrate the central origin of these findings. The histological alterations in the central nervous system are not caused by the pulmonary edema but they are direct or indirect effects of the cerebral hyperoxia. The particular localization of these alterations correlate to neurophysiological results of other investigators. (Authors' abstract)

1375.
NORTHWAY, W.H., L. Rezeau, R. Petriceks, R. Dorsett and T. Roberts.
Pulmonary oxygen toxicity: adaptive response in the newborn mouse.
Invest. Radiol. 8:281-282;July/Aug. 1973.

Abstract only. Examination of lungs of 368 newborn mice, some of which were exposed to 100% oxygen and some to air for up to 14 days, indicated marked inhibition of DNA synthesis in those exposed to oxygen up until the sixth day of exposure. Spontaneous deaths occurred from the fourth day through the eighth day. With the drop in mortality, DNA synthesis increased, indicating an adaptive growth response. Although all pulmonary cells demonstrated inhibition of DNA synthesis, the bronchiolar mucosal cells were affected most strongly. Findings suggested a local membrane toxic effect of oxygen aside from any general metabolic effect on these cells. (MFW/BSCP)

1376.
NOVAK, L. and Y. Cesnak.
Dynamic katathermometer for measuring the cooling effect of the environment.
Space Biol. Med. 7:85-90;May 15, 1973.
(JPRS 59015)

The instrument proposed is designed on the principle of a biophysical model of a warm-blooded organism. [The authors have] attempted to preserve small size of the sensor and also adhere to the automatism principle in its operation with maintenance of a constant sensor temperature in the range of 37 + 0.1%. Sensor design was selected in such a way as to eliminate heat losses by its holder. Its principal advantage is the possibility of rapid dynamic measurement of the cooling action of the environment in the selected place in experimental space. The instrument consists of a sensor and regulator into which a measuring device is incorporated. The sensor ensures a rigorously constant temperature and it measures the heat released into the surrounding medium. The sensor is placed on the compensation part, which limits heat transfer by the holder and by the conductors of the lead-in cable. It has the configuration of a cylinder 2 cm in diameter and 6 cm high. The total length of the detector part, consisting of the sensor, compensation part, and holder with its base, is 11 cm. Sensor design also makes possible its use for a study of the dynamics of changes in heat-insulating properties of different materials under unusual conditions, in the air or water. It is also feasible to use it in small cabins occupied by human beings or in which nonuniform external heating substantially changes the cooling effect of the medium. These changes can be registered using our katathermometer more rapidly and graphically than on the basis of registry of changes in ambient temperature. This has been demonstrated by tests of the dynamic katathermometer in a temperature and pressure chamber. (Authors)

1377.
NOVIKOVA, I.S., I.V. Pervukhina, L.A. Slonova and I.K. Ryzhova.
Khromatograficheskii metod opredeleniya dvuokisi ugleroda v vozdukhe.
[Chromatographic method of determining carbon dioxide in air].
Gig. Sanit. 38(11):77-78; 1972.

A comparison of the titrometric and gas chromatographic methods showed that in the case of large CO_2 concentrations in the air the titrometric method gives underestimated results, and thus the gas chromatographic method is preferred owing to its high sensitivity, specificity and accuracy. Air samples can be stored 4-5 days. (MDS) (© BA)

1378.
NOWLIS, D.P., H.H. Watters and E.C. Wortz.
Habitability assessment program.
In: Miller, J.W., J.G. Van Derwalker and R.A. Waller, eds. Tektite 2: Scientists-in-the-sea, p.VIII-68-VIII-89. Washington, D.C., U.S. Department of the Interior, August 1971.

This paper summarizes the results of an attempt to develop and apply evaluation techniques to measure parameters that affect the perception of life quality in an isolated habitat. Methods, procedures, and results of the program are discussed. The objectives of development and evaluation of methods for measuring habitability were met during this program. In addition, much was learned about the problems of designing habitable structures for occupancy during long periods in isolation. A series of conclusions are drawn from the data and inferences are made concerning habitat design factors such as privacy, food, task support, recreation, stimulus variety, and duration of isolation. (Authors' abstract)

1379.
NOWLIS, D.P., E.C. Wortz and H. Watters.
Tektite 2 habitability research program.
Los Angeles, Cal., AiResearch Mfg. Co., Rep. 71-6192-1, 121p. Jan. 14, 1972.
(N72-15,069)

Multi-level parameters relating to perceived life quality in an isolated research and residence quarters, were measured using a variety of tests. The habitat under study, emplaced beneath the sea off the coast of St. John's Island as a part of the Tektite II program was being used for marine research. The crew for each of the ten missions consisted of one engineer and four scientists. One mission had an all-female crew. Mission length was either 14-20 days and four engineers, in covering six missions, stayed in the habitat for periods of 30 days each. A personality test was taken before confinement in the habitat. Two attitude tests were filled out by the aquanauts while they were still in the habitat. Daily moods were monitored during all missions. Special observations were made of leisure time use. Standardized private debriefings were administered at the end of each mission to each aquanaut. Other behavioral observations made by another research team were intercorrelated with the other measures described above. (Author) (STAR)

1380.
NOWLIS, D.P.
Tektite 2 habitability research program: day-to-day life in the habitat.
Los Angeles, Cal. AiResearch Mfg. Co., Rep. 71-6192-2. (NASA-CR-130034) 130p. Mar. 1972. (N73-16094)

Because it is widely agreed that the field of environmental psychology is quite young, it was determined that a sample of recorded observations from a representative mission should be included in the report on Tektite to give the professional reader a better feeling of normal day-to-day life in the isolated habitat. Names of the crew members have been replaced with numbers and some off-color words have been replaced by more acceptable slang; some remarks have been omitted that might lead to easy identification of the subjects. Otherwise, the following pages are exactly as transcribed during the late afternoons and the evenings of the mission. (Author) (STAR)

1381.
NUYTTEN, P.
Deep helium diving in the high Arctic.
In: 1973 Offshore Technology Conference, April-May, 1973, Houston, Texas. Preprints, Vol. I, p.497-504. Published by the conference.

One of the most significant problems currently facing the tri-faceted (commercial, scientific and military) diving communities is the necessity to carry out deep, manned operations in water temperatures equal to those found in the Arctic circle. The problems of respiratory heat loss, and diver protective garments are well known, but most prevalent solutions are largely based on laboratory acquired data and interpolation of traditional intemperate water techniques. This paper outlines parameters of the problem, methodology of approach and evaluation of some solutions. The research and testing took place in facilities in California and western Canada, under actual operating conditions in the sub Arctic, through the ice in the high Arctic, and finally culminated in hyperbaric tests at 1,000' in 32° water. (Author's abstract)

1382.
NYSTROM, D.J. and J.L. Stortz.
Hotline — a communications system for diving research.
Sea Technol. 14:18-20;Sept. 1973.

[Hotline] is an audio telephone system linking divers within hyperbaric chambers to external experimenters and topside control. Individual station preamplification is provided for high gain, provision is made for helium unscrambling for deep helium dives, and sector isolation with override is available for complex experimental procedures. Redundancy, modular construction and backup communication systems reflect a design dedicated to safety and extreme operational flexibility. (Author)

1383.
O'BRIEN, F.R.
Design of the environmental gas system for a High Pressure Life Laboratory.
Eng. J., p.20-24;July/Aug. 1973.

The facility here discussed is under construction; it is designed for hyperbaric research with small animals, the purpose of which is to further knowledge and understanding of the problems incurred in underwater habitats. The High Pressure Life Laboratory consists of two carbon steel spheres of 7 ft. internal diameter which will have an operating pressure of 700 psi, equivalent to 1340 fsw. Attached to the spheres are subchambers, which can be maintained at the same atmosphere as the central chamber. The two spheres with their subchambers can operate at different atmospheres from one another, but each chamber complex must be uniform within itself. Methods of gas circulation and of contamination control are described; both cryogenic and adsorption methods are used. Control of the system by a computer has led to interface problems in the humidification and reheat systems; these are described. Decompression methods, both with and without animals, are described. One chamber complex was in operating condition at the time of writing and by the end of 1973, the complete facility is expected to be operative. The facility is located at the University of North Dakota. (MFW/SCD)

1384.
OBRIST, W.D., H.A. Saltzman, I.A. Sulg, L.W. Thompson and R.E. Townsend.
The quantitated EEG in hypoxic and hyperbaric conditions.
In: Hesser, C.M. and D. Linnarsson eds. Proceedings of the first annual scientific meeting of the European Undersea Biomedical Society, Stockholm, 13-15 June 1973. Forsvarsmedicin 9:466-471;July 1973.

These studies were made during a 1970 saturation dive designed to study the effects of pressure and breathing mixtures on respiratory gas exchange, arterial pressure, pulse, EEG, and reaction time. An increased mean alpha frequency, concomitant with prolonged reaction time and increasing failure of response, was noted when subjects breathed nitrogen under increased pressure in normoxic conditions. Various possible explanations are suggested, and it is stated that further investigation is warranted since these alpha changes might act as a predictor of behavioral impairment. It is concluded as a result of these studies that the quantitated EEG is a valuable measure of the metabolic and functional state of the brain under these conditions. It is stated that "a combined period and voltage analysis of the EEG, as well as a continuous monitoring of average values offers here an adequate information about the most meaningful single parameters of the EEG. At the same time a considerable data reduction is achieved — an important aspect of EEG quantitation." (MFW/UMS)

1385.
O'DONNELL, R.D., P. Chikos and J. Theodore.
Effect of carbon monoxide exposure on human sleep and psychomotor performance.
J. Appl. Physiol. 31:513-518;Oct. 1971.

Recent studies have indicated that human performance degrades after exposure to small amounts of carbon monoxide (CO) while other studies have found no decrement. To further test the effect of such exposure, four subjects were exposed to 75 and 150 parts per million of CO during sleep for 9 hr, producing mean carboxyhemoglobin levels of 5.9 and 12.7%. Sleep was monitored continuously through electro-physiological recording. Upon waking, subjects were given mental arithmetic, time estimation, tracking, monitoring, and visual tests. No performance decrements or differences from control conditions were found in any of the tests used. With respect to sleep patterns, it was found that subjects under CO had more deep sleep and less light sleep than in the control condition. Rapid-eye-movement sleep was not affected. It was concluded that, although certain CO effects occur in sleep, these are not great enough to affect performance and that for healthy well-motivated human subjects these levels of CO do not produce performance decrements in the tasks used. (Authors' abstract)

1386.
OHIWA, H. and H. Kita.
Adaptive changes in ventilation to increased work of breathing at scuba diving.
In: Wada, J. and I. Takashi, eds. Proceedings of the fourth international congress of hyperbaric medicine, Sapporo, Japan, Sept. 1969, p.141-145. Baltimore, Williams, and Wilkins, 1970.

The authors note that the hypoventilation of trained scuba divers may be considered as a form of adaptive change. By this change of ventilatory pattern, they combat the increase of ventilatory work under pressure, thus arriving at an optimum respiratory rate. This adaptive change brings on carbon dioxide accumulation, even at shallow depth. (MFW/BSCP)

1387.
OHRESSER, P., J. Tassy, J.F. Amoros and J. Dor.
Les accidents de plongee: A propos de 75 observations recueillies en 3 ans.
[Diving accidents: 75 cases collected in three years].
Maroc Med. 52:445-447; 1972.

The author discusses the frequency and general characteristics of various types of diving accidents, including cerebral accidents, pneumothorax, bends, and neurological accidents, and recommends treatment procedures. Since most diving accidents can be traced to disregard or misuse of the decompression tables, the author recommends a strict adherence to the appropriate decompression procedures, and applauds the educational work undertaken by the diving clubs in this regard. (MEMH/SCD)

1388.
OHRESSER, P.
A propos de la table ronde sur la therapeutique de decompression.
[Concerning the round table on decompression therapy].
Bull. Medsubhyp 8:3;Nov. 1972.

After a survey of the 120 observations accumulated over six years, the author emphasizes the following points: (1) No cerebral injury has been observed. In two cases in which neurological symptoms appeared to indicate brain injury, the diagnosis was erroneous. In order to prove brain injury, it is necessary to have (a) EEG anomalies; (b) the opinion of a qualified neurologist; (c) the testimony of a credible witnes of the dive. (2) The GERS tables are probably efficacious, but the relative importance of pressure and of oxygen is difficult to determine. (3) The efficacity of the GERS tables is only partial in serious neurological injuries; oxygen therapy cannot be augmented, because the maximum safe limit is now indicated. (4) Oxygen therapy being thus limited, other therapeutic methods must be investigated. Findings of Cockett and of Ricci indicate a connection between decompression accidents and fat embolisms. After the 48th hour, abnormal coagulation factors have been observed, which probably result from a failure of lipid metabolism. These findings indicate the advisability of the use of low molecular weight Dextran and of injectable aspirin. Heparin will be used immediately upon any sign of abnormal coagulation. (MFW/BSCP)

1389.
OHTA, Y., T. Kawashiro and T. Yokoyama.
Tissue gas tensions of the rat's subcutaneous gas pockets and the oxygen intoxication.
In: Wada, J. and I. Takashi, eds. Proceedings of the fourth international congress on hyperbaric medicine, Sapporo, Japan, Sept. 1969, p.32-36. Baltimore, Williams and Wilkins, 1970.

Incidence of oxygen intoxication was experimentally studied on the THAM-treated rats as well as on the control. Changes in the tissue gas tensions to be occurred under hyperbaric conditions were discussed in terms of the gas tensions in the subcutaneous pockets. Oxygen consumption of rats was measured under both ambient and hyperbaric conditions. The changes in the blood perfusion were estimated from the calculated arterial-venous oxygen content difference and the overall oxygen consumption. The THAM-treated rats revealed significantly lower incidence of oxygen intoxication than that of the control. These rats demonstrated lower oxygen tension and higher carbon dioxide tension in the gas pocket. Oxygen consumption of the THAM-treated rats was decreased significantly under ambient environmental condition as well as under hyperbaric condition. The estimated arterial-venous oxygen content difference was decreased under hyperbaric environment. (Authors' summary)

1390.
OHTA, Y. and H. Matsunaga.
Bone lesions in divers.
In: United States-Japan conference on natural resources development. Proceedings of the first joint meeting of the U.S.-Japan panel on diving and technology, Tokyo, 1972, p.136-141. Japan, Ministry of Agriculture and Forestry, 1972.

Radiological data collected from 301 divers over a period of three years revealed evidence of osteonecrosis in 50.5%. Of these, 14.6% were juxta-articular, most of which were in the humeral head. Most of the head, neck and shaft lesions were found in the lower extremities. Length of diving experience was related positively to incidence of osteonecrosis. The sites of bone lesions were in the following order: upper humerus 92 cases; lower femur 72 cases; upper femur 58 cases; upper tibia 9 cases. Of the 152 men afflicted, 60 had solitary lesions and 92 had multiple lesions. There was greater incidence among divers with a history of decompression sickness, but there was no relationshnip between the location of bends pain and the site of the lesions, and no relation between spinal paraplegia and bone lesions. There was a relation between depth of diving and incidence of lesions. (MFW/UMS)

1391.
OHUCHI, T., S. Meyer and T. Teraura.
Catheter-mounted oxygen electrode for monitoring oxygen tension.
Cardiovasc. Res. Cent. Bull. 10(4):111-122; 1972.

A new monopolar oxygen electrode mounted at the tip of a catheter connected to an IBC oximeter was used in both in vitro and in vivo studies. Good correlation was found between the values obtained with the catheter-mounted electrode and those obtained with the bipolar oxygen electrode for arterial and venous PO_2. Calculated from PO_2 values recorded with the monopolar electrode, the A-V [arteriovenous] O_2 content was in good agreement with the values obtained with the Guyton analyzer provided the arterial PO_2 did not exceed 90 mm Hg. Below this point, measurement of A-V O_2 content was reliable. (AFK) (© BA)

1392.
OLINGHOUSE, L.
Shark sense.
Skin Diver 22:46-49;July 1972.

This is a generally informative article about the nature and habits of the shark, and ways in which to guard against or ward off shark attack. It is noted that shark's teeth, in addition to being extremely sharp, also are contaminated with harmful microscopic bacteria of the genus Paracolon, which can cause death as the result of even minor wounds, if proper antibiotics are not immediately administered. Of nearly 300 species, only ten are known to be man-eaters: the great white, the tiger, the blue, the largest of the hammerheads, the mako, the bull, the lemon, the dusky, the whitetip, and the Pacific Ocean gray shark. The Navy has developed an effective shark repellant in the form of a combination of black dye, which conceals the diver, and 20% copper acetate. Another successful device to be used in connection with survival equipment, is a black plastic bag with inflatable rings for buoyancy. Lacking means of repelling a shark, the underwater swimmer should keep moving in a steady manner, since thrashing movements are known to attract sharks. If attack does occur, the shark can frequently be driven off by a sharp blow on the nose. (MFW/BSCP)

1393.
OLSON, G.M. and K. Laxar.
Performance on the expanded time bearing plot as a function of bearing accuracy.
U.S. Nav. Submar. Med. Res. Lab., Rep. NSMRL 716, 32p. June 26, 1972.

Two experiments analyzed the effects of statistical noise in raw sonar bearings on performance in a laboratory version of the expanded time bearing plot. Accuracy of faired bearings and bearing rate estimates were taken as the measure of performance. Greater amounts of noise led to poorer performance, but these decrements were smaller when the noise was random than when it was correlated. Human performance was contrasted with that of an orthogonal polynomial curve-fitting routine designed to do the same task. The mathematical routine was affected by the noise in the same way as humans were. However, on simple plots the mathematical routine provided superior solutions while on curves of more complex shapes or at the ends of curves humans were superior. Thus, in certain situations the human's perceptual and cognitive abilities gave him a distinct advantage over the mathematical routine. (Authors' abstract)

1394.
OLSON, G.M. and K. Laxar.
Speed of comprehending submarine fire control displays: II. Further evidence of right-left differences.
U.S. Nav. Submar. Med. Res. Lab., Rep. NSMRL 758, 21p. plus append. Sept. 14, 1973.

[The problem was] to examine man's ability to make quick decisions based on displays containing information about "right" and "left". [It was found that] subjects took longer to interpret displays involving the direction left than displays involving right in two extensions of previous research. How these asymmetries emerged depended in part on the details of subjects' strategies in interpreting and responding to complex displays. These studies provide evidence of limitations of man's ability to think about space. Such limitations are relevant to tasks like submarine fire control or navigation, where indirect information must be used to derive spatial representations. Further, since tasks similar to these reported have been used as indices of performance in hyperbaric environments, and the kind of analysis provided here could prove useful in pinpointing the nature of performance deficits in such environments. (Authors' summary)

1395.
OLSON, G.M. and K. Laxar.
Speed of comprehending submarine fire control displays: III. Processing information about "right" and "left" — a note on left-handers.
U.S. Nav. Submar. Med. Res. Lab., Rep. NSMRL 760, 4p. Sept. 14, 1973.

[The problem was] to examine the ability of left-handed subjects to make quick decisions based on displays containing information about "right" and "left". [It was found that] left-handed subjects did not show the right-left processing asymmetries characteristic of right-handers, although in all other respects their performance was comparable to that of right-handers. This finding provides limits on the generalizability of earlier research by showing that left-handed subjects have a different, possibly more complex cognitive model for the directions right and left. This study provides evidence of differences between right and left-handed subjects in their ability to think about space. Such limitations are relevant to tasks like submarine fire control or navigation, where indirect information must be used to derive spatial representations. (Authors' summary)

1396.
O'NEILL, W.J.
Integrated breathing apparatus for dives to 1500 feet.
In: Professional diving symposium, New Orleans, Nov. 1972. Mar. Technol. Soc. J. 7:17-24; Mar./Apr. 1973.

The SIMBA (system of integrated modular breathing apparatus) system is an integrated modular family of diving equipment. Its four main gas supply modules are designed to cover the full spectrum of diving throughout the water column to 1500 feet employing a minimum of modules. The first module functions as a surface-supplied air or mixed-gas open-circuit free-flow unit with a demand over-ride. The second module will facilitate 90 percent of deep work through bell, habitat or submersible-supplied closed circuit "Arawak" push-pull system. Exterior mounted submersible pumps enable the diver to breathe chamber gas. Significant benefits are derived from this system over contemporary deep working apparatus. The third module covers the tethered or free swimming closed or semi-closed circuit scuba capability. The fourth module is a tethered backpack of the Venturi or powered circulator principle sometimes used without breathing bags as we know them. All are served by a single human engineered innovative helmet which may be served by any of the four-mentioned breathing gas supplies. The probability of underwater mission or task accomplishment can be improved by considering some psychological aspects of wet human engineering in system conceptual design. Stress induced performance degradation in normally motivated divers is reduced in the second mode, using the Arawak system. Natural human instincts are complied with to assure increased diver productivity. An argument is given in favor of extending our bottom horizontal ranging capability with movable bells rather than longer hoses or tethers. Throughout this paper emphasis is placed on the second mode of breathing gas supply (Arawak) since it is the least understood in the industry. Open circuit helmets and bag type counterlung apparatus are in current use and thus bear less definition. The term module used here implies a set of equipment designed to supply gas to a diver in the "mode" specified. (Author's introduction)

1397.
O'REILLY, J.P.
Behavioral effectiveness at 16 ATA.
Honolulu, Univ. Hawaii, Rep. UNIHI-SEAGRANT-TR-73-01, NOAA-73051504, 80p. Apr. 1973.
(COM 73 10920)

The existence of helium narcosis at 16 ATA was supported, where narcosis was defined as a reduction in behavioral effectiveness. Moderate loss in cognitive ability was noted at maximum pressure, while little decrement was evidenced in behaviors requiring less cognitive involvement. This result is in agreement with Bennett's hypothesis that narcosis is a function of synaptic blocking in the CNS. While moderate performance loss was experienced — up to 25% decrement in associative memory ability — divers' capacity to function effectively was not seriously impaired. Motor coordination, vigilance responding, and sensory mechanisms appeared to be minimally affected by He-O_2 exposure. The possibility of performance alteration due to increased arousal exists, particularly during a stressful decompression; the direction of change appears a function of task complexity. Divers may be able to function adequately to depths of 2000 feet, but there is some question as to the degree of task complexity they are capable of performing correctly at that depth. Until more precise measurements of the narcotic effect of helium are secured, there is still some reservation possible concerning man's ability to function at peak effectiveness in a hyperbaric environment. (Author's abstract modified by GRA)

1398.
ORIOL, P. and J. Chouteau.
Le controle de l'atmosphere des maisons sous-marines.
[Atmosphere control in underwater habitats].
In: CIESM. Rapports et proces-verbaux des reunions, No. 22(4), p.769-771. Monaco, Commission Internationale pour l'Exploration de la Mer Mediterranee, 1972.

Regulation of oxygen supply, removal of carbon dioxide, and humidity control are discussed. It is stated that the most difficult problem in a closed environment is the control of contaminants produced by man and by the habitat itself, which are malodorous, irritating, and sometimes toxic. The chemical measures used in regulating the partial pressures of the components of the atmosphere are discussed. Mass spectrometry and gas chromatography are briefly mentioned as being useful. It is stated that underwater habitats are at present safe for use at moderate depths (up to 100 m), both for research and for education and training. At greater depths, their use is still within the domain of the specialist. (MFW/BSCP)

1399.
ORRIS, W.L.
Diving doctors.
Skin Diver 22:40-41, 60-61, 63, 78;July 1972.

The author, a physician, points out the lack of dissemination of knowledge regarding the nature of accidents and illnesses relating to diving. Underwater medicine has emerged as a recognized specialty. With the prevalence of jet travel, it is now possible for a doctor in any location to be faced with a patient suffering from an underwater-related injury or illness, and it is therefore necessary for all doctors either to have sufficient knowledge of the field or to have access to those doctors who do, so that proper treatment can be given with the greatest possible speed. The author lists the names, addresses and phone numbers of 85 doctors who are willing to act as consultants in such cases. In many instances, the field of underwater medicine in which the doctor is specially qualified is also indicated. (MFW/BSCP)

1400.
ORSI, E.V.
The role of hyperbaric oxygen in changing response to virus infection.
In: Abstracts of BuMed-ONR sponsored Navywide workshop in high pressure biomedical research, U.S. Submarine Base, Groton, Conn., May 1971, p.16. Published by the Naval Submarine Medical Research Laboratory, 1971.

Abstract only. Entire item quoted: During the past three years the author has been studying the role of hyperbaric oxygen in changing host response to virus infection. His system has consisted of Coxsackievirus B-1 (one of the human enteroviruses CFW mice, and cell cultures of human and mouse origin. Initially he found that exposure to 100% oxygen at 3 ATA enhanced cell pathology, mouse mortality and increased the amount of virus in the heart and brown fat tissues particularly if exposure preceded infection. Subsequently, evidence for lysosome involvement in hyperbaric oxygen enhanced infected cell damage was obtained with cell cultures. Reports of adrenal mediated hyperbaric toxicity, by other Navy supported investigators directed his attention to adrenal-lysosome interaction in hyperbaric stressed viral infections in both animal and cell culture systems. Current studies have concentrated on lysosomal enzyme leakage following virus infection with prior hyperbaric oxygenation. Results show that combined infection and high pressure oxygen or the administration of adrenochrome prior to infection diminishes lysosomal leakage of RNA-ase and is accompanied by higher amounts of virus in the heart tissue. In addition, it has been found that adrenalectomy reverses the interferon level depletion associated with hyperbaric oxygen. Extralysosomal activity of heart tissue RNA-ase and Betaglucuronidase of these animals are currently under study.

1401.
OSBORNE, C.K., R. Carolla, D. Jefferson and C.E. Mengel.
Effect of methemoglobin on in vivo RBC lipid peroxidation.
Aerosp. Med. 44:62-67;Jan. 1973.

Hyperoxia has been shown to cause in vivo lipid peroxidation and hemolysis. The present study was undertaken to explore a possible protective effect of methemoglobin (MET) on this process. Tocopherol deficient mice were given $NaNO_2$ (.01 to .09 mg/Gm. B.W.) prior to exposure to 100% O_2 at 5 Atm. P. (OHP) for 45 min. The MET formed was dose related (0 to 43%). Control mice (0% MET) exposed to OHP developed lipid peroxides (29 muM/ml RBC) and evidence of hemolysis (hct 45% to 31%, hemoglobin visible in plasma and urine). In contrast mice with 43% MET exposed to OHP developed no lipid peroxides and no hemolysis (hct 45 to 46, no hemoglobin in plasma or urine). Inhibition of RBC catalase activity (.201 + .010 to .164 + 0.16 meq/ml perborate reduced) following treatment of mice with amino-triazole (AT) was seen after OHP, indicating H_2O_2 excess. MET (60%) in AT-treated mice prevented catalase inhibition (H_2O_2 excess) during OHP (.197 + .021). In vitro RBC suspensions with 90% MET and washed of excess $NaNO_2$ developed less lipid peroxides (20) than controls (116) on exposure to UV light. Similarly, RBCs developed less lipid peroxides (48) than controls (199) on in vitro exposure to OHP. These data show that MET prevents in vivo and in vitro RBC lipid peroxidation and hemolysis by oxidant stress. They are consistent with the hypotheses that (1) irrespective of the O_2 tension around the RBC oxyhemoglobin is required for lipid peroxidation to occur, and (2) H_2O_2 excess, the predominant mediator of lipid peroxidation, is prevented by MET. (Authors' abstract)

1402.
OSER, H.
Medizinische Erfahrungen beim Einsatz des Unterwasserlaboratoriums 'Helgoland' im Herbst 1971.
[Medical observations during the use of the underwater laboratory 'Helgoland' in autumn, 1971].
DFVLR-Nachrichten, p.307-308;Aug. 1972.

The laboratory remained under water for almost a week. The aquanauts lived continuously under conditions involving a pressure of 2.0 atm. The pressure corresponds to the environmental pressure at a depth of 10 m. The state of health of the aquanauts was medically supervised. Infections involving parts of the ear made necessary almost daily medical inspections. A new oxygen control device used is considered together with decompression times required for various environmental conditions. (Aerosp. Med.)

1403.
OSTACHKOV, K.V., V.V. Larin, V.S. Sokozovs'kii, V.A. Savits'kii and S.I. Byutner.
Termotopografiya tila ta deyaki pokazniki obminnikh protsesiv u legovogolaziv za umov riznikg rezhimiv pidvodnikh zanuren'.
[Body thermography and some indices of metabolic processes in light divers under conditions of different regimens during underwater immersions].
Fiziol. Zh. 18:614-620;Sept./Oct. 1972.

The immersion of light divers under water is followed by the development of the stress reaction which is manifested in a change of the body thermotopography at the expense of increasing loss of warmth, some clotting, leucocytosis and inhibition of serum hydrolases activity. The degree of the body cooling oxygen expense and changes in respiratory and pulse frequency and blood pressure depend on the depth of immersion, water temperature, the diving dress type and respiratory apparatus as well as on the intensity of physical loading. (English summary)

1404.
OTT, J.A.
Concepts of underwater experimentation.
Helgolander Wiss. Meeresunters. 24:54-77; 1973.

Recent advances in underwater research are reviewed and critically discussed. New technologies include deep-sea diving apparatus, saturation diving from underwater habitats, submersibles and remote-controlled vehicles. The fields of application include increasingly ecology and animal behavior. The term "underwater experimentation" is defined and examples provided to illustrate pertinent research. Underwater experimentation is compared to laboratory experimentation. The latter is restricted to a limited set of suitable organisms, which are subjected to "controlled" but frequently quite "artificial" conditions. Furthermore, only systems of a very low degree of complexity can be studied in the laboratory. Underwater experimentation is limited by the restricted performance of man under in situ conditions. Automatisation of experimental units and use of remote-controlled vehicles are proposed to enhance man's underwater capacity. The need for the design of underwater experiments, especially for system analysis, is emphasized. There is an increasing demand for predictive models to anticipate the potential impacts of civilisation on the marine environment. (Author's summary)

1405.
OTT, N.T., R.R. Lorenz and J.T. Shepherd.
Modification of lung-inflation reflex in rabbits by hypercapnia.
Amer. J. Physiol. 223(4):812-819; 1972.

The effects of vagal afferents on hindlimb and renal vascular beds were studied in anesthetized, artificially ventilated rabbits with sinus and aortic nerves cut. To assess changes in vascular resistance, the hindlimb and kidney were perfused at constant flow. The increase in resistance caused by vagal cold block (VCB) reflected the activity of vagal afferents prior to the block. Either tidal volume (V_T) was varied and endtidal CO_2 was held constant or V_T was held constant and end-tidal CO_2 was varied. The increase in hindlimb resistance with VCB became greater as V_T or end-tidal CO_2 increased. The increase in renal resistance with VCB became greater as end-tidal CO_2, but not as V_T, increased; this increase was greater than that seen in the hindlimb, was accompanied by increased activity in renal sympathetic nerves and was unaffected by local PCO_2 changes. During hypercapnia, the lung-depressor reflex probably serves to counteract the increase in renal and hindlimb vascular resistance caused by the action of CO_2 on the vasomotor centers and acts more so on the kidney vessels. (© BA)

1406.
OWEN, D.M.
Heart attack at 110 feet.
Skin Diver 20:22-23, 24, 26, 26-28;Nov. 1971.

The author describes what was later determined to be a mild heart attack which occurred during a working dive in cold water. The normal sensations of shallow and rapid breathing which occur in cold water seemed more acute and prolonged, and a feeling of apprehension was strong. The task performed during the dive was an unusually strenuous one, and when unfamiliar sensations of chest discomfort persisted, accompanied by extreme fatigue, the author decided to seek medical advice. The day following, an ECG revealed myocardial infarction. A week in intensive care, two more weeks in hospital, and two and one-half months of rest at home restored the patient to normal. The purpose of writing this account is to alert divers to this possibility; symptoms of a heart attack could easily be attributed to the discomfort caused by diving equipment, and by cold water, and might thus be ignored. It is emphasized that diver examinations should include large chest X-ray, lung volume, ECG, and analyses of serum cholesterol, total lipids, glucose, and uric acid. (MFW/BSCP)

1407.
OWEN, T. and P.W. Hochachka.
Aspartate and alanine aminotransferases. Role in muscle of diving mammals.
Fed. Proc. 33(5,pt.2):1431;May 1971.

Abstract only. Entire item quoted: Mitochondrial and supernatant glutamate-oxalacetate transaminase (GOT) and supernatant glutamate-pyruvate transaminase (GPT) were purified 89, 204, and 240-fold respectively, from dolphin muscle. Starch gel electrophoresis of crude and purified preparations revealed that all three enzymes exist as single forms. K_m values of α-ketoglutarate, alanine, pyruvate and glutamate for GPT are 0.45, 8.2, 0.87, and 15 m$\underline{M}$, respectively. For GOT the K_m values of α-ketoglutarate, aspartate, oxalacetate and glutamate are 0.76, 0.50, 0.10 and 9.4 m$\underline{M}$, rspectively, for the mitochondrial form and 0.13, 2.4, 0.06, and 3.2 m$\underline{M}$, respectively, for the supernatant form. In all cases, as the assay pH decreases from pH 7.3, the K_m values of the α-keto acids decrease while those of the amino acids increase. The apparent equilibrium constants for the glutamate-oxalacetate transaminases are independent of pH. Studies of the inhibition of the glutamate-oxalacetate transaminases by dicarboxylic acids indicated that these enzymes may be controlled by pools of metabolic intermediates. Three key roles for the transaminases in the energy metabolism of the diving mammal are considered.

1408.
OWENS, G. and M. Roberts.
Continuous, simultaneous and instantaneous tissue gas and blood flow measurements using the mass spectrometer.
J. Surg. Oncol. 4(4):363-368; 1972.

Using a membrane permeable to gases, it was shown that partial pressures [p] of O_2, CO_2 and N_2 can be monitored continuously, simultaneously and instantaneously using a mass spectrometer. In physiologic studies in experimental animals [dogs], tissue gases from kidney, liver, skin and brain were recorded. Responses in these organs to changes in blood flow, blood gases, surgical trauma and isolated perfusion were conducted. Blood flow can be calculated by adding an inert gas (Ar) to the ventilation mixture and recording its washout time. Simultaneous PO_2, PCO_2 and P [pressure] Ar permits focal metabolic studies previously impossible to record. [Data on humans are referred to.] (© BA)

1409.
OYAMA, Y. and M.P. Spencer.
Cardiopulmonary effects of intravenous gas embolism; with special reference to fate of intravascular gas bubbles.
Jap. Circ. J. 35:1541-1549;Dec. 1971.

To determine the graded cardiopulmonary effects and fate of pulmonary gas embolism, 11 sheep (with chronically implanted Doppler ultrasonic flow probes on pulmonary and brachiocephalic arteries) were subjected to experimental intravenous injection of nitrogen, oxygen and carbon dioxide. Three different rates of injection of each gas (0.03, 0.09 and 0.15 ml/kg/min) were used for 30 minutes. Doppler ultrasonic flow probes were found to be very sensitive to the injected intravascular gas and produced characteristic "chirps." The electromagnetic blood flowmeter was insensitive to the passage of these gases. Cardiopulmonary responses include elevation of pulmonary arterial pressure, diminished cardiac output and arterial hypoxemia. Nitrogen produced the greatest response and carbon dioxide the least, correlating with differences in solubility and diffusion rates. These responses developed with a one-half time of 15-20 minutes, with recovery, following cessation of injection, at the same rate. No statistically significant changes occurred in heart rate, systemic arterial pressure, pH or PCO_2. Passage of intravenous gas through the pulmonary vasculature to the systemic circulation occurred only at the 0.15 ml/kg/min dosage rate. The opening of the intrapulmonary arteriovenous shunts was primarily responsible for the decrease in arterial oxygen tension and passage of gas through the lung. (Authors' abstract)

1410.
PADDEN, J.B. and M.G. Jacko.
Breathing-air oil-mist monitor.
In: Battelle Columbus Laboratories. Proceedings, 1973 divers' gas purity symposium, November 27-28, 1973, p.XVI-1-XVI-22. U.S. Navy Supervisor Diving, Nav. Ships Syst. Comm., Rep 2-73, 1973.

A simple and low-cost oil-mist monitor suitable to detect and determine the oil-mist concentration in divers' breathing air was developed. An oil-sensitive membrane undergoes permeability change, after a brief induction, as the oil droplets clog the very fine pore openings. The final form of the test system worked well and the general approach is recommended for future work on respirable air testing. The oil-sensitive membrane was shown to function predictable and with great sensitivity. The oil-mist concentration in the sample line was found to be a fraction of the concentration in the main line. For example, at 5 mg/m^3. This indicates that the final form of the monitor would have to be calibrated in the system where it is used. The disposable cassette feature of the monitor appears to be unworkable in its present state. Therefore, it is recommended that in further work the oil-sensitive membrane be supported by a commercially available, high-pressure, membrane holder. (Authors)

1411.
PAEGLE, R.D.
Prevention of pulmonary oxygen toxicity.
New York, St. Vincent's Hosp., Med. Cent. N.Y., Dept. Pathol., Final Rep. on Contract N00014-72-C-0141, 19p. Oct. 31, 1972.

Increasing the O_2 concentration in steps (40%, 70%, 80%) not only markedly enhanced the survival of rats when they were finally exposed to 95% and 100% oxygen but frequently also resulted in marked scarring of lungs. The CFE strain rats demonstrated a third (chronic) phase of pulmonary oxygen toxicity, which was characterized by scarring and emphysema. This stage has not been delineated previously. The adaptation had to be started at relatively low concentrations, i.e. 40% or 70%. The survival in 95% or 100% oxygen was equally brief. In a colony of Sprague-Dawley rats, where some animals have subclinical chronic respiratory disease, the administration of 100% oxygen may evoke or exacerbate acute bronchitis or even acute bronchopneumonia. The rats from a chronic respiratory disease free colony (CFE) of Sprague-Dawley rats were more susceptible to oxygen toxicity than those from another colony with sporadic endemic respiratory disease. The variability in individual susceptibility to O_2 toxicity was marked. Some CFE strain rats died after exposure to relatively low concentrations of oxygen: 2% died after exposure to 70% and 14% after 80% O_2. Although BHA appeared to have a mildly beneficial effect, none of the drugs tested significantly prolonged the survival of the rats in 100% O_2. (Author's conclusions)

1412.
PAIK, K.S., B.S. Kang, D.S. Han, D.W. Rennie and S.K. Hong.
Vascular responses of Korean ama to hand immersion in cold water.
J. Appl. Physiol. 32:446-450;Apr. 1972.

Peripheral vascular responses to immersion of one hand in 6°C water for 30-60 min were studied in eight ama and eight nondivers in both summer and winter. Slight increases in systolic and diastolic blood pressures observed during the early phase of immersion were not different between the groups or between seasons. In both seasons, ama tended to maintain higher muscle and skin temperatures and skin heat flux as compared to the controls, but a significant difference between the two groups was noted only in winter for muscle temperature ($P < 0.01$). Measurements of finger temperature and blood flow indicated the presence of hunting reactions in the controls but not in the ama. The occlusion of venous return from the hand had no detectable effect on the lower arm muscle temperature but either increased (in ama) or prevented further reduction (in the controls) of the lower arm skin temperature. These results may suggest that during immersion of the hand in 6°C water the degree of vasoconstriction of finger blood vessels is significantly greater while a greater fraction of hand blood flow returns via superficial veins, in ama as compared with the controls. Such a greater vasomotor tone in ama was demonstrable even during hyperemic phase following arterial occlusion. (Authors' abstract)

1413.
PAKMAN, L.M.
Inhibition of pseudomonas aeruginosa by hyperbaric oxygen. 1. Sulfonamide activity enhancement and reversal.
Infect. Immun. 4(4):479-487; 1971.

To elucidate an explanation for in vitro sulfonamide enhancement with in vivo therapy, P. aeruginosa cultures were exposed to selected antifolate antimicrobials in the presence of 1.87 atm absolute of O_2 and compared with non-HPO treated controls. Under these conditions, HPO alone retarded growth. Trimethoprim, a nonsulfonamide which inhibits dihydrofolate reductase, was not bactericidal, nor did HPO enhance existent bacteriostatic activity. The sulfonamide, sulfisoxazole, was not bactericidal, but HPO enhanced bacteriostatic activity two-fold; bacteriostasis was mitigated in HPO-treated and control cultures by p-aminobenzoate but not by a mixture of compounds involved in folate-mediated "1-C" biosynthesis. Mafenide, a unique sulfonamide, at high concentrations with HPO, was synergistically bactericidal; non-HPO-treated cultures were bacteriostatically inhibited. Bacteriostatic activity of lower mafenide concentrations was also enhanced at least twofold by HPO. These inhibitory effects of mafenide, acting with or without HPO, were mitigated by the above mixture, but not by p-aminobenzoate. This may explain the lack of in vivo HPO mafenide enhancement in burn-wound sepsis where exudates would contain such a mixture. Lastly, HPO itself was largely bactericidal at 2.87 atm absolute of O_2. This was reversed to various degrees by the above mixture, or its components, or by folic, folinic or p-aminobenzoic acids. These in vitro interactions suggest HPO per se may act at the same site as some sulfonamides to inhibit folate synthesis (nor primarily at the dihydrofolate reductase level), coenzyme functions or both. (© BA)

1414.
PALLOTA, R.
La terapia della malattia da decompressione.
[Therapy of decompression sickness].
Clin. Ter. 61:249-71;May 15, 1972.

Various aspects of the treatment of decompression sickness are discussed. Factors governing the choice of recompression programs for different symptomatologies are considered, and a number of recompression tables are reproduced. The author comments on the advantages, contraindications, and dangers of the various procedures based on his experience with more than 200 cases. The use of medication in conjunction with recompression therapy is also discussed. Safety precautions related to the transfer of the patient from one hyperbaric chamber to another, and to the use of medical equipment under hyperbaric conditions are outlined. In conclusion, it is pointed out that hyperbaria may be used in the medical treatment of a number of disorders, although exploitation of this possibility has scarcely begun. The establishment of an (Italian) Institute for Hyperbaric Medicine is urged. (MEMH/BSCP)

1415.
PANNIER, J.L., E. Lacroix and I. Leusen.
Effects of adrenergic blockade on the hemodynamic response to acute experimental hypercapnia.
Arch. Int. Physiol. Biochim. 80(4):761-774; 1972.

The hemodynamic effects of acute experimental hypercapnia were studied on anesthetized dogs under artificial ventilation in control conditions and during blockade of the adrenergic receptors. The hemodynamic effect of respiratory acidosis (10% or 16% CO_2) in control conditions varied considerably: cardiac output was either increased, decreased, or unchanged; variations in total circulatory resistance were opposite to the alterations in cardiac output, and mean arterial blood pressure [MABP] was generally unchanged. Left ventricular end-diastolic pressure [LVEDP] increased and heart rate decreased in all experiments. During the administration of propranolol, respiratory acidosis produced always a marked decrease in cardiac output, no change or a slight increase in total peripheral resistance, a decrease of MABP. LVEDP increased very importantly and heart rate was generally unchanged. During the administration of azapetine, a respiratory acidosis produced always a marked increase in cardiac output and a decrease in total circulatory resistance while MABP was not systematically influenced and LVEDP was unchanged or increased only slightly. During the administration of both azapetine and propranolol, cardiac output was not modified during CO_2 inhalation while total circulatory resistance and MABP decreased. There was always a marked rise in LVEDP and a decrease in heart rate. These studies indicate the importance of the orthosympathetic neurohumoral support for the hemodynamic response to an acute hypercapnia. (DTS) (© BA)

1416.
PANNIER, J.L. and I. Leusen.
Circulation to the brain of the rat during acute and prolonged respiratory changes in the acid-base balance.
Pfluegers Arch. 338(4):347-359; 1973.

The fraction of the cardiac output distributed to the brain was studied with a particle distribution method at different acutely induced arterial PCO_2 levels in control rats and in rats kept during 24 h before the experiment in an atmosphere containing either 10% CO_2 in air (prolonged hypercapnia) or 10% O_2 in N_2 (hypoxic hyperventilation producing prolonged hypocapnia). The curve relating the fraction of the cardiac output distributed to the brain and the Pa CO_2 (arterial blood CO_2 tension) is shifted upwards and to the left after prolonged hypocapnia and downwards and to the right after prolonged hypercapnia. A similar shift is observed when orthosympathetic vasoconstrictor activity is eliminated in the three groups of rats by alpha-adrenergic receptor blockade. The changes in the fraction of the cardiac output perfusing the brain are essentially due to modifications in the cerebral blood flow, since the cardiac output was not significantly influenced by the alterations in the $PaCO_2$. The results are discussed in relation to the changes occurring in the CO_2/HCO_3-dissociation curve in blood and brain during prolonged respiratory changes in the acid-base balance. (© BA)

1417.
PANNIER, J.L.
Fractional distribution of the cardiac output to the brain of rats during acute and prolonged hypercapnia.
Arch. Int. Physiol. Biochim. 81:153-155;Feb. 1973.

The present study was designed to investigate further the relationship between cerebral blood flow (CBF) and brain tissue pH in anesthetized rats during prolonged (24 hr) respiratory acidosis and alkalosis. . . In anesthetized rats, the curve relating the fraction of the cardiac output distributed to the brain and the $PaCO_2$ is shifted upwards and to the left after prolonged hypocapnia, and downwards and to the right after prolonged hypercapnia. The results are discussed in relation to the changes occurring in the CO_2 HCO_3-dissociation curve in blood and brain during prolonged respiratory changes in the acid-base balance. They lend further support to the hypothesis that pH changes in the brain tissue influence the cerebrovascular resistance. (Author)

1418.
PAPPAS, M. and A. Allentuch.
Structural synthesis of frame reinforced submersible, circular, cylindrical hulls.
Newark, N.J., Newark Coll. Eng., Dept. Mech. Eng., Rep. NCE-NV-5, 91p. May 1972.
(AD 763 400)

The report describes an automated computer synthesis capability for the preliminary design of circular, cylindrical, "T" frame, stiffened hulls subject to hydrostatic pressure. (GRA)

1419.
PAPPAS, M. and A. Allentuch.
Optimal design of submersible frame stiffened, circular cylindrical hulls.
Newark, N.J., Newark Coll. Eng., Dept. Mech. Eng., Rep. NCE-NV-6, 89p. July 1972.
(AD 761 643)

The report presents the results of a series of optimal hull design studies performed using an automated optimum design capability program and procedures. The procedures generate the optimal design of a submersible, "T" frame stiffened, circular, cylindrical hull segment. (GRA)

1420.
PARC, J., A. Michaud, J. Le Chuiton and A. Michel.
Experimentation sur porcs miniatures de plongees fictives a 400, 600, 750, et plus de 1000 meters.
[Experiments with miniature pigs of simulated dives to 400, 600, 750 and over 1000 meters].
Bull. Medsubhyp 8:12-17;Nov. 1972.

The animals were kept in the chamber at atmospheric pressure for 24 hours before each dive. During this time a short dive to 30 meters was made. The breathing mixture was helium-oxygen with a trace of nitrogen. In the first series of dives, which did not exceed 750 meters, the chief aims were to test various combinations of tissues and coefficients of supersaturation and to investigate the importance of humidity. One hundred and eighty minute tissue and 1.53 coefficient of supersaturation were found satisfactory. It was established that low humidity had a beneficial effect. It was found that compression in stages was preferable to continuous compression. Homogenization of the breathing mixture was found to be extremely important; when this technical problem was overcome, the threshold of compression symptoms was pushed back from 600 meters to 800 meters. The compression was carred out in jumps of 100 meters in four to five minutes, with rests of 30 minutes, up to 500 meters. From 500 to 1000 meters, jumps of 50 meters were made, with rests of 30 minutes or more, depending on the condition of the animal. Beyond 1000 meters, the protocol of compression was extremely varied, depending upon circumstances. In the last experiments, stops of two hours were always made at 500 and at 750 meters. The oxygen partial pressure was elevated progressively and linearly in different degrees during the experiments, in order to determine at what point high oxygen partial pressures are best tolerated by the lungs at great depths. The final experiment was made at 111 b, with PO_2 kept at .21 b. The animal appeared in better condition than those of previous experiments; however fatigue became more and more apparent, and at the sixtieth hour at depth dyspnea became apparent, at the same time that the CO_2 level was raised due to technical problems. The animal died shortly after decompression began. Only one animal was brought back alive from 1100 meters; decompression was based on 180 minute tissue and 1.30 coefficient. Certain symptoms were observed during these experiments which resembled the hpns syndrome demonstrated by human subjects: nervousness, motor dysfunction, epileptiform crises. It is stated in conclusion that these experiments were limited and imperfect, and that findings must be verified and consolidated. (MFW/BSCP)

1421.
PARIENTE, R. and G. Brouet.
Modifications ultrastructurales pulmonaires induites par l'oxygene. Consequences physiopathologiques.
[Pulmonary ultrastructural modifications induced by oxygen. Physiopathologic consequences].
Rev. Eur. Etud. Clin. Biol. 16:379-385;Apr. 1971.

The authors study the ultra-structural effects of oxygen intoxication in rats. The animals were subjected for periods of variable length to pure oxygen at atmospheric pressure in a water vapour saturated atmosphere and subsequently to 80% and 65% oxygen enriched atmospheres. The authors then compared these effects to those caused when exposing rats to pure oxygen at 580 and 480 mm Hg pressures, well below atmospheric pressure. Tests were also made in mixed, oxygen + helium, atmospheres. Finally, the authors study the effects of chronic intoxication and examined sections of specimens taken at various stages of intoxication. Reproducible fixation and colouring methods were used. They enabled demonstrating that: Interstitial oedema is the first symptom of oxygen intoxication, it is followed by the exfoliation of endothelial capillary cells and membraneous (type I) pneumocytes, finally, there occurs a hyperplasia of the myelinic elements and of the surfactant. Oxygen at 715 mm Hg causes lesions starting from the 24th hour of exposure. The largest number of lesions was recorded at the 72nd hour, death occured shortly after. The threshold of toxicity seems to be a 65% oxygen content atmosphere at 480 mm Hg pressure. Nitrogen and helium have a small protection effect, if any, Chronic intoxication causes collagenous interstitial lung fibrosis. (MEMH/BSCP)

1422.
PARK, S.S.
Effect of superimposed metabolic alkalosis on CO_2 acclimatization in cats.
In: Abstracts of BuMed-ONR sponsored Navywide workshop in high pressure biomedical research, U.S. Submarine Base, Groton, Conn., May 1971. p. 21. Published by the Naval Submarine Medical Research Laboratory, 1971.

Abstract only. Entire item quoted: In order to evaluate the effect of superimposed metabolic alkalosis on CO_2 acclimatization, cats were exposed to varying concentrations of CO_2 for a period of 5 to 14 days. In ten experiments, the cats were fed a regular diet. In the other ten experiments the animals were placed on bicarbonate-enriched diet. In cats fed the regular diet the total CO_2 content and PCO_2 in the arterial blood and CSF increased progressively with the increase of partial pressure of CO_2 in the chamber ($PICO_2$). The compensatory increase of arterial or CSF $[HCO_3]$ was, however, incomplete, resulting in a linear increase of $[H^+]$ in both arterial blood and CSF. In cats fed bicarbonate, a greater increase of CO_2 content and reduction of $[H^+]$ were noted in the blood at each level of $PICO_2$. The arterial PCO_2, however, was little influenced by the alkalotic regimen except on three occasions when the increase of arterial bicarbonate was extreme. The influence of the alkalotic regimen on the CSF $[HCO_3^-]$ and $[H^+]$ was also very slight in the majority of experiments. On three occasions of extreme alkalosis, there was a marked increase of CSF $[HCO_3^-]$ which was associated with a nearly complete compensation of CSF pH and respiratory suppression evidenced by marked increase of arterial PCO_2. These results suggest that an effective but limited regulatory mechanism exists for the transport of bicarbonate ions across the blood-brain barrier and prevents an excessive increase of CSF $[HCO_3^-]$ under these conditions. Such a regulation of $[HCO_3^-]$ is predictable from the hypothesis recently proposed by Siesjo et al (Scand. J. Clin. Lab. Invest. 24:1, 1969) and is considered to play an important role in preventing the severe respiratory suppression which would otherwise occur if the CSF pH were completely compensated.

1423.
PARK, S.S. and A. D'Orazio.
Effect of superimposed metabolic alkalosis on the chronic acclimatization to a CO_2-rich atmosphere.
New York, Yeshiva Univ., Albert Einstein Coll. Med., Fin. Rep. On Contract N00014-68-A-0302-0001, 4p. Oct. 31, 1972.

The effect of superimposed metabolic alkalosis on the cerebrospinal fluid acid-base balance and respiratory control during chronic acclimatization to a CO_2 rich atmosphere was studied in cats. . . . [As a result of these investigations] a theory of combined transport mechanisms has been proposed. According to this theory, the active transport mechanism is arterial pH dependent in cats, and functions as the principal stabilizer of CSF pH, while the passive transport mechanism is determined by the PCO_2 dependent shift of the CSF/blood electric potential difference and modifies the effect of the pH stabilizing active transport mechanism. The concerted action of these two processes is considered responsible for the prevention of excessive increase of CSF $[HCO_3^-]$ in our experimental condition. Such regulation of CSF $[HCO_3^-]$ may play an important role in maintaining the effectiveness of respiratory regulation through the central chemoreceptor. The use of THAM as an alkalizing agent, however, appears to defy such a regulatory mechanism, resulting in further respiratory suppression. (Authors)

1424.
PARKER, G.
The buddy buoy.
Skin Diver 20:31-32;May 1971.

The buoy can be a combination of safety float to rest on, flag buoy, repository for equipment, and trap to hold a catch of marine life. There is a 10 to 15 foot line descending from the buoy, at the edge of which there is a ring to which each diver attaches his line. The two divers can then play out as much line as they have and have freedom to explore without losing contact with one another. If one puts his anchor down, the other will immediately know. A system of signals can also be worked out. The type of buoy illustrated here consists of an inner tube with a basket attached to it underwater, and a garbage pail lid which is held on the inner tube by rubber strips. The flag is also held on the tube by a rubber strip. The divers' lines are on simple reels with small anchors attached. [It should be noted here that in subsequent issues of Skin Dver (August 1971 and October 1971) this device is attacked and defended. The criticism is that this system is extremely dangerous, particularly for inexperienced divers, since it permits the divers to get too far away from one another. The original concept is defended by the author and also by a former student of his, who points out that in the case of a cave diver who had been trapped in a crevice, if a buddy buoy had been in use, his partner would have known he was in trouble]. (MFW/SCD)

1425.
PARKER, J.F., Jr. and M.G. Every.
Habitability issues in long-duration undersea and space missions.
Falls Church, Va., BioTechnology, Inc., Rep. on contract N00014-71-C-0397, 52p. July 1972.

Habitability issues are coming increasingly to the fore as U.S. technology continues its rapid advancement. Many now must live and work in small habitats, both for undersea and space exploration, for extended periods of time. His well-being and productivity during the long missions of the future will be greatly affected by the extent to which proper habitability principles are incorporated into the design of the systems. This report reviews a number of studies in the area of habitability. Emphasis was placed on extracting from these studies that information most relevant to any long-term mission in confinement. It is concluded that, whereas the basic laws of habitability are known, there is much yet to be learned concerning development of social structures in small groups in relative isolation, planning for necessary hygiene needs, development of proper work spaces, and construction of internal and external communications systems. With respect to testing for habitability and the documentation of habitability principles, the space program was found to be considerably more advanced than was the program for undersea missions. (DCD abstract)

1426.
PARKER, J.W.
Perceptual and motor effects of air at 2-9 ATA (category: hyperbaric pressure).
In: Abstracts of BuMed-ONR sponsored Navywide workshop in high pressure biomedical research, U.S. Submarine Base, Groton, Conn., May 1971, p.32. Published by the Naval Submarine Medical Research Laboratory, 1971.

Abstract only. Entire item quoted: Eight subjects were exposed to hyperbaric conditions at 50, 100, 150, 200 and 250 feet of sea water in a man-rated chamber. Each subject made two dives to each depth in a random order. Subjects were tested with a single digit addition test, a cancellation test and the Response Analysis Tester (RATER), a choice reaction-time test in two modes, self- and auto-paced. Data also were collected on the surface before and after the series of chamber dives. Results with the addition test showed a decline in the number of problems attempted and a decrease in accuracy as pressure increased. Cancellation accuracy also was affected by increased depth. RATER scores showed a decrease with increased pressure especially in the self-paced mode. Auto-paced scores as well as number of errors of omission and commission did not demonstrate as great an effect. Noteworthy is the fact that great variability among subjects was found. Pre- and post-experimental surface data covered a relatively narrow range, while at the various depths subjects varied widely in their performance. It was concluded that with the short bottom times used, the effects of inert gas narcosis can be demonstrated with the tests employed and that decrement in performance increases with the increase in ambient pressure of air.

1427.
PARRISH, B.B., E.F. Akyuz, J. Anderson, D.W. Brown, W.L. High, J.M. Peres and J. Piccard.
Submersibles and underwater habitats:a review.
Underwater J. 4:149-167;Aug. 1972.

This comprehensive report is the result of three years' study by a working party appointed by the FAO Advisory Committee on Marine Resources Research to review the state-of-the-art in the use of submersibles and underwater habitats in fisheries and marine research. Bathyscaphs, tethered submersibles, free, self-propelled submersibles and diver lock-out submersibles are discussed. The section on habitats is confined mainly to Tektite 2. In the authors' conclusion, they evaluate the situation as follows: "The application of "on the spot" observation and, where necessary work techniques, using, according to the nature of the research problem and the working conditions, either scuba divers, working from the surface or underwater habitats, or an appropriate submersible, provide the most direct and effective way of tackling many of these problems. It is, of course, of major importance that in choosing the most effective technique to use in an investigation these techniques must be viewed objectively alongside other less direct, sampling and/or recording techniques, in terms of both cost and potential pay-off in scientific results. This however, must be done for each major research project and not in a generalized, subjective way for all research projects combined, as both the major proponents and the critics of "man in the sea" techniques have tended to do in the past. It is important to recognize that submersibles and underwater habitats are not ends in themselves, as some critics infer, but research tools the usefulness of which for any investigation must be subjected to the same objective assessment as other tools." There is a long list of references. Table 1b lists habitats from Precontinent I, in 1962, through Tektite 2, in 1970. Table 1a, a separate fold-in, classifies all underwater vehicles, the earliest of which is the Russian Hydrostat (1944) and the latest, Johnson-Sea-Link (1971). The table gives present status, present owner and basic specifications and equipment for each vehicle. (MFW/BSCP)

1428.
PATERSON, N.R. and A. Rossfelder.
Application of manned submersibles to geophysical surveying in the Arctic.
Can. Petrol. 12:43-49;July 1971.

After discussing the practicability of using the small manned submersible in geological and geophysical exploration, the author describes the development of NARWAL, a two-man submersible designed for use in the Arctic, where surface operation is greatly limited. In the design of this vessel, care has been taken to provide for the particular hazards of Arctic operation. It incorporates "(1) redundancy of vital components such as propulsion and power source; (2) redundancy of de-ballasting means; (3) detachable appendages; (4) structural and component protection from impact, collision, or temperature effects; particularly over thick windows with protective dome; (5) emergency beacons markers and icecrossing snorkel; (6) secondary escape hatch through front window, allowing for underwater exit or access; and (7) enduring life-support, with a minimum of two days and a maximum of four days depending upon mission and availability of pay load. A long-lasting heat source, independent from all power sources, is planned. Procedures for freeing the crew and the submarine from the ice-canopy in case of entrapment have been devised and they include access and escape hole blasting and coring at safe distance from the vessel." The author believes that for Arctic operations the small, manned submersible is more adaptable, efficient and economical than a large-size submarine or unmanned instrumented vehicles transported by larger vessels. (MFW/BSCP)

1429.
PATON, W.D.M. and E.B. Smith.
Decompression sickness and inert gas narcosis.
Oxford, U.K., Dept. Pharmacol. Phys. Chem. Lab., Final report on contract N00014-69-C-0037, 6p. Oct. 1972.

This report lists the research areas covered during the years 1967-72. Under decompression sickness they are: arterial bubbles, decompression characteristics of various inert gases; the role of separated gas in decompression procedures. Under inert gas narcosis, they are: effects of anesthetic gases on mice; physiological effects of high pressure on mice and newts; pressure reversal. Other research described bears no relation to hyperbaric problems. Articles and papers are listed. (MFW/BSCP)

1430.
PATTE, M.
Medecine de plongee sous-marine.
[Medical aspects of diving].
Brux. Med. 53:237-266;Apr. 1973.

On the physiology of diving, the author discusses the following: (1) The physical laws applicable to diving (Boyle, Henry, Dalton etc.); penetration of light and propagation of sound underwater; (2) Effects of pressure on organisms: mechanical, biophysical; decompression schedules, tissue saturation, repetitive diving, breathing mixtures. (3) Biochemical phenomena: oxygen toxicity, blackout from carbon dioxide, increased toxicity of carbon monoxide at high pressure, inert gas narcosis; (4) Modifications of the ECG and of the cardiovascular system. (5) Modifications of the EEG. (6) Thermoregulation: caloric consumption; minimizing of cutaneous heat loss. (7) Increased diuresis. (8) Very deep dives and intervention dives: cold, regulation of oxygen partial pressure; HPNS, changes in blood chemistry; respiratory function. (9) Breathhold diving:physiological adaption; time and depths limits. (10) Psychology of the diver. (11) Possible chronic disorders resulting from diving: toxic effects of dysbarism; emphysema; nervous system disorders; fatty degeneration of the liver; osteonecrosis; hearing loss. On incidents and accidents of diving, the following are discussed: (1) drowning from: both submersion and syncope, athe latter brought on by trauma, emotion, shock, or thermo-differential factors; salt water and fresh water drowning; therapy. (2) Suffocation: either from carbon dioxide or increased respiratory resistance. (3) The pathology of the ear: barotrauma of the middle ear; deafness; decompression accidents of the ear. (4) Pulmonary barotrauma. (5) Violent abdominal gas pains. (6) Squeeze. (7) Inert gas narcosis. (8) decompression sickness: symptoms, etiology and treatment; recompression tables for both air and oxygen. (9) Dangers of breath hold diving. (10) Sequence of treatment. First aid station, equipped with oxygen and drugs, transportation to a recompression center (locations of which are listed); specific treatment for different types of accidents. In a section on physical fitness, contraindications are listed; age limit is discussed, as are asthma and diving and proper diet. An appropriate physical examination is described. (MFW/SCD)

1431.
PAUL, K.L. and R.Y. Morita.
Effects of hydrostatic pressure and temperature on the uptake and respiration of amino acids by a facultatively psychophilic marine bacterium.
J. Bacteriol. 108(2):835-843; 1971.

Studies of pressure and temperature effects on glutamic acid transport and utilization indicated that hydrostatic pressure and low temperature inhibit glutamate transport more than glutamate respiration. The effects of pressure on transport were reduced at temperatures near the optimum. Similar results were obtained for glycine, phenylalanine, and proline. Pressure effects on the transport systems of all four amino acids were reversible to some degree. Both proline and glutamic acid were able to protect their transport proteins against pressure damage. The data presented indicate that the uptake of amino acids by cells under pressure is inhibited, which is the cause of their inability to grow under pressure. (Authors' abstract)

1432.
PAULEV, P.E. and H.G. Hansen.
Cardiac response to apnea and water immersion during exercise in man.
J. Appl. Physiol. 33:193-198;Aug. 1972.

Seven subjects held their breath in the supine position in air and in water in three different situation: 1) breath holding at steady-state cycling, 2) short periods of exercise during breath holding, and 3) breath holding at rest. In steady-state exercise (450 kpm/min) apnea elicited a small fall in heart rate ("bradycardia") in the fittest subjects. When subjects started to exercise (750 kpm/min) in air or in water while holding their breath the heart rate rose, both when measured as the number of heart beats/15-sec intervals and as indicated by the cardiotachogram. The fall in heart rate during breath holding (apnea) when immobile is explained as the result of: 1) a high pressure baroreceptor reflex ("apnea bradycardia"), 2) a "temperature bradycardia" which is found to augment this "apnea bradycardia" in a low-temperature environment, and 3) psychological factors. Apnea-induced bradycardia was also found to occur during exercise, especially in individuals with a high maximal oxygen uptake. Change in heart rate for each individual is dependent upon the ratio between the absolute work load and the aerobic working capacity of the subject. (Authors' abstract)

1433.
PAULEY, S.M., J.C. Saunders, F.L. Depenbusch and A.T.K. Cockett.
Unusual experiences in the hyperbaric chamber.
In: Wada, J. and I. Takashi, eds. Proceedings of the fourth international congress of hyperbaric medicine, Sapporo, Japan, Sept. 1969, p.495-499, Baltimore, Williams and Wilkins, 1970.

One case discussed is that of a 26-year old woman diver who made a fast ascent while holding her breath. Bloody froth was apparent, and partial paralysis immediately ensued. By the time she reached a recompression chamber, 3½ hours later, during which time she had been given 100% oxygen, paralysis was complete except for the left leg. She was recompressed to 165 feet in 6 minutes, and 1000 ml 6% dextran in saline was given. After two hours, she was taken to 140 feet and given 1000 ml of 5% dextrose in DW. At 60 feet she was given 30 minutes of 100% O_2, and more was given intermittently. Before being taken to 50 feet she was given 5000 U of heparin. Two subsequent doses of heparin, eight hours apart, were given. She was able to walk after 20 hours, while at 40 feet. She was hospitalized 38 hours later, where she gradually recovered, with one setback of pain in the right chest and arm. She was discharged 17 days after the accident, with minor sequelae of diminished sensation in the right arm and hand and mild aphasia. The unique feature of this case was the combined use of heparin and dextran during recompression. (MFW/BSCP)

1434.
PAULEY, S.M., N. Alazraki and J. Chandler.
Use of fluorine-18 bone scans to detect aseptic bone necrosis in U.S. Navy divers.
In: Aerospace Medical Association. 1972 annual scientific meeting Bal Harbour, Florida, May 1972. Preprints, p.257. Published by the Association.

The major problems in the recognition and control of this disease have been; 1) difficulty in determining what is and what is not ABN on radiographs, 2) the insidious onset of ABN; the disease often not clinically apparent months to years after exposure to a hyper or hypobaric environment, 3) failure to set rigid standards for periodic radiographic long bone studies in groups of hyperbaric and hypobaric workers, 4) the reluctance of hyper and hypobaric medical personnel to send radiographs to special diagnostic committees rsulting in missed diagnoses, both false positive and false negative, and 5) the reluctance to subject persons to the high radiation levels resulting from frequent long bone roentgenograms. Hyperbaric and hypobaric researchers and clinicians have not yet widely used the relatively new photoscintillation scanning techniques which enable one to detect bone lesions before they are apparent on the roentgenogram. Bone must lose 30% to 50% of its calcium before a lesion will be evident on x-ray. Bone scans give us the advantage of detecting pathology before it is apparent on the x-ray, and in some cases, before the onset of pain. It is of interest to note that a single AP view of the pelvis using x-ray gives 1.1 rads to the whole body. A complete ^{18}F bone scan, however, gives only .07 rads to the whole body. This scanning dose is fifteen times less radiation than an AP radiograph of the pelvis. (Authors)

1435.
PEMBERTON, C.E., Jr.
Harassment.
Skin Diver 21:16, 18, 93;June 1972.

The need for a period of harassment as a routine part of a training course is asserted. It is important not to inflict on the student forms of harassment with which he is not fairly likely to be able to cope. All situations presented should simulate emergencies that could be expected to occur during a dive. The following forms of harassment are acceptable: turn air off, pull face mask off, pull regulator off, entangle student in net, hook hose on tank, invert the student, or drop his weight belt. A student should always be warned in advance of the sort of thing to expect. If he fails to pass the harassment test, he should always be given a second chance, if only to demonstrate with finality his unsuitability for diving. (MFW/UMS)

1436.
PENTELIUS, T.
Ljudabsorptionskoefficienten i havet foer freekvensomraedet 0.1-50khz som funktion av temperatur och salthalt.
[Absorption coefficient in the sea over the frequency range 0.1-50 khz, as a function of temperature and salinity].
Stockholm, Sweden, Res. Inst. Nat. Def., Rep. FOA-3-C-3620-57, 11p. Jan. 1970.
(N71 35 861)

A summary of certain experimental results concerning the absorption of sound at low frequencies is presented. Experiments show that the absorption at low frequency is higher than that obtained by extrapolation from measurements carried out at higher frequencies. Nomograms and tables for the determination of the absorption coefficient are presented. (Author) (STAR)

1437.
PENZIAS, W. and M.W. Goodman.
Man beneath the sea. A review of underwater ocean engineering.
New York, Wiley-Interscience, 1973. 831p.

This book is a wide-ranging survey of the subject, covering past accomplishments, current problems and future prospects. It is copiously illustrated, and much of the data is presented in tabular form. Each chapter is followed by an extensive list of references, and, in some cases, a bibliography. The chapter headings are: (1) Introduction, (2) A technical history of diving; (3) Design concepts for diving systems; (4) Review of diving systems; (5) Manned submersibles; (6) Communications, navigation and sonar; (7) Gas storage, mixing and distribution; (8) Life support systems; (9) Pressure vessels and hatches; (10) Underwater electrical connections and penetrators; (11) Umbilicals; (12) Underwater breathing apparatus; (13) Diver dress; (14) Wrenches and robots; (15) Power in a nutshell; (16) The ocean environment; (17) Introduction to the physiology of diving and subsea work; (18) The man in the sea; (19) Performance in the ocean environment; (20) The future. There is a subject index, and an insert consisting of a list of submersibles throughout the world. (MFW/BSCP)

1438.
PEPELKO, W.E. and S.M. Cain.
Cooling of anesthetized paralyzed dogs during hypercapnia and B-adrenergic blockage.
Aerosp. Med. 43:287-290;Mar. 1972.

Oxygen consumption and body temperature were measured in male mongrel dogs, anesthetized, paralyzed, artificially ventilated and cooled in a water bath at 34° C. Treatments included inspiration of 10% or 20% CO_2 β-adrenergic blockade (propranolol) and β-blockade plus 10% CO_2. Oxygen consumption in ml/kg/min STPD after water immersion showed an average increase of 0.41 in air breathing controls but decreased an average of 0.31 with β-blockade, 0.69 with 10% CO_2 inspiration, 0.76 with 10% CO_2 plus β-blockade and 1.35 with 20% CO_2 inspiration. All experimental groups had a lower post-treatment oxygen consumption than controls, ($P < .05$) with the 20% CO_2 group exhibiting a greater depression than the other three experimental groups ($P < .05$). The rate of decline in body temperature was greater while breathing 20% CO_2 than room air ($P < .05$). It was concluded that hypercapnia inhibits β-adrenergic calorigenic mechanisms while having little apparent effect upon heat loss. (Authors' abstract)

1439.
PEPELKO, W.E.
Interaction of chronic hypoxia and hypercapnia upon blood gases and acid base status.
Proc. Soc. Exp. Biol. Med. 140:628-632;June 1972.

Rats were exposed for four days to inspired carbon dioxide levels of 0, 30, 60, and 90 torr combined with inspired oxygen levels of 70 or 140 torr. The purpose of the experiment was to measure the partial pressures of oxygen and carbon dioxide in the arterial blood as well as the pH and standard bicarbonate in the arterial blood of rats chronically exposed to these levels of CO_2, combined with oxygen. Results show that the arterial blood levels of oxygen increased up to an inspired CO_2 of 60 torr in the normoxic rats. At the three levels of inspired CO_2, the increased arterial CO_2 partial pressure was not influenced by hypoxia to a noticeable degree. Standard bicarbonate increased with increasing inspired CO_2 levels in all groups. However, it was consistently lower in the low-oxygen breathing rats than in the normoxic animals. Arterial partial CO_2 pressure was markedly lower in the hypoxic rats only when inspired CO_2 levels were zero. This resulted in a lower arterial blood pH in the hypoxic than in the nonhypoxic rats inspiring comparable CO_2 levels. (Aerosp. Med.)

1440.
PEPELKO, W.E.
Elimination of nonshivering thermogenesis by hypercapnia.
Tex. Rep. Biol. Med. 31:115-116;Spring 1973.

Abstract only. Excerpts quoted: The present experiment was designed to measure the effect of CO_2 upon nonshivering thermogenesis in 24 young adult rats previously acclimated for 30 days or longer at a temperature of 5°C.

The animals were anesthetized, paralyzed with succinyl chlorine to prevent shivering, artificially respired with either room air, 5%, 10% or 20% CO_2 and cooled in double walled chamber with cold water. All three levels of CO_2 resulted in a significant depression of VO_2 at room temperature ($P < .001$). During cold exposure VO_2 increased 50% or more. This increase in nonshivering thermogenesis was partially inhibited by 5%, 10% or 20% CO_2 and cooled in a double walled chamber with cold water. All three levels of CO_2 resulted in a significant depression of VO_2 at room temperature ($P < .001$), although oxygen consumption remained above control levels. With 10% CO_2 inspiration, VO_2 was not significantly different from that of thermoneutral controls and with 20% CO_2, VO_2 declined to a level significantly ($P < .001$) less than controls. The data clearly indicate that inspiration of 10% CO_2 or greater completely eliminates non-shivering thermogenesis in cold-adapted, cold-stressed rats.

1441.
PEPELKO, W.E. and G.A. Dixon.
Arterial blood gases in unanesthetized rats exposed to hypoxia, hypercapnia or both.
Physiologist 16:420;Aug. 1973.

Abstract only. Entire item quoted: Catheters were implanted into the caudal arteries of 120 adult male rats under anesthesia. Upon awakening, an animal was placed in a restrainer and exposed individually to the experimental environments in a small, thermally controlled, cylindrical chamber. Catheters were ducted through the end of the chamber to permit arterial blood collection. Blood samples were collected and analyzed for pH, PO_2, and PCO_2 prior to and during exposure to 20 different experimental gas mixtures. The PIO_2 levels were controlled at 146, 122, 98, 79 or 63 mm Hg. These were combined with PIO_2's of 0, 30, 60 or 90 mm Hg. Six animals were exposed to each gas mixutre. During air breathing pH averaged 7.466 $\pm$ 0.020 S.E., PaO_2 91.8 $\pm$ 3.46 mm Hg and $PaCO_2$ 41.2 $\pm$ 1.87 mm Hg. During exposure to the experimental gases the mean arterial pH ranged from 7.150 $\pm$ 0.020 to 7.604 $\pm$ 0.039, PaO_2 ranged from 30.8 $\pm$ 2.03 mm Hg to 140.8 $\pm$ 5.10 mm Hg and $PaCO_2$ ranged from 25.8 $\pm$ 2.77 mm Hg to 102.0 $\pm$ 1.81 mm Hg. It was concluded that the rat differs from man in that bicarbonate buffering is greater in the rat, resulting in a higher pH during air breathing and smaller decrease in pH with increasing $PaCO_2$. Differences between arterial and inspired CO_2 were very small at 60 and 90 mm Hg and were not influenced by PIO_2 at these CO_2 levels. This suggests that respiration may not be increased further by increasing the $PICO_2$ above 60 mm Hg or by decreasing the PIO_2 at 60 or 90 mm Hg $PICO_2$.

1442.
PERKINS, G.F. and C.D. Wood.
Response of the cardiovascular system in oxygen toxicity.
In: Aerospace Medical Association. 1973 annual scientific meeting, Las Vegas, Nevada, May 1973. Preprints, p.155. Published by the Association, 1973.

In previous investigations with hyperbaric oxygen, rats had developed pulmonary edema that was secondary to acute hypertension. In this experiment, animals were exposed to 100% oxygen at atmospheric pressure for 56 to 72 hours; this resulted in pulmonary edema and pleural effusion, but no hypertension occurred. It was also noted that ATP content of the heart decreased, which might have caused the heart to weaken sufficiently to bring abut these lung changes. The authors state in conclusion that "ATP changes observed here apparently represent only a part of the disruption of metabolic pathways by increased concentration of oxygen; however, it does suggest a possible mechanism for some of the responses to oxygen toxicity." (MFW/BSCP)

1443.
PERRAULT, G.L., T.L. Roess and F.D. Powell.
Submarine parameter identification.
Buffalo, N.Y., Bell Aerospace Co., Rep. 9500-920237, 123p. June 1972.
(AD 747 315)

Research was conducted to determine the feasibility of adaptively identifying the values of the hydrodynamic parameters of a submarine or model from submerged free-flight trajectory data. The modified Kalman filter approach which was used was based on the equation-error parameter identification principle instead of the more conventional response error method, resulting in a relatively modest computational requirement. If the controls are driven by appropriate pseudo random noise sequences, it is possible to determine almost all the parameters to good accuracy from a five minute trajectory sample which is contaminated by realistic additive noise plus bias. Several configurations of suitable instruments for measuring the trajectory are described and the algorithms for processing the trajectory data are discussed. (Authors) (GRA)

1444.
PFEIFFER, R.E.
Remote monitoring of critical physiological factors of the saturated diver.
IEEE international conference on engineering in the ocean environment, Panama City, Florida, September 1970. Digest of technical papers, p.32-37. Published by the conference.

Hard copy not available.

1445.
PFISTER, A. and C. Nogues.
Determinisme des lesions pulmonaires provoquees par l'oxygene ou l'ozone chez le rat.
[Lung lesions induced by oxygen or ozone in the rat].
Pathol. Biol. (Paris) 22:89-98;Jan. 1974.

The experiments carried out at the L.C.B.A. on O_2 and O_3 poisoning in the rat are reviewed and compared with various publications. The modifications observed at the pulmonary level are essential and consist of opposite phenomena of alteration and reaction. Lesions are characterized by necrosis and by exudative inflammation which are caused by oxidative metabolic modifications of the pulmonary cells. The regenerative process consists of a reepithelialization from type II pneumocytes and of a renewal of interstitial tissue. Prognosis depends to a certain degree on the extent of the regnerative process but, if it is exaggerated, it can bring about a diffuse interstitial fibrosis or even a progressive fibrosing alveolitis. (English summary)

1446.
PHILLIPS, J.D.
Near bottom magnetics studies using a deep submersible.
In: Woods Hole, Mass., Woods Hole Oceanogr. Inst., Rep. Wh01-72-90, p.21-26, Nov. 30, 1972.

The towed magnetometer system using the interim Varian 4937A magnetometer was found to be totally useful for scientific observation aboard ALVIN. The normal ambient noise level of the system is less than ± 2 gammas. Maneuvering and heading effects are less than 10 gammas. The later effects can be eliminated by a small increase in tow cable length. While the operational feasibility of the system was also judged to be very good,several improvements must be made, namely: the tow fish/cable must be made more buoyant and streamlined so as to ascend faster than ALVIN's maximum ascent rate; the magnetometer electronic circuitry must be redesigned so as not to use a chassis ground configuration in order to allow direct connecting to ALVIN's 28 volt power supply. A new type safety cable disconnect system is required for routine use of the towed sensor system. (Author's summary)

1447.
PHILP, R.B., K.N. Ackles, M.J. Inwood, S.D. Livingstone, A. Achimastos, M. Binns-Smith and M.W. Radomski.
Changes in the hemostatic system and in blood and urine chemistry of human subjects following decompression from a hyperbaric environment.
Aerosp. Med. 43:498-505;May 1972.

Sixteen human subjects were exposed to a total pressure of 10 ATA for 10 min breathing air and were then decompressed accordingly to a continuous profile. Blood and urine parameters before and after the dive were compared for each subject. Four persons were asymptomatic and 12 reported symptoms including pruritus in all 12, Type 1 bends requiring recompression in three, swollen auxilliary lymph nodes in two and joint pain several hours later in one. The following statistically significant changes were noted in all divers: increased packed-cell volume, hemoglobin concentration, plasma free fatty acids and prothrombin time; decreased platelet counts (-10-12%), plasma cortisol (-30%), complement activity (-20%), serum lactate, euglobulin lysis time and prothrombin consumption time. The group with symptoms showed statistically significant increases in reticulocyte count, megathrombocyte index, fibrin degradation products and platelet adhesiveness and significant decreases in serum sodium and Antithrombin III activity. The results indicate that compression-decompression alters physiological parameters even in the absence of decompression symptoms and it is possible that even mild symptoms may be associated with intravascular bubbles which effect the hemostatic process. (Authors' abstract)

1448.
PHILP, R.B., M.J. Inwood and B.A. Warren.
Interactions between gas bubbles and components of the blood: implications in decompression sickness.
Aerosp. Med. 43:946-953;Sept. 1972.

Light and electron microscopy was done on the vasculature of stage- or explosively-decompressed rats using techniques which preserved the conformation of intravascular bubbles. Observed were (1) deposition of an electron-dense layer, approximately 200 A thick, at the blood-gas interface, (2) adherence of numerous platelets to this layer with formation of pseudopodia, (3) platelet aggregation at the interface and in the interstices between coalesced bubbles, (4) the occurrence of lipid-like masses at the gas interface in some sections, (5) a significant increase in the numbers of free, circulating endothelial cells and (6) adherence of leukocytes to the bubble or its coating. A review of the literature pertaining to interactions between blood and foreign surfaces including gas bubbles indicated the occurrence of similar phenomena and suggested to us that intravascular bubbles act as foreign surfaces to cause denaturation of plasma proteins, platelet adhesion and aggregation, and coalescence and adhesion of plasma lipids. The observations offer an explanation for the post-decompression thrombocytopenia which has been observed in experimental animals and in man. (Authors' abstract)

1449.
PHILP, R.B.
Blood-bubble hypothesis re decompression sickness.
Hyperbaric Med. Newsletter, p.3:Mar./Apr. 1973.

The author summarizes the current state of knowledge on the blood-bubble interaction resulting from inadequate decompression precautions, as demonstrated in the recent (February 1973) conference in Toronto. In man, the following usually (but not always) happen: (1) the development of a pathological syndrome; (2) the development of detectable bubbles; (3) hematological changes associated with hemoconcentration; (4) reduction in circulating platelet count; (5) increase in blood enzymes of a type usually associated with tissue damage; (6) increased clotting activity; (7) relief of symptoms and disappearance of bubbles upon recompression; (8) effectiveness of low molecular weight dextran, which has plasma expanding, anti-sludging and anti-platelet adhesive properties. In animals, alterations of plasma proteins, adherence and aggregation of platelets, increased clotting, and sludging, following rapid decompression, have been observed. Less widely established and accepted findings are: (1) The intravascular injection of air into anesthetized animals causes a loss of circulating platelets; (2) Protective drugs are those which have antithrombotic properties or surface activity, and, to a lesser degree, anticoagulants; (3) Elevated plasma lipids apparently increase susceptibility to bends. It is pointed out that new evidence presented at the symposium, such as inhibition in man of the post-dive fall in platelet count by dipyridamole derivatives, and the effectiveness of anti-coagulant and anti-inflammatory drugs in retarding post-dive acceleration of fibrinogen and platelet turnover in animals, indicate that further studies of blood-bubble interaction, and of the effects of drugs, are needed. (MFW/BSCP)

1450.
PHILP, R.B.
Historical evolution of the blood-bubble interaction hypothesis in the pathogenesis of decompression sickness.
In: Ackles, K.N., ed. Blood-bubble interaction in decompression sickness. Proceedings of an international symposium held at Defence and Civil Institute of Environmental Medicine, Downsview, Ontario, Canada p.5-18. Published by the Institute, December 1973. (DCIEM Conference Proceedings 73-CP-960)

This research began with observations by Swindle (1937) and End (1938) of the sludging of red cells in fine vessels of decompressed rats, and the formation of emboli and petechial infarcts. Jacobs and Stewart observed the aggregation of platelets around bubbles in 1942. In 1961 and 1962 in France, heparin was demonstrated as protective against bends in animal studies (Laborit) and in treatment of divers (Barthelemy). Malette, Fitzgerald and Eisman demonstrated that methysiloxane reduced mortality, and attributed this to the inhibition of the development of a protective envelope around the bubble. The author carried further the work of the French with heparin and other anticoagulants indicating that protection might stem from the antilipemic effect, or from some surface action, rather than from anticoagulation per se. Extensive work was done with dextran, which indicated inhibition of platelet aggregation and red-cell agglutination. Rat lung studies indicated that fatal bends were usually accompanied by sludging in the microcirculation of the lungs. Further research by the author demonstrated the formation of a capsular structure around bubbles, and the presence of free endothelial cells in the blood of explosively decompressed rats. The capsule was later discovered to consist of densely packed platelets. Sicardi, in France, reported a 37% reduction in mean platelet count of divers decompressed after an exposure to 200 m. in a hyperbaric chamber. Studies carried out by the author revealed that the fall in platelet count of divers with symptoms of decompression sickness was twice that of those without symptoms. Other studies have demonstrated the adhesiveness of platelets and the reduction of platelet count after even very safe dives. (MFW/UMS)

1451.
PICKWELL, G.V. and W.E. Evans, eds.
Handbook of dangerous animals for field personnel.
U.S. Nav. Undersea Cent., Rep. NUC-TP-324, 124p. Dec. 1972.
(AD 754 069)

The handbook describes the appearance, habits and distribution of some of the more common sea snakes, land snakes, and crocodiles of southeast Asia. Color photographs and paintings of these animals are included as aids to recognition. A section on the American honeybee is included as a general guide to dealing with venomous insects; future, additional sections will cover southeast Asian insects, spiders and scorpions. A medical section describes tests of the potency of antivennins for the bites of the Malayan pit viper, common cobra, and blue krait, and suggests a dose schedule for treatment. Revisions and additions to this handbook are expected in response to readers' comments and descriptions of encounters with dangerous animals; to this end, questionnaires and encounter description forms are included at the end of the handbook. (Author) (GRA)

1452.
PIERCE, A.K.
Oxygen toxicity.
Basics of RD 1:1-4;Dec. 1972.

Continuous breathing of high concentrations of inspired oxygen leads to a diffuse parenchymal injury manifested by a decreased compliance and marked right-to-left shunting, causing hypoxemia. The exact time-dose relationships are not well defined. Treatment at present is ventilatory support with the reduction of inspired oxygen to as low a concentration as is compatible with prevention of marked hypoxemia. The serious, often fatal, nature of this syndrome, requires that every physician treating patients with oxygen be aware of the potential hazard and maintain the inspired oxygen concentration at as low a level as possible in order to minimize the likelihood of development of oxygen toxicity. (Author's summary)

1453.
PIIPER, J., P. Dejours, P. Haab and H. Rahn.
Concepts and basic quantities in gas exchange physiology.
Resp. Physiol. 13:292-304;Dec. 1971.

The amount of a gas species is dimensionally considered not as a volume, but as a quantity of substance M, expressed in moles, but also, less appropriately, in volumes STPD. The transfer rate of a gas species (M), with dimension (quantity of substance) $(\text{time})^{-1}$, may thereby be clearly distinguished from the volume flow rate (V) which has the dimension (volume)·$(\text{time})^{-1}$. The concentration (C), defined as quantity of substance per volume, is used for all media (blood, water, and gas). For the gas phase, C is proportional to the fractional concentration, F. and is dependent on temperature, pressure and water vapor pressure. For the increment of concentration in liquid or gas phase of a gas species per increment of its partial pressure, $\Delta C/\Delta P$, the term "capacitance coefficient" is proposed. In respect to gas transfer, it is a measure of the carrying capacity of a medium for a given gas species. It is usefully applied not only to water and to blood (slope of CO_2 and O_2 dissociation curves), but also to the gas phase, for which it is identical for all ideal gases at a given temperature. Some basic equations of gas transfer by blood, air and water convection and by diffusion have been rewritten according to these concepts. (Authors' abstract)

1454.
PILMANIS, A.A. and J.P. Meehan.
Central venous pressure and heart rate changes during apnea and apneic water immersion.
In: Abstracts of the Twenty-fifth Congress of Physiological Sciences Satellite Symposium. Recent progress in fundamental physiology of diving. Marseille, France, July 1971, p.13-15. (Proceedings unpublished).

Abstract only. Excerpt quoted: A preliminary series of 16 dives (13 subjects) using compressed air to depths ranging between 100 and 200 feet was recently completed off Catalina Island, California, Heart rate, respiration rate, water temperature and depth were recorded during all dives. No central venous pressures were recorded in this series of dives. The water temperature at these depths ranged between 10°C and 11°C. Breath-holding was performed at depth. Pronounced apneic bradycardia was present in all subjects to depths of 200 ft. There was no significant difference between apneic bradycardia at 100, 125, 150, 200 ft in depth. The composite results showed apneic heart rate reduction in air (up right posture) reaching 20%. The composite results of breath holding at depths of 100 to 200 ft showed heart rate levels reaching 40% below control levels. Recovery of the heart rate to pre-apnea control levels at the termination of apnea was gradual, on the average lasting 50 sec. There were no significant differences between the heart rate levels and respiratory patterns with light swimming activity during the 100, 125, 150 and 200 ft dives. The heart and respiratory rates showed no significant differences between the control levels in air and the levels at depth. The composite heart rate at the four depths was 98 (control rate of 92) and the composite respiratory rate was 12 (control rate of 13). However, there was a significant difference in the ratio of inspiratory time to expiratory time. The control in air figure was 1.0 This ratio increased to 1.8 at depth, i.e. the inspiratory phase of respiration at these depths was almost twice as long as the expiratory phase. In some individuals this ratio was consistently as much as 3 or 4 to 1.

1455.
PIRNAY, F., R. Marechal, R. Dujardin, M. Lamy, R. Deroanne and J.M. Petit.
Exercise during hyperoxia and hyperbaric oxygenation.
Int. Z. Angew. Physiol. 31:259-268;July 20, 1973.

Physiological reactions during exercise were tested under hyperoxic and hyperbaric conditions. In 6 subjects walking and running at increasing speeds on a treadmill, maximum performance showed little change when the respired air was enriched with O_2. Maximum metabolism, measured by CO_2 production, increased by 3.2%. During the exercise on a bicycle ergometer, maximum O_2 uptake increased by 3% in 5 subjects breathing pure O_2 at 1 ATA. During hyperoxia the maximum O_2 consumption measured at 2 and 3 ATA did not differ significantly from that measured at 1 ATA. Heart rate showed highly comparable maximum values under the various experimental conditions. During submaximal exercise, heart rate was consistently lower when the subjects breathed O_2. The O_2-linked difference became slighter with every increase in work load. Under hyperbaric and hyperoxic conditions, ventilation was invariably reduced during exercise. (Authors' abstract)

1456.
PIRUZYAN, L.
The laser in experimental biology.
Moscow, Academy of Science of the USSR, [1972].

[This volume contains] 20 scientific articles dealing with [the author's] biophysical work in laser and magnetic field research during the past five years under the auspices of the USSR Academy of Sciences. Dr. Piruzyan and his colleagues have reviewed the foreign literature on the use of the laser in experimental biology. . . Dr. Piruzyan and his collaborators report that biopotentials are caused not only by the concentration gradient of specific ions but may be connected with some free-radicle states and semiconductivity phenomena occurring in biostructures. They have studied the effect of hyperoxia and hypoxia on free radicle generation in mouse organs, and have stated that antioxidants appear to protect animals from hyperoxia by diminishing free radicle activity in all organs but the brain of the exposed mouse. (From a review by D.E. Busby and J.H. Brown in Aerosp. Med. 43:1270, Nov. 1972)

1457.
PLANEY, A.H.
Predicting deep ocean performance at Navy simulation facility.
UnderSea Technol. 13:30-31;June 1972.

Man's ability to cope with the hostile undersea environment will be considerably enhanced with the operation of the $7.4 million Ocean Simulation Facility nearing completion at the Naval Coastal Systems Laboratory in Panama City, Fla. This huge hyperbaric complex will enable the U.S. Navy and the nation to develop, test and evaluate underwater man-in-the-sea systems to depths of 2,250 feet, with particular emphasis on the man-equipment interface. It is expected to be in operation by mid-1973. The largest man-rated facility of its type in the world, the OSF complex, will be capable of simulating under laboratory control nearly all environmental conditions found in the ocean. This unique facility will serve as a national center available to government, academic and industrial laboratories for research, development, test and evaluation of hardware and systems related to man's performance in the ocean environment. . . In the areas of deep submergence and swimmer-diver operations there are critical needs for advanced engineering research and development of undersea equipment. (Author)

1458.
PLANTE-LONGCHAMP, G. and Blanchi.
Deux nouveaux cas de lesion labyrinthique apres plongees et leur traitement.
[Two new cases of labyrinth lesions after diving and their treatment].
Bull. Medsubhyp 7:20-21;Oct. 1972.

The authors note the frequent occurrence of isolated vestibular lesions, and also their absence in the literature. Two cases are described in which vertigo and nausea occurred after what should have been safe dives. One case was successfully treated by vasodilators and antivertiginous drugs. Some labyrinth damage and hearing loss was still present after three weeks. The second case was treated by recompression, apparently with success. An intratissular bubble in the labyrinth fluids seemed to the authors a more likely cause of these accidents than barotraumatism, but it is difficult to explain bubble formation in dives so far within safety limits. It is suggested that the special nature of the arteries in the labyrinth might make it possible for a spasm to isolate the labyrinth fluids, so that bubbles could form even during a dive of short duration. The fact that one diver was completely cured by recompression used together with vasodilators would confirm this hypothesis. It is also possible that gas formations in the inner ear might have a more or less harmful effect, mechanically, on the various membranes, in which case recompression might not be completely successful. The authors plan to experiment further and report their findings. (MFW/BSCP)

1459.
PLANTE-LONGCHAMP, G., J. Wolkiewiez and C. Prim.
Bilan des evacuations sous reanimation medicale des victimes d'accidents de plongee-amateur.
[Report on the evacuation of divers under medical treatment].
Bull. Medsubhyp 10:10-14;Dec. 1973.

The authors report their one year old experience in the treatment of accidents that had occurred to non professional skin-divers who had to stand long delays in being transported to the Hyperbaric Oxygen Center. While being transported, the injured persons are treated with oxygen — aspirin — rehydration — vessel dilator — corticosteroides and perfusion of macromolecules solution. Among eight patients showing real neurogenic accidents and evacuated under that treatment within two hours, none had to be subjected to a therapeutic recompression. Repeated applications of hyperbaric oxygen therapy at 1.7 bar have been sufficient to cure them. (English abstract)

1460.
POCIDALO, J.J.
Sur quelques effets physiologiques et biochimiques de l'hyperoxygenation.
[Some physiological and biochemical effects of hyperbaric oxygen].
Rev. Tuberc. (Paris) 35:713-720;Nov. 1971.

The authors study various effects of hyperbaric oxygen including: (1) oxygen transport, external ventilation, pulmonary volumes, the transfer capacity and the alveolo-arterial oxygen gradient; (2) the general circulation and various visceral circulations, including brain, kidney and retina; (3) the cytotoxicity of oxygen, especially on enzymes with SH groups, such as succinate dehydrogenase, and oxidation of pyruvate by way of a possible inhibitory effect on coenzyme A. (English summary)

1461.
PODLESCH, I. and G.E. Herpfer.
Coronary blood flow under high oxygen pressure.
In: Wada, J. and I. Takashi, eds. Proceedings of the fourth international congress of hyperbaric medicine, Sept. 1969, Sapporo, Japan, p.231-235. Baltimore, Williams and Wilkins, 1970.

It was the purpose of this study to measure coronary sinus blood outflow in lightly anesthesized spontaneously breathing, closed chest dogs undergoing hyperbaric oxygenation both before and after receiving a coronary artery dilatating agent. . . It was found that arterial PCO_2 did not change significantly, indicating that the known influence of PCO_2 upon coronary artery perfusion can not be responsible for the decrease in coronary sinus blood flow as consistently found under hyperbaric oxygenation. The remarkable increase of coronary sinus blood flow after a coronary artery dilating agent has been administrated has so far not been reported. The reason for that particular response can not be given definitely since many parameters determining cardiac dynamics and thus influencing coronary artery perfusion have not been determined strict enough to allow for definite conclusion. (Authors)

1462.
PODRASHANDKI, A. and G. Stefanow.
Entwicklung von Unterwassersystemen in der UdSSR
[Development of underwater systems in the USSR].
Meerestechnik 3:224-226;Dec. 1972.

After presenting a survey of various stationary and mobile underwater systems the authors examine the basic requirements which in part were decisive in influencing the design of the 'Benthos-300' diving apparatus. In addition, the development of automatic systems which have already translated theory into practice in space flight technology should confirm that unmanned remote-control systems offer advantages, particularly in respect of certain sectors of marine research. [The photographs which illustrate the article show the underwater laboratory "Tschernomor", the hydraulic manipulator from "Sever-2" and the unmanned remote-control underwater system "Crab".] (English summary expanded by MFW/BSCP)

1463.
POLVANI, D.G.
Predicting underwater acoustic volume reverberation at megahertz frequencies.
In: 1973 Offshore Technology Conference, May 1973, Houston, Texas. Preprints, Vol. II, p.245-258. Published by the conference.

Recently, close range, high resolution sonars and acoustic Doppler current meters have created a need for understanding underwater acoustic volume reverberation at frequencies greater than 500 KHz. The cause of signal dropout in Doppler current meters must also be determined. At the high frequencies and close ranges involved, traditional volume reverberation results are inappropriate. Several scattering models are described which predict volume reverberation at frequencies up to 10 MHz and ranges down to 12 inches. A coherent scattering explanation of signal dropout has also been developed. Numerical results for representative conditions in the world's oceans are given. Sensor parameters for maximum return signal are described. Suggestions are offered for applying the analytical results to the improvement of Doppler current meters and the development of acoustic fish counters, pollutant monitors, ship's speed logs, and oceanic thermal fluctuation spectral analysis. (Author's abstract)

1464.
PONOMAREV, V.P.
A self-evaluation test — a functional test for selection and monitoring of training in underwater swimmers.
Sportsmen-Podvodnik 35:27-33; 1973.

A method of training an individual to accurately monitor the level of decrease in the oxygen content of his own arterial blood is described. This method (formulated by Z.B. Gandel'sman) can only be used with individuals already trained in some form of respiration control, e.g., underwater diving, etc. The subject is made to breathe alternately into two bags while oxygen content in the blood is monitored by the instructor. The subject is notified each time oxygen content decreases by 2%. The training session is continued until oxygen has decreased to 70%. The following sessions, the subject must indicate each 2% decrease himself; these are then compared to the actual levels. Out of 100 persons, 96-97 are generally capable of learning to evaluate oxygen decrease in arterial blood. (S & T Alert)

1465.
POOCK, G.K.
Underwater display visibility as influenced by turbidity, viewing distance, and color of illumination.
U.S. Nav. Postgrad. Sch., Rep. NPS-55-PK-72051-A, 23p. May 1972.
(AD 752,031)

The purpose of the study was to determine the effects of illumination, color, viewing distance, and turbidity on a visual reading task in a totally dark, flooded environment. The reading task was to read a voltmeter and make a correct oral report of the reading. A total of 180 data points spread over 18 viewing conditions were taken for each subject. Seventeen military officers were used as subjects. Experimental conditions were presented in a random manner to all subjects. As statistical examination of the results showed that white or green illumination is better than red in reducing reading response time. Turbidity levels were significant in affecting response time showing an increased response time as the attenuation coefficient increased. There was no difference in the effect of an eight inch viewing distance versus a thirteen inch viewing distance. The error rate was constant, with no variable having a greater effect on the error rate than did other variables. The expected error rate over all variable was .037 errors per each trial taken. (Author) (GRA)

1466.
POOCK, G.K.
Underwater display visibility as influenced by turbidity, display background color, and the color and intensity of illumination.
U.S. Nav. Postgrad. Sch., Rep. NPS-55-PK-72071-A, 36p. July 1972.
(AD 752,028)

The purpose of the study was to determine the effects of water turbidity, display background color, and the color and intensity of illumination on a visual reading task in a dark, flooded environment. The reading task was to read a voltmeter and make a correct oral report of the reading. The sixteen subjects used in the study were allowed to set the intensity at a level which they felt was the minimal needed without sacrificing accuracy or speed in the reading task. As was expected, the results show do difference in the effects of the other variables since subjects apparently adjusted the intensity to a level which equalized the effects of the other variables in any given condition. There was a significant statistical difference in the response times under the two water turbidities used but this difference was only .07 seconds. (Author) (GRA)

1467.
POPE, D.H. and L.R. Berger.
Algal photosynthesis at increased hydrostatic pressure and constant PO_2.
Arch. Mikrobiol. 89(4):321-325; 1973.

Rates of O_2 evolution, $^{14}CO_2$ uptake, and growth were measured in several species of algae and diatoms exposed to hydrostatic pressures up to 600 atm. All of the parameters measured decreased approximately linearly with increased pressure over the range tested. Oxygen evolution appears to be less sensitive to increased pressure than CO_2 fixation or growth. (© BA)

1468.
POPE, D.H. and L.R. Berger.
An apparatus to measure the rate of oxygen evolution while maintaining PO_2 constant during photosynthetic growth in closed culture vessels capable of operation at increased hydrostatic pressures.
Biotechnol. Bioeng. 15:505-518;May 1973.

A double polarographic device is described which permits regulation of dissolved oxygen concentration at any preset PO_2 in suspensions or cultures of photosynthetic algae. It also simultaneously permits measurement of the rate of oxygen evolution during photosynthesis. The apparatus is designed to operate in closed vessels in the absence of a gas phase, and may be used at increased hydrostatic pressures. The device operated successfully at all hydrostatic pressures tested up to 500 atmospheres. Regulation of oxygen levels was maintained constant at various preset concentrations equivalent to atmospheric PO_2 values ranging between 0.02 and 0.21 at 25°C. (Authors' summary)

1469.
POPOV, V.N. and V.I. Chernyshov.
Equation of the state of a helium and nitrogen mixture.
Akad. Nauk, SSSR Izvest. Energet. Transp. 3:162-165; 1971.
(Translation Wright-Patterson AFB, Foreign Technol. Div., Rep. FTD-HT-23-956-72)
(AD 753-964)

The equation of state describing the experimental data within the temperature range of 273.15 to 773.15K and a pressure up to 400 bars was obtained with respect to the compressibility of helium, nitrogen, and mixtures of them. Comparison of the calculated values of the coefficients of compressibility and density of the mixture of helium with nitrogen calculated by the proposed equation of state with the experimental values demonstrates satisfactory comparison in the entire temperature and pressure range encompassed by the experiment. (Authors)

1470.
POPOVIC, V.P. and J.E. Baughman.
Fifty times longer survival of animals which breathe organic liquid after profound body cooling.
In: Aerospace Medical Association. 1971 annual scientific meeting. Houston, Texas, April 1971. Preprints, p.110. Published by the Association, 1971.

During circumstances of rapid decompression, as in escape from a submarine, fatal decompression sickness due to gas bubbles may occur. It is thought possible that under such emergency conditions, this might be prevented by the heating of liquid fluorocarbon. In order to extend the survival time of experimental animals, the authors have combined hypothermia with fluorocarbon breathing. The first group, submerged at 37°C, survived only six to 14 minutes after removal. The second group, at 23°C survived for nine hours. The third group, at 11°C, "survived eight hours of fluorocarbon breathing." It is not made clear whether these animals "permanently" survived. (MFW/BSCP)

1471.
PORCELLI, R.J. and E.H. Bergofsky.
Adrenergic receptors in pulmonary vasoconstrictor responses to gaseous and humoral agents.
J. Appl. Physiol. 34:483-488;Apr. 1973.

A significant role for adrenergic mechanisms in the mediation of pulmonary pressor responses to infused humoral agents (histamine, serotonin, epinephrine, and norepinephrine) and gaseous agents (hypoxia and hypercapnia) is demonstrated in the present study in the perfused left lower lobe of the living cat. Alpha-blockade virtually abolished the pulmonary pressor responses to hypoxia, hypercapnic acidosis, histamine, and norepinephrine but never produced reversal of the pressor response (i.e. vasodilation) to these agents. Reversal of the pulmonary pressor response to epinephrine did occur after alpha-blockade, but the vasodilation was slight and consistent with previous observations of meager vasodilations with isoproterenol without blockade. The data suggest that betaadrenergic mechanisms are not only relatively scarce in the pulmonary circulation but also are not directly stimulated by hypoxia, hypercapnic acidosis, or histamine. Nonetheless, enhanced pulmonary pressor responses to hypoxia, hypercapnia, and histamine occurred during beta-blockade and may be due to the unmasking of additional, but previously antagonized, alpha-receptors. Since no significant effect on the pressor response to serotonin was evident from either alpha- or beta-blockade, a different mechanism mediating the pressor response to this agent is suggested. (Authors' abstract)

1472.
PORTER, R.B. and R.H. Banks.
Electrical-electronic equipment in high-pressure HeO environments.
In: 1970 IEEE international conference on engineering in the ocean environments, Panama City, Florida, 21 September. Digest of tutorial papers. p.6-11. New York Lewis Winner, 1970.

The characteristics of the environment with its high pressure and high helium content forces the designer to consider its effect on the performance of practically all mechanical, electrical and electronic equipment. . . . The equipment operates in a closed environment. Many commonplace materials. . . out-gas solvent vapors and may be toxic or noxious; they represent no problems in normal usage, but many of them become intolerable in a closed environment. The physiologists do not yet know man's capacity for toxicity levels at increased pressures. This is very important to the designer since the material he desires to use for potting or insulation may produce intolerable toxic gases. A great deal more study and research is required in this area. . . The authors believe that the ingenuity of the engineering community can meet the challenge of inner space as it has in outer space. As research and development continues it is believed that in the future there will be available for the designer a list of components certified for use in the environment discussed. (Authors)

1473.
POWELL, M.R.
Mechanism and detection of decompression sickness.
Tarrytown, N.Y., Ocean Systems, Inc., Tech. Mem. UCRI-673, 66p. Dec. 15, 1971.

The authors discuss the theoretical and experimental basis of through-transmission ultrasound detection of bubbles in a biological system and compare this method to Doppler, pulsed-echo, and acoustic-optical imaging techniques. Specifically, they have followed ultrasound signal attenuation as a function of pressure and as a function of time during the following controlled decompression from depth (pressure) exposures. Measurements were made using the foot and also the thigh muscle of the rat as the site of detection. The course of development of decompression sickness symptoms and of visible bubbles in the circulatory system were compared to ultrasonic signal attenuation measurements for similar decompression conditions. Animals [Wistar rats] were compressed in air to 6 ATA and decompressed at 2 atm/min after variable exposure of 15-75 min. at depth. Parameters of ultrasound signal attenuations — time to attain an effect, rate of change to maximum effect, magnitude of maximum effect, and time to recover the original signal — parallel the manifestation of corresponding parameters of decompression sickness symptoms. Visible intravascular bubbles, primarily in the venous system, were found in animals exhibiting a range of decompression symptoms from mild or none to severe or death, but were seldom seen after about one hour past decompression. Arterial bubbles on the other hand, were often seen in animals which died from decompression and only occasionally in animals which survived. These overall results are consistent with a working hypothesis which considers bubbles to be a necessary and sufficient mechanism for the several pathophysiological manifestations of decompression sickness and death. Three bubble "types" differing in anatomic location and size are postulated as occurring sequentially: capillary bubbles in localized tissues, bubbles released into the venous circulation, and bubbles later entering into the arterial circulation. There appear to be two distinct phases or mechanisms of pathophysiological response to decompression: one primarily involving capillary bubbles and leading to pain and paralysis, and the other involving arterial bubbles and leading to death. Bubbles may be seen in the venous system in the absence of observable signs of decompression sickness. (From author's summary)

1474.
POWELL, M.R.
Leg pain and gas bubbles in the rat following decompression from pressure: monitoring by ultrasound.
Aerosp. Med. 43:168-172;Feb. 1972.

Through-transmission mode ultrasound, at a frequency of 5.7 MHz, has been employed to study gas-liquid phase separation in rats resulting from decompression. The time course for this separation was compared to the time course for development of decompression sickness signs in rats exercising on a treadmill. The parameters of ultrasound signal attenuation, i.e., time to attain an effect, rate of change of effect and magnitude of effect, parallel the manifestations of corresponding signs of decompression sickness. The results are discussed in terms of a working hypothesis which considers bubbles to be the necessary and sufficient mechanism for the several pathophysiological manifestations of decompression sickness and death. Three bubble "types" differing in anatomic location and size are postulated. (Author's abstract)

1475.
POWELL, M.R.
Gas phase separation following decompression in asymptomatic rats: visual and ultrasound monitoring.
Aerosp. Med. 43:1240-1244;Nov. 1972.

We have made studies of the distribution of the gas phase in the venous and arterial system of the rat following decompression from pressure. A Doppler ultrasound flowmeter, operated in the transcutaneous mode, was employed to detect the presence of bubbles before a surgical manipulation was performed. By visual inspection of the major venous and arterial tracts we determined the size, number and anatomical location of bubbles. Inspections were made on groups of rats decompressed on profiles which produced 100% mortality. The profiles were then reduced in severity, by reducing the time spent at pressure to a point where individual rats were free of signs of decompression sickness. Even in this group bubbles could easily be found to come from tissue areas not usually associated with decompression sickness in the rat (e.g., abdominal tissue). (Author's abstract)

1476.
POWELL, M.R., R.W. Hamilton, Jr. and G.F. Doebbler.
Mechanism and detection of decompression sickness.
Tarrytown, N.Y., Ocean Systems, Inc., Final report on Contract N00014-69-C-0346, 7p. Apr. 25, 1973.

This report describes the work and results found during studies conducted to elucidate the basic physiology, biochemistry, and biophysics involved in the etiology of decompression sickness. The authors have investigated gas transport in living tissue by means of in vivo probes and mass spectrometric analysis, bubble growth in the tissue microcirculatory system using through-transmission ultrasound, bubble distribution in the major circulatory pathways with both doppler ultrasound flowmeters and visual inspection, and the changes in serum biochemistry following varying degrees of decompression injury. Experiments have been conducted on rats, miniature pigs, and men as the subjects. The principal methodology employed has been to use dive profiles which result in minimal to no observable signs of decompression sickness in our animal subjects to approximate the situations which obtain in manned diving. This allows an easier transcription of results found from animal experimentation to man; death is not used as an endpoint in animals, since that data would not apply generally to man. . . . [In vivo tissue gas analysis indicated] that the elimination rate was not equal to the uptake rate for decompressions which would not produce signs of decompression sickness. This could be explained as a change in the perfusion rate for the whole tissue as a result of blockage of capillaries by a separated gas phase. . . . Changes in the serum levels of creatine phosphokinase and lactate dehydrogenase were sought. No difference in enzyme levels between pre-dive and after short air bounce dives were found. Large elevations of these two enzymes were found when nitrogen-oxygen was used as the compression gas and where mild symptoms developed. However, no changes were found when helium- or neon-oxygen mixtures were used even if definite severe signs of decompression sickness ("limb bends") were evident. . . Three of the Hormel miniature pigs used in these and other decompression studies have been autopsied and examined for evidence of bone necrosis. . . If lesions are found they will be correlated with the diving history of the animals. (Authors)

1477.
POWELL, M.R.
Tissue gas uptake at elevated pressures determined in vivo by mass spectrometry.
In: Aerospace Medical Association. 1973 annual scientific meeting, Las Vegas, Nevada, May 1973. Preprints, p.237-238. Published by the Association, 1973.

The author describes the methodology of the experiment, which combines the technique of mass spectrometry and gas permeable probes to measure tissue and blood gas tensions. The subjects were Wistar rats. In some experiments, through-transmission ultrasound monitoring was employed to detect gas-liquid phase separation. Nitrogen uptake in the rats' thigh muscles increased exponentially with a single time constant. In rats decompressed rapidly from 3.7 ATA, elimination half-time was equal to uptake half-time. In experiments in which greater pressure was used (4.3 ATA and 5.7 ATA) the elimination time was considerably slower than the uptake time. The uptake half-times varied considerably in individual subjects; this indicates that the assigning of a "tissue half-time" to a given tissue in compiling decompression tables should be approached with caution. (MFW/BSCP)

1478.
POWELL, M.R., R.W. Hamilton, Jr. and G.F. Doebblen.
Biochemical indicators of decompression sickness.
In: Ackles, K.N., ed. Blood-bubble interaction in decompression sickness. Proceedings of an international symposium held at Defence and Civil Institute of Environmental Medicine, Downsview, Ontario, Canada, p.34-35. Published by the Institute, December 1973. (DCIEM Conference Proceedings 73-CP-960)

These experiments were undertaken to study the effects of increasing the degree of decompression on serum enzyme levels. Rats, guinea pigs, and rabbits, were used. From these studies, it appears that decompression sickness does not alter plasma enzyme levels. Moderate injury elevates plasma levels of LDH and CPK, and sometimes GOT, but not GPT. Injury severe enough to cause paralysis brings about a large increase in all four enzyme levels. After decompression from air, the enzyme levels rose. This did not occur after decompression sickness occurred. In these experiments, there is possibly a cardiac origin for CPK and LDH changes, since the other enzyme levels did not rise unless paralysis occurred. Venous bubbles too small to be detectable by methods other than ultrasound can form in adipose tissue from which they would be released into venous circulation. If sufficiently numerous, they would cause cardiac stress. The change in plasma CPK and LDH levels, therefore, do not parallel the degree of decompression sickness as indicated by limb pain, but probably reflect a cardiac disturbance. (MFW/UMS)

1479.
POZDNYAKOVA, R.Z., N.N. Shchupakov and V.I. Kopylov.
Nekotorye pokazateli dykhatel'noi funktsii krovi u zdorovykh lyudei v usloviyakh izmenennoi gazovoi sredy.
[Certain indices of the blood respiratory function in healthy persons under conditions of an altered gas environment].
Nauch. Rab. Inst. Okha. Tr. Vses. Tsentr. Sovet. Prof. Soyuzov 73:57-61; 1971.

Placement of healthy persons in a barochamber at 3 atm with a partial O_2 pressure of 420-430 mmHg for one hour caused arterial pressure to increase four times; saturation of the arterial blood with O_2 reached 100%, the O_2 content in the arterial blood increased from 10.14 to 20.85% of volume, and the arteriovenous difference increased from 5.66 to 7.71% of volume. In all cases, the total amount of O_2 transported by the blood decreased: in the arterial blood by an average of 111 ml/min. and the venous blood with O_2 decreased from 68 to 67%. The Hb content, O_2 content and partial O_2 pressure in mixed venous blood and the acid-base balance of the blood did not change. The decrease in the hemodynamic equivalent (1 1. of O_2 was extracted from 12.5 1. of blood as opposed to the normal 16) indicated the increased effectiveness of the blood flow. After hypoxia ended saturation with O_2 and its content in the arteries were normalized. The amount of O_2 transported by arterial and mixed venous blood, saturation of the venous blood with O_2 and its partial O_2 pressure remained decreased by 106 and 85 ml/min, 7% and 5 mm Hg respectively. (NLG) (© BA) (Translated from Ref. Zh. Biol. 1972, No. 4N782)

1480.
POZDNYAKOVA, R.Z., N.N. Shchupakov and V.I. Kopylov.
K voprosu o sdvigakh nekotorykh pokazatelei gemodinamiki u lyudei, nakhodyashchikhsya v usloviyakh izmenennoi gazovoi sredy.
[A study on changes of some hemodynamic indices in people in conditions of changed atmospheric gas].
Nauchn. Rab. Inst. Okhr. Tr. Vses. Tsentr. Sov. Prof. Soyuzov 70:48-54; 1971.

Safety of medical personnel in hyperbaric rooms is emphasized. Healthy subjects were submitted to increased air pressure (3 absolute atm) for 1 hr. A 13-25% decrease in pulse was observed. Arterial blood pressure did not change. Blood systolic volume decreased insignificantly and minute volume decreased 13-28% on the average. The minute volume normalized in 30-40 min after decompression. The observed changes are considered to be adaptive response in hyperbaric conditions. (KP) (© BA) (Translated from Ref. Zh. Biol. 1971, No. 9N79)

1481.
PRAZIC, M. and B. Salaj.
Audiologiczny aspekt dyscypliny sportowej nurkowania.
[Audiologic aspects of diving as a sport].
Autolaryngol. Pol. 25:605-607; 1971.

It is being thought that barotraumatic lesions are caused by sudden changes in the environmental pressure, leading to structural lesions in the sound-conducting apparatus. Tests were conducted on divers aged 18-38 years. All were in good physical condition, disclaiming any hearing or equilibrium disorders. The tests included audiometry and thermal stimulus tests. 62% of the divers showed no deviation from the normal, either in the hearing tests or in the vestibular function tests. The rest showed hearing disorders or lack of thermal sensitivity in various degrees. Since all changes were bilateral, it is concluded that the lesions affect the middle ear. The middle ear's blood supply is poor, therefore any further impairment of the blood circulation may lead to serious consequences. One in every four divers showed some functional disorder of the vestibular apparatus. Since these divers did not have any subjective symptoms, it is indicated that all divers must be subjected to regular audiologic control examinations for early diagnosis of any possible disorders. (OLC/BSCP)

1482.
PREFAUT, C.
Impressions d'un medecin participant a une plongee en saturation: Sagittaire III.
[Impressions of a physician who participated in a saturation dive: Sagittaire III].
Bull. Medsubhyp 10:28-31;Dec. 1973.

The author relates his impressions as a member of the Sagittaire III team during the three-week period of a saturation dive to 300 m. He describes the chamber and its facilities, the daily schedule of experimental activities, the medical problems which arose, and the psychological reactions of the divers to their situation. The psychological benefits of a busy schedule, and the banal nature of the medical difficulties encountered (primarily otitis and transient neurological disturbances) are noted. The author concludes that "there is no real physiological limitation for a depth of 31 Ata even for a non-professional," and that if technical difficulties are resolved, human life is possible for prolonged periods under the sea. (MEMH/UMS)

1483.
PREFAUT, C., D. Prosperi and G. Chardon.
Note preliminaire sur la determination de la ductance globale du Co en condition hyperbare.
[Preliminary note on the determination of overall CO ductance under hyperbaric conditions].
Bull. Medsubhyp. 10:35-37;Dec. 1973.

In order to investigate possible changes in pulmonary exchange efficiency under hyperbaric conditions, the authors studied variations in the overall ductance of CO. The investigation was carried out during the Sagittaire III experiment (3-week saturation dive to 300 meters), on four male subjects, three of whom were professional divers. Analyses of expired air were done by gas chromatography. Although values obtained before the diver were 18% above Lacoste's lower limits for normal, at 31 Ata these values fell by 23% and remained low in three of the four subjects two days after the conclusion of the experiment. The relationship of factors such as oxygen partial pressure, humidity, and the effects of atmospheric pressure on pulmonary circulation are discussed. (MEMH)

1484.
PRESTON, F.S.
Water hazards, or how to avoid a watery grave.
Practitioner 211:209-219;Aug. 1973.

This is an article directed to the diving population and to the medical practitioner with scant knowledge of diving dangers and problems. The following subjects are dealt with: hypothermia — its diagnosis, its prevention, its treatment, and complications during treatment (hypotension, "after-drop", and cardiac arrest); drowning — causes, pathology, clinical picture, treatment, and prevention; accidents and hazards — blackout from anoxia, barotrauma, both of the ear and of the lung (resulting in air embolism), pneumothorax; decompression sickness and its treatment; and nitrogen narcosis. Of necessity, each subject is rather briefly dealt with, but the article represents an effective and clearly written review for the reader who is unfamiliar with the subject area. (MFW/UMS)

1485.
PRISTROM, S.L.
Vliyanie oksigenoterapii na soderzhanie kaliya i natriya v syvorotke krovi i eritrotsitakh u bol'nykh koronarnym aterosklerozom.
[Effect of oxygen therapy on the potassium and sodium content in blood serum and erythrocytes of patients with coronary atherosclerosis].
Zdravookhr. Beloruss. 18(10):37-39; 1972.

Patients (148) with coronary atherosclerosis were investigated. Under the influence of the O_2 therapy Na content in blood serum and erythrocytes decreased, K contents in erythrocytes increased and K concentration in serum slightly changed. Eliminating the phenomena of hypoxemia, O_2 therapy normalizes K and Na contents in erythrocytes and blood serum. (SS) (© BA)

1486.
PRITZLAFF, J.A.
Submersible safety through accident analysis.
Mar. Technol. Soc. J. 6:33-40;May/June 1972.

Some 20 submersible incidents are discussed. Considering that these incidents cover 14 vehicles over the span of five years and several thousand dives, the safety and operational record of manned submersibles is extremely good. A review of the various incidents shows that most of them are connected with handling and at-sea use where seamanship, operational planning, and nautical skill are the key factors. In gathering background data for this paper, all of the vehicle operators indicated that pre-dive and post-dive checklists were vital to the safe operation of their submersible. A typical checklist set from Deepstar 2000 is included for general information and guidance. In only one-third of the reported incidents did submersible equipment designs play a significant part. It must be recognized while a submersible is a specialized type of vessel and that care and expertise must be used in its design and construction, it is still a vessel to be used at sea by seamen. The need for good seamanship in its truest sense of the word must be realized and practiced. (Author's conclusions)

1487.
PROCTOR, L.D., C. Carey, E. Lee, H. Van Den Ende and K.E. Schaefer.
EEG changes during saturation excursion dives to 1000 feet depth.
In: Abstracts of the Twenty-fifth Congress of Physiological Sciences Satellite Symposium: Recent progress in fundamental physiology of diving. Marseille, France July 1971, p.49-51. (Proceedings unpublished)

Abstract only. Excerpts quoted: During saturation-excursion dives to 1000 feet depth four channels of EEG were recorded on two subjects. Most sessions were 6.0 min. long and consisted of alternating 1.2 min. periods with eyes open and eyes closed. Several EEG sessions included 10 min. periods of exercise (100 watts) and recovery at 800 and 100 feet depth and also periods in which different gas mixtures with higher nitrogen and oxygen partial pressures were inhaled during the decompression period. . . Subject A showed a pattern consisting predominantly of a low amplitude fast frequency pattern, about 20 μ V in amplitude, opening or closing of the eyes had little or no effect on the basic pattern. Subject exhibited — with eyes closed — a continuous 10-11 herz alpha pattern in the parietal areas with an amplitude from 50-70 μV. There was an unusual feature to the alpha activity from the left hemisphere. Most of the time it showed a notch at the peak of the wave and could be called an alpha variant. This was not present in the right hemisphere. On occasion the alpha was replaced by a rhythmic 20-22 hz rhythm of about 20-30 μ V. When the eyes were opened the alpha activity disappeared and was replaced by a low amplitude fast frequency pattern. This subject showed a seizure discharge at one occasion during the whole experiment when the 800 ft level was reached. While the eyes were open there abruptly appeared two Hz slow waves of 200-300 μ V amplitude in the left parietal region. After 6 sec. these increased in frequency to 5 hz and then slowed to 3 hz over a period of 14 sec. During the first few sec. of the EEG seizure the right hemisphere became nearly isoelectric but after a few seconds it also showed a 4 hZ activity but an amplitude of 5 μ V. The EEG seizure ceased abruptly and simultaneously in both hemispheres and was not again observed through the remainder of the experiment. During the compression period both subjects showed a pronounced tendency to decrease the mean frequency, greater depth also correlated with fewer high amplitude waves and lower band 18-50 hz while the 6-8 hz band tended to increase. During the saturation period the mean frequency returned again to the initial level in both subjects. During the decompression period it began to decline in subject B simultaneously with an increase in the percentage of waves in 6-8 hz range. These changes in the EEG pattern of subject B also appeared to show a relation to the urinary CO_2 excretion which increased during the saturation and decompression period. The inhalation of gas mixtures during the decompression period (3.5 ATA N_2 and 1.4 ATA O_2) which had slight effects on performance (rater score) produced marked changes in the EEG of the two subjects. There was a definite increase in the amount of alpha activity in subject A and pronounced decrease in alpha activity in subject B as well as a high percentage band 0-2 hz. Exercise of 100 watts carried out at 800 and 1000 feet depth had no measurable effects on the EEG pattern.

1488.
PROCTOR, L.D., C.R. Carey, R.M. Lee, K.E. Schaefer and H. Van den Ende.
Electroencephalographic changes during saturation-excursion dives to a simulated sea water depth of 1,000 feet.
Aerosp. Med. 43:867-877;Aug. 1972.

. . . Subject D.F. showed an EEG consisting predominantly of a low amplitude fast-frequency pattern, about 20 uV in amplitude opening or closing of the eyes had little or no effect on the basic pattern. Subject C.D. exhibited — with eyes closed — a continuous 10-11 Hz alpha pattern in the parietal areas with an amplitude from 50-70 uV. During the compression period both subjects showed a pronounced tendency toward a decrease in mean frequency, greater depth was also correlated with fewer high amplitude waves and lower band 18-50 Hz while the 6-8 Hz band tended to increase. During the saturation period the mean frequency returned again to the initial level of both subjects. During the decompression period it began to decline in subject C.D. simultaneously with an increase in the percentage of waves in 6-8 Hz range (theta w.). These changes in the EEG pattern of subject C.D. also appeared to show a relation to the urinary CO_2 excretion which increased during the saturation and decompression period. The inhalation of gas mixtures during the decompression period (3.5 Ata N_2 and 1.4 Ata O_2) which had slight effects on performance (rater score) produced marked changes in the EEG of the two subjects. There was a definite increase in mean frequency in subject C.D. associated with a high percentage of 18-50 Hz waves and a higher percentage of 0-2 Hz waves. The other subject, D.F. showed a prominent decrease in mean frequency, reduction in the percentage of 18-50 Hz waves and a general shift to a lower frequency range. (From authors' abstract)

1489.
PRUSZYNSKI, B., H. Chlebus, M. Jarecki, J. Preibisz and T. Tolloczko.
Arteriography and analysis of hemodynamic changes in experimental pulmonary artery embolism.
Pol. Rev. Radiol. Nucl. Med. 36(5):515-522; 1972.

The results of arteriography and measurements of pressure in the pulmonary artery in an exeperimental model of multiple embolism in medium and small-caliber vessels induced by autogenous thrombi formed in vitro and in vivo, and single emboli induced by means of a polyvinyl sponge in large branches of the pulmonary artery, allow the following conclusions: 1. The hemodynamic disorders in the pulmonary circulation in multiple embolism of the segmental and smaller arteries differ distinctly from the disorders accompanying single emboli in large branches. 2. In the group of multiple emboli in medium and small-caliber vessels, pulmonary pressure increases very markedly. Vasoconstriction plays a role in pulmonary hypertension. 3. The radiologic expression of pulmonary hypertension consists in dilatation of the pulmonary artery and its large branches. The vascular dilatation is not correlated with the degree of increase in pressure. 4. Winding course of the lobar arteries is probably a sign of markedly diminished capacity of the pulmonary vascular bed. 5. In single emboli of a large artery induced by means of a polyvinysponge, signs of vasoconstriction of the pulmonary arterioles are absent. On the other hand, in the venous bed, flow of contrast medium from all the pulmonary veins on the side of embolism to the left atrium is impaired. (Authors' conclusions)

1490.
PUCHELLE, E. and E. Reichart.
Electrolytes plasmatiques et globulaires du rate en hypercapnia de longue duree.
[Red cells and plasmatic electrolytes in the rat exposed to long-term hypercapnia].
C.R. Soc. Biol. 164(12):2618-2621; 1970.

The technique of inducing hypercapnia is described and the plasmatic K and Na variations of the hematocrits and renal Cl elimination are discussed. Hypochloremia and hyperkalemia are noted in many experiments of breif hypercapnia. They also occur during induced long-term hypercapnia in the rat. Plasma Cl and K varied. (DL) (© BA)

1491.
PUELO, L.E. and H.H. Sobel.
Oxygen-modified collagen and its possible pathological significance.
Aerosp. Med. 43:429-431;Apr. 1972.

Acid soluble collagen isolated from the skin of mice was exposed to 150 psi of oxygen at 37°C for four weeks in pH 8.0 buffer. The product was considerably modified from its native state, becoming insoluble in dilute acetic acid, exhibiting reduced ability to form gels in hot water and reduced digestibility by bacterial collagenase. The action of the latter on oxygen-modified collagen results in a soluble fraction which exhibits marked fluorescence at 425 nm after activation at 350 nm. Approximately 10% of a brown collagenase-insoluble product results. The collagenase-soluble fraction yields a fluorescent peptide which contains most or all of the tyrosine in this fraction. Oxygen-modified collagen might be formed in vivo during exposure to high oxygen tension and results in certain pathological changes, such as aseptic necrosis of bone which is observed in diving personnel. (Authors' abstract)

1492.
PUGLIA, C.D., E.M. Glauser and S.C. Glauser.
Core temperature response of rats during exposure to oxygen at high pressure.
J. Appl. Physiol. 36:149-153;Feb. 1974.

Rats exposed to oxygen at high pressure (50, 60, 70 psig) undergo a lowering of their core temperature during exposure. This hypothermic response occurs prior to the onset of the convulsions generally observed in such an environment. This response was of relatively immediate onset, beginning with the first 5 min of exposure and was continuous up to the onset of the convulsions. Oxygen pressure dependence was observed since the rate of change of core temperature increased with increased oxygen pressure. This temperature response was significantly less in a compressed air environment (60 psig), indicating an oxygen pressure dependence rather than pressure alone. It is suggested that this phenomenon may represent a continuously monitorable manifestation of oxygen toxicity. (Authors' abstract)

1493.
PULLEN, F.W.
Round window membrane rupture: a cause of sudden deafness.
Trans. Amer. Acad. Ophthalmol. Otolaryngol. 76:1444-1450;Nov./Dec. 1972.

The diagnosis of round window membrane rupture and fistula may not as yet be established by any known clinical examination and is possible only by direct visualization of the round window. Clues to the diagnosis appear to be a history of exertion, the suddenness of the hearing loss, and the lack of vestibular signs. Three of four patients with sudden hearing loss [one of whom was a scuba diver] were found to have round window membrane fistulas and the hearing improved after closure. It would behoove the otolaryngologist to consider carefully the patient's history and the vestibular and audiologic evaluation before undertaking surgical exploration of the ear afflicted with sudden deafness. [In the discussion following, the author states that in the case of divers, tissue is preferable to gelfoam as graft material]. (Author's summary)

1494.
PURER, A.
Reducing errors in gas mixing and sampling.
In: Battelle Columbus Laboratories. Proceedings, 1973 divers' gas purity symposium, November 27-28, 1973, p.IV-1-14. U.S. Navy Supervisor Diving, Nav. Ships Syst. Com., Rep 2-73, 1973.

Gas mixtures are a very important aspect in diving since the toxic effect of oxygen and nitrogen limits the use of air to shallow depths; for deeper dives one is forced to use gas mixtures. In such mixtures helium is preferred as the inert gas since it is nontoxic and its low density reduces breathing effort. The upper and lower acceptable oxygen limit of these mixtures becomes extremely narrow at greater depth. Critical requirements such as these allow little margin for error. Two sources of error that are often overlooked are sample contamination due to improper sampling techniques and nonhomogeneous gas composition in high pressure cylinders. These errors can invalidate cylinder analysis or instrument calibration. This gas mixing investigation provides a practical approach to eliminating errors in gas mixing, sampling and analysis. (Author's abstract)

1495.
PURSER, P.
The electrical energy required to produce ignition.
In: Innes, G.S. ed. The production and hazards of a hyperbaric oxygen environment. Proceedings of a symposium held at University College, London, January 1968, p.57-58. Oxford, Pergamon Press, 1970.

[The author investigated] electrical causes of ignition in order to prevent any fire ever happening. The investigation was restricted to the ignition of solid materials in oxygen at one and three atmospheres pressure; the method used was to mock-up possible ignition situations in a small pressure chamber. . . Electrostatic sparking is not a hazard provided that simple precautions are taken, e.g. earthing the patient by antistatic rubber on the couch, or by the monitoring indifferent lead. Current electricity should not be a hazard at currents less than 0.5A and power transfer less than 0.5W. (Author)

1496.
QUIST, A.B. and T.G. Phillips.
MK VI MOD XI control block bench test.
U.S. Navy Exp. Diving Unit, Rep. NEDU-8-72, 16p. May 1972.

The MK VI MOD XI Mixed Gas, Semi-Closed Circuit SCUBA control block assembly was bench tested by the Navy Experimental Diving Unit during the period 21-25 February 1972. The purpose of testing was to evaluate modifications which were incorporated into the control block assembly as a result of discrepancies noted during Fleet OPEVAL completed in March 1971. Test results indicate that the equipment now meets the necessary certification requirements for service approval of the MK VI MOD XI SCUBA. (Authors' abstract)

1497.
QUIST, A.B. and T.C. King.
Westinghouse CCM-1 mixed-gas, closed-circuit, underwater breathing apparatus.
U.S. Navy Exp. Diving Unit, Rep. EDU 7-72, 51p. May 1972.

The Westinghouse CCM-1 closed-circuit, mixed-gas, underwater breathing apparatus was evaluated to determine its suitability for use by Naval Inshore Warfare Forces. More than forty-seven hours of diving time was spent objectively and subjectively testing this equipment for that purpose. The longest dive of the evaluation was six hours and 35 minutes. The deepest dive was to 150 feet. Two dives were conducted in 43° water. During the early stages of the evaluation, repeated maintenance problems became apparent. However, once corrected, the CCM became quite easy to maintain and was found to be an easy to operate, reliable diving apparatus which appears suitable for use by Naval Inshore Warfare Forces. As a result of these tests, it is recommended that further testing, under operational conditions, be conducted to more fully identify the reliability, maintainability and supportability of this equipment. (Authors' summary)

1498.
RACE, G.J., J.L. Matthews, J.W. Finney and J.H. Martin.
Ultrastructural changes in rat adrenal cortex following hyperbaric oxygen (OHP).
In: Wada, J. and I. Takashi, eds. Proceedings of the fourth international congress of hyperbaric medicine, Sapporo, Japan, Sept. 1969, p.170-178. Baltimore, Williams and Wilkins, 1970.

Adrenal cortical cells when studied by electron microscopy and exposure to increased oxygen levels, whether from in vivo specimens or in vitro specimens, show a number of prominent changes. These include a mitochondrial dissociating effect consisting of ballooning and degeneration of mitochondria with vesicular degeneration of endoplasmic reticulum. Also, in the nucleus, peripheral chromatin location is seen with occasional nuclear pores being present. Mitochondrial membrane changes can be demonstrated in the in vitro preparation in the absence of stress of ACTH stimulation. Initiation and repair of mitochondrial membranes appear to occur within a matter of 1 or 2 hours following removal from the OHP environment. Responses to oxygen stress are more marked than responses to sham stress, suggesting that oxygen per se exhibits a mitochondrial dissociating effect. (Authors' conclusions)

1499.
RADCLIFFE, S.V., E. Aladag, J.F. Wallace and G. Das.
Effects of high pressure on deformation characteristics. Part I. The mechanical behavior of beryllium at high pressure. Part II. Measurement of redundant work with hydrostatic extrusion.
Cleveland, O., Case West. Reserve Univ., Div. Met. Mater, Sci., Rep. AFML-TR-69-17, 51p. Apr. 1970.
(AD 868 334)

The study was undertaken with the principal objectives of elucidating the mechanical behavior of well-characterized polycrystalline beryllium as a function of pressure at room temperature in order to facilitate understanding of the factors controlling plastic flow and fracture under ambient conditions and to assist in optimizing the application of forming processes to this metal at high pressure, e.g. hydrostatic extrusion. (GRA)

1500.
RADOMSKI, M.W.
Protection against oxygen induced convulsions and lung damage by metallic cations.
In: Fructus, X., Ed. Third international conference on hyperbaric and underwater physiology, p.184-187. Paris, Doin, 1972.

Rats were given intraperitoneally, aqueous solutions of Mg, Ca, Co, Mn, Zn, K and Li prior to being exposed to 6 ATA of oxygen for 60 minutes. Control rats were treated with water. Li was found to afford the most effective protection against both forms of oxygen toxicity. The order of protection against convulsions was Li $>$ Mg $>$ Zn $>$ Mn, with the others not effective. Li, Mn and Zn prevented lung damage. Since it is doubtful that Mg enters into the brain in pharmacologically effective quantities, its protection against convulsions possibly stems from a curare-like effect at the neuromuscular junction. The therapeutic effect of Li is not understood, although it is known that this cation does accumulate in the CNS and exerts a central action on brain functions. (MFW/UMS)

1501.
RADOMSKI, M.W. and W.J. Watson.
Effect of lithium on acute oxygen toxicity and associated changes in brain gamma-aminobutyric acid.
Aerosp. Med. 44:387-392;Apr. 1973.

Lithium, which has been used in the treatment of certain hyperexcitable states in humans, was tested at various doses and pretreatment times for its effectiveness against the convulsions and lung damage induced by hyperbaric oxygen (OHP) (5.5 ata). Changes in brain gamma-aminobutyric acid (GABA) prior to the onset of OHP convulsions were also monitored. Lithium at 9.4 mmol/kg proved to be highly effective in inhibiting the development of OHP-induced convulsions and lung edema in rats. Lithium also prevented the decrease in brain GABA which invariably precedes convulsions in control animals. Protection was evident only at peak serum levels of lithium (15-60 min postinjection) but was absent 24 hours postinjection at which time brain levels of lithium were maximal. Convulsions induced by strychnine, picrotoxin, and thiosemicarbazide were also delayed by lithium whereas metrazol-induced convulsions were not affected. The evidence suggests that the anti-convulsive property of lithium in the animal exposed to OHP is related to its effects on central neuroinhibitory processes and on brain GABA metabolism. (Authors' abstract)

1502.
RAHE, R.H., W.B. McHugh, N. Kaplan, R. Rimon and R.J. Arthur.
Serum lactic acid variability in subjects experiencing stressful training.
U.S. Navy Med. Neuropsychiat. Res. Unit, Rep. NMNRU-72-10, Jan. 1972.
(AD 754,489)
(Also published in Dis. Nerv. Syst. 33:403-408;June 1972)

Eighty-four U.S. Navy enlisted men enrolled in Underwater Demolition Team (UDT) training were investigated as to serum lactic acid variability surrounding a selected portion of their stressful training. In contrast to reports by other authors, no significant correlation was seen between subjects' serum lactic acid levels and a psychological questionnaire's indices of psychoneurotic symptomatology. A significant correlation was seen between a measure of physical fitness of the men and their serum lactic acid concentrations. (Authors) (GRA)

1503.
RAHE, R.H., R.J. Biersner, D.H. Ryman and R.J. Arthur.
Psychosocial predictors of illness behavior and failure in stressful training.
U.S. Navy Med. Neuropsychiat. Res. Unit, Rep. NMNRU-71-46, 8p. Apr. 1971.
(AD 757 290)
(Also published in J. Health Soc. Behav. 13:393-397;Dec. 1972)

The total score of the Cornell Medical Index (CMI) and a unit scale developed from the Schedule of Recent Experience (SRE) were found to be valid predictors of dispensary visits made during stressful Underwater Demolition Team (UDT) training. The CMI and SRE scores were cross-validated and when combined, were found to significantly increase prediction of dispensary visits. The SRE was found to be more highly associated than the CMI with dispensary visits made by those who eventually quit training because of medical problems, while the CMI was more related to dispensary visits made by those who later voluntarily dropped from training. Those who were medically dropped from training made significantly more dispensary visits and had illnesses and injuries which were nearly twice as severe as those who passed or voluntarily quit training. (Authors) (GRA)

1504.
RAHN, H., O.D. Wangensteen and G.J. Crowley.
Tissue O_2 and CO_2 tensions of trout in high altitude lakes.
Trans. Amer. Fish. Soc. 102(1):132-134; 1973.

Preliminary studies of the relationship between the water O_2 tension (or content) and the tissue O_2 tensions (PO_2) of trout living in waters of intermediate (7200 ft.) and high (>10,000 ft.) altitude of the Sierra Nevada range of East-Central California are described. The tissue O_2 tensions of free-swimming fish, the ultimate factor determining the limits of aerobic metabolism, were assessed. (JEL) (© BA)

1505.
RAINNIE, W.O. and L.A. Shumaker.
ALVIN progress report.
In: Marine industries: problems and opportunities. Proceedings of the ninth annual conference of the Marine Technology Society, p.459-460. Washington, D.C. Marine Technology Society, 1973.

Abstract only. Excerpt quoted: The hull [ALVIN's titanium hull] was designed by the Naval Ship Research and Development Center (NSRDC) and constructed at Mare Island Naval Shipyard. After a thorough ultrasonic and radiographic inspection, the assembled hull was pressure tested at NSRDC, Carderock, to 13,200 feet. It was then shipped to Woods Hole where the ALVIN personnel incorporated it into the ALVIN vehicle during the period March through June 1973. In July of 1973 the entire vehicle was tested in the pressure tank at NSRCD, Annapolis to a pressure equivalent of 12,000 feet. This test consisted of four cycles unmanned and finally a single cycle fully manned and operational. During this final test all systems including life support, propulsion, ballasting and trimming were tested. In addition strain gages on the hull and electrical penetrators were monitored and movement of the windows, hatches and penetrators were measured by the operators. All of these tests verified the design calculations. When shallow water trials and initial deep ocean tests are completed this year, a new ALVIN will commence operations with increased depth, payload and versatility to carry out Navy and civilian research programs in the deep oceans.

1506.
RANDALL, D.J., D. Baumgarten and M. Malyusz.
The relationship between gas and ion transfer across the gills of fishes.
Comp. Biochem. Physiol. (A) 41:629-637;Mar. 1972.

The relationship between perfusion pressure and flow of saline through the gills of an isolated head of rainbow trout (Salmo gairdneri) was determined. Noradrenaline, adrenaline and isoprenaline decrease the vascular resistance to flow through the gills in the isolated head preparation, indicating the presence of both alpha and beta-adrenergic receptors in the gills. The rate of Na loss across the gills of intact trout was determined in fish with ligated urogenital papillae. The rate of Na loss was higher in "active" than in "quiet" fish. Adding noradrenaline or isoprenaline to the water containing the fish also increased the rate of Na loss across the gills. The significance of these observations is discussed. (Authors' abstract)

1507.
RASMUSSEN, J.E.
Man in isolation and confinement.
Chicago, Aldine Publishing Co., 1973.

Some of the research presented (The work of Radloff, Haythorn and Altman) was actually conducted in an undersea environment. The book as a whole has application to this area of activity in that it deals with the ability of man to cope with sensory, perceptual, and social stress arising from an abnormal environment. In particular, studies dealing with sensory deprivation (Zubek) and biological rhythms (Fraisse) are relevant. The emphasis is social-psychological rather than biomedical, with much attention given to selection criteria both for individuals and for groups with relation to satisfactory performance in confined and isolated environments. (MFW/UMS from review by P.D. Nelson in Undersea Biomed. Res. 1:114-115;Mar. 1974)

1508.
RAUTMANN, J.
Sound dispersion and phase fluctuations in the upper ocean.
Nav. Postgrad. Sch., Thesis, 91p. Dec. 1971.
(AD 741 148)

In-situ measurements of the speed of sound in the upper ocean have revealed the existence of significant dispersion and large fluctuations over the frequency range 25-80 kHz. The near-surface values of c ranges from +6 M/sec to -3 M/sec relative to the bubble-free values with a maximum estimated error of 0.5 M/sec. It was possible to identify bubbles of 'surface' radius centered around 54 microns down to 4.3 meter depth as well as a population centered around 124 microns (at 4.3 M) found at all depths. The speed fluctuation showed near-Gaussian probability density functions except at the dispersion center frequencies. The standard deviation of the speed varied from 0.27 M/sec for 58.0 kHz to 0.52 M/sec at 69.6 kHz. (Author) (GRA)

1509.
RAVIN, M.B.
Effects in goats of acute hypercarbia on body oxygen stores.
Br. J. Anaesth. 45:869-873;Aug. 1973.

Eight anesthetized and paralysed goats were ventilated for 2 hours with 100% oxygen. By mechanically increasing the deadspace, the level of PaO_2 was acutely elevated to an average of 62 mm Hg. During the final 30 min of ventilation, the inspired mixture was altered from oxygen to air. The rates at which the arterial and mixed venous oxygen concentrations approached their new steady state values were represented by half-times (tl/2) of 0.43 and 1.04 min, respectively. The turnover rate in cisternal spinal fluid proceeded at a considerably slower rate, tl/2=3.2 min. Acute hypercarbia does not significantly alter the oxygen turnover rate, nor significantly affect the oxygen stores in the cisternal fluid. (Author's abstract)

1510.
RAWLINS, J.S.P.
Diver heating: progress and problems.
In: Fructus, X., Ed. Third international conference on hyperbaric and underwater physiology, p.109-112. Paris, Doin, 1972.

The Environmental Stress Division of the US Navy Medical Research Institute has developed mathematical models, based on physiological premises, to predict the insulative and heat requirements necessary to maintain a diver in thermal balance under various conditions of depth and water temperature. The theoretical predictions have been checked experimentally and are found to correlate well with the observed results. Prototype diver-heating systems have been developed which will maintain a diver in thermal balance at depths down to 600 ft. and temperatures down to 32°F. However, there are still a number of physiological problems to be resolved before this capability can be extended to greater depths, or a system developed suitable for introduction into the Services. This report summarizes those problems and discusses plans for the future. (Author's summary)

1511.
RAWLINS, J.S.P.
Thermal balance in divers.
In: Cold/wet survival symposium. J. Roy. Nav. Med. Serv. 58:182-188;Winter 1972.

The author reviews early cold studies, in which it was learned that thermal balance could not be maintained even in 75°F water. The author and colleagues worked out thermal balance equations which predict heat replacement requirements with suits of known thermal conductivity at various work rates, depths, and temperature, using various breathing mixtures. These predictions were checked out by means of "steady-state" experiments. The relative advantage of dry and wet suits, incompressible suits, and heat replacement systems are discussed. The last consist mainly of (1) a wet suit containing electrical wiring, (2) an undergarment containing a closed-circuit warm water heating system, and (3) a suit with a free-flooding warm water system. The last, of 1/4 inch neoprene, was the most satisfactory under most conditions. Other subjects briefly discussed are power sources, habitats, helium, gas movement, humidity, radiant heat loss and respiratory heat loss. Tests confirmed that (1) respiratory heat loss approximated metabolic heat output at 600 feet in 34°F water; (2) at 800 feet, excessive deep body heat loss occurred even in 86°F water; (3) reactive tissue response, such as massive muco-serous exudation can force the diver to discard his mouthpiece. The response to cold is widely variable in different individuals. For this reason, a very conservative approach to the maintenance of thermal balance is imperative, particularly since the means now exist to make this possible. (MFW/BSCP)

1512.
RAYMOND, L., R.B. Weiskopf, M.J. Halsey, A. Goldfein, E.I. Eger, III and J.W. Severinghaus.
Possible mechanism for the antiarrhythmic effect of helium in anesthetized dogs.
Science 176:1250-1252;June 16, 1972.

Breathing a mixture of 75 percent helium and 25 percent oxygen instead of 75 percent nitrogen and 25 percent oxygen reduced the occurrence of dangerous cardiac arrhythmias after ligation of the circumflex coronary artery in open chest dogs anesthetized with pentobarbital. In dogs not subjected to circumflex ligation, the sensitivity of blood pressure, heart rate, and extrasystoles to epinephrine injected intravenously was not altered by the substitution of helium for nitrogen; however, helium did reduce the baseline heart rate and the concentration of endogenous plasma catecholamines. The antiarrhythmic effect of helium may thus be mediated by changes in sympathetic activity. (Authors' abstract)

1513.
REBUCK, A.S., M. Kangalee, L.D. Pengelly and E.J.M. Campbell.
Correlation of ventilatory responses to hypoxia and hypercapnia.
J. Appl. Physiol 35:173-177;Aug. 1973.

Ventilatory response to isocapnic hypoxia and to CO_2 under hyperoxic conditions were measured in 11 normal subjects, using a rebreathing technique. During hypoxia studies, end-tidal PCO_2 was kept constant at the mixed venous level ($P\bar{V}CO_2$) by varying expired gas flow through a CO_2-absorbing bypass. Initial bag PO_2 ranged from 140 to 160 mm Hg, and rebreathing was continued until PAO_2 had fallen to between 30 and 40 mm Hg. Hypoxic responses were calculated by (a) the slope of the reciprocal of ventilation against PAO_2 (rSO_2) and (b) the slope of ventilation against $1/(PAO_2\text{-}32)$ (A) to obtain linear functions. For rSO_2, responses ranged from 2.67×10^{-4} to 7.59×10^{-4} min liter/mm Hg PO_2 (mean $= 4.39 \times 10^{-4}$, SE $= 0.15 \times 10^{-4}$), and for A, from 19 to 270 liters mm Hg PO_2/min (mean = 144, SE = 9.3). Ventilatory response to CO_2 ranged from 1.17 to 3.11 liters/min per mm Hg PCO_2 (mean = 1.94, SE = 0.05). There was a significant correlation between rSO_2 and SCO_2 ($P < 0.01$) and between A and SCO_2 ($P < 0.01$), such that subjects with a higher ventilatory response to hypoxia also had more marked sensitivity to CO_2. The $P\bar{V}CO_2$ was inversely related both to CO_2 and hypoxic sensitivity ($P < 0.05$), suggesting that the control mechanisms have functionally related sensitivities, in turn related to mixed venous CO_2 tension. (Authors' abstract)

1514.
REDDING, R.A.
Oxygen toxicity and lung lipid metabolism.
Pawtucket, R.I. Memorial Hosp., Rep. NIH-NHLI-71-2153, 32p. Aug. 8, 1972.
(PB 222078/8)

The effect upon rats exposed to 40 and 70% O_2 appears to be a similar pattern of response, but of different severity and pace suggesting that the response is dose-dependent. In 14 days in the 40% O_2 series, and within seven days in the 70% O_2 series, total body weight loss occurred with an increase in lung tissue phospholipid content. At 70% O_2 exposure over ten days, developing lung oedema was suggested by a decreasing dried/fresh lung weight ratio, increased alveolar protein content, and a fall in lung compliance. There were slight decreases in the quantity of alveolar phospholipids, but they remained highly desaturated. Ultrastructural changes occurring after the peak of the pulmonary oedema, initially consisted of widening and fragmentation of the alveolar-capillary membrane. The results suggest that initial physiological and morphological events may be related to lung oedema, rather than changes in lung surfactant. The lungs may be participating in phospholipid synthesis secondary to fat mobilization and general body weight loss. (GRA)

1515.
REDDING, R.A.
O_2 toxicity and lung lipid metabolism.
Pawtucket, R.I., Memorial Hospital, Rep. PHS-71-2153, 31p. Sept. 20, 1973.
(PB-225,527/1GA)

The effect of 100% O_2 exposure appears similar to 40% and 70% O_2 exposure previously reported but more intense and rapid in pace again suggesting a dose dependent response. Within three days of 100% oxygen exposure, 50% of the rats died. In the survivors sacrificed at intervals within this time frame, massive pleural effusion and pulmonary edema was suggested by a falling dried/fresh lung weight ratio, increasing alveolar protein content, and marked alterations in lung compliance configuration. The alveolar phospholipids, dominated by lecithin, increased with interval of exposure, as did whole lung lipids. Ultrastructural fragmentation of endothelial cell walls, with subsequent edema of interstitium and alveoli confirmed biochemical data. The results suggest that initial pathophysical, biochemical, and morphological evidence for edema is not accompanied by physico-chemical changes in lung surfactant. The latter does not appear to play an important role in the pathogenesis of O_2 lung toxicity. (GRA)

1516.
REEKS, T.
Disposal of oxygen from hyperbaric chambers.
In: Innes, G.S. ed. The production and hazards of a hyperbaric oxygen environment. Proceedings of a symposium held at University College, London, January 1968, p.117-118. Oxford, Pergamon Press, 1970.

It is recommended that hyperbaric chambers be vented into the open air and not into a room. . . Other sources of ignition in a hyperbaric chamber should be considered [such as] ignitions from the oxygen supply system. . . The risks from this source may well be greater than from more apparent factors. (Author)

1517.
REESE, K.M.
GE divers come up with antibends device.
Chem. Eng. News, p.32;Nov. 12, 1973.

Two scuba diving scientists from General Electric have invented a wrist computer that replaces tables currently used to avoid bubble formation while ascending. The computer device calculates decompression schedules continuously over variations in depth and time, while the U.S. Navy decompression tables are limited to specific depths and durations. The computer device, it is claimed, permits longer dives and faster decompressions. The computer simulates the different absorption rates of muscle, fat, and cartilage in the body, and indicates when a decompression stop is required, and when the ascent can continue to the next level. At present the device weighs nine ounces, is 2.75 inches in diameter, and 2 inches thick. With design refinement, it is believed possible to reduce the size by half. (MFW/SCD)

1518.
REEVES, E., A.E. McKee, J.A. Stunkard and P.W. Schilling.
Radiographic and pathologic studies for aseptic bone necrosis in dogs incurring decompression sickness.
Aerosp. Med. 43:61-66;Jan. 1972.

A group of 19 mongrel dogs have been compressed to their "bends threshold" depth for at least five hours and then brought to sea level pressure with "no-stop" decompression. Such procedures have resulted in signs of decompression sickness 50% of the time. Recompression with dog treatment tables has resolved all signs of decompression sickness in all but two of the 361 cases of decompression sickness. Radiography of the limbs, shoulder and hip joints of these animals was made yearly for five years. Necropsy was performed at the end of the five year period on 18 animals with histologic sections made of the organs, limbs, shoulder and hip joints for microscopic examination. Bone changes seen radiographically consisted of hip and elbow dysplasias and exostotic changes in shoulder and knee joints. The predominant pathologic bone lesions seen in this study were erosion and necrotic foci of the articular cartilage. Erosion of the surface cartilage and denudation altered the shape of the femoral head, leading to dense sclerosed bone, but there was no evidence of necrosis of cortical or cancellous bone. (Authors' abstract)

1519.
REICH, T.
Pathogenesis of pulmonary oxygen toxicity.
In: Abstracts of BuMed-ONR sponsored Navywide workshop in high pressure biomedical research, U.S. Naval Submarine Base, Groton, Conn., May 1971. p.5. Published by the Naval Submarine Medical Research Laboratory, 1971.

Abstract only. Entire item quoted: The purpose of this study was to determine whether pulmonary oxygen toxicity is a reaction to local hyperoxia or an effect — possibly neurohumeral or systemic hyperoxygenation. To produce severe local reaction without marked systemic hyperoxia, isolated chronic broncho-cutaneous fistulas were constructed to the right lower lobe in dogs allowing selective ventilation of this segment. Animals were studied in the conscious state at 5 ATA for five hours or until death. It was found that ventilation with 100% O_2 in five unoperated controls (Group I: arterial PO_2 $\pm$ 3100 mmHg) and via both trachea and fistula in five operated dogs (Group II: PaO_2 $\pm$ 2800 mmHg) produced gross signs of pulmonary oxygen poisoning (atelectasis not inflatable with air under 40 cms water pressure, edema, hepatization) and death frequency in less than five hours; 100% O_2 fistula and air via trachea (Group III: 8 dogs PaO_2 $\pm$ 500 mmHg) produced no gross evidence of lung damage in any portion of the lungs; 100% O_2 via trachea and air via fistula (Group IV: 7 dogs, PaO_2 $\pm$ 2100 mmHg) produced diffuse pulmonary damage predominantly but not exclusively in the oxygen ventilated segments; damage was less severe than in Groups I and II. Convulsions occurred with increasing frequency in Groups III, IV, and I and II. Whole lung sections (per Gough-Wentworth) are being analyzed and appear to agree with gross findings. In view of the fact that lung damage did not occur in the absence of marked elevation of PaO_2 it is concluded that systemic hyperoxia plays a major role in the pathogenesis of pulmonary oxygen toxicity.

1520.
REICH, T., J. Tait, T. Suga, N.E. Naftchi and M. Demeny.
Pathogenesis of pulmonary oxygen toxicity: role of systemic hyperoxia and convulsions.
J. Appl. Physiol. 32:374-379;Mar. 1972.

The effect of systemic hyperbaroxia in the pathogenesis of pulmonary oxygen toxicity was studied at 4.7 atmospheres absolute (Ata) for five hr. or until earlier death in awake dogs with isolated chronic diaphragmatic bronchocutaneous fistulas. Ventilation with 100% O_2 via both trachea and fistula (group I, seven animals, PaO_2 2m903 $\pm$ 86 mm Hg) produced lung damage and convulsions in all animals and death before five hr in two; 100% O_2 via trachea and 10% O_2 $\pm$ 90% N_2 via fistula, (Group II, twelve animals, PaO_2 1,999 $\pm$ 65) produced damage in all lobes in each animal, convulsions in five, and death before five hr in two of these; 100% O_2 via fistula and 10% O_2 $\pm$ 90% N_2 via trachea (group III, twelve animals, PaO_2 795 $\pm$ 82) and air via trachea and fistula (group IV five animals, PaO_2 574 $\pm$ 23) produced no macroscopic and significantly less microscopic damage, no convulsions and no deaths. Thus, it is concluded that pulmonary oxygen toxicity can result rapidly from systemic hyperbaroxia alone, that convulsions are not necessary for lung to be damaged by OHP, and that the postcapillary pulmonary vessels are not involved primarily in the pathogenesis of this injury. (Authors' abstract)

1521.
REICHART, E. and E. Puchelle.
Influence de la duree de l'hypercapnie sur les electrolytes plasmatiques et globulaires.
[Influence of the duration of hypercapnia on the plasma and red cell electrolytes].
C.R. Soc. Biol. 165(6):1416-1419; 1971.

After two weeks or more of hypercapnia, the plasma K in rats significantly increased compared to that in controls. There was a non-significant variation in the red cells. The relation $K_{external}/K_{internal}$ increased to 0.058 after three weeks of hypercapnia. Plasma chlorine fell, after the second week. The total blood CO_2 was 82.2% by volume at two weeks, compared to the controls with 70.2%. The plasma hypochloremia is explained by the passage of Cl into the erythrocytes, while the K passes from cells (probably of liver and skeletal muscle) to the plasma. (MDS) (© BA)

1522.
REICHART, E., O. Cogniel, G. Brother, M. Marchand and T. Colas.
Bilan acido-basique sanguin chez le rat au cours des deux premiers moix d'hypercapnie.
[Blood acid-base status in the rat during two months of exposure to hypercapnia].
Pfluegers Arch. 334(2):253-263; 1972.

Acid base disturbances were studied in rats exposed for eight weeks to 8 $\pm$ 1% CO_2 in normoxic condition (20-23%). After acclimatization, the $\Delta PvCO_2$ [venous O_2 pressure] was 34-38 torr and the $\Delta PaCO_2$ [arterial O_2 pressure] was 32-30 torr. No significant changes were observed in PCO_2 [CO_2 pressure] which remained relatively constant during all experiments. The acidosis induced by hypercapnia increased during the first two weeks but then largely regressed. Siesjo's formula was used to express pH regulation. The percentage of metabolic bicarbonates rose with increasing length of exposure to hypercapnia. (© BA)

1523.
REILLY, R.E.
Annotated bibliography. Human performance in the undersea environment.
Falls Church, Va., BioTechnology Inc., Rep. on Contract N00014-70-C-0052, 84p. Jan. 1970.

The purpose of this effort was to review technical literature concerning human mental and perceptual-motor performance in wet and dry hyperbaric environments. Recognizing that active researchers in this area span the globe and that publication lags are so great, a direct request was made to those individuals and agencies who it was thought might provide up to date information and references which might not be identified through normal data retrieval channels. The response to this request was far beyond expectations. Consequently, despite severe time and fiscal constraints, it was decided to incorporate as much of this literature as possible into a bibliography in the hope that through rapid preparation and circulation, it would serve as a contribution to the research community. [The bibliography contains 149 references and abstracts, plus a list of other bibliographies, a list of scientists engaged in underwater research, and a subject index.] (Author's introduction expanded by MFW/BSCP)

1524.
REIMERS, S.D.
Atmospheric control in the hyperbaric environment.
U.S. Navy Exp. Diving Unit, Rep. NEDU-26-72, 9p. 1972.
(Also published in Nav. Eng. J., p.50-65;June 1971)

Careful control of the atmosphere in a hyperbaric facility is necessary to protect the health and well-being of the occupants. In this paper total environmental control in the hyperbaric chamber is broken down into eight subareas of control: total pressure, oxygen partial pressure, CO_2 partial pressure, fire prevention, temperature, humidity, trace contaminants, bacteria, and noise. For each subarea an assessment is given of the difficulty and degree of control required and its importance to the divers' well-being. Also discussed for each subarea are the state of the art, and the areas of greatest technological need. Control of oxygen and CO_2 partial pressure in breathing circuits of diving equipment is described. Methods of heating the diver and his inspired gas are also briefly discussed. (Author's abstract)

1525.
REIMERS, S.D. and O.R. Hansen.
Environmental control for hyperbaric applications.
U.S. Navy Exp. Diving Unit, Rep. NEDU-25-72, 5p. 1972.

Careful control of the environment in a hyperbaric facility is necessary to protect the health and well-being of the occupants. In this paper total environmental control in the hyperbaric chamber is broken down into eight categories of control: total pressure, O_2 partial pressure, CO_2 partial pressure, temperature and humidity, trace contaminants, fire detection, bacteria and noise. For each category an assessment is given of the difficulty and degree of control required and its importance to the occupants' well-being. For a diver in the water the special problems encountered in O_2 partial pressure control, CO_2 partial pressure control, and temperature control are also discussed briefly, each in its respective category. For each category the state of the art is discussed and the requisites for technological advancement are identified. (Authors' abstract)

1526.
REIMERS, S.D. and B.S. Lebenson.
KMB-8 band mask evaluation. Final report.
U.S. Navy Exp. Diving Unit, Rep. NEDU-17-72; 45p. Aug. 1972.

The Kirby-Morgan KMB-8 band mask was tested and evaluated for comfort and its ability to supply a diver's respiratory demand. Tests were run at various work rates and depths from 10 fsw to 650 fsw. The mask was found to meet the respiratory pressure requirements of MIL-R-24169A. It was found to be satisfactory for fleet use provided certain recommended minor changes in the mask design and bail-out bottle configuration are carried out. Recommended depth limits for air and HeO_2 diving are also established. (Authors' abstract)

1527.
REIMERS, S.D.
Simulation testing of divers' breathing apparatus.
U.S. Navy Exp. Diving Unit, Rep. NEDU-2-73, 19p. Mar. 14, 1973.

The development of human simulation and physiologic testing methods is greatly altering the development cycle for military diver life support equipment. The relationships of both testing methods to each other and to the complete development cycle are discussed. The state of development of the NEDU "human simulator" and the measuring techniques needed to support it are discussed in detail. Areas needing further work are identified. (DCD abstract)

1528.
REIMERS, S.D. AND J.K. Summitt.
Sound level testing of the standard USN MK V air and helium-oxygen diving helmets.
U.S. Navy Exp. Diving Unit, Rep. NEDU-4-73, 94p. June 8, 1973.
(AD 764 528/6)

Nine standard USN Mark V air diving helmets and two standard USN Mark V helium-oxygen diving helmets were subjected to sound level testing on two specially built acoustical manikins at the Navy Experimental Diving Unit. The sound levels existing in the helmets were found to be into the hearing damage risk levels under nearly all the conditions tested. Wide variability in the measured sound levels was found to exist from helmet to helmet. The relationship of the test results to other similar work is discussed. Several possible ways of reducing the measured sound levels are presented. (Authors) (GRA)

1529.
REIMERS, S.D.
Sound level testing of the Yokohama helium-oxygen diving helmet.
U.S. Navy Exp. Diving Unit, Rep. NEDU-6-73, 19p. June 20, 1973.

A helium-oxygen diving helmet manufactured by the Yokohama Diving Apparatus Company, Ltd., of Yokohama, Japan, and distributed in the U.S. by J & J Marine Diving Company of Pasedena, Texas, was subjected to sound level testing on a specially built acoustical manikin at the U.S. Navy Experimental Diving Unit. Ten manned test dives were also conducted. The sound levels existing in the helmet were found to be into the hearing damage risk levels, but not so far as to preclude normal helium-oxygen diving operations with the helmet. Subject to certain restrictions, the sound levels existing in the helmet were judged to be safe for exposures of up to 4-1/2 hours per 24-hour period. (Author's abstract)

1530.
REIMERS, S.D., H.C. Langworthy and J. Hesket.
Evaluation of the advanced (Swindell) air diving helmet.
U.S. Navy Exp. Diving Unit, Rep. NEDU-7-73, 67p. July 13, 1973.

The Advanced (formerly Swindell) Series 2000 Model Open-Circuit Air Diving Helmet manufactured and distributed by the Diver's Exchange, Inc. of Harvey, La. was subjected to evaluation testing at the Navy Experimental Diving Unit. The helmet was tested for sound levels and ventilation efficiency using specially built test manikins. It was tested for diver comfort in a series of 36 manned dives. Since many of the testing methods used were new, a discussion of the procedures used as well as the results obtained is presented. The sound levels existing in the helmet were found to be into the damage risk levels under all of the conditions tested, but not so far as to preclude its use provided appropriate precautions are taken. The ventilation efficiency of the helmet was found to be generally adequate provided the air supply pressure is maintained at sufficient levels. The helmet was found to be comfortable for work rates up to and including moderate work. (Authors' abstract)

1531.
REIMERS, S.D., H.C. Langworthy and J. Hesket.
Evaluation of the advanced (Swindell) helium-oxygen diving helmet.
U.S. Navy Exp. Diving Unit, Rep. NEDU-10-73, 107p. Aug. 14, 1973.

The advanced (formerly Swindell) Model 3610 Mixed Gas Diving System manufactured and distributed by the Diver's Exchange, Inc. of Harvey, LA was subjected to evaluation testing at the Navy Experimental Diving Unit. The Model 3610 System consists primarily of a Model 3000 Mixed Gas Helmet used with a neckseal and a Model 3700 Back Pack Scrubber. The system was tested for sound levels and ventilation efficiency using specially built test manikins. It was tested for diver comfort in a series of 20 manned dives. Since many of the testing methods used were new, a discussion of the procedures used as well as the results obtained is presented. The sound levels existing in the helmet were found to be into the damage risk levels under many of the conditions tested, but not so far as to preclude risk of the system provided that appropriate precautions are taken. The ventilation efficiency of the system was found to be generally adequate for diving in the depth range of 0 to 300 fsw provided the gas supply pressure is maintained at sufficient levels. The system was regarded by the divers as generally more comfortable than the standard USN $He\text{-}O_2$ diving outfit. Nonetheless diver complaints of helmet and jock strap discomfort became common at work rates approximating moderate work. (Authors' abstract)

1532.
REIMBERS, S.D., H.C. Langworthy and J.W. Lewis.
An evaluation of the Desco air diving helmet.
U.S. Navy Exp. Diving Unit, Rep. NEDU-13-73, 71p. Sept. 18, 1973.

The DESCO Air Diving Helmet manufactured and distributed by the Diving Equipment and Supply Co., Inc. of Milwaukee, Wisconsin was subjected to evaluation testing at the Navy Experimental Diving Unit. The helmet was tested for sound levels and ventilation efficiency using specially built test manikins. It was tested for diver comfort in a series of 40 manned dives. Since many of the testing methods used were new, a discussion of the procedures used as well as the dives. Since many of the testing methods used were new, a discussion of the procedures used as well as the results obtained is presented. The sound levels existing in the helmet were found to be into the damage risk levels under al! of the conditions tested, but not so far as to preclude its use provided appropriate precautions are taken. The ventilation efficiency of the helmet was found to be generally adequate even though the maximum helmet flow rate fell below the desired maximum level of 4.5 acfm at depths below 100 fsw. The helmet was found to be comfortable for work rates up to and including moderate work. (Authors' abstract)

1533.
REIMERS, S.D., J.K. Summitt, W.F. Aichele and T.W. James.
Evaluation testing of the David Clark Model S-5005 Air and Mixed Gas Diving System.
U.S. Navy Exp. Diving Unit, Rep. NEDU-14-73, 49p. Oct. 2, 1973.

The David Clark S-5005 Air and Mixed Gas Diving System was subjected to evaluation testing at the Navy Experimental Diving Unit. The system was tested for diver comfort in the open circuit air mode in a series of 25 manned dives. The helmet used with the system was tested for sound levels in both the open circuit air and semi-closed circuit mixed gas modes by means of a specially constructed test manikin. The helmet was found to be uncomfortable in the water due to extreme noise and excessive buoyancy. Manned diving with the system in the open circuit air mode was suspended when one of the test divers complained of abnormal hearing subsequent to his dive and audiometric examinations performed on him and the preceding test diver revealed significant temporary hearing losses in both men. Further evaluation of the system in the open circuit air mode was terminated when the sound level tests revealed that the sound levels in the helmet in the open circuit air mode were so far into the damage risk levels that safe use of the helmet was judged impractical. All evaluation efforts were subsequently terminated when it was learned that David Clark was discontinuing its line of diving equipment. (Authors' abstract)

1534.
REIMERS, S.D.
Mixtures and the Kirby-Morgan KMB-8 Bandmask.
U.S. Navy Exp. Diving Unit, Rep. NEDU-17-73, 42p. Oct. 10, 1973.

The Kirby-Morgan KMB-8 Bandmask (mid-1972 version) used with a U.S. Divers Conshelf XII first stage regulator was subjected to a series of breathing pressure tests at the Navy Experimental Diving Unit using a breathing machine and a specially constructed test manikin. The mask was tested using a 80% sulphur hexafluoride, 20% oxygen gas mixture at the surface. It was also tested on air and on a variety of helium-oxygen mixtures at the depths where their densities equalled that of the surface SF_6O_2 mixture. The equal density testing technique was determined not to be a valid method of predicting the inhalation performance of a KMB-8 Bandmask and other similar open-circuit demand systems. The over bottom pressure existing at the inlet to the second stage regulator under peak respiratory flow rate conditions was found to be the parameter most critically affecting the inhalation performance of the mask. The primary cause of the loss of over bottom pressure of the inlet to the second stage under flowing conditions was found by both experimental data and analytical calculations to be flow resistance in the components between the first stage outlet port and the second stage inlet port. (Author's abstract)

1535.
REIMERS, S.D.
Performance characteristics and basic design features of a breathing machine for use to depths of up to 3000 feet of sea water.
U.S. Navy Exp. Diving Unit, Rep. NEDU-20-73, 34p. Nov. 20, 1973.

Breathing machines have been a central part of the equipment used to evaluate respiratory protective devices and underwater breathing apparatus for several years. The leading breathing machines in use today are surveyed. A set of specifications are proposed for the development of a breathing machine for use in the testing of underwater breathing apparatus to depths of 3000 feet of sea water. Based on the breathing machines surveyed, a basic design for the 3000 fsw breathing machine is proposed. (Author's abstract)

1536.
REINS, D.A. and J.C. Shampine.
Evaluation of heat loss from Navy divers' wet suit.
U.S. Navy Clothing Textile Res. Unit, Rep. Nos. TR-102, 4-70, 24p. July 1972.
(AD 747 276)

In a series of over 200 tests, subjects wore standard, 3/16 inch, closed-cell neoprene-foam, air-sea rescue suits in water of 55, 45, and 35 deg. F. The tests were designed to identify areas of the body where major heat losses occur. Other physiological parameters were monitored to assure the physical safety of test subjects while body temperature and metabolic rates were measured. Recommendations are made as to areas in which insulative value could be increased without hampering free movement of the wearer, and design modifications are suggested to limit free movement of water into and out of the suit. (Authors) (GRA)

1537.
RENTZ, F.P.
A review of available heated wet-suit protection for divers and swimmers.
U.S. Nav. Submar. Med. Res. Lab., Rep. NSMRL 739, 15p. Feb. 28, 1973.

It is evident that heated wet suits are required for long underwater missions in temperate water and for short excursions in cold water. Several diver heating systems have already been developed and are in use, such as the free-flooding umbilical supplied suit and the battery powered, electrically heated suit. These are adequate for most underwater tasks today. A diver working from a personnel transfer capsule or a deep habitat is usually tethered for safety. An umbilical carrying heated water or electrical power would not be much added encumbrance. A combat swimmer could use the battery-powered suit for his free-swimming mission of two to three hours, drawing power from the larger, swimmer delivery vehicle battery during the longer trip to and from the area. Thus, he would not really be limited by the relatively short free excursion time permitted by today's batteries. Improvements in these systems are to be expected, as well as eventual development of a successful, practicable, isotope-fueled heating unit. With their low cost and high energy-to-weight ratio, the combustion heating devices may soon achieve prominence. A system which will keep a free-swimming diver comfortable in cold water for periods of six to eight hours has yet to be perfected, and represents a challenge for future development. (Author's conclusion)

1538.
RESCHKE, M.F., D.E. Parker and H.E. Von Gierke.
Stimulation of the vestibular apparatus in the guinea pig by static pressure changes: head and eye movements.
J. Acoust. Soc. Amer. 48:913-923;Oct. 1970.
(Also published Oxford, Ohio, Miami Univ., Dept. Psychol., Rep. AMRL-TR-70-100, Jan. 5, 1970)
(Ad 754 825)

Head and eye movements elicited by static pressure increases of up to 1-min duration in the external auditory meatus were recorded using guinea pigs as subjects. The minimum stimulus intensity required to produce a response was 1.5 - 2.0 cm Hg. Observations were made of response latencies, durations and amlitudes as a function of stimulus intensities, durations and onset rates. Head and eye movements elicited by the pressure stimulation were found to be significantly correlated. The results of this investigation are interpreted as supporting the hypothesis that stapes footplate displacement, and consequently perilymph/endolymph displacement, produce direct mechanical stimulation of the semicircular-canal receptors. Moreover, these results suggest that the same mechanism might be responsible for stimulation of the vestibular system by low-frequency inaudible sound and for the vestibular effects observed in response to audio-frequency high-intensity sound. In the latter case, vestibular stimulation is hypothesized to occur as a result of a shift in the average position of the stapes footplate owing to overdriving the ossicular chain. (Author) (GRA)

1539.
RESNICK, J.S., D.M. Brown and R.L. Vernier.
Oxygen toxicity in fetal organ culture. I. The developing kidney.
Lab. Invest. 28:437-445;Apr. 1973.

Toxic effects of increased oxygen concentrations were evaluated in an organ culture system using fetal mouse kidney of 11 to 13-1/2 days gestation. Normal nephrogenesis and ureteral branching were observed with oxygen concentrations of room air (PaO_2 = 139 to 141 mm Hg), while severe cell necrosis, absence of nephrogenesis, and abnormal ureteral branching were observed with high oxygen concentration (PaO_2 = 695 to 720 mm Hg). Intermediate oxygen concentration (PaO_2 = 470 to 500 mm Hg) resulted in intermediate toxicity which was most evident in abnormal ureteral branching and abnormal nephrogenesis with less evidence of necrosis. The separate effects of potassium concentration in the medium was also evaluated and no evidence of abnormal nephrogenesis was observed despite potassium levels as low as 1.8 mEq. per liter. It is concluded that the oxygen concentration used in organ culture experiments is an important variable. There is also an age-dependent variable in evaluation of toxic substances in fetal organ cultures that must be considered. This experimental system allows a more precise in vitro evaluation of a variety of developing fetal organs. (Authors' abstract)

1540.
REUTER, S.H.
95% of divers' ear problems start in eustachian tube.
Clin. Trends 10:8;Oct./Nov. 1971.

The author urgently recommends the "feet-first" position in diving, because the head-first position brings on vascular congestion in the membranes of the eustachian tubes, thus increasing the danger of middle-ear barotrauma. Also, divers should be trained to inflate the eustachian tube every two or three feet, during descent, instead of waiting until the inequality of pressure becomes great enough to force the divers to exercise the Valsalva maneuver, at which time "the shearing of force of this pressure wave [the sudden inward pressure change on the footplate], combined with possible hemorrhage from torn blood vessels. . . causes permanent damage to the sensory receptors of the cochlea." The author disagrees with the widely held belief that the high-tone hearing loss common in experienced divers is due to thickening of the ear drum as a result of frequent exposure to cold and to pressure change. (MFW/BSCP)

1541.
REYNOLDS, W.J., H.T. Milhorn, Jr. and H. Holloman, Jr.
Transient ventilatory response to graded hypercapnia in man.
J. Appl. Physiol. 33:47-54;July 1972.

The transient ventilatory responses of a group of normal male volunteers to mixtures of 3, 5, 6, and 7% CO_2 in air were determined by continuous recording of expiratory flow, PO_2 and PCO_2 with an FM magnetic tape recorder. The analog data were then digitized and calculations performed by a digital computer to yield breath-by-breath values for tidal volume respiratory frequency, minute ventilation and alveolar PO_2 and PCO_2. Each experiment consisted of 20 min breathing room air, a 25-min stimulus period, and another 20-min period on room air. Minute ventilation was observed to increase smoothly at all stimulus levels. Tidal volume underwent a rapid on-transient and maintained a stable plateau thereafter, while respiratory frequency increased much more slowly. Alveolar PO_2 underwent a fast on-transient and a slow two component off-transient. The fastest on- and off-transients were those for alveolar PCO_2 which was also the only variable observed to undershoot its control value upon removal of the stimulus mixture. (Authors' abstract)

1542.
REYNOLDS, W.J. and H.T. Milhorn, Jr.
Transient ventilatory response to hypoxia with and without controlled alveolar PCO_2.
J. Appl. Physiol. 35:187-196;Aug. 1973.

The transient ventilatory responses of a group of normal male volunteers to step inputs from room air to mixtures containing 9, 8, and 7% oxygen were determined by continuous recording of expiratory flow, PO_2, and PCO_2 with a FM magnetic tape system. The analog data were then digitized and calculations performed to yield breath-by-breath values for tidal volume, respiratory frequency, minute volume, and alveolar PO_2 and PCO_2. In one experimental series the subject's alveolar PCO_2 was allowed to fall, and in another it was held constant by a rapidly responding external control system (capnostat). Small overshoots in the ventilation on-transient were observed in approximately half of the subjects during the hypocapnic experiments but were not present at all in the isocapnic series. The ventilation on-transient was noted to lag behind that of the alveolar PO_2 at all stimulus concentrations with a larger lag seen in the isocapnic series. Small undershoots in the ventilation off-transient were observed in both series, in each case resulting from an undershoot in the respiratory frequency off-transient. (Authors' abstract)

1543.
RHEINWALD, V.
Untersuchungen uber den Einfluss des Pervitins auf die Gasblasenbildung nach Dekompression aus Uberdruck.
[Studies on the influence of pervitin on the incidence of gas bubbles in blood after decompression].
Bad Godesberg, West Germany, Deutsche Forschungs-und Versuchanstalt fuer Luftund Raumfahrt, Inst. Fuer Flugmedizin, Rep. CLR-FB-72-66, 49p. 1972.
(NAVSHIPS TRANSL. 1429;Oct. 1973)

The influence of the drug Pervitin on the incidence of gas bubbles in blood during quick decompression was proved in experiments with albino rats. The starting point of this study was the fact that the blood circulation determines the elimination of gas under decompression. Opposed results show the theoretical supposition that Pervitin improves elimination of N_2 during decompression because of its effect on circulation, is not well founded. Preventive treatment of rats with Pervitin medication led to no significant reduction of mortality. (Author's abstract) (STAR)

1544.
RHODES, H.L., L. Stroud and P.C. Tully.
Vapor-liquid equilibria data for two helium-nitrogen-methane mixtures from 76.5 to 164 k and pressures to 1200 psia.
Washington, D.C., Bureau Mines, Rep. BuMines-RI-7598, 34p., 1972.
(PB 208 004)

Vapor-liquid equilibria data for two helium-nitrogen-methane mixtures are presented for 12 temperatures from 76.5 to 164 K and pressures from 100 to 1200 psia. Gas mixtures of 65-34-1 and 25-27-48 percent helium-nitrogen-methane were studied in a windowed phase equilibria cell equipped with vapor recirculating pump. Isobaric and isothermal k-values are plotted for both mixtures. Two isometric plots are included. (Authors) (GRA)

1545.
RICCI, G.C.
Newer pathophysiologic orientations and newer therapeutical approach on systemic syndromes related to scubair decompression sickness.
In: Fructus, X., Ed. Third international conference on hyperbaric and underwater physiology, p.145-153. Paris, Doin, 1972.

The numerous elements gathered on the pathogenesis of D. S., may be summarized as follows: (a) D. S. leads to a morbid, complex phenomenon, variable from one subject to another and from one particular moment to another and is not necessarily bound to the course of an erroneous dive. (b) In the etiology of D. S. we must consider fatigue, cold, muscular work, tachypnea, training, emotions, dyslipemia, fat meals, atherosclerosis, decreased elasticity of the circulatory apparatus and spinal arthritis, at all levels, but in particular in the cervical region. (c) The General Adaptation Syndrome [metabolic and circulatory changes] produced by cold, emotions, hyperbaric respiration, lack of gravity, unusual underwater work, with its hemodynamic and endocrino-metabolic reactions, can favor D. S. (d) Lastly, before and after treating decompression accidents, perhaps not sufficient attention was given to their bio-humoral component and to the fact that serious accidents can often be followed by hypovolemic shock and fatty embolism. In conclusion, it is without a doubt that all these remarks open new horizons on the treatment of D. S. — without abandoning recompression therapy, especially in its present state, which gives much more importance to hyperbaric oxygen therapy than to air barotherapy alone. Within the picture of a well-performed medical resucitation, the pharmacodynamic action of oxygen to different drugs permits us to tend towards a much more efficient D. S. therapy. (Author)

1546.
RICCI, G.C.
New concepts on the pathophysiology and treatment of scubair decompression sickness.
In: Aerospace Medical Association. 1972 annual scientific meeting, Bal Harbour, Florida, May 1972. Preprints, p.254. Published by the Association.

The author reports the first therapeutical results of 13 cases of severe Decompression Sickness and/or lung overpressure. He reports on clinical, X-ray and laboratory findings and data and the effects of the therapy based on drug treatment (plasma expanders, Heparin and different anticoagulant and antithrombotic agents, antiproteinases, corticoids, chlorpromazine, Diazepam) associated to a non-high recompression therapy with air-oxygen and/or oxygen alone. The clinical results also give the author the opportunity of underlining, "a posteriori", the new orientation on the above-mentioned pathophysiology of these syndromes related to volemic changes, biophysical and biochemical lipid modifications, platelet clumping and sludging of blood, connected to the effects of gas emboli or gas in solution (osmosis) in the elicitation or precipitation of such a systemic clinical picture. (Author)

1547.
RICCI, G.C. and E. Massa.
Pathophysiology and treatment of dysbaric accidents and of air decompression sickness.
In: Ackles, K.N. ed. Blood bubble interaction in decompression sickness. Proceedings of an international symposium held at Defence and Civil Institute of Environmental Medicine, Downsview, Ontario, Canada, p.211-217. Published by the Institute, December 1973. (DCIEM Conference Proceedings 73-CP-960)

Specifically [the authors] recommend: 1) To treat each case individually according to clinical and laboratory data rather than to rely on assumptions deriving from the type of dive and the depth of diving. 2) To administer treatment by: a) plasma expanders especially with anti-sludging effects (low molecular weight dextran); b) anticoagulant and agents that would prevent or combat platelet aggregation and thrombosis (heparin, ASA associated with depyridamole; c) Corticoids, often at strong doses, against oedema or oedematous reactions at any level; d) hyperbaric treatment with choice of air, air — O_2 mixtures or pure oxygen, according to the relative need of each subject; e) other supportive collateral agents (protease inhibitors for general metabolic support, diazepam or chlorpromazine for psychomotor agitation.) (Authors)

1548.
RICCI, C.G.
Detresse respiratoire et atteinte medullaire dans la maladie de la decompression. Hypotheses pathogeniques et observations cliniques.
[Respiratory distress and medullary impairment in decompression sickness. Pathogenic hypotheses and clinical observations].
Bull. Medsubhyp 10:32-34;Dec. 1973.

Blood-bubble interactions not only seem to develop in the lung as a target oragan or as a primum movens, but many types of "lung dysbarism" — including breathhold diving — can lead to pulmonary distress, i.e., pulmonary hypertension and stasis with venous repercussion on the venous medullary plexus. Consequently, in some cases, the pathophysiology of medullary impairment can be related to a similar mechanism which can be favored by local hemodynamic modifications due to lack of gravity, i.e., immersion blood-shift from the forearms. (Authors's abstract)

1549.
RICCIUTI, E.R.
Killers of the seas. The dangerous creatures that threaten man in an alien environment.
New York, Walker and Co., 1973. 308p.

An interestingly written survey of the sea creatures that may be dangerous to man. The dust cover indicates that it is written for "the sailor, swimmer, diver, fisherman, and armchair naturalist." It is largely anecdotal but contains enough scientific information to make it reasonably authentic. The book supports its title by perhaps over-emphasizing the viciousness of the creatures in the waters of the world. The chapter titles are as follows: The shark: an ancient horror; A mixed bag (bluefish, barracuda, moray, etc.); The sting of the sea (stonefish, rays, sea urchins, etc.); The poisoners (puffer, shellfish, red tides, etc.); Seagoing mammals; The hazards of reptiles; and sea monsters — past, present, and future. (CWS/UMS)

1550.
RICHARDS, E.L.
Certifying hyperbaric chambers.
Professional diving symposium, New Orleans, Nov. 1972, Mar. Technol. Soc. J. 7:28-31; Mar./Apr. 1973.

In February of 1968 the U.S. Navy initiated a system certification program for certification of test chambers and diver equipment. The effort will lead to the requirement that any chamber or diver equipment used by Navy personnel must be Navy certified. The U.S. Coast Guard has established a similar certification program. This paper presents a brief discussion of the certification procedure. Further discussion of some of the more important design considerations is given as an aid to anyone intending to build and certify a chamber system. (Author's abstract)

1551.
RICHARDSON, B., S.R. Jaskunas and E.J. Stork.
Effects of hyperoxic breathing gases on blood cell formation.
In: Aerospace Medical Association. 1972 annual scientific meeting, Bal Harbour, Florida, May 1972. Preprints, p.122-123. Published by the Association.

A series of experiments using rats was designed to examine possible mechanisms of oxygen-induced suppression of erythropoiesis. The results of these studies suggest the following conclusions: 1. As anticipated, hyperoxia suppresses the production and repopulation of RBC's following blood loss. 2. Hyperoxia suppresses the production of the erythropoietin hormone. That the effect is on production rather than activity of degradation of circulating hormone is evinced by the fact that administration of exogenous erythropoietin stimulates RBC production regardless of oxygen tension. Thus it appears that the primary mechanism by which hyperoxia suppresses erythropoiesis and the consequent decline in RBC mass are due primarily to suppression of the hormone production, rather than to any direct effect of oxygen on bone marrow stem cells. (Authors)

1552.
RICHMOND, D.R., J.T. Yelverton and E.R. Fletcher.
Far-field underwater-blast injuries produced by small charges.
Albuquerque, N. Mex., Lovelace Found. Med. Educ. Res., Rep. DNA-3021 T, 100p. July 1, 1973.
(AD 763 497)

Underwater blast injuries, at increasing ranges beyond the lethal zone from small charges, were studied using animals. The study was conducted in an artificial pond that measured 220 by 150 ft at its surface. The pond was 30 ft deep over its 30- by 100-ft center portion. Sheep, dogs, and a few monkeys were exposed to the blast oriented vertically in the water (long axis perpendicular to the surface). Most were exposed to the blast at 1-ft depths, heads above the surface, and a limited number at 2- and 10-ft depths. Explosive charges were mostly bare spheres of Pentolite weighing 0.5, 1, 3, and 8 lb. All charges were detonated at 10-ft depths. The immersion-blast injuries were of minor severity and consisted mainly of lung hemorrhages and small areas of contusions in the gastrointestinal tract. The incidence and severity of the injuries were correlated with the impulse in the underwater blast wave. Based on the results of the study, a safe impulse level of 2 to 3 psi. msec for unprotected swimmers, head above the surface, was proposed. This safe impulse level was discussed in relation to the underwater blast-wave parameters in the test pond and existing response data for personnel. (Authors' abstract modified by GRA)

1553.
RIEGEL, P.S. and J.S. Glasgow.
Improvements to the control block of the Mark VI MOD 2 scuba.
Columbus, Ohio, Battelle, Columbus Labs, Rep. SupDive-TR-3-72, 18p. June 30, 1972. (AD 744 235)

A program was conducted to improve certain deficiencies associated with the control block of the Mark VI Mod 2 scuba, a semiclosed-circuit rebreather. The areas to be improved included the bypass valve, the gas metering system, and the differential-pressure gauge. After computation of flows and laboratory testing of components and orifices was performed, a prototype embodying improvement in the problem areas was fabricated and delivered to the Navy. (Authors) (GRA)

1554.
RIEU, M., J.F. Dessanges and D. Lemaigre.
Influence de l'inhalation de melanges gazeux hypercapniques sur l'evolution de l'equilibre acido-basique au cours de l'hypothermie profonde chez le chien.
[Influence of the inhalation of hypercapnic mixtures on the evolution of acid-base equilibrium during profound hypothermia in the dog].
C.R. Soc. Biol. 165(11):2054-2057; 1971.

Dogs were cooled in ice and artificially ventilated. Arterial pressure and ECG were recorded. Blood samples were taken from the carotid artery at intervals during cooling and rewarming. The pH, the PCO_2 and HCO_3^- of the blood were measured as well as lactic and pyruvic acids. In some animals, hyperventilation using air enriched with O_2 was done, while in others CO_2 was used. In hyperventilation, blood alkalosis increased in cooling to 20°. On rewarming, the alkalosis decreased and was replaced by acidosis. There was a decrease of PCO_2 and of HCO_3^- on cooling. This was associated with an increase of blood lactic acid. At 25° there was an association between lactic and pyruvic acids but excess lactate occurred on further cooling and rewarming. Breathing of CO_2 produced a constancy of pH, HCO_3^-, pyruvic and lactic acids without the appearance of excess lactate. It is possible to have profound hypothermia without disturbance of blood pH during rewarming. (MDS) (© BA)

1555.
RIJNJA, H.A.
Small sensitive hydrophones.
Acustica 27(4):182-188; 1972.

Guide lines are given for optimum choices of sensitivity and capacity of piezoelectric hydrophones of small size, suitable to detect extremely weak signals. The sensitivity level of such a hydrophone shall be higher than -180 dB below 1 V/uPa. The frequency of mechanical resonance of the hydrophone can be chosen as high as 60 kHa and its capacitance of the order of 50 pF or more.The required load resistance will be not higher than 1000 MΩ . The frequency range of these hydrophones extends easily downward to below 10 Hz. The capacitance of a hydrophone shall preferably be equal to its external load capacitance caused by the cable or the input circuit of the preamplifier. (Author's summary)

1556.
RIND, H.
Parametric analysis of submersibles.
Mar. Technol. Soc. J. 6:37-40;Sept./Oct. 1972.

The oceanographic industry is at a turning point in its history. Of the submersibles built over the past several years, a large number are sitting idle because funds are not available for cost effective missions within their capabilities. At the same time, new submersibles are being built with insufficient study of the functions which they can perform economically. At this time it is appropriate to review from an engineering viewpoint existing vehicles to determine if it is possible to design the next generation of submersibles with greater efficiency. This paper develops an empirical equation relating six mission/submersible variables. This equation was developed from data on 33 submersibles built between 1960 and 1970. It can be applied to preliminary designs of new vessels, and thereby enable mission/design tradeoffs to be made sufficiently early to optimize the usefulness of the submersible. (Author's abstract)

1557.
ROBERTS, A.J., T.F. Bobbitt and S.R. Jaskunas.
Effects of hyperoxia on heme biosynthesis.
In: Aerospace Medical Association. 1972 annual scientific meeting, Bal Harbour, Florida, May 1972. Preprints, p.120-121. Published by the Association.

The results of these studies suggest that oxygen has little or no effect on amino-levulinic acid (ALA) synthesis under the conditions tested. Instead, the effect of oxygen on heme synthesis appears to occur at some step between ALA formation and the insertion of iron into protoporphyrin. Landaw *et al.* (Aerosp. Med. 41:48-55;Jan. 1970) have reported evidence that the *in vivo* incorporation of glycine-14C into heme under hyperoxia may be reduced through dilution caused by an increase in plasma free glycine levels. If such dilution effects were to account for the results observed here, they would have to arise from intracellular sources and apply not only to glycine incorporation, but also to the incorporation of ALA and iron into heme. Globin synthesis is controlled by heme levels; i.e., globin molecules are synthesized 1:1 for heme molecules present. Thus, any prolonged exposure to anoxia or hyperoxia could be expected to cause a reduction in both heme and globin synthesis. In the reticulocyte system used here for globin trials, iron and heme were abundant in the initial preparation and never limited globin formation. (Authors)

1558.
ROBERTS, A.J., T.F. Robbitt, S.R. Jaskunas and B. Richardson.
Effects of hyperoxia on heme biosynthesis.
Brooks AFB, Texas, Sch. Aerosp. Med., Rep. SAM-TR-73-2, 15p. Feb. 1973.
(AD 756 836)

In vitro suspensions of chicken erythrocytes, rabbit reticulocytes and rat bone marrow cells have been used to examine the effects of oxygen tension of heme synthesis. The data indicate that heme synthesis is maximal at 10% O_2 at approximately 745 torr (mm Hg). Lesser O_2 levels (0%, 3%, 5%, and 7%) greatly reduce heme synthesis, while higher levels (20% and 100%) moderately reduce it. Hemoglobin (i.e. globin) synthesis, as measured by the incorporation of He-leucine, is unaffected by O_2 tension. Although the synthesis of aminolevulinic acid (ALA) from glycine and succinate is considered the rate-limiting step in heme synthesis, the effects of O_2 on the incorporation of glycine-C14 and ALA C14 into heme are simlar. Since 10% O_2 at 745 torr approximates mean tissue PO_2 at seal level, the suppression of heme synthesis at O_2 levels greater than 10% may indicate the effect of hyperoxia on heme synthesis in the intact animal. (Authors' abstract modified by GRA)

1559.
ROBERTS, D.G., ed.
Diving applications in marine sciences research. Proceedings of a seminar held at the National Institute of Oceanography, December 1971.
Published by the Institute. 1972. 174p.

Successful completion of any research project involving diver support is dependent on and limited by a number of inter-related factors. These vary according to the nature of the research and the environment but include the nature of the tasks required by the research; the environment including depth, water temperature, currents, visibility, etc.; diver training and safety; the safe physiological and psychological limitations of the diver and the available safety and logistics support. There is therefore some interest in examining and discussing the different approaches used by oceanographers, geologists and biologists and also the important limitations and necessary prerequisites imposed by diver training, safety and physiology. As an informal forum for discussion of these problems, a seminar was held at the National Institute of Oceanography. [Individual papers will be found under the following author entries: Bellamy, D.; Eastaugh, R.W.; Flemming, N.C.; Gill, J.S.; Hemmings, C.C.; Hempleman, H.J.; Kelland, N.C.; Willis, S.; Woods, J.D.]. (From editor's introduction)

1560.
ROBINSON, A.Z., R.J. Bobber and C.L. Buchanan.
Proposal for a deep-sea system for evaluating acoustic transducers (Deepseat).
U.S. Nav. Res. Lab., Rep. NRL-MR-2514, 38p. Sept. 1, 1972.
(AD 750,666)

A program for solving the problem of evaluating transducers at elevated hydrostatic pressure when existing facilities are not adequate for that purpose is proposed. The program would develop a calibration platform to be lowered to the required depth in the deep ocean. The calibration experiments would be controlled from the ocean surface by means of a hardwire telemetry link. Measurement data would be telemetered back to the surface by the same link for processing and interpretation. Emphasis is placed upon the use of a minicomputer for control of the measurement procedures and for processing and display of the results. (Authors) (GRA)

1561.
ROCCO, R.M.
Passively insulated diving suit.
In: The working diver, 1972. Symposium proceedings, February 1972, Columbus, Ohio, p. 191-196. Washington, D.C., Marine Technology Society, 1972.

Development has been completed on a new, passively insulated diving suit for use in cold and deep waters. The insulating material consists of glass microspheres in a mineral oil matrix. With a compression of only 3 percent at 1000 ft, the material maintains its insulating characteristics as well as its buoyancy at depth. The suit, designated the NON-COMP suit, is a laminate with the insulation being sandwiched between an abrasion resistant outer liner and a soft, conforming inner liner. Seals are provided at the face, neck, waist, wrists, and ankles, to prevent the exchange of water with the environment. The most extensive cold water diving with the NON-COMP suit has been during the recovery of a B-52 in Lake Michigan in the spring of last year. Water temperature was 39.1°F at a working depth of 246 feet. The suit accomplished its task of keeping the divers comfortable, and in addition provided excellent mobility. Most significantly, it was the preferred suit for the divers who swam it. (Author's abstract)

1562.
ROCKERT, H.
Oxygen toxicity during anaemia.
In: Hesser, C.M. and D. Linnarsson, eds. Proceedings of the first annual scientific meeting of the European Undersea Biomedical Society, Stockholm, 13-15 June 1973. Forsvarsmedicin 9:257-259;July 1973.

Acute experimental anaemia was induced on 19 male rats weighing 150 g by bleeding 1 ml followed by an immediate injection of the same amount physiological NaCl into the vascular system. The mean haemoglobin content was reduced from 13.3 to 9.6 g/100 ml. The rats were exposed to OHP (100%) under 6 atmospheres absolute pressure and the time to the onset of convulsions was measured. The anaemic rats got convulsions after 650 seconds as compared to the control group for which the corresponding value was 1300 seconds. The difference is highly significant. (Author's abstract)

1563.
ROCKWELL, P.K., R.E. Elliott and M.R. Snoey.
NEMO, a new concept in submersibles.
Nav. Civ. Eng. Lab., Rep. NCEL-TR-49, 73p. Nov. 1971.
(AD 735 103)

Experimental and analytical studies, conducted to evaluate continental shelf depth performance of a spherical acrylic plastic hull, have led to the design and construction of NEMO (Naval Experimental Manned Observatory). NEMO consists of an acrylic plastic pressure hull with a 61-inch inside diameter and a 66-inch outside diameter, plus life support and operational subsystems. The life support system, which consists of an oxygen supply, CO_2 scrubber, closed-circuit emergency rebreathers, and atmosphere monitoring equipment, provides 8 hours of life support, plus an additional 24 hours emergency backup for two men. (Authors) (GRA)

1564.
ROCKWELL, P.K. and H.J. Migliore.
Operational evaluation of NEMO, an acrylic-hulled submersible.
U.S. Nav. Civil Eng. Lab., Rep. TR-778, 18p. Nov. 1972.
(AD 753,190)

The Naval Civil Engineering Laboratory has conducted an operational evaluation of NEMO (Naval Experimental Manned Observatory), an acrylic-hulled submersible. The objectives of the program were to determine the benefits of the panoramic visibility afforded by the transparent acrylic plastic hull, to evaluate the overall design and modes of operation of NEMO, and to judge the potential application of NEMO-type vehicles to the Navy's oceanographic and ocean engineering needs. It is concluded that (1) visibility through the hull is free from shape distortion, making NEMO an excellent observation platform, (2) objects look smaller and closer than actual, (3) operator comfort is good, (4) design of the vehicle is basically sound, simple, and reliable, (5) vehicle operation has been demonstrated to be safe, and (6) NEMO's versatility and usefulness are hampered by the lack of a true hovering/flying capability. It is recommended that future transparent-hulled vehicles have more mobility than NEMO and that a manipulation arm be added. (Authors' abstract)

1565.
RODARTE, J.R. and R.E. Hyatt.
Effect of acute exposure to CO_2 on lung mechanics in normal man.
Resp. Physiol. 17(2):135-145; 1973.

The effect of CO_2 on lung mechanics was examined in ten healthy men at rest. Measurements were begun after each inspired an air mixture containing 6% CO_2 for five min. Lung volumes, expiratory flow-volume curves, static pressure-volume curves of the lung, and pulmonary conductance were measured. CO_2 breathing produced a small but statistically significant increase in total lung capacity. Pulmonary conductance measured by a flow-interruption technique increased markedly in one subject but decreased in all others. The decrease in conductance was not prevented by treatment with a bronchodilator and was considered the result of an increase in laryngeal resistance. There was no consistent effect of CO_2 breathing on any other parameter. (© BA)

1566.
RODINA, A.G.
Methods in aquatic microbiology.
(Translated, edited and revised by R.R. Colwell and M.S. Zambruski)
Baltimore, University Park Press, 1972. 461p.

A timely text dealing with all aspects of microbiology as it relates to the aquatic world. As pointed out in the introduction, the development of microorganisms is closely related to a variety of factors involving the medium: oxygen content; mineral and organic nutrient; pH; temperature; and the development of phytoplankton and zooplankton. On the other hand the character and intensity of bacterial metabolism are the basis of nutrient cycles which occur in bodies of water. Microorganisms play a significant role in the corrosion of metal and concrete structures and in the fouling of water pipes and the bottom of ships. The problem of productivity in the aquatic environment is based on a knowledge of microbiology. Thus, microbiological studies of fertilized ponds used for fish culture are valuable in determining appropriate times of fertilizer application and the quantities to be applied. Sanitary and public health bacteriology is essential to a pure water supply. The entire problem of pollution requires a knowledge of the bacterial content of the water. Microorganisms serve as the index for all changes which arise in the aquatic environment. This book in its 15 chapters covers all of this and much more, and anyone interested in the aquatic environment should read it. (CWS/UMS)

1567.
RODKEY, F.L.
Significance of endogenous carbon monoxide production by crew members in confined pressurized spaces.
In: Abstracts of BuMed-ONR sponsored Navywide research in high pressure biomedical research, U.S. Submarine Base, Groton, Conn., May 1971, p.43. Published by the Naval Submarine Medical Research Laboratories, 1971.

Abstract only. Excerpt quoted: The rate of CO production by man was measured in a closed rebreathing system where CO excretion was prevented. The average rate of production observed in eight normal men was 8.1 $\pm$ 2.9 (S.D.) μM of CO per kilogram body weight per day or about 12.7 ml of CO per day for a 70 kilogram man. The mean and standard deviation for eight measurements on one subject were 5.2 $\pm$ 0.9 μM/Kg.day, or 8.1 ml of CO per day for this 70 kilogram subject. The larger mean and standard deviation for the eight subjects compared to a similar number of measurements on a single individual suggest that there is a real difference in endogenous CO production by different subjects. The interaction of CO, oxygen, and hemoglobin at total pressures up to 21 atmospheres absolute was studied. The relative affinity of adult human hemoglobin for CO and oxygen was shown to be independent of total pressure, nature of the inert gas, hemoglobin concentration, and pH. These data permit accurate calculation of the CO-O_2-hemoglobin equilibrium at any given oxygen tension and CO contamination of the inspired air. The effect on the hemoglobin-oxygen equilibrium of progressive increase of CO contamination due to endogenous CO formation by crew members in confined spaces can be accurately predicted.

1568.
ROLF, L.L. and D.M. Travis.
Pleural fluid-plasma bicarbonate gradients in oxygen-toxic and normal rats.
Amer. J. Physiol. 224:857-861;Apr. 1973.

Acid-base and electrolyte measurements were made on pleural fluid from normal rats and on the pleural effusion produced by oxygen toxicity. The bicarbonate concentration in the pleural fluid was 5-8 mM higher than venous plasma, and the fluid was more alkaline than plasma. The excess bicarbonate was greater than anticipated on the basis of the accepted mode of formation of pleural fluid and the contribution of anion excess due to the Donnan factor. When unilateral artificial pleural effusions of distilled water were produced, electrolyte equilibrium between pleural fluid and venous plasma was reached in about 40 min. Sampling after this time indicated that a pleural fluid-plasma bicarbonate gradient was established and persisted during maneuvers that lowered plasma bicarbonate. It is concluded that a plasma-dependent pleural fluid-plasma bicarbonate gradient exists in the rat in health and disease. Although explicit mechanisms that control this gradient are unknown, these studies suggest that catalysis by carbonic anhydrase is not prerequisite for generation and maintenance of this gradient. (Authors' abstract)

1569.
ROLLE, A.L.
Focussed or lens-type ultrasonic imaging for small deep-diving submersibles.
In: Ocean 73. 1973 IEEE international conference on engineering in the ocean environment, p.284-300. IEEE publication 73-CHO-7740-OCC.

This paper summarizes the results of an investigation into the critical problems of developing a practical focussed or lens-type ultrasonic image converter for small submersibles capable of operating to 20,000-foot depths. The problem of specular reflections, lens depth of field, and acoustic absorption are described. Trade offs between information rate, complexity, and imaging performance are discussed. A simple, partially filled rotating array converter is proposed as the most cost effective approach for an operational system using current technology. Results from high-pressure tests of experimental array elements are presented. (Author's abstract)

1570.
ROSENBAUM, R.M.
Cellular and systemic aspects of oxygen toxicity and the induction of tolerance to oxygen.
In: Abstracts of BuMed-ONR sponsored Navywide workshop in high pressure biomedical research, U.S. Naval Submarine Base, Groton, Conn., May 1971. p.8. Published by the Naval Submarine Medical Research Laboratory, 1971.

Abstract only. Excerpts quoted: At concentrations equal to 3 atm. (abs.) oxygen interferes with the nuclear-cytoplasmic transfer of 28S r-RNA, thereby resulting in incomplete ribosome formation as determined in a model cell system. This defect results in failure to produce a complete ribosome formation as determined in a model cell system. This defect results in failure to produce a complete ribosome, and hence appears to explain why protein synthesis in O_2-poisoned lungs is limited. The restricted uridine-H^3 and palmitate-C^{14} incorporation into such O_2-exposed lungs from intact animals suggests a plausible mechanism whereby O_2 toxicity interferes with secretion of pulmonary surfactant. Animals rendered O_2-tolerant survive well at 1 atm (760 mmHg) O_2 but are susceptible to higher O_2 levels. Surviving tolerant animals show characteristic mitochondrial conformational changes with increases in mitochondrial protein but stable levels of enzyme activity such as SDH. This suggests adaptive mechanisms such as increased numbers of enzymatically active sites on hypertrophied mitochondrial structural protein able to compete selectively with the inhibitory effects of high concentrations of O_2. . . . Studies of O_2 effects on two distinct pathways of tryptophan metabolism show O_2 enhancement of heme-dependent enzyme systems in the major nicotinic acid pathway, while the rate-limiting enzyme of the minor pathway is inhibited by O_2 and is SH dependent. O_2 effects on these pathways may account for the increased vascular resistance observed during the hyperoxic states as mediated by the minor pathway of tryptophan metabolism involving production of serotonin.

1571.
ROSENBAUM, R.M. and M. Wittner.
Mechanisms of structural-functional defects in pulmonary oxygen toxicity.
Bronx, N.Y., Albert Einstein Coll. Med., Rep. NIH-NHLI-71-2152, 21p. July 10, 1972. (PB 222 151/3)

The means by which hyperbaric oxygen causes pulmonary damage is being studied at the ultrastructural and molecular biological level. The effect of increased oxygen concentrations on the metabolic and synthetic activities of the pulmonary alveolar component with special emphasis on the synthesis of surfactant, and how this may relate to adaptation to high PO_2 levels has been a primary concern of this project. Studies of synthesis of RNA during increased PO_2 have shown a reversible inhibition of overall RNA synthesis. A more specific inhibition of ribosomal-RNA processing, which leads eventually to cell death since new protein synthesis is blocked, has been detected and would account for fatal O_2 toxicity resulting from prolonged exposure. Studies attempting to elucidate the mechanism of tolerance or adaptation to a toxic O_2 environment have demonstrated proliferation of alveolar type II cells and an increase in overall pulmonary phospholipid synthesis including surfactant. (GRA)

1572.
ROSS, H.C. and W.D. Won.
Susceptibility of mice to airborne Klebsiella pneumoniae infection in helium-oxygen atmospheres.
Aerosp Med. 44:1009-1012;Sept. 1973.

Exposure of mice to a 97% helium-3% oxygen environment at 100 psig (8 ata) and 22°C induced a rapid rise in plasma cortisol and whole blood 5-hydroxtryptamine levels, as well as lymphopenia, weight loss and a 2-3° drop in body core temperature. The respiratory LD_{50} for Klebsiella pneumoniae under these conditions, was 2 x 10^2 organisms/mouse with median mortality on Day 4. When the environmental temperature was raised to 35°C there were slight elevations in plasma cortisol and 5-hydrostryptamine, and LD_{50} became 3 x 10^2 organisms with median mortality occurring on Day 8. Lymphopenia and eosinopenia were not significant. It appears that the effect of helium-oxygen environment at a pressure equivalent of 200 ft of sea water on host resistance to Klebsiella pneumoniae infection is similar to, but greater than, the effect of near freezing temperature. (Authors' abstract)

1573.
ROSS, H.E.
Spatial perception under water.
In: Woods, J.D. and J.N. Lythgoe, eds. Underwater science: An introduction to experiments by divers, p.69-101. London, Oxford University Press, 1971.

The author divides perceptual errors underwater into two categories: constant errors and variable errors: "Constant errors are due to the consistent misinterpretation of a sensory cue, and they disappear fairly readily with experience. Variable errors are inconsistent and impredictable. They are probably due to a reduction of the usual sorts of sensory information, aggravated by underwater stresses such as cold, anxiety and nitrogen narcosis. Variable errors also decrease with practice, except where the sensory information is irretrievably lost." The following are discussed: visual judgments of size, shape and distance underwater: curvature distortion relation between size and distance, distance judgments, size judgments, judgments in the vertical plane, spatial judgments involving proprioceptive information, knowledge of the vertical, weight perception and motor skills, geographical orientation, bodily movement and visual movement, and vertigo. Stereoscopic acuity is clearly worse under water, and deteriorates with distance. Experiments indicate that adaptation occurs, and that experienced divers tend to compensate for incorrect size and distance estimations. (MFW/BSCP)

1574.
ROSS, H.E. and M.H. Rejman.
Adaptation to speed distortions under water.
Br. J. Psychol. 63(2):257-264; 1972.

A diver's face-mask normally makes close objects in clear water appear both enlarged and too near. Objects travelling across the line of sight therefore appear to move faster than in air, and objects moving along the line of sight slower. Subjects estimated the speed of a moving rod in air and water, before and after a 10 min. period spent swimming and playing a pegboard game under water. Twenty subjects were tested with the rod moving across, and 20 with it moving along, the line of sight. In both conditions subjects showed the expected directions of speed distortion in water, with significant adaptation and after-effects after 10 min. submersion. The results are consistent with the assumption that the type of speed perception measured here is largely dependent on size and distance perception, and that speed adaptation follows automatically from the correction of the spatial metric. (Authors' abstract)

1575.
ROSS, H.E. and P. Lennie.
Cues for perceptual adaptation.
Br. J. Psychol. 63(1):38-40; 1972.

The completely adapted diver responds to some cue other than sensory information about the nature of the distortion, and that cue is the knowledge that he is looking from air into water through a flat glass surface. Experiments on learning to switch from 1 type of distortion to the opposite produce varied results. The subject relies on veridical information about the distorting system, by head and body movements, mistakes in eye-hand coordination and changes in the apparent size and shape of familiar objects. As the eye moves behind a flat glass plate, the pupil accepts a slightly different bundle of rays from the same point of an object in water; as the angle of refraction varies non-linearly with the angle of incidence, there is a change in the optical location of the point, giving a small deformation with eye movements, particularly when looking to the periphery of the face-mask. The distortion is gaze-contingent, in the same way as that produced by wedge prisms. Models for perceptual adaptation should account for both normal and distorted vision, and for all degrees of adaptation. The brain probably always applies some kind of transformation to the retinal image, and checks whether any discrepancies arise from that transformation, and changes them. The experienced diver learns what type of transformation to apply when looking into water. Adaptation occurs rapidly during the first minute in water, and thereafter more slowly. Some subjects do consciously correct. This could account for some of the differences between novice and experienced divers. The appropriate factor of magnification varies with the angular size of the object; with the distance of the object from the face-plate and the eye; with the apparent distance of the object; with the way in which the subject trades off size-distortion against distance-distortion; and with the extent to which the subject has perceptually adapted. (FW) (© BA)

1576.
ROSTAIN, J.C.
Travaux de recherches sur l'utilisation de divers melanges gazeux pour les plongees tres profondes.
[Study of the effect of various breathing mixtures and of high pressures on the baboon (Papio papio)].
Marseille, France, CNEXO/COMEX, Rep. 69/89-II, 24p. Apr. 1971.

The author's conclusions are based on experiments carried out between May 1969 and December 1970. Trembling, paroxystic discharges, and epileptic seizures occur at comparable depths in both helium-oxygen and hydrogen-oxygen breathing mixtures. These phenomena apparently depend on the rate of pressurization and first appear at greater depths when the rate of pressurization is slowed. Although EEG patterns are unchanged to 650m with "heliox", patterns characteristic of "hydrox" were observed; the anomalies disappeared after the breathing mixture was changed to "heliox", and did not reappear in air at atmospheric pressure. Oxygen partial pressure seems to be responsible for EEG abnormalities during decompression with PIO_2 at 500-600 mb; the abnormalities did not occur when PIO_2 was around 300 mb. The factor of confinement, which cannot be considered responsible for the EEG abnormalities observed, nor for the deaths of some animals, should not be neglected. Isolation, too, seems to affect baboons psychologically. The water and food dispensing systems were not ideal. Psychological stress, due to the frightening preparations (installation of electrodes, etc.) must also be taken into account. Most of the deaths which occurred in helium-oxygen and hydrogen-oxygen mixtures were due to decompression accidents or technical failures. (MEMH/UMS)

1577.
ROSTAIN, J.C. and R. Naquet.
Resultats preliminaires d'une etude comparative de l'effet des melanges oxygene-helium et oxygene-hydrogene et des hautes pressions sur le babouin Papio papio.
[Preliminary results of a comparative study of the effects of oxygen-helium and oxygen-hydrogen mixture and of high pressures on Papio papio].
In: Fructus, X., ed. Third international conference on hyperbaric and underwater physiology, p.44-49. Paris, Doin, 1972.

Adolescent, non-photosensitive baboons (Papio papio) were used as subjects in a series of simulated dives using oxygen-hydrogen and oxygen-helium breathing mixtures. EEG and EKG were recorded continuously during all experiments. With the helium-oxygen mixture, trembling was noted during compression in all animals between 300 and 450 m. Paroxystic manifestations were observed in the EEG around 650 m, and convulsive seizures around 700 m. With slower pressurization greater depths were attained before similar phenomena were noted. With the hydrogen-oxygen breathing mixture, trembling was also noted around 450 m. EEG patterns presented a number of modifications, varying in intensity with the individual animal; these modifications may be related to oxygen partial pressure. Complementary experimentation will be needed to elucidate questions concerning the roles of the rate of pressurization, oxygen concentration and partial pressure, and pressure itself. (MEMH/UMS)

1578.
ROSTAIN, J.C. and C. Lemaire.
Evolution du tremblement au repos et pendant l'effort au cours de plongees profondes en atmosphere helium-oxygene.
[Evolution of tremor at rest and during exertion during deep dives in a helium-oxygen breathing mixture].
Rev. EEG (Paris) 3(2):203-206; 1973.

The characteristics of the tremor observed during the High Pressure Nervous Syndrome were studied in six subjects during dives to 500, 520, and 610 m. Modes of pressurization differed from dive to dive. Tremor was measured in the upraised right hand by accelerometry, both with and without a load of 1 or 2 kg. Results were subjected to computer analysis. Tremor appeared during all three dives at depths between 200 and 300 m, and was observed throughout the dive, disappearing during decompression. Tremor was more pronounced in the extremities. Although professional activity was little affected, handwriting was disturbed. The cause and origin of the tremor have not yet been determined. (MEMH/UMS)

1579.
ROSTAIN, J.C.
L'effet des haute pressions avec divers melanges gazeux chez le singe Papio papio.
[The effect of high pressures with different gas mixtures in the monkey Papio papio].
Thesis presented to the University of Provence, May 1973. 131p.

The purpose of this study was to further the understanding of the factors contributing to the high pressure nervous syndrome manifested in human divers in recent years, as dives went deeper. After some generalized introductory material, a brief review of previous work in the field, and a description of the materials and techniques employed in these experiments, the author describes, in part one, the physiological characteristics of the baboon Papio papio at atmospheric pressure. In part two, the effects of nitrogen-oxygen, helium-oxygen, and hydrogen-oxygen at various pressures and durations of exposure are described. Part three concerns the role of physical parameters, i.e., confinement at atmospheric pressure, compression rate, and oxygen partial pressure. Part four consists of a discussion of the above and an attempt to evaluate the roles of the various parameters. It is noted that experiments with a species less sensitive to convulsions might lead to different conclusions. (MFW/UMS)

1580.
ROSTAIN, J.C.
Evolution des potentiels evoques visuels moyens chez l'homme au cours de sejours prolonges en atmosphere helium-oxygene a 300 et 500 m.
[Evolution of mean visual evoked potentials in man during a prolonged sojourn in a helium-oxygen atmosphere at 300 and 500 m].
In: Hesser, C.M. and D. Linnarsson eds. Proceedings of the first annual scientific meeting of the European Undersea Biomedical Society, Stockholm, 13-15 June 1973. Forsvarsmedicin 9:459-465;July 1973.

Series of visual evoked potentials were recorded during saturation dives in a helium-oxygen environment (Sagittaire I, 8 hours at 300 m and Sagittaire II, 100 hours at 500 m). A stroboscope lamp was placed in the interior of the chamber at a distance from the eyes at not more than 20 cm. There were six subjects aged 20-30 years. The mean visual evoked potentials obtained from 50 responses showed a certain number of modifications persisting during the compression. It was mainly a matter of variations of amplitude: the amplitude of certain components increased, while others diminished. These modifications became accentuated with depth. They were not noticeably improved during the stay of 100 hours at 500 m. On the contrary, at 300 m, the dissociation between the various components regressed from the sixth day on. The role of the hyperbaric environment in these modifications is discussed. (Author's abstract translated by MFW-UMS)

1581.
ROSTAIN, J.C. and J.P. Charpy.
Evolution of anterior slow EEG activities during psychometric tests in deep dives in an oxy-helium atmosphere.
Electroenceph. Clin. Neurophysiol. 34:788;Sept. 1973.

Abstract only. Entire item quoted: Psychometric and EEG correlations carried out during a dive to 520 m (Physalie V) showed that preexisting theta activities were reinforced in the fronto-central regions while Rey's numerical analysis tests were being conducted. It seemed interesting to: (1) confirm these results and determine their significance by means of more precise procedures and (2) identify the variables linked with the psychometric activity which could be responsible for the changes that occurred. Tests were selected and classified according to the psychometric questions posed by the execution of the task (sensory-motor tests, e.g., reaction time and manual dexterity; vigilance and intellectual efficiency tests, e.g., Rey's numerical analysis, paper form board, Catell's factor G test). EEGs were carried out continuously (before, during and after the tests) with magnetic tape recording on which spectral analyses were based (power spectra). Reinforcement of fronto-central theta activities was observed, starting at 300 m, during the numerical analysis tests. Similar but less important EEG changes occurred during three other tests (Zacco's 2 barrier test, paper form board and Catell's factor G test). However, as compared with resting records, no EEG changes occurred during the sensory-motor tests. The results are discussed in relation to the hyperbaric conditions and to the procedures used to carry out the tests.

1582.
ROSTAIN, J.C., G. Regesta and R. Naquet.
Study of the organization of sleep of divers staying at 300 meter depths in oxy-helium atmosphere.
Electroenceph. Clin. Neurophysiol. 34:788;Sept. 1973.

Abstract only. Entire item quoted: EEG recording of sleep was carried out on several subjects during saturation dives to 300 meter depths in a slightly hyperoxic oxy-helium atmosphere (300 bm O_2). The EEGs, done every night during the entire dive (almost 4 weeks), showed some disturbances of the organization of sleep in the divers. Thus, in most of the subjects, during the night, the periods of awakening, stages I and II, increased more or less significantly (duration and frequency of occurrence); on the other hand, stage IV decreased and even disappeared. Stages III and REM varied more or less significantly according to the subject. Numerous intermediate phases were counted. The EEG characteristics of the different stages may be slightly different from those seen on the surface in the controls. These morphological differences may be related to changes of the waking EEG record which appeared during compression and which persisted more or less continuously during the stay at the bottom.

1583.
ROSTAIN, J.C., C. Lemaire and C. Agarate.
Physiological results of experimental dives down to 610 meters with human subjects.
Paper presented at the scientific meeting of the World Confederation of Underwater Activity, London, October 1973. 11p.

This paper was accompanied by slides showing the compression curves for Physalie V, Sagittaire II, and Physalie VI. In the last, the compression rate was much slower, and a two-day stop was made at 350 m. Tremor was greatly reduced and somnolence disappeared more rapidly during Physalie VI. Also, EEG modifications were much less pronounced. Manual dexterity was less impaired. Visual choice reaction time increased 100% in Physalie VI, 10 to 25% between 300-500 m in Sagittaire II and improved during bottom time. Mental agility was constant in Sagittaire II and decreased 14% in Physalie VI. Monitoring indicated no undesirable cardiovascular effects. In Sagittaire II, there was a significant increase in the red cell count, while it remained constant during Physalie VI, during compression. In both dives, red cell count decreased during decompression. The authors believe that working dives of the future can go to 600 m. The limit will probably be set by respiratory limitations due to the density of the breathing mixture. (MFW/UMS)

1584.
ROTH, S.H., R.A. Smith and W.D.M. Paton.
Pressure antagonism of anesthetic-induced conduction failure in peripheral nerve.
Proc. Can. Fed. Biol. Sci. 16:7; 1973.

Abstract only. Entire item quoted: A specially constructed nerve bath and pressure chamber enabled recordings of the action potential of an electrically stimulated nerve in the presence of various anesthetics to be observed on an oscilloscope and recorded on film. Dose response curves for the effects of gaseous, volatile and local anesthetics on the action potential height, strength-duration and conduction velocity were obtained for frog sciatic nerve. It was observed that the depression of the action potential induced by gaseous anesthetics (e.g. nitrous oxide, cyclopropane) was reversed with the addition of the gas helium at non-anesthetic pressures, (50-100 atm). This observation was similar to the reversal of anesthesia recently reported by K.W. Miller et al. on newts. The anesthetic effect of volatile agents (e.g. chloroform, ether) was only partially reversed; and the effects induced by local anesthetics (e.g. nupercaine, pentobarbital) were not reversed. The results suggest that the mechanism of action of all anesthetics may not be similar; that the hypothesis of membrane expansion by anesthetic agents proposed by Miller et al. and by Roth and Seeman may not be the only contributing factor involved in anesthesia of peripheral nerve; and that the mechanism of action of general and local anesthetics may be different.

1585.
ROTHMAN, H.B. and H. Hollien.
An investigation of HeO_2 speech unscramblers under controlled conditions.
In: Sergeant, R.L. and T. Murry, eds. Processing helium speech: proceedings of a Navy-sponsored workshop, August 1971, U.S. Nav. Submar. Med. Res. Lab., Rep. NSMRL 708, p.39-52. May 22, 1972.

The authors report the results of evaluating tests of unscramblers, as well as of masks and microphones, at the time of the preparations for SeaLab III, and in the summer of 1970. Detailed results of these tests are presented in tabular form. Schematic diagrams of the recording set-ups at the Navy Experimental Diving Unit, and at Westinghouse are given. Procedures are described in detail. The results of these tests indicated that (1) none of the devices provided adequate speech improvement; (2) the Industrial Research Products Inc. (IRPI) unscrambler performed best; (3) The IRPI and the Singer/G-P microphones were similar in performance and superior to the EV-664, Mark 8 and Mark 11 models; (4) for future evaluations, rigorous and exacting procedures must be followed. More basic research in this field is required. A new aspect in the overall program is the study of the human as a helium speech decoder; it is indicated that with practice over a period of time, the individual listener can be trained to become an efficient decoder. (MFW/BSCP)

1586.
ROTHMAN, H.B. and H. Hollien.
Further evaluation of HeO_2 unscramblers under controlled conditions.
Gainesville,Fla., Univ. Fla., Commun. Sci. Lab ., Rep. CSL-ONR 47, 16p. July 1, 1972.

This paper, the last of a series of reports dealing with helium speech unscramblers, data are presented on relative speech intelligibility as processed via unscramblers under two conditions: on-line and off-line. The on-line test was conducted at the Westinghouse Ocean Research and Engineering Center; three subjects read Campbell PB_{25} word lists at a depth of 600 feet through four unscramblers and five microphones. Results indicate that the Raytheon and IRPI unscramblers improved speech intelligibility by substantial amounts and that the IRPI and G-P/Singer microphones provided mean scores approximately double those of the other three. The off-line test, conducted at the Communication Sciences Laboratory evaluated the same four unscramblers plus a fifth; further, two of the units had been somewhat modified during the interval between tests. The CSL off-line test is comprised of 57 separate word lists representing various talkers, depths and conditions. Results indicate that the RELA unscrambler consistently outperformed the other with the G-P/Singer and IRPI units providing somewhat greater intelligibility improvement than did the other two unscramblers. Finally, this report provides a discussion of the strengths and weaknesses of current approaches to HeO_2 speech processing and makes recommendations for the improvement of these devices. (DCD abstract)

1587.
ROUX, M., H. Legait and E. Reichart.
Activite de la cortico-surrenale et de l'appareil hypothalamo-hypophysaire chez le rat maintenu en hypercapnia de longue duree.
[Activity of the adrenal cortex and the hypothalamo-hypophysis apparatus in the rat maintained in hypercapnia of long duration].
C.R. Soc. Biol. 165(5):1159-1164; 1971.

The female rats were kept under aseptic conditions in an atmosphere containing 8% CO_2 during 15 days. The total volumes of cortical and medullary regions of the adrenal were measured and the activity of the regions was evaluated by measuring the mean nuclear diameter in the cells. The weight of the adrenal was significantly increased in the hypercapnic animals. There was no volumetric difference or change in nuclear diameter. The different lobes of the adenohypophysis showed no significant volumetric differences between hypercapnic animals and controls. There were no differences in nuclear diameter. However, there was involution of the pars nervosa. Cytological differences in the hypophysis were observed. There were chromophobic hypertrophied cells sometimes vacuolized with fine erythrosinophilic granulations in the cytoplasm. These cells are corticotropic. (MDS) (© BA)

1588.
ROWLANDS, J.R., R.E. Linder and R.M. Estefan.
A theoretical and experimental evaluation of a proposed concept for the deep scattering layer.
San Antonio, Tex., Southwest Res. Inst., Final report on contract N00140-70-C-0275 72p. Jan. 27, 1971.
(AD 739 558)

An experimental apparatus has been designed, constructed and utilized for electron spin resonance studies of spin labeled proteins and membranes at simulated ocean depths up to 5,000 feet. Hemoglobin, hemocyanin and albumin have been labeled with at least two different nitroxide spin labels and subjected to temperatures ranging between 0 and 43°C and pressures up to 2500 psig and studied by electron spin resonance. The effects of salts, hydrogen ion concentration and organic solvents, upon spin labeled biopolymers have also been studied as a function of temperature and pressure. (Authors) (GRA)

1589.
RUBISSOW, G.J. and R.S. MacKay.
Bends studies and control using ultrasonic imaging of body bubbles.
In: Proceedings of the 1973 Ultrasonics Symposium, p.537-539. New York, Institute of Electrical and Electronics Engineers, 1973.

Single bubbles down to one micron diameter are noticeable in intact animal and human subjects using 7.5 MHz sound thus allowing study of decompression sickness. Diverse structures are observed by both continuous Doppler and pulsed imaging systems during pressure changes. A fast sector scan is employed with combined brightness and deflection display. For many dives bubbles first appear in the blood in fat, though in fast dives they may first appear in muscle. We have demonstrated bubbles to exist and appear at the site of discomfort, recompression bubble showers, silent or preclinical bubbles, and safe decompression by adjusting ascent to control bubble size without tables. One can measure degree of super-saturation in a given tissue by adjusting ambient pressure so bubbles there neither grow nor shrink. (Authors' abstract)

1590.
RUCCI, F.S., G. Grasso and P. Consorti.
Ossigeno iperbarico e fosfatasi acida nel fegato di ratto.
[The effects of hyperbaric oxygen on acid phosphatase in the rat].
Boll. Soc. Ital. Biol. Sper. 47(23):785-787; 1971.

Twelve male rats were exposed to 3 or 5 ATA of oxygen for periods of one-half to three hours. At the end of the exposure period the animals were decapitated and acid phosphatase levels in the liver were determined. An equal number of rats served as controls. The only significant difference between experimental and control animals concerned the rats subjected to 5 ATA for three hours. In a second experiment, adrenalectomized rats were exposed to 5 ATA of oxygen for three hours and acid phosphatase levels in the liver and spleen were noted. The authors conclude that adrenalectomy seems to protect the lysosomal membrane from the effects of hyperbaric oxygen, which confirms the importance of the lysosomes in the appearance of acute oxygen poisoning. (MEMH/SCD)

1591.
RUCKNER, E.A., Jr.
Parameters affecting underwater vision.
U.S. Nav. Postgrad. Sch., Thesis, 24p. Mar. 1972.
(AD 743,756)

The purpose of this study was to determine the effects of illumination color, viewing distance, and turbidity on a visual reading task in a totally dark, flooded environment. The reading task was to read a voltmeter and make a correct oral report of the reading. A total of 180 data points spread over 18 viewing conditions were taken for each subject. Seventeen military officers were used as subjects. Experimental conditions were presented in a random manner to all subjects. A statistical examination of the results showed that white or green illumination is better than red in reducing reading response time. Turbidity levels were significant in affecting both increasing as the Attenuation Coefficient increased. (Author) (GRA)

1592.
RUFF, S.
Experimental and theoretical investigation of the decompression problem.
Bad Godesberg, West Germany, Deutsche Forschungs- und Versuchsanstalt fur Luft- und Raumfahrt, Rep. DLR-FB-71-48, 101p. Oct. 7, 1971.
(N72-20075)

The bubble in the organism is recognized as the governing quantity for the construction of safe decompressions. On this basis and using the empirical material, a set of allowed gas tensions in the tissue is proposed. From this, decompression schedules for arbitrary dives in helium-nitrogen mixtures can be calculated. An expression for the bubble growth in the organism during a decompression is developed and applied to the discussion of the allowed gas tensions proposed here. In the appendix dives of the institute and the decompression schedules of the U.S. Diving Manual are analyzed. (Author) (STAR)

1593.
RUIZ, B.C., H.W. Calderwood, J.H. Modell and J.E. Brogdon.
Effect of ventilatory patterns on arterial oxygenation after near-drowning with fresh water. A comparative study in dogs.
Anesth. Analg. 52:570-576;July/Aug. 1973.

The purpose of this experiment was to determine whether positive end-expiratory pressure (PEEP), combined with intermittent positive pressure ventilation (IPPV) will increase PaO_2 in the treatment of near-drowning in dogs. It was found that there was a significant rise in PaO_2 during treatment, but there was a return to pre-treatment level once treatment was discontinued. In order to maintain the increased PaO_2 beyond the treatment period, the surface-active material must be regenerated, a process that would be expected to require approximately 20 hours. It is believed that these findings could have a direct application in the treatment of hypoxia after near-drowning. (MFW/SCD)

1594.
RUSSELL, C.J., A. McNeill and E. Evonuk.
Some cardiorespiratory and metabolic responses of scuba divers to increased pressure and cold.
Aerosp. Med. 43:998-1001;Sept. 1972.

Some cardiorespiratory and metabolic responses of 10 scuba divers during a short period of rest and moderate exercise were studied under field conditions at 1.2 and 3 atmospheres absolute. The data were collected in a fresh water lake which has a constant temperature of 5.5°C below a depth of 1 m and is located at an altitude of 915 m. The results indicated that at greater depths, both during rest and exercise, the VO_2, VCO_2, V_T, O_2 pulse, and heart rate increased significantly ($P < 0.05$), while the respiratory frequency progressively decreased. The V_E decreased significantly ($P < 0.05$) only during the resting test periods. At greater depths the progressive increase in VO_2 and VCO_2 can be attributed primarily to the increased work of breathing air of greater density and to the responses induced by exposure to cold water. The elevation in heart rate may have been caused by a release of catecholamines into the general circulation due to the cold stress, while the greater O_2 pulse may reflect the individual or combined contributions of a larger stroke volume or an increased oxygen extraction from the blood. (Authors' abstract)

1595.
RUSSELL, F.E.
Some chemical and zootoxicological properties of stingray venom.
Los Angeles, Cal., Univ. South Cal. Med. Cent. Rep. PSA-9-108-0-0, 5p. Mar. 31, 1972.
(AD 741 220)

A definitive chemical and pharmacological study has been carried out on the venom of the stingrays, particularly the round stingray Urobatis halleri, common to the Southern California coast. The lethal fraction of the venom is a protein of medium molecular weight, but apparently bound with an enzyme, or some other substance, which makes its separation as a pure substance very difficult. Pharmacological studies indicate that in severe envenomation, secondary shock can occur and can lead to death. A series of studies on the in vitro neutralization of Urobatis halleri venom with antivenins prepared against the bat stingray Myliobatis californicus and the round stingray U. castexi were carried out. One ml of the M. californicus antivenin neutralizes the lethal activity of 10 mg of bat stingray venom. One ml of the U castexi antivenin neutralizes the lethal activity of 5 mg of this stingray's venom. The M. californicus antivenin provided little protection against the lethal activity of U. halleri venom. The U. castexi gave some protection at the 0.20 level, the 0.50 level and the 1.00 level. It is apparent that there is some significant cross protection between the antivenins of these two si stingray species. Further immunochemical work is in progress on the venoms of four Urobatis species. (GRA)

1596.
RUSSELL, F.E.
Behavior, ecology and toxicity of venomous marine fishes.
Los Angeles, Cal., LAC/USC Med. Cent., Prof. Staff Ass., Rep. 22, 9p. Sept. 30, 1972.
(AD 749 375)

The present experiments were designed to define the hemodynamic alterations produced by the venom of S. guttata in the dog. The effects of atropine upon the action of venom were studied in three dogs. The effects of venom upon systemic venous return were studied in two open chest dogs. In animals pretreated with atropine the initial arterial hypotension is inhibited and the number and severity of ECG changes are reduced. The arterial hypotension produced by S. guttata venom represents a distributive defect in circulating blood volume which may be due to the release of endogenous acetylcholine. The venom causes the release of acetylcholine in vitro, and the hemodynamic changes are reminiscent of those produced by the injection of acetylcholine. The effects of venom upon the packed cell volume, return of blood to the right heart, and the appearance of the spleen at necropsy may be due in part to splenic constriction, with its consequent autotransfusion of venous blood with a high red cell mass. (Author) (GRA)

1597.
RUSSELL, F.E.
Behavior, ecology and toxicity of venomous marine fishes.
Los Angeles, Cal., LAC/USC Med. Cent., Prof. Staff Ass., Rep. 24, 15p. Mar. 31, 1973.
(AD 759 063)

Labile components of California scorpionfish venom produce marked respiratory and hemodynamic changes in cats, rabbits, and dogs. The venom affects respiratory rate, causes bronchoconstriction and pulmonary edema; large doses cause respiratory arrest. The venom produces arterial hypotension within 15 sec, followed by a period of increased pressure. The hypotension represents a major distributive defect of blood in arterial resistance most likely due to the release of endogenous acetylcholine. This effect can be inhibited by pretreatment with atropine. Other prominent alterations include pulmonary artery hypertension, elevation of L.V.E.D.P., portal venous hypertension, ECG changes, elevation of the packed cell volume and initial augmentation of systemic venous return. The venom most likely acts through a combination of direct actions, neurogenic reflex mechanisms and effects induced by the liberation of autopharmacological substances. (Author) (GRA)

1598.
RUSSELL, G.M. and A.J. Kemmerer.
Surface exhaust system for scuba regulators.
UnderSea Technol. 14:21;June 1973.

This article describes a system designed to eliminate scuba exhaust bubbles. . . The exhaust system consists of an ambient pressure valve placed between a standard 2-hose demand regulator and a surface exhaust hose. . . . [It] has been tested and used successfully at depths to 37 ft. with both scuba tank and surface supplied air. . . The principal advantage of this system over others is that it can be fabricated easily with sophisticated ship equipment. Its usefulness probably falls primarily into the area of underwater scientific work when the maintenance of a bubble-free environment is important. Additional uses may be in commercial diving operations where the return of helium/oxygen gas mixtures to the surface is desirable for possible recycling. (Authors)

1599.
RUSSOTTI, J.S. and R.L. Sergeant.
Design considerations for a microphone-equipped mouthpiece for Navy diver communication.
U.S. Nav. Submar. Med. Cent., Rep. NSMRL 695, 4p. Jan. 14, 1972.

A safe microphone-equipped breathing mouthpiece is essential for effective verbal communication under water. The conventional safe swimmer mouthpiece is unsuitable for speech production because of its restrains to articulatory movement and the restricted volume of air into which the speech is radiated. This paper describes a communication mouthpiece, the design of which provides full consideration of the mechanics and mechanisms of speech production and eliminates inherent deficiencies found in conventional models. Crucial to the design is the inclusion of a self-equalizing flexible diaphragm which reduces the residual volume of dead air in the breathing manifold by separating it from the rest of the mouthpiece. This then permits a larger extrabuccal space for improved speech production while minimizing the dangers of CO_2 build-up in the breathing mixture. Design considerations presented are of value to speech communications systems designers, manufacturers of diver/swimmer equipment, and engineers interested in the mechanisms of speech production including factors critical to intelligible speech production in confined cavities. (Authors' summary)

1600.
RUSSOTTI, J.S. and Ronald E. Greeb.
Aural detection performance over a 129 minute simulated sonar watch.
U.S. Nav. Submar. Med. Res. Lab., Rep. NSMRL 754, 7p. Sept. 12, 1973.

The problem of operator fatigue and its possible effects in reducing the detection performance of the man-machine system was investigated during the course of a 129-min simulated sonar watch. Successive measurements on the same non-alerted contact taken 43, 86 and 129 min into the detection period showed no significant change in initial detection from one another, nor from pretest values taken the day before. These results indicate that under conditions where the operator's vigilance is maintained by a not-unusual frequency of contact (operators were presented six contacts at random intervals during each 43 min-period), and where operators are not aware of actual elapsed time, no change in operator initial detection performance is encountered. The information presented in this report will be useful to all personnel involved in sonar watchstanding and researchers concerned with sonar operator aural detection. (Authors' summary)

1601.
RYACK, B.L., G.B. Walters and R.L. Rodensky.
Submarine escape: side, tube, and top egress with alternative escape appliances and team sizes.
Hum. Factors 14:249-258;June 1972.

Egress capability with the British Mark VII Submarine Escape Immersion Suit (SEIS) and the Steinke Hood was evaluated for one, two and three-man teams from side, tube, and top-egress escape trunks. Top egress was considerably more rapid than either tube or side egress; tube egress was superior to side egress. Egress time increased linearly as a function of team size for both escape appliances. For tube and side egress, escape with the Steinke Hood was more rapid than with the SEIS: the SEIS was superior for top egress. Escape position of a subject within a team had no effect on egress time. When compared to side and tube egress, top egress results in a substantial reduction of total bottom time. (Authors' abstract)

1602.
RYACK, B.L. and G.B. Walters.
Human factors evaluation of submarine escape IV: evaluation of submarine escape and survival equipment Mark 1 Mod 0 for side and top egress with two disconnect systems.
U.S. Nav. Submar. Med. Res. Lab., Rep. NSMRL 752, 16p. Sept. 12, 1973.

A newly developed submarine escape appliance, Escape and Survival Equipment, Mark 1, Mod 0 (EASE), which provides exposure protection for the escapee was evaluated for side egress and top egress escape trunk configurations. Two systems for rapid separation of the escape appliance from the escape trunk air supply, automatic disconnect and manual disconnect, were also evaluated. Escape capability with the EASE was found to be comparable to that with other escape appliances. Although the automatic disconnect was more rapid than the manual disconnect, the difference was not significant. However, the magnitude of this difference might be expected to increase under the stressful conditions of an actual escape. As reported in previous studies, top egress was superior to side egress. Adoption of the EASE for use in submarine escape systems is recommended. (Authors' abstract)

1603.
RYCKEWAERT, A. and D. Kuntz.
Les osteonecroses aseptiques de la tete femorale chez l'adulte.
[Aseptic osteonecrosis of the femoral head in adults].
Acquis. Med. Recent., p.167-177; 1970.

A brief general discussion of aseptic osteonecrosis of the caput femoris in the human adult is presented. Lesions of the bone and their development, radiological appearance, and clinical symptoms are detailed. The etiology of the disorder is traced to ischemia of the caput resulting from injury or compression of the capillary arteries supplying its circulation. Secondary and primary forms of osteonecrosis, correlated mechanical and metabolic-biochemical factors, and their possible pathogenic mechanisms are described. Treatment possibilities are briefly mentioned. The author's discussion of barotraumatic osteonecrosis is limited to the following remarks: Secondary forms are less frequent. They include: (1) Osteonecroses due to microparticular vascular obturation; the particles in question may be intravascular or peri-vascular, causing obturation by compression. Within this group we may include: (a) barotraumatic osteonecroses, observed in subjects who work in compressed air after a too-rapid decompression. They result from the liberation within the bone marrow of bubbles of nitrogen which obstruct or compress the small vessels of the femur head. (MEMH/BSCP)

1603.1.
SACCO, A.M., R.A. Gussman and C.E. Billings.
Aerosol generation in high-pressure environments.
Amer. Ind. Hyg. Ass. J. 33:170-177;Mar. 1972.

Man has demonstrated his ability to withstand environmental pressures up to 500 psia. In so doing he comes closer to making routine excursions on the Continental Shelf 1000 feet beneath the sea. In view of the extremely limited information available on the behavior of aerosols under high pressures, a series of studies was undertaken to evaluate potential problems. One phase of this investigation has dealt with the generation of both solid and liquid aerosols at high pressures. Initial results have yielded evidence of a general increase in particulate diameter with increasing pressure from the sources evaluated. Results of both solid and liquid aerosol experiments are presented. (Authors' abstract)

1604.
SAFAR, P., E.M. Nemoto and J.W. Severinghaus.
Pathogenesis of central nervous system disorder during artificial hyperventilation in compensated hypercarbia in dogs.
Critical Care Med. 1:5-16;Jan. 1973.

An animal model and experimental protocol were developed to elucidate the pathogenesis of coma and convulsions observed during artificial hyperventilation of patients with chronic hypercarbia. Compensated hypercarbia was simulated by sustained elevation of $PaCO_2$ to 80 torr and normalization of pHa by bicarbonate given i.v. . . . . The results indicate that CNS failure during rapid normalization of $PaCO_2$ in compensated hypercarbia is due to cerebral hypoxia, which is caused by cerebral vasoconstriction from CSF alkalosis and a shift of the hemoglobin oxygen dissociation curve to the left from alkalemia; both effects result in impaired oxygen delivery to brain cells. Thus, to avoid these dangerous effects in patients with chronic hypercarbia and acute decompensation, oxygenation should be prompt,but $PaCO_2$ should be corrected gradually to avoid alkalemia; base excess, hypochloremia and hypokalemia also should be corrected. (From authors' abstract)

1605.
SAFONOV, V.A., E.B. Velikanov, V.M. Nekroasova and Y.N. Ivanov.
O'vozmozhnom mekhanzme vliyaniya uglekislogo faza na dykhanie.
[The possible mechanism of action of carbon dioxide on respiration].
Biol. Nauk. 112(4):40-47; 1973.

The purpose of the present study is to create a model for the determination of the effect of hypercapnia on the respiratory center. Fifty cats were used in this experiment. Hypercapnic gas mixture, consisting of 3% CO_2, 20% O_2 and 77% N, was administered to the lungs of the animals through a valve system distributor allowing the animals to inhale alternately the atmospheric air of the gas mixture from the bag and exhale into the atmosphere. Electric activity of the respiratory neurons was measured by means of extracellular glass electrodes. Electric discharge and impulse activity of 126 neurons, synchronous with the phases of the respiratory cycle, were registered by an electronic computer. The authors found that hypercapnia causes acceleration of the respiratory rate dominated by a distinct shortening of the expiratory phase. They also noted decreased duration of discharges and number of impulses, with simultaneous increase of the average frequency of impulses in the discharges. The authors postulate that elevated CO_2 content in the inhaled air suppresses the threshold potential of the early and late respiratory neurons. Consequently, the duration of discharges is decreased, thus shortening the entire expiratory cycle. (OLC/UMS)

1606.
SAGA, S., J.H. Modell, H.W. Calderwood, A.J. Lucas, M.K. Tham and E.W. Swenson.
Pulmonary function after ventilation with fluorocarbon liquid P-12F (Caroxin-F).
J. Appl. Physiol. 34:160-164;Feb. 1973.

Eleven dogs were ventilated with Caroxin-F fluorocarbon liquid for 1 hr and then reconverted to breathing gas. Pulmonary function studies were done before and 1, 3, 7, 14, 28, 84, and 168 days after liquid ventilation. All dogs survived the experiment. They maintained adequate levels of arterial oxygenation during liquid breathing. There was an increase in $PaCO_2$ and decrease in pH_a during liquid ventilation, but they returned to control values when the animals were reconverted to breathing gas. The mean PaO_2 was 84 $\pm$ 11 torr (mean $\pm$ SD) and $PaCO_2$ 34 $\pm$ 4 torr (at $FIO_2 = 0.21$) 24 hr after liquid breathing. An increase in pulmonary resistance and a decrease in compliance and lung volumes were observed 24 hr after liquid ventilation. These values returned toward normal at 72 hr. We demonstrated that dogs can be ventilated with oxygenated Caroxin-F fluorocarbon for at least 1 hr and returned to breathing gas. The temporary aberration in pulmonary function can be attributed to the presence of residual fluorocarbon in the lung, rather than a pathophysiologic alteration caused by the fluorocarbon. (Authors' abstract)

1607.
SAHEBJAMI, H., G. Gacad and D. Massaro.
Influence of corticosteroids on recovery from O_2 toxicity.
Clin. Res. 21(1):73; 1973.

Abstract only. Entire item quoted: We studied the effect of 9-fluoroprednisolone (9-Fl) on descending pressure-volume (P-V) relationships of rat lungs during recovery from exposure to 100% O_2 administered at 1 atm for 96 hrs. Some rats were killed immediately after exposure (Gr. 1). Gr. 2 were given 9-Fl in alcohol, Gr. 3 were given alcohol alone, and Gr. 4 were given saline intramuscularly immediately after removal from O_2, and then all were allowed to breathe room air for 48 hrs before sacrifice.

Volume (ml/g)	Pressure (cm H_2O) 0	5	10	15	20	30
Gr. 1	1.4 $\pm$ .1	2.6 $\pm$ .2	3.2 $\pm$ .2	3.4 $\pm$ .2	3.6 $\pm$ .2	3.4 $\pm$ .3
Gr. 2	2.5 $\pm$ .2	5.1 $\pm$ .3	6.4 $\pm$ .4	6.9 $\pm$ .5	7.2 $\pm$ .5	7.6 $\pm$ .5
Gr. 3	2.0 $\pm$ .2	3.5 $\pm$ .2	4.5 $\pm$ .3	4.9 $\pm$ .3	5.1 $\pm$ .3	5.5 $\pm$ .3
Gr. 4	1.9 $\pm$ .2	3.9 $\pm$ .2	4.8 $\pm$ .2	5.1 $\pm$ .2	5.4 $\pm$ .2	5.8 $\pm$ .2

The differences between Gr. 1 and Gr. 2, 3, 4 and between Gr. 2, and Gr. 3 and Gr. 4 are significant ($P = 0.025$). There were no differences between Gr. 2, 3 and 4 when the P-V relationships are expressed as a percent of the air volume at 30 cm H_2O. We found no differences in compliance between Gr. 2, 3 and 4 when saline was used to fill the lungs. We conclude that 9-Fl accelerates recovery of lung compliance from O_2 toxicity.

1608.
ST. CLAIR, J.C.
Cleaning of breathing gas systems.
In: Battelle Columbus Laboratories. Proceedings, 1973 divers' gas purity symposium, November 27-28, 1973, p. VI-1-VI-10. U.S. Navy Supervisor Diving, Nav. Ships Syst. Comm., Rep 2-73, 1973.

Contaminants of diving systems and their components include grease, oil, rust, scale, corrosion, filings, and burrs. Chemicals generally used for cleaning are solvents, alkaline detergents, and acids. The drying medium is filtered nitrogen. Instructions are given as to the methods of cleaning the following: carbon steel high pressure flasks; piping to high pressure flasks; valves, regulators and manifold blocks; pressure and vacuum gauges; gas mixing consoles; hoses; filters; general inplace piping. (MFW/UMS)

1609.
SAITO, T.
Effect of hyperbaric oxygenation on the coronary circulation — a preliminary report.
In: Wada, J. and I. Takashi, Proceedings of the fourth international congress of hyperbaric medicine, Sapporo, Japan, Sept. 1969, p.122-127. Baltimore, Williams and Wilkins, 1970.

The coronary vessels were tonified through oxygen inhalation especially with the hyperbaric oxygenation, and the increase in the vascular tone continued considerably long after complete decompression and start of room air inhalation. Complete recovery of the coronary vascular tone to the control level was attained within 30 to 60 minutes of room air inhalation. Mean aortic pressure was maintained at steady level in most cases throughout compression, maintenance and decompression periods. Slight reduction in cardiac output (-13.7 $\pm$ 13.4%) and small increment of the total peripheral vascular resistance (+8.3 $\pm$ 19.9%) were also observed. There were no remarkable hemodynamic changes besides the above mentioned in the study. (Author)

1610.
SAKURAI, K., H. Kashiwagi, M. Kasamatsu, T. Sato and Y. Suzuki.
Laser scanner and its application.
In: Ocean 73. 1973 IEEE international conference on engineering in the ocean environment, p.31-34. IEEE publication 73 CHO 774-0 OCC.

Large angle laser beam scanning was achieved by using holographic technique, and applied to a range finder system. The holographic scanner consists of the rotating drum (1200 rpm) and 50 hologram plates with it and deflects light beam in 14° horizontally and in 6°40' vertically at 1000 scans per se. Deflected laser beam is reflected back from the target and detected by photomultiplier with the gate circuit. Finally the detected signal is displayed on the cathode ray tube (20 frames/sec). Laser TV system is also constructed using the vibrating mirror scanner. This system is simple, compact and obtainable of clearer pictures. (Authors' abstract)

1611.
SALTZMAN, H.A. and I. Fridovich.
Oxygen toxicity: introduction to a protective enzyme: superoxide dismutase.
Circulation 48(5):921-923; 1973.

The primary defense appears to be an enzyme which catalyzes the reaction $O_2^- + O_2^- + 2H+ \rightarrow H_2O_2+O_2$ and which was named superoxide dismutase. This enzyme is ubiquitous among O_2-metabolizing cells but is lacking in obligate anaerobes. Superoxide dismutase is an enormously efficient catalyst which operates at rates approaching the theoretical limit set by rates of diffusion. Raising the concentration of O_2 induces increased accumulation of this enzyme in micro-organisms and cells which contain high concentrations of superoxide dimutase are more resistant to the lethality of hyperbaric O_2 than comparable cells which contain lower levels of this enzyme. It was possible to prepare mutants of Escherichia coli which exhibited a temperature-dependent defect in their ability to accumulate superoxide dismutase. These mutants had a parallel, temperature-dependent inability to grow in the presence of O_2. Work currently underway suggests that mammalian cells are just as dependent on superoxide dismutase for their ability to tolerate exposure to O_2 as the microorganisms investigated. (ES) (© BA)

1612.
SALTZMAN, H.A.
Oxygen toxicity. Introduction to a protective enzyme: superoxide dismutase.
Circulation 48:921-923;Nov. 1973.

The manifestations of the neurological and pulmonary forms of oxygen toxicity are briefly discussed. A brief review of oxygen toxicity research, going back to Paul Bert, is given. It is noted that the onset of toxicity is considerably delayed by the intermittent use of low-oxygen breathing mixtures. Among the protective agents are vitamin E, succinate, gamma aminobutyric acid, glutathione, disulfiram, and certain nonamine oxidase inhibitors. These are not at present in general clinical use. The hydrogen peroxide theory of oxygen toxicity is discussed, and declared to be not entirely satisfactory because it does not take into consideration reduction products of oxygen which are even more harmful than hydrogen peroxide. The first reduction product of oxygen, O_2^-, known as the superoxide radical, is generated by a variety of biochemical events, both enzymatic and nonenzymatic. The primary defense against the superoxide radical is the enzyme superoxide dismutase. The attempt must now be made to learn how to reduce production of superoxide radicals hyperoxygenated cells, or to increase levels of superoxide dismutase. (MFW/BSCP)

1613.
SALVADORE, C., C. D'Auria and G. Visciani.
Note di fisiopathologia, prevenzione e terapia degli accidenti morbosi da attivita subaquea.
[On physiopathology, prevention and therapy of morbid complications of underwater activity].
Rass. Int. Clin. Ter. 51:1076-1080;Sept. 1971.

After brief remarks on the history of diving, the authors describe, in varying detail, a number of dysbaric syndromes associated with diving, including thoracic compression, aerosinusitis, conjunctival hemorrhaging, edema, decompression sickness ("caisson sickness" or "bends"), pulmonary rupture, hyperbaric oxygen poisoning, and nitrogen narcosis. Clinical symptoms, etiology, prevention, and treatment are touched upon. Although medical and surgical therapies exist for many of these syndromes (most notably recompression for decompression sickness) education in the self-discipline of strict observance of safety precautions represents the most effective counter-measure, in the author's opinion. They outline several very general counsels for prospective divers, as well as contraindications. (MEMH/BSCP)

1614.
SALZANO, J.V., H.A. Saltzman and J.A. Kylstra.
Effects of pressure on ventilation and gas exchange in man.
In: Abstracts of the Twenty-fifth Congress of Physiological Sciences Satellite Symposium. Recent progress in fundamental physiology of diving. Marseille, France, July 1971. p.29-30. (Proceedings unpublished)

Abstract only. Excerpts quoted: Three resting subjects breathed O_2-N_2 and/or O_2-He mixtures at 1, 4.02, and 7.05 ATA and O_2-He at 8.57 ATA in a dry compression chamber. The fraction of O_2 in each gas mixture was adjusted to maintain the PIO_2 constant at approximately 150 mmHg. At 7.05 ATA the subjects breathing a normoxic nitrogen mixture were exposed to the maximum inspired gas density encountered in this experiment, almost seven times that of air at the surface and comparable to the relative density of 0.3 ATA O_2 in He breathed by divers at a depth in the ocean of 1,534 ft (472 m or 47.5 ATA). Under these same conditions the lowest kinematic viscosity was also present. No significant change in heart rate or blood pressure occurred with exposure to inspired pressure of helium, neon and nitrogen in excess of 5000 mmHg. The effects of ambient pressure and density of inspired gas on ventilation and gas exchange is shown in Table 1 by coefficients of correlation between the environmental parameters and group means of the respiratory variables. The group mean (A-a) DO_2 was not affected by changes in ambient pressure but a suggestion of an inverse relationship with density was indicated by a negative correlation coefficient of 0.65 ($P = 0.08$), table 1. The transfer of oxygen from the environment to arterial blood was not adversely affected by the viscosity of the inspired medium.

1615.
SALZMAN, G.
Physiologische Barrieren auf dem Weg ins Meer.
[Physiological barriers on the way into the sea].
Meerestechnik 4:99-101;June 1973.

When proceeding into the depth of the sea, human beings can choose between two environmental conditions: either within the accustomed 'atmosphere', protected by pressure tanks or, without restricting their freedom of movement, being exposed to the ambient pressure, by gradual adjustment. The adjustment is made more difficult by mechanical, narcotic and physical hurdles. Scientists in the USSR investigated to what extent the human organism can be loaded under the conditions of the 'inner space', and what means can be used to proceed beyond the limits found. (English abstract)

1616.
SAND, R.F.
Compressor accident investigation.
In: Professional diving symposium, New Orleans, Nov. 1972. Mar. Technol. Soc. J. 7:25-27; Mar./Apr. 1973.

The failure of an air filter canister on a portable diving air compressor involved so many possible causes that a number of engineering and safety specialists were consulted before the cause was identified. No one specialist identified all factors which contributed to the unsafe condition. The complexity and interdependence of high pressure technology used in diving apparatus is not a matter of routine capability even in academic or research institutions where the urge to redesign, modify or adjust is particularly evident. What is required for effective accident prevention in the academic diving communty is a safety program with at least the following elements. First, the adoption of standards for all diving and diving support equipment to cover the basic equipment design, accessories, fittings, and fabrications. Second, the development of equipment operational procedures including instruction in high pressure mechanics to prevent the practice of unsafe improvisation to solve the problem at hand. Third, training in first aid and emergency care for all diving and support personnel. Fourth, an organizational structure to provide for administrative control for safe operations. (From author's abstract and conclusions)

1617.
SANDERS, A.P.
Untitled:
In: Abstracts of BuMed-ONR sponsored Navywide workshop in high pressure biomedical research, U.S. Naval Submarine Base, Groton, Conn., May 1971, p.9. Published by the Naval Submarine Medical Research Laboratory, 1971.

Abstract only. Entire item quoted. Succinate effectively protects against oxygen toxicity in rats exposed to 5-11 ATA oxygen pressure. Succinate infusion in dogs protects against oxygen toxicity at 3 2/3 - 5 ATA — particularly when a tranquilizer (Compazine) is used, and movement is not restricted. Pharmacological studies were performed in dogs receiving IV sodium succinate (8 mM/kg/hr., pH6.4, 0.4 molar) for two hours. Blood chemical analyses (ph, PO_2, PCO_2, O_2 saturation blood sugar, BUN, serum Na+m K+, Ca++, Cl+, PO_4 and total protein) were obtained during 72 hours after start of infusion. Other than hypernatremia in the initial six hours, no major abnormalities were observed. Succinate in the diet is being investigated as a protectant in oxygen toxicity. Standard rat chow containing 8% or 16% succinate is fed rats before and during oxygen exposures (1-4 ATA). Controls receive standard rat chow and identical exposures. Succinate stimulus of energy production in normal tissues led to the investigation of succinate usage in facilitating brain recovery post ischemia. Succinate infusion increases dog brain ATP 21% and facilitates brain recovery after circulatory arrest. Decreased brain ATP precedes onset of convulsions induced by hypoxia, metrazol, and hydrozylamine. The efficacy of succinate as a protectant has been studied in theosemicarbizide, metrazol, or hyperbaric oxygenation induced convulsions and found effective. Studies comparing protective agents in convulsions led to the hypothesis, and gave indirect proof that a Clutathione-Glutamate-GABA-Succinate shunt functions as secondary support in maintaining brain ATP. Detailed tracer biochemical studies are in progress to test this hypothesis. Succinate infusion has a marked effect on the cardiovasculature in dogs (increased potential of QRS wave, increased arterial pressure and systolic-diastolic pressure difference in hypovolemia, and more rapid, recovery of blood pressure after cardiac arrest). The therapeutic use of succinate in hypovolemic, endotoxic, or anaphylactic shock is being studied.

1618.
SANDERS, A.P., R.M. Gelien, Jr., R.S. Kramer and W.D. Currie.
Protection against the chronic effects of hyperbaric oxygen toxicity by succinate and reduced glutathione.
Aerosp. Med. 43:533-536;May, 1972.

A comparison of data from control and experimental animals injected with succinate or GSH and chronically exposed to 5 ATA of 100% O_2 was plotted as cumulative % convulsed, cumulative % paralyzed, and cumulative % dead. These data were subjected to statistical analysis by the Kolmogorov-Smirnov Two Samples Statistic of Absolute Values of Maximum Difference Between Two Independent Sample Cumulative Percentages. The statistical analysis indicated that the succinate and GSH curves had a probability of less than 0.01 ($P < 0.01$) of being the same as the control curves for each of the observations. Kowalski et al reported in this journal that sodium succinate failed to protect rats from the chronic effects of hyperbaric oxygen. The results of the statistical analyses of the data of Kowalski et al and the data in this report indicate that succinate and GSH protect rats from the chronic effects of hyperbaric oxygen toxicity. (Authors' abstract)

1619.
SAPOV, I.A. and A.S. Solodkov.
Rezul'taty izucheniyz funktsii organizma podvodnikov vo vremya pokhodov.
[Results of studying the bodily functions of submariners during cruises].
Voennomed. Zh. (10):69-72;Oct. 1971.

The authors studied the physiological functions in submariners during underwater expeditions. The effects of such expeditions on the organism depends on various factors, mainly the length of underwater stay and the general physical condition of the individuals prior to the expedition. During underwater expedition various changes were noted in skin temperature and body temperature regulation depending on the temperature of the surrounding area. Thermoregulatory disorders may affect vegetative functions. Body temperature may rise as high as 38-38.5°C, leading to occasional heat strokes. During long-term expeditions air conditioning of the submarine environment is an absolute necessity. In some cases disturbed function of the cerebral cortex was manifested by neurologic symptoms, such as headache, sleep disorders, general weakness, etc. Impaired ocular adaptation, as well as heightened auditory threshold were also observed. Prolonged submarine expeditions may interfere with circulatory and respiratory functions, as well as basal metabolism. Digestive disorders, manifested by nausea, constipation, meteorism, appetite disorders and symptoms of vitamin deficiency were also among the findings. The secretory function of the stomach was affected in some cases; gastric acidity changes ranged from hyperacidity to extreme hypoacidity, even total absence of hydrochloric acid. The authors point out that the most important aspects of the harmful effects of underwater expeditions are the changes in the hematologic indices. They found a great variation in blood cell count, blood gas levels, blood sedimentation and chemical composition of the blood. Lability of the hematologic indices may be related to the degree of pollution of the atmosphere inside the submarine. Blood chemistry changes involved blood sugar, cholesterol, bilirubin, phosphorus and steroid levels, as well as some serum enzymes. The authors found that most of the physiological and biochemical changes were of temporary nature, disappearing spontaneously shortly after the expedition. Only in exceptional cases was special medical attention required. (OLC/BSCP)

1620.
SAPOV, I.A., V.K. Abrosimov and I.S. Karev.
Obzhim vodolaza.
[Diver's squeeze].
Voennomed. Zh. (11):71-74;Nov. 1972.

In order to assure free and even breathing for deepsea divers the air cushion inside the diving suit should reach down to the level of the waist. This way the pressure inside the diving suit remains equal to the outside pressure of the water at any given depth. If for some reason (e.g. defective equipment) the pressure in the air cushion is decreased below the pressure of the surrounding water, this difference in pressure causes thoracic compression in the diver, a pathological condition called Diver's Squeeze. The authors tested in animal experiments the functional changes in divers during thoracic compression, using cats in a specially designed chamber. Changes in hemodynamics and respiratory indices were observed. ECG studies revealed cardiovascular changes, occasionally even atrioventricular block. In order to prevent compression sickness in divers, careful inspection of all diving gear before each submersion is mandatory. The authors describe safety measures to be strictly observed by submarine crews during deep sea diving expeditions. In case of thoracic compression the affected diver must be immediately returned to the surface and therapeutic measures initiated. If compression occurs at the depth of 12 m or more, the diver must be immediately placed in a decompression chamber for therapeutic recompression. This is not needed when returning from depth less than 12 m. In these cases oxygen inhalation therapy is indicated. In more serious cases involving cerebrovascular complications the patient should be hospitalized. (OLC/SCD)

1621.
SASS, D.J., E.L. Ritman, P.E. Caskey, J. Greenleaf and N. Banchero.
Effects plus GY acceleration on blood oxygen saturation and pleural pressure relationships in dogs breathing first air, then liquid fluorocarbon in a whole body water immersion respirator.
Rochester, Minn., Mayo Clin., Rep. NASA-CR-127 262, 16p. 1972.
(N72 27078)

A total body water immersion, mechanical respiration, body support assembly has been used with dogs on the human centrifuge to compare effects of +1 Gy and +6 Gy acceleration on cardiovascular and respiratory function in dogs under three conditions: (1) normal respiration in air; (2) totally immersed in a saline-filled respiratory chamber providing control of respiratory rate, tidal and residual volumes when breathing air or oxygen; and (3) when respired in the same manner with oxygenated liquid fluorocarbon. Intrathoracic pressures were recorded by strain-gauge manometers connected to fluid filled catheters introduced without thoracotomy into the thoracic aorta, pulmonary artery, right and left atria, left pulmonary vein, and right and left pleural spaces. Three curvette oximeters measured oxygen saturation of blood continuously withdrawn from the thoracic aorta, pulmonary artery, and left pulmonary vein. Oxygen saturation measurements and intrathoracic pressures were analyzed on-line by a CDC 3000 digital computer. Results are included. (Authors) (STAR)

1622.
SASS, D.J., E.L. Ritman, P.E. Caskey, N. Banchero and E.H. Wood.
Liquid breathing: prevention of pulmonary arterial-venous shunting during acceleration.
J. Appl. Physiol. 32:451-455;Apr. 1972.

Dependent pulmonary atelectasis, arterial-venous shunting, and downward displacement of the heart caused by the gravitational-inertial force environment were prevented in dogs breathing oxygenated liquid fluorocarbon in a whole-body water-immersion respirator. Partial closure of the major airways during part of the expiratory phase of liquid respiration was a significant problem initially but was minimized in subsequent studies. (Authors' abstract)

1623.
SASS, D.J.
Roentgenographic study of relative heart motion during vibration in water-immersed cats.
U.S. Nav. Med. Res. Inst., Med. Res. Prog. Rep., 10p. Sept. 24, 1972.
(Also published in J. Biochem. 6:219-225;May 1973)
(AD 765-044/3)

Anesthetized cats were subjected to constant-amplitude (10 mm peak-to-peak) whole-body vibration in either the prone, left lateral decubitus, or upright positions to determine whether or not the heart could be forced to undergo large-amplitude translational motion relative to other intrathoracic structures and show resonance phenomena as described by others. The animals were totally immersed in water within a rigid transparent assembly to minimize vibratory motion of the chest wall and abdominal viscera which could transmit translational forces to the heart. Radiopaque 2 mm beads were implanted in the cardiac apex, domes of the diaphragm, and in the chest wall, and the amplitude of motion of each bead was measured in serial roentgenograms as the frequency and peak acceleration of the vibration were increased step-wise from 3 Hz to 20 Hz. In contrast to the results of roentgenographic studies of heart motion due to vibration reported by others in animals less well restrained, in the present study, motion of the heart due to whole-body vibration was minimal, less than 3 mm at the cardiac apex, and resonance was not detected. (Author's abstract modified by GRA)

1624.
SASS, D.J., E.H. Wood, J.F. Greenleaf, E.L. Ritman and H.C. Smith.
Effects of breathing liquid fluorocarbons on regional differences in pleural pressures and other physiological parameters.
Rochester, Minn., Mayo Clinic, Rep. SAM-TR-72-15, 171p. Dec. 1972.
(AD 763092)

Contents: Effects of Gy acceleration on blood oxygen saturation and pleural pressure relationships in dogs breathing first air, then liquid fluorocarbon in a whole-body water-immersion respirator; Respiratory variations in left ventricular stroke volume during liquid breathing; Effects of +Gy acceleration on the regional distribution of pulmonary blood flow in dogs breathing organic liquids in a whole-body water-immersion respirator; Study of acidemia in dogs breathing oxygenated FC 80 liquid fluorocarbon; Computer processing of physiological data; Effect of inflation levels and body position changes upon regional pulmonary parenchymal movements in dogs at IG; Effects of changes in the magnitude and direction of the force environment on regional distortion of lung parenchyma in dogs; Gas embolism due to intravenous injection of FC 80 fluorocarbon. (GRA)

1625.
SAUER, J.A. and K.D. Pae.
Effect of high pressure on properties of polymers.
New Brunswick, N.J., Rutgers, State Univ., Bu. Eng. Res., Rep. AROD-7928:6-C, 6p. Oct. 1972.
(AD 750,731)

The report briefly summarizes the results of the research studies carried out during the last three and a half years concerning the effects of hydrostatic pressure on the mechanical behavior and mechanical properties of polymers. This research is summarized by briefly stating the problems studied and the general results obtained, and then listing the papers published, the progress reports submitted, the technical papers presented at conferences, the theses completed or partially completed, and the faculty directly or indirectly involved. (Authors) (GRA)

1626.
SAUMAREZ, R.C., J.F. Bolt and R.J. Gregory.
Neurological decompression sickness treated without recompression.
Br. Med. J. (1):151-152;Jan. 20, 1973.

A case of combined type I and type II decompression sickness is described, in which severe neurological symptoms were present. Treatment was not started until 16 hr after the dive had terminated. Examination indicated hemoconcentration and cerebral edema. Treatment consisted of penatzocine 100 mg intramuscularly and 100% oxygen, followed in 15 min by 500 ml dextran 40 in saline; 12,500 IU heparin and 40 mg frusemide were given intravenously, 500 ml, and 500 ml 8.4% sodium bicarbonate solution, also 500 ml 20% fructose to sober the patient, who was drunk at the time of his arrival at the hospital. As broncho-constriction and arterial hypoxemia persisted, 500 mg aminophylline was given intravenously, followed by 250 mg every four hours. Neurological symptoms regressed rapidly; the patient continued to receive dextran 40 and heparin, and was sedated with chlorpromazine, and breathed pure oxygen for 28 hr. followed by 28% for 20 hrs. The patient was discharged in four days with only a slight right-sided nystagmus. (MFW/SCD)

1627.
SAUNDERS, K.B., D.M. Bank, P. Ebden, J.P. Van der Hoff, D.J. Maberley and S.J.G. Semple.
Acid-base status and gas exchange in the anesthetized dog breathing pure oxygen.
Respiration 29(4):305-316; 1972.

Michel proposed in 1968 that the arterial and mixed venous blood are linked through the lungs by the in vitro buffer line. In anesthetized greyhounds, the relation between simultaneous arterial and mixed venous samples was examined, assuming reasonable values for the Haldane effect. The results agree with Michel's hypothesis. The effect of O_2-breathing on arterial and mixed venous acid-base status was calculated. No measurable steady-state effect is predicted in arterial blood, and none was found. In mixed venous blood, a small fall in pH (0.02U) and rise in PCO_2 (2.4 mm Hg) are predicated; similar changes were found in two dogs, but might be explained by simultaneous changes in CO_2 output, arterial PCO_2, and cardiac output. (© BA)

1628.
SAUNDERS, W.
Submersibles as sample-collecting devices and as possible platforms for in situ experiments.
In: Brauer, R.W. ed. Barobiology and the experimental biology of the deep sea, p.188-196. Chapel Hill, N.C. North Carolina, University of North Carolina, Sea Grant Program 1972.

The submersible has made great progress since the early days of the bathyscaph and bathysphere. The difference between the bathyscaph and what is designated here as a "submarine", is similar to that between a dirigible and a free balloon. Cousteau's Diving Saucer made the transition between the "elevator" approach and that of a maneuverable vessel with propulsion. The specific submersible discussed here is Lockheed's Deep Quest. It can accommodate four, for 48 hours at 2400 m. After launching it is autonomous, operating on lead acid batteries, at a speed of up to 4 knots. Two highly versatile manipulators can be exchanged for special purpose tools as needed. Deep Quest is capable of performing many tasks: search and recovery, trap laying, coring, sampling, measurement of optical, chemical and acoustic properties of the ocean. It can cruise, hover, or lie motionless on the bottom. Methods of underwater viewing and recording are briefly discussed. (MFW/SCD)

1629.
SAUNIER, C., A. Rizzo, R. Hennequin, B. Hannhart and P.Horsky.
Modifications de l'equilibre acido-basique et du lactate du sang arteriel pendant la recuperation en air apres trois jours d'hypercapnie.
[Modifications of acid-base balance and of arterial blood lactate during recuperation in air after three days of hypercapnia].
C.R. Soc. Biol. 167(2):315-319; 1973.

The appearance of hyperlactatemia during spontaneous recuperation in atmospheric air after prolonged respiratory acidosis seems certain to be brought on by extracellular alkalosis, which remains moderate, and also by rapid variation of intracellular pH following the rapid return to normal PCO_2. This phenomenon seems to be terminated after half an hour of recuperation, giving way to the phenomenon of redistribution of bicarbonates which brings on an increase in the base excess. (Authors' conclusion translated by MFW/UMS)

1630.
SAWYER, R.N.
Some aspects of scuba in college health.
J. Amer. Coll. Health Ass. 20:323-327;June 1972.

The author describes the scuba training program at Yale, which has been available for the past 11 years, to all members of the University community. Table 1 lists the injuries facing the scuba diver; Table 2, the factors contributing to these injuries; Table 3, the essential factors for safe scuba diving, Table 4 outlines the program of medical qualification and training, and Table 5 reviews the experience during 1970 and 1971 as the percentages disqualified both medically and because of inadequate watermanship. Part of the training program is required attendance at lectures on barotrauma and air embolism. Examinations on these lectures must be passed before any actual training in the use of scuba equipment at depth is undertaken. The emphasis in the physical examination, after minute scrutiny of chest X-rays is directed toward the central nervous system, the cardiovascular system, pulmonary function and the ENT system. (MFW/BSCP)

1631.
SAWYER, R.N. and J.H. Baker.
The longitudinal health survey. I. Description.
U.S. Nav. Submar. Med. Res. Lab., Rep. NSMRL 733, 90p. plus appendices. Dec. 14, 1972.

A multiphasic medical screening program has been developed for randomly selected submarine and diving personnel. Each individual passes through twelve phases of data collection: a statement of personal background and history, psychological testing, selected anthropometry, roentgenography, dental evaluation, pulmonary ventilation tests, audiometry, electrocardiography, vision tests, selected blood chemistry analyses and physical examination. The accumulated data is coded on Holerith cards for ease of storage, retrieval and ultimate computer analysis. The present report defines the scope and objective of each of the measured parameters as well as the computer programs developed for the processing of these parameters. It is intended that data shall be collected for 2,000 individuals and that follow-up data will be obtained at periodic intervals. (Authors' abstract)

1632.
SCAGLIONE, G.C., M. Mazzone, G. La Monaca and G. Albano.
Ruolo dei fattori individuali nell'etiologia della malattia da decompressione. Nota I — Importanza dell aquantita di gas assorbito sulla morbilita dell'animale normale e surrenectomizzato.
[List of individual factors in the etiology of decompression sickness. Note 1. Importance of the quantity of gas absorbed in the morbidity of normal and adrenalectomized animals].
Med. Sport 23:236-242; 1970.

Four series of experiments were run on normal and adrenalectomized animals. These were exposed to hyperbaric conditions with various gas mixtures designed to cause generalised forms (due to circulating emboli) or local nerve forms (due to topical emboli) of compression disease. The results indicate that biophysical factors, such as the volume of gas dissolved in the tissues (generalised forms) or its tensive level (local forms), play an outstanding part in the etiopathogenesis of the disease, whereas biohumoral factors are of secondary importance. Hyperbaric acclimatization would also seem to be biophysical, since the effects of training are not influenced by prior adrenalectomy. (English summary)

1633.
SCHAEFER, G. and J.C. Delhaze.
Influence of exposure to compulsive locomotion and of hyperbaric oxygenation to gamma-aminobutyric acid levels in mice.
Aerosp. Med. 43:209-210;Feb. 1972.

In OHP (oxygen high pressure) experiments parenteral administration of GABA leads to a new increase and/or to only a very slight depression of the GABA level in the brain and to a weakening convulsion intensity. This observation confirms the idea of a protective function of GABA against intoxication of the nerve cell induced by OHP. . . . Findings with regard to relationships between GABA level and "paradoxic" sleep have been completely confirmed by the observation that intraperitoneal administration of GABA increases the level of serotonin in the brain. The cause of the change in GABA metabolism induced by hyperbaric oxygenation is not clear. As prophylactic administration of GABA, however, is able to suppress convulsions induced by OHP, it is conceivable that the increase in the GABA level in the brain induced by hyperbaric oxygenation for 72 hrs functions as a protective mechanism against O_2 intoxication of the nerve cells. (Authors)

1634.
SCHAEFER, K.E., H. Niemoeller, A.A. Messier, E. Heyder and J. Spencer.
Chronic CO_2 toxicity: species difference in physiological and histopathological effects.
U.S. Nav. Submar. Med. Res. Lab., Rep. NSMRL 656, 26p. Mar. 4, 1971.

Guinea pigs and rats were exposed for prolonged periods of time to CO_2 concentrations ranging from 1.0-1.5% CO_2 to 20% CO_2. Rats tolerated these exposures well, in contrast to guinea pigs, 30-50% of which died during exposure to 15% CO_2. Growth curves and organ/body weight ratios obtained in guinea pigs showed marked effects during prolonged exposure to CO_2 concentration as low as 3% CO_2. According to data in the literature, organ weight/body ratios of rats are not affected by prolonged exposures to 11% CO_2 and normal growth is only slightly reduced at these CO_2 levels. Further species differences in the response to CO_2 were observed in serum enzyme responses. GOT and GPT concentrations increased greatly in guinea pigs during exposure to 3% and 15% CO_2 while the enzyme levels in rats were not affected even at 20% CO_2. Since there was no incidence of tissue necroses, the increased serum enzyme levels in guinea pigs have been interpreted as signs of increased permeability caused by hypercapnia. Studies of acid-base balance showed that guinea pigs had higher levels of hydrogen ion concentration than rats for every arterial CO_2 level investigated. The time course of adaptation to CO_2 was, however, similar. The differences in tolerance to CO_2 between guinea pigs and rats has been related to their differing buffer capacity. No species differences were observed with regard to histopathological effects. There was a lack of severe tissue damage during exposure to 15% CO_2. No necroses in liver, heart or muscles were found in guinea pigs or rats under these conditions, although lungs, spleen, intestine and kidneys exhibited hemorrhages during the first 24 hours. Exposure to 15% CO_2 caused an inhibition of mitosis in liver cells of rats and an arrest in spermatogenesis in both guinea pigs and rats. An organ specific pattern of fat accumulation was observed in chronic hypercapnia. (Authors' abstract)

1635.
SCHAEFER, K.E.
The role of CO_2 in confinement.
In: Fructus, X., ed. Third international conference on hyperbaric and underwater physiology, p.76-79. Paris, Doin, 1972.

Twenty-one subjects were confined in a submarine and exposed to 1.5% CO_2 over a period of 42 days with nine-day control periods prior to and following exposure. The results showed no significant changes in performance or in basic physiological parameters, such as blood pressure, pulse rate, weight, and body temperature. However, studies on respiration, acid-base balance, and calcium phosphorus metabolism exhibited some remarkable adaptive changes. The changes in the blood pH and urinary CO_2 clearly indicate the existence of a phase of uncompensated respiratory acidosis lasting for 23 days, which was followed by a phase of compensated respiratory acidosis from the 24th to the 42nd day of exposure. Pulmonary CO_2 excretion and respiratory exchange ratio also exhibit the two phases of respiratory acidosis. The respiratory minute volume was increased 38% and 34% respectively during the described two phases of CO_2 exposure and decreased immediately on return to air. Alveolar CO_2 tension was elevated approximately 3 mm Hg throughout exposure and during the nine-day recovery period. (Author)

1636.
SCHAEFER, K.E. and R.D. Allison.
The effects of simulated breathholding dives in the dry and wet chamber on blood shifts into the thorax.
In: Aerospace Medical Association. 1972 annual scientific meeting, Bal Harbour, Florida, May 1972. Preprints, p.181. Published by the Association.

Studies were done on 5 divers in a wet and dry chamber during simulated breathholding dives to 25, 50, and 90 feet to determine whether 1) the blood shifts are only caused by hydrostatic pressure and 2) whether there is an increasing blood shift with increasing depth above the level at which the thorax is compressed to residual volume. . . A decrease in thoracic resistance indicating a blood shift into the thorax was never found during the simulated dives in the dry chamber. During the breathhold dives in the wet chamber the thoracic resistance decreased 13% during submersion of the head and breathholding for about 2 minutes. Duration of breathhold dives to all depths were about 2 minutes. Thoracic resistance decreased 26% at 25 feet, 28% at 50 feet and 32% at 90 feet depth. These findings clearly demonstrated that major bloodshifts occur before the diver's thorax has been compressed to residual volume. (Authors)

1637.
SCHAEFER, K.E., R.D. Allison, C.R. Carey and R. Strauss.
The effects of simulated breathholding dives in the dry and wet chambers on blood shifts into the thorax.
U.S. Nav. Submar. Res. Lab., Rep. NSMRL 729, 14p. Oct. 26, 1972.
AD 761 146)

Heart rate, blood pressure and transthoracic resistance changes were measured in five trained divers during simulated breathhold dives to 25, 50, and 90 feet in a wet and a dry chamber. During the 'wet' dives heart rate fell significantly below control values and the transthoracic resistance changes provided evidence for blood shifts into the thorax. Reverse blood shifts out of the thorax developed at the end of breathholding on return to the normal atmospheric pressure. The 'dry' dive on the other hand did not show any systematic changes in transthoracic resistance and the heart rate did not decrease significantly below control levels. The results of these studies clearly indicate that the hydrostatic effect of immersion on legs and abdomen forces the blood into the thorax. Blood shifts amounted to about 500 ml during breathholding when immersed on the surface and were in excess of one liter during breathhold dives to 25, 50 and 90 feet. (Authors' abstract modified by GRA)

1638.
SCHAEFER, K.E.
Involvement of CO_2 and calcium stores in decompression sickness.
U.S. Nav. Submar. Med. Res. Lab., Rep. NSMRL 738, 9p. Feb. 12, 1973.

Analysis of urine electrolytes obtained during saturation excursion divers of four divers to depths equivalent to 800 to 1000 feet of sea water showed in all cases during decompression an increase in urinary CO_2 excretion and calcium excretion. In two subjects who developed symptoms of decompression sickness manifested in poorly localized muscle aches and stiffness of joints which did not respond to recompression and oxygen treatment, the carbon dioxide excretion in the urine was more pronounced and was preceded or followed by a calcium tide. These observations point to the bone with its large CO_2 and calcium store as a target organ in decompression sickness. The hypothesis is presented that during compression a greater influx of calcium and carbon dioxide occurs, into the fast exchanging bone carbon dioxide and calcium stores related to an increase in bone-blood flow. During decompression a greater outflow of calcium and carbon dioxide seems to develop corresponding with a decreased bone-blood flow. Recent advances in bone physiology appear to provide a fitting framework for this hypothesis. The hypothesis appears to offer new avenues of approach to the study of decompression sickness and aseptic bone necrosis. (Author's abstract and application)

1639.
SCHAEFER, K.E. and J.H. Dougherty, Jr.
A new physiological sign of impending decompression sickness: nitrogen bursts in the expired air during oxygen breathing in decompression.
In: Aerospace Medical Association. 1973 annual scientific meeting, Las Vegas, Nevada, May 1973. Preprints, p.243. Published by the Association, 1973.

Three experiments were conducted during which data on inert gas exchange were collected by means of breath by breath monitoring with a mass spectrometer. In the first experiment, 23 dives were made to 2 and 7 ATA, there were three cases of bends and bursts of nitrogen in the expired air following complete initial washout during oxygen breathing. In the second experiment, three subjects made excursion dives to 150 FSW (simulated) from saturation at 30 FSW. In one case, bends occurred together with nitrogen bursts; bubbles were detected ultrasonically. In the third experiment, three subjects were exposed to 120 FSW (simulated;) and carried excursion dives to lower and higher pressure; there were four cases of skin bends (itching and tingling) with nitrogen bursts occurring simultaneously. The finding of nitrogen bursts following washout would indicate improper nitrogen elimination. (MFW/BSCP)

1640.
SCHANBERG, S.M., G.D. Blenkarn and H.A. Saltzman.
Monamine oxidase inhibitors, cerebral amines and acute neural toxicity from hyperbaric oxygen.
In: Wada, J. and I. Takashi, eds. Proceedings of the fourth international congress on hyperbaric medicine, Sapporo, Japan, Sept. 1969, p.55-60. Baltimore, Williams and Wilkins, 1970.

Neurologic toxicity from hyperbaric oxygen occurred without significant alterations in brain levels of norepinephrine and serotonin. Certain monoamine oxidase inhibitors, pargyline and iproniazid, provided significant protection from the neurologic manifestations of toxicity induced by exposure to hyperbaric oxygen. Isoniazid, an analog of iproniazid without monoamine oxidase-inhibiting activity, was ineffective. The administration of α-methyl-p-tyrosine and dl-p-chlorophenylalanine inhibited synthesis of norepinephrine and serotonin, respectively, but did not alter either tolerance to oxygen or the protective action of pargyline. Similarly, administration of dopa or 5-HTP, precursors of these cerebral amines, was ineffective in modifying tolerance to oxygen. These studies suggest that both the central nervous system toxicity induced by hyperbaric oxygen and the protection from toxicity afforded by certain monoamine oxidase inhibitors are not mediated through alterations in the brain metabolism of norepinephrine and 5-hydroxytryptamine. (Authors' conclusions)

1641.
SCHATTE, C.L., J.B. Simmons II, D.P. Clarkson and J.P. Jordan.
Predictability of PaO_2 in different inert gas-oxygen environments.
Space Life Sci. 3(3):206-209; 1972.

Recent experimentation with metabolic changes in rats exposed to thermally isoconductive environments has involved the use of inert gas-oxygen mixtures with different total pressures (PT) and inspired oxygen fractions (F_IO_2). To determine the F_IO_2 for each mixture that would result in similar arterial oxygen pressures (PaO_2) and saturations (OS), arterial blood of dogs breathing the mixtures through a mask was analyzed for pH, PO_2, PCO_2, and OS. Using P_IO_2's calculated from the alveolar gas equation as a theoretical basis, the oxygen partial pressure for the helium mixture had to be increased by 5.6% while that in argon decreased by 10.2% below the computed values to obtain PaO_2's acceptably similar to those resulting from air exposure. No consistent variation in pH, $PaCO_2$ and OS were apparent. Based on the data presented, which were obtained under highly specialized conditions, it appears that the use of helium and argon as diluent gases may significantly affect arterial oxygen tension. (Authors' abstract)

1642.
SCHATTE, C.L., J.P. Jordan, R.W. Phillips, D.P. Clarkson and J.B. Simmons II.
Nonthermal metabolic response of rats to He-O_2, N_2-O_2, and Ar-O_2 at 1 atm.
Amer. J. Physiol. 225:553-558;Sept. 1973.

Experiments were performed to describe qualitatively and quantitatively the nonthermal metabolic response of rats to normoxic mixtures of helium, nitrogen, or argon at 1 atm ambient pressure. Ambient temperatures were maintained within the thermal neutral temperature range determined for each gas mixture, thereby minimizing thermal conductive effects. Hypoxic mixtures were similarly tested to determine any differences in hypoxic responses as a function of the diluent gas. Rats exposed to argon for 5 days had a reduced metabolic rate relative to nitrogen, as evidenced by oxygen and food consumption, CO_2 production, and the catabolism of radiosubstrates. While some parameters indicated that helium increased metabolic rate, oxygen consumption did not significantly differ from that in nitrogen. The physiologic and metabolic response to an imposed hypoxia varied among the different environments. Certain indices suggested that the hypoxic effects were less severe in helium and more pronounced in argon than in nitrogen. The mechanisms by which the diluent gases produced the observed changes could not be identified, but some possibilities are discussed. (Authors' abstract)

1643.
SCHATTE, C.L. and P.B. Bennett.
Acute metabolic and physiologic response of goats to narcosis.
Aerosp. Med. 44:1101-1105;Oct. 1973.

The metabolic response of goats was assessed during a one hour exposure of 97% N_2-3% O_2, 97% He-3% O_2 or air at 7 atmospheres absolute (ata) and to 75% N_2O-25% O_2 at sea level. Physiologic and metabolic parameters measured included heart rate. EEG, visual evoked cortical response, ECG, body temperatures, oxygen consumption, CO_2 production, the uptake and oxidation of CO_2 of infused glucose-UL-^{14}C, the blood levels of glucose, pyruvate, lactate, and free fatty acids. Hyperbaric nitrogen caused an increase in metabolic rate and a general decrease in blood constituent levels which was interpreted as reflecting a shift toward fatty acid metabolism at the expense of carbohydrate. A similar but more pronounced pattern was observed with hyperbaric helium. Breathing N_2O at sea level resulted in a substantially depressed metabolic rate and an apparent shift toward greater carbohydrate catabolism. It is considered that the effects at raised pressure were primarily the result of stress whereas the effect of N_2O was typical of a volatile anesthetic. (Authors' abstract)

1644.
SCHATZ, R.A. and H. Lal.
Elevation of brain GABA by pargyline: a possible mechanism for protection against oxygen toxicity.
J. Neurochem. 18:2553-2555;Dec. 1971.

Pargyline caused an elevation of brain GABA in normal mice and prevented the OHP-induced decline in GABA content. It also provided marked protection against OHP convulsions. Furthermore, there was a significant correlation between susceptibility to OHP convulsions and brain levels of GABA in pargyline or saline-treated mice. Previously, phenelzine and iproniazid, two inhibitors of monoamine oxidase structurally unrelated to pargyline, were reported to elevate brain GABA. These drugs also protect against OHP convulsions. Reserpine decreases both brain GABA and the latency of OHP convulsions. Iproniazid prevents both the decrease in the threshold to electroshock seizures and the decrease in brain GABA caused by reserpine. Tranylcypromine, another MOA inhibitor, also reverses the reserpine-induced decrease in the latency to OHP seizures. The results of this investigation suggest that the protective effect of pargyline against oxygen toxicity may be a consequence of its ability to prevent the OHP-induced decrease in the brain GABA. (Authors)

1645.
SCHATZ, R.A. and H. Lal.
Effect of succinic acid, pargyline or L-ascorbic acid on brain ammonia and glutamine: A mechanism of protection against oxygen (OHP) toxicity.
Toxicol. Appl. Pharmacol. 25(3):486; 1973.

Abstract only. Entire item quoted: Since increased levels of brain ammonia and decreased levels of glutamine have been implicated in OHP toxicity, we investigated the effects of pargyline, succinic acid and ascorbic acid on brain ammonia and glutamine in relation to OHP toxicity. Intraperitoneal administration of pargyline (100 mg/kg), succinic acid or ascorbic acid (12 mmol/kg) provided protection against OHP toxicity (convulsions, pulmonary edema and hemorrhage, post-exposure mortality). All three agents prevented the OHP-induced elevation in brain ammonia levels and the OHP-induced decrease in brain glutamine. Further, there was a significant correlation between seizure susceptibility and brain ammonia and glutamine level in pargyline, succinic acid or ascorbic acid-treated mice. It is suggested that the protective effects of these three agents is mediated via effects on ammonia metabolism.

1646.
SCHEID, P. and J. Piiper.
Theoretical analysis of respiratory gas equilibration in water passing through fish gills.
Resp. Physiol. 13:305-318;Dec. 1971.

In order to evaluate the significance of diffusion resistance inside the water passing through fish gills for respiratory gas transfer, calculations were performed on simplified gill models of varied shape and flow velocity patterns. The degree of equilibration inefficiency, equivalent to a functional water shunt, was shown to depend upon the shape of the lamellae and on the flow velocity profile. For identical shape of the lamellae and flow velocity profile, the equilibration inefficiency increased with the parameter $(b^2 \cdot \bar{v})(l^0 \cdot d)$ ($\bar{v}$, mean water velocity; d, diffusion coefficient of gas in water; l_0, length of the lamellae; b, half distance of the lamellae). By applying the theory to literature data on gill water flow and morphometrics in teleosts, it was estimated that, in basal conditions, about 10%, and with increased gill water flow (hypoxia, activity), about 50% of the respiratory water flow might be functionally shunted, and that about ¼ of the experimentally determined total O_2 uptake resistance might be attributed to diffusion resistance of gill water. (Authors' abstract)

1647.
SCHENCK, H.V., Jr., J. McAniff, M.-L. Schenck and H. Schenck.
Diving accident survey, 1946-1970, including 503 known fatalities.
Kingston, R.I., Univ. R.I., Dept. Ocean Eng., Scuba Safety Rep. 5, 39p. Jan. 1972.

A group of 274 fatal diving accident cases from the years 1946-64, 1966-69 are analyzed and compared with the more complete data from the years 1965 and 1970. All three data groups give similar percentages of skin and scuba diving deaths, accident locations, and age groups of victims. There is some suggestion that older and female divers make up a greater percentage of the 1970 fatal census. Beginning divers make up a significantly larger proportion of the 1970 group (25%) when compared with the earlier data (13%). The great majority of cave diving fatalities involve equipment that is totally inadequate to the environmental challenge, and this group of fatalities occur in deeper water. The majority of divers use, or attempt to use, the buddy system. A group of 24 fatal cases involving buddy-breathing are analyzed and show the weaknesses and problems with this method in deep water emergencies. Various rescue failures are also discussed. Various types of accidents: boat run-downs, fish attacks, spear-gun accidents, and others are related to the total census. Equipment and investigation defects are also discussed. (Authors' abstract)

1648.
SCHENCK, H.V., Jr. and J. McAniff.
Mortality rates for skin and scuba divers.
Kingston, R.I., Univ. R.I., Dept. Ocean Eng., Scuba Safety Rep. 7, 11p. Apr. 1972.

The Underwater Society of America has determined that out of a group of 40,328 man-years of memberships, 12 divers perished while following diving activity. Since the reporting of such casualties resulted in the payment of a $500 death benefit to the beneficiaries, it is assumed that this represents the total diving casualty figure from this group. Based on assumed age distributions for divers and mortality rates for U.S. white males, this diving mortality represents a ten percent increase over the expected mortality from all causes and a one-third increase over expected accident mortalities. Although diver age is not important in assessing relative diving risk, experience of the scuba diver is a critical factor. It is estimated that beginning divers may have a diving mortality rate six times that of experienced persons. . . . Table II gives ground rules for fair overall, insurance premium increases for divers based on the Underwater Society data and the U.R.I. fatality studies. For straight-life coverage, at all ages, an increase of more than 10% would seem to be unjustified. For accidental death benefits, an increase of about one third is suggested by Table II. However, if the insured diver agreed to complete a scuba course which had "several" or "an adequate number" of openwater training dives these premium increases should be reduced by one-third or more. Cave diving should be permitted under standard diving rates providing the diver uses the additional safety equipment and training suggested by experts in this phase of diving sports. When the diving industry produces a life vest with proper flotation and corrosion-free fittings, which is fool-proof and dependable, we believe these extra premiums could be reduced greatly and perhaps eliminated. (Authors' abstract and conclusions)

1649.
SCHENCK, H.V., Jr. and J. McAniff.
An analysis of fata skin and scuba diving accidents.
Mar. Technol. Soc. J. 6:41-48;May/June 1972.

A total of 503 diving fatalities occurring from the years 1946 through 1970 were investigated. In only two years, 1965 with 94 cases and 1970 with 135 cases, was the accident census reasonably complete. In general, scuba diving contributed from 70 to 80% of the total sample and the 16 to 25 year age group contained more than half of the victims. Experience of the victims was variable, but between 8 to 13 percent were on their first scuba dive. Most cave diving fatalities involved failure to use proper equipment and this accident group generally involved deeper dives. The majority of divers used the buddy system, but failures of both buddy-breathing and buddy-rescue attempts are discussed. Most autopsy reports gave "drowning" as the cause of death, but there was some indication that up to 25 percent of the cases may have involved lung over-pressures. Regulator failure and impure air were not detected as important problems in diving safety. Major equipment failures involved poor design and lack of performance of life vests and the difficulties attendant on assisting an injured diver out of his straps, buckles and belts. Various ways of improving the safety of diving and the training of divers are revealed by the statistical analysis. (Authors' abstract)

1650.
SCHENCK, H.V., Jr. and J. McAniff.
Skin and scuba diving fatalities involving U.S. citizens, 1971, including a complete summary of fatal accidents for 1970.
Kingston, R.I., Univ. R.I., Dept. Ocean Eng., Scuba Safety Rep. 6, 42p. Sept. 1972.

During 1971 there were 115 fatal accidents involving compressed air, non-military diving by U.S. citizens, compared with 116 fatal cases in 1970. Sixteen skin divers died in 1971 as against 27 in 1970. New York and Hawaii showed substantial increases in diving deaths with Florida and Washington showing large reductions. Accident distributions by weekday and month were similar for the two years, Saturday and Sunday having almost two-thirds the case totals and the four summer months (May through August) having well over half the case load. The bulk of victims were drawn from the age range, 16 to 30 years. Twenty percent of all scuba victims were on their first dive or first open dive compared to 16% in these categories in 1970. Fifteen novices died undergoing instruction, eight of these in a "regular" or professional program. The bulk of the victims were lost in the water for periods in excess of ten minutes. Resuscitation was attempted in almost all cases where some chance of success existed. The Coast Guard was involved in 36 cases in 1971 compared with 32 in 1970. No major equipment defects emerged from the study with the exception of the small inflatable vests, which often failed to inflate or to support the diver properly when they did. Primary causes of accidents are varied, with inexperience and panic, lung over-pressure, and diving in dangerous areas being important problems. Instructor groups, Skindiver Magazine, and some maufacturers believe that 1971 involved more diving activity than did 1970. If this is correct, then it appears that civilian diving was somewhat safer in 1971 than in 1970. (Authors' abstract)

1651.
SCHENCK, H.V., Jr. and J.J. McAniff.
United States underwater fatality statistics—1972.
Kingston, R.I., Univ. R.I., Rep. URI-SSR-73-8, 39p. Dec. 1973.
Available from U.S. Government Printing Office.

This report includes: Part 1 — History and source analysis. Part 2 — General scuba fatality statistics. Part 3 — The scuba victim: training and medical aspects. Part 4 — Equipment aspects. Part 5 — Fatal and nonfatal scuba case summaries. Part 6 — General summary of skin diving fatalities. Part 7 — References. There are four figures and 28 tables. The most common course of scuba fatalities were (1) possible emoblism, panic, or exhaustion; (2) out of air in cave; (3) diving in rough or dangerous water. There were 118 scuba fatalities and 16 skin diver fatalities. Salt water deaths far outnumbered fresh water deaths, California and Florida led geographically, and the under-30 age group was affected more than the older group. (MFW/UMS)

1652.
SCHETTINI, A., L. McKay, J. Mahig and J.H. Modell.
The response of brain surface pressure to hypercapnic hypoxia and hyperventilation.
Anesthesiology 36:4-12;Jan. 1972.

Intracranial pressures (cisternal cerebrospinal fluid and brain surface pressures) were measured in nine anesthetized dogs during and after experimental hypercapnic hypoxia. Both pressures increased significantly after 20 min. of hypoventilation with the hypoxic mixture (PaO_2 20 $\pm$ 7.3 torr; $PaCO_2$ 87 $\pm$ 7.9 torr). When the dogs were subsequently hyperventilated with oxygen, the cerebrospinal fluid pressure rapidly declined, but pressure at the brain surface remained twice the control value. This pressure dissociation was even more striking when the dogs were then given an infusion of distilled water intravenously. These findings suggest that swelling of the brain occurs during hypercapnic hypoxia and is not reversed by an hour of hyperventilation. The lack of correlation between cisternal CSF and brain surface pressures suggests that CSF was displaced from the cranium while brain volume expanded. CSF pressure did not, therefore, reflect the actual pressure of the brain. (Authors' abstract)

1653.
SCHIBLI, R.A. and A.A. Buhlmann.
The influence of physical work upon decompression time after simulated oxy-helium dives.
Helv. Med. Acta. 36:327-342; 1972.

The effect of physical work on decompression was examined by determining the minimal decompression time of simulated He/O_2 diving procedures in 82 different subjects. At a bottom time of 60 min at 10 ATA He/O_2, the minimal decompression time without work was 250 min; if work was performed by bicycling during bottom time the minimal decompression time was 360 min. Similarly, the minimal decompression after a bottom time of 120 min without work was 475 min; however, with work 565 min at least were required. In a bottom time of 180 min at 4.5 ATA with He/O_2 the minimal decompression time without work was 150 min; with work 180 min. The results demonstrate that minimal decompression after a 60 or 120 min dive with work must be longer than the minimal decompression time after a similar dive without work. It is suggested that primarily "slow tissues" become more saturated. We now compute decompression time after work using virtual bottom times. For the He half times of 2-105 min the virtual bottom times are set 100% of the real bottom time, for 120 min half time it is 120%, for 150 it is 125%, for 180 it is 133%, for 210 it is 140%, and for 240 it is 145%. (Authors' summary)

1654.
SCHIMPF, K.
Experimentelle dekompressionskrankheit des kaninchens. Gerinnungsveranderungen und therapeutische beeinflussung.
[Experimental decompression sickness in rabbits. Coagulation changes and therapeutic influencing].
Verh. Dtsch. Ges. Inn. Med. 77:1027-1029; 1971.

Blood coagulation changes in rabbits were studied during the first few hours after decompression. The animals were compressed to 4 ata in 22 min., and decompression was begun after 75 min. at 4 ata and accomplished in times varying from one to 81 min. (A group of control rabbits was not subjected to compression.) The animals received via catheter heparin, trasylol, AMCHA, or physiological saline solution immediately after decompression, or aspirin 12 hours before compression. Blood samples were taken before and at intervals after decompression, and were tested for coagulation factors VIII, V, II and I, thrombocyte count and thrombin time. Thrombocyte counts were highest in animals receiving heparin, and lowest in those receiving AMCHA. Coagulation factors and plasma changes could not be interpreted because of wide variations; a larger experimental population is necessary. Impressions of organ pathology are also noted. (MEMH/SCD)

1655.
SCHLAMM, N.A.
Effect of elevated atmospheric pressure and normoxic helium-oxygen gas on microorganisms.
In: Abstracts of BuMed-ONR sponsored Navywide workshop in high pressure biomedical research, U.S. Submarine Base, Groton, Conn., May 1971. p.14. Published by the Naval Submarine Medical Research Laboratories, 1971.

Abstract only. Excerpt quoted: It was found that pressurization to 68 atm with a gas of 0.3% O_2 in He results in altered antibiotic susceptibility of certain bacteria. Three strains of Staphylococcus aureus, for example, showed decreased susceptibility to penicillin, cephalotin, vancomycin, and bacitracin, but increased susceptibility to colistin sulfate. Escherichia coli and Pseudomonas aeruginosa showed similar but less pronounced alterations. By contrast, there were not pressure effects on antibiotic susceptibility of three strains of Streptococcus pyogenes. Further tests on microbial properties also showed that elevated pressure caused a significant reduction in the lag phase of several E. Coli strains, thereby reducing the time required for maximum growth. However, total cell yield was not affected by pressurization. Continuing tests designed to explain mechanism involved in such alterations are now in progress. In these studies, tests with radioactively labelled compounds have shown for example, that pressurization reduced adsorption of penicillin by S. aureus, suggesting an effect on the enzyme D-alanine transpeptidase, to which the antibiotic binds It was similarly shown that total accumulation, as well as the uptake rate, of 2 galactosides in E. coli were increased by pressurization. A pressure effect on permease activity was thus indicated. The findings with permeases and a bacterial enzyme represent phenomena which could account for alterations in antibiotic susceptibility and growth rate discussed above.

1656.
SCHLAMM, N.A.
Effect of elevated atmospheric pressure on antibiotic susceptibility of Staphylococcus and Streptococcus pyogenes.
Antimicrob. Agents Chemother. 1:512-513; 1972.

Staphylococcus aureus showed decreased susceptibility to penicillin, vancomycin, sodium cephalothin, and tetracycline, but increased susceptibility to sodium colistimethate, at a pressure of 68 atm in helium or helium-oxygen gas. Susceptibility of Streptococcus pyogenes was unchanged by pressurization. (Author's abstract)

1657.
SCHLAMM, N.A. and O.P. Dailey.
Effect of hyperbaric atmospheres on beta-galactoside transport in 'Escherichia coli'.
U.S. Nav. Med. Res. Inst., Rep. 3, 6p. Apr. 12, 1972.
(AD-750,454)
(Also published in Can. J. Microbiol. 18(7):1162-1164; 1972)

The rates of transport of two beta-galactosides by whole cells of Escherichia coli were elevated by pressurization to 68 atm with helium or helium-oxygen gases. Kinetic analyses showed that the high atmospheric pressure caused an increase in V max values of some 20 to 48% whereas K sub m values were unchanged. (Authors) (GRA)

1658.
SCHLAMM, N.A. and O.P. Daily.
Effect of elevated atmospheric pressure on penicillin binding by 'Staphylococcus aureus' and 'Streptococcus pyogenes'.
U.S. Nav. Med. Res. Inst., Rep. 4, 7p. Nov. 20, 1972.
(Also published in Antimicrob. Agents, Chemother. 3:147-151;Feb. 1973.)
(AD 761 231)

A gas pressure of 68 atm, elicited by helium-oxygen gas mixtures, reduced the susceptibility to penicillin of Staphylococcus aureus but not of Streptococcus pyogenes. The elevated pressure also caused a reduction in the binding of 14C-penicillin to S. aureus, but not to S. pyogenes. When these studies were extended to glycine incorporation, it was shown that, even without penicillin, pressurization reduced glycine incorporation into the cell wall of S. aureus. Incorporation into other cellular components was not altered by pressurization. Cells grown in a pressurized environment were slightly more susceptible than those grown at 1 atm to rapid change in osmotic pressure. In the presence of penicillin, glycine incorporation into the cell wall was reduced to the same low level at 68 atm and at 1 atm. These results suggest that pressurization renders S. aureus less susceptible to penicillin because it reduces the enzymatic activity of the binding component on the cell, a penicillin-sensitive transpeptidase. (Author) (GRA)

1659.
SCHMID-SCHONBEIN, H., G. Gallasch, E. Volger and H.J. Klose.
Microrheology and protein chemistry of pathological red cell aggregation (blood sludge) studied in vitro.
Biorheology 10:213-227;June 1973.

After decades of indirect studies about the phenomenon of pathological red cell aggregation (RCA), a method was developed which allows the photometric quantification of the kinetics of this most important hemorheological abnormality in viscometric flow in vitro. When compared to physiological RCA, the shear resistance is increased, the rouleaux are clumped due to side-to-side attachment and the aggregate grows in size during viscometric flow. Since only small volumes (5-10μl) are required for microrheological tests, the serum proteins responsible for pathological RCA in myetoma patients were analyzed. So far, a_2M and I_gM could be identified as globulins producing RCA, however with distinct differences. The effect of high molecular weight dextran and of changes in hematocrit value are also studied. (Authors' abstract)

1660.
SCHMIDT, R.J., Jr.
Mark X closed circuit rebreather training course.
In: Miller, J.W., J.G. Van Derwalker, and R.A. Waller, eds. Tektite 2: Scientists-in-the-sea, p.IV-7-IV-14. Washington, D.C., U.S. Department of the Interior, August, 1971.

During the Tektite 2 Man-In-The-Sea Program, 48 aquanaut scientists were exposed to a seven day training course in the use and maintenance of the Marx X Closed Circuit Rebreather. This course included 30 hours of classroom instruction on the use and maintenance of the Mark X and at least 10 hours of in-water use of the unit. A sample training schedule and written test are included in this report. The major conclusion reached from the rebreather training course on TEKTITE II is that it safely fulfilled its primary purpose to train aquanauts in the maintenance and use of a closed circuit diving apparatus. More divers spent more in-water hours on a closed circuit diving unit than ever previously recorded. This feat alone speaks very highly of the training and of the reliability of the Mark X rebreather. Although the units suffered from the problems associated with the introduction of any new gear, the problems that did arise were diagnosed and corrected by the aquanauts. Their training and personal diving capability are what kept malfunction from becoming serious problems. [As an appendix, the GE Rebreather quiz is reproduced]. (Author's abstract)

1661.
SCHMIDT, T.C., D.J. Kenyon, M. Freitag and R.W. Hamilton, Jr.
Recovery and reuse of diving gases.
In: Battelle Columbus Laboratories. Proceedings, 1973 divers' gas purity symposium, November 27-28, 1973, p.XV-1-XV-12. U.S. Navy Supervisor Diving, Nav. Ships Syst. Comm., Rep 2-73, 1973.

In its role with oxygen as a breathing gas, an inert carrier gas is neither consumed nor structurally changed. If this inert gas could be recovered and impurities removed after a diving operation, it could be used over and over again for an indefinite period of time. Although cryogenic helium reclamation systems exist which re-refine the recovered gas to its pure form, their employment is not mandatory to the recovery and reuse of diving gases. By the use of various buffering and recompression procedures, the gas exhausted from a diving system during decompression can be recovered and stored. The contaminants present in the recovered gas are those produced by the divers and by the introduction of air into the system. The contaminants produced by the divers can easily be removed by the use of appropriate absorbent beds, and those due to air contamination can be kept to acceptable levels by the choice of compression techniques; by using admixture of some new gas, the recovered mixture can be made ready for the next dive. This simple concept has been shown to be feasible and its cost effectiveness has been validated by a working prototype. (Authors' abstract)

1662.
SCHMIDT, T.C.
The psycho-physiological effects of compressed air (a literature review).
Hoboken, N.J., Stevens Inst. Tech., Thesis, Feb. 1973.

The psycho-physiological effects of hyperbaric air are a syndrome of physiologic and neurologic dysfunction manifested primarily as cognitive and psychomotor impairments and behavioral changes. That nitrogen plays a primary role is undisputed. The body is being affected though by simultaneously increased levels of nitrogen, oxygen, carbon dioxide, and pressure, and cycles of interaction are possible. The net effect of these factors upon the EEG is unlike that produced by narcotic agents and is unique from that produced by any of them alone, and more closely resemble that due to certain psychotropic drugs. Certain pharmacologic agents which reduce the effects of compressed air potentiate the action of narcotics, and those which act in opposition to narcotic agents potentiate the effects of compressed air. The same pharmacologic agents which afford some protection from the effects of compressed air block the action in certain psychotropic drugs, and serotonin, a central neurohormone localized in certain areas of the brain. It is suggested that the syndrome of dysfunctions due to hyperbaric air may be better explored by the study of the neurochemical effect of the total compressed air environment, rather than by the effect of nitrogen upon isolated cellular function. (Author's abstract)

1663.
SCHMIDT, T.C., V.A. Dorr and R.W. Hamilton, Jr.
Chamber fire safety.
Tarrytown, N.Y., Ocean Systems, Inc., Res. Devel. Lab., Rep. UCRI-721, 30p. Mar. 15, 1973.

Because hyperbaric diving, decompression, and treatment chambers may involve atmospheres enriched in oxygen and in their nature make quick escape of occupants impossible, special precautions are needed to assure safe operations. All of the traditional aspects of fire safety are involved: sources of ignition, fuel, and oxygen as well as detection and extinguishing. Significant factors are that materials normally considered flameproof may burn fiercely in the presence of extra oxygen or compressed air; that electrical power represents the major source of ignition while sparks — a serious threat where there are flammable vapors — are relatively innocuous; that atmospheres containing less than 5% oxygen will not support combustion (even of hydrogen) and yet may be safe to breathe; and that a deluge of water represents the best compromise for extinguishing. [This report and the six following were prepared for inclusion in a handbook on underwater bioengineering which is being produced by the Science Communication Division of The George Washington University Medical Center, scheduled for publication in early 1975 by Plenum Publishing Corp.] (MFW/UMS)

1664.
SCHMIDT, T.C. and R.W. Hamilton, Jr.
Electric shock hazards.
Tarrytown, N.Y., Ocean Systems, Inc., Res. Devel. Lab., Rep. CRL-T-746, 19p. Dec. 21, 1973.

Other than fire hazard the chief electrical related hazard is that of electrocution. In a dry diving chamber potential electrocution is ever-present during the use of instrumentation and current consuming devices. Sea water and perspiration increase the shock hazard potential, and in a "wet chamber" the hazard becomes even more significant. Persons in a diving or decompression chamber are generally well grounded, crowded, and confined. In cases of severe electrical shock requiring immediate treatment, rescue is difficult or impossible.

1665.
SCHMIDT, T.C. and R.W. Hamilton, Jr.
The "high pressure nervous syndrome" and other high pressure effects.
Tarrytown, N.Y., Ocean Systems, Inc., Res. Devel. Lab., Rep. CRL-T-745, 41p. Dec. 21, 1973.

The high pressure nervous syndrome is described — tremor, convulsions, somnolence, EEG changes, dizziness and nausea. Hyperbaric arthralgia (joint pain and the "no joint juice" sensation) and hyperbaric bradycardia are also discussed. Etiology, mechanisms, and therapy for all three conditions are discussed. Slow compression rate has a preventive effect. The pharmacologic use of inert gases and barbituates is effective against tremor and convulsions. (MFW/UMS)

1666.
SCHMIDT, T.C. and R.W. Hamilton, Jr.
Inert gas narcosis and compressed air dysfunction.
Tarrytown, N.Y., Ocean Systems, Inc., Res. Devel. Lab., Rep CRL-T-744, 41p. Dec. 21, 1973.

Quantitative changes in performance, behavioral effects in chamber diving and open sea diving are discussed. Nitrogen as the principal cause of compressed air narcotic effects, interactions with carbon dioxide and with hypoxia and hyperbaric oxygen, neurologic measurements, predisposition, and adaptation, length of exposure and narcotic potency are also discussed. Methods of alleviation include the preventive measures of carbon dioxide control, slow compression rate, exercise regulation, protective drugs (Frenquel, chlorpromazine) and the use of alternative breathing mixtures in which the diluent gas is less dense (helium, neon, hydrogen). (MFW/UMS)

1667.
SCHMIDT, T.C. and R.W. Hamilton, Jr.
Oxygen toxicity.
Tarrytown, N.Y.: Ocean Systems, Inc., Res. Devel. Lab., Rep. CRL-T-743, 44p. Dec. 21, 1973.

Prolonged exposure to increased partial pressure of oxygen can result in toxic effects which become progressively more severe as the inspired partial pressure and/or duration of exposure is increased. The most dramatic of these are toxic effects upon the respiratory system (The Lorraine-Smith Effect) and upon the central nervous system (The Paul Bert Effect); as well as other toxic effects upon the body including destruction of red blood cells and the neurosensory tissues of the eye. . . . In continuous exposure of many hours at partial pressures not exceeding 2.0 atm, the respiratory system is the first to be affected. Oxygen at partial pressure less than about 0.5 atm is unlikely to have a toxic effect regardless of the percentage composition in inhaled mixtures; but from about 0.5 atm, the symptomology is a function of the partial pressure of the oxygen and the duration of exposure. . . . On exposures to partial pressures of several atmospheres and higher, the central nervous system (CNS) is the first to be affected. (From author's introduction)

1668.
SCHMIDT, T.C.
Physiology of drowning.
Tarrytown, N.Y., Ocean Systems, Inc., Res. Devel. Lab., Rep. CRL-T-746, 7p. Dec. 21, 1973.

Most of the fatal casualties among divers and underwater swimmers are due to drowning. This number could be reduced by the proper practice of resuscitation and post-resuscitation treatment. To this end, a knowledge of the pathogenesis of drowning is indispensible. Books on forensic medicine usually define drowning as an 'asphyxial death due to submersion in water', but this is by no means adequate. In addition to asphyxia, the effects of water inhaled into the lungs is of major importance; a minute and a half of complete submersion will kill a dog whereas recovery will occur after four minutes of complete deprivation of air by other means. There is also a considerable difference in both patho-physiology and treatment depending upon whether the drowning occurs in fresh or salt water. Finally, the treatment of the patient after resuscitation has been achieved is crucial to his survival. It is not uncommon for a person to be discharged in an apparently symptom free condition, only to succumb a short time later. (From author's introduction)

1669.
SCHMIDT, T.C.
Underwater blast.
Tarrytown, N.Y., Ocean Systems, Inc., Res. Devel. Lab., Rep. CRL-T-747, 22p. Dec. 21, 1973.

Underwater blast constitutes an important problem to swimmers and divers alike. During World War II, underwater blast was a far greater cause of casualties than air blast. A man who would be unharmed by an air explosion of a hand grenade at 15 feet distance (providing he is out of direct line of schrapnel) would undoubtedly be killed if a similar charge was exploded at the same distance underwater. The hazard of underwater blast has escalated with the greater use of underwater swimmers for underwater demolition work, in both military and commercial applications.If such an operation is properly carried out, the risk of hazardous exposure is small. However, this is not always the case in work with underwater ordnance, or where explosives are used as a deterrent to the offensive operations of self-contained divers. (Author)

1670.
SCHNEIDER, R.S.
Lakelab.
Sea Grant 70's 3:4-5;Sept. 1972.

LAKELAB is hexagonal in shape, ten feet across at its widest dimension and seven feet high inside, allowing freedom and comfort to the diver-scientists who inhabit it. The habitat rests approximately eight feet off the bottom on three adjustable legs. It has two 16-inch acrylic plastic viewports and one 30-inch port. The larger port is designed as a hatch to mate with future habitats now in the planning stage. LAKELAB weighs 9,000 pounds, including a six-inch-thick concrete floor which helps it remain stable when storms roil the water. Divers enter through a large (30" x 60") rectangular hatch in the bottom, by climbing up a ladder. The habitat is situated in 35 feet of water, with the entrance hatch at a depth of 27 feet. (Author)

1671.
SCHOCKET, S.S., J. Esterson, B. Bradford, M. Michaelis and R.D. Richards
Induction of cataracts in mice by exposure to oxygen.
Israel J. Med. Sci. 8:1596-1601;Aug./Sept. 1972.

Manifestations of toxic effects of hyperbaric oxygen on the eye in various species, including man, have been widely reported in the literature. The authors present here an account of their investigations with mice, which have demonstrated mitotic abnormalities of lens epithelium following hyperbaric oxygenation, and, for the first time recorded the formation of cataracts as a result of such exposure. The authors suggest that the presence of lysosomes in the cytoplasm of the lens epithelium may be a factor in the production of cataracts following repeated hyperbaric oxygen exposures, since oxygen is known to liberate the lysosomal enzyme deoxyribonuclease, which could attack both strands of the DNA double helix, causing cell degeneration sufficiently widespread to result in a cataract. (MFW/SCD)

1672.
SCHOENFISCH, W.H. and J.A. Kylstra.
Maximum expiratory flow and estimated CO_2 elimination in liquid-ventilated dogs' lungs.
J. Appl. Physiol. 35:117-121;July 1973.

Volume-flow characteristics of saline and FC-80 fluorocarbon-filled excised dogs' lungs were determined by volume displacement plethysmography. In all experiments, flow started from a lung volume at which the static recoil pressure of the same lung filled with air had been 20 cm H_2O. Maximum flows of saline and fluorocarbon were compared over the first 50% of the total volume expired. For the four saline-filled lungs this volume averaged 308 $\pm$ 112 ml and for the three fluorocarbon-filled lungs 265 $\pm$ 120 ml. The mean flows were 121 $\pm$ 32 ml/sec for the saline filled lungs and 104 $\pm$ 46 ml/sec for the fluorocarbon-filled lungs. At these flow rates, a respiratory frequency of five breaths/min, and a $PaCO_2$ = 40 mm Hg, the estimated $\dot{V}CO_2$ is 56 ml/min for saline-ventilated lungs, 127 ml/min for fluorocarbon-filled lungs and 850 ml/min for dogs' lungs ventilated with 0.3 M tris (hydroxymethyl) aminomethane (Tris) solution.

It is concluded that respiratory homeostasis can be maintained in dogs ventilated with FC-80 fluorocarbon liquid or Tris solutions. (Authors' abstract)

1673.
SCHREINER, H.R., R.W. Hamilton, Jr. and T.D. Langley.
Neon: an attractive new commercial diving gas.
In: 1972 Offshore Technology Conference, May 1-3, Houston, Texas. Preprints. Vol I, p-501-516. Published by the Conference, 1972.

As requirements for deeper and deeper dives come up, the current techniques using helium are fast becoming inadequate. This paper presents a new approach toward solution of some of the problems involved in the type of deep commercial diving on which the offshore oil industry relies. The proposition is that mixtures containing neon as the main inert ingredient offer a cost/effective way to improve underwater operations at continental shelf depths. [The two chief disadvantages of helium, heat loss and unintelligible speech are thought to be avoided by the use of neon]. (From authors' introduction)

1674.
SCHULZ, H.
Elektronenmikroskipisch Grundlagen bei Hyperoxie.
[Electron microscope findings in hyperoxia].
Pneumonologie 149:181-192;Dec. 19, 1973.

Electron microscopic examinations during hyperoxia and hyperbaric oxygenation confirm the exudative changes in the lung in the early stages, with endothelial swelling and latent interstitial edema. Because of marked spreading of the blood-air pathways, a reduction occurs in the diffusion capacity. Disturbances in the premeability of the cell membrane involve the capillary endothelium initially more than the alveolar epithelium. The level of the O_2 partial pressure is more decisive than hyperbaric oxygenation for the appearance of cell damage. Inspiration of pure O_2 at excess pressure also causes neurochemically induced acute hypertension with pulmonary edema due to an increase in the partial pressure CO_2 in tissues. Several pathogenic pathways are probably involved in the formation of pulmonary edema in hyperoxia and hyperbaric oxygenation. In hyperoxia atelectases are probably produced by the exudation of blood plasma containing fibrin monomer with subsequent inactivation of the surface activity present and by the blockade of the intracellular synthesis of surfactant. Direct damage to cell enzymes after O_2 poisoning, especially the effect of peroxidation of the mitochondrial membranes, must be considered. The degree of severity of diffusion disturbance depends on the O_2 partial pressure and on the duration of exposure. Hibernation delays O_2 toxicity. The lungs of smaller laboratory animals react more quickly and sensitively to the harmful effects of O_2 than the lungs of larger laboratory animals and man. Short periods of artificial respiration at intervals, with 40% O_2 in the inspiration mixture, are harmless and cause no changes in the lungs. If hyperoxia is used for a longer period, on a previously damaged lung, e.g., in shock, fat emoblism or lung trauma, the damage becomes worse and may end in death resulting from progressive dyspnea. In hyperoxic lung damage, several months are required for anatomical cure; the restoration of lung function precedes the anatomical cure. (© BA)

1675.
SCHULZE, W.
Adsorptionsgleichgewichte von Helium, Wassertoff und Neon an festem Kohlendioxid.
[Adsorption equilibria of helium, hydrogen and neon on solid carbon dioxide].
Berlin, West Germany, Technische Univ., Thesis, 72p. 1971.
(N72-31162)

Adsorption equilibria for helium, hydrogen, and neon on carbon dioxide layers and the effects of carbon dioxide condensation conditions on the absorption process are studied. The dependence of gas adsorption temperatures in effective deposition is described with isotherms obtained through the Dubinin-Raduschkevich equation. It is shown that the adsorption behavior of the CO_2 layer depends as well on the temperature as on the mass of the condensed CO_2 and the condensation velocity. The inner surface layer increases up to temperatures of about 20 K, reaches a maximum of 368 sq m/g in the temperature region from 10 to 20 K, and decreases again at lower production temperatures. This effect is attributed to the formation of layers containing cyrstals of differing dimensions. (Transl. GG.) (STAR)

1676.
SCHUSTERMAN, R.J.
Mammal underwater acoustics.
Menlo Park, Cal., Stanford Res. Inst., Final Rep. on contract N00014-71-C-0173, 27p. July 18, 1972.
(AD 746 520)

Underwater signal-detection performance of sea lions was influenced by changes in the probability of signal presentation in both acoustic and visual tasks. Normally, marine mammals in a signal-detection task maintain a low level of false alarms while attempting to maximize their correct detections or hits. It was shown that such an objective in a marine mammal (the California sea lion) can be changed without, in some instances, changing the animal's sensitivity. Thus, by changing response criterion as a function of varying the probability of signal presentation, a set of probability limits could be induced into a sea lion regarding the acceptance or rejection of signal presence or signal difference. By relating the probability of hits to false alarms for several signals of varying magnitude, one can plot the "receiver-operating-characteristic" (ROC) curves for sea lions. (Author) (GRA)

1677.
SCHWINGHAMER, R.J.
Impact sensitivity of materials in contact with liquid and gaseous oxygen at high pressure.
Huntsville, Ala., NASA Marshall Space Flight Cent., Rep. NASA-TM-X-64634, 24p. Jan. 4, 1972.
(N72-16437)

As a result of the Apollo 13 incident, increased emphasis is being placed on materials compatibility in a high pressure GOX environment. It is known that in addition to impact sensitivity of materials, approximately adiabatic compression conditions can contrive to induce materials reactivity. Test runs at high pressure using the ABMA tester indicate the following: (1) The materials used in the tests showed an inverse relationship between thickness and impact sensitivity, (2) several materials tested exhibited greater impact sensitivity in GOX than in LOX. (3) The impact sensitivity of the materials tested in GOX, at the pressures tested, showed enhanced impact sensitivity with higher pressure. (4) The rank ordering of the materials tested in LOX up to 1000 psia is the same as the rank ordering resulting from tests in LOX at 14.7 psia. (Author) (STAR)

1678.
SCIARLI, R., J.M. Feliciano, J. Mayol, H. Regis, C. Andrac and P. Laval.
Physio-pathological results (electroencephalogram, electrocardiogram, blood gasometry) during an apnea undertaken by an international free diving recordman (depth).
In: Abstracts of the Twenty-fifth Congress of Physiological Sciences Satellite Symposium. Recent progress in fundamental physiology of diving. Marseille, France, July 1971, p.21. (Proceedings unpublished)

Abstract only. Entire item quoted: The authors relate the experimental procedure followed by a free diving world recordman. The subject first underwent a complete respiratory examination during rest. After his warming up process consisting of movements, he carried out an apnea, during which the following data were recorded: hemoglobin saturation (continuous); electroencephalogram (continuous); frequent blood test (PaO_2-$PaCO_2$-pH). Two identical tests were made — 13 June 1969, 8 July 1969. These simulated free dives lasted 3 min, 32 sec. and 3 min 45 sec., respectively. Presentation of results and graphic recordings. Commentary on the extraordinary stamina shown during these long simulated free dives resulting from long methodical training.

1679.
SCIARLI, R., F. Sicardi, C. Lemaire and D. Prosperi.
Mycobacteriologie et plongee a saturation.
[Mycobacteriology and saturation diving].
Bull. Medsubhyp 9:15-21;Mar. 1973.

Mycobacteriological investigations were carried out during Sagittaire I, a saturation dive which took place in November and December 1971. The ultimate depth was 300 meters; the four divers lived at this depth for eight days. The atmosphere of the chamber was disinfected by a device of the Aerovap type, and the divers used a preventive local disinfectant. The following were observed: pustules, ear-aches, conjunctivitis, and skin rash. The most common problem was painful inflammation and secretion in the auditory canals, without involvement of the tympanum, and usually in the absence of pathogenic bacteria. Discomfort of the external ear became more severe during the latter part of the dive, to such an extent that it interfered with sleep. It is believed that the increased humidity (86%) was responsible for this condition. It did not occur during the subsequent Sagittaire II and Physalie VI dives, in which the humidity was kept between 40 and 50%. (MFW/SCD)

1680.
SEALEY, J.L.
Minimal recompression, hyperbaric oxygen treatment of decompression sickness in tunnel workers.
In: Wada, J. and I. Takashi, eds. Proceedings of the fourth international congress on hyperbaric medicine, Sapporo, Japan, Sept. 1969, p.100-104. Baltimore, Williams and Wilkins, 1970.

The author presents data on treatment of bends during the construction of the Lake City Tunnel in Seattle, Washington. The "minimal recompression, oxygen breathing" method of Goodman and Workman was used in 136 cases, only one of which was not relieved by oxygen at 28 psig. The author concludes that the use of hyperbaric oxygen during the final 30 to 60 minutes of decompression, particularly with "bends susceptible" individuals, would greatly improve the decompression sickness statistics. (MFW/BSCP)

1681.
SEARLE, K.
The engineering problems in handling diving gases.
In: The working diver, 1972. Symposium proceedings, February 1972, Columbus, Ohio, p.93-107. Washington, D.C., Marine Technology Society, 1972.

From the amateur weekend diver through to the Navy's professional deep saturation diver, a requirement for the storage and delivery of breathing gas is involved. Between the doctor specifying the gas and the diver inhaling it, the engineer is required to maintain its purity, compress, filter and deliver it. In doing so, he must study materials to contain the gas at pressure without contamination and in some applications, to withstand rough handling in a hostile salt water environment. Special rules and precautions must be observed when handling high pressure oxygen. When considering a large saturation chamber complex, the pipe-work, control valves and processing plant become a major part of the system. The sheer volume of gas required to pressurize the chambers, replenish the food locks, allow for mixing adjustments etc. and provide a reasonable safety margin of gas storage becomes a real ship fitting problem. A main control valve manifold for gas distribution becomes necessary. The siting of these major items relative to the control console and chamber assembly is most important in providing an efficient system layout readily accessible by the dive control team. This paper covers these aspects of handling diving gases in general and also refers to the application of these principles to a new Saturation Deep Diving Complex currently being designed for the Royal Navy. (Author's abstract)

1682.
SEGUI, G. and V. Conti.
Comportement alimentaire de trois oceanautes au cours d'une experience de vie a saturation. [Alimentary behavior of three aquanauts during a saturation experiment].
Bull. Medsubhyp 7:15-18;Oct. 1972.

During the Janus II experiment, a study was made (1) of the alimentary behavior of three divers, and (2) as precisely as possible, of calcium content. The normal 3500 calorie intake of the athlete was increased to 4000 calories for divers, because of the heat loss factor. This diet is composed of 120 gr protide, 160 gr. lipids and 500 gr. glucides. Green vegetables were limited to 200 gr. and fruits to 400 gr., because of the variability of their calcium content; more cereals and potatoes were included than would normally be the case, in the interests of stabilizing the calcium intake. Four meals were given — breakfast, lunch, a snack at 6 P.M. and dinner at 10 P.M. Breakfast, and the snack, which were given one hour before a working dive, contained high proportion of glucides. The diet was simple, containing no sauces or fried foods except for an occasional tomato sauce, fried potatoes or sauteed fish. Alcoholic beverages were eliminated, since they contributed neither energy nor thermal balance, and might aggravate narcotic phenomena or hpns. Carbonated beverages were also eliminated, because of the gas. A minimum of two liters of liquid was recommended because of increased diuresis. During decompression, a slightly lighter diet was consumed (3000 calories). It was found, contrary to expectation, that the food lost little of its taste, and the sense of taste of the divers remained acute enough so that they refused soup which had accidentally been oversalted. However, textures changed noticeably: bread became elastic, thick soup coagulated, fried foods diminished by one third in volume, rice became lumpy, apples and pears became bruised, bananas spoiled at once, oranges underwent little change. During decompression, these changes lessened. It was found that circumstances prevented as accurate a calcium study as had been intended, but studies of blood and urine indicated that phosphocalcic metabolism was not disturbed during the experiment. Appetites remained good, and weight was about the same at the beginning and at the end of the experiment. (MFW/BSCP)

1683.
SEIPLE, R.L.
Hardware development for Project Quick Find, the sea lion object recovery system.
U.S. Nav. Undersea Cent., Rep. NUC-TP-304, 31p. July 1972.
(AD 746 486)

The hardware program for Project Quick Find involved the development of a variety of training devices, grabber recovery units, and other related hardware. This report describes the development, test, and evaluation of a sea lion nose-carried grabber device used to effect the recovery of bottom-sitting test ordnance. The primary grabber developed was deployed by a sea lion against a Fleet-fired ASROC missile and was instrumental in its recovery, unassisted by diver personnel. (Author) (GRA)

1684.
SEM-JACOBSEN, C.W. and O.B. Styri.
ECG arrythmias monitored from free swimming scuba divers at various depths.
In: Fructus, X., Ed. Third international conference on hyperbaric and underwater physiology p.130-136. Paris, Doin, 1972.

The authors have monitored 50 divers below 200 feet, 25 divers below 300 feet, three below 400 feet and two below 600 feet since 1965. The three most common ECG irregularities are extrasystoles, irregular heart rate, and immediate bradycardia similar to the diving reflex in diving mammals, and unrelated to the bradycardia observed in most divers after prolonged exposure. These irregularities wre idiosyncratic, and could contribute to the individual's biological signature. There was an unexplainable case of ventricular fibrillation recorded in a fatigued diver. The authors hope to detect biological signatures that will facilitate the prediction of stress tolerance in divers. (MFW/UMS)

1685.
SEM-JACOBSEN, C.W. and O.B. Styri.
Uptake and clearance of hydrogen gas in the human brain.
In: Fructus, X., ed. Third international conference on hyperbaric and underwater physiology, p.124-129. Paris, Doin, 1972.

Measurements of saturation and clearance of three per cent H_2 gas in the human brain have revealed increase, decrease or lack of change in blood flow and in gas exchange rates under a variety of conditions. The reproducible data give a picture of the complex, simultaneous focal changes in the blood flow in the various areas and systems of the brain. Mass Spectrometer analysis is planned to be used in comprehensive tests to validate the data and to provide greater accuracy in their interpretation. The data illustrate the complex, focal changes in the uptake and clearance of an inert gas such as H_2 in the brain. These data from the brain as well as from other tissues in the human body are badly needed. The results may improve our knowledge and understanding of tissue gas exchange and decompression problems. The treatment of decompression sickness may also benefit from this type of study. (Authors' summary)

1686.
SENGERS, J.M.H.L., M. Klein and J.S. Gallagher.
Pressure-volume-temperature relationships of gases: virial coefficients.
In: American Institute of Physics Handbook, third edition, p.4.204-4.221. New York, McGraw-Hill, 1972.
(COM 73-50034)

Tables of second virial coefficients as functions of temperature are presented for 14 gases. These gases are mainly noble gases and constituents of air. In most cases, these are based on a reexamination of the original P-V-T data. Where necessary and possible, these data have been refitted and improved experimental virials determined. In the case of eight of these gases, it has been possible to fit the experimental second virials to those predicted by the (m,6) potential function and potential parameters determined. In almost all cases an optimum fit was obtained for m+18. Experimental third virial coefficients are presented at the experimental temperatures. A table of Boyle and Joule-Thomson inversion temperatures is also presented. (GRA)

1687.
SENIOR, J.R.
Studies on the effect of hyperbaric oxygen breathing on the rate of ethanol metabolism in man.
U.S. Nav. Submar. Med. Res. Lab., Rep. NSMRL 717, 21p. July 7, 1972.
(AD 761, 144)

The initial step in the metabolism of ethyl alcohol in man is the oxidative removal of two hydrogen atoms from the hydroxy-methyl group of the compound, which is accomplished almost exclusively in the liver, and is catalyzed by the well-studied enzyme, alcohol dehydrogenase. The hydrogen removed, along with other hydrogen or equivalent reducing substances from subsequent oxidative reactions on the derived acetaldehyde and acetate, is eventually transferred from the cell sap into the mitochondria where the electrons from the hydrogen are transported to combine ultimately with oxygen; the hydrogen-derived protons then are used to form water. It has never been determined whether the overall rate of ethanol oxidation might be accelerated by increasing the whole body, and presumably intrahepatic, PO_2 to the maximal tolerable level. In two healthy male subjects, exposed twice for one hour to 100% oxygen at three atmospheres absolute pressure, no consistent or impressive acceleration in the disappearance of ethanol from whole blood and body water could be demonstrated. This work provides a significant clue in understanding the mechanism of ethanol-induced liver injury, and represnts a merging of the disciplines of underwater physiology and biochemistry-cell biology. (Authors' abstract modified by GRA)

1688.
SERAFETINIDES, E.A., J.T. Shurley, R. Brooks and W.P. Gideon.
Sensory versus perceptual isolation: a comparison of their electrophysiological effects.
Aerosp. Med. 44:539-541;May 1973.

Sixteen volunteer normal females, ages 18-19, were randomly assigned to Condition A (water-tank type of sensory isolation), or Condition B (bed-type of perceptual isolation). Each subject experienced both condition A and B with an interval of one month and order effects were controlled for. A battery of concurrently taken electrophysiological measurements revealed significantly higher values in Condition A (water tank) for EEG frequency, eye movements, heart rate and some — but not all — of electrodermal events. The differences are discussed in terms of varying input of different sensory modalities and degree of stimulus familiarity involved in the two experimental conditions under study. (Authors' abstract)

1689.
SERGEANT, R.L.
Untitled.
In: Abstracts of BuMed-ONR sponsored Navywide research in high pressure biomedical research, U.S. Submarine Base, Groton, Conn., May 1971, p.52. Published by the Naval Submarine Medical Research Laboratories, 1971.

Abstract only. Entire item quoted: This talk outlines objectives of ongoing research in verbal communications in hyperbaric environments at the Naval Submarine Medical Research Laboratory. Data are presented from several specific studies covering the following areas of research: A primary method of calibrating microphones under high ambient pressure for use in psychoacoustic experimentation, effects of the diver's mouthpiece on the intelligibility of his speech, the use of specialized vocabularies during operations in deep sea environments to improve upon communicability, the evolution of techniques to process helium-speech, and relationships between speech produced while breathing air, heliox, and hydrogen-rich mixtures under pressure conditions of 103 pounds per square inch absolute. Application of research results to Navy operational tasks within hyperbaric environments are discussed.

1690.
SERGEANT, R.L. and T. Murry.
Reciprocity calibration of microphones under high ambient pressures.
U.S. Nav. Submar. Med. Cent., Rep. NSMRL 671, 7p. July 21, 1971.

The purpose of this study was to demonstrate a technique for primary calibration of microphones under high ambient pressures and various gas mixtures. The reciprocity calibration technique was chosen for calibrating a piezoelectric microphone to 600 feet in a helium-gas mixture. Corrections for gas mixture and depth changes were applied to the basic reciprocity formula. Using the reciprocity calibration technique with a piezoelectric microphone, it was found that sensitivity decreased at frequencies below 2000 Hertz as pressure increased. At the pressures encountered from 300-600 feet, the sensitivity of the microphone was stable from 3000 to 8000 Hertz. Betwen the surface and 600 feet depths, there was approximately a 15 to 18 dB loss in sensitivity. (Authors' abstract)

1691.
SERGEANT, R.L.
The intelligibility of hydrogen-speech at 200 feet of seawater equivalent.
U.S. Nav. Submar. Med. Cent., Rep. NSMRL 701, 9p. Mar. 1, 1972.

The purpose of this study was to evaluate the effect of breathing hydrogen on the intelligibility of speech. Taped recordings were made of a talker breathing normal air within one atmospheric pressure absolute (ATA) and also breathing successively, hydrogen, helium and air, at 7 ATA. Responses to the recordings by six panels of listeners were analyzed. As expected, the speech in air at 1 ATA was the most intelligible, and the speech in air at 7 ATA was next best. There was no appreciable difference in mean intelligibility between the helium and hydrogen gas mixtures. These results indicate that any decision in favor of using either hydrogen or helium mixtures in deep sea diving should not depend upon differences in intelligibility of unprocessed helium-versus hydrogen-speech. (Author's abstract)

1692.
SERGEANT, R.L.
Problems of undersea communication by voice.
In: Sergeant, R.L. and T. Murry, eds. Processing helium speech: proceedings of a Navy-sponsored workshop, August 1971. U.S. Nav. Submar. Med. Res. Lab., Rep. NSMRL 708, p.2-3. May 22, 1972.

The author summarizes briefly the problems confronting the diver. In hard hat diving, the transducer used is adequate for shallow air dives, but was not designed to cope with helium distortions of speech. Also, reverberance within the helmet interferes with intelligibility. In the case of scuba divers, different types of masks have been developed to permit voice communication; speech intelligibility depends on the design of these masks (how much freedom is given to lips, jaws and cheeks, size of speaking cavity, etc.) as well as on other factors to do with the equipment and the environment, chief of which is distortion from helium. Speech processors should be incorporated into the communication system, and should be carried by the diver. In hyperbaric pressure chambers, noise interference is an important problem in most cases. At helium depths, signal processing is required. (MFW/BSCP)

1693.
SERGEANT, R.L. and T. Murry, eds.
Processing helium speech: proceedings of a Navy-sponsored workshop, August 1971.
U.S. Nav. Submar. Med. Res. Lab., Rep. NSMRL 708, 68p. May 22, 1972.

This report is a detailed summary of the proceedings of a workshop held during August 1971 on helium-speech processing. The meeting was jointly sponsored by the Office of Naval Research and the Bureau of Medicine and Surgery. It was held at the Naval Submarine Medical Research Laboratory in Groton, Connecticut. Approximately 40 participants were brought together, including foreign scientists, U.S. Navy scientists, operational personnel, Naval and independent contractors, and speech scientists in the academic world, all who have been active in underwater communications. Formal papers were presented and discussed, a forum and discussion period was held, and a summary and comments were presented. Progress and future developments toward reliable speech communication under hyperbaric helium-oxygen conditions were assessed. Concepts of helium-speech processing were advanced from the need of an unscrambler unit to one which includes the understanding and nature of the constraints allied to the unscrambler; that is, talker, listener, face mask and transducer. It was concluded that after a decade of research the ability to correct hyperbaric helium speech finally exists. Now a system that is small, inexpensive, rugged and reliable must be designed and incorporated into diving operations. [Abstracts of individual papers will be found under the following author entries: Coleman, R.F.; Elkins, J.H.; Flower, R.A.; Gill, J.S.; Lindqvist, J.; Morrow, C.T.; Murray, T.; Rothman, H.B. and H. Hollien; Sergeant, R.L.; Tolhurst, G.C. (2); Wathen-Dunn, W.]. (Authors' abstract)

1694.
SERGEEV, E., G.I. Kurenkov and A. Sterlikov.
Some aspects of heat exchange in man under hyperbaric pressure in the O_2-N_2 environment and diving under sea.
Abstract submitted to first annual scientific meeting of the European Undersea Biomedical Society, Stockholm, 13-15 June 1973. (Paper not published).

Abstract only. Entire item quoted: The study of influence of high pressure chamber and undersea laboratory microclimate on aquanauts showed the zone of comfortable microclimate to be used at the depth of 40 m in N_2-O_2 environment is in the range 25 - 26.5 degrees of resultant temperature (RT), which integrates dry bulb temperature, humidity, mean radiant temperature and mobility of gas medium. The zone thus is defined as high and narrow in comparison with normal atmospheric pressure in air (16 - 20.3°RT). The study of divers heat exchange in the Black Sea showed that it is necessary to use the winter type equipment, at depths below 12 m and temperatures of 8 - 12°C during work. The divers' loss of heat with expired gas at 50 m comprises 22 kcal/h. The main part of heat (96.5%) was lost through evaporation of moisture from the surface of the respiration system. Contribution to the increased convective heat loss is made by reduction of isolating features of woolen (to 26% at 5 ATA) and fur (to 89% at 5 ATA) underwear.

1695.
SERRILL, W.S., C.E. Mengel and D. Jefferson.
Effects of hyperoxia and tocopherol deficiency on nitrite-induced methemoglobinemia.
In: Aerospace Medical Association. 1971 annual scientific meeting. Houston, Texas, April 1971. Preprints, p.66. Published by the Association, 1971.

In the present studies the authors examined the effects of hyperbaric oxygen and tocopherol deficiency on nitrite induced methemoglobinemia. Tocopherol variability was used because of its potential biochemical role as an antioxidant. . . In summary, OHP has a beneficial effect in this drug induced methemoglobinemia (decreased formation, earlier clearance). Tocopherol deficiency increases sensitivity to this drug induced oxidant stress. The data imply that tocopherol may play a role in biologic redox-systems other than its one as a lipid antioxidant. (Authors)

1696.
SEYMOUR, G.
The concurrent validity of unobtrusive measures of conflict in small isolated groups.
U.S. Navy Med. Neuropsychiat. Res. Unit, Rep. NMNRU 71-16, 7p. 1971.
(AD 739 005)

Six unobtrusive measures of group behavior (type of response to a conflict criterion item) and response or not to a sociometric questionnaire were correlated with three criteria reflecting a concurrent validation procedure. Results supported the general hypothesis that the unobtrusive measures used were indicative of conflict in small isolated groups. An unexpected finding indicated that response to stress or conflict may be characterized by apparently opposite types of behavior within groups — either withholding information or making strong negative statements about another. (Author) (GRA)

1697.
SHAKOVA, V.I. and S.A. Mitronova.
Vpliv fizichnogo navantazhennya na stan vi shchor nervovoi diya l'nosti lyudini v umovakh roboti pid vodoyu.
[The effect of physical loading on the state of the higher nervous system activity in man during underwater working].
Fiziol. Zh. 19:541-542;July/Aug. 1973.

Correction tests and determination of the latent period of visual-motor reactions were given to volunteer young athletic adults to evaluate higher nervous activity under various conditions. Results of the study showed that the execution of simple tasks, such as weight lifting on dry land, swimming with fins, swimming at 5 m under water, improved the condition of the higher nervous activity in all subjects. More complicated tasks, however, (underwater weight lifting, expander exercises at the depth of 5 m, swimming and weight lifting at the underwater depth of 14 m) resulted in individual differences between the participants. In subjects having strong nervous systems and good adaptability of neural processes all tests showed improved indices. In subjects with weaker nervous systems, on the other hand, all indices were considerably lower. (OLC/UMS)

1698.
SHAMEEL, M.
Untersuchungen ueber den Einfluss des hydrostatisc-en Druckes auf den O_2-Gaswechsel mariner benthischer Algen.
[Investigations concerning the influence of hydrostatic pressure upon the O_2-exchange of marine benthic algae].
Int. Rev. Gesamten Hydrobiol. 58(5):741-782; 1973.

Several species of marine benthic algae were subjected to artificial hydrostatic pressures from 10-800 atm. for varying time periods. Subsequently the O_2 gas exchange (both during assimilation and respiration) was examined using the Winkler technique. Between 10 and 60 atm., exerted for 10 h, there was little effect on several of the algae, including the more sensitive species. High pressures, however, such as those over 100 atm., caused either an increase of gas exchange (stimulation) or a reduction (damage). The tested algae can be listed in order of the increasing susceptibility to pressure as follows: *Fucus vesiculosus, Ulva lactuca, Membranoptera alata, Caulerpa prolifera, Valonia macrophysa, Delesseria sanguinea, Phycodrys sinuosa.* This order does not depend upon the depth at which the algal species normally live, but more upon their ecological resistance to extreme conditions. Thus F. vesiculosus is intertidal, whereas D. sanguinea lives in relatively deep water where environmental conditions change comparatively little. Portions of the thallus of *Laminaria saccharina* where the metabolic rate was higher showed less resistance to pressure than portions where the rate was lower. In some species (*Delesseria*) resistance increased with increasing temperature up to 30°C, whereas other species (*Fucus*) exhibited no such effect. In general, resistance decreased at salinities above or below normal environmental salinities. (CCD) (© BA)

1699.
SHANE, S.L.
The wet suit strangler.
Skin Diver 20:51, 85;June 1971.

It is stated that one medical problem that can occur in diving, and which is frequently ignored during diver training courses, is carotid sinus reflex. It is caused by apparel that is too tight around the neck, thus causing pressure on the carotid sinuses. The human system possesses pressure sensors to sense the pressure in the carotid arteries and to regulate the flow of blood to the brain by speeding up or slowing down the heart rate. If the sensor detects pressure caused from without, it acts in the same way; as a result the heart ceases to pump an adequate supply of blood to the brain, thus bringing on an impairment of function. Treatment consists of first removing the constricting garment, and getting the diver out of the water as soon as possible. Administration of oxygen helps relieve discomfort. While this problem is a potentially dangerous one, it is easily avoided if understood. (MFW/SCD)

1700.
SHANE, S.L.
How they do it in England.
Skin Diver 21:70-71, 91;June 1972.

The British methods of scuba training, operated almost entirely under the supervision of the British Sub-Aqua Club, are described. Training of each student is carried on by the same instructor, on a one-to-one basis. It is considered important that a student qualify as a snorkel diver before undertaking scuba training, so that he will be accustomed to open sea conditions. The classifications are snorkel diver, then 3rd, 2nd and 1st class diver. The instructor has great discretionary power over whether or not a student passes, even though he may have technically passed the required tests. To pass from 3rd class to 2nd class, the student must complete 20 supervised open water dives, during which various emergency drills are exercised. On acquiring this classification, he becomes a fully qualified diver, entitled to make unsupervised dives. To become a 1st class diver, he must have logged at least 100 open water dives, a portion of which must have been below 100 feet. To retain this classification, ten dives a year, under varying conditions, must be made. This type of training system is feasible in England, where the total number of divers is only a small percentage of the number in the United States. (MFW/UMS)

1701.
SHANE, S.L.
Problems with a nitrogen high.
Skin Diver 22:26-27;May 1973.

The symptoms of nitrogen narcosis, from euphoria at about 100 feet through mental confusion and loss of judgment to unconsciousness, which may come at 350 feet, are described. The chief danger is that mental function is affected more quickly than motor function; at 100 feet, the diver will have only about two-thirds of his normal reasoning power and about four-fifths of his normal reaction time, while mechanical dexterity deteriorates by only 7.9%. It is believed that narcosis is brought on by interference with the transmission of impulses among the nerve cells. Factors that predispose toward nitrogen narcosis are anxiety, fatigue, alcohol consumption before a dive, and carbon dioxide retention, which can be caused by rapid descent, dense breathing mixture, high oxygen partial pressure and physical exertion.

1702.
SHANKLIN, D.R. and E.P. Lester.
On the pulmonary toxicity of oxygen. II. The effect of the second gas.
Biol. Neonate 20:140-158; 1972.

Oxygen injury to the lung is proportional to percentage O_2 content in O_2-N_2 binary mixtures. N_2, He, Ne, Ar, and SF_6 have differing effects on the toxicity of constant O_2 content. The lung apparently is capable of distinguishing between inhaled gases including those ordinarily considered to be "biologically inert". Examination of basic attributes of the gases used and the extent of lung injury suggests that the molecular dimensions of mass and size make a major contribution to the variation in the extent of the lesion. (Authors' summary)

1703.
SHAPUNOV, V.M.
Otsenka ekonomichnosti i effektivnosti vneshnego dykhaniya del'fina Phocaena phocaena. [Evaluation of economy and effectiveness of external respiration in the dolphin Phocaena phocaena].
Zh. Evol. Biokhim. Fiziol. 7(4):392-397; 1971.

Studies were made on some of the indices of external respiration (composition of expired and alveolar air, O_2 utilization, etc.) in resting Black Sea dolphins. Due to large respiratory volumes, high degree of O_2 utilization in the lungs, high O_2 effect of the respiratory cycle and favorable relation between alveolar and lung ventilation, the animals may have an effective supply of O_2 during prolonged respiratory pauses. These features account for prolonged diving and swimming of dolphins at high rates. (SB) (© BA)

1704.
SHAW, R.F.
New non-invasive continuous blood oxygen monitoring using eight waveband photometry.
Circulation 48 (Suppl. 4):IV-13;Oct. 1973.

Abstract only. Entire item quoted: Technically practical and reliable continuous arterial O_2 saturation (OS) measurement has been attained with a new technique utilizing eight radiant spectral bands transilluminating the ear (or other body surface). The device uses an earpiece of fixed geometry which need not contact the ear. Neither ear compression nor calibration is required, since all operating coefficients are stored within the instrument. The technique compensates for patient motion, variability of skin colors, ear sizes and shapes. To assess accuracy, 530 body surface measurements of OS from 55 to 100% were performed on 80 adult caucasians, negroes and orientals of various ages, sizes and smoking habits, and compared with measurements of arterial blood samples simultaneously obtained. Standard deviation was less than 2% OS and maximum difference was less than 4% OS. Good accuracy can be maintained even in the presence of severe peripheral vasoconstriction associated with shock or total body hypothermia by applying an alpha-adrenergic blocking agent to the ear. Ongoing adaptation to flow-directed central-venous fiber optic catheters should furnish capability for continuous monitoring of mixed-venous O_2 and arterio-venous O_2 difference and frequent determinations of cardiac output by Fick or dye dilution methods.

1705.
SHEAR, L. and I.S. Brandman.
Hypoxia and hypercapnia caused by respiratory compensation for metabolic alkalosis.
Amer. Rev. Resp. Dis. 107:836-841;May 1973.

Two patients with metabolic alkalosis manifested compensatory hypoventilation severe enough to cause hypoxia and hypercapnia. These changes could not be attributed to a coexisting, independent pulmonary problem; evidence for pulmonary disease was not found, and blood gas values gradually returned toward normal with correction of the alkalosis. Available data are too limited to define 95% confidence limits for the respiratory response to metabolic alkalosis of the severity observed; however, when previously established limits for less severe alkalosis were extrapolated upward, they included the blood gas values obtained in these patients and similar ones reported by others. This study indicates that metabolic alkalosis in patients without pulmonary disease can cause compensatory hypoventilation, hypercapnia and hypoxia. The magnitude of change in blood carbon dioxide and oxygen tensions is directly proportional to the serum bicarbonate concentration. (Authors' abstract)

1706.
SHEFFIELD, J.R. and R.A. Masonheimer.
An acoustic-mechanical method for re-establishing communications with subsea systems.
In: 1973 Offshore Technology Conference April/May 1973, Houston, Texas, Preprints, Vol. II, p.387-396. Published by the conference.

To establish communications between a vessel and a subsea system, whether operation is active or suspended, requires three steps: (1) locating the general area by navigational techniques, (2) locating the exact point of entry and (3) completing the process by mechanically establishing physical communications. This discussion is limited to the details of Steps 2 and 3; however, an inaccurate navigating system could require long-range acoustic devices (step 2) that are not commercially available and would have to be built. [The authors conclude that] 1. Fully developed acoustic equipment for finding and entering subsea locations is commercially available. 2. Mechanical equipment, combined with commercial acoustic devices, can be designed to remotely establish all four guidelines and retrieve the corrosion cap on suspended subsea wellheads. 3. For special jobs, various configurations of mechanical equipment, combined with commercially available acoustic devices, can be used to establish communication with subsea systems. However, care should be taken in mating the acoustic and mechanical equipment so that a simple field technique for using the combined equipment can be developed. (Authors)

1707.
SHENTON, E.H.
Diving for science. The story of the deep submersible.
New York, U.U. Norton and Company, Inc., 1972, 267p.

The author discusses the history, development, and potentialities of research submersibles. The design and construction of many types of submersibles, with specific examples, are described. Although scientific research and salvage operations carried out by manned submersibles are proof of their value, investigation reveals the fact that nearly half of the 66 submersibles, specifications for which are given here, are currently idle. The state of the art is at present undergoing an evolution, and it is believed that many of these will not be reactivated, but that with improving economic conditions new submersibles will be built that will take advantage of the trials and errors of recent years. (MFW/BSCP from review by JCS in Sea Frontiers 18,377-378;Nov./Dec. 1972)

1708.
SHERWOOD, W.G.
Operational evaluation of a deep ocean search and recovery ship.
In: Applications of marine technology to human needs. Preprints, 8th annual conference and exposition, Marine Technology Society, September, 1972, Washington, D.C., p.521-542. Published by the Society, 1972.

A deeep ocean search and recovery ship has been designed and built by Aluminum Company of America. This 243 foot all-aluminum ship, owned and operated by Ocean Search, Inc., is currently undergoing operational evaluation of its capabilities in the Atlantic. For search, identification and recovery, the ship employs an unmanned search vehicle on the end of a drill pipe string. The drill pipe with its sensors and recovery tools can be deployed using conventional seagoing drilling ship techniques through a center well down to a depth of 8000 feet. For recovery, the pipe system is capable of heavy lifts up to 200 tons at 6000 feet. This paper discusses the overall program objectives and design criteria for the ship's hull, arrangements, structural considerations, propulsion machinery, and corrosion protection. Sensor systems with their controls and displays are described. Ship response and pipe dynamics are discussed and analytical results given. Preliminary results of the initial six months operational evaluation of search, identification and recovery operations in water depths up to 6000 feet are presented. (Author's abstract)

1709.
SHERWOOD, W.G.
Surface support vessel for subsea operations.
In: 1973 Offshore Technology Conference. April/May 1973, Houston, Texas, Preprints, Vol. II, p.173-184. Published by the conference.

A new deep ocean search and recovery ship has been designed and built by Aluminum Company of America. The 243 foot vessel, the largest aluminum structure afloat, has recently completed its operational evaluation. Among its recent accomplishments was the location and recovery of a 15-ton acoustical array from a depth of 2257 ft. Targets have been identified and recovered from 6350 ft. In the design of this vessel, drill ship configurations and techniques have been combined with the state-of-the-art acoustic and visual sensors. The sensor and recovery systems are deployed through a 12 x 36 ft. center well. Omni-directional thrust propulsion units are provided for dynamic ship positioning. It is visualized that this type of vessel will function as a surface support vessel for sub-sea operations including the lowering of a Personnel Transfer Chamber. Installed sensor systems with their controls and displays are described. Ship response and pipe dynamics are discussed and analytical results are given. Recently, shallow water trials have been conducted with an underwater work chamber for diver support. In these tests, it was possible to accurately implant large, heavy structures on predetermined bottom target sites. Using its dynamic ship positioning along with both acoustic and underwater TV sensors, the vessel was able to position a diver support chamber over the bottom work site. The diver support chamber contains hydraulic tools, jet pumps, welding and cutting leads, and a heavy lift capability as well as emergency lift support backup. (Author's abstract)

1710.
SHIBATA, J., M. Kimura, K. Ueda and Y. Seika.
Ship hull anti-fouling system utilizing electrolyzed sea water.
Tokyo, Japan, Mitsubushi Heavy Ind., Ltd., Rep. MTB-80, 9p. Sept. 1972.
(PB 212,700)

Mitsubishi Heavy Industries, Ltd., has recently developed a new anti-fouling system for protection of ships' hulls. In this system, electrolyzed sea water is mixed with air and released from nozzle pipes which are fitted to the bilge parts of a ship's hull, so that the mixture of electrolyzed sea water and air rises up to the water surface along the ship's side shells. A test unit with a capacity large enough to cover a 100 m long ship's shell plate was built and operated continuously for five months producing and issuing the electrolized sea water over a 4 m x 10 m steel plate immersed in sea water for confirmation of its efficiency and durability. On the basis of the above test results and the preliminary designs of the system worked out for several different ship applications, it is confidently believed that the system offers a great benefit to shipowners. (Authors) (GRA)

1711.
SHIKANOV, Y.P.
Spravochnik vodolaza.
[Diver's handbook].
Moscow, Izd-vo "Voyenizdat," 1973. 470p.

This compact, but informative reference work gives concise information on the construction, use and repair of the basic types of diver's equipment, mechanisms, and clothing, which permit diving, surfacing, decompressing, air- and gas-supply to divers, telephone communication, and underwater lighting and television. Included are the fundamentals of the organization and technique for safety during divers' descents. Instructive cases with divers given, as well as practical advice to divers during emergency situations under water. Medical support to diver descents is also discussed. Specific ailments of divers and steps for their prevention are reviewed. Decompression and recompression tables are included. Physiological problems listed in the index include: barotrauma of the lungs, decompression disease, oxygen starvation, gas pressure, narcotic action of nitrogen, diver work-and-rest schedule, breathing device minimum-pressure gages, gas analyzers, underclothing, and a 20-page categorized table on advice during emergency situations. (S&T Alert)

1712.
SHILLER, W.R.
Dental services for personnel in extended high pressure living.
In: Abstracts of BuMed-ONR sponsored Navywide workshop in high pressure biomedical research, U.S. Submarine Base, Groton, Conn., May 1971, p.12. Published by the Naval Submarine Medical Research Laboratory, 1971.

Abstract only. Excerpts quoted: The most recent dental problem incidence studies on isolated FBM submarine personnel have indicated that about 65% of the problems which occurred could have been prevented by greater attention to preventive practices and treatment on the part of the individual and the Dental Corps. These data also present specific areas to pay greatest attention in providing dental support for high pressure living. Data secured for submarine studies concerning dental tissue reactions have been used to set up study outlines for high pressure dental tissue monitoring. Gingival tissues in particular are amenable for such assessment. Well-calibrated indices for expressing gingival disease states are being employed. The dental pulp is known to react to high pressure effects. Cases have been accumulated on this effect; however, the analyses of these data have shed no new light on the problem of dental barotrauma.

1713.
SHILLING, C.W.
Information processing for underwater activity.
In: Abstracts of BuMed-ONR sponsored Navywide workshop in high pressure biomedical research, U.S. Submarine Base, Groton, Conn., May 1971, p.33. Published by the Naval Submarine Medical Research Laboratory, 1971.

Abstract only. Entire item quoted: The Biological Sciences Communication Project (BSCP) completed a review of the literature covering the period, Jan. 1, 1962 through Sept. 30, 1969, with a few areas going back to earlier years. This book, An *Annotated Bibliography on Submarine Medicine and Deep Sea Diving*, has been published by Gordon and Breach and is available at this meeting. In order to keep up to date with present research, the BSCP, under contract with the Office of Naval Research, is issuing a set of approximately 50 cards per month which contain the complete citation, informative abstract, and key words. It is the plan that, after appropriate accumulation of these, another book will be published bringing them all together under one cover. For the future we plan to add to the card collection each month by including the psychological aspects, i.e. selection, training, man-machine relationships, and efficiency. Also, it is planned to add material dealing more directly with underwater habitats, vehicles, and all types of gear and equipment. In addition, as support is obtained, it is planned to develop, with the assistance of the *Undersea Medical Society*, a microthesaurus in the field of underwater activity. A more ambitious activity is planned for the development of a data book on submarine and deep sea diving medicine and human performance in the undersea environment.

1714.
SHUBROOKS, S.J., Jr. and S.D. Leverett, Jr.
Effect of the Valsalva maneuver on tolerance to $+G_Z$ acceleration.
J. Appl. Physiol. 34:460-466;Apr. 1973.

Systemic arterial pressure (Psa) response to the Valsalva maneuver and its effects on acceleration tolerance were studied in ten healthy men during exposure to positive ($+G_z$) radial acceleration. For rapid onset (1 G/s) exposures of both 15 s and 45 s duration, large increases in $+G_z$ tolerance were found to occur during performance of a Valsalva maneuver accompanied by vigorous voluntary muscular tensing either with or without use of an anti-G suit. This effect was seen with single prolonged (up to 15 s) maneuvers as well as with repeated maneuvers. Systolic, diastolic, and pulse pressures were in all cases maintained at levels far greater than those which would have occurred during acceleration without the Valsalva; with repeated maneuvers Psa rose progressively often to levels greater than control. These responses were shown to be equivalent to those accompanying the M-1 maneuver, the generally accepted means of increasing $+G_z$ tolerance. The increased intrathoracic pressure, whether produced by the Valsalva or the M-1, is combined with muscular tensing or use of an anti-G suit, resulted in an elevation of Psa and an increased tolerance even during sustained high $+G_z$ exposures. (Authors' abstract)

1715.
SHVARTZ, E. and N. Meyerstein.
Relation of tilt tolerance to aerobic capacity and physical characteristics.
Aerosp. Med. 43:278-280;Mar. 1972.

Thirty-four normal men, aged 17-30, were tested for physical characteristics, maximal aerobic capacity (VO_2 max) and orthostatic tolerance. VO_2 max was predicted from sub-maximal heart rates on a bicycle ergometer, and orthostatic tolerance was determined by a 20-min tilt table test. Four subjects fainted during the tilt table test. The results showed small and insignificant relationships between weight, surface area and tilt table responses. Some relationship was found between height and orthostatic heart rate (r = -0.320), the fainters being slightly taller than the non-fainters. The same degree of relationship existed between VO_2 max and orthostatic heart rate. The best indicator of orthostatic response was reclining heart rate. It had a correlation coefficient of r = 0.180 with orthostatic heart rate, the fainters displaying higher orthostatic values than the non-fainters by 11.8 and 15.5 beats/min respectively. Reclining heart rate is therefore a useful indicator of orthostatic tolerance. (Authors' abstract)

1716.
SICARDI, F. and C. LeMaire.
Evolution des capacites vitales et de la numeration des hematies.
[Evolution of vital capacity and of the number of erythrocytes].
Bull. Medsubhyp 8:18-21;Nov. 1972.

The data here presented were taken from Sagittaire I and II, Swecom, and Physalie VI. These dives were to 300, 500, and 610 meters, with PO_2 ranging from .30 ATA to .65 ATA. The authors conclude that the use of elevated oxygen partial pressures in these experiments has made it possible to establish the absence of alterations in the pulmonary alveoli, since the vital capacity, considered an excellent criterion of pulmonary irritation, did not vary. The passage of oxygen across the alveolar-capillary membrane was not changed and appeared to bring about in the circulating blood a hyperoxic response (decrease in erythrocytes) the more marked as the PO_2 was the more elevated. (MFW/BSCP)

1717.
SIESJO, B.K., J. Folbergrova and V. MacMillan.
The effect of hypercapnia upon intracellular pH in the brain, evaluated by the bicarbonate-carbonic acid method and from the creatine phosphokinase equilibrium.
J. Neurochem. 19(11):2483-2495; 1972.

Intracellular pH in the brain was evaluated by the bicarbonate-carbonic acid method and from the creatine phosphokinase equilibrium, in rats exposed to 6-40% CO_2 for 45 min. There was agreement between the two methods, indicating that the creatine phosphokinase equilibrium in vivo showed the pH dependence predicted from previous in vitro studies. The stepwise increase in the tissue CO_2 tension from 45 to 265 mm Hg lowered the intracellular pH from 7.04 to 6.68. The regulation of intracellular pH in hypercapnia was better than that which was predicted from physiochemical buffering alone, and calculations indicated that the intracellular buffer base concentration increased by more than 10 mg/kg at maximal CO_2 tension values encountered. (© BA)

1718.
SILL, V., H.C. Siemensen, H. Morr, N. Volkel and M. Menge.
Pulmonalarteriendruck, Plasma-Kateocholamine und Renin-Aktivitat wahrend akuter Hyperkapnie.
[Pulmonary artery pressure, plasma catecholamines, and renin activity during acute hypercapnia].
Z. Kardiol. 62:1085-1089;Dec. 1973.

In 6 subjects the influence of acute hypercapnia (mean PCO_2:50.27 torr) on the pulmonary artery pressure and on vasoactive substances epinephrine, norepinephrine and plasma renine activity was studied. The PCO_2-dependent pressure elevations in the pulmonic artery are not the result of an activation of the sympathetic system. While the pulmonary artery pressure documents significant elevation, the plasma catecholamines with a PCO_2 of 50.27 torr show no alteration in comparison with normal air breathing. The increase in plasma renin activity was significant. With hypercapnia as with low oxygen breathing the elevated pulmonary artery pressure can be normalized by intravenous administration of aminophyllin. (English summary)

1719.
SILVERMAN, M.N.
An introductory study on the effects of two-way closed circuit television on a small crew of aquanauts living in an isolated and stressful environment.
In: Miller, J.W., J.G. Van Derwalker and R.A. Waller, eds. Tektite 2: Scientists-in-the-sea, p.VIII-63-VIII-67. Washington, D.C., U.S. Department of the Interior, August, 1971.

The study was based on the author's belief that all manned space and manned undersea missions should include two way closed circuit television, or video phone, as a primary means of communication. To that end a video phone link was established between the habitat and the command van on the surface. Three measures were taken to determine the aquanauts' attitude and use of the video phone: (1) Pre and post mission questionnaires; (2) forty hours of random video taping showing the use of the video phone; (3) daily recording of communications behavior on computer cards. The results indicated that the video phone provided: (1) a valuable means of communication between the aquanauts and the command center; (2) facilitated equipment troubleshooting; (3) increased the aquanauts' feeling of confidence in the surface crew; (4) reduced feelings of isolation. (Author's abstract)

1720.
SIMON, L.M., E.D. Robin, R. Elsner, A.L.G.J. Van Kessel and J. Theodore.
A biochemical basis for differences in maximal diving time in aquatic mammals.
Comp. Biochem. Physiol. (B) 47(1):209-215; 1974.

Pyruvate kinase activities and cytochrome oxidase activities in 5 tissues (heart, brain, skeletal muscle, liver, lung) were measured in 3 species of diving mammals (sea lion [*Zalophus californicus*], harbor seal [*Phoca vitulina*], Weddell seal [*Leptonychotes weddelli*]) with widely varying maximal diving times. There was increased pyruvate kinase activity in heart and brain with increasing maximal diving times. This suggests the enhanced glycolysis as reflected in increased pyruvate kinase activities may be important in permitting cell survival in the face of prolonged O_2 depletion. No similar relation was found with respect to cytochrome oxidase activity. The biosynthesis of key glycolytic enzymes may be geared to an increasing requirement for ATP generated by anaerobic glycolysis in aquatic mammals. (© BA)

1721.
SINCLAIR, R.D.
Evaluation of a high oxygen — low carbon dioxide breathing atmosphere.
In: Aerospace Medical Association. 1973 annual scientific meeting, Las Vegas, Nevada, May 1973. Preprints, p.153-154. Published by the Association, 1973.

The purpose of this experiment was to "evaluate the physiological responses to submaximal, provocative exercise tests both before and after a period of physical conditioning. The subjects completed an 8-week training period, at the beginning and end of which treadmill tests to determine maximal aerobic capacity and submaximal exercise tests to evaluate the low CO_2-high O_2 breathing mixture. Table 1 shows responses to exercise under each breathing gas condition (air, low O_2, high O_2, and CO_2-O_2, before and after training. Minute ventilation (L/min) was from 83.7 in high O_2, 122.8 in CO_2-O_2 before training, minute ventilation for low O_2 was close to that for CO_2-O_2, with that for air midway between. In the post-training period all values were slightly lower, but bore the same relation to each other. The author concludes "that while the presence of a high background of O_2 may slightly reduce the ventilatory effort associated with a given combination of exercise and hypercapnia in air, this advantage may be offset by CO_2 retention and corresponding increases in arterial PCO_2 and hydrogen concentration." (MFW/BSCP)

1722.
SKURATOVS'KII, A.S. and P.V. Gubatiuk.
Pristrii dlia shtuchnogo dikhannia v barokomeri pid pidvishchenim gazovim tiskom pri ozhivlenni organizmu, shcho zaginuv vid shvidkoi dekompresii.
[Device for artificial respiration at elevated gas pressure in a pressure chamber when reviving an organism that succumbed from rapid decompression].
Fiziol. Zh. 17:276-277; 1971.

Description of equipment for conducting artificial respiration in a pressure chamber when reviving an organism after clinical death caused by rapid decompression. All resuscitative operations are performed without removing the subject from the chamber. The equipment consists of a collar drawn over the subject's chest; the collar is inflated and deflated with the aid of electromechanical regulating valves. (Aerosp. Med.)

1723.
SLACK, D.S.
Recycling systems for helium.
In: Professional diving symposium, New Orleans, Nov. 1972. Mar. Technol. Soc. J. 7:13-16; Mar./Apr. 1973.

Reclaiming helium from diving bells, chambers etc. after use results in considerable operational cost savings as well as reducing logistics requirements and savings of a rare natural resource. Recent developments in small helium reclaim systems make this possible. This paper covers these developments in compact, simple, helium reclaim systems for diving operations. Included is performance data and characteristics of reclaim systems supplied by Airco to the Navy's Mark I dive system and the USS PIGEON ASR 21. Since these are among the first units designed specifically for diving operations, theory of operation and reasoning behind selecting the process used are discussed. System design and use in commercial diving complexes are also discussed. (Author's abstract)

1724.
SLACK, D.S.
A diver chemical-powered wet suit heater.
Mar. Technol. Soc. J. 7:35-37;July 1973.

The author describes his design for a compact diver-carried heater which pumps hot water into a tubing vest. The energy source is the calcium metal/water reaction (Ca : $2H_2O$ = Ca $(OH)_2$ + H_2). The high heat input into the torso area utilizes the diver's circulation system to carry heat to the extremities. The heater has been tested in 35°F water. One diver, wearing the heater and a one-quarter inch wet suit was kept cmfortable for one hour, while his companion, wearing the same type of suit but no heater, became chilled after 15 minutes. Water must be occasionally fed to the reaction by means of a hand-pump operated by the diver. (MFW/SCD)

1725.
SLACK, W.K., G.C. Hanson, H.E.R. Chew, G. Cockerill and R. O'Connor.
Analysis of complications of hyperbaric oxygen therapy in 455 patients treated in single-person hyperbaric oxygen chambers.
In: Wada, J. and I. Takashi, eds. Proceedings of the fourth international congress of hyperbaric medicine, Sapporo, Japan, Sept. 1969, p.505-509, Baltimore, Williams and Wilkins, 1970.

Four hundred and fifty-five patients received treatment with hyperbaric oxygen in single-person hyperbaric oxygen chambers. Some of the adverse effects were ear ache in 29.7% of the cases; temporary deafness in 3%; gastrointestinal (nausea, vomiting) in 1%, increase in bronchospasm in 0.8%; and neurological complications in 3%. Convulsions occurred in only 13 patients, most of whom were very ill and in a highly toxic state as a result of the disorders for which they were being treated, so that it was impossible to tell to what extent the hyperbaric oxygen itself was responsible. It is concluded that hyperbaric chambers are safe, useful and effective. (MFW/BSCP)

1726.
SLAYMAN, K.E.
Activities in marine science at the Swedish Board for Technical Development.
London, Off. Nav. Res., Rep. ONRL-R-3-782, pp p. Feb. 10, 1972.
(AD 740 095)

The Swedish Board for Technical Development (STU) is the central government agency for support of technical research and development in Sweden. Within STU, the Marine Technology Group (HTG) is responsible for initiation and support of research projects in marine science. HTG is currently engaged in four items of R and D in marine science — Development of Instruments and Methods for their Use; Platforms and Service Systems; Diving Technology; and Exploitation of the Marine Environment. (Author) (GRA)

1727.
SLEIGH, M.A. and A.G. MacDonald.
The effects of pressure on organisms.
London, Cambridge University Press, 1972. 516p.

Recommendations concerning pressure units. The physics and chemistry of high pressures. Effects of pressure on the dissociation of weak acids. Effects of pressure on the structure of water in various aqueous systems. Effect of pressure on biopolymers and model systems. Effects of deep-sea pressures on microbial enzyme systems. Role of pressure in the stabilization and destabilization of bacterial spores. Effects of pressure on the metabolic processes of plants. The adaptation of enzymes to pressure in abyssal and midwater fishes. Comparative investigations on the pressure tolerance of marine invertebrates and fish. The role of high hydrostatic pressure in the physiology of marine animals. Gas-filled structures providing buoyancy in photosynthetic organisms. Buoyancy mechanisms of cephalopods in relation to pressure. Swim-bladder organization and depth ranges of deep-sea teleosts. The energetics of vertical migration by fishes. Deep diving behaviour and effects of pressure in reptiles, birds and mammals. Some mechanisms involved in the cardio-vascular adaptation to diving. Some problems of human diving. Importance for mammals of rate of compression. Inert gas narcosis and animals under high pressure. Human respiration under increased pressures. Pressure and the rhythmic behaviour of inshore marine animals. Pressure discrimination in teleost fish. Detection of small changes in hydrostatic pressures by Crustacea and its relation to electrode action in the cuticle. The effects of pressure on organisms: a summary of progress. Abstracts of papers read at a discussion section: Hydrostatic pressure and membrane permeability. Effects of high hydrostatic pressure on transformation in Naegleria gruberi. In vitro and in vivo studies of the effects of high hydrostatic pressures on chick embryonic organs. (Announcement in Underwater J.)

1728.
SLISKOVIC, Z.
Znacaj faringotimpanalne tube u ronilastvu.
[The behavior of the pharyngotympanic tube during diving].
Vojnosanit. Pregl. 29:237-241;May 1972.

The author studied the otorhinolaryngologic implications of deepsea diving. He observed the effects of the oscillation of hydrostatic pressure on the paranasal sinuses, nose, inner ear and tympanic membrane with special emphasis on the reaction of the eustachian (pharyngotympanic) tube. Under simulated diving conditions at the depth of 4 m a group of 20 healthy divers reported sensations of fullness in the ear, stuffiness in the sinuses and, at a later stage, even pain. All these symptoms were caused by sudden changes in the pressure on the eustachian tube and the tympanic membrane. Subjective and objective barotraumatic lesions were found in 14 divers, 7 of which cases are discussed in this paper, with detailed data in Table 1. Under the same experimental conditions as the 20 healthy subjects, these divers developed acute and chronic barotraumatic symptoms of various degrees. They reported the same subjective sensation of fullness, pressure and pain; objective examination revealed various lesions. The most frequent otoscopic findings were redness of the tympanic membrane with occasional perforation and bleeding, catarrhal changes in the sinuses with edema and hyperemia of the torus tubarius. Occasional acute otitis media, sinusitis, tonsillitis were additional findings. Frequent acute exposure to barotrauma often resulted in chronic lesions to the tubes and tympanic membrane. Functional changes, such as hearing loss and equilibrium disorders were detected by audiometry and vestibular function tests. Treatment consisted of ephedrine solution instilled into the ear, nose and sinuses, supported by antibiotic (penicillin) therapy and suspension of diving activities for 5-12 days. The author emphasises the importance of the intact conditions of the otorhinolaryngeal system in divers, controlled by frequent follow-up examinations. (OLC/BSCP)

1729.
SLOAN, R.E.G. and W.R. Keatinge.
Cooling rates of young people swimming in cold water.
J. Appl. Physiol. 35:371-375;Sept. 1973.

Body temperature of the younger and thinner members of a group of boys and girls aged 8-20 years fell by up to 3.2°C when they swam for up to 40 min in water at 20.3°C, at an energy expenditure of about 4.8 kcal/min. The rate of cooling correlated well regardless of age or sex with the individual's overall surface fat thickness on both trunk and limbs; the correlation was improved by making allowance for differences in surface area/mass ratio. Fat thickness was less and fall in body temperature more rapid in young than older swimmers, and in boys than girls, even after correction for surface area/mass ratio. Regional differences in fat distribution were less important, but older swimmers and boys, of given trunk fat thickness generally had less limb fat and cooled faster than younger swimmers and girls, of similar trunk fat thickness and surface area/mass ratio. (Authors' abstract)

1730.
SMALL, A.
Research in hyperbaric pharmacology.
In: Abstracts of BuMed-ONR sponsored Navywide research in high pressure biomedical research, U.S. Submarine Base, Groton, Conn., May 1971. p.46. Published by the Naval Submarine Medical Research Laboratories, 1971.

Abstract only. Entire item quoted: The effect of hyperbaric helium on drug action has been investigated in small laboratory animals exposed to 19.0 ata helium/0.2 ata oxygen, equivalent to a depth of 600 feet. Anesthetized or unanesthetized animals in a hyperbaric chamber were injected by means of a remotely actuated infusion that delivered drug through an indwelling jugular vein catheter, and effects of the drugs on the animals were monitored by direct observation or by electrical recording. Acute toxicity was studied either by determining the median lethal dose (LD-50) or by measuring the dose necessary to produce death when the drug was administered by slow intravenous infusion. Control animals were treated in exactly the same manner as pressurized animals but were exposed only to air at 1 ata. These methods were used to measure acute toxicity of aspirin in mice and the toxicity of morphine, tripelennamine, pentobarbital, lidocaine, and ethanol in rats, as well as the effects of ouabain and digoxin in rats, guinea pigs, and cats. In the case of ouabain and digoxin, there were some differences in the chronotropic response of guinea pigs to the drugs at pressure, but these effects were considered to be unimportant. In general, it was found that hyperbaric helium does not alter the acute toxicity of any drug studied. In future work, the toxicities of several other compounds will be determined in pressurized animals using modifications of methods described here. In addition, studies will be initiated to determine if hyperbaric helium has any effect on the therapeutic efficacy of drugs.

1731.
SMALL, A., H.W. McElroy and R.S. Ide.
Studies of the elctrocardiogram and the toxicity of cardiac glycosides in animals exposed to hyperbaric helium.
Toxicol. Appl. Pharmacol. 20(1):44-56; 1971.

The rapid growth of deep saturation diving has increased the possibility that drugs will have to be used in underwater habitats or manned hyperbaric chambers, where men are saturated with helium at a high partial pressure. The effects of hyperbaric He on the toxicity of cardiac glycosides were investigated in animals equilibrated with 19.0 ata (atmospheres absolute) He/0.2 ata O_2 in a hyperbaric chamber. Control animals were exposed to air at 1 ata, but otherwise were treated the same as pressurized animals. Restrained, unanesthetized rats with indwelling jugular vein catheters were infused with ouabain until cessation of respiratory movements occurred. Guinea pigs, anesthetized with Dial-urethane, received a slow i.v. infusion of either ouabain or digoxin, and the toxic effects of these drugs on the ECG were monitored until asystole ensued. Studies with cats were essentially the same as those in guinea pigs, but only ouabain was infused. The ECG and heart rate were also observed during compression and throughout the equilibration period. Results of these experiments showed that pressurization alone had virtually no effect on heart rate or ECG in guinea pigs and cats. In addition, pressure did not alter the lethal dose in the rat or the doses required to elicit specific ECG disturbances in guinea pigs and cats. An effect of pressure on the chronotropic response to ouabain and digoxin was observed in guinea pigs, but this was considered to be relatively unimportant. Hyperbaric He does not affect the toxicity of cardiac glycosides. (© BA)

1732.
SMALL, A., H.W. McElroy and R.S. Ide.
Acute toxicity of histamine and tripelennamine in animals exposed to hyperbaric helium.
Toxicol. Appl. Pharmacol. 26(3):418-425; 1973.

The effects of hyperbaric He on the acute toxicity of tripelennamine and histamine were studied. Pressurized animals were equilibrated with an atmosphere consisting of 19 atmospheres absolute (ata) He plus 0.2 ata O_2 in a hyperbaric chamber; control animals were treated in an identical fashion, but were exposed only to air at 1 ata. Restrained, unanesthetized rats and guinea pigs with indwelling jugular vein cannulas were injected i.v. with tripelennamine and the acute toxicity determined as the LD50 after 3 hr. Acute toxicity of histamine was determined in anesthetized guinea pigs. The animals were given a slow i.v. infusion of histamine via a jugular vein cannula until asphyxia-induced cardiac arrhythmias occurred. The results of these experiments revealed no effect of hyperbaric helium on the toxicity of tripelennamine in rats or on the toxicity of histamine in guinea pigs. The toxicity of tripelennamine in pressurized guinea pigs was significantly lower than in controls. (Authors' abstract)

1734.
SMIT, P.
Heart rate of exercising divers.
In: Fructus, X., ed. Third international conference on hyperbaric and underwater physiology, p.113-117. Paris, Doin, 1972.

Some general observations stand out: heart rate level is higher in exercising divers than in divers at rest, and it is lower during apnoeic diving manoeuvres than during scuba dives. The latter, during the exercise dives, is slightly lower than the snorkel breathing heart rate level. The standard deviations are always wider during exercise dives than during motionless dives. Not all stages of the activities at 1 1/3 atmospheres absolute are marked by the characteristic bradycardia. Further experiments are necessary to show whether the heart rate of human divers remains at a plateau when they stay submerged for periods longer than 10 minutes. (Author's summary)

1735.
SMITH, A.H. and D.V. Tappan.
High pressure reaction vessel system I. Installation, modification and initial experiments.
U.S. Nav. Submar. Med. Res. Lab., Rep. NSMRL 713, 9p. June 9, 1972.

[The problem was] to modify an existing high pressure vessel system for the satisfactory analysis of reactions carried out in metabolizing biological systems under conditions simulating pressures down to 1,000 feet of sea water. A series of modifications was developed for precise control of reaction conditions and times to safely allow injection of reaction components into the pressure vessels after pressurization. Additional modifications were also required and devised for enabling rapid and efficient cleaning of reaction vessels and attendant components. Appropriate sampling devices have been fabricated and installed to allow analyses of products of reaction mixtures by standard laboratory methods such as gas chromatography, spectrophotometry, and radioisotopic analysis. In order to properly understand the biological effects of high pressures on human tissues it is necessary to be able to study simplified biological systems exposed to increased pressures under laboratory conditions. The system that we now have available allows observations on the influence of varying pressures or temperatures or varying solution components on tissue preparations from animals, on appropriate human tissues such as blood or on single-celled organisms. (Authors' summary)

1736.
SMITH, A.L.
Hyperbaric chamber design factors. Pt. 1.
Hydrospace 4:34-36;Apr. 1971.

The author discusses configuration, materials, electrical and communication systems, hull penetrations and life support systems. Configuration is divided into capacity and shape. The major limiting factor is the diving cycle. The author defines hyperbaric chamber as a vessel "designed to accommodate men under varying pressure, as distinct from one-atmosphere observation chambers", and includes the chamber used in connection with a lock-out submersible, the submersible diving chamber, transfer chambers, deck decompression chambers, work chambers and medical chambers. The design requirements of the various types are discussed from the point of view of habitability, cost, and safety. (MFW/BSCP)

1737.
SMITH, A.L.
Hyperbaric chamber design factors. Pt. 2.
Hydrospace 4:38-41;June 1971.

In this section, the author discusses materials, and lists the criteria as: strength, strength-to-weight ratio, fatigue characteristics, galvanic compatibility, corrosion resistance, fabricatability, availability and cost. The newer materials now being evaluated are acrylic plastic, concrete, and glass. High strength steels are the materials most widely used. The problem of fire hazard is discussed in relation to materials and to breathing mixtures, as well as to electrical power distribution systems. The basic design considerations of hull penetrations are strength and seal integrity. The design of the life support system of a chamber that is the final test; one choice of type of life support system depends on the diving cycle and the number of personnel, and will affect the interior and exterior design of the chamber. Sensors must affectively monitor pressure, CO_2, O_2 and inert gases. Humidity and temperature control are extremely important in dives of long duration. Drawings show a life support plan for a closed circuit system within a chamber. (MFW/BSCP)

1738.
SMITH, A.L.
How this new Act affects you.
Hydrospace 5:39;Feb. 1972.

The mandatory clauses of the new [Mineral Workings (Offshore Installations)] Act will be limited and the main provision could be in a clause that will insist on an approved set of codes of practice being observed. It is expected that the revised Code of Practice for Diving Operations, as brought forward under the auspices of the Underwater Engineering Group will become an approved document. There presumably will be no reason why suitable and competent company instructions in large firms may not also get Government approval to use their own set of rules. It is at this stage that the Act may become too loose and there is a real danger that the Regulations will be manipulated to suit employers and contractors. This must not be allowed to happen. There has been an alarming increase in diving accidents recently which could have been avoided if even the bare accepted practices had been observed and enforced. The Regulations must be a positive instrument, otherwise it will be misused and men will continue to be lost and maimed underwater. (Author)

1739.
SMITH, C.J. and I.L. Manning.
Research at the Naval Undersea Center.
Nav. Res. Rev. 26:1-21;July 1973.

The three areas of research going forward at the Naval Undersea Center which are discussed in this article are (1) mammal training, (2) oceanographic vehicles, and (3) the simulation facility. (1) Sea lions have been trained, in Project Quick Find, to assist in the recovery of submerged objects. Any submerged object equipped with a pinger device can be recovered. The sea lion attaches a grabber device to the target. A similar project, Deep Ops makes use of pilot whales, which can go to much greater depths (at least 1600 ft) than the sea lion. In this case, the device carried and positioned by the whale inflates a balloon which raises the submerged object. (2) Deep View, manned untethered, a glass submersible, is capable of operating at 1500 feet. In Makakai, manned untethered transparent acrylic submersible, has been tested to 600 feet. It consists of a spherical hull attached to two pontoons. The Remote Unmanned Work System (RUWS) is designed to operate at 20,000 feet; it is controlled by cable from a surface ship, and will be used in recovery, survey, and research. An underwater television system, Snoopy, is small, light and maneuverable. It is equipped with a grabber, a compass, and an automatic depth control. Work is being done in the use of concrete as a structural material for underwater aircraft carriers and underwater helicopter carriers. An underwater simulation facility evaluates torpedo performance and ASW exercises. (MFW/CSD)

1740.
SMITH, G., K.M.S. Dewar and A.A. Spence.
The effect of high inspired partial pressures of oxygen on conscious volunteers.
Br. J. Anaesth. 43:1199; 1971.

This experiment compares airway resistance measurements before and after breathing 100% oxygen at 2 ATA for five hours. There was a rise in airways resistance of 30%, a rise in thoracic gas volume of 25%, and a fall in specific airways conductance of 41%. High oxygen tension apparently produced a rise in airways resistance due to broncho-constriction; the rise in thoracic volume was compensatory. Alveolar collapse and gross cellular disturbance did not occur at this exposure. (MFW/BSCP)

1741.
SMITH, G. and I.M.A. Ledingham.
The effect of prolonged hyperoxia on the cardiovascular system of anaesthetized dogs.
Br. J. Anaesth. 44:469-472; 1972.

Six dogs have been anaesthetized with trichloroethylene and ventilated with 100% oxygen at 2 atmospheres absolute for 8 hours followed by a 2-hour period of ventilation with 15% oxygen/85% nitrogen. A fall in cardiac output of approximately 30% occurred within 4 hours of commencing 100% oxygen ventilation, accompanied by a fall in left ventricular dp/dt (max), a 70% increase in systemic vascular resistance and a rise in left ventricular end-diastolic pressure. On resumption of oxygen/nitrogen at the end of 8 hours there was a rapid restoration of all parameters towards the initial values. It would appear that the changes in cardiac output and vascular resistance with oxygen are not progressive within an 8-hour period and that myocardial oxygen toxicity is reversible in this time. (Authors' summary)

1742.
SMITH, G., P.M. Winter and R.F. Wheelis.
Delayed rate of development of pulmonary oxygen toxicity following oleic acid induced lung damage.
Br. J. Anaesth. 45:641;June 1973.

Oleic acid was injected into rabbits to determine its protective effect against oxygen toxicity. The mean survival time of treated animals exposed to 100% oxygen at one atmosphere was 164 + 17.6 hours, as compared with 81 + 6.2 hours for controls. Histological examination of animals injected with oleic acid and exposed to air revealed focal fibro proliferative changes similar to the generalized changes of the proliferative phase of oxygen toxicity. In oxygen-exposed animals, these changes were also observed, together with the generalized features of oxygen toxicity. Further experiments revealed that the adrenal response to oxygen was reduced by oleic acid. Possible mechanisms of this protective effect include (1) increased tolerance of the fibro proliferative lung elements, (2) a reduction in the arterial PO_2, and (3) a reduction in the sympathoadrenal response to oxygen. (MFW/SCD)

1743.
SMITH, G.
Hyperoxy and hyperbaric oxygenation: Influences on the lungs.
Pneumonologie 149:49-53;Oct. 31, 1973.

The rate of development of pulmonary oxygen toxicity is species dependent and affected by the partial pressure of inspired oxygen. Low doses of oxygen are associated with a chronic response whilst high doses are associated with the acute response which comprises an early exudative phase followed by a proliferative phase comprising fibrosis and hyperplasia of type II cells. Measurements of lung function have recorded that pulmonary oxygen toxicity may be associated with changes in compliance, airways resistance, diffusing capacity and capillary blood volume. The effect of intra-pulmonary shunting on oxygen tolerance is discussed. (English abstract)

1744.
SMITH, J.G.
Low temperature performance of CO_2 scrubber systems.
In: Battelle Columbus Laboratories, Proceedings, 1973 divers' gas purity symposium, November 27-28, 1973, p. II-1-II-34. U.S. Navy Supervisor Diving, Nav. Ships Syst. Comm., Rep 2-73, 1973.

The course and extent of CO_2 removal are compared quantitatively for soda lime and barium lime over a temperature range just below the freezing point to 85°F. Increases in gas temperature have also been measured and are correlated with CO_2 absorption. Conditions of gas composition, flow rate and absorbent loading are held constant to minimize extraneous variables. Moisture generation and its distribution in the bed are quite important. Proper adjustment of these variables is required to achieve optimum performance in different temperature ranges. Some attempt is made to understand and explain the role of water in relation to CO_2 removal. (Author's abstract)

1745.
SMITH, K.H.
Application of Doppler ultrasound to the objective detection of decompression sickness and etiology and pathogenesis of aseptic bone necrosis.
In: Abstracts of BuMed-ONR sponsored Navywide workshop in high pressure biomedical research, U.S. Submarine Base, Groton, Conn., May 1971. p.25. Published by the Naval Submarine Medical Research Laboratory, 1971.

Abstract only. Entire item quoted: The Hyperbaric Laboratory at the Virginia Mason Research Center is presently conducting two areas of investigation for the United States Navy. One deals with the application of Doppler ultrasound to the objective detection of decompression sickness in animals and men exposed to increased pressure atmospheres. Decompression is monitored by examining the signal from an ultrasonic Doppler blood flowmeter placed on the experimental subject. The results of this study have shown that bubbles can be detected in the cardiovascular system on ascent prior to onset of decompression sickness. Changes in the Doppler flow signal which are indicative of bubble formation continue to be present for many hours after surfacing. Although attempts have been made to correlate the appearance of Doppler indicated bubbles with tissue supersaturation, non-uniformity of data has not allowed us to predict allowable tissue supersaturations without bubble formation. For the future it is proposed to ascertain those entities in the biological system which are affecting a shift in the Doppler signal and which remain present over 72 hours following decompression. In addition, it is planned to investigate the physiologic effect of bubbles in the circulatory system. Another area of investigation is the search to find the etiology and pathogenesis of aseptic bone necrosis. In the study to evaluate an animal species most suitable as an animal model for the production of aseptic bone necrosis, a detailed investigation of the circulatory anatomy of the femoral head in a variety of laboratory animal species was made. This study culminated in the selection of the miniature pig. The future plan is to use every available diagnostic and investigative means to evaluate the health of the femoral head following exposure to long term residence and decompression from increased pressure atmospheres.

1746.
SMITH, K.H., P.J. Stegall, L.A. Harker and S.J. Slichter.
Possible effects of bubble — induced coagulation following decompression.
In: Ackles, K.N. ed. Blood bubble interaction in decompression sickness. Proceedings of an international symposium held at Defence and Civil Institute of Environmental Medicine, Downsview, Ontario, Canada, p.260-271. Published by the Institute, December 1973. (DCIEM Conference Proceedings 73-CP-960)

Platelet and fibrinogen survival were measured following hyperbaric exposures in minipigs and in divers. In the pigs, one decompression from 80 fsw for four hours at 30 fpm was followed by a marked decrease in both survival times. A combination of heparin and platelet function inhibitors ameliorated the hemostatic survival, but neither drug alone was effective. This would indicate that more than one mechanism was involved. Fibrinogen survival returned to normal much more quickly (one week) than did platelet survival (three weeks). In the human subjects, no significant changes followed a 100 fsw dive of one hour. Platelet survival time decreased significantly following two 150 fsw dives of 10 and 15 minutes. In two 200 fsw dives, two subjects had bends, but in only one dive was there a significant decrease in platelet survival. Findings indicate that a condition of intravascular consumption is produced by diving. It is suggested that the persisting shortened platelet survival may be the result of vessel damage, since there would be increased platelet adherence to the site of the injury. (MFW/UMS)

1747.
SMITH, M.C., Jr., C.S. Huber, G.A. Swaney and C. Stadler.
Tektite 2 food system.
In: Miller, J.W., J.G. Van Derwalker and R.A. Waller, eds. Tektite 2: Scientists-in-the-sea, p.VIII-90-VIII-95. Washington, D.C., U.S. Department of the Interior, August 1971.

Food systems were designed for Dives 2, 3, 4, 6, 8, 9, 10, 11, and 12 in the Tektite 2 program. Seven hundred twenty six man days of food were required to support this series of dives. The core menu for the first series of dives (2, 3, and 4) was composed primarily of precooked frozen food. Core menus for subsequent dives had an equal mixture of pre-cooked frozen, dehydrated, and thermostabilized foods. Food systems which included a variety of food types, i.e., frozen, dehydrated and thermostabilized, had a significant effect on food monotony — longer periods of time were required to detect food monotony. Food preference data were collected from 39 aquanauts, which will be useful in the design of food systems for Skylab and subsequent manned spaceflight programs. Age distribution, technical training, and the fact that Tektite 2 subjects were highly motivated offered some similarity to the present population of astronauts. (Authors' abstract)

1748.
SMITH, P.F.
Research on underwater hearing by free-swimming Navy divers.
In: Abstracts of BuMed-ONR sponsored Navywide research in high pressure biomedical research, U.S. Submarine Base, Groton, Conn., May 1971, p.53. Published by the Naval Submarine Medical Research Laboratories, 1971.

Abstract only. Entire item quoted: Research on underwater hearing by free-swimming Navy divers executed at the Naval Submarine Medical Research Laboratory has been concerned with three broad areas. First experiments were conducted on underwater auditory thresholds to obtain normative data and to obtain evidence concerning the mechanism of underwater hearing. It has been found that divers with deficient air conduction hearing but normal bone conduction levels hear as well underwater as do divers exhibiting normal air conduction levels. However, the tympanic cavity does seem to play an important role in underwater hearing. Second, the effects of intense sound sources on the hearing of Navy divers has been of concern. Experiments were conducted in which the temporary threshold shifts resulting from exposure to intense underwater sounds were measured. Results indicated that for the frequency regions explored the dynamic range of the ear underwater is comparable to its dynamic range in air. Divers' wet suit hoods serve as rather good underwater ear defenders. Third, studies, have been initiated on acoustic orientation and navigation by free-swimming divers. At present only preliminary data have been obtained. To date we have learned that some divers can locate some underwater sound sources some of the time but underwater sound localization lacks both the precision and reliability of sound localization in air. Explanatory hypotheses have been formulated and remain to be tested.

1749.
SMITH, P.F.
Mobile psychoacoustic laboratory.
U.S. Nav. Submar. Med. Res. Lab., Rep. NSMRL 699, 7p. Feb. 8, 1972.

A mobile laboratory that provides an adequate environment for a variety of psychoacoustic measurements has been constructed. The mobile unit is used for psychoacoustic and bioacoustic field studies. This laboratory houses a 10-man audiometric booth. In addition to space within the booth, there are in excess of 120 square feet of floor space available for installation of equipment. Most clinical or experimental autiometric and otologic procedures and group audiometric tests can be administered within the laboratory. Cables may be run to apparatus set up away from the trailer permitting detailed environmental noise analyses, acquisition of bioacoustic data, conducting underwater hearing and communications experiments, etc. (Author's abstract)

1750.
SMITH, R.A., J.H. Cole, R.L. Johnson and P.G. Bhuta.
Feasibility demonstration of low frequency acousto-optical imaging for sonar applications.
Redondo Beach, Cal., TRW Syst. Group. Interim Rep. AT-SVD-TR-73-10, 100p. July 12, 1973.

The technical problem addressed under this program is the extension of acousto-optical imaging techniques to the frequency range of interest for DoD underwater applications. Previous investigations of acousto-optical imaging have been carried out with objects insonified by sound at frequencies of 4 MHz or greater. Under this contract TRW has formed good optical images of targets insonified with sound at frequencies as low as 280 KHz. In addition, imaging by using light heterodyne pickup was conceived and demonstrated using a single detector scan. This technique, when developed, should permit the formation of acousto-optical images at frequencies as low as 25 KHz. This constitutes a major breakthrough in the technology of forming optical images from acoustic wave fronts. . . The DoD implications of this work are as follows. The High Resolution Sonar Study Panel of the Mine Advisory Committee considered the value of two dimensional imaging for Naval underwater applications and concluded that the capability would provide tactical advantage for several applications if it could be performed at ranges of from 100 to 500 yards. The principal application at these ranges is mine hunting and swimmer detection. In addition there are short range applications (object identification, ship hull inspection) which can be performed at higher frequencies. As a result of this project, the feasibility of forming two dimensional images acousto-optically on long ranges has been demonstrated. (From authors' introduction and summary)

1751.
SMITH, W.J., Jr.
Amplitude modulation of an acoustic wave propagating near the ocean surface.
Nav. Postgrad. Sch., Thesis, 87p. Dec. 1971.
(AD 741 108)

Sixty kHz CW sound was propagated parallel to and near the ocean surface adjacent to an array of four thermistors, a salinometer, a sound velocimeter, a turbulent velocity probe, and a wave-height probe in order to investigate the statistics and environmental causes of amplitude modulation. The temporal variations of the sound amplitude were studied during four twenty-minute runs over a range of 2 meters at varying depths from near the surface to 14 meters during sea-state one conditions in water of 16 meters-depth. Analysis indicated mean percentage amplitude modulation of approximately 5% with a variance of approximately 10-3. (Author) (GRA)

1752.
SMOLIN, J.J. and T.G. Oparina.
Unikal'nyi eksperiment po dlitel' nomu prebyvaniyu cheloveka pod povyshennym davleniem.
[Unique experiment of a prolonged stay of man in a hyperbaric environment].
Voennomed. Zh. 9:58-60;Sept. 1973.

The authors discuss the saturation chamber dive made at the University of Pennsylvania Institute for Environmental Medicine (See Covey, C.W., UnderSea Technol. 12:19-20;Sept. 1971). In this experiment, a simulated depth of about 5,000 feet was attained by substituting neon for helium in the breathing mixture at about 1,200 feet. That is, density of the neon mixture at 1,200 feet was equivalent to what the density of a helium mixture would be at 5,000 feet. These authors do not accept the conclusions of the conductors of the experiment, i.e., that men could work safely at 5,000 feet breathing helium oxygen, since these conditions were simulated, and the physiological effect of helium at such a depth is not known. Certain advantages of neon over helium, such as its lower thermoconductivity, are acknowledged. (OLC/UMS)

1753.
SNIVELY, W.K., Jr. and J. Thuerbach.
Voluntary Hyperventilation as a cause of needless drowning.
J. Kansas Med. Soc. 70:289-292;June 1972.

It is stated here that hyperventilation may well be the cause of many drownings in which the victims are young, healthy, and competent swimmers, and for which there is no discernible cause. Hyperventilation causes the lowering of carbon dioxide tension, which brings on respiratory alkalosis, resulting in numbness and tingling. Low carbon dioxide levels also cause constriction of blood vessels that supply the brain. The oxygen content of the blood becomes exhausted before the carbon dioxide level can raise sufficiently to trigger the impulse to breathe. Several case histories of underwater swimmers who hyperventilated, lost consciousness, and survived, are described, as are some drowning incidents apparently resulting from the effects of hyperventilation. It is noted that the Korean amas seem to have developed a technique of hyperventilating within safe limits. (MFW/UMS)

1754.
SOBEL, H.
High pressure oxygen and age changes.
In: Abstracts of BuMed-ONR sponsored Navywide research in high pressure biomedical research, U.S. Submarine Base, Groton, Conn., May 1971, p.51. Published by the Naval Submarine Medical Research Laboratories, 1971.

Abstract only. Excerpt quoted. There are reasons to believe that high oxygen tension could affect the quantity and physical-chemical characteristics of the fibrous constituents and the ground substance constituents of connective tissue. It could do so by direct action on molecules, through effects on enzymes and metabolic channels, by the formation of H_2O_2 and free-radicals. Mice exposed to 1.08 atm of oxygen in nitrogen for 72 hours each week exhibited 20% increase in fluorescence of collagen and a decrease in sale soluble collagen. However, no other changes consistent with accelerated aging were present. Mice exposed to this environment for an average of 12% of lifespan exhibited no evidence of life shortening. Furthermore, the changes in fluorescence were apparently repaired. A study of the molecular aspects of fluorescence in collagen are underway. It is expected that information acquired will permit a measurement of the amount of previously accrued exposure to high oxygen tension. A procedure has been developed for keeping mice indefinitely for 12 hours each day under 100% O_2 at 632 mm. We will study problems of mortality and morbidity, and life-long effects of O_2 on the connective tissues of skin, bone and lung. In the earlier study no specific effect of O_2 on protein metabolism was found; the observed changes resulted from reduced intake of food. In addition, there was some preliminary observation that a learning deficit appeared in mice previously exposed to high oxygen tension.

1755.
SOCHIVKO, V.P.
Chelovek i avtomat v gidrosfere.
[Man and machine in the hydrosphere].
USSR, Izd-vo Sudostroyeniye, 1974. 198p.

The contents of this monograph are as follows: Ways and problems of mastering and exploiting the hydrosphere; Systems analysis; Psychophysiological barriers and overcoming them; A robot in the hydrosphere; Man-machine systems in the hydrosphere; Engineering use of organic systems; Programming methods to conquer the hydrosphere. (From S & T Alert)

1757.
SOCIETY FOR UNDERWATER TECHNOLOGY
Report by the committee on diver training and performance standards.
Guildford, U.K., IPC Science and Technology, 1972. 15p.

This committee was set up for the purpose of drawing up standards of training and performance for commercial divers. In this report the following subjects are concisely dealt with: selection criteria; medical examination requirements; elements of basic training; additional skills going beyond basic training; standards to be set; currently existing diving schools; record keeping; qualifications for diving instructors; manuals and regulations; legal questions involved in the implementation of the recommendations made. The appendices give such data as medical examinations, syllabus for basic training course, equipment and buildings essential to a diving school, and a list of references of official and non-official publications dealing with diving. (MFW/BSCP)

1758.
SODE, J., E.T. Flynn, R. Bower and W.H. Spaur.
Glucose (Glu), insulin (IRI), cortisol (F) and growth hormone (HGH) during saturation diving.
U.S. Navy Med. 59:20;June 1972.

Abstract only: The authors measured F by fluorometry, IRI and HGH by radioimmunoassay and Glu, BUN (Blood urea nitrogen) and electrolytes by autoanalyzer in ten subjects making a shallow HeO_2 saturation dive; fasting blood samples were obtained just prior to the dive and after one full day's exposure at 75 feet. Whole blood was decompressed, and the serum separated and frozen until analyzed. At 75 feet, serum sodium (Na) was slightly lower ($p < .05$) but other parameters remained unchanged. All HGH values were under 5 ng/ml. Mean values $\pm$ SEM (standard error of the mean) for serum Glu (Mg%), IRI (mcU/ml) and F (mcg%) were: 103 $\pm$ 3.3, 4.4 $\pm$ 0.3, and 22.9 $\pm$ 2.0 respectively before the dive, and 102 $\pm$ 1.8, 4.6 $\pm$ 0.4 and 23.2 $\pm$ 1.3 at 75 feet. Before the dive and at 75 feet, mean values for Glu and F were higher; for IRI and IRI/Glu, ratios were lower than those of fasting basal subjects. This was consistent with the expected adaptive response to the stress of the experiment. The factors contributing to the development of "hyperbaric hypoglycemia" and the role of immersion, depth and saturation exposure require further study.

1759.
SOKOLIANS'KII, I.F.
Vpliv bagatorazovoi dii giperoksii na PO_2 v skeletnikh m'yazakh bilikh shuriv.
[The effect of multiple action of hyperoxia on the PO_2 in the skeletal muscles of albino rats].
Fiziol. Zh. 18:367-371;May/June 1972.

Effect was studied of single and multiple action of hyperoxia up to 4 ata on dynamics PO_2 in skeletal muscles of albino rats. Oxygen tension was determined by means of vitrified electrodes of open type which were calibrated relative to PO_2 of physiological solution. Experiments showed that PO_2 in muscles reaches great values when O_2 pressure in gas phase is 2-4 ata. A gradual decrease of PO_2 in muscles is observed during animals staying on the "ground" for 40 min. With oxygen pressure 4 ata 40 min after PO_2 in muscles decreased by 47.7% of its maximum increasing. After preliminary adaptation to hyperoxia a decrease in oxygen consumption and haemoglobin content in blood was observed. Adaptation to hyperoxia conditioned a lower increment of PO_2 in muscles at oxygen pressures from 1 to 4 ata. (English summary)

1760.
SOLODKOV, A.S. and G.L. Apanasenko.
Osobennosti fiziologicheskikh reaktsii u podvodnikov v poslepokhodovom pernode. [Characteristic physiological reactions in submarine crew members].
Voennomed. Zh. (1):78-80;Jan. 1973.

Physiological changes manifested in submarine personnel during the post-expedition recovery period are fairly constant and can be observed for a considerable length of time following prolonged deepsea expeditions. During expeditions they are exposed to a different regimen of work and rest; cardiac rhythm and metabolic rate are slowed down and muscle tonus is weakened by limited physical activity. A certain degree of fatigue at the end of the trip, return to normal activities and readaptation to a different circadian rhythm during the recovery period are considered by the authors as the main factors. The authors classify their findings into three groups of symptoms, corresponding to three subsequent phases of the recovery period. During the first period immediately after their return to surface the submariners manifest slight tachycardia, mild hypotension, lowered excitability of the parasympathetic nervous system and reduced muscle tonus. More pronounced, and sometimes opposite, reactions characterize the second phase. Increased tachycardia, hypertension, increased excitability of the sympathetic nervous system, tremor, myalgia and edema of the legs were observed, and disappeared during the third stage of the readaptation period. A organized rest and recreation regime aids readaption. (OLC/UMS)

1761.
SOLOWAY, A.H.
Oxygen metabolism — metabolic implications in hyperbaric systems.
Boston, Mass., Northeastern Univ., Final rep. on contract N00014-68-A-0207-0001, 7p. Sept. 7, 1972.
(AD 749 381)

There is the potentiality that hyperbaric oxygen systems accentuate the production of certain oxygenated metabolites and their percursors and these compounds per se may be noxious and capable of causing pathological changes. Certain metabolic pathways have been examined to establish whether in these sequences labile oxygen intermediates such as peroxides and epoxides are formed. This research would serve as the basis for determining whether hyperbaric conditions promote elevated amounts of such compounds. Such a finding would raise distinct long term hazards to hyperbaric conditions in view of the fact that peroxides and epoxides have been shown to be mutagenic and even carcinogenic. (GRA)

1762.
SOMERO, G.N. and P.W. Hochachka.
Biochemical adaptation to the environment.
Amer. Zool. 11:157-165; 1971.

Biochemical adaptation to environmental parameters such as temperature appears to involve two distinct types of changes in the organism's chemistry. On the one hand, the quantities of certain molecular species present in the cells may change. Alternatively, the actual types of molecules present may vary. Rainbow trout (Salmo gairdneri) acclimated to warm and cold temperatures exhibit a striking example of this latter type of adaptation. For all enzymes we have examined in this species, distinct "warm" and "cold" isozymes are present. The isozymes found in warm-acclimated (18°C) trout function well only at temperatures above 10-12°C. The isozymes present in cold-acclimated (4°C) trout function optimally at 2-5°C, temperatures this species normally encounters in winter. These data, plus information on comparable changes in membrane lipids, lead us to propose that adult poikilotherms may undergo a considerable degree of "biochemical restructuring" on a seasonal basis. The factors which control this "restructuring," and the rates at which the process occurs at high and low temperatures, are topics for future investigation. (Authors' abstract)

1763.
SOMERS, L.H.
Research diver's manual.
Ann Arbor, Mich., Univ. Mich., Sea Grant Tech. Rep. 16, MICHU-SG-71-212, 289p. + Append. Aug. 1972.

This manual is directed toward the undergraduate level, covering in clear and concise terms the following subject areas; diving physics, physiological and medical aspects of diving, diving procedures, diving without breathing apparatus, self-contained diving, surface-supplied diving, diving environment. It is illustrated with drawings and photographs and much of the data is tabulated. Appendices present such items as questionnaires, medical examination forms, description of courses, emergency procedures for accidents in the Michigan area, conversion tables and equipment lists. (MFW/SCD)

1764.
SOMERS, L.H.
Selection and training of aquanauts for Hydro-Lab type saturation dives.
Hydro-Lab J. 2(1):97-103; 1973.

Professionally supervised saturation dives at a depth of approximately 50 feet may be successfully and safely undertaken by scientist-divers of limited diving backgrounds. Elaborate aquanaut selection criteria are not deemed necessary for shallow, short-duration saturation dives. In most cases, scientist-divers who have received high-quality basic scuba diver training and acquired a reasonable amount of diving experience, 50 dives or more under all conditions, perform safely and satisfactorily. The diver must be medically qualified and in fairly good physical condition. Personal psychological conditioning to overcome the natural instinct of surfacing in an emergency is probably the most important aspect of individual preparation. A 3-5 day period of habitat and seafloor orientation diving prior to saturation is deemed necessary. (Author's abstract)

1765.
SONNENSCHEIN, R.R.
Symposium on the effects of pressure on organisms.
London, Off. Nav. Res. Rep. ONRL-C-5-72, 12p. Feb. 22, 1972.
(AD 740 094)

At the symposium on the Effects of Pressure on Organisms, held in Bangor, Wales, on 6-10 September 1971, effects of high pressure on physio-chemical systems and on a wide variety of plant and animal forms were discussed as well as anatomical and physiological adaptations of living forms to pressure and submersion. (Author) (GRA)

1766.
SOMOGYI, E.
Clinical and medico-legal aspects of hyperbaric oxygenation.
Z. Rechtsmed. 71(2):79-90; 1973.

Hyperbaric oxygenation as a therapeutic procedure gained considerable popularity during the last decade. It is increasingly applied to severe cases of respiratory and circulatory diseases as well as to cases of poisoning such as with CO and cyanide, and in the course of radiation and tumor therapy. The limitations of the method involve not only technical but also physiological factors. Apart from caisson disease, O_2 toxicity is the most frequent complication. Oxygen toxicity may result from extreme increase of O_2 saturation or air pressure. The sensitivity to O_2 depends to a large extent on the age of the patient and the presence of diseases. The effect of hyperbaric oxygenation is measurable experimentally. Detailed experimentation is indicated prior to clinical application by this method. Widespread application of hyperbaric oxygenation requires detailed investigation of related clinical and morphological problems from a medico-legal aspect. (© BA)

1767.
SOPOV, I.A., G. Apanasenko, Yu. M. Bobrov and V.S. Shchegolev.
Adaptation of submarine crewmen to increased carbon dioxide concentration.
Voennomed. Zh. (7):71-74;July 1973.

The authors briefly summarize previous research, including foreign, with submarine crewmembers and discuss shifts in body function that are primarily due to increased CO_2 concentration in the atmosphere; e.g. bradycardia, increasing delay in inspiration and expiration etc. They state that the organism also has the capability to adapt to increased CO_2; an important factor in adaptation is alkaline reserves in the blood. Their analysis concludes that prolonged stays in an atmosphere of weak CO_2 concentration helps to adapt the body to minor physical stress. Intermittent increases in CO_2 concentration are more effective in this respect than a constant atmosphere of increased CO_2 concentration. However, this effect is apparently short-term, and the authors agree that minor physical stress cannot be used to study working capacity in submarine crewmen. Although improved living quarters in submarines have led to changes in previously recorded body function shifts, an overall decrease in working capacity is still observed. Two tables and a graph are included. (S&T Alert)

1768.
SORKIN, G. and D.H. Kallas.
Hydrospace materials.
J. Hydronautics 5:79-84;July 1971.

The performance under high hydrostatic pressure of the most important deep submergence materials is covered by the paper. Special attention is given to materials with meaningful applications such as titanium, high strength steels and filament wound plastics for structures; buoyancy materials for use external to the pressure capsule and encapsulating materials for external machinery and components. Several novel approaches such as new techniques for welding and fabrication, methods for encapsulation and a new concept for deep submergence buoyancy systems are covered. The fabrication of high strength and exotic metals under field conditions is discussed in detail and several examples of innovative fabricating techniques are illustrated. The paper includes a look at the decade which follows and a prognosis of what can be expected from materials during this period. (Eng. Index)

1769.
SOSS, S.L.
Sensorineural hearing loss with diving.
Arch. Otolaryngol. 93:501-504; 1971.

Sensorineural hearing loss was associated with skin diving in three men. There appeared to be similarities between losses due to barotrauma and noise in one case, suggesting that perceptive losses with diving may not follow a single pattern. [In one case a vigorous Valsalva maneuver was performed prior to hearing loss]. (Author's abstract)

1770.
SOUTHCOTT, R.V.
The effects of the southern Australian marine stinging sponges, Neofibularia mordens and Lissodendoryx sp.
Med. J. Aust. 58-2(18):895-901; 1971.

Injuries from both accidental and experimental contact with the southern Australian marine stinging sponges *N. mordens* Hartman and *Lissodendoryx* sp. are reported. Contact with fresh *Neofibularia* causes a high incidence of dermatitis, the lesions usually lasting weeks or longer, to a maximum of 9 mo. After freezing for 4 yr, thawed *Neofibularia* remains quite toxic. Some toxicity remains after drying for 4 yr; 78-yr-old specimens toxic in 1890 are no longer toxic. Dry sponge, whether fresh or old, is non-toxic; wetting is necessary to activate the toxic agent. The toxic agent is partially resistant to boiling or immersion in soap or formaldehyde solution. An attempt to demonstrate circulating antibody to the sponge by enhancement of response on skin contact after intradermal injection of serum from a sensitive subject into 2 volunteers was unsuccessful. Thawed *Neofibularia* (frozen 4 yr) on the rabbit eye causes acute inflammation of the conjunctiva and periorbital tissues, leading to iritis, corneal clouding and ultimate blindness. It is considered that *Neofibularia* is potentially dangerous to the human eye, e.g., by accidental rubbing by divers or beachcombers. *Lissodendoryx* sp. is also a contact irritant, but causes lesser lesions both to human skin and rabbit eye. In rabbit eye it causes only transient conjunctivitis without permanent effect. Another irritant sponge genus, *Tedania*, also occurs in Australian and New Zealand waters. (JWS) (© BA)

1771.
SPALSBURY, D., Ed.
The working diver, 1972. Symposium proceedings, February 1972, Columbus, Ohio. Washington, D.C., Marine Technology Society, 1972. 300p.

This symposium considers the various practical problems with which operational diving is confronted. These include breathing mixtures, diving systems, the problems of cold, the development of methods of heating divers' suits and breathing mixtures, power sources, and safety precautions. Specific papers will be found under the following author entries: Banks, R.H.; Bentz, R.L.; Bilodeau, D.E.; Bright, C.V.; Delauze, H.G.; Edel, P.O., J.M. Holland, C.L. Fischer and W.B. Fife; Gilardi, G.C.; Green, G.C.; Henkener, J.A. and D.E. Adkins; Jegou, A.; Liffick, G.L. and S.A. Black; Long, R.W.; MacInnis, J.B.; Milweek, W.I., Jr.; Morrissey, G.R.; Rocco, R.M.; Searle, K.; Vaughan, R.W.; Wide, P. (MFW/BSCP)

1772.
SPAUR, W.H.
Dive 1600 feet, 20 April-21 May 1973.
U.S. Navy Exp. Diving Unit, U.S. Nav. Med. Res. Inst., Bur. Med. Surg., Rough draft, 21p. May 20, 1973.

The dive was conducted at the Hyperbaric Research Facility of Taylor Diving and Salvage Company, Inc., New Orleans. It was found that in the chamber, pulmonary ventilation measurements, such as maximum voluntary ventilation, were reduced to 55% of surface value. Most of the impairment occurred between the surface and 1000 feet; however, divers were conscious of breathing with exertion from 1300 feet down, but not at shallow depths. Blood tests revealed no abnormalities of CO_2 partial pressure. The MK10-MOD 4 closed circuit underwater breathing apparatus was used successfully at 1600 feet. Neuromuscular changes were evident below 1000 feet; intention tremor occurred, and fine motor tasks were imperfectly performed. However, no decrement in multi-limb coordination finger dexterity and manual dexterity were observed in tasks with SINBAD. Balance loss was evident and could pose a serious hazard. It is considered likely that, given present procedures and equipment, 1600 feet represents the safe effective depth limit. (MFW/SCD from author's summary)

1773.
SPAUR, W.H., W.R. Braithwaite and W.B. Wright.
Physiological testing — a method for evaluating underwater breathing apparatus.
In: Aerospace Medical Association. 1973 annual scientific meeting. Las Vegas, Nevada, May 1973. Preprints, p.244-245. Published by the Association, 1973.

The testing apparatus consists partly of a fiberglass tank filled with six feet of water. The diver is placed in this "wet pot", on a bicycle ergometer. Before entering the chamber, the diver is prepared by percutaneous cannulation of the radial artery. The cannula is protected until the diver is in position in the tank, then his hand and wrist are put through a water-tight sleeve in the wall of the tank. The cannula is then connected to other apparatus which enable measurements of arterial blood pressure, ECG, inspired oxygen, inspired carbon dioxide, respiratory rate and breathing apparatus pressures. Blood is drawn from the radial artery and tested for oxygen partial pressure, carbon dioxide partial pressure, pH, serum pyruvate and serum lactate. Two types of diver equipment were evaluated in this manner. A prototype hard hat and constant volume dry suit was tested to 200 feet in open circuit air mode and to 300 feet in helium-oxygen recirculating mode. The subjects were able to perform the assigned work tasks, but the CO_2 level became dangerously high at 200 feet. The second type of equipment, a self-contained, closed-circuit, mixed gas underwater breathing apparatus, was tested on three subjects at 1000 feet. Work periods were not completed, CO_2 levels rose excessively, dyspnea occurred, with respiratory rates of up to 36 per minute. The data on the hard hat equipment made it possible to estimate safe working depths for this rig as it now stands. Results of the other test brought about corrective design changes. (MFW/BSCP)

1774.
SPENCER, M.P., N. Simmons and H.P. Clarke.
A precordial transcutaneous cardiac output and aeroemoblism monitor.
Fed. Proc. 30:703; 1971.

Abstract only. Entire item quoted: A 5 mHz CW Doppler ultrasonic unit was developed for use in Dx and Rx on divers for venous gas emboli formed during decompression, as well as monitoring craniotomies and other patient Dx and Rx procedures where there is danger of aeroembolism. The pulmonary blood flow signal is clearly separated from most cardiac motion signals. The sensor employs half-inch square resonant transmitting and receiving crystals, separated by 2 cm, focused at the pulmonary artery 3-7 cm retrosternal, thus avoiding nearfield pickup. In the electronics, one tuned stage followed by two video stages provides 90 db of RF gain, allowing decreased bulk and use of lower transmitter power, while increasing battery life, detector efficiency and safety to the patient. Heart motion signals are further reduced by high-pass filters (cutoff frequency of 500 Hz and attenuation of 35 db at .067 cutoff frequency), installed immediately following the detector, to prevent blocking of the audio by large amplitude, low frequency signals. Low noise transistor stages are used at the inputs of both the RF and the audio section.

1775.
SPENCER, M.P. and H. Okino.
Venous gas emboli following repeated breathhold dives.
Fed. Proc. 31:355;Mar./Apr. 1972.

Abstract only. Entire item quoted: The presence of intravascular gas emboli during decompression of humans after respiration in hyperbaric atmospheres has been established (Occup. Med. 11(5):238,1969). The earliest ultrasonic detectable gas emboli presage decompression illness and the lungs have the capacity to dissipate large volumes of gas. (Aerospace Med. 42(8)822, 1971). Reported cases of breathhold bends have been in association with hyperbaric exposures. We tested for the presence of cardiovascular emboli in a Funado Ama of Japan with the precordial detector (Fed. Proc. 30:703, 1971). It was applied over the left sternal border after a 51 minute period of 30 successive open ocean dives to 15 meters. Descent and ascent required 12 seconds each and dives averaged 53.3 seconds. Besides the usual cardiac signals bubble chirps and clicks were heard, enhanced in numbers by movements of the limbs and lasting one hour without symptoms. These findings though in keeping with asymptomatic bubbles detected on some standard compressed air tables, are surprising considering that presently accepted no-decompression tables allow 100 minutes at 15 meters, and suggest that much smaller super saturation of blood gases than previously recognized may give rise to blood bubbles.

1776.
SPENCER, M.P. and H.F. Clarke.
Precordial monitoring of pulmonary gas embolism and decompression bubbles.
Aerosp. Med. 43:762-767;July 1972.

A 5 mHz cw Doppler ultrasonic detector was developed for use in diagnosis and treatment of venous gas emboli formed in the blood of divers during decompression — or subjects at high altitudes, as well as for monitoring craniotomies and other closed chest procedures where there is danger of aeroembolism. The sensor employs 1/2 inch square resonant transmitting and receiving crystals, separated by 2 cm and focused at the pulmonary artery, 3 to 7 cm retrosternal. In the electronics one turned stage is followed by two video amplifiers providing 90 db of RF gain, allowing decreased bulk and use of lower transmitter power while increasing battery life, detector frequency and safety to the patient. Results with this detector to date indicate decompression venous gas emboli form before arterial embolization and are asymptomatic when first detected by the present unit. (Authors' abstract)

1777.
SPENCER, M.P., D.C. Johanson and H.F. Clarke.
Instruction manual for the IEMP doppler ultrasonic precordial blood bubble detector.
Seattle, Wash., Inst. Environ. Med. Physiol., Final Report on Contract N00014-72-C-0095, 48p. Feb. 15, 1973.
(AD 765 369/4)

A report detailing the operation of a 5 MHz Doppler ultrasonic bubble detector developed for use in detection of venous gas emboli formed in the blood of divers during decompression as well as for monitoring craniotomies, cardiopulmonary bypass equipment and other medical procedures where there is danger of aeroembolism. A precordial sensor employing 1/2 inch square resonant transmitting and receiving crystals separated by 2 cm and focused 2-7 cm retrosternal is employed for the detection of all gas emboli returning in the veins to the right heart and lungs, the precordial sensor, being positioned to the left of the midsternal border over the pulmonary artery and right ventricle. Additional monitoring of the peripheral vasculature through the use of specialized probes is also described. (Authors) (GRA)

1778.
STACHIW, J.D.
Spherical acrylic pressure hulls for undersea exploration.
J. Eng. Ind., p.731-750;May 1971.

The exploratory phase of the research program into the applicability of acrylic to the construction of spherical pressure hulls for undersea exploration has been completed. The findings show that acrylic pressure hulls are as reliable as hulls made from conventional materials if the viscoelastic temperature-dependent properties of the acrylic are taken into account during its design, fabrication and operational service in the sea. The design data and information from the exploratory phase of the R & D program have been already applied to the fabrication of the NEMO Model 600 acrylic capsules with 66-in OD x 61-in ID for 600-ft-depth service. (Author's abstract)

1779.
STACHIW, J.D.
Acrylic pressure hull for submersible NEMO.
Presented at the American Society of Mechanical Engineers meeting September 1971, Houston, Texas, as paper No. 71-UnT-2, 8p.

The acrylic submersible NEMO has been certified by the U.S. Navy for manned operations to 600-ft depth on the basis of an extensive experimental test program for spherical acrylic pressure hulls. This discussion of the NEMO acrylic capsule design is presented because, if other submersible systems incorporating an acrylic spherical pressure hull are of identical or similar design to the NEMO capsule, the existing experimental data can be applied equally well to the other systems. . . If greater operational depths than provided by NEMO capsule (max. 1000 ft) are desired, linear extrapolation of hull dimensions will provide a satisfactory solution for the 1000- to 2000-ft depth range. (Author)

1780.
STACHIW, J.D. and K.O. Gray.
Procurement of safe viewports for hyperbaric chambers.
J. Eng. Ind., p.943-951;Nov. 1971.

Lack of ASME Pressure Vessel Code standards for the selection of material, designs, fabrication techniques, and proof-testing methods for viewports in hyperbaric chambers makes it mandatory that engineering judgement be exercised to the fullest in the procurement of such viewports. Based on the experience gained by the authors in past experimental programs dealing with design criteria and procurement of acrylic viewports for major Navy hyperbaric chamber installations, practical guidelines are proposed for specifying such viewports. The guidelines contained in this paper address themselves to selection of viewport shape, safety factor, material, fabrication, quality control, proof-testing and periodic inspection. (Authors' abstract)

1781.
STACHIW, J.D. and J.R. McKay.
Windows for external or internal hydrostatic pressure vessles. Part VII. Effect of temperature and flange configurations on critical pressure of 90-degree conical acrylic windows under short-term loading.
U.S. Nav. Civil Eng. Lab., Rep. NCEL-TR-773, 55p. Aug. 1972.

Conical acrylic windows of 90-degree included angle and 0.083 to 0.775 thickness-to-minor-diameter (t/D) ratios have been tested to ultimate failure under short-term hydrostatic loading. The ambient temperature was varied from 32F to 90F and the relationship between minor window diameter (D) and minor window cavity diameter in the flange (Df) varied from 0.970 to 1.500. The test results show that the critical pressure of identical windows at 90F is approximately 10% to 20% less than at 70F and at 32 F it is approximately 15% to 25% more than at 70F. To improve the critical pressure of 90-degree conical acrylic windows, it is recommended that such windows be designed with a window/flange mismatch ratio of D/D greater than 1.00, the exact magnitude depending on the window's t/D ratio, service, and design considerations. (Authors) (GRA)

1782.
STACHIW, J.D.
Acrylic plastic hemispherical shells for NUC undersea elevator.
U.S. Nav. Undersea Cent., Rep. NUC-TP-315, 35p. Sept. 1972.
(AD 749 029)

Free-formed, flanged, acrylic hemispherical shells with a nominal 27-in median radius have been experimentally evaluated for service as external pressure hulls with a nominal 56-ft depth. Because the free-forming fabrication technique produces hemispheres with significant variation in thickness, and sphericity, uneven stress distribution results during external hydrostatic loading. As a result, extreme care must be exercised when utilizing free-formed acrylic hemispheres because their elastic instability pressure and magnitude of stresses cannot be predicted on the basis of equations for ideal acrylic spheres. Using an experimental approach to the evaluation of 54-in-median-diameter hemospheres, it was found that nominally 1-in-thick acrylic plate stock is adequately thick for free-forming of shells that will be utilized as pressure hulls for an operational depth of 56 ft. (Author) (GRA)

1783.
STACHIW, J.D.
Transparent materials in the sea.
Prepared for the second international ocean development conference and exhibition, October 1972, Tokyo. NUC TN 732, 33p.

The significance of man's extension into the ocean depths lies not in his mere presence there, but in his ability to perform useful work in an environment to which by his nature he is ill adapted. Still, to successfully complete a majority of undersea missions man must rely on sight, his most acute and versatile sense in an atmospheric environment. To afford himself the utilization of this sense in the new environment he interposes a transparent pressure resistant barrier between his eyes and the hydrospace. The transparent barrier may take the form of a submersible viewport or an all enclosing transparent capsule. With the air of such transparent pressure barriers, he can in comfort visually explore hydrospace, or observe and control work-oriented functions of underwater equipment in his charge. The purpose of this paper is to collect under one cover a summary of all the basic information pertinent to windows and transparent hulls. The first section of the paper concerns itself with the history of viewports and the properties of standard viewport materials; the second, with research in the hydrospace window field; the third, to a summation of viewports in actual use, and the last, on transparent hulls and what can be expected in the future for observation systems. (Author's abstract)

1784.
STACHIW, J.D. and J.R. Maison.
Flanged acrylic plastic hemispherical shells for undersea systems.
U.S. Nav. Undersea Cent., Rep. NUC-TP-355, 104p., Sept. 1973.
(AD-769,213/OGA)

The effects of an equatorial flange and a nonuniform wall thickness upon the critical pressure and stress distribution in acrylic plastic hemispheres were investigated by experimental and analytical methods. Forty acrylic hemispheres were fabricated and tested to destruction under short-term hydrostatic pressure applied on the convex surface. Dome apex displacements were obtained from each specimen and strains were obtained from a selected few. A finite-element elastic analysis was performed on one window configuration for two different boundary conditions and the experimentally derived stresses were used to determine which assumed boundary condition was best for analysis. It appears that in acrylic plastic hemispheres with t/R sub i = or $<$ 0.200 an integral equatorial flange has no deleterious effect on the critical pressure of the hemisphere. Reduced wall thickness at the apex, however, significantly reduces the critical pressure of flanged and flangeless hemispheres. Critical pressures of hemispheres with varying wall thickness correlate well with the mean wall thickness. Axial displacements of the apex under hydrostatic loading were found to be approximately of the same magnitudes for both flanged and flangeless shells of constant thickness. The displacements of flanged shells with variable thickness were significantly higher than of flanged shells with constant thickness when the comparison was made at the same nominal t/R sub i ratio. (Authors) (GRA)

1785.
STARK, E.F., R.Y. Nishi, J.L. Babcock, W.H. Daley and R.W. Turner.
Operation and calibration manual for the Mark VIS Pneumatic Analogue Decompression Computer.
Downsview, Ontario, Canada, Def. Div. Inst. Environ. Med., Def. Res. Board, Rep. DCIEM 939, 29p. May 1973.

The Mark VIS Pneumatic Analogue Decompression Computer is used for controlling decompression of subjects in an hyperbaric chamber or of divers in the open ocean. This manual describes the operation, calibration and maintenance procedures for the pneumatic and mechanical sections of the computer. (Authors' abstract)

1786.
STEES, J.L. and O.R. Brown.
Effects of hyperoxia on sulfhydryl concentration of "Escherichia coli".
Columbia, Mo., Univ. Mo., Space Sci. Res. Cent., Rep. TR-4, 26p. July 1972.
(AD 746 193)

The concentration of reduced sulfhydryl (SH) in cell-free extracts of Escherichia coli grown with air as the gas phase was 26.8 plus or minus 1.2 mnoles SH/mg soluble protein. Exposure of bacteria to 1 ata of oxygen where growth continued but at a reduced rate, or to 6.2 ata of oxygen where growth was completely stopped, did not result in significant changes in intracellular SH concentration. Cell-free extracts exposed to 1.2 ata of oxygen resulted in SH oxidation at 0.5%/min, compared to 0.75%/min for reduced glutathione at 4.2 ata. Fractionation of cell-free extracts by ultrafiltration indicated that approximately 92% of the measurable SH-groups were protein-related. These data indicate that neither oxidation of intracellular SH, nor the relatively slow oxidation of surface SH-groups is a significant factor in the rapid growth inhibition of E. coli by hyperoxia. Bacteria reversal of possible intracellular SH oxidation during the interval between decompression and extraction was not excluded. (Authors) (GRA)

1787.
STEES, J.L. and O.R. Brown.
Stability of yeast fatty acid synthetase component enzymes to irreversible inactivation by hyperbaric oxygen.
Microbios 8(31/32):247-256; 1973.

Fatty acid synthetase, purified 120-fold from bakers' yeast, was exposed to O_2 at 40.2 atm absolute pressure for 1 h at 20 C. Optical assays, containing mercaptan and based on rates of oxidation of NADPH, were used to measure the activities of the complex with the following substrates: acetyl-CoA and malonyl-CoA and malonyl-CoA for measuring the complete reaction sequence; acetoacetyl-CoA; acetoacetyl-CoA, plus malonyl-CoA, and cortonyl-CoA only, for the 2nd reduction. The condensation step was estimated separately by a radioactive assay. None of the component enzyme activities were detectably reduced by hyperoxic exposure. (© BA)

1788.
STEFANELLI, A.
L'effetto biologico delle elevate pressioni idrostatichei realizzazione di alcuni apparecchi per l' osservazione diretta del materiale.
[The biological effect of high hydrostatic pressures: Construction of apparatus for direct observation of the material].
Atti Acad. Naz. Lincei Rend. Cl. Sci. Fis. Mat. Nat. Sez III 52(4):569-572; 1972.

Experimental data of Marsland and Pease on the inhibitory effects of hydrostatic pressure (about 300-400 atm) on cell division, as observed in segmenting eggs of various animal species, prompted an investigation of embryonic morphogenesis in which cell division occurs with cell degeneration and movements. To this aim, three pressurized chambers were devised: twoof them allow for direct observation of specimens, one being suitable for pressure values up to 600 atm, the other for values up to 1500 atm, while in the third chamber it is possible to fix specimens under pressure, either by means of a fixative or by freezing. (© BA)

1789.
STEGALL, P.J., K.H. Smith and J. Hildebrandt.
Aseptic bone necrosis and hematologic changes in miniature pigs as the result of compression/decompression exposures.
Fed. Proc. 31:653;Mar./Apr. 1972.

Abstract only. Entire item quoted: Aseptic bone necrosis was produced in one of five miniature pigs exposed to a combination of decompression profiles varying in rate from fast (65.5 fpm) to slow (5-1.3 fpm). A suspicious area in one of the femoral metaphyses found three months after the pig's initial dive became more radiolucent in the following three months, and additional radiolucencies were noted in the other femur and bilaterally in the humeri. A diagnosis of aseptic bone necrosis was confirmed by biopsy. "Bends" thresholds fell in each pig with successive stress; one possible explanation for this induced sensitivity may be the presence of gas nuclei persisting from one exposure to the next, initiating bubble formation at lower degrees of supersaturation. After each exposure, significant decreases in fibrinogen concentration and thrombin times were noted. Platelet adhesiveness was elevated 25% immediately post-dive, but platelet counts were maximally decreased ($>$50%) 24-48 hours later. Reticulocyte counts fell significantly as well. CPK levels increased markedly in samples drawn after both fast and slow decompression rates, while LDH values fell by $>$30% in the same samples. Serum lipid levels rose $>$ 30%, with the greatest changes being in triglycerides and phospholipids. Hematologic and chemical changes were not always accompanied by observable symptoms, suggesting that disseminated intravascular coagulation (consistent with this picture) may occur without clinical evidence of decompression sickness.

1790.
STEGALL, P.J., K. Smith and J. Hildebrandt.
Selective platelet destruction and dysbaric osteonecrosis in miniature pigs after decompression. Fed. Proc. 32(3,pt.1):835;Mar. 1973.

Abstract only. Entire item quoted: Of 11 pigs chronically exposed to hyperbaric pressure (60 fsw for 6 hrs.) with fast decompression (30 fpm), 3 died of decompression sickness or "the bends". The remaining developed dysbaric osteonecrosis within 6 weeks to 1 year, seen by biopsy or radiographically. Osteonecrosis here is due to occlusion of bone blood flow as seen histologically. To better explain the observed thrombocytopenia and bone infarcts, a kinetic study of platelet and fibrinogen survival and turnover times was done. While fibrinogen values remained essentially unchanged, platelet survivals shortened from a normal 5 days ($\pm$ .5 days) to 1 day ($\pm$ .2 days) following single exposures with fast decompression. These values remained shortened up to 6 weeks at which time a progressive return to normal baseline was documented. Platelet plugs, bubbles and probable endothelial damage were seen histologically. Either abnormal surfaces (e.g., bubbles) or endothelial injury may be responsible for this predominant platelet destruction; because [the shortening of the survival time] persists, however, we interpret the data as disseminated vessel damage. Present studies will determine if platelet function inhibitors are able to interrupt the increased rate of consumption, and in turn lead to prevention of osteonecrosis.

1791.
STERK, W.
Effect of SCUBA diving on pulmonary compliance.
In: Abstracts of the Twenty-fifth Congress of Physiological Sciences Satellite Symposium. Recent progress in fundamental physiology of diving, Marseille, France, July 1971, p.27-28. (Proceedings unpublished)

Abstract only: Dynamic pulmonary compliance in shallow water was measured (in 1/cm H_2O) for five divers. During half an hour in prone position the mean value went from 0.123 to 0.105; in the upright position, for 15 minutes, mean values were 0.098 at one minute, 0.096 at five minutes, and 0.101 at 15 minutes. These values compare with 0.211 at surface pressure without equipment. The author believes that prolonged pulmonary vascular congestion could play a role in compliance reduction; another explanation is that since the respiratory muscles do not relax on expiration, due to negative pressure, the level of breathing decreases and the compliance is reduced. Recordings of the quasi-static lung compliance show that the expiratory reserve volume is largely decreased during diving. This may be due to a craniad displacement of the abdomen-diaphragm. The vital capacity decrease during diving, of 22% in the prone position and 25% in the upright position may result from the closure of lung units, the hydrostatic forces, and the diving equipment working against the respiratory muscles, and also to the possible increase of intrathoracic blood volume. (MFW/BSCP)

1792.
STERK, W.
Respiratory mechanics of diver and diving apparatus.
Utrecht, Netherlands, Drukkerij Elinkwijk, 1973. 129p.

The author was asked to advise on the physiological aspects of a semi-closed circuit breathing apparatus being developed for the Royal Netherlands Navy. In order to do this, he studied the lung mechanics involved in the interrelationship of the diver and the apparatus as tested in a wet hyperbaric chamber. Only resting conditions were studied; the exercise fact will have to be considered separately. One chapter deals with measurements made on recording instruments, the next describes the apparatus itself, the next two concern the diver's pulmonary dynamics and energetics and his pulmonary compliance. The final short conclusive chapter sums up the physiological relationship between the diver and his breathing apparatus. The author notes the need for accurate recording instruments with which to monitor the diver's respiratory mechanics during actual diving. It is only by such means that the physiologist can determine the depth limits of current breathing equipment, and obtain the data necessary to enable the equipment designer to improve breathing apparatus. (MFW/UMS)

1793.
STERN, S.A. and H.L. Frisch.
Dependence of inert gas narcosis on lipid "free volume".
J. Appl. Physiol. 34:366-373;Mar. 1973.

This paper suggests that the anesthetic (or narcotic) potency of metabolically inert gases is due to their effect on the "free volume" of a bulk lipid phase, possibly in the cell membrane. According to this hypothesis, narcosis occurs when the inert gas dissolved in the lipid phase causes the free volume to exceed a specific threshold value. The anesthetic potency of a gas depends not only on its lipid solubility, as postulated by the Meyer-Overton hypothesis, but also on the thermal expansivity and compressibility of the lipid phase as well as the environmental temperature and hydrostatic pressure. The new hypothesis is expressed in quantitative terms and shown to be in good agreement with experimental data from the literature for both pure gases and gas mixtures. In particular, the theory offers an explanation for the reported pressure reversal of inert gas narcosis and predicts that it should be possible to reverse this type of narcosis also by a change of temperature. Experimental approaches for further testing of the free-volume hypothesis are outlined. (Authors' abstract)

1794.
STETSULA, V.I., I.I. Tal'ko and V.M. Krivenko.
E sperimental'noe obosnovanie primeneniya khimotripsina pri lechenii ascepticheskogo nekroza kostei.
[Experimental study of chymotrypsin in the treatment of aseptic necrosis of bone].
Ortop. Travmatol. Protez. 34:72-74;Jan. 1973.

The authors studied the action of chymotrypsin on experimental aseptic necrosis in dogs. Development by radiographic and histological methods. In the chymotrypsin-treated animals regenerative processes in the bone tissue and bone marrow were observed. Chymotrypsin enhanced blood circulation by speeding up revascularization in the necrotic tissues. Fresh erythrocytes, macrophages and neutrophilic leukocytes were detected in the necrotized zone, proving that chymotrypsin stimulated the hematopoietic activity in the regenerating bone marrow. The dogs were observed for three to four months following the initial induction of thrombosis. Chymotrypsin was administered in repeated ten-day courses. On the 180th day the bone structure was found to be completely regenerated, regardless of the extent of the necrosis. The authors theorize that parenterally administered chymotrypsin stimulates local blood circulation by depolymerizing proteins in the necrotic inflammation zone. Blood circulation enhances bone regeneration as well as the hematopoietic activity of bone marrow. Based on experimental results, the authors recommend repeated doses of chymotrypsin in the treatment of aseptic necrosis in man. (OLC/UMS)

1795.
STETZNER, L.C. and B. De Boer.
Thermal balance in the rat during exposure to helium-oxygen from 1 to 41 atmospheres.
Aerosp. Med. 43:306-309;Mar. 1972.

Changes in temperature, heart rate, and respiration rate were recorded for control rats at 1 ATA in air at 76°F or He-O_2 at 86°F, and for experimental animals in He-O_2 at 86° during compression to 41 ATA, maintenance at this pressure for 4 hours, and decompression. Comparisons showed that surface, subcutaneous, and rectal temperatures decreased during compression but returned to normal upon decompression. Heart rate, respiration rate, O_2 consumption increased during exposure and returned to normal levels when the animals were decompressed. In a second experimental group, core temperature was maintained at the control level by increasing the chamber temperature to approximately 94°F during compression, maintaining it at this level during exposure to 41 ATA, and decreasing the chamber temperature during decompression. When the decompression core temperature was maintained, other temperature parameters, heart and respiratory rates, and oxygen consumption remained at control levels. Weight increase for rats in He-O_2 at 1 ATA was less than for the air controls. Rats exposed to 41 ATA with variable chamber temperature lost weight during the experiment, but less than those maintained at 86° during exposure to 41 ATA. (Authors' abstract)

1796.
STETZNER, L.C. and B. DeBoer.
A comparison of helium, nitrogen, and nitrous oxide on rat rectal temperature under normobraic and hyperbaric conditions.
Fed. Proc. 31:549;Mar./Apr. 1972.

Abstract only. Entire item quoted: The use of artificial environments in the study of animal and human adaptability has resulted in some concern about temperature regulation during exposure to gases at high pressure. Male rats were placed in plexiglass housings and a YSI 402 thermistor probe was inserted 6.0 cm. to obtain rectal temperature (R.T.). Groups of 6 rats were placed in a hyperbaric chamber controlled throughout all the experiments at 86°F. The effects of nitrous oxide (N_2O) in concentrations of 7, 14, and 21 psi were compared with nitrogen (N_2) controls. Six and 21 ATA of N_2 were compared with 21 and 41 ATA Helium (He). (6ATA N_2 is nearly equidense to 41 ATA He). A mixture of 10.5 psi N_2O and 21 ATA He was compared with 21 ATA N_2. The effects of 41 ATA He combined with 21 psi N_2O are reported. Our results indicated: R.T. N_2O, 14, and 21 psi, no change; R.T. with 6 ATA N_2, little change. Significant decreases occurred in order with 21 ATA He $<$ 21 ATA $N_2 \ll$ 21 ATA (He + 10.5 psi N_2O) $\ll$ 41 ATA He $\ll$ 41 ATA (He + 21 psi N_2O). All temperatures returned to normal at the end of decompression. These changes are interpreted for a combination of gas properties — lipid solubility (narcosis), conduction, convection and density.

1797.
STETZNER, L.C. and B. De Boer.
Changes in rats during exposure to nitrous oxide at 7, 14, and 21 psi with physiologic levels of oxygen and nitrogen to a total pressure 36 psi.
Aerosp. Med. 43:729-731;July 1972.

Rectal temperature (RT), heart rate (HR), and respiration rate (RR) were recorded for control rats at 36 psi (absolute) N_2-O_2 and for experimental nitrous oxide (N_2O) groups with dilutions of 7, 14 and 21 psi. (Total exposure at 36 psi was four hours, and chamber temperature was 86°F) RT showed little change. Slight increases in HR occurred with 7 and 14 psi N_2O and were maximal with 21 psi. There was no difference in RR with 7 psi, but significant increases at both 14 and 21 psi. O_2 consumption showed increases of 20% at 7 and 40% at 14 psi but little change at 21 psi. A slight increase in activity was observed at 7 psi. A decrease in coordination and an increase in irregular bursts of activity were observed throughout the four hours of exposure at 14 psi. Animals subjected to 21 psi N_2O were anesthetized (AD_{100}). All animals recovered rapidly upon removal of the N_2O by decompression and flushing with N_2-O_2. (Authors' abstract)

1798.
STEWART, J.R.
Marine technicians handbook: Procedures for shipboard diving.
The University Guide for diving safety.
San Diego, Cal., Univ. Cal., Inst. Mar. Resources, Rep. IMR-TR-23, 35p. Nov. 1971.
(COM 72-10,699)

The first part of this handbook provides a university guide for diving safety. It contains information on the policy on diving, training, certification, scuba equipment and diving rules. The second part presents emergency procedures for university divers in the La Jolla, California area and recompression chamber listings. Procedures for shipboard diving are given in the third part. (Author) (GRA)

1799.
STILES, R.E.
Submarines for deep water pipelining.
Pipe Line Ind. 38:64-66;June 1973.

The International Hydrodynamics Co., Ltd., has been awarded a contract to assist in the laying of cable on the Canadian continental shelf, using the new submersible Pisces V, now under completion at North Vancouver. A drawing shows a submersible as it might appear if designed especially for pipelining. Pipe aligners consist of hydraulic pistons protruding from the bottom of the sub. A habitat is built into the sub amidships, and extends over the pipe ends to be joined. A life support system, connected to the outer shell of the habitat, will permit divers to work at depths of 600 feet for six hours. The living compartments contain six bunks, two fresh water systems, sanitary facilities, heat and air-conditioning. All compartments have instrumentation, communication systems, closed circuit television cameras and viewing ports. Depth pressure, breathing mixture, and atmosphere control are automatic but can also be operated manually. The methods by which the pipe would be carried, laid, and welded are described in some detail. (MFW/BSCP)

1800.
STOLL, A.P.
Purification of helium-oxygen diving mixtures for recirculation.
Underwater J. 4:124-126;June 1972.

In this technical note, the author describes and explains a closed helium-oxygen purification system. Helium is a very expensive gas, and must be re-used if an operation is to be economically feasible. The principle here is cryogenic purification, by which method oxygen, nitrogen and most other impurities such as carbon monoxide and methane are separated out of the mixture, with very little loss of helium. The system described is one developed and constructed by the British Oxygen Company. Detailed drawings and diagrams accompany the article. (MFW/BSCP)

1801.
STONE, H.L., K. Gray, R. Stabe and J.M. Chandler, Jr.
Renal blood flow in a diving trained sea lion.
Nature 242:530-531;Apr. 20, 1973.

The authors investigated the peripheral circulation of a sea lion by measuring the renal flow response to face immersion in water. Previous investigations had indicated cessation of flow to the kidney. However, these studies had been carried out with restrained and frightened animals. In the present study, a trained, unrestrained animal was used. Apparently, inflow to the kidney did not cease, but was reduced along with the cardiac output, as in the duck. The authors suggest that "oxygen may be conserved in the kidney by shunting blood around highly metabolic areas such as cortex, and simultaneously these shunts may be used to adjust vascular resistance to ensure adequate O_2 to the heart and brain and to reduce the work of the heart specifically. (MFW/SCD)

1802.
STRAUSS, M.B.
The challenge of cold water.
Skin Diver 20:66-67;Mar. 1971.

The author discusses the medical effects of reduction of core temperature: (1) shunting of blood; the blood is shunted from the extremities to the trunk; (2) metabolism; shivering increases body heat production five to seven-fold and exercise ten to twenty-fold. However, the demands made overhsadow the beneficial effects. Divers conditioned to cold have a shivering threshold of a much lower temperature. (3) Insulation; subcutaneous fat is the most effective insulator. (4) Body shape; when the ratio of surface area to body mass is lower, heat loss is reduced. As to methods of conserving the body's heat under water, the wet suit conserves the body's own metabolic heat, but does not provide any supplemental heat. Electrical, nuclear and chemical sources of heat have been found unsatisfactory and dangerous. The hot water circulatory system seems at this time to be the most satisfactory method of providing heat. The answer to the need for noncompressible material still remains to be found. Cold makes the diver more susceptible to decompression sickness, nitrogen narcosis and oxygen toxicity, and reduces the quality of his performance, both manual and mental. (MFW/BSCP)

1803.
STRAUSS,M.B., W.S. Lee and R.W. Cantrell.
Serous otitis media in divers breathing 100% oxygen.
In: Aerospace Medical Association. 1973 annual scientific meeting, Las Vegas, Nevada, May 1973. Preprints. p.149. Published by the Association, 1973.

Underwater Demolition Team, SEAL trainees were observed to develop serous otitis media after diving with high concentration of oxygen. They were not manifested until after a night's sleep. Although a cause of oxygen otitis media had been hypothesized previously, the possibility that elevated oxygen partial pressures produce a toxic effect on the mucosa of the middle ear is raised. (Authors' summary)

1804.
STRAUSS, R.H. and L.D. Prockop.
Decompression sickness among scuba divers.
JAMA 223(6):637-640; 1973.

Severe deficits, including paraplegia, may be avoided if hyperbaric therapy is begun soon after the onset of neurological symptoms of decompression sickness. (© BA)

1805.
STREDA, A.
Participation of osteonecrosis in the development of severe coxarthrosis.
Acta Univ. Carol. Med. Monogr. 46:9-166; 1971.

This extensive monograph is divided into two sections: (1) Detailed analysis of the x-ray picture of osteonecrosis of the hip joint; (2) Participation of osteonecrosis in the development of severe coxarthrosis. There is a short discussion devoted to hyperbaric osteonecrosis, in which it is stated that "extensive necrotic change in the hip joint was first described in caisson workers." It is attributed to gas embolism. The differences between necrosis from caisson disease and that caused by infarction are discussed, both as to developmental characteristics and location. (MFW/BSCP)

1806.
STREIMER, I.
Human performance characteristics in a complex manual task underwater.
Hum. Factors 14:95-99;Feb. 1972.

Five subjects executed a complex maintenance task at a pool depth of six feet. Heart rate, oxygen uptake, and task accomplishment times were continuously monitored. The results indicate that significant performance degradations may be anticipated during the performance of manual work under water. (Author's abstract)

1807.
STREIMER, I., D.P.W. Turner, L. Volkmer and P. Pryor.
A study of forced-pace work characteristics at a 33-foot working depth.
San Diego, Cal., Man Factors, Inc., Rep. MFI 72-123, 52p. Sept. 1972.

Certain human performance characteristics developed during the execution of simple repetitive manual work at a depth of 33 feet were studied in the open sea. The task examined was the counterclockwise rotation of a crank for a period of 10 minutes. Cranking radius was nine inches and cranking resistance level was six pounds. This task was executed in the following modes: 1. Self-paced, self-selected rest modes. 2. Work rates 10, 20 and 30 percent greater than that selected in the self-paced mode. 3. Work rates 10, 20 and 30 percent greater than that selected in the self-paced mode performed in two work-rest cycle formats: (a) three 30-second rest periods, equally spaced in the ten minute work cycle; (b) ten nine-second rest periods, equally spaced in the ten minute work cycle. Performance measurements included work output (horsepower), breathing gas consumption (liters air/min), standard temperature pressure, dry (STPD), oxygen uptake (liters oxygen/min, STPD), pulmonary efficiency (percent oxygen removed from air), heart rate, and carbon dioxide production (CO_2 percent). The obtained values are discussed with respect to the results of previous studies performed at working depths of 5, 33 and 66 feet. The principal findings may be summarized thus: 1. In the self-selected rest work mode statistically significant differences were found as follows: (a) Breathing gas consumption increased in positively accelerating fashion with increased work load. (b) Oxygen uptake increased linearly with increased work load. (c) Pulmonary efficiency decreased linearly with increased work load. 2. No significant differences attributable to work-rest periods — work load interactions were found. 3. Traditional ergonomic relationships such as oxygen/pulse ratios, work pulse index were found applicable to evaluation of worker effort/task difficulty interactions. (Authors' abstract)

1808.
STRICKLAND, C.L. and R.L. Hittleman.
Analysis of three lighting sources.
Offshore 32:72, 75-76, 79;Aug. 1972.

The purpose of this paper is not to concentrate on any one problem but to provide, through a series of controlled experiments, more data to the system engineer to help him overcome some of the many problems involved in the application of underwater light sources. These lights are the three most common underwater sources in use today. They are: the tungsten quartz iodide light; the mercury vapor, and the mercury-thallium iodide light. . . . Each of the three lights have distinct advantages for certain specialized applications, but as a general light source, the thallium lamp appears to have a significant advantage for most applications. And as smaller and more efficient ballast transformers are developed and design improvements are made to the thallium lamp to increase its operating life, this light should become the primary underwater light source in the next few years. (Authors)

1809.
STRICKLAND, C.L.
Underwater television — its development and future.
Underwater J. 5:244-249;Dec. 1973.

In the past ten years, underwater television systems have evolved from bulky, unreliable studio-type cameras mounted in watertight housings to miniature, highly portable units capable of extending man's vision into the most rugged environments. The reason for this evolution has been the development of cameras designed specifically for use underwater and their acceptance as useful tools for virtually any application where man must extend his visual capability in order to do useful work. This evolution process is continuing towards highly sophisticated underwater television systems designed for specialized work such as offshore drilling in deep water, underwater mining, sewer and pipeline inspection, ship-hull inspection and many others. (Author's abstract)

1810.
STROME, S.B., M.W. Kalland and H.D. Meen.
Potentiation of diving bradycardia during exercise.
In: Abstracts of the Twenty-fifth Congress of Physiological Sciences Satellite Symposium. Recent progress in fundamental physiology of diving. Marseille, France, July 1971, p.8-9; (Proceedings unpublished)

Abstract only. Excerpts quoted: Fifteen healthy subjects ranging in age from 21 to 37 years were exposed to face immersion superimposed on various states of apneic rest and exercise. The exercise was performed on a bicycle ergometer and face immersion accomplished by elevating a water-filled container. The following test maneuvers were conducted: (1) Face immersion during rest after apnea for respectively 10, 20, 30 and 40 sec. (2) Face immersion during exercise after apneic exercise for respectively 5, 10, 15 and 20 sec. Results showed a significant potentiation of the diving bradycardia occurred when approximately 10 sec of apneic exercise preceded the face immersion. Face immersion superimposed on 15 or 20 sec of apneic exercise did not further enhance the bradycardia. Based on these results it was reasonable to hypothesize that diving bradycardia possibly is potentiated when some level of hypercapnia is established, in our experiments, the state of hypercapnia reached after approximately 10 sec of apneic exercise prior to face immersion. In order to examine this possibility, five subjects were exposed to face immersion superimposed on steady state of exercise while breathing air containing various concentrations of carbon dioxide (2, 4, 6 and 8%). Blood samples were drawn from a prewarmed fingertip at rest (breathing normal air), and immediately prior to face immersion, which was initiated after 6-8 min of steady state exercise (breathing carbon dioxide). The results show that while breathing the various concentrations of carbon dioxide the subjects exhibited PCO_2 values in the blood ranging from 41 to 70 mm Hg (pH 7.38 to 7.23) prior to face immersion. However, no potentiation of the diving bradycardia could be detected under these conditions. Thus, it appears that hypercapnia per se cannot be held responsible for the observed potentiation of diving bradycardia.

1811.
STRUMZA, M.-V.and J. Hainaut.
Facteurs impliques dans les variations de la coagulation en fonction de la baisse de la pression d'oxygene dans le sang arteriel.
[Factors implicated in clotting changes as a function of the decrease of oxygen pressure in arterial blood].
C.R. Soc. Biol. 165(6):1229-1232; 1971.

Coagulability of dog blood was determined by the Howell test in a siliconized tube, by thromboelastography (TEG) on platelet-rich plasma and on platelet-free plasma with dilute cephalin and Ca. The value of r+k [clotting time] in the TEG was 14.2 in normoxic animals. In moderate hypoxia above an arterial O_2 partial pressure [PaO_2] of 35 torr, coagulability diminished regularly, and r+k was 24.4. For PaO_2 between 10-35 torr, there was a shortened clotting time (r+ k = 13.6). This was accentuated in extreme hypoxia (r+k = 8.2). There is thus a clotting delay in moderate hypoxia. In moderate hypoxia, the constant "a" of the TEG, which reflects fibrinogenemia and the thrombodynamic function of the platelets, is decreased. In severe hypoxia, it is increased to 70 mm (normal 63 mm). That platelet factors must intervene in these effects and is suggested also by the cephalin test, which shows a progressive increase in clotting time with hypoxia; platelet factors overwhelm the effect in severe hypoxia to produce hypercoagulability. (MDS) (© BA)

1812.
STUART, D.L. and A.A. Arseneaux.
New gas mixtures allow deeper diving.
Offshore 33:130,132,135;May 1973.

The authors discuss the development of breathing mixture technology, noting the increasing accuracy with which mixtures are prepared, thanks to such techniques as gas chromatography, infrared-spectrography, polarography and micro-fuel cell oxygen analysis. When large quantities of helium must be transported over large distances, it can be converted into liquid form. Air Products and Chemicals, Inc. is the company whose accomplishments in the field of manufacturing, storing, and shipping breathing mixtures under conditions of ever-increasing quality control are discussed here. (MFW/SCD)

1813.
STUCKER, F.J. and W.B. Echols.
Otolaryngic problems of underwater exploration.
Milit. Med. 136:896-899;Dec. 1971.

The popularity of underwater activity by the scientist and sportsman is constantly increasing, and the ENT problems associated with diving need to be understood by the general practitioner. The most common complaints stem from the diver's inability to equalize pressures in his middle ear and sinuses, and prevention as well as therapy are directed at clearing the natural ostia and aerating passages. This may be done by the use of decongestants, nose drops, and patience, while allowing the upper respiratory infection to clear. Complications of pressure differentials, such as acute sinusitis or otitis media, are treated with appropriate antibiotics in addition to the preceding means. The most serious problems arise from Boyle's Law of pressure-volume changes, and primarily affect the deep water diver. The rapid expansion of intrapulmonary gases will rupture the lung if the glottis is closed, and bubbles forming in the blood stream and tissues will produce vascular occlusion and tissue destruction, if the schedule for resurfacing is not adhered to. Therapy of these problems lies primarily in recompressing the victim as soon as possible. (Authors' summary)

1814.
STUTZER, H. and H.W. Buchholz.
Operative behandlung der Socarthrose bei Caissonkrankheit.
[Surgical treatment of coxarthrosis in caisson disease].
Mschr. Unfallheilk. 76:524-527;Nov. 1973.

A total hip prosthesis in a case of coxarthrosis following decompression sickness is described. The importance of this method is discussed. (From English summary)

1815.
SUDBURY, J.D.
Cotrolled depth, submerged barge for Arctic transport is feasible and economical.
Offshore 32:47-50;Aug. 1972.

A new concept, which should extend the conditions under which barges are economically attractive, will involve towing a submerged barge at a controlled depth below the ocean surface. . . This is primarily a description of Continental Oil Company's efforts to develop a system for hauling 2-million barrels per day of crude from the North Slope of Alaska to the East Coast of the U.S. . . . Designs for an icebreaker, submersible barge and control systems to traverse these Northwest Passage conditions were completed. Cost analysis shows that the towed barge system should be able to haul crude oil from Prudhoe to the East Coast of U.S. for $1.50/barrel with a 19% return on investment. Design and construction of a 1/10 scale model is proposed before any final conclusions about feasibility of this system. (Author)

1816.
SUGIURA, H., S. Suzuki and S. Kato.
Investigations on the fibrinolytic activity of human urine. Effects of hyperbaric oxygen on the fibrinolytic activities in blood and urine.
Jap. J. Urol. 63:43-56;Jan. 1972.

Exposure of subjects to oxygen at increased pressure has lately been found of several clinical applications. Hyperbaric oxygen has been advocated in the management of certain medical and surgical conditions. However, the effect of oxygen at high atmospheric pressure (OHP) on the living body, especially on fibrinolytic activity remains unknown. This study was undertaken to determine, in 20 cases of urological diseases with hematuria, the effect of oxygen at 3 atmospheres absolute (3 ATA) on the fibrinolytic activities of circulating blood and urine. Whole plasmin activity was found to be increased but activities of proactivator, plasminogen activator and antiplasmin were not found to be changed. These changes are believed to be caused by stress brought about by oxygen at increased tensions. On the other hand, oxygen at 3 atmosphere pressure produced a decrease in the fibrinolytic activities of urine (fresh urine and extract of urine prepared with 2M-KSCN). It is suggested that this change may in part be caused by renal vasoconstriction brought about by oxygen at increased tensions and by oxygen poisoning of the renal tubular cell enzyme systems. These seem to indicate that the kidneys act not as regulators of circulating fibrinolytic activity but as independent contributors to this activity and that the quantities provided so far as at present is known are determined by the rate of blood flow through the kidneys. (English summary)

1817.
SUSHKOV, F.V., V.V. Portugalov, L.N. Smolenskaya, Z.L. Sorvacheva, R.LL Arndt, A.G. Dianov and V.V. Isayenko.
Biologicheskaya otsenka vliyaniya gelio-kislorodnoi sredy na kul'tury I letok mlekipitayushikh. [Biological evaluation of the effect of the oxygen-helium atmosphere on the mammalian cell culture].
Kosm. Biol. Med. 7:38-43;July/Aug. 1973.

The cultivation of animal and human cells in vitro in the oxygen-helium atmosphere induced no noticeable changes in the morphological and physiological parameters of the tested cultures. No changes were observed in 10 subsequent generations during the successive passages of the cultures under the conditions studied. (English summary)

1818.
SUTTON, D. and E.M. Taylor.
A research program on hyperbaric environmental effects upon primates and other animals.
Tempe, Ariz., Ariz. State Univ., Rep. 71-F, Nov. 1, 1971.
(AD 735 117)

The contract developed and tested sensitive methodologies for measuring sensory and motor impairment in hyperbaric environments. The measures are generally applicable to various animal species, and their results are similarly generalizable. (Author) (GRA)

1819.
SUZUKI, J.
Intelligibility of helium speech.
In: United States-Japan conference on natural resources development. Proceedings of the first joint meeting of the U.S.-Japan panel on diving and technology, Tokyo, 1972, p.55-59, Japan, Ministry of Agriculture and Forestry, 1972.

Syllable articulation and confusion in the perception of helium speech are measured and discussed. It is revealed that the intelligibility of speech decreases when the pressure increases, and verbal communication will be lost under high pressure. Data on the confusion will be utilized for designing an unscrambler translating helium speech into intelligible speech, and for selection or synthesis of understandable words in underwater speech communication. Moreover, analysis of confusion gives some suggestion for the mechanism of speech perception in human. Physical and perceptual analysis of helium speech are being carried out because unknown problems still remain and helium voice unscramblers are being developed by several methods. (Author's conclusions)

1820.
SWAN, J.W.
Glass-reinforced plastics under high pressure.
Underwater J. 5:101-109;June 1973.

Of all the materials for possible use in construction of deep submersibles, glass-reinforced plastic has some undoubted attractions including high specific strength, resistance to corrosion and fouling, ease of construction and more. Some of its drawbacks, however, include weakness in bonded joints and low interlaminar shear strength. The experiments described here study the performance of small-scale GRP cylinders under high pressures. Problems of long-term creep, osmosis, response to vibratory loads, installation of machinery, damage repair — to name but a few — have not been assessed, while other important factors affecting the construction and future life of a full-scale submarine have been only summarily treated. With regard to the evaluation that has taken place, however, some success can be claimed. The double-wall construction, while only partially successful, could possibly be improved. For example, a low-weight filling in the core structure, rather than air, might be considered with compensation for the additional weight imposition being realized by reduced thickness of shell. It should be possible to reduce the high void content, which in some specimens reached 5-6% by volume (2% maximum would be more acceptable), even to using the more expensive polar-type laminate (void was undetectable in many of the polar single-wall specimens). In spite of all this, however, the same design of model gave one highly satisfactory performance, that is 27 100 cycles to collapse. The ring-stiffened design also seems to warrant further investigation. And to further the scope of GRP as a submarine material, computer-aided design programs based on realistic orthotropic material concepts are essential. (Author)

1821.
SWARTZ, H.M.
Toxic oxygen effects.
Int. Rev. Cytol. 35:321-343; 1973.

Several different toxic "oxygen effects" are known, including those associated with ionizing radiation, lyophilization, drying, freezing, and exposure to above-normal oxygen pressures (abbreviated here as OHP for oxygen high pressure). These effects are generally considered separate and unrelated, although various investigators have commented on similarities among some of them: radiation and OHP (Gerschmann et al., 1954); freezing and radiation (Ashwood-Smith, 1964); lyophilization and drying (Benbough, 1967; Cox and Baldwin, 1967); lyophilization and radiation (Kirby-Smith and Randolph, 1961); and drying, lyophilization, and OHP damage (Benbough, 1969; Hess, 1965). (Author's summary)

1822.
SYLVESTER, J.T., B.J. Whipp and K. Wasserman.
Ventilatory control during brief infusions of CO_2-laden blood in the awake dog.
J. Appl. Physiol. 35:178-186;Aug. 1973.

CO_2-equilibrated blood was briefly infused at constant rates into the ascending aorta (AA) and superior vena cava (SVC) of unanesthetized dogs and the ventilatory responses ($\dot{V}_E$, V_T, f) determined breath by breath. Responses to SVC infusions did not begin until the infused stimulus reached the systemic arterial circulation. Responses to AA infusion had an average latency of 6.6 sec and a peak response time of 18.6 sec. A linear relationship was found between peak $\dot{V}_E$ and $PaCO_2$ with slope (S) = 0.58 liter/min per mmHg. $\dot{V}_E$ increased with stimuli as small s as 1 mmHg Δ $PaCO_2$. Pentobarbital markedly depressed ventilatory responses. Bilateral carotid body resection (CBR) doubled latency but did not affect peak response time or S. When CBR-animals were vagotomized, peak response time and S remained unaltered and latency was not further changed. The duration of response, however, was significantly prolonged. These results demonstrate the presence of a ventilatory control component capable of triggering rapid changes in ventilation in response to brief, "physiologic" changes in arterial PCO_2 and pH. The carotid and aortic bodies proved not to be the unique chemoreceptors responsible for these rapid responses. (Authors' abstract)

1823.
SYROVEGIN, A.V.
Vliyanie povy shennogo davleniya vozdushnoi sredyna vozbridimost, neiromotornogo aparata u cheloveka.
[Effect of hyperbaria of air on the excitability of the neuro-motor apparatus in humans].
Byull. Eksp. Biol. Med. 75(3):23-26; 1973.

Reflex activity of spinal motor neurons and excitability of the neuro-muscular apparatus was studied in 10 persons under conditions of hyperbaria of the air medium. An increase in pressure to 6 atm. caused a reduction of the reflex excitability of the spinal cord motor neurons, accompanied by an increase in the activity of the neuro-muscular apparatus. Continuous 18-min. exposure to the mentioned pressure failed to arrest the processes causing a change in excitability of the motor cells of the spinal cord and of the neuromuscular system during increase of pressure to 6 atm. A reduction of pressure to 2.2 atm. during decompression did not significantly alter the excitability of the neuromuscular apparatus recorded during the 18th min. under pressure of 6 atm. (JPK) (© BA)

1824.
SYROVEGIN, A.V., G.I. Kurenkov and V.V. Kutepoo.
Reflektornaya vozbudimost' spinal'nykh motoneironov u chel oveka v usloviyakh giperbarii vozdushnoi sredy.
[The reflex excitability of the spinal motor neurons in humans during high atmosphere pressure].
Fiziol. Zh. SSSR 59(1):344-348; 1973.

A study on the reflex excitability of human spinal motor neurons under increased atmospheric pressure revealed an increase in the excitability during pressure increase from 1-3 atm. A further increase of pressure to 9 atm. resulted in a subsequent decrease in the reflex excitability. (MDS) (© BA)

1825.
SYROVEGIN, A.
Effect of hyperbaric N_2-O_2 on arbitrary and induced human muscular activity.
Abstract submitted to first annual scientific meeting of the European Undersea Biomedical Society, Stockholm, 13-15 June 1973. (Paper not published).

Abstract only. Entire item quoted: Several tests were carried out in a dry recompression chamber. Intermuscular relations of divers in respectively simple arbitrary movements under the pressure of 5-6 ATA were studied by the electromyographic method. The failure of muscular interactions and increase of latent time of motor reaction were recorded. The reflex stimulation spinal motorneurons testing by the H-reflex method revealed that motor coordinations failure with the pressure increase of air-medium up to 9 ATA is accompanied by the decrease of spinal reflex stimulation. The increase of brake-system activity may be observed under 5 ATA pressure in N_2-O_2 medium and complete saturation of organism, as well as time decrease of motor "preadjusting" may be observed during a simple arbitrary movement (e.g., bend of foot). This fact makes it possible to suppose that under test, when organization of a simple movement is taking place, the commands, to be conducted by extrapyramidal system to spinal monomeurons, reduce or even stop, while pyramidal effects remain.

1825.1
TAFT, C.K.
Submersible maneuvering.
Durham, N.H., Univ. N.H., Rep. on contract N00014-67-A-0158-0006, 30p. Sept. 1, 1972.
(AD 750 002)

The wake steering shroud is a method of steering marine vessels which uses a shroud surrounding a propeller to accelerate the fluid and cause a low pressure region inside the shroud downstream from the propeller. The shroud shape is such that the wake is attached to the inside of a shroud under these conditions. Control ports are provided in the side of the outside and this causes separation of the wake from the inside of the shroud downstream of the propeller. The resulting separation causes an asymmetrical pressure distribution inside the shroud and provides a radial steering force. The concern of the report is to gain a better understanding of this phenomena and develop the concept to the point where it can be applied to marine vessels for steering and propulsion. (Author) (GRA)

1826.
TAFT, C.K.
Submersible maneuvering.
Durham, N.H., Univ. N.H., Rep. on contract N00014-67-A-0158-0006, ARPA Order 1958, 30p. Feb. 1, 1973.
(AD 757 096)

The report presents experimental data obtained from tests performed on various configurations of a shrouded propeller used for submersible propulsion. (GRA)

1827.
TAILLEUR, J.
Plongee sousmarine et resistance capillaire: Interet de Cyclo-3.
[Underwater diving and capillary resistance: The value of Cyclo-3].
Med. Sport. 45(3):286-289; 1971.

Capillary resistance was measured by an angiosterometer in subjects treated with Cyclo-3 and in untreated subjects. Experiments were conducted in swimming pools and in the open sea. Results indicated that this treatment is helpful in preventing the mild hemorrhaging and the pseudo-hemorrhagic syndromes that are apprarently connected with diving. The work performance during prolonged deep dives, such as those undertaken in underwater habitats, would be improved by this treatment. (MFW/BSCP)

1828.
TAKUMI, Y. et al.
[Duration and clinical significance of posthyperventilation hypoxaemia].
Jap. J. Anesthesiol. 22:348-355;Apr. 1973.

Depression of alveolar PO_2 induced by the fall in gas exchange ratio after hyperventilation was studied in men. Patients were anesthetized with neuroleptoanalgesia and air during operations (on extremities or lower abdomen) and were ventilated mechanically so much that $PACO_2$ fell to about 25mmHg. At the end of the operations, they were disconnected from the ventilator and allowed to breathe spontaneously normal room air and 15, 30 and 60 minutes after the onset of spontaneous respiration, mixed respiration, mixed expiratory air and arterial blood were sampled and analyzed with Scholander microgasanalyser and PO_2- and PCO_2 electrodes. The fall in expiratory gas exchange ratio was significant 15 minutes after the onset of spontaneous respiration but 30 minutes later it improved almost to the control level. On the other hand, changes in PO_2 in arterial and superior vena cava bloods were observed 10, 20 and 30 minutes after the cessation of hyperventilation with ether-air or fluorthane-air mixtures. PO_2 in the superior vena cava fell to under 40mmHg during first 10 minutes but it elevated rapidly so that no significant falls in PVO_2 were found 20 minutes later. Hence it may be concluded that the danger of tissue hypoxia can persist for about 15 minutes after the onset of spontaneous respiration during the recovery from hyperventilation. (English summary)

1829.
TANSEY, W.A.
Medical aspects of cold water immersion, a review.
U.S. Nav. Submar. Med. Res. Lab., Rep. NSMRL 763, 15p. Sept. 19, 1973.

Whole body hypothermia is an acknowledged cause of death in victims of cold water immersion. Survivors of submarine escape must contend with this physiologic stress in the open sea. This report contains a concise statement of basic physiologic principles and modes of treatment and is considered a timely adjunct to training programs for submarine escape so that victims may better cope with hypothermic environments, and medical personnel may be better able to revive victims rescued from such accidents. (Author's abstract)

1830.
TAPPAN, D.V.
Biochemical-physiological responses to hyperbaric stress.
In: Abstracts of BuMed-ONR sponsored Navywide workshop in high pressure biomedical research, U.S. Submarine Base, Groton, Conn., May 1971, p.20. Published by the Naval Submarine Medical Research Laboratory, 1971.

Abstract only. Entire item quoted. Several aspects of the work conducted at the Naval Submarine Medical Research Laboratory on biochemical and physiological modifications in the blood and other tissues of laboratory animals and men exposed to hyperbaric situations are reviewed. Enzymic responses, alterations in several tissue metabolites including phosphate esters, as well as pH, gas exchange and hemoglobin responses to pressure combined with various gaseous environments are discussed. Alterations in pulmonary mechanics, with reduction and partial recovery of flow rates are also described. Consideration is given to the metabolic response of subjects to the increased oxygen pressures required by Navy standard diving decompression tables. Comparison is made with the effects of normobaric oxygen and with increased pressure without high oxygen levels. Efforts toward the evaluation of stresses related to diving situations through the analysis of several urinary metabolites are discussed and the utility of some routine clinical measures as estimators of hyperbaric and other stresses is considered.

1831.
TAPPAN, D.V., R.O. Madden and M.J. Jacey.
Urinary indicators of stress: effects of exposure to simulated sonar noise for 8 to 23 days.
U.S. Nav. Submar. Med. Res. Lab., Rep. NSMRL 766, 11p. Oct. 15, 1973.

Studies have been made of the relationship among excretion rates of urinary steroid hormones (indicators of stress) and a variety of other urinary metabolites in healthy young men subjected to mild laboratory-controlled stress consisting of simulated sonar noise and continuous confinement for 8 to 23 days. The objective of the study was to evaluate the stress of an increased noise component in the environment of Naval personnel living on submarines. An approach to the problem has been to utilize orderly means for evaluation of the several kinds of urinary data commonly obtained for stress analysis. Significant correlations among the excreted hormones and accompanying metabolic components make possible an estimate of steroids, and thus of stress from any of several combinations of metabolic data. Using the techniques proposed, it is possible to evaluate stress responses from information more readily available than from the more complex and protracted steroid measurements. It is anticipated that these techniques might be applied to the estimation of stress in operational situations in which human or material damage might be averted by prompt evaluation of the degree of accumulated personnel stress. (Authors' abstract)

1832.
TAYLOR, J.G.
Underwater distortion: and plain distortion.
Br. J. Psychol. 63(1):31-38; 1972.

In a paper on underwater distortion of size (Ross et al), results are reported which claim to be at variance with a theory attributed to Taylor. The so-called theory is actually a deduction from Taylor's theory of perception and, when it is correctly stated, it is confirmed by the reported results. The use of objective methods for the study of perceptual adaptation is criticized and it is argued that subjective reports give a more accurate account not only of perceptual adaptation but of the adaptation of the behavioral system that is disrupted by any transformation applied to the retinal input. (© BA)

1833.
TEAL, J.M.
Pressure effects on the respiration of vertically migrating decapod crustacea.
Amer. Zool. 11:571-576; 1971.

The respiration of five species of North Atlantic decapods was measured under conditions of pressure and temperature which allow calculation of the metabolism of these animals in the oceans. The species were: Systellaspis debilis, Acantherphyra purpurea, Oplophorus spinosus. Parapandalus richardi, and Sergestes crassus. Results indicate a tendency for metabolism to remain relatively constant with depth, the decrease due to lower temperature offset by an increase due to rising pressure. This contrasts with previous work with epipelagic euphausids which tended to have greatly reduced metabolism with increasing depth. Perhaps the metabolic rate of decapods must remain high enough for them to remain effective predators throughout their depth range, by day as well as night. (Author's abstract)

1834.
TEMPEL, G.E. and X.J. Musacchia.
Renal function in helium-cold hypothermic hamsters.
Physiologist 16:468;Aug. 1973.

Abstract only. Entire item quoted: Renal function in a depressed metabolic state was studied. Plasma and urine concentration of Na^+, K^+, and urea; and renal corti-medullary concentration gradients of Na^+ and urea were examined. Hamsters were studied as follows: (C) control (T_{re}37°C); (H) hypothermia, 48 hrs (T_{re}7°C); (R1) rewarming from hypothermia (T_{re}18°C); and (R2) rewarmed from hypothermia (T_{re}37°C for 2 hrs). Plasma Na and K appear unaffected by 48 hrs of hypothermia. In normothermia mean concentrations were 117.4±7.0 and 6.5± 0.8 mEq/l for Na and K respectively. Mean values for H animals were 110.3±12.6 mEq Na/l and 5.5±0.7 mEq K/l. By contrast, plasma urea levels increased from 0.5±0.05 mM/l for (C) animals to 0.8 mM/l for the (H) group. Urinary Na showed little difference between (C) and (H) hamsters. Mean concentrations were 99.4±45.2 for the former and 80.4±37.7 for the latter. However, concentrations of K and urea were both reduced in samples obtained after 48 hrs T 7°C. (C) hamsters demonstrated a K concentration of 299.2±90.8 mEq/l which declined to a value of 78.3±45.9 in (H) animals. Likewise, urea concentration declined from a control value of 98.1±16.5 mM/l to levels of 1.8±1.2 mM/l for the (H) group. Tissue slice analysis showed no solute gradient for either Na^+ or urea in hamsters hypothermic for 48 hrs. (R1) animals sacrificed at T_{re}18°C also lacked a gradient. However, the normal gradients returns in (R2) animals.

1835.
TENNEY, J.B., Jr.
Habitat engineering.
In: Miller, J.W., J.G. Van Derwalker and R.A. Waller, eds. Tektite 2: Scientists-in-the-sea, p.II-31-II-42. Washington, D.C., U.S. Department of the Interior, August 1971.

This report describes the engineering and field support role of the General Electric Company during the TEKTITE II program. Initial activities include planning and habitat refitting in Philadelphia. Habitat engineers were trained during this period. Work in conjunction with habitat emplacement and startup is described. After the habitat became fully operational, a field support team provided a 24-hour watch on the habitat. Between scientific missions, maintenance tasks were performed and the habitat was secured and recovered upon completion. (Author's abstract)

1836.
THALMAN, E.D.
Freon contamination at 400 feet during a saturation dive.
In: Battelle Columbus Laboratories, Proceedings, 1973 divers' gas purity symposium, November 27-28, 1973, p.IX-1-IX-8. U.S. Navy Supervisor Diving, Nav. Ships Syst. Comm., Rep 2-73, 1973.

During a 1600' saturation dive done by the Navy Experimental Diving Unit, the chamber was inadvertently contaminated with Freon 113 at the 400 foot stop during descent. Gas chromatography was used to determine the extent of the contamination which was 30 ppm. The chambers were ventilated and the contamination was eliminated in a very short period of time. Although 30 ppm of Freon 113 is not considered a hazard at atmospheric pressure, the length and depth of the dive dictated that all the contaminant be eliminated from the chamber before the dive progressed. Once the contaminant was eliminated, the dive proceeded on schedule. (Author's abstract)

1837.
THOMAS, A.N., S.A. Ketchum III, A.D. Hall and J.R. Zubrin.
A protective effect of venous admixture on chronic pulmonary oxygen toxicity.
In: Wada, J. and I. Takashi, eds. Proceedings of the fourth international congress on hyperbaric medicine, Sapporo, Japan, Sept. 1969, p.22-28. Baltimore, Williams and Wilkins, 1970.

The extent of chronic pulmonary oxygen toxicity is closely correlated with the PO_2 of the blood perfusing the lung when PO_2 of the inspired gas is kept constant. The severity of pulmonary oxygen toxicity as manifested by histologic changes and increasing surface tensions is proportional to the level of the pulmonary venous PO_2. This experiment demonstrates that chronic pulmonary oxygen toxicity is probably caused primarily by hyperoxic perfusion and not by the direct topical effect of oxygen on respiratory epithelium. (Authors' conclusion)

1838.
THOMAS, C.
Sampling analysis methods to test breathable air.
In: Battelle Columbus Laboratories. Proceedings, 1973 divers' gas purity symposium, November 27-28, 1973. p.III-1-III-14. U.S. Navy Supervisory Diving, Nav. Ships Syst. Comm., Rep 2-73, 1973.

A sampling system and analytical techniques have been developed to monitor particulate material, oil mist, carbon dioxide, carbon monoxide, and oxygen in breathing air. The sampling system is designed to accept the entire flow from a compressor or diving station, thus circumventing the problem of isokinetic sampling for solid particles and oil mist contaminants. The sampling system is easily transportable and air shippable and designed for use by the average diver or his mechanical support personnel. Analysis of the sample can be performed by a moderately well-equipped laboratory, either afloat or ashore. Routine sampling and analysis of breathing air can be standardized and performed simply, quickly, cheaply, and reproducibly. In addition, sufficient sample remains for analysis of nonroutine vapors, gases, and particulate material, where these may be suspected or questioned. (Author's abstract)

1839.
THOMAS, J.R.
Auditory discrimination under increased pressures of helium-oxygen and air.
U.S. Nav. Med. Res. Inst., Rep. 4, 8p. Oct. 4, 1972.
(Also published in Psychol. Rep. 32:159-164; 1973)
(AD 760 591)

Rats were trained on a conditional discrimination task to differentially respond to the presence or absence of an auditory stimulus in a background of noise. Performance on the discrimination task was impaired during exposure to increased pressures of simulated depths in a hyperbaric chamber. The extent of performance impairment was determined by the particular depth. No systematic differences on the discrimination task were found between compressed air and helium-oxygen as the breathing mixtures at depth. (Author) (GRA)

1840.
THOMAS, J.R.
Amphetamine and chlordiazepoxide effects on behavior under increased pressures of nitrogen.
Pharmacol. Biochem. Behav. 1(4):421-426; 1973.

Rats trained on a multiple fixed-ratio (FR) spaced-responding (DRL) schedule for food reinforcement were exposed to hyperbaric pressures (equivalent to 100, 200, 250 and 300 feet of sea water) breathing compressed air. High rates of responding on the FR schedule decreased under pressure and low rates on the DRL schedule increased. Amphetamine and chlordiazepoxide produced dose related accentuation of some rate change effects at depth and changes in performance at depth that were not predictable from the effects of the drugs at ambient pressure. (© BA)

1841.
THOMAS, J.R.
Auditory discrimination under increased pressure.
Psychol. Rep. 32:159-164; 1973.

Rats were trained on a conditional discrimination task to differentially respond to the presence or absence of an auditory stimulus in a background of noise. Performance on the discrimination task was impaired during exposure to increased pressures of simulated depths in a hyperbaric chamber. The extent of performance impairment was determined by the particular depth. No systematic differences on the discrimination task were found between compressed air and helium-oxygen as the breathing mixtures at depth. (Author's summary)

1842.
THOMAS, J.R.
Nitrogen, helium, and neon effects on timing behavior at increased pressures.
Aerosp. Med. 44:45-48;Jan. 1973.

Rats trained on a schedule involving a temporal discrimination were exposed to nitrogen, helium, and neon at 7.1 ata and 8.6 ata. The timing behavior was differentially affected by the three gases. Nitrogen completely disrupted the temporal discrimination and increased response rates. Helium produced only a small change in the timing behavior. Neon was quite different from nitrogen or helium in that it decreased response rates while still maintaining the temporal discrimination. The schedule of reinforcement was demonstrated to be quite sensitive to different gas effects. (Author's abstract)

1843.
THOMAS, W.G., M.J. Preslar and J.C. Farmer.
Calibration of condenser microphones under increased atmospheric pressures.
In: Thomas, W.G. and J.C. Farmer. Psyychoacoustic and electrophysiologic studies of hearing under hyperbaric pressure, p.1-22. Chapel Hill, N.C., Univ. N.C. Med. Sch., Auditory Res. Lab., Rep. on Contract N00014-67-A-0321-0005. June 1, 1973.
(Also published in J. Acoust. Soc. Amer. 51(1, Pt.1):6-14; 1972)

The sensitivity and frequency response characteristics of Type L Standard Laboratory microphones were measured with an electrostatic actuator at surface and at twelve different levels to 31 ATA in a hyperbaric chamber. The microphones were measured in compressed air and a helium-air environment, with and without the capillary pin. In addition, one microphone remained at a depth of 31 ATA for twenty-four hours to measure its stability under pressure. Results indicated a loss in sensitivity in compressed air and helium-air as a function of pressure. In a compressed air environment a resonant peak occurred at 4000 Hz, which shifted to 8000 Hz in the helium-air environment. The microphones showed extremely close agreement between compression and decompression, between different pressurizations, and between different microphones. Also, there was no change in sensitivity over a twenty-four hour period of pressurization at 31 ATA. Calibration data at several pressures are given. (Authors' abstract)

1844.
THOMAS, W.G., M.J. Preslar and J.C. Farmer.
Calibration of earphones under increased atmospheric pressures.
In: Thomas, W.G. and J.C. Farmer. Psychoacoustic and electrophysiologic studies of hearing under hyperbaric pressure, p.23-39. Chapel Hill, N.C., Univ. N.C. Med. Sch., Auditory Res. Lab., Rep. on Contract N00014-67-A-0321-0005. June 1, 1973.

The sensitivity and frequency response characteristics of TDH-39 earphones were measured at surface and eleven different depths to 31 atm absolute (ATA) in a hyperbaric chamber. Measurements were made in compressed air and a helium-air environment. The earphones showed a general increase in sensitivity with a relatively flat response to 1000 Hz. Sensitivity in higher frequencies was frequency selective. The earphones exhibited great variability between phones and within the same phone during different pressurizations. In addition, differences were noted between compression and decompression. (Authors' abstract)

1845.
THOMAS, W.G., J. Summit and J.C. Farmer.
Human auditory thresholds during deep, saturation helium-oxygen dives.
In: Thomas, W.G. and J.C. Farmer. Psychoacoustic and electrophysiologic studies of hearing under hyperbaric pressure, p.46-55. Chapel Hill, N.C., Univ. N.C. Med. Sch., Auditory Res. Lab., Rep. on Contract N00014-67-A-0321-0005. June 1, 1973.

Air conduction and bone conduction thresholds were derived on thirty-three different divers on eight saturation dives in helium-air between 300 ft. and 1000 ft. A total of 400 air conduction and 300 bone conduction audiograms were given at twenty-six different depths during compression and decompression. The results indicate a reversible, depth related conductive hearing loss. The shape of the audiometric function and absolute amount of hearing loss are somewhat different from data reported in hyperbaric air. (Authors' abstract)

1846.
THOMAS, W.G. and J.C. Farmer.
Psychoacoustic and electrophysiologic studies of hearing under hyperbaric pressure.
Chapel Hill, N.C., Univ. N.C. Sch. Med., Auditory Res. Lab., Rep. on Contract N00014-67-A-0321-0005, 55p. June 1, 1973.

This Summary Report covers work performed under Contract N00014-67-A-0321-0005 from June 1, 1970, to May 31, 1973. Work performed includes: (1) calibration of laboratory standard Type-L condenser microphones to a simulated depth of 990 feet (31 ATA); (2) calibration of standard audiometric earphones to a simulated depth of 990 feet (31 ATA); and, (3) measurement of human auditory thresholds during deep, saturation dives in helium-air. Human threshold data have been collected at numerous depths during compression and decompression for air conduction and bone conduction to a simulated depth of 990 feet (31 ATA). Electrophysiological measurements have been recorded from experimental animals under similar conditions. These data have been analyzed and the results will be reported in the Annual Report at the end of the current Contract period. [The specific sections are treated separately and will be found under the following author entries: Thomas, W.G., M.J. Preslar and J.C. Farmer (2); Farmer, J.C., W.G. Thomas and M.J. Preslar; Thomas, W.G., J. Summit and J.C. Farmer]. (Authors' abstract)

1847.
THOMPSON, A.
Personal flotation device maintenance.
Skin Diver 20:75-76;Dec. 1971.

The author estimates that 50% of flotation vests now in use would not inflate if the lanyard was pulled. This is due to the fact that the passages through which the CO_2 must pass become clogged — sometimes by the powder used during manufacture, sometimes by salt. When the oral inflator is used, a small amount of salt water always gets into the vest. If this has been done, the vest must be thoroughly rinsed with warm water. The passage between the CO_2 cartridge and the vest bladder must be kept clear, also. The Schroeder valve in the CO_2 detonator is a likely seat of corrosion and malfunction. The exterior of the vest should also be thoroughly rinsed with warm water, with special care being given to the CO_2 mechanism, the oral inflator, and the knurled locking nut (which prevents water from accidentally entering the vest through the oral inflator). (MFW/BSCP)

1848.
THORLING, E.B. and A.J. Erslev.
The effects of some erythropoietic agents on the "tissue" tension of oxygen.
Br. J. Haemotol. 23(4):483-490; 1972.

The effects of erythropoietin, hemolysate, cobalt chloride and testosterone proprionate in the 24-hr Fe utilization of hypertransfused male rats and on the O_2 tension [PO_2] in a subcutaneous air pocket were studied. Only testosterone propionate failed to increase the 24-hr Fe utilization of hypertransfused rats. Only cobalt chloride altered the PO_2 in the gas pockets. A striking increase in PO_2 was observed with cobalt chloride suggesting a block in O_2 utilization with intracellular hypoxia. Using more intense treatment of female hypertransfused rats with various androgen preparations, namely, testosterone propionate, norethandrolone and nandrolone decanoate, only the latter had significant erythropoietic effect. This was apparently not mediated by tissue hypoxia, since the PO_2 in subcutaneous air pockets did not change. (© BA)

1849.
THORNSTEDT, H.
Legal and ethical considerations in hyperbaric research.
In: Hesser, C.M. and D. Linnarsson, eds. Proceedings of the first annual scientific meeting of the European Undersea Biomedical Society, Stockholm, 13-15 June 1973. Forsvarsmedicin 9:379-381;July 1973.

The position of Swedish law can be summarized in the following way: Consent to grave injuries does not exempt from criminal liability. However, consent to light injuries and pain does. Consent even to light injuries and pain is obligatory. Consent must be given freely. No special form for consent is prescribed. Consent in writing is accordingly not required. The subject must be informed before he gives his consent. Very little is known about how detailed the information must be. The consent must be given beforehand. It can be withdrawn at any time. Consent does not under all conditions exempt the research leader from liability even if the injury is slight or only pain appears. When a court has to decide whether a research leader has acted negligently or not, it most certainly will take into consideration if he has followed the rules which have been decided within the medical profession. (From author's abstract)

1850.
THYS, J.P., A. Gallez, D. Blum and P. Paulet.
Nonsinusal arrhythmias and atrioventricular conduction during hyperbaric oxygenation.
Amer. Heart J. 83:433-434;Mar. 1972.

Cardiac rhythm was monitored during the exposure of a three-year old boy to 2 ATA of pure oxygen. After fifteen minutes, increasing arrhythmias were absorbed. These consisted of "nonrespiratory sinus bradycardia (50 beats per minute) episodes of shifting and wandering pacemaker, first degree atrioventricular block, second degree atrioventricular block with Wenskesbach phenomenon, sinoatrial block with nodal rhythm." The authors believe that this is the first occasion on which such severe, though reversible, abnormalities had been observed in the course of hyperbaric therapy. (MFW/BSCP)

1851.
TIKHONOV, M.A.
Mechanics of respiration during simulation of weightlessness in an immersion medium.
Space Biol. Med. 6:63-87;Jan. 18, 1973.
(JPRS 58010)

Changes in lung capacity, air passage resistance and dynamic compliance during water immersion were investigated in six healthy male test subjects. At the beginning of the immersion experiment the functional residual capacity of the lungs decreased by an average of 7% and remained at that level until the end of the experiment. At the onset of the experiment lung compliance also decreased by an average of 20% but tended to recover by the end of immersion. At the beginning of the experiment air passage resistance increased by 65-80% and decreased slightly by the end of immersion. These changes may be caused by shifts in intrathoracic pressure and redistribution of the circulating blood volume. (Author's abstract)

1852.
TIMBAL, J., H. Viellefond, H. Fuenard and P. Varene.
Determination du coefficient d'echange thermique par convection entre l'homme et l'environnement en milieu $He-O_2$ jusqu'a 31 bar.
[Determination of the coefficient of thermal exchange by convection between man and the environment in a $He-O_2$ medium to 31 bars].
J. Physiol. (Paris) 65 (Suppl. 3):512A; 1972.

Four nude, prone subjects were studied for body heat loss in a $He-O_2$ atmosphere at six levels of pressure between 1.5 and 31 bars at a constant oxygen partial pressure. (300 mb $\pm$ 10). Heat loss through respiratory convection increases as the pressure is increased. Heat loss through evaporation, calculated on the basis of the subject's weight loss, did not vary with pressure. Heat loss through radiation decreased passively as pressure was increased because of the progressive heat rise in the environment. (MEMH/UMS)

1853.
TIMME, R.W., R.L. Davidson and A.C. Tims.
Expendable hydrophone for sonobuoy application.
U.S. Nav. Res. Lab., Underwater Sound Ref. Div., Rep. NR7-7644, 45p. Sept. 17, 1973.
(AD 766 786/8)

A low-cost, low-noise, high-sensitivity hydrophone has been developed for possible application in an expendable air, deployable, passive sonar array system. An acoustic element consisting of two Type III ceramic radially poled cylinders was combined with a low noise, high-gain preamplifier to produce a hydrophone with a sensitivity of -149 dB re 1 V/micro Pa, operating frequency range of 10 Hz to 3 kHz, and depth capability of 4500 m. In addition to a description of the hydrophone and its operating specifications, a discussion of design criteria and prototype selection is included. (Authors) (GRA)

1854.
TIMS, A.C.
A new capped-cylinder design for an underwater sound transducer (USRD Type F50).
J. Acoust. Soc. Amer. 51(5, pt2):1751-1758; 1972.

A small broad-band transducer has been developed primarily for use as a receiver in the frequency range 1 Hz to 70 kHz, but it can be used also as a sound source in the frequency range 10-70 kHz. The nominal free-field voltage sensitivity at the end of a 30.5-m cable is -205.9 dB re 1 V/ μ Pa at frequencies below 10 kHz. The sensitivity changes by less than 1 dB with hydrostatic pressure change from atmospheric to 6890 kPa and with temperature change from 3° to 30°C. As a sound source, the transducer is linear with driving voltage to 200 V CW at frequencies from 10 to 60 kHz. The broad-band characteristics are attributed to the novel design of the sensor element — a design that is applicable to a variety of cylindrical sensor configurations. (Author's abstract)

1855.
TITCOMBE, R.M.
Handbook for professional divers.
Philadelphia, J. B. Lippincott Co., 1973. 294p.

This book is intended as an instructive manual which sets forth the currently accepted practices observed in professional diving. Its chief function is to reduce the number of disabling accidents. The chapter headings are as follows: (1) Personnel. (2) Communication and safety instructions. (3) Decompression. (4) Decompression sickness — treatment. (5) Accidents and incidents. (6) First aid. (7) Underwater physics. (8) Underwater physiology. (9) Principles of self-contained diving. (10) Equipment specifications. (11) Maintenance of plant and equipment. (12) Medical requirements. (MFW/BSCP)

1856.
TITOV, A.P.
Utoplenie plovtsov v vodolaznom snaryazhenii.
[Drowning of swimmers wearing diving gear].
Sud. Med. Ekspert. 16:54;July/Sept. 1973.

The most simple Soviet-made diving gear, Model No. 1, is being widely used by amateur sport swimmers. It consists of a half-mask, goggles, breathing tube and fins. It can be used for surface swimming with the head under water, breathing atmospheric air through the tube. It also serves for diving. The authors report two cases of drowning while victims were wearing this equipment. The first case was an experienced swimmer in excellent health when he started out for underwater hunting. One hour later his body was found under 3 meters of water. Death by drowning was verified by autopsy findings: livid cadaveric ecchimoses covering his shoulder region, Paltauf's spots on the pleura, inflated, edematous lungs with uneven distribution of blood, and brain edema. The second case was similar; the body of this swimmer was found 24 hours later at the depth of 12 meters. The mechanism of drowning is explained by primary loss of consciousness, caused by acute O_2 deficiency, combined with excess CO_2 accumulation, as a result of voluntary withholding of breath. (OLC/UMS)

1857.
TJERNSTROM, O.
On alternobaric vertigo: experimental studies.
In: Hesser, C.M. and D. Linnarsson, eds. Proceedings of the first annual scientific meeting of the European Undersea Biomedical Society, Stockholm, 13-15 June 1973. Forsvarsmedicin 9:410-415;July 1973.

It is concluded that alternoberic vertigo is induced during the period of unequal middle ear pressure, when pressure in the uncleared ear has reached a certain level, rather than at the moment of pressure regulation. Individuals who have high forcing pressures at one side, are more susceptible to alternobaric vertigo. Examination of diver candidates to reveal unequal forcing pressures would be useful in eliminating such individuals. (MFW/UMS)

1858.
TODD, G.P.
An electronic decompression analog alternative to the Haldane model.
In: Abstracts of BuMed-ONR sponsored Navywide research in high pressure biomedical research, U.S. Submarine Base, Groton, Conn., May 1971, p.48. Published by the Naval Submarine Medical Research Laboratories, 1971.

Abstract only. Entire item quoted: The aim of work to be reviewed is development of reliable, standardized measures of well-understood behavioral functions for assessment of human performance capabilities in hyperbaric environments. At this time, efforts are concentrated on obtaining a better understanding of some tasks often used in studies of diver integrity under hyperbaric conditions. In addition, attempts to define behavioral analogs of those tasks for primates and to relate performance therein to the complex of biomedical events found under high pressure have been initiated. Implications of NAVSUBMEDRSCHLAB studies of mental arithmetic, the Stroop test, and tracking (simulated vehicle control) for identification of behavior functions tapped by those tasks and for improved experimental control of task performance measurement in hyperbaric studies will be described. The effects of repeated measurement, variation in task characteristics, and tactics of task performance on the stability and sensitivity to stress of task performance are reviewed.

1859.
TOLAND, C.
Treatment of a case of near-drowning in chlorinated fresh water.
Br. J. Anaesth. 44:616-619; 1972.

This report describes the management of a case of near-drowning in chlorinated fresh water. The patient recovered fully, both physically and mentally. Complications involving the major systems of the body had developed prior to admission to hospital. Treatment included controlled ventilation via a cuffed nasotracheal tube, steroids, antibiotics and digoxin. Intravenous fluids given, and considered beneficial in influencing the prognosis, were plasma, blood, mannitol and sodium bicarbonate. The patient's condition was evaluated by frequent blood-gas analysis and appropriate adjustment of inspired oxygen concentration and ventilator settings made. High pressures were required to ventilate the patient because of the low compliance of his lungs. (Author's summary)

1860.
TOLHURST, G.C.
History of helium speech processing instrumentation.
In: Sergeant, R.L. and T. Murry, eds. Processing of helium speech: proceedings of a Navy-sponsored workshop, August 1971, U.S. Nav. Submar. Med. Res. Lab., Rep. NSMRL 708, p.4-10. May 22, 1972.

The author traces the development of various types of helium speech processors. The first instrument operated by heterodyning downward the output of two broad-bandpass filters by a factor of 1.5. This instrument, in improved forms, was used in SeaLabs I, II and III, and a similar instrument is now marketed by the Integrated Electronics Corporation as Model 702B. Under a Navy contract which ran for two years, HRB-Singer explored the principle of pulse encoding the initial portion of each phoneme, decoding the pulse trains and reading out at a slower rate. This did not work for voiceless consonants. Westinghouse, also under a Navy contract, worked on the short-time, periodic sampling of helium speech, discarding the nonsampled time periods and reading out of storage the sampled time periods at a slower rate. The instrument developed as a result of these studies disappeared at the time of the dissolution of SeaLab III and was never adequately tested. A third Navy contract was awarded (1968) to Kearfott Division of Singer-General Dynamics, to develop a processor operating on the principle of selective time sampling, with major differences from the Westinghouse instrument. Other devices subsequently developed in the U.S., France, and the U.K., are briefly mentioned, some of which are described in detail in other papers presented at this workshop. The chief requirement from the Navy's point of view is that the device be small enough to be diver-carried; this requirement has hampered research. Other theories and proposals not pursued for various reasons are briefly described. (MFW/BSCP)

1861.
TOLHURST, G.C.
Open forum and discussion period, chairman's summary.
In: Sergeant, R.L. and T. Murry, eds. Processing helium speech: proceedings of a Navy-sponsored workshop, August 1971, U.S. Nav. Submar. Med. Res. Lab., Rep. NSMRL 708, p.39-52. May 22, 1972.

In summary, the discussion in open forum seemed to indicate that the Navy should soon know whether it will have an interim all-diver speech communication system. If the systems now under test are not adequate, suggestions were made as to several "next steps", including: personnel selection and training; speech preprocessing methods; and alternative helium-speech translating methods. Suggestions were made by which information feedback to management, operations and science could be accelerated and utilized in planning and problem solution. (Author)

1862.
TOMASI, G. and B. Tomasi.
Why gamble with the bends?
Skin Diver 20:8-9;Oct. 1971.

The three factors involved in computing no decompression repetitive dives are: (1) depth and duration of first dive, (2) surface interval, and (3) depth and duration of second dive. The authors explain how to make use of the Navy tables 1-11, 1-12, and 1-13 in the revised edition of the diving manual, to determine the no decompression bottom times, or to determine the required surface interval, whichever information is desired. These tables can also indicate when the diver has overstayed his no-decompression time in repetitive diving; table 1-10 shows the mechanics of computing stops. It is strongly emphasized that sport divers should never undertake decompression dives unless they are diving in an area equipped with a recompression chamber. (MFW/BSCP)

1863.
TORBATI, D., D. Harel and S. Lavy.
The time of appearance of paroxysmal electrical discharges in normal and hypophysectomized rats under hyperbaric conditions.
Israel J. Med. Sci. 8(1):39-42; 1972.

The sensitivity of the hypophysectomized adult rat to the toxic effect of O_2 under high pressure on the CNS was studied. The appearance of the 1st paroxysmal electrical discharges was considered to be the initial sign of an adverse effect of the O_2 on the brain. No statistically significant difference in the time of appearance of the 1st generalized electrical discharge between hypophysectomized and normal rats was found. (© BA)

1864.
TRAPP, W.G., T.R. Patrick and P.A. Oforsagd.
Cardiac support with hyperbaric oxygen.
In: Wada, J. and I. Takashi, eds. Proceedings of the fourth international congress of hyperbaric medicine, Sapporo, Japan, Sept. 1969, p.205-211. Baltimore, Williams and Wilkins, 1970.

A review of clinical and experimental studies with hyperbaric oxygen at 3 atmospheres absolute reveals that this atmosphere is a strong stabilizer and strengthener of myocardial function. The study includes experiments using the Duke University model hyperbaric pump-oxygenator, experimental cardiac transplants, closed heart surgery in cyanotic infants, low cardiac output in post-operative open-heart surgery, defibrillation in experimentally fibrillated animals, and severe exercise in trained athletes. In addition, pulmonary changes previously attributed to the toxic effect of high pressure oxygen now appear to be responsible to inadequate respiratory excursion, dehydration and other factors. (Authors' abstract)

1865.
TRAVIS, D.M., L.L. Rolf and K.A. Berdick.
Respiratory failure in oxygen-induced lung disease: A study of survival, development of hypoxemia, and response to benzolamide.
Amer. Rev. Resp. Dis. 106(5):740-751; 1972.

A form of acute respiratory failure was produced in rats to study hypoxemia resulting from lung disease and response to drugs. Graded lung damage was induced in Wistar rats by exposure to O_2 at a pressure of 1 atm for intervals varying between 50 and 65 hr. Abrupt removal from O_2 to air then resulted in acute respiratory distress. In adult rats, the duration of O_2 exposure was related to increasing severity of respiratory difficulty and shortened survival. Respiratory failure did not develop in new born rats even after nine days in O_2, but localized edema and atelectasis appeared in the lungs after three days. Rats dying in O_2 showed progressive hypoxemia and terminal hypercapnia and acidemia. Rats dying in air after induction of lung disease by O_2 often hyperventilated and showed alkalemia before the terminal phase of hypoxemia, acidosis and death. Benzolamide, a renal carbonic anhydrase inhibitor, was given four hr before the end of O_2 exposure to produce mild metabolic acidosis. This treatment resulted in increased survival during the subsequent exposure to air and minimized the alkalemia associated with hyperventilation. The experiments showed that O_2 at atmospheric pressure can be combined with air exposure after development of graded amounts of lung damage for convenient study of acute respiratory failure and demonstrated the response to benzolamide in the hypoxemia of lung disease. (© BA)

1866.
TRAVIS, D.M., M. Green and H. Don.
Simultaneous comparison of helium and nitrogen expiratory "closing volumes".
J. Appl. Physiol. 34:304-308;Mar. 1973.

We measured 81 closing volumes (CV) by a bolus method (He) and a resident gas method (N_2) simultaneously on the same breaths in 15 healthy adults. The pairs of such tracings were usually similar in appearance and in CV. The overall He-N_2 CV difference of 0.9% vital capacity (VC) was not significant ($P > 0.05$). Differences were observed in individual tracings. When a difference in CV by the two methods was significant in a subject, the N_2CV was smaller than the HeCV. This occurred in three subjects, all with a moderate or heavy cigarette smoking history, who had a N_2 CV 2-4% VC smaller than He CV ($P < 0.02$). The results reflect the mechanisms underlying the bolus and resident gas methods. Consideration of these mechanisms suggests that closing volumes are similar in healthy subjects but may differ in the presence of regional abnormalities of airways or lung parenchyma. Simultaneous use of a bolus and a resident gas method may give useful information in addition to that obtained from one method alone. (Author's abstract)

1867.
TRESANSKY, G.J.
The NMRI Mark III Mod I tremor device.
U.S. Nav. Med. Res. Inst., Rep. 2, 22p. May 1973.
(AD 763 343)

A muscle force transducer was developed as a research tool to detect and quantify tremors in divers working under hyperbaric conditions. The tremor device measures microtremor superimposed upon a neuromuscular response maintained within a specific force band. It incorporates a simple motor skill task, which requires the diver subject to maintain, for a predetermined number of seconds, a constant downward pressure with the tip of the middle finger upon a lever which is preset to a specific force. Variations in the subject's ability to maintain the zero reading are considered tremor. Measurement of tremor against an established baseline of an individual diver can provide an indication of neurological change, which may interfere with underwater work performance. (Author) (GRA)

1868.
TRIFONENKOV, A.M.
Opodgotovke khirurgicheskikh brigad podroknykh lodok.
[The training of surgical brigades for submarines].
Voennomed Zh. (12):64-65;Dec. 1972.

The author emphasizes the importance of adequate training for members of the submarine surgical team. He outlines the three stages in the training of the ship surgeon. The first stage is his specialization which should begin immediately after medical school. During the second stage he will be assigned to a hospital surgical department and the third and final stage consists of group training for teamwork of the entire surgical brigade of the submarine. The surgeon's assistant has to perform duties of the scrub nurse and has to undergo training in a hospital surgical department under the supervision of the head surgical nurse. His duties on board will include the preparation of the operating area, preparing the patient for surgery, assisting the surgeon during operation, suturing the incision, etc. The most frequently occurring surgical emergencies on board ship are injuries and acute abdominal diseases. In order to keep them in constant training, naval surgical brigades, while on shore, are assigned to base hospitals and medical stations. (OLC/SCD)

1869.
TRIGGER, A.W.
Divers' air filter testing.
In: Battelle Columbus Laboratories. Proceedings, 1973 divers' gas purity symposium, November 27-28, 1973. p.XVIII-1-XVIII-28. U.S. Navy Supervisor Diving, Nav. Ships Syst. Comm., Rep 2-73, 1973.

A comprehensive program to evaluate air filters for compressors that supply air for Navy divers is described. Oil challenge concentrations of up to 775 micrograms per liter (calculated at working pressure and temperature) were utilized to determine the efficiency of present filtration systems. Conformance of the filters to the proposed revised Mil Spec MIL-F-24152 (Ships), which requires a maximum output of 5 micrograms per liter in the effluent air when operated at challenge levels up to 100 hours, is assessed. Test oil characteristics with respect to concentration, mean particle size, and particle size distribution are stated. Filter unit performance was quantified by both gravimetric methods and light-scattering photometry. A proposed continuous monitor for effluent particulate content is described. No single filter element tested to date will give both the purity of air and the longevity of operation required by the proposed specification. Deficiencies of filter housing design are illustrated and corrective actions proposed. The ultimate goal is to provide the Navy with a rigid specification for the purchase and testing of air compressor filter units that will conform to OSHA and Navy requirements. A secondary goal is to establish a test technique and/or specification conformance. Final results will be utilized to develop an understanding of the air filtration process and to optimize filter unit performance. (Author's abstract)

1870.
TRIPATHI, B., N. Ashton and G. Knight.
Effect of oxygen on the developing retinal vessels of the Rabbit. III. Mode of growth of rabbit retinal vessels in tissue culture.
Exp. Eye Res. 15:321-351;Mar. 1973.

This paper is the third (see Ashton et al. 1973) in a series reporting studies on the effect of hyperoxia on the growing retinal vesels of the rabbit. It deals with the in vitro behaviour of the rabbit retinal complex in a normal tissue culture environment, a necessary preliminary to an investigation of the effect of hyperoxia on such cultures, which is reported in the fourth and last paper of this series. An account is given of the materials and methods employed, including time-lapse cinephotomicrography, phase contrast light microscopy, conventional light microscopy and electron microscopy. The origin and mode of growth of the cells composing the vascular complex, their differentiation and formation into capillaries, and the behaviour of their associated cells are described. It was found that growth began both as a bidding of mesenchymal-like cells, arising from endothelium and pericytes, and as a direct growth of endothelial growth with the formation of interlacing cords or strands which very occasionally differentiated into capillaries. The outgrowth was associated with an active proliferation of macrophages, but there was no evidence that these arose from the mesenchymal or endothelial cells or vice versa. Since this is the only reported work on tissue cultures of retinal endothelium the findings are compared and contrasted with tissue culture studies of endothelium from other tissue sources. (Authors' abstract)

1871.
TROCINO, J.L. and H.S. Weisbrod.
Pyrotechnic illumination in the underwater enviroment.
In: Duntley, S.Q., J.J. Lones and H.S. Weisbrod, eds. Proceedings of the society of photo optical instrumentation engineers. Underwater photo optical instrumentation applications, March 1971, Honolulu, p.85-88, Published by the Society, 1972.

A series of design and formulation improvements by various contributers during the last decade have produced a family of pyrotechnic flare devices which are compact, comparatively inexpensive, and simple for the amateur or professional diver to use. The new devices are based upon a high-intensity composition which burns inside a clear lucite plastic chamber. The pyrotechnic material produces intense light, but only a small amount of gas. The gas that is generated is confined within the plastic chamber where it escapes slowly through a small orifice. The entrapped gas easily isolates the comparatively small burning surface from the water while the light produced passes without serious loss through the sides of the plastic chamber. (Authors)

1872.
TROSHIKIN, G.V.
Respiration in an atmosphere under high pressure.
Fiziol. Zh. SSSR 57(12):1808-1812; 1972.
(Translation NASA TT-F14,258. May 1972).

The electrical activity of the external intercostal muscle and the time of the respiratory cycle were investigated in adult Wistar rats during exposure to various gas mixtures at increased pressure. Increased density of inspired gas mixture, due either to an increase in external respiration or physical characteristics of the inert gas, used for dilution of the oxygen, produces an increase in the amplitude of the electrical pulses in the respiratory volleys and the time of the respiratory cycle. A reaction of this kind in a dense medium is the consequence of an increase in the resistance to respiration and a rise in the load on the respiratory musculature. The paper also considers the mechanism of the increase in resistance to respiration in a pressurized atmosphere. (Author's abstract)

1873.
TROSHIKIN, G.V.
Termoregulyatsionnye reaktsii u zhivotnykh v gelio-kislorodnoi srede.
[Thermoregulation reactions of animals in an oxygen-helium atmosphere].
Kosm. Biol. Med. 6(5):84-86; 1972.

Rats of the Wistar breed were placed in a hermetically sealed chamber and successively exposed for a period of 1 hr each to atmospheres containing: air, a mixture of He and O_2 (21% O_2), and air again. In a He O_2 atmosphere at a temperature of 20-28°C, the heat emission of rats increased due to the high heat conductivity of He. This led to an increase in the intensity of chemical thermo-regulation in comparison with such reactions under the same temperatures in an air atmosphere. At a temperature of 30°C chemical thermoregulation became minimal. (MDS) (© BA)

1874.
TROSHIKIN, G.V.
Termoregulyatsionnye reaktsii u krys v gipolsicheskoi atmosfere s axotnym i gelierym razbarleniem.
[Thermoregulation reactions of rats in the nitrogen and helium hypoxic atmospheres].
Meditsina 6:23-27;Dec. 1972.

Thermoregulation reactions (gas exchange, thermoregulation activity of muscles and rectal temperature) of 60 rats exposed for 1 hour to nitrogen and helium atmospheres containing 20.9, 11.4 and 7.4% of oxygen at t=25°C were investigated. As compared with the controls (breathing air), the test animals exposed to a helium-oxygen (21%) atmosphere displayed an increase of the gas exchange and thermoregulation activity of muscles and a decrease of the rectal temperature, thus indicating the cooling effect of helium. An exposure of rats to a hypoxic helium-oxygen (11.4%) atmosphere as compared with the similar nitrogen-oxygen gas mixture brought about a less distinct decline of the gas exchange and a more marked decrease of the body temperature the thermoregulation tone varying insignificantly and tending to increase in the helium-oxygen atmosphere. An exposure of rats to a hypoxic helium-oxygen (7.4%) atmosphere as compared with the similar nitrogen-oxygen gas mixture induced a more noticeable decrease of the gas exchange and body temperature, the thermoregulation activity of muscles changing insignificantly and tending to decrease in the nitrogen-oxygen atmosphere. The above functions, except the rectal temperature, recovered faster after an exposure to a hypoxic helium atmosphere. The difference in the effect of hypoxic nitrogen and helium-oxygen atmospheres is related to the helium cooling action. (English summary)

1875.
TROWBRIDGE, T.
Optical properties of a spherical plastic underwater observatory NEMO.
Contributed for publication (without presentation at the American Society of Mechanical Engineers), as paper No. 70-UnT-A, 7p. 1970.
(Published by the J. Eng. Ind., date unknown)

The optical effects occurring during observation from within a transparent spherical underwater observatory are analyzed. Quantitative results are presented for the NEMO observatory. These results include location, size, and shape discrepancies for the entire range of possible object locations, for the entire range of possible eye locations, and for "best" and "worst" cases of eye orientation. Results were obtained from ray tracing computed in accordance with Snell's law by using an iterative numerical procedure. The distance and size discrepancies were found to be severe; however, the distortions in shape and the discrepancies in the subtended angles were remarkably mild. It may be that for reasonable eye locations, observations in all directions from spherical observatories will present a much more realistic scene than observations through a planar interface, even for viewing normal to the planar interface. (Author's abstract)

1876.
TROY, S.S. and D.H. Ford.
Hormonal protection of rats breathing oxygen at high pressure.
Acta Neurol. Scand. 48:231-242; 1972.

Sex differences in susceptibility to high pressure oxygen (OHP)-induced convulsions were observed in mature rats. Male rats convulsed significantly earlier than did females. After adrenalectomy, seizures disappeared in most females and some male rats. The number of adrenalectomized male rats which resisted OHP-induced convulsions increased from 40% to 91% when they were treated with estradiol subcutaneously. Rats which do not convulse during the exposure to OHP eventually develop pulmonary edema and congestion and die. Strain variations in respect to susceptibility to oxygen poisoning and the controversial nature of OHP and electroshock-induced convulsions in response to steroid hormones are discussed. (Authors' abstract)

1877.
TRUDELL, J.R., W.L. Hubbell and E.N. Cohen.
Pressure reversal of inhalation anesthetic-induced disorder in spin-labeled phospholipid vesicles.
Biochim. Biophys. Acta 291:328-334; 1973.

The effects of anesthetics in luminous bacteria, newts, tadpoles, and mice are reversed by application of 150-200 atm of helium or hydrostatic pressure. The disorder induced by the inhalation anesthetic halothane in spin-labeled phospholipid vesicles is also reversed by similar pressures of helium. If pressure reversal of anesthesia occurs in intact nerve systems, then all theories of anesthesia must accomodate the phenomenon and nerve membrane model systems demonstrate it as well. The occurrence of pressure reversal in spin-labeled phospholipid vesicles supports their use as models for the hydrophobic region of nerve membrane. This finding is in agreement with the theory that anesthetics act by disordering the lipid region of the membranes. (Authors' summary)

1878.
TRUSHIN, A.I.
Primenenie apparatury dlya markoza i iskusstvennoi ventilyatsii ligkikh v barokamerakh.
[The use of an equipment for anesthesia and artificial respiration in the hyperbaric chamber].
Med. Tekh. 3:11-15;May/June 1973.

Hyperbaric oxygenation is used in modern medicine for therapeutic purposes as well as during complicated surgical procedures. The present communication describes various Soviet-made appliances used for anesthesia and artificial respiration under hyperbaric conditions. The most important part of the equipment is the distributor of the anesthetic. The anesthetic to be used in the chamber must be carefully chosen in order to prevent explosion. The author recommends fluothane as the least explosive of anesthetic materials. The most important factor in the prevention of explosion during anesthesia in the barochamber is the right dosage and concentration of the anesthetic. The author describes two different systems of vaporizers for the distribution of liquid anesthetics: (1) with laminar (streamline) flow, (2) with turbulent flow. Depending on the type of the vaporizer and the hydraulic resistance of the spray nozzle, the anesthetist may determine the concentration of the anesthetic administered to the patient. Experimenting with liquid fluothane in both types of vaporizers (laminar and turbulent), the author devised a mathematical method for the calculation of the concentration of the anesthetic. Factors to be considered are: the partial pressure of fluothane, size of the spray nozzle of the vaporizer, elasticity and resistance of its valves, and the viscosity of the anesthetic mixture. The relationship between the concentration of the anesthetic in the vaporizer (with laminar or turbulent flow; and the pressure inside the chamber is illustrated in figure 1. For therapeutic hyperbaric oxygenation the author considers "Pneumat-1" as the best Soviet-made equipment. Experimental calculations on the relationship between respiratory parameters and pressure inside the barochamber are shown on figure 3. (OLC/SCD)

1879.
TU, A.T.
Sea snake venom.
Fort Collins, Colo., Colo. State Univ. Dept. Biochem., Final Rep. on Contract N00014-67-A-0299-0005, 16p. Oct. 31, 1970.
(AD 754 455)

The chemical properties of sea snake venoms and pure toxins from these venoms are investigated. Collections of sea snakes studied were from Japan, Formosa, Hong Kong, Thailand, Malaysia, and the Philippines. (GRA)

1880.
TUNNICLIFF, G. and J.D. Wood.
The inhibition of mouse brain neurotransmitter enzymes by mercury compounds and a comparison with the effects of hyperbaric oxygen.
Comp. Gen. Pharmacol. 4(13):101-105; 1973.

Exposure of mouse brain homogenates to hyperbaric O_2 (OHP) at 30 lb/in.^{2} gauge results in a 39.6% inhibition of glutamic acid decarboxylase activity. 5-HTP [5-hydroxy-tryptamine] decarboxylase, dopa decarboxylase, and choline acetyltransferase are inhibited to a lesser extent, 10.5%, 5.0% and 4.6% respectively. Tyrosine hydroxylase, catechol-O-methyltransferase, monoamine oxidase and acetylcholinesterase (AChE) are unaffected by the OHP. Except for AChE each of the above brain enzymes is inhibited by the 3Hg compounds: mercuric acetate, p-chloromercuribensoate and methyl mercuric chloride at a concentration of 10^{-4} M, the degree of inhibition being greatest with mercuric acetate and least with methyl Hg. In contrast to the situation with hyperbaric O_2, γ-aminobutyric acid metabolism is not preferentially altered by Hg compounds. (© BA)

1881.
TUNNICLIFF, G., M. Urton and J.D. Wood.
Susceptibility of chick brain L-glutamic acid decarboxylaze and other neurotransmitter enzymes to hyperbaric oxygen in vitro.
Biochem. Pharmacol. 22:501-505;Feb. 5, 1973.

Homogenates from chick whole brain were exposed to oxygen at 30 psi gauge pressure for 20 min at 25°. Controls were similarly incubated, but under a continuous flow of nitrogen at ambient pressure. The activities of the following neurotransmitter enzymes were then assayed in the homogenates: L-glutamic acid decarboxylase (GAD), 4-aminobutyrate-alpha-oxoglutarate aminotransferase (GABA-T) choline acetyltransferase (ChAc) acetylcholinesterase (AChE), tyrosine hydroxylase, dihydroxyphenylalanine decarboxylase (dopa decarboxylase), tryptophane hydroxylase, 5-hydrosytryptophan decarboxylase (5-HTP decarboxylase), monoamine oxidase (MAO) and catechol-O-methyl transferase (COMT). The activity of each of the biosynthetic enzymes, except that of the tyrosine and tryptophan hydroxylases, was inhibited by the high pressure oxygen (OHP), with that of GAD displaying the largest percentage decrease (GAD, 51%; Dopa decarboxylase, 12%; 5-HTP decarboxylase, 10%; ChAc, 7% inhibition). The four degradative enzymes were not inhibited by OHP. In a second experiment, homogenates were exposed to oxygen at 90 psi gauge pressure. Again GADshowed the greatest decrease in activity (GAD, 66%; Dopa decarboxylase, 18%; 5-HTP decarboxylase, 24%; and ChAc, 12% inhibition). The relatively high sensitivity of GAD to inhibition by OHP was in harmony with the hypothesis that a deranged gamma-aminobutyric acid metabolism plays a major role in the etiology of OHP-induced seizures. (Authors' abstract)

1882.
TURNER, H.C.
A design for a hydrostatic pressure chamber for calibrating piezoelectric pressure transducers.
Waltham Abbey, U.K., Explos. Res. Devel. Estab. Rep. ERDE-TN-20, DRIC-BR-21258, 12p. May 1970.
(AD 767 626/5 GA)

The measurement of the intensity and duration of underwater shock waves uses piezoelectric transducers permanently sealed to one end of a coaxial cable. A hydrostatic pressure chamber with a fast pressure release for the calibration of these transducers is described. The chamber has been designed to operate at pressures up to 10.4 MN/sq. m. Pressure is obtained from a built-in manual hydraulic screw pump and the pressure is released by a specially designed quick acting valve. (GRA)

1883.
TZIMOULIS, P.J.
Bombs away.
Skin Diver 20:3, 8, 10;Feb. 1971.

The greatest danger of damage in scuba equipment is inside the tank. Current DOT regulations for checking compressed gas cylinders is not adquate for scuba tanks. Sea water is more damaging than fresh water. There are many ways in which water can get into a scuba tank; one of the most common is pumping in air which has been insufficiently dried. This is particularly likely to happen with portable compressors. Other ways in which water can get into a tank are discussed. One form of corrosion is pitting, in which a hole is worn into the wall of the tank; ultimately, a weakened area results, through which compressed air is blown. To avoid this danger, the following steps may be taken: (1) Have an internal visual inspection of the tank once a year; (2) If corrosion has started, the cylinder should be steam cleaned, tumbled, and warm-air dried; where pitting is seen there should be a hydrostatic test; (3) whenever a tank becomes completely empty in sea water, the interior should be thoroughly inspected; (4) tanks should not be stored fully charged, should be stored in an upright position, and not in a very hot place. (MFW/SCD)

1884.
TZIMOULIS, P.J.
It takes more than a card.
Skin Diver 22:4;July 1973.

The author emphasizes the point that the basic scuba training course is but the beginning of a diver's education. Dr. Glenn Egstrom of UCLA is quoted as saying that upon completion of such a course, the next ten to 12 open water dives should be made under supervision of an instructor or an experienced diver. Another year of diving, at an average of at least two dives per month, is needed to gain the necessary confidence and experience. It generally requires 40 to 50 open water dives over a period of two years or more to make an experienced diver. The British Sub-Aqua Club requires over 100 dives for a First Class rating. In judging the extent of a diver's experience, number of dives is a much bertter indication than time span. The ultimate measurement of a diver's qualification will probably be the mastering of a given list of skills and accomplishments. Standardization along this line may come about as training methods become more developed and more exact. (MFW/SCD)

1885.
UCHUPI, E. and R.D. Ballard.
Bottom reconnaissance and detailed site survey by research submersibles.
In: Woods Hole, Mass., Woods Hole Oceanogr. Inst., Rep. WHO1-72-90, p.17-20; Nov. 30, 1972.

The geological bottom reconnaissance program is aimed at developing a series of instrument systems for the DSRV ALVIN and its support ship LULU which will significantly improve the ability of deep submersibles to carry out meaningful geologists in three major areas: the investigation of dynamic processes and structural features through detailed surveys, the collection and description of important bedrock exposures, and the placement of large bottom mounted instruments for short and long term measurements. (Authors)

1886.
UDDIN, D.E. and E.T. Flynn.
Serum enzyme studies during hyperbaric exposure.
In: Abstracts of BuMed-ONR sponsored Navywide workshop in high pressure biomedical research, U.S. Submarine Base, Groton, Conn. May 1971, p.17. Published by the Naval Submarine Medical Research Laboratory, 1971.

Abstract only. Entire item quoted: Serum enzyme levels have been frequently used as diagnostic aids to determine the site and extent of tissue damage. During a series of dives in helium-oxygen atmospheres, measurements of enzyme activity have been made before, during and after the hyperbaric exposure. The type of profiles that have been used include sub-saturation, saturation, and saturation-excursion types. Serum creatine phosphokinase (CPK), lactic dehydrogenase (LDH), glutamate-oxalacetate transaminase (GOT) and glutamate pyruvate transaminase (GPT) were measured by spectrophotometric methods. CPK levels appear to be the most sensitive indicator that was assayed. Increases of CPK occurred during saturation-excursion dives and during certain subsaturation dives. An increase of 5 to 10 fold over pre-dive control levels occurred in some divers. Generally, large increases in CPK were mirrored by delayed increases in LDH, GOT and occasionally GPT. Increases in serum CPK are generally attributed to muscle damage, either cardiac, or skeletal muscle. In addition to increases in serum CPK caused by pathological conditions, physical exercise has been shown to elevate serum CPK levels. Since swimming and weight lifting exercises were performed by the divers, it is conceivable that the increases observed are due to exercise rather than some factor in the high pressure environment. Another alternative is that repeated cycles of compression and decompression caused the increases in CPK.

1887.
UDDIN, D.E., R.E. Danziger, T.L. Sallee, J.M. Alexander and E.T. Flynn.
Biochemical studies during saturation diving: a comparison of a saturation dive with saturation-excursion dives.
U.S. Nav. Med. Res. Inst., Rep. on NAVMED-MF12.524.014-1005B.2, 47p. Oct. 12, 1971.
(AD 740 508)

A number of serum constituents were measured before, during and after one saturation-excursion dive to 300 feet of sea water (FSW), two saturation-excursion dives to 600 FSW, and one saturation dive to 1000 FSW. Significant increases in creatine phosphokinase (CPK) and lactate dehydrogenase (LDH) activity were noted on both saturation-excursion profiles, however, there were essentially no changes in serum enzyme activity during the saturation dive to 1000 FSW. On all three profiles, serum lactic acid was elevated with the largest increase occurring on the 1000 FSW dive. No changes were noted in the serum lipid constituents on any of these dives. These changes in serum biochemistries are discussed in relation to the differences in environmental conditions. (Authors) (GRA)

1888.
UHL, R.R., C. Van Dyke, R.B. Cook, R.A. Horst and J.M. Merz.
Effects of externally imposed mechanical resistance on breathing dense gas mixtures during exercise: I. Mechanics of breathing.
In: Aerospace Medical Association. 1971 annual scientific meeting. Houston, Texas, April 1971. Preprints, p.74-75. Published by the Association, 1971.

The authors have developed tests by which underwater breathing apparatus can be evaluated with regard to the effects of increased gas density and exercise on its performance. They developed a test protocol, and developed a prototype breathing system which simulates the effects of increased respiratory resistance. The following parameters were measured: tidal volume, rate, minute ventilation, alveolar ventilation, work and power of breathing, and compliance and resistance during inspiration and expiration. Arterial and expired gases were measured to assess alveolar ventilation. Five subjects were studied on a bicycle ergometer, using air and an SF_6-O_2 mixture, exercising and not, and being subjected to no resistance, one resistance or both (inspiratory and expiratory) resistances. It was found that when both resistances were added, during exercise, breathing the dense mixture, the subjects were stressed to their maximal tolerance. Hypoxemia and hypercarbia was present in all subjects. The most sensitive parameters were found to be power requirements of ventilation and work per liter of alveolar ventilation. (MFW/BSCP)

1889.
UHL, R.R., P.L. Hendricks, J. Merz, D.B. Arlin and E.L. Miller.
Cardiorespiratory response to breathing dense gas at exercise with imposed mechanical airway resistance.
In: Aerospace Medical Association. 1972 annual scientific meeting, Bal Harbour, Florida, May 1972. Preprints, p.174-175. Published by the Association.

Extremely well trained athletes could tolerate the combined effects of 500 kgM/work, breathing 80%SF_6/20%O_2 and moderate mechanical airway resistance, but one subject who was in apparently good physical shape, and rather representative of the diver community, sustained respiratory failure, due to increased dead space effect. When ventilatory failure occurs from these causes the heart is required to compensate, and the presence of a high myocardial metabolic demand in the face of hypercarbia and acidosis is not healthy. The implications to divers who are in the coronary prone group are not reassuring. (Authors' conclusions)

1890.
UHL, R.R., C. Van Dyke, R.B. Cook, R.A. Horst and J.M. Merz.
Effects of externally imposed mechanical resistance on breathing dense gas at exercise: mechanics of breathing.
Aerosp. Med. 43:836-842;Aug. 1972.

The effects of increased gas density, exercise and imposed mechanical resistance to respiration on breathing mechanics were studied in five subjects. 80% sulfur hexafluoride, 20% oxygen, a gas mixture 4.7 times as dense as air, was breathed to simulate increased density of the hyperbaric environment. Subjects were studied at rest and pedaling a bicycle ergometer at 500 Kgm/min. Mechanical resistance during inspiration, expiration or both was imposed. Subjects experienced progressive ventilatory requirement, and, finally, respiratory failure. Minute ventilation and alveolar ventilation increased with increasing stress. Alveolar ventilation became fixed at a mean value of ca 35 LPM, while carbon dioxide production rose rapidly. Ventilatory power requirement progressively increased to 40 times control values. Respiratory work per liter alveolar ventilation increased to 15 times control values. Frictional resistance increased markedly, and when respiratory failure occurred, compliance fell. This objective protocol is recommended for use in evaluation of underwater breathing apparatus. (Authors' abstract)

1891.
UHLIG, G. and G. Haux.
Report on the experiences with the underwater laboratory, Helgoland.
In: Fructus, X., ed. Third international conference on hyperbaric and underwater physiology, p.95-98. Paris, Doin, 1972.

The underwater laboratory Helgoland is 9 m long with a 2.5 meter diameter, consists of a wet room, a dry room which can be used as a decompression chamber, a system of atmosphere control which absorbs carbon dioxide by soda-lime, removes contaminants by charcoal filters, and constantly replenishes oxygen. It can accomodate four men. In spite of the unfavorable underwater conditions in the North Sea, of low temperature, poor visibility, and unfavorable sea states, underwater tasks were performed successfully. Each succeding team carried out longer working dives. The third team in the series of dives discussed here performed three hours daily, with some individual dives of four hours. (MWF/UMS)

1892.
UHRICH, R.W.
Terminus controlled deep ocean manipulator.
In: Ocean 73. 1973 IEEE international conference on engineering in the ocean environment, p.301-304. IEEE publication 73-CHO-7740-OCC.

The Naval Undersea Center has designed and built eleven different manipulative devices having up to seven independent functions. The most sophisticated of these devices is the Remote Unmanned Work System manipulator which is an all-purpose, seven function master-slave manipulator for light work at depths to 20,000 feet. The master or controller for this manipulator is a 3/4 scale analog. The operator grasps the "hand" or terminus of this device and moves it to a desired location and orientation; the hand of the manipulator or slave follows to a corresponding position. Forces encountered by the manipulator are stimulated in the controller giving the operator a form of force feedback. This type of terminus controller possesses several distinct advantages over exoskeletal "strap-on" manipulator controllers. (Author's abstract)

1893.
ULEWICZ, K.
Einfluss der Hyperbarie auf die immunologische Reaktionen des Organismus.
[The effect of hyperbaria on the immune response of an organism].
Ann. Immunol. Hung. 15:121-128; 1971.

To study the effect of hyperbaria on the immunological response, rabbits were exposed in a pressure chamber to O_2 hyperbaria of from 1.8 - 3.1 atm O_2 for a period of one hour. One to two days after exposure the opsonin index rose up to 4.8 with the degree of hyperbaria playing no role; normalization was in all cases achieved in ten days. Rabbits immunized with a killed Salmonella typhi suspension exposed to similar conditions manifested 24 hr to ten days later a titer decrease determined by the hemagglutination reaction. Simultaneously 1-14 days following exposure a quantitative decrease of IgG immunoglobulins and a lesser decrease of IgA and of IgM immunoglobulins was observed in the blood serum with no noticeable difference between animals exposed to normobaria or to hyperbaria. (RK) (© BA)

1894.
ULEWICZ, K. and P. Michniewski.
Untersuchungen zum Verhalten einiger seroligischen Reaktionen bei Kaninchen nach Oxygen-Hyperbarie.
[Studies on the relationship of some serological tests in rabbits to hyperbaric oxygen].
Ann. Immunol. Hung. 15:129-136; 1971.

Changes in serological tests were observed in rabbits exposed to hyperbaria (O_2) for a period of one hour. Changes indicated alterations in the immunological response of the organism. Immunized rabbits exposed to O_2 normobaria or hyperbaria for one hour manifested a decreased hemagglutination titer after 24 hr. Immunoelectrophoretic studies indicated that in almost all rabbits exposed to O_2 a quantitative decrease of immunoglobulin G (IgG) occurred one to ten days later. IgA and IgM levels dropped to a lesser degree. In humans the reaction is similar. (RK) (© BA)

1895.
ULEWICZ, K., P. Michniewski, B. Lokucijewski and T. Doboszynski.
Badania nad zachowaniem sie odezynow zlepnych oraz obrazu elektroforetyeznego bialek surowicy krwi u krolikow poddanych dzialaniu hiperbarii tlenowej.
[Agglutination tests and the electrophoretic picture of blood proteins of rabbits subjected to hyperbaric oxygenation].
Przegl. Lek. 27:581-584;Sept. 30, 1971.

The influence of oxygen hyperbaria within the range of 1.8 to 3.1 atm O_2 for a single 1-hour exposure on agglutination tests for the antigens of S. typhi O and S. Typhi H was studied on a material of 25 immunized rabbits, as was also the electrophoretic picture of the blood serum proteins. A certain tendency to fall in the titres of agglutination tests was found, but the shifts observed were not statistically significant. (Authors' abstract)

1896.
ULRICH, W.D., B.E. Smith and R.M. Fine.
Acoustic-optical detection of decompression sickness in hamsters.
U.S. Nav. Med. Res. Inst., Med. Res. Prog. Rep. 3, 23p. Mar. 1, 1972.
(AD 743,475)

Severe decompression sickness was produced by explosive decompression in twenty-three of forty-one anesthetized hamsters. Analysis of the post-decompression respiration pattern and ultrasonic transmission led to two observations: (1) animals without apnea never demonstrated macroscopic bubbles, and (2) animals which gasped always demonstrated macroscopic bubbles. The ultrasound attenuation generally preceded gasping but did not precede apnea unless more than ten minutes had elapsed since decompression. The respiratory signs were considered to be a consequence of pulmonary aeroembolism. Pilot studies with 2-(4-phenyl-piper-azinylmethyl) cyclohexanone HCL, showed that it decreased mortality in unanesthetized hamsters but increased mortality in animals anesthetized with chloralose-urethane. Pilot studies with piphenhydramine in anesthetized hamsters showed no change in mortality rates. (Authors)(GRA)

1897.
UNDERSEA MEDICAL SOCIETY.
U.S. Navy Supervisor of Diving, Dive — 1600 feet.
Pressure Med. Physiol. 2(Spec. Insert 2):1-4;July/Aug. 1973.

The April-May 1973 dive was designed to document the diver's ability to perform useful work at depth, using U.S. Navy apparatus and procedures. Six U.S. Navy divers, including two medical officers, participated. The compression rate was 0-14 fsw at 14 fpm, 14-400 fsw at 5 fpm, 400-1000 at 400 fph, 1000-1300 fsw at 30 fph, and 1300-1600 fsw 20 fph with stops at 400, 1000, and 1300 feet for studies. At 1600 feet, the MK10 MOD4 closed circuit breathing apparatus was tested, and it was found that light work could be accomplished, but increased work loads brought on respiratory distress which differed from that observed at shallower depths in that no significant carbon dioxide retention was detected. No EEG abnormalities were observed. Otitis externa was prevented by prophylactic use of 2% acetic acid in aluminum acetate in the ear and twice daily and immediately following each immersion. Subjective mood checklists revealed an increase in anxiety and hostility during compression, which remained slightly above normal until the eighth day of decompression. Mood fluctuated and appeared to be related to success or failure in performance tests. The ARL Helium Speech Converter from the U.K. was successfully used. Thermal comfort was achieved apparently at the expense of increased oxygen consumption. A higher than normal caloric intake was recorded though all divers lost weight. The decompression schedule was 10 fph for the first 30 f, then 1600-200 fsw at 6 fph, 200-100 fsw at 5 fph, 100-50 fsw at 4 fph, and 50 fsw-surface at 3 fph. For additional findings, see Spaur, W.H., Rough draft, May 20, 1973. (MFW/SCD)

1898.
UNITED STATES-JAPAN CONFERENCE ON NATURAL RESOURCES DEVELOPMENT.
Proceedings of the first joint meeting of the U.S.-Japan panel on diving and technology, Tokyo, 1972.
Japan, Ministry of Agriculture and Forestry, 1972, 196p.

The papers dealt with diving technology, equipment, and physiology and the development of diving technology for the advancement of marine science, with emphasis on cooperation and exchange between the two countries. Specific papers will be found under the following author entries: Beckman, E.L.; Fagan, C.J. and E.L. Beckman; Lefant, C.; Mano, T. and I. Nashimoto; Matsuda, M.; Miller, J.W.; Moore, T.O.; Nashimoto, I. and Y. Baba; Nashimoto, I. and Y. Mano, (two); Ohta, Y. and H. Matsunaga; Suzuki, J. (MFW/UMS)

1899.
UNITED STATES NAVAL COASTAL SYSTEMS LABORATORY.
Scientist in the Sea 1973.
Announcement, 1973.

The SITS program is designed to provide students with the breadth and depth of scientific diving information and skill to meet the growing demands of the marine science community. The curriculum is designed to provide advanced scientific diving technology for 16 scholars in graduate training and post-doctoral studies. Students will receive training in navigation and search, communications, semi-closed and open circuit scuba, advanced umbilical diving techniques, planning and implementation of diving programs, exposure to saturation diving principles and equipment, relevant scientific principles and methods from oceanography, biological sciences, geology, engineering science, behavioral sciences, diving medicine and archeology. Students completing the program will receive 12 quarter hours graduate credit and SUSIO certification in academic scientific diving. [The deadline for applications for the June 13 to August 22, 1973 course was April 16, but any one wanting further information on other courses may contact Dr. R. Smith, State University System Institute of Oceanography, 830 First Street, South, St. Petersburg, Florida]. (Author)

1900.
UNITED STATES NAVAL OCEANOGRAPHIC OFFICE.
Manned submersibles and underwater surveying. (SP-153)
Washington, D.C. Government Printing Office, 1970, 156p.

This report is based on the results of the U.S. Naval Oceanographic Office (NAV-OCEANO) operations with various manned submersibles through December 1969, but also includes the work of other agencies where their results are pertinent. The purpose of this report, and the objective of the Deep Oceanographic Survey Vehicle (DOSV) Project, are to define the state-of-the-art and availability of submersible instrumentation to conduct an undersea survey, the capability for conducting surveys with available Navy and commercial submersibles, the operational performance and design criteria, as deduced from operational experience, for a near-optimal DOSV, and to show those areas of ocean surveying where the manned submersible is best applied and has demonstrated its unique capability. (Author)

1901.
UNITED STATES NAVAL SUBMARINE MEDICAL RESEARCH LABORATORY.
Abstracts of BuMed-ONR sponsored Navywide workshop in high pressure biomedical research, U.S. Naval Submarine Base, Groton, Conn., May 1971.
Published by the Naval Submarine Medical Research Laboratory, 1971. 54p.

This workshop was composed of the following sessions: (1) Pulmonary function. (2) Oxygen toxicity. (3) Dental and microbiological aspects (4) Biochemical effects. (5) Membranes, bubbles and bones. (6) Performance. (7) Compression/decompression. (8) Environmental effects. (9) Bioengineering. (10) Hearing and vision. This publication consists of abstracts of the papers presented, which will be found under the following author entries: Adams, G.M.; Bachrach, A.J.; Berghage, T.E.; Brauer, R.M.; Chryssanthou, C.P.; Danziger, R.E.; DuBois, A.B. and A.B. Fisher; Elliott, D.H.; Farhi, L.E.; Hackney, J.D.; Hamilton, R.W., Jr., H.R. Schreiner, M.R. Powell and G.F. Doebbler; Heckley, R.J.; Hill, T.A.; Hills, B.A.; Hoke, B.; Houlihan, R.T.; Howe, G.R.; Knox, C.; Koski, W.S. and K.M. Wilson; Kunz, A.L.; Kylstra, J.A.; Lambertsen, C.J.; Langley, T.D. and R.W. Hamilton, Jr.; Lanphier, E.H.; Luria, S.M.; Malecki, G.S.; Martin, J.L. and R.M. Jacobs; Mazzarella, M.A.; McSherry, C.K.; Moeller, G. and J.R. MacKinnon; Moritz, W.E.; Neptune, E.M.; Orsi, E.V.; Park, S.S.; Parker, J.W.; Reich, T.; Rodkey, F.I.; Rosenbaum, R.M.;

Sanders, A.P.; Schlamm, N.A.; Sergeant, R.L.; Shiller, W.R.; Shilling, C.W.; Small, A.; Smith, K.H.; Smith, P.F.; Sobel, H.; Tappan, D.V.; Todd, G.P.; Uddin, D.E. and E.T. Flynn; Vail, E.G.; Wilson, R.H. and F.R. O'Brien. (MFW/BSCP)

1902.
UNITED STATES NAVAL SUBMARINE MEDICAL RESEARCH LABORATORY.
Cumulative bibliography and index of research reports and publications originating in the submarine medical research laboratory 1942 through 1971.
Groton, Conn., U.S. Nav. Submar. Med. Cent., Dec. 31, 1971, 120p.
(AD 758 988)

A cumulative bibliography and index of research reports and publications on submarine medicine is presented. The index contains a chronological list of SMRL reports and an index of authors. (GRA)

1903.
UNITED STATES NAVY
U.S. Navy diving manual.
Washington, D.C., United States Navy Department, Supervisor of Diving, 1973.
(NAVSHIPS 0994-001-9010).
(Available from the Government Printing Office, Washington, D.C.)

The manual has been rewritten, and its format changed. Volume 1 deals with air diving, and its contents are: (1) History of diving; (2) Underwater physics; (3) Underwater physiology; (4) Operations planning; (5) Air diving operations (scuba); (6) Surface-supplied air diving operations; (7) Air decompression; (8) Diving emergencies; (App. A) Formulas and conversion factors; (App. B) Record keeping and reporting; (App. C) Sea state chart; (App. D) U.S. Navy-approved diving equipment; (App. E) Selection, qualification and training of personnel; (App. F) Ship repair safety checklist; (App. G) Navship Publicatins; (App. H) Gage calibration procedures; (App. I) Dangerous marine animals; (App. J) General safety checklist: (App. K) Surface-supplied diving operations pre-dive checklist; (App. L) Pressure test for USN recompression chambers. Volume 2 concerns mixed gas diving, and its contents are: (9) Mixed-gas diving theory; (10) Mixed-gas underwater breathing apparatus; (11) Surface-supplied mixed gas diving operations; (12) Deep diving systems; (13) Oxygen diving operations; (14) Mixed-gas decompression (App. II-A) Diving gases; (App. II-B) Cleaning oxygen systems; (App. II-C) Safe handling of gases; (App. II-D) U.S. Navy-approved mixed-gas diving equipment; (App. II-E) Mk 6 Mod 0 mixed-gas scuba; (App. II-F) Mk 10 Mod 4 mixed-gas UBA; (App. II-G) Mk II Mod 0 mixed-gas UBA; (App. II-H) Surface-supplied mixed-gas diving operations — predive checklist. (MFW/UMS)

1904.
UNITED STATES NAVY SUPERVISOR OF DIVING.
Directory of world-wide, shore-based hyperbaric chambers. Volumes I and II.
Washington, D.C., Department of the Navy, Naval Ship Systems Command, 1971.
(NAVSHIPS 0994-010-4012)

This publication lists hyperbaric facilities of all kinds, such as the research facility at the Experimental Diving Unit, facilities designed for medical treatment in hospitals, and small chambers designed primarily for emergency use. Complete descriptive data are given when available — working pressure, size, heating gas, occupancy, etc. Also given are the nearest airport, helipad and boat dock. Volume I contains facilities in the United States and Canada, Volume II contains all others. No attempt is made to evaluate the facilities or the quality of their operation. (MFW/BSCP)

1905.
UNITED STATES NAVY SUPERVISOR OF DIVING.
Diver equipment. General requirements for material certification.
Washington, D.C., Department of the Navy, Naval Ship Systems Command, 1971. 62p.
(NAVSHIPS 0994-012-3010)

This publication describes the general requirements that a designer or manufacturer must meet to obtain material certification of diver equipment. These requirements are intended to serve as guidelines and not as restrictions on the development or use of new ideas and equipment. Material certification requirements are discussed throughout ten chapters. However, the bulk of material requirements is contained in Chapter 3, "Diver Equipment Design Criteria". Specific components and systems are covered in Section 2 of this chapter, "Design Acceptance Criteria". Recordable evidence of compliance with certification requirements in the form of documentation is stressed. [The table of contents is as follows: 1. Purpose and applicability; 2. Material certification scope; 3. Diver equipment design criteria; 4. Fabrication and assembly processes; 5. Quality assurance; 6. Testing; 7. Operation and maintenance; 8. Survey of the diver equipment; 9. Material certification application; 10. Tenure of material certification.] (Author's abstract and contents)

1906.
UNITED STATES NAVY SUPERVISOR OF DIVING.
Handbook: U.S. Navy diving operations.
Washington, D.C., Department of the Navy, Naval Ship Systems Command, 1971, 197p.
(NAVSHIPS 0994-012-3010)

As part of a continuing effort to maximize the availability of useful information for the fleet diver, the Office of The Supervisor of Diving has prepared this concise guide for the conduct of diving operations. Its content is based upon the most frequently used information from the Diving Manual and also introduces several new types of equipment and previously unpublished information on diving. The handbook has been designed for quick reference by the diver "on station" and features many new visual forms of information display. Throughout the handbook, illustrations, charts, and diagrams have been used in place of text matter. Rotary selector charts and calculators have been employed to condense information into compact forms and minimize the need for computations and cross-referencing to other sources of information. Color printing has been used to highlight and separate various sections. Areas, such as recompression treatment, have been reorganized to simplify instructions. (From preface)

1907.
UNITED STATES NAVY SUPERVISOR OF DIVING.
U.S. Navy recompression chamber operator's handbook.
Washington, D.C., Department of the Navy, Naval Ships Systems Command, 1973. 68p.
(NAVSHIPS 0994-014-5010)

This concise publication is intended as a quick reference on-station guide, and not as a substitute for the U.S. Navy Diving Manual section on this subject, which is more complete. This well-organized, pocket-size handbook discusses chamber operation, recompression treatment, installation and maintenance, and other uses (such as surface decompression, omitted decompression, and diver candidate tests for selection). (MFW/UMS)

1908.
UNSWORTH, I.P.
Case report: Pulmonary barotrauma in a hyperbaric chamber.
Anaesthesia 28:675-678;Nov. 1973.

The author describes a case of tension pneumothorax, which occurred during decompression of a 55-year-old woman being treated with hyperbaric oxygen for cancer. Upper abdominal pain occurred at 1.3 ATA, and disappeared following recompression to 1.5 ATA. Within two minutes of completion of the second decompression, cyanosis, a drop in blood pressure to 90/50 mm Hg, and apparent loss of consciousness occurred. The patient had previously undergone a permanent tracheostomy, through which oxygen was administered. External cardiac massage was performed. X-ray revealed complete collapse of the right lung, a shift of the mediastinum to the left and a lowering of the right diaphragm. Treatment consisted of the release of gas through a wide-bore underwater drainage and pulmonary reinflation. The patient had been suffering from a chronically obstructive airway, with neoplasm in the right lobe, which was thought to have caused the pneumothorax. (MFW/BSCP)

1909.
URGENA, R.B.
Oxygen toxicity: Basic and clinical considerations.
J. Iowa Med. Soc. 12:583-587;Nov. 1972.

This is a review article on oxygen toxicity with references made to numerous investigations in the field. It is noted that with divers the CNS type of oxygen toxicity, which starts with muscular twitches around the face and culminates in convulsions, is the most frequent. Morbidity is minimal, and retrograde amnesia the only sequela. The clinical type of pulmonary oxygen toxicity, which apparently consists of an early exudative phase and a late proliferative phase, is discussed at some length. The mechanism is not clear, but the toxic effect of oxygen on many enzyme systems is believed to be involved. It has been demonstrated that partial pressure of oxygen and the actual concentration of oxygen in the breathing mixture, are more significant than atmosphere pressure in oxygen toxicity. Duration of exposure, temperature and humidity play important roles. Clinical studies have shown that an extrapulmonary factor depending on arterial oxygen tensions is involved. Patients with high A-a oxygen gradients are more resistant. Hypercarbia enhances toxic reactions. Adrenocorticoid hormones appear to aggravate toxicity. Safety measures to be observed when oxygen is used therapeutically are delineated. Close monitoring of the inspired oxygen concentration, and the arterial oxygen tension should be maintained when long term therapy is undertaken. (MFW/BSCP)

1910.
URICK, R.J.
Some perspectives and recent findings in shallow water acoustics.
U.S. Nav. Ord. Lab. Rep. NOLTR 71-204, 36p. Nov. 1971.
(AD 735 108)

Shallow water acoustics has had in this country a long, though sporadic history dating back to World War II, when the acoustic mine stimulated feverish activity in the subject. Yet, many aspects of this most difficult branch of underwater acoustics are not understood. Many of its complications are due to the temporal and spatial variability of the shallow water medium and its boundaries. For example, it was found that the transmission of shallow water sound will vary with direction and time at one location and to be different at apparently similar locations. Such variations make acoustic prediction difficult, and necessitate on-the-spot measurements at the place and time that data is required. To this end, the author had developed and tried out at a number of coastal locations an airborne method of data collection using sonobuoys, explosive sound signals, and simple, portable recording equipment. The transmission results have been summarized by loss contour charts showing the transmission environment around a receiving point in shallow water. (Author) (GRA)

1911.
URICK, R.J., G.R. Lund and T.J. Tulko.
The depth profile of ambient noise in the deep sea north of St. Croix, Virgin Islands.
U.S. Nav. Ord. Lab., Rep. NOL-TR-72-176, 30p. Aug. 1972.
(AD 750,693)

The deep sea appears to be quieter at mid-depth than at greater or lesser depths. This was found in a series of measurements of the ambient noise background at a location north of St. Croix, V.I., using hydrophones suspended from a cable at intervals of 2000 feet down to 8100 feet. The noise profiles show a sharp decrease of noise from the surface down to 6100 feet and a reversal of the profile below. The measurement site is an active, dynamic one, and shows a large variability in noise level from hour to hour. (Authors) (GRA)

1912.
URICK, R.J.
Coherence of ambient noise and the signal from a steady source at different depths at a deep sea location.
U.S. Nav. Ord. Lab., Rep. NOLTR-74-68, 40p., Apr. 18, 1973.
(AD 763 334)

A 200-ft vertical array of six irregularly spaced hydrophones has been used to obtain coherence information on the ambient sea noise and the sound from a distant 1120 Hz source. Data was recorded at different depths down to 12,000 ft in 13,600 ft of water. Time delay correlograms substantiate a binary ambient noise model consisting of a low frequency component of horizontally travelling noise from distant sources and a high frequency component of vertically arriving noise from local noise sources on the sea surface. The coherence at all frequencies was found to decrease with increasing frequency and hydrophone spacing. On the other hand, the coherence of the 1120 Hz signal was independent of spacing and was higher and less variable in the direct sound field from the source than it was in the more distant bottom-reflected field. The results apply to the optimum design of vertical arrays in the deep sea. (Author) (GRA)

1913.
VAIL, E.G.
Hyperbaric respiratory mechanics.
In: 1970 IEEE international conference on engineering in the ocean environment, Panama City, Florida, 21 September. Digest of tutorial papers, p.30-36. New York, Lewis Winner, 1970.

1. Primary airway collapse occurs in the subsegmental bronchi at critical collapse pressure up to 140 mm Hg. Maximum expiratory flow peak is always limited by the critical collapse pressure of the subsegmental bronchi. 2. There is no such physiological phenomena as "inert gas narcosis" or "nitrogen narcosis." Such phrases imply a biochemical action on the physiological system. Since the physiological condition results from the physical effects of the density of the breathing gas mixture, more appropriate phrases as "hyperbaric hypoxia" for the saturation diver and "normobaric hypoxia" for the emphysema patient. Both individuals suffer concurrent hypoxia and carbon dioxide retention as a result of inadequate alveolar ventilation in their respective environments. 3. There is no saturation diving system or respirator device presently in use which is capable of resolving the relationships of critical collapse pressure, expiratory flow rate, expiratory resistance, and expiratory time which cause airway collapse, and maintain a proper physiological level for alveolar ventilation. Any system which contributes to an increased expiratory resistance will only shorten the onset of airway collapse earlier in the expiratory phase. 4. A new philosophy in establishing bioengineering design criteria for respiratory devices is required. These design criteria must include a full appreciation of the science of fluidics and elastic tube theory, as well as the anatomical and physiological characteristics of respiratory mechanics. 5. Empirical graphs which depict the critical collapse pressure based entirely on the maximum expiratory flow rate can be used for every individual to establish an expiratory flow and time cycle to assure adequate alveolar ventilation. Divers and patients can be trained to use the expiratory flow rate required to obtain optimal alveolar ventilation for the selected diving depth or relief of the hypoventilation condition. (Author's conclusions)

1914.
VAIL, E.G.
Respiratory mechanics — airway collapse.
In: Abstracts of BuMed-ONR sponsored Navywide workshop in high pressure biomedical research, U.S. Naval Submarine Base, Groton, Conn., May 1971, p.4. Published by the Naval Submarine Medical Research Laboratory, 1971.

Abstract only. Entire item quoted: Pulmonary function tests were conducted on 37 healthy adults. The experimental data indicate that maximum expiratory flow rates are limited by collapse of the segmental bronchi. Maximum inspiratory flow rates are limited, during performance of maximum breathing capacity (MBC), by closure of the subsegmental bronchi. Maximum expiratory flow rates during MBC are also limited by collapse of the subsegmental bronchi. If airway closure/collapse occurred in the small bronchi, bronchioles, terminal bronchioles, or respiratory bronchioles, then the flow rate would have to exceed 18 liters per second.

1915.
VALIMAKI, M. and J. Niinikoski.
Development of reversibility of pulmonary oxygen poisoning in the rat.
Aerosp. Med. 44:533-538;May 1973.

Acute pulmonary oxygen poisoning was studied in rats by exposing them to 90-95% O_2 at 1 atm for 24, 48, or 72 hours. Progressive pulmonary oedema developed within 48 hours, and approximately 40% of the rats died during the third day of exposure. Pulmonary surfactant was extracted from the rats by endobronchial washing with saline, and the composition of endobronchial extracts was analysed. When acute pulmonary oedema occurred, a simultaneous increase took place in the amounts of lipid phosphorus, DNA, nitrogen, protein and hexosamines in the endobronchial washings. The most sensitive indicators of O_2-induced pulmonary damage were the amounts of peptide-bound hydroxyproline and uronic acids which increased sharply after 24 hours of O_2 breathing. Recovery from oxygen poisoning was studied in rats breathing air for 1-14 days after the 3-day exposure to oxygen. One day after resumption to air breathing the amount of DNA in the endobronchial extract returned to normal while lipid phosphorus, nitrogen, protein, peptide-bound hydroxyproline, hexosamines and uronic acids remained pathologically high. After five days of air breathing the composition of endobronchial extracts was entirely normal indicating a recovery from the exudative phase of oxygen poisoning. During the 15-day recovery period the amounts of collagen hydroxyproline and uronic acids increased progressively in the lung tissue. This may indicate development of fibrosis occurring after oxygen-induced pulmonary trauma. (Authors' abstract)

1916.
VAN DEN BRENK, H.A.S.
The hazards of oxygen toxicity in a hyperbaric environment.
In: Innes, G.S., ed. The production and hazards of a hyperbaric oxygen environment. Proceedings of a symposium held at University College, London, January 1968, p.42-52. Oxford, Pergamon Press, 1970.

The author discusses the effects of increased oxygen partial pressure on the cell reproduction cycle, primarily in relation to its use in cancer therapy, and concludes that under clinical conditions it is unlikely that HPO would damage the proliferative capacities of cellular systems. He then discusses the somatic effects of oxygen toxicity, which occur chiefly in the central nervous system (causing convulsions and brain damage) and the lungs (causing pulmonary hemorrhagic consolidation, edema and atelectasis). The author presents the theory that the pulmonary lesions result not directly from the effect of oxygen on the lungs but indirectly from damage caused by oxygen in the central nervous system. Various experiments along these lines conducted by the author and other investigators have indicated that convulsions brought on by agents other than oxygen will bring about lung lesions indistinguishable from those associated with oxygen toxicity. This line of experimentation also points up the possibility that such a "stressor" action of oxygen could upset neuroendocrinologic balance and produce other adverse sequelae. Used with proper care, it is unlikely that therapeutic HPO will produce harmful effects. However, it must be kept in mind that hypersensitivity to HPO exists in some individuals. The author concludes that "oxygen may be regarded as a biological stressor which places a load on the antioxidative defense mechanism of cells and tissues, to which neurones of the CNS appear most intolerant." (MFW/BSCP)

1917.
VAN DYKE, C., R.R. Uhl, R.B. Cook, R.A. Horst and J.M. Merz.
Effects of externally imposed mechanical resistance on breathing dense gas mixtures during exercise: II. Alveolar ventilation and acid-base metabolism.
In: Aerospace Medical Association. 1971 annual scientific meeting. Houston, Texas, April 1971. Preprints, p.78-79. Published by the Association, 1971.

Breathing with an underwater breathing apparatus (UBA) at 1000 feet in the ocean was simulated by having five subjects breathe a dense gas (SF_6/O_2) against imposed mechanical resistances. Results indicated that during moderate exercise there was retained carbon dioxide, acidosis, and ominously reduced arterial oxygen tensions. (Authors' summary)

1918.
VAN KEMPEN, L.H.J., H. Deurenberg and F. Kreuzer.
The CO_2 pressure in gases and liquids.
Resp. Physiol. 14(3):366-381; 1972.

An electrode is described consisting of a combined Pt-calomel electrode (or Ag/AgCl electrode) immersed in 0.1 N KCl solution with 10^{-3} M/l quinhydrone and separated from the medium by a CO_2 permeable membrane. The whole system is thermostated. The resulting electrode potential is linearly related to the logarithm of the CO_2 partial pressure of the medium. From 25 E[internal energy] vs. pH curves at 25$\pm$0.1°C with quinhydrone concentrations ranging from 1-25 10^{-3} M/la- $\Delta E/\Delta pH$ value of 58.2$\pm$2.7mV/pH was derived and EO was 700 $\pm$ 4mV. Addition of 0.25 M/l $NaHCO_3$ to the electrode fluid changed $\Delta E/\Delta \log PCO_2$ [CO_2 tension] from 29.7-57.2. The effect of Cl ions and O_2 on the electrode potential and the influence of time and light on the spectral properties of quinhydrone were studied. Stability, response time, and error of PCO_2 in this electrode system are of the same order of magnitude as in the Stow electrode. (© BA)

1919.
VAN LIEW, H.D.
Diffusion limitation of nitrogen washout: studies with subcutaneous gas pockets.
In: Abstracts of the Twenty-fifth Congress of Physiological Sciences Satellite Symposium. Recent progress in fundamental physiology of diving. Marseille, France, July 1971, p.57-58. (Proceedings unpublished)

Abstract only. Excerpts quoted: In experiments with unanesthetized rats, rates of volume decrease were compared in nitrogen-filled pockets and oxygen-filled pockets (Van Liew, Resp. Physiol. 12(2):163-168, 1971). The large capacity for carriage of oxygen on hemoglobin means that diffusion limitation has relatively little effect on the amount of O_2 picked up by blood. Therefore, oxygen provides a baseline for establishing the degree of diffusion limitation for N_2. Use of a mathematic technique that accounts for differences in solubility and diffusivity of O_2 and N_2 and for the hemoglobin carriage of O_2 led to the conclusion that nitrogen comes about 75% of the way to equilibrium in capillary blood. That is, each unit of blood leaving the tissue carried about 3/4 as much nitrogen as it would if the diffusion of nitrogen was infinitely rapid. In other words, the blood flow is 75% effective for nitrogen washout. This same conclusion was reached earlier in comparisons between N_2, He and H_2 in gas pockets when the latter two gases were assumed to have no diffusion limitation.

1920.
VAN LIEW, H.D.
Gas pocket oxygen and carbon dioxide in rats in normoxic hyperbaric environment.
Aerosp. Med. 44:371-373;Apr. 1973.

The gas pocket technique indicated that subcutaneous tissue PO_2 was approximately normal and tissue PCO_2 was at most 10 mm Hg above normal in unanesthetized rats exposed to normoxic gas mixtures at 4.4 and 7.8 Ata. (Author's abstract)

1921.
VAN LIEW, H.D., R.D. Rodner and A.L. Olszowka.
Steady-state compositions of tissue gas pockets in rats in hyperoxic environments.
Aerosp. Med. 44:499-504;May 1973.

This is a study of composition and rate of N_2 exchange of artificially-formed gas pockets in unanesthetized rats exposed to O_2-enriched environments up to 6 ata. Despite limitations of the technique, the following conclusions were reached: (1) The maximal rise of tissue PCO_2 attributable to the hyperoxia was 11 mm Hg except in rats severely afflicted by oxygen toxicity. (2) High pocket PO_2 in hyperoxic environments is partly artifact, perhaps partly a reflection of better arterial oxygentation, and probably not due to increased blood flow to the tissue. (3) Tissue PCO_2 was above 100 mm Hg in rats that had convulsed due to O_2 toxicity, and was about 6 mm Hg below normal the day following exposure to toxic levels of O_2. (Authors' abstract)

1922.
VANROUX, R.
Effects of metabolic acidosis on ventilation during muscular exercise.
Bull. Physiolpathol. Resp. (Nancy) 9(3):807-813; 1973.

When the work load reaches a certain level, ventilation increases asymptotically. This slope is examined in this study. The author discusses ventilation and metabolic acidosis during increasing load, and during an exercise with steady load. A significant relationship exists between the evolution of metabolic acidosis and ventilatory equivalent for oxygen. It is concluded that ventilation increases as the load increases (1) to meet the greater oxygen requirement and (2) to compensate for metabolic acidosis. (MFW/UMS)

1923.
VANUXEM, P., S. Delpierre, Y. Jammes, D. Vanuxem and C. Grimaud.
Barosensibilite sinusal et mechanique ventilatoire: influence de la gazometrie sanquine.
[Sinusal barosensitivity and ventilatory mechanics: influence of bloos gastrometry].
J. Physiol. (Paris) 65 (Suppl. 3):515A; 1972.

The effects of brief sinusal hyperpressure (150-200 mm Hg) on various ventilatory parameters were studied in anesthetized rabbits under normal gasometric conditions and in normoxic and hyperoxic hypercapnia. Under normal conditions, sinusal hyperpressure tends to depress respiratory parameters; this respiratory response always precedes the circulatory response slightly. In normoxic hypercapnia, only some of the respiratory response always precedes the circulatory response slightly. In normoxic hypercapnia, only some of the respiratory parameters are affected, while in hyperoxic hypercapnia, there is no change after 15 minutes; a significant decrease in transpulmonary inspiratory pressure is noted after 20 minutes. (MEMH/UMS)

1924.
VARENE, P.
Les facteurs limitants de la plongee profonde. 1. Les troubles de la ventilation pulmonaire.
[Limiting factors of deep diving. 1. The problems of pulmonary ventilation].
Gaz. Med. France 78:4099-4106;July 9, 1971.

These physiological data show the relative inadaptability of human ventilatory mechanics to dense environments, and account for the fact that, after a more or less brief period, the diver finds limitations placed on his performance. If, in this respect, we are still far from having reached the absolute limit of possibility, it appears certain that, at the present stage in the development of experimental diving, the threshold of relative limitations has been crossed, particularly when muscular exercise is involved, with the breathing mixtures now used. Technological solutions to be attempted in the future must certainly take into account these findings. Under present conditions, it appears that such solutions might be found at the equipment level, where the energy process is involved. But the difficulties to be surmounted will doubtless be much greater with regard to purely ventilatory limitations. (Author's summary translated by MFW/BSCP)

1925.
VARENE, P., C. Jacquemin and J. L'Huillier.
Les performances ventilatoires en plongee.
[Ventilatory performance in diving].
In: Fructus, X., ed. Third international conference on hyperbaric and underwater physiology, p.88-94. Paris, Doin, 1972.

It is concluded that comparative studies of the functioning of the pulmonary exchange from the aspects of ventilation and of energy make it possible to place different limits on these performances. During muscular exercise, this limit is of ventilatory origin, the convection mass becoming insufficient to assure exchange. Inversely, the regulatory system of these exchanges conditions these performances by the energetic parameters of the ventilation. Taking these findings into account, the adaptation of the diver will result in pushing farther back the ventilatory limit to the detriment of the exchanges. The disturbance of the exchanges will be concerned chiefly with CO_2, oxygen generally being superabundant in the environment. (Authors' conclusion translated by MFW/UMS)

1926.
VARENE, P., H. Viellefond, H. Guenard and J. L'Huillier.
Experience Sagittaire I: Le bilan thermique des plongeurs en atmosphere helium oxygene.
[Sagittaire I experiment: Thermal evaluation of divers in a helium-oxygen atmosphere].
Contract CEV/CNEXO 70/244, Cent. Essais Vol, Lab Med. Aerosp., Rep. CEV 71/506, 85p. Oct. 1972.

Thermal evaluation was carried out during the Sagittaire I experiment on 4 nude, resting subjects in a helium-oxygen atmosphere at pressures between 1.5 and 30.79 ATA. An increase in respiratory quotient is due to increased exhalation of CO_2 with increases in pressure; alveolar CO_2 partial pressure is also increased. Evaporation due to skin perspiration does not vary greatly from normobaric values. Radiation heat loss diminished with the rise in pressure and the concomitant rise in ambient temperatures. Heat loss due to respiration increased as a function of ambient pressure and of the temperature of the breathing mixture. Heat loss due to skin convection increases as a function of the composition of the breathing mixture and of the ambient pressure. (MEMH/UMS)

1927.
VAUGHAN, R.W.
Modification of the YFNB-43 barge to support the Mark I Deep Dive System.
In: The working diver, 1972. Symposium proceedings, February 1972. Columbus, Ohio, p.53-84. Washington, D.C., Marine Technology Society, 1972.

A description of the significant tasks involved in the modification of the YFNB-43 Barge to accommodate the MK Deep Dive System so as to produce an integrated self-sufficient diving platform is presented herein. The main theme of the presentation is the utilization of available existing equipment and the design problems associated with installing this equipment on the barge. Significant items discussed are selection of a barge, positioning of MK I DDS modules, handling system, mooring equipment, gas supply, power supply, habitability, waste treatment system. (Author's abstract)

1928.
VAUGHAN, W.S., Jr. and A.S. Mavor.
Diver performance in controlling a wet submersible during four-hour exposures to cold water.
Hum. Factors 14(2):173-180;Apr. 1972.

Six 4-hr., open-sea test trials were conducted with a wet submersible. The purpose of these trials was to assess the effects of long exposure to cold (16.4°C) water on man's ability to perform basic submersible control tasks. The subjects were experienced submersible pilots who had a minimum of 20 hours training prior to the experimental trials. Skin and rectal temperatures were continuously recorded from both the pilot and rider of the submersible. A continuous record of vehicle depth and water temperature was also obtained. The pilot's task was to mantain a prescribed depth while performing a sequence of course changes for a 4-hr. period of submergence. Depth error variance was correlated with pilot core and skin temperature changes over time, and although pilot core temperature fell as much as 1.83°C, no degradation in depth control performance was apparent. (Authors' abstract)

1929.
VEENKANT, R.L.
Underwater sound propagation in the Straits of Florida. The MIMI Lunar-cycle receptions.
Ann Arbor, Mich., Mich. Univ., Cooley Electron Lab., Rep. TR-219, 156p. Jan. 1972.
(AD 736,229)

The study is part of a continuing program of underwater sound propagation research called project MIMI. The report covers reception and processing and a limited number of analytic comments. The test timing and duration were chosen to allow closer examination of propagation anomalies previously observed during the early winter and to obtain continuous data on an entire lunar-tide cycle (approximately 28 days). The major objectives were to provide data for the design of more extensive experiments and to test the programs and techniques associated with the LINC-8 computer. Signal processing was designed to yield both multipath information and data on anomalous path conditions. The principal success of the study has been in the improvement of processing programs and experiment design. (Author) (GRA)

1930.
VEGHTE, J.H. and F.K. Klemm.
Cold water evaluation of environmental marine diving suits.
Wright-Patterson AFB, Aerosp. Med. Res. Lab., Rep. AMRL-TR-72-65;22p. 1972.
(AD 754 278)

The 24-hour cold water immersion-life raft exposures were conducted in our laboratory test facility involving three subjects in each exposure. Physiologic data were obtained during these exposures to discern the better cold water protective capabilities of two environmental marine diving suits. The Swedish Unisuit proved thermally superior to the Dunlop suit. Several recommendations are made. (Authors) (GRA)

1931.
VEGHTE, J.H.
Cold sea survival.
Aerosp. Med. 43:506-511;May 1972.

Two prototype three-man life rafts were evaluated during the winter months in Arctic waters off Kodiac Island, Alaska, to assess potential survival problems and determine tolerance limits. Each raft incorporated thermal characteristics specifically designed for cold water. Water and air temperatures varied from 0 to +2C and -5 to +1C respectively. Surface and core temperatures of each of the three subjects were monitored continuously during the 22-hr exposure in the TUL raft and the 6-hr exposure in the P-B raft. Each subject wore a different clothing assembly: a full pressure suit, light flight clothing and the ventile anti-exposure suit. All subjects were removed upon reaching subjective tolerance. The results showed that none of the clothing assemblies was adequate to maintain a person in comfort even with dry boarding. No significant biochemical shifts in the blood or urine were found. The TUL raft was found to be superior in its thermal characteristics and afforded better subject protection. General tolerance for cold water immersion, wet and dry and cold water raft exposures are depicted graphically, based on previously reported data. (Author's abstract)

1932.
VERLANDER, J.M. and S.E. Huggins.
Alteration in central nervous activity of *Caiman sclerops* during voluntary diving.
Fed. Proc. 31:378;Mar./Apr. 1972.

Abstract only. Entire item quoted: Certain aspects of the diving reflex, notably extreme bradycardia, have been demonstrated in a wide variety of vertebrate species, including crocodilian reptiles. Alterations in other physiological parameters during diving have been less intensively studied. This investigation sought to amplify knowledge of physiological changes contingent with diving using unrestrained animals diving voluntarily in shallow water. In particular, possible alterations in CNS activity were sought, employing the EEG as the indicator of such changes. Five pair of epidural electrodes implanted over the forebrain were employed. Power spectral density analysis indicated a lowering of frequency and an increase in relative power during diving, comparable to that seen in this group of animals during sleep and in the supine trance-like state. Careful observation of the entire physiological picture indicates that the act of submersion or of emergence does not directly initiate or terminate the reflex, but that the diving complex may be instituted or terminated through the intervention of the forebrain.

1933.
VERUNAC, J.J.
Recurrent severe facial emphysema in a submariner.
J. Amer. Dent. Ass. 87:1192-1194;Nov. 1973.

A young submariner, in good health, repeatedly suffered severe facial swelling within a few hours of submergence on submarine patrol. Examination revealed an exposed root canal, through which air entered when the air pressure increased. Air passed through the thin bucal bone into the interstitial spaces of the head and neck. The resulting emphysema would greatly increase until it became incapacitating. Removal of the tooth ended the condition. (MFW/UMS)

1934.
VIELLEFOND, H., G. Saumon, J.L. Huillier and P. Varene.
Etude, en fonction de la pression ambiante, des relations existant entre les debits, les pressions, et les volumes pulmonaires.
[Study of the relationships among debits, pressures, and pulmonary volumes, as a function of ambient pressure].
J. Physiol. (Paris) 65:312-A - 313-A; 1972.

The influence of ambient pressure on respiratory parameters was studied by calculating total lung conductance and lung compliance from a series of curves representing six volumetric values. Results of these calculations show that total lung conductance, vital capacity, respiratory volume, and lung compliance do not vary systematically with ambient pressure. Relationships between total lung conductance and vital capacity were found for values between 20% and 50% of total vital capacity. (MEMH/UMS)

1935.
VIELLEFOND, H., G. Saumon and P. Varene.
Exploration mechanique ventilatoire de l'homme en hyperbarie prolongee.
[Investigation of the ventilatory mechanics of man under prolonged hyperbaric exposure].
J. Physiol. (Paris) 65(Suppl.1):173A; 1973.

It has been found that maximum voluntary ventilation decreases with pressure because of an increase in total resistance and a decrease in maximum expiratory debit. These findings were verified in a simulated dive to 52 ATA, of three days duration, using a breathing mixture of helium and oxygen. Results showed that pulmonary compliance did not change, that total resistance increased, and maximum expiratory debit decreased, with pressure. It is concluded that if respiratory parameters undergo such noticeable changes in subjects at rest, that a purely ventilatory limitation exists for muscular exercise at depths below 500 meters using helium oxygen. (MFW/SCD)

1936.
VILYUNOV, G.A., Yu.N. Osherovskni, B.R. Glants, A.A. Rafal'skni, A.F. Litavrin and V.M. Kalinarzh.
Klinicheskoe primenenie baroterapii.
[Clinical use of barotherapy].
Voennomed. Zh. (8):73-76;Aug. 1973.

The authors list the following cases in which hyperbaric oxygenation proved to be successful: Treatment and prevention of decompression sickness in divers and submariners, therapy of various wounds and injuries complicated by gas gangrene, hypoxia in severe head injuries, reanimation in drowning, therapy of toxic pulmonary edema and, most effectively, in the treatment of carbon monoxide poisoning. Barotherapy was administered at military base hospitals in standard recompression chambers used for divers, or portable recompression chambers used in mobile units. All barochambers were equipped with automatic devices for continuous registration of pulse frequency, oxyhemogram, respiratory, ECG and EEG indices during treatment. The authors recommend that medically supervised barotherapy should be available not only at major military base hospitals but also as part of emergency first aid services for submarines. (OLC/UMS)

1937.
VIND, H.P., C. Mathews and O.R. Hansen.
On site testing of divers' compressed air.
In: Battelle Columbus Laboratories. Proceedings, 1973 divers' gas purity symposium, November 27-28, 1973, p.XI-1-XI-26. U.S. Navy Supervisor Diving, Nav. Ships Syst. Comm., Rep 2-73, 1973.

According to the U.S. Navy Diving Manual, almost all of the air supplied to helmeted Navy hard hat divers is pumped by oil lubricated compressors and may be contaminated by unacceptable amounts of oil, hydrocarbon vapors, carbon monoxide, and carbon dioxide. The divers' air can also be contaminated by organic solvent vapors from their hoses and by hydrogen sulfide fumes from polluted harbors. At the request of the Navy's Supervisor of Diving (SUPDIV), the Naval Civil Engineering Laboratory (NCEL) conducted a nationwide survey of commercially available instruments for analyzing divers' air. Numerous sensitive and readily portable instruments were found for measuring the concentration of specific contaminants such as carbon monoxide, chlorinated solvents, sulfur compounds, and hydrocarbons. A commercially available portable infrared gas analyzer was found that scans the entire infrared spectrum and can therefore be used to test for numerous impurities. However, because of their simplicity, low price, portability, and convenience, colorimetric chemical detector tubes are perhaps the most suitable devices for the on-site analysis for gaseous impurities in divers' air. A simple and inexpensive instrument for in-line monitoring of oil aerosols in divers air was assembled at NCEL from commercially available components. It was in essence a heavy-duty Fram Fluidic monitor. (Authors' abstract)

1938.
VOGLIS, G.M.
Unterwasser-"Sehen" mit Schallwellen.
[Underwater-"viewing" with sonar radiation].
Meerestechnik 3:237-239;Dec. 1972.

A new sonar viewing device that has undergone extensive tests in Britain has broken new ground in practically every sector of underwater work. It will give hydrographers, fishermen and salvage workers an "eye" which can image almost simultaneously an area of more than two acres with sufficient detail to enable an operator to detect a small fish shoal. Here one of the scientists who developed the device outlines the research and the uses of the super scanner. (English summary)

1939.
VOLOZHIN, A.I. and T.I. Lemetskaya.
Izenenie kal'tsievogo i belkovogo obmena v kostayakh i zubakh pri giperkapnii.
[Changes in calcium and protein metabolism in the bones and teeth during hypercapnia].
Byull. Eksp. Biol. Med. 75(5):42-43; 1973.

The rate of Ca^{45} loss from the bones and teeth increased in rats under the effect of 2 gradual increases in hypercapnia (3-5% CO_2). Suppression of synthetic processes in the bone tissue was accompanied by a considerable dilation and congestion of bone marrow and periodontium vessles. (JPK) (© BA)

1940.
VON DIRINGSHOFEN, H.
The effects of the hydrostatic pressure of the water bath on the capillary blood pressure and on the dehydration of the connective tissue.
Z. Krieslaufforsch. 37:382-390; 1948.
(Translation NASA-TT-F-14894, May 1973). (N73-23052)

Schade's observations on water exchange between blood and connective tissue dehydration are used to study the effect of water bath hydrostatic pressure on blood pressure. It is found that increased water level in the bath shifts the fluid exchange between blood and connective tissue. Therapeutic possibilities are discussed. (STAR)

1941.
VON LIEVEN, T. and G. Walther.
Zum Nachweis einer Myokardschadigung bei der hyperbaren Oxygenation (Tierexperimentelle Untersuchungen).
[Demonstration of myocardial lesions due to hyperbaric oxygenation (animal experiments)].
Med. Welt. 23:200-202;Feb. 5, 1972.

The author has attempted to determine with enzyme histochemical methods whether there is demonstrable early damage to the heart muscle under oxygen intoxication. Rats were subjected to an atmosphere of 97-98% O_2 under 3.8 ata pressure at temperatures of 24-29°C for four hours. Animals were autopsied after decompression and the behavior of certain enzymes was noted. After two hours of compression, most of the rats became restless, and cramping was observed in six animals toward the end of the compression period. Only one animal had no symptoms of oxygen poisoning during decompression. Histochemical examination revealed areas of precipitated succinate dehydrogenase, isocitrate dehydrogenase, and malate dehydrogenase in the heart muscle and a general reduction of the enzyme reaction products. In his discussion, the author relates these findings to disturbances in cellular breathing and in the permeability of the cell membrane and points to possible applications of these findings in the hyperbaric oxygen treatment of coronary insufficiency and infarcts. (MEMH/BSCP)

1942.
VON NIEDING, G., H. Krekeler, W. Liese and H . Oser.
Effect of different ambient gas composition and pressures on nitrogen elimination.
In: Abstracts of the Twenty-fifth Congress of Physiological Sciences Satellite Symposium. Recent progress in fundamental physiology of diving, Marseille, France, July 1971, p.67. (Proceedings unpublished)

Abstract only. Entire item quoted: Previous short term (1 hr) investigations have demonstrated a considerable nitrogen excretion through the lungs, which could not be explained by nitrogen diffusion through the skin. The latter amounts to only 10% of the nitrogen elimination through the lungs. Extending the studies to 24 hr nitrogen excretion was measured during breathing of ambient air at 1 and 2 atmospheres, during exposure to 1 ata (80% helium, 20% oxygen), and 2 ata (0.2 ata O_2, 0.8 N_2, and 1.0 He). Average nitrogen excretion observed during 24 hr was 5 ml/min which corresponds to the values previously obtained during 1 hr studies. At 2 ata air the nitrogen excretion increased. After 24 hr of exposure to 80% He and 20% O_2 at 1 ata nitrogen excretion was still present, but reduced compared to the values at 1 ata air. To clarify the effect of skin diffusion a second series of studies was undertaken, in which the subjects were enclosed with gas tight bags while breathing room air. The gas tight bags were ventilated with either air, 100% nitrogen, helium or oxygen. The nitrogen elimination through the lungs was again 5 ml/min while the bag was ventilated with room air and increased slightly when the ambient gas was changed to pure nitrogen and decreased during ambient helium or oxygen ventilation.

1943.
VON SCHNAKENBURG, K. and H. Nolte.
Results of electron microscopic studies in the rat brain under oxygen at high pressure.
Aerosp. Med. 44:259-264;Mar. 1973.

As has been previously shown, nerve cell alterations in the CNS of the rat were found after a generalized tonoclonic seizure caused by high oxygen partial pressure. Two different types of lesions were seen in typical predilection sites: The reticular substance of the medulla, the pericentral area of the cervical spinal grey matter, the ventral cochlear nuclei, the corpus mamillare, and, in particular, the colliculi inferiores. By means of electron microscopy, the differentiation into two types of nerve cell alterations has been confirmed. Type A lesions are characterized by pycnosis and hyperchromatosis of the nerve cells, vacuolisation of the cytoplasma, and simultaneous swelling of the perineural glial processuses. In contrast, type B lesions revealed lysis of the cytoplasma and karyorrhexis. As demonstrated before, both types have to be considered as a direct effect of the experimental hyperoxia. They are most likely to be regarded as two different morphological lesions by the severely disturbed cellular metabolism. (Authors' abstract)

1944.
VOROSMARTI, J., Jr., M.E. Bradley and N. Anthonisen.
The effects of increased gas density on pulmonary dynamics.
In: Abstracts of the Twenty-fifth Congress of Physiological Sciences Satellite Symposium. Recent progress in fundamental physiology of diving, Marseille, France. July 1971, p.31-32. (Proceedings unpublished)

Abstract only. Excerpts quoted: During two dry saturation dives preliminary to Sealab III, the ventilatory dynamics of seven normal male divers were studied; two subjects to a depth of 600 ft and five subjects to a depth of 825 ft.). . . Measurements were obtained in the seated subjects while breathing quietly, during deep fast respirations and while performing three forced maximum expirations. Breathing mixtures used pre-dive were 30% oxygen-balance helium, 30% oxygen-balance nitrogen and 30% oxygen-balance sulfur hexafluoride. At depth the breathing mixtures were 0.3 atm oxygen, 1.2 atm nitrogen, balance helium, or pure neon with 0.35 atm oxygen. Measurements were obtained on the surface and at 600, 750 and 825 ft. The gas densities (relative to air at 1 atm) provided by these gas mixtures and depths were 0.43, 1, 3.2, 3.9, 4.25, 9.5 and 15. Work of breathing was calculated by constructing pressure-volume loops and measuring appropriate areas with a planimeter. There was a small (1-4%) decrease in the vital capacity at depth, the FEV_1 as percent of vital capacity, fell from a value of 88% at a relative gas density (RGD) of 0.43 to 43% at RGD = 15. The PEFR dropped from a value of 12.85 L/sec to 3.1 L/sec at the highest density. The expired volume at which PEFR occurred decreased to about half the surface volume at an RGD of 5 with no further decrease at the higher densities. The MMEFR values decreased in a curve similar to the PEFR, but it appeared there was no continuing decrease at densities higher than RGO 9. The calculated MBC at RGD of 15 was 34.4% of the surface value. During quiet respiration the work of breathing expressed at kg-m/L at surface, 0.125 at RGD of 15. The work of breathing during deep, fast respirations was more variable. The surface value was 0.2 kg-m/L and the value at RGD of 15 was 0.34 kg-m/L.

1945.
VOTH, R.O.
Safety of hydrogen pressure gauges.
In: Advances in cryogenic engineering. A collection of invited papers presented at national technical meetings, 1970-71, p.182-187. Washington, D.C., National Bureau of Standards, 1972.

To determine the relative safety of various gauge case designs, thirty-five pressure gauges were purchased and intentionally ruptured using high pressure hydrogen gas. Fire was emitted from nearly all gauges; however, gauges with solid fronts and plastic crystals emitted the fire and debris out the rear of the case making them safer for use in a hydrogen system. One brand of gauge ruptured at reduced pressure when tested with hydrogen. The reduced rupture pressure indicated possible hydrogen embrittlement of the pressure sensing element. (Author) (GRA)

1946.
VROEGOP, P.
[Psychodiagnostic selection of divers: study review, 1972].
Netherlands, Hilversum Diving Medical Center, Jan. 1973.

A program of more careful psychodiagnostic examination of diver-training candidates was inaugurated in 1967, since which time the training results have greatly improved. The effectiveness of the program is demonstrated in a diagram, which shows that after the inauguration of these examinations there was a much higher percentage of rejections as well as a lower percentage of drop-outs and a high percentage of candidates successfully completing training. Age was found to be an important factor also, in that divers near the maximum age limit (28 for diver officers and 24 for divers) underwent training more successfully. Examination included interviews, careful survey of the anamnesis, and various questionnaires and tests, the nature of which is not made very clear in this report. (MFW/SCD)

1947.
VROMAN, L., A.L. Adams, M. Klings and G. Fischer.
Blood and air.
In: Ackles, K.N. ed. Blood-bubble interaction in decompression sickness. Proceedings of an international symposium held at Defence and Civil Institute of Environmental Medicine, Downsview, Ontario, Canada, p. 49-70. Published by the Institute, December 1973. (DCIEM Conference Proceedings 73-CP-960)

We are trying to identify proteins absorbed out of and then interacting with blood plasma at various interfaces; for example by observing their subsequent interaction with specific antisera, using recording ellipsometers, anodized tantalum sputtered glass interference colors, water vapor condensation patterns, and a Coomassie Blue staining technique. Adhesion of platelets to the adsorbates is also observed. To study the air interface, in one series of experiments intact plasma and fibrinogen were allowed to form films on buffer in a recording surface film balance, and the films, before or after compression, were transferred to an ellipsometer for study. In another series, intact plasma and whole blood were allowed to roll over a hydrophobic solid substrate on which the films of protein and platelets that may have formed at the liquid/air interface could be printed out and further analyzed. The present preliminary data, combined with previous ones, suggest but do not prove that fibrinogen is at least one of the proteins deposited by blood within 2 sec. at its air interface; that this fibrinogen is less rapidly converted by the plasma into harmless matter than it will be when absorbed at some other interfaces; that intact factor XII cofactor may be involved in this conversion; and that, in presence of calcium ions, platelets will adhere to the fibrinogen film at the air interface within a few seconds, and will undergo rapid viscous metamorphosis. If our conclusions are correct, urokinase may be useful in the treatment of decompression sickness — but further study is needed. (Authors' summary)

1948.
WADA, J. and I. Takashi, eds.
Proceedings of the fourth international congress of hyperbaric medicine, Sapporo, Japan, September, 1969.
Baltimore, Williams and Wilkins, 1970.

The first two sessions of the symposium were on oxygen toxicity; Session III — Problems of increased atmospheric pressures; Session IV — Physio-pathology in hyperbaric oxygenation; other sessions were devoted to purely therepeutic aspects of hyperbaric oxygen, in the treatment of various diseases. Specific papers relating to the more general aspects of hyperbaric oxygen and oxygen toxicity will be found under the following author Entries: Ajiki, H., J. Wada, K. Ikeda, S. Sugii, K. Karino and T. Iwa; Bennett, P.B., and K.N. Ackles; Buckles, R.G. and E. Hardenbergh; Chouteau, J., G. Imbert, J.C. Le Pechon and J. Alinat; Clarke, G.M.; A.T. Sandison and I.McA. Ledingham; Crockett, A.T.K., J.C. Saunders, F.L. Depenbusch and S.M. Pauley; Dorr, V.A. and H.R. Schreiner; Horne, T.; Houlihan, R.T., M.D. Altschule, Z.L. Hegedus and M.H. Cross; Ishizuka, R., K. Miyakawa, T. Maekawa, B. Imamura, T. Akashi, N. Tanaka, Y. Kasai, H.C. Jockin and W.F. Bernhard; Ishizuka, R., K. Miyakawa, T. Maekawa, K. Tajima, T. Nagao, I. Onodera, T. Sato and Y. Kasai; Ledingham, I. McA. and J.K. Davidson; Matsuda, M., Z. Ito, T. Kaminaga, H. Nakayama and A. Morita; McBride, T.I., J.P. Vance and I.McA. Ledingham; McSherry, C.K. and H. Gilder; Nashimoto, I.; Ohiwa, H. and H. Kita; Ohta, Y., T. Kawashiro and T. Yokoyama; Pauley, S.M., J.C. Saunders, F.L. Depenbusch and A.T.K. Cockett; Podlesch, I. and G.E. Herpfer; Race, G.J., J.L. Matthews, J.W. Finney and J.H. Martin; Saito, T.; Schanberg, S.M., G.D. Blenkarn and H.A. Saltzman; Slack, W.K., G.C. Hanson, H.E.R. Chew, G. Cockerill and R. O'Connor; Sealey, J.L.; Thomas, A.N., S.A. Ketchum III, A.D. Hall, J.R. Zubrin; Trapp, W.G., T.R. Patrick and P.A. Oforsagd; Watanabe, I., K. Miyake, T. Yoshida, K. Kojima, Y. Miyake, T. Asano, K. Sakakibra, B. Sakakibara, T. Washizu, H. Takahashi, M. Kobayashi, M. Kawamura and S. Knoishi; Winter, P.M., FT. Oliver and E.A. Jacobs; Winter, P.M., B.T. Williams, B. Roding and Y.G. Schenk; Yasuda, K., H. Takeya, T. Yoshida and K. Furukawa; Youdin, M., T. Reich. (MFW/BSCP)

1949.
WADE, N.J.
The effect of water immersion on perception of the visual vertical.
Br. J. Psychol. 64(3):351-361; 1973.

Judgments by 4 human subjects of the apparent verticality of a single visible line of light were compared under normal support conditions and under water. During head, body and trunk tilts up to 40° the visual vertical was not influenced by water immersion. Great degrees of lateral body tilt (up to 180°) resulted in slightly greater departures of the visual from the gravitational vertical during immersion relative to terrestrial performance. This was apparently due to the reduction of information from surface pressure receptors in the trunk. The mean visual aftereffects following head, body and trunk tilts were not affected by water immersion in any consistent manner. Visual orientation constancy was only marginally reduced by immersion in water. (© BA)

1950.
WAGNER, P.D., R.B. Laravuso, R.R. Uhland and J.B. West.
Effects of breathing enriched O2 mixtures on the distribution of ventilation-perfusion ratios in dogs and normal human volunteers.
J. Clin. Invest. 52(6):86a-87a; 1973.

Abstract only. Entire item quoted: Continuous distributions of ventilation-perfusion ratios ($\dot{V}A/\dot{Q}$) were measured in 17 dogs and 9 normal human volunteers breathing both air and added O_2. We used a new technique (Fed. Proc. 31:347; 1972) employing the intravenous infusion of a mixture of dissolved inert gases. The dogs were studied after inducing acute respiratory failure by injection of small glass beads or oleic acid into the venous blood. O_2 breathing increased the blood flow to areas in which the $\dot{V}A/\dot{Q}$ ratio was low (< 0.1) and also resulted in shunts ($\dot{V}A/\dot{Q}$ of O). These changes generally occurred within 30 min. In one apparently normal subject, a shunt of 10.7% developed, and in the dogs, the shunt increased by up to 16%. In the dogs, changes were seen with inspired O_2 concentrations as low as 50%. On returning to room air, shunts were completely reversed in the human subjects (awake, semirecumbent) but this was not the case with the dogs (supine, anesthetized, not periodically hyperinflated). These changes with O_2 could be explained by two processes resulting from the large rise in alveolar PO_2 in units with low $\dot{V}A/\dot{Q}$ ratios. First, expired ventilation falls due to the increased O_2 transfer, and this may be so marked as to result in alveolar collapse. The second mechanism is an increase in perfusion due to the release of hypoxic vasoconstriction. Two clinical implications of these studies are: (a) some atelectasis rapidly occurs during O_2 breathing even in health and especially in disease: (b) in the measurement of shunt by the traditional method of breathing 100% O_2, much of the shunt may be an artifact of the method, particularly in patients with lung disease.

1951.
WAKEHAM, W.A., J. Kestin and E.A. Mason.
Viscosity and thermal conductivity of moderately dense gas mixtures.
J. Chem. Physics 57:295-301;July 1, 1972.

This paper presents a simple, semitheoretical expression for the initial density dependence of the viscosity and thermal conductivity of gaseous mixtures in terms of the appropriate properties of the pure components and of their interaction quantities. The derivation is based on Enskog's theory of dense gases and provides an equation in which the composition dependence of the linear factor in the density expansion is explicit. The interaction quantities are directly related to those of the mixture extrapolated to zero density and to a universal function valid for all gases. The reliability of the formulation is assessed with respect to the viscosity of several binary mixtures. The method developed allows the calculation of the viscosity and thermal conductivity of moderately dense binary and and multicomponent mixtures of gases. (GRA)

1952.
WALLER, J.R. and C.A. Zogg.
The growth of microorganisms in helium-oxygen environments of ambient and eleven atmospheres absolute (ATA).
Aerospace Medical Association. 1971 annual scientific meeting. Houston, Texas, April 1971. Preprints, p.71-72. Published by the Association, 1971.

This report summarizes studies on the growth of various microorganisms in a pressurized He-O_2 atmosphere. . . The maximum growth responses of the bacteria tested in broth cultures were unaffected by He-O_2 environments at ambient or 11 ATA. No blanket statement can be made regarding the effects of He-O_2 environments at ambient or 11 ATA on actively growing bacteria in broth cultures, since representatives of the bacteria tested exhibited various responses, from none to inhibition or stimulation. The most consistent result was the inhibition of all but two organisms, E. coli and Cl. perfringens, by the ambient He-O_2 atmosphere. Some bacteria which were inhibited by the application of ambient pressure He-O_2 environments exhibited stimulation of growth at 11 ATA. Other bacteria exhibited growth inhibition in He-O_2 under pressure as well as at ambient pressure. (Authors)

1953.
WALLER, R.A.
Facilities.
In: Miller, J.W., J.G. Van Derwalker and R.A. Waller, eds. Tektite 2 Scientists-in-the-sea, p.II-1-II-18. Washington, D.C., U.S. Department of the Interior, August 1971.

The author describes the habitat used in the Tektite 2. Drawings and a photograph of a cutaway model are given. It was the same habitat, with some modifications, that was used in the Tektite-1 experiment. The atmosphere control system is described. A 92/8 nitrogen-oxygen mixture was maintained; the PO_2 was corrected by replacing air with nitrogen after the habitat was in place. CO_2 was removed by a Baralyme scrubber. Table 1 lists the monitoring parameters and equipment. The thermal control system, emergency air systems, communication, electrical and sanitary systems and the alarm system are described. The decompression facility was mounted on a pontoon catamaran; it consisted of a Mark IV Personnel Transfer Capsule, a gantry handling system, a Mark III Deck Decompression Chamber, and a decompression console and gas monitoring equipment which were housed in a metal shed on the barge. The dive platform for support divers and extra equipment, and the surface support center, both of which were on shore, are described. The surface support center was comprised of the command van, the utilities trailer, a tube trailer, and a small park trailer. A cutaway model of the command van and a photograph of its interior are given as well as a diagram of the utilities trailer layout. Facilities at the base camp are also described. (MFW/BSCP)

1954.
WALLER, R.A.
Minitat project.
In: Miller, J.W., J.G. Van Derwalker and R.A. Waller eds. Tektite 2: Scientists-in-the-sea, p.III-1-III-16. Washington, D.C., Department of the Interior, August 1971.

It became apparent during TEKTITE I that the advantages of a movable underwater habitat which could be easily and quickly moved from site to site during a single dive or a series of dives would provide far more flexibility than a fixed habitat. An additional incentive to this approach was provided by the speculation on the part of several physiologists that saturation diving with oxygen/nitrogen mixtures should be possible to depths in excess of 100 feet. If the speculation proved to be true, extended depth capability in saturation diving would render large portions of the shallow continental shelf accessible to exploration and study through *in-situ* techniques without invoking the expense and other problems associated with helium gas mixtures. Thus, the rationale for a movable habitat which could be relocated between an established vertical gradient as well as along a horizontal plane appeared to offer a logical course to follow beyond TEKTITE I. Within this framework a prototype habitat project was scheduled as an adjunct to the TEKTITE II program early in the planning. These sections describe the habitat, its support vessel, and the results of the effort. The scaled-down habitat, illustrated in figures 1 and 2, is a vertical cylinder mounted on a pontoon catamaran which provides flotation during surface transport and a self-raising/lowering capability. An ambient pressure wet room is connected to the underside of the pressure vessel and slightly recessed in the open work deck of the catamaran. Primary services, such as power, atmospheric gas, and fresh water were supplied from the surface support vessel R/V UNDAUNTED. [The Minitat project was delayed due to technical difficulties consisting of, first, a lack of stability when passing through the air-water interface, and, second, a miscalculation regarding the flooding and venting sequence. There were also delays due to weather conditions. When the operational phase was finally reached, an accident due to a breakdown in communications caused flooding. Although all systems were restored to working order, it was too late in the life of the Tektite 2 project to plan another dive in Minitat]. (Author and MFW/BSCP)

1955.
WALLER, R.A.
Operations.
In: Miller, J.W., J.G. Van Derwalker and R.A. Waller, eds. Tektite 2: Scientists-in-the-sea, p.II-19-II-30. Washington, D.C., Department of the Interior, August, 1971.

The operational phase of TEKTITE II consisted of: the various tasks necessary to maintain and support an underwater habitat and its rotating crews of scientists and engineers; the training and housing of the aquanaut crews and program support personnel; adequate procedures to insure the safety and well-being of program personnel and site visitors; and, related activities associated with logistics, transportation, and communications. This section treats each of these tasks in order and also describes other tasks including site preparation, installation of major equipment, and site evacuation. (Author's introduction)

1956.
WALROD, R.A.
Computer aided design of a tethered vehicle for deep ocean viewing.
In: Applications of marine technology to human needs. Preprints, 8th annual conference and exposition, Marine Technology Society, September 1972, Washington, D.C., p.699-712. Published by the Society, 1972.

A highly maneuverable unmanned tethered submersible has been designed to provide real time viewing at ocean depths up to 20,000 feet. The design goal is to allow an operator aboard a surface vessel or manned submersible to conduct a precisely controlled remote inspection with the freedom and maneuverability of a diver. To increase operator endurance and maintain his sense of spacial orientation during an inspection mission, the viewing system line of sight is servo coupled to the operator's head position. A math model is formulated to relate all relevant design parameters to vehicle performance and is the basis for an interactive digital computer program. The vehicle configuration program (VECON) enables the engineer to control the direction and scope of the design study in real time from a time-sharing terminal. A vehicle configuration is derived that achieves the required performance and minimizes vehicle size. An instrumented test bed vehicle has been constructed. Test results validate VECON as a design tool and demonstrate the capabilities of the vehicle. (Author's abstract)

1957.
WALSH, J.M., J.R. Thomas, D.R. Thorne and A.J. Bachrach.
Differential performance changes under hyperbaric conditions.
Aerosp. Med. 43:623-625;June 1972.

Albino rats breathing compressed air at a pressure equivalent to 200 feet of sea water performed on behavior schedules generating either high or low, or combined high and low response rates (FR, DRL and FR-DRL). High rate performance decreased under pressure while low rate performance increased. Results indicate the applicability of behavioral technology in hyperbaric medicine, and demonstrate that the effects of high pressure on performance may be determined by rather specific aspects of the performance itself. (Authors' abstract)

1958.
WALSH, J.M.
Effects of amphetamine on hyperbaric behavior.
In: Aerospace Medical Association. 1973 annual scientific meeting, Las Vegas, Nevada, May 1973. Preprints, p.263-264. Published by the Association, 1973.

The purpose of this study was twofold: (1) to utilize a well-established behavioral baseline to derive dose-effect relationships for amphetamine at surface and at increased pressure; (2) to evaluate concurrently the capability of amphetamine to reduce behavioral deficits associated with nitrogen narcosis. Results indicate that amphetamine induced stimulation of CNS activity is not effective in reducing or protecting against performance decrements under increased pressures of nitrogen. In fact amphetamine appears to act synergistically with pressure. The magnitude of behavioral disruptions at relatively low dosages (1.0 mg/kg) indicates that caution should be exercised in the use of amphetamine-type compounds under hyperbaric conditions. (Author)

1959.
WALTERS, G.B. and B.L. Ryack.
Human factors evaluation of submarine escape. III The effects of three types of charging connectors on disconnect time.
U.S. Nav. Submar. Med. Cent., Rep. NSMRL 688, 11p. Nov. 24, 1971.

Three types of connectors utilized in charging submarine escape appliances in simulated submarine escapes were evaluated with respect to speed of disconnect in a dry environment. Statistically significant differences in disconnect time were found between the various types of connectors; however, the magnitude of these differences is so small that they are of practical significance in the submarine escape evaluation. It is recommended that the study be repeated in a wet environment, more closely simulating actual submarine escape conditions. (Authors' abstract)

1960.
WALTERS, G.B. and B.L. Ryack.
Human factors evaluation of submarine escape.
U.S. Nav. Submar. Med. Res. Lab., Rep. NSMRL 753, 12p. plus append. Sept. 12, 1973.

Utilizing a simulated Escape and Survival Equipment, Mark 1, Mod 0 (EASE) escape appliance, four arrangements of the standard Schrader quick-disconnect air fitting and two escape trunk hose positions, fixed and floating, were evaluated with respect to speed and reliability of disconnect in a dry environment. The results indicated that the most desirable arrangement of the Schrader connector is one in which the female part of the connector is attached at a 90° angle with respect to the charging hose of the EASE, while the male connector is attached at a 0° angle with respect to the air hose in the escape trunk. Hose position was not significant for this arrangement. Since the connector is intended to be used in a wet environment, and this research was performed in a dry environment, it is recommended that the study be repeated in a wet environment before final conclusions are drawn. (Authors' abstract)

1961.
WALTHER, G.
Uber den Reaktionsverlauf der Sauerstoffvergiftung.
[Reactions involved in oxygen toxicity].
Beitr. Gerichtl. Med. 24:321-326; 1972.

On the basis of presently available biochemical studies as well as his own histochemical investigations, the author proposes a three-stage series of mechanisms to explain hyperbaric oxygen poisoning. The three stages involve, respectively, the chemical effect of hyperbaric oxygen (oxidation and the formation of radicals), disturbances of cell metabolism, and organ-specific changes which have been reported, especially in the brain, lungs, and blood. (MEMH/UMS)

1962.
WALTHER, G.
Uber pathologische Veranderungen der Lunge bei der intermittierenden hyperbaren Sauerstofftherapie.
[Pathological changes in the lung during intermittent hyperbaric oxygen].
Acta Med. Acad. Sci. Hung. 30(1-2):149-152; 1973.

Rats were subjected to two hours of hyperoxia at 3.8 ATA every six hours for two days. (The fourth exposure was carried out at 2.8 ATA due to the poor condition of the animals). Lung tissue showed extensive inflammation after the third and fourth exposures, in addition to typical alveolar and edematous changes. Osmotic resistance of erythrocytes was unchanged with respect to controls. In the author's veiw, the lung changes noted are linked to the metabolic (not respiratory) acidosis caused by hyperbaric oxygenation; enzyme investigations suggests that cell membrane damage may be involved. (MEMH/UMS)

1963.
WALTZ, A.R.
An improved light source for underwater illumination.
In: Ocean 73. 1973 IEEE international conference on engineering in the ocean environment, p.4-6. IEEE publication 73 CHO 774-O OCC.

An improved underwater light system developed at the Naval Undersea Center is described. This light system has been designed for use with underwater television cameras on deep-diving submersibles. There are several features unique to this light system which improve its performance over existing underwater lights; among these are: short start and restart times, two different light sources for use in different spectrally selective waters, closed reflector design, and adjustable projection beam angle to complement different camera viewing field angles. The electronic and optical design considerations of the light system are described. (Author's abstract)

1964.
WANDEL, A.
Diving, its dangers and treatment possibilities after diving accidents.
Tauchtechnik Inf. 8:10-17;Mar. 1972.

Immediate recompression is urgently required for treating pressure drop illness or caisson illness and for treating overextension of the lungs with air embolism. Since in these cases the symptoms may very often be most serious with the patient being unconscious, a one-man pressure chamber is not sufficient for optimum treatment. In serious cases of pressure drop illness or caisson illness and overextension of the lungs with air embolism, it must, at any rate, be possible for a diver physician or an assistant to enter the pressure chamber together with the victim during pressure chamber treatment (recompression). Since very long recompression periods (up to 49 hours) are required for treatment of pressure drop illness or caisson illness and air embolism, it must also be possible to move the pressure chamber to a pressure chamber system to connect it to that system, and to transfer the victim and the physician or an assistant accompanying him to the pressure chamber system without reducing the pressure. A portable pressure chamber, spacious enough to accommodate the victim and a physician or an assistant, is the ideal solution and should be designed in such a way that its maximum operating pressure is 5 atm g. and that this operating pressure including flushing of the chamber can be maintained for more than three hours. In addition to the normal compressed air supply, there should be a possibility for supplying oxygen to two persons in order to shorten the treatment times. These requirements could be met in an optimum manner by a portable two-man pressure chamber. A portable one-man pressure chamber does not meet these requirements to the same extent. It is quite sufficient in less serious cases of pressure drop illness (caisson illness) and air embolism if the victim is not unconscious and still cooperative. If purchase of a pressure chamber should be decided upon, no compromise should be accepted which could be harmful to the patient. (Author's conclusions)

1965.
WARDLE, H.
A matter of principle.
Hydrospace 5:19;June 1972.

The author discusses the controversy that has arisen as a result of the inclusion in the Mineral Workings (Offshore Installations) Act of proposed diving regulations following the recommendations set forth in the Underwater Engineering Group's "Principles of safe diving practice." The author states that "the real issue is directly connected with the depth where it is necessary to use mixed gas diving to minimize the narcotic effect when deep diving on air, and when such a decision has been made, whether the diver should operate from a diving bell or from surface supply." Historically, diving operations in the United States have tended to favor the hard hat, surface operated, stage decompression technique. Although in recent years the U.S. Navy has done considerable work using bells, commercial diving operations continue to depend largely on the former technique. The British point of view is that the bell, or submersible decompression chamber, technique is safer, although it may have certain operational or commercial weaknesses. The author emphasizes the prime importance of the establishment of safety procedures, and urges that any interested person who has constructive suggestions should communicate them to Mr. Don Lennard, Underwater Engineering Group, 6 Storey's Gate, London SW 1. (MFW/SCD)

1966.
WARREN, B.A., R.B. Philp and M.J. Inwood.
The ultrastructural morphology of air embolism: platelet adhesion to the interface and endothelial damage.
Br. J. Exp. Pathol. 54(2):163-172; 1973.

The pathogenesis of the ill effects following air embolism [bubbles related to decompression sickness rather than what is generally referred to as air embolism, which is brought on by discharge of gas into the blood stream through lung rupture] cannot be attributed solely to the space occupying and surface tension effects of the air bubbles altering the normal flow of blood through the vasculature. Decompression sickness was induced in rats and the following features of this process observed by electron microscopy in the vessels of the mesentery; imprisonment of blood elements (especially platelets) took place within the various enclosures created by the boundaries set up by different sized air bubbles between the layers of blood and the vessel walls, and the air/blood interface. Air bubble size and the thickness of the film of blood between bubbles varied enormously. The air/blood interface had the following characteristics. A surface associated protein layer measuring 20 nm coated the air bubbles and could slide off the bubble of origin and float freely in the blood. Material morphologically similar to the surface layer was found away from the surface and included small lipid droplets between its layers, and platelets adhered to this to form small aggregates suspended from the interface. The surface layer fused with like laminae and was found within the fluid blood in the vessel, sometimes with adherent platelet aggregates. Platelet adhesion to the bubble interface with the formation of platelet aggregates of an early type i.e. without gross fibrin formation within the aggregates. Pressure damage to underlying endothelial cells by the passage of air bubbles under pressure resulted in herniation of the endothelial cells through fenestrations in the more rigid structures of the vessel wall. Deposits of fibrin on the walls of the vessels were noted after endothelial damage. Lipid droplets were attached to the surface associated protein on the air side of the air/blood interface and also incorporated within it, i.e., covered by this layer on both sides, in which case they took on an ellipsoidal shape. These alterations account for certain features of decompression sickness, such as the drop in platelets, even when the mechanical blockage by air bubbles is not significant. (© BA)

1967.
WARREN, B.A.
The ultrastructure of the blood-bubble interface and related alterations in the blood and vessel walls in the air embolism.
In: Ackles, K.N. ed. Blood bubble interaction in decompression sickness. Proceedings of an international symposium held at Defence and Civil Institute of Environmental Medicine, Downsview, Ontario, Canada, p.104-124. Published by the Institute, December 1973. (DCIEM Conference Proceedings 73-CP-960).

The ultrastructure of the air bubble/blood interface and the related phenomenon including endothelial damage in vessels in rats and rabbit was examined. The air bubbles were surrounded by a dense osmiophilic surface layer or "skin" about 200°A thickness. Platelets adhered to this "skin" and underwent shape change with the formation of dendritic pseudopodia along the surface. In the typical aggregate no fibrin was formed. Air clefts with this layer on either side were found extending into the plasma and platelets were noted attached to these clefts. A floculent form of fibrin was occasionally associated with platelets at the surface. Lipid droplets were attached to the surface layer on the air side of the interface and occasionally incorporated within the layer. The complex of lipid droplets and surface layer was found on occasion separated from the air bubble. Damage to the endothelium due to pressure occurred with disruption of the cells and exfoliation from the vessel wall. Platelet thrombi formed over these sites. (Author's summary)

1968.
WATANABE, I., K. Miyake, T. Yoshida, K. Kojima, Y. Miyake, T. Asano, K. Sakakibra, B. Sakakibara, T. Washizu, H. Takahashi, M. Kobayashi, M. Kawamura and S. Konishi.
Ocular manifestation under hyperbaric oxygenated condition.
In: Wada, J. and I. Takashi, eds. Proceedings of the fourth international congress on hyperbaric medicine, Sapporo, Japan, Sept. 1969, p.67-73. Baltimore, Williams, and Wilkins, 1970.

The atuhors report the changes of the ERG (electroretinagram), of the retinal and choroidal vessels, and histological changes in the retina while under hyperbaric oxygen and during recovery following return to atmospheric pressure. Amplitude of the ERG decreased to extinction under hyperbaric oxygen. In these experiments, the ERG recovered after the animals (rabbits) were returned to atmospheric pressure; this fact did not agree with earlier findings of irreversible changes. Histochemical changes and biochemical changes coincided with the electrical changes. In these experiments, reduced glutathione was used effectively as an antioxidant. (MFW/BSCP)

1969.
WATANABE, I., Y. Miyake, T. Asano and T. Sakai.
[Hyperbaric oxygen and ERG].
Folia Opthalmol. Jap. 22(6):384; 1971.

The experiment was undertaken to examine the effect of hyperbaric oxygen on the retina in vivo using the ERG [electroretinogram]. The EEG was extinct under 2.5 hr 4 atmospheres absolute oxygenation. However, the amplitudes of the ERG under the same condition were variable depending upon the premedication. The drugs used were -SH group inhibitors or those with -SH or those of a similar kind. It was concluded that the primary points of O_2 poisoning of the retina are -SH groups. (JWS) (© BA)

1970.
WATANABE, I., Y. Miyake and T. Asano.
The electro-physiological study of -SH groups under hyperbaric oxygen.
Acta Soc. Ophthalmol. Jap. 76(3):122-125; 1972.

In this experiment, the ERG was used as a testing method to demonstrate the effect of hyperbaric oxygen on the retina. Contrary to previous findings that had indicated that the ERG changes under hyperbaric oxygen were irreversible, the authors report the reversibility of these changes, as well as of changes of the retinal and choroidal vessels, and histochemical and morphological changes of the eye under hyperbaric oxygen. It had been assumed that there was a critical point in the compression-decompression schedule at which irreversible changes occurred. The present investigators employed a new schedule (changes not specified). The mechanism of the oxygen effect on the retina lies in its effect on -SH groups. The protective effect of cystein in vitro had previously been reported by other investigators. The present investigators injected other drugs before compression: IAA, parachloromercuric benzoate (PCMB), Iodeacetamide, Glutathion (GSH), $Na10_3$, water and physiological saline. Unanesthetized adult rabbits were compressed to 4 ata and kept there for 25 hours, after which the ERGs were extinct. After decompression, the ERG recovered, in different degrees depending on the drug used, even in animals that were kept at 1 ata for an additional hour. In a table, it is indicated that the most successful premedications were: IAA at 15 mg/kg, $NaIO_3$ (dose not specified), GSH at 400 and 800 mg/kg, cystine and glycine (dose not specified). (English summary modified by MFW/BSCP)

1971.
WATANABE, S. and T. Homma.
System design of ocean space robots for measurement.
In: Ocean 73. 1973 IEEE international conference on engineering in the ocean environment, p.265-268. IEEE publication 73-CHO-7740-OCC.

The Ocean Space Robot system described here was planned by MITI in April 1971 and have been under development at the Japan Society for the Promotion of Machine Industry. The primary objective of this project is to develop an ocean space measuring system comprised mainly of unmanned vehicles and mooring buoys. This system can measure and analyse multiple parameters in an ocean area by obtaining space distributions and time variations of the parameters in this area. The vehicle is capable of traveling under water at moderate speeds for long distances along the preselected trajectory while making measurements and recording them internally. When the vehicle merges from water, the data are telemetered to the land base and stored in the computer there. The role of the mooring buoy is to survey time variations of ocean parameters at its location. Furthermore, the mooring buoy acts to relay between the land base and each vehicle. (Authors' abstract)

1972.
WATHEN-DUNN, W.
Workshop summary and comments.
In: Sergeant, R.L. and T. Murry, eds. Processing helium speech: proceedings of a Navy-sponsored workshop, August 1971, U.S. Nav. Submar. Med. Res. Lab., Rep. NSMRL 708, p.39-64. May 22, 1972.

The author describes in some detail the normal speech generation process. He then discusses the ways in which helium and pressure affect this process. The contributions of some of the participants in this workshop are summarized: the compensating function of the microphone; the three different methods of unscrambling helium speech (heterodyning, vocodering and time-domain processing); two other means for dealing with helium speech-digital processing (homomorphic processing, which includes cepstral processing), and a method based on predictive coding, which appears to yield a simple algorithm for getting the inverse filtering characteristic of the vocal tract. It is pointed out that computers are useful only if they are fast enough to accomplish the required processing in real time, and small and cheap enough to be practical. This is a real possibility for the future. The author points out that in communication, mere intelligibility is not enough. To be considered really satisfactory, a speech signal must also reveal the identity of the speaker and the emotional content of the speech. As to closed message sets, it is noted that, while intelligibility may be thus increased, it is the unexpected message that carries the greatest amount of information. This should be born in mind when constructing closed message sets. (MFW/BSCP)

1973.
WATSON, A.G. and D.A. Dowd.
The azygos veins of the Weddell seal, Leptonychotes weddelli (Lesson).
Can. J. Zool. 50(12):1583-1587; 1972.

Both left and right azygos trunks were present with segmental anastomoses between them. The right azygos trunk was the larger and opened into the anterior vena cava; the left azygos trunk terminated in the left costocervical vein. At each segmental level the azygos trunks communicated with collecting sinuses into which drained blood from intercostal spaces and the extradural intravertebral vein. These collecting sinuses were themselves connected to each other by longitudinal anastomoses. The relationship of this system to blood flow during diving is briefly discussed. (© BA)

1974.
WATTERS, H.H.
Training.
In: Miller, J.W., J.G. Van Derwalker and R.A. Waller, eds. Tektite 2: Scientists-in-the-sea, p.IV-1-IV-6. Washington, D.C., U.S. Department of the Interior, August 1971.

There were three primary training efforts associated with Tektite 2: A habitat systems course in Philadelphia, Pa. for engineer aquanauts, premission aquanaut training on St. John, and watch director training, also conducted on St. John. These programmed sessions were supplemented by written familiarization materials, previously distributed to participants. Instructors for St. John training were drawn from the operational organization; training activities were coordinated by the NASA onsite representative. In addition to a cursory description of aquanaut selection procedures, each training effort is discussed. (Author's abstract)

1975.
WEBB, P.
Body heat loss determined calorimetrically during cold underwater swims.
In: Aerospace Medical Association. 1973 annual scientific meeting, Las Vegas, Nevada, May 1973. Preprints, p.15-16. Published by the Association, 1973.

Three subjects swam underwater in a tank at temperatures of 5, 10 and 15°C. The exposures were to have lasted 60 minutes, but frequently they were shortened at the requests of the subjects. Mean voluntary exposure time at 5°C was 45 minutes, at 10°C, 48 minutes, and at 15°C, 58 minutes. They wore dry rubber suits and thick long cotton underwear. Rewarming was accomplished by passing warm water through the tubes in the underwear and gradually lowering the water temperature as thermal balance was restored. Mean estimated heat loss in Kcal was 210 at 5°C, 216 at 10°C and 203 at 15°C. The degree of heat loss was considerably higher than was expected from prevous studies in cold air. Changes in surface and deep body temperatures could not be used to estimate heat loss. This was done by adding the heat input from warm water and the metabolic heat generated during rewarming. (MFW/BSCP)

1976.
WEBB, P.
The thermal drain of comfortable hyperbaric environments.
Nav. Res. Rev. 26:1-7;Mar. 1973.

The author describes cold discomfort experienced by divers in various saturation dive experiments in which the temperature was thought to be kept at an adequate level. Two major points are brought out: (1) that thermal comfort requires gas temperature to be kept above normal, and (2) that divers compensate for heat loss by increased metabolism, which brings about weight loss. A diagram illustrates the fact that the temperature of comfort increases as the pressure increases. It has been demonstrated that increased metabolic rate results in increased oxygen consumption. In hyperbaric helium, the blood glucose level decreases, the serum lactic acid increases, and the serum free fatty acids increase; these changes are consistent with increased carbohydrate metabolism. Experience indicates that subjectively comfortable temperatures in a hyperbaric environment can actually bring on heat loss. During the 1200-ft saturation dive at the University of Pennsylvania, although the divers consumed 3500 calories a day, they demonstrated a caloric deficit. Possibly a 4500 calory diet is a minimum daily requirement at this depth, and under more severe conditions even 6000 calories a day may be required. The problem of getting divers to consume sufficient calories as dives become deeper and of longer duration is considered by the author to be an increasing one. (MFW/BSCP)

1977.
WEBB, P.
Rewarming after diving in cold water.
Aerosp. Med. 44:1152-1157;Oct. 1973.

Rewarming was studied in three lightly clothed divers who had swum submerged in water of 5°, 10°, and 15°C for 45 to 60 minutes, reaching the limit of subjective tolerance to cold. Heat for rewarming the men after the dive came from warm water being circulated through a water cooling garment, plus their own metabolic heat. Both of these heat quantities were measured, and it was found that an average of 210 kcals (range of 165-292 kcals) was needed to replace the heat lost during the dives. The completion of rewarming was signalled by: the release of body heat when previously it had been conserved by the cold subject; a rise in heart rate and the return of cutaneous vasomotor control of body heat loss; and a restoration of the normal balance between heat produced and heat lost. Over-warming led to sweating. None of the following body temperatures reliably indicated completion of rewarming: rectal, ear canal, esophageal, skin (mean or any of 8 sites), calf or chest subcutaneous temperature, or calculated mean body temperature. (Author's abstract)

1978.
WEBSTER, I. and L.J. Blum.
Traumatic lung.
Forensic Sci. 1(2):167-178; 1972.

Injuries to the lung can be due to many causes such as blast injury, fat embolism or injury to the thoracic cage. Traumatic lung refers to changes in the lung which occur in trauma elsewhere in the body such as head injuries or associated with shock. The lung parenchyma can show edema, hemorrhage, or desquamative alveolitis or a combination of any of these. Electron microscopy may show granularity of the endothelial cells of the capillary with widening of the canal between the cells. There may also be edema of the basement membrane and regenerative changes in the alveolar epithelium followed by swelling and desquamation. Trauma can be the sole cause of these changes as a similar picture can be produced by other conditions such as O_2 toxicity, viral infections and toxins, and a full clinical history is important in diagnosis. (© BA)

1979.
WEEKS, A.
Ten marine teams call mini habitat home.
Mar. Technol. Soc. J. 6:6-13;July/Aug. 1972.

The author gives an account of the marine research program carried out by the small habitat Edelhab and its mother ship, the catamaran Lulu. The NOAA project, called FLARE (Florida Aquanaut Research Expedition) lasted three months and was carried out by seven teams of scientists. The two objectives of the project were to explore coral reef ecology, and to evaluate the movable habitat with surface support vessel as an effective laboratory facility. The habitat with surface support vessel as an effective laboratory facility. The habitat was anchored at a depth of 45 feet, and the divers were able to use compressed air. They were returned to the surface for a 19-hour decompression at the end of four days. (MFW/BSCP)

1980.
WEISSMAN, B., R.S. Green and P.T. Roberts.
Frontal sinus barotrauma.
Laryngoscope 82:2160-2168;Dec. 1972.

Rapid descent in an aircraft or rapid ascent during scuba diving can result in sinus barotrauma. We have recently evaluated 14 Air Force pilots and one scuba diver demonstrating the spectrum of complications that can occur with aerosinusitis. Although sinus barotrauma has been recognized since the Second World War, very little has appeared in the American literature since 1944. . . . Obstruction of the sinus ostium may be due to tenacious mucus, edematous tissue or anatomical deformity. Upon descent, a relative negative pressure occurs in the sinus, and a plug of mucus or swollen and redundant nasal mucosa may act as a cork occluding the sinus orifice. Negative pressure in this sealed sinus is resolved by filling the cavity with fluid (transudate) or blood. With rapid or extreme pressure changes, the mucosa can be ripped from the sinus wall resulting in a hematoma in the sinus. [No specific data is given on the diver]. (Authors)

1981.
WELFLING, J. and S. De Seze.
Necrose de la tete humerale.
[Necrosis of the humerus head].
Nouv. Presse Med. 2:2311-2312;Oct. 6, 1973.

The diagnosis and etiology of humerus head osteonecrosis are discussed. Humerus head osteonecrosis is diagnosed radiologically. X-ray photographs show lesions similar to those of femur head necrosis. The first radiological signs generally precede clinical symptoms, and the disease may have an evolution of several years. Like femur head necrosis, humerus head necrosis is usually associated with some other disorder, such as disseminated lupus erythematosus, decompression sickness, hemoglobinopathies, hyperlipidemic obesity, and long-term corticotherapy. The microembolisms occurring during these conditions are thought to be responsible for the bone ischemia which is the cause of the disease. (MEMH/UMS)

1982.
WESSMAN, E.E.
Analysis and simulation of a submarine steering control system.
U.S. Nav. Postgrad. Sch. Thesis, 75p. June 1972.
(AD 745 146)

An existing computer simulation of a hydraulic submarine steering control system was analyzed to determine the source of its unrealistic behavior, which included verifying mathematical equations and numerical parameters, duplicating and simulation on another computer, and investigating the validity of the assumptions made in its development. Rudder turning rate and load pressure drop oscillations which were thought to be unrealistic were caused by the neglect of significant rudder moments related to the control surface turning rate. Knowledge of actual system performance was found to be incomplete and further research was suggested. Potentially beneficial modifications in the servo-valve and actuator simulators were identified. Continuing work in the field of unsteady rudder behavior was suggested in order to improve simulator and actual system designs. (Author) (GRA)

1983.
WEST. V.R. and J.F. Parker, Jr.
A review of the influence of physical condition parameters on a typical aerospace stress effect: decompression sickness.
Falls Church, Va., Biotechnology Inc., Final Rep. on contract N00014-72-C-0263, 53p. June 1973.
(AD 763 453)

The study examines data on episodes of decompression sickness, particularly from recent Navy work in which the event occurred under multiple stress conditions, to determine the extent to which decompression sickness might be predicted on the basis of personal characteristics such as age, weight, and physical condition. Such information should ultimately be useful for establishing medical selection criteria to screen individuals prior to participation in activities involving extensive changes in ambient pressure, including those encountered in space operations. The main conclusions were as follows: There is a definite and positive relationship between increasing age and weight and the likelihood of decompression sickness. However, for predictive purposes, the relationship is low. To reduce the risk of bends, particularly for older individuals, strenuous exercise should be avoided immediately after ambient pressure changes. Temperatures should be kept at the low end of the comfort zone. For space activities, pressure changes of over 6-7 psi should be avoided. Prospective participants in future missions such as the Space Shuttle should not be excluded on the basis of age, certainly to age 60, if their general condition is reasonably good and they are not grossly obese. (Authors' abstract modified by GRA)

1984.
WEYBREW, B.B. and E.M. Noddin.
Psychological effects of prolonged exposure to sonar signals at an elevated intensity. II. Twenty-four days' exposure to signals at 85 dB.
U.S. Nav. Submar. Med. Cent., Rep. NSMRL 691, 24p. Dec. 6, 1971.

The problem was to design and implement a multidisciplinary study to assess the biomedical and psychological effects of 24 days' continuous exposure to an intermittent sonar "beep" at 85 dB. Eight of the ten male subjects (5 civilians and 5 Navy sonar-men) while showing a moderate increase in depressive symptoms early in the second exposure phase, demonstrated no remarkable degradation in vigilance, muscle tension, or mood. One civilian subject manifested an anxiety reaction sufficiently acute to warrant his disqualification as an experimental subject about 60 hours after the onset of the sound. Similarly, anxiety symptoms requiring tranquilizer medication occurred in a second civilian subject five days before the termination of the "beep". Whereas, the subject selection data argue that this psychopathology existed in these two men prior to the sound exposure, the experimental design does not allow for an unequivocal causal statement. This study presents data bearing on the question of whether a nuclear submarine may employ the active sonar mode continuously during prolonged submerged missions without, at the same time, undergoing some degree of degradation in crew member performance and overall quality of adjustment to the submerged conditions. (Authors' summary)

1985.
WEYBREW, B.B., J.A. Gessler and E.M. Noddin.
Factors related to drug abuse in the submarine service. I. Selected demographic and psychometric data.
U.S. Nav. Submar. Med. Res. Lab., Rep. NSMRL 726, 15p. Aug. 30, 1972.

Approximately 70 drug abuse cases originating from the submarine fleet were compared to a matched control group of like size with a view toward identifying some of the major causes of drug abuse in this population. The drug abuse group were younger, more were high school dropouts, and tended to earn poorer grades in submarine school. The drug abuse group also received lower ARI scores, but showed no differences in GCT or MECH scores. Too, there were no between-group differences found for test scores purported to measure emotional stability, depression, or motivation for the submarine service. While the data in the present study were too sparse to make any meaningful inferences regarding the incidence of drug abuse in the submarine service, there was nonetheless ample evidence that there are a multiplicity of etiological factors involved and that the present psychiatric screening approach is not very effective for identifying the potential drug abuse cases. The results of an attempt to integrate and classify the many and varied causal factors for drug abuse found in the voluminous literature is contained in Appendix A of the report. (Authors' abstract)

1986.
WEYBREW, B.B. and E.M. Noddin.
Factors related to drug abuse in the submarine service. II. Personality trait patterns as delineated by the Minnesota multiphasic personality inventory.
U.S. Nav. Submar. Med. Res. Lab., Rep. NSMRL 737, 11p. Feb. 2, 1973.

The Minnesota Multiphasic Personality Inventory (MMPI) subtest profiles for 20 enlisted submarier candidates who had admitted drug abuse (DA) were compared with a matched sample of 20 enlisted men without any DA history and with two similar civilian DA samples. In general, the mean profiles for the Navy DA sample were quite similar to the civilian DA groups showing "peaks" on Depression (D), Psychopathic deviate (Pd), Psychasthenia (Pt) and on the validity or F-scale. The Navy DA group mean was higher than the civilian DA means on the F-scale, and on the clinical scales, Paranoia (Pa), Schizophrenia (Sc) and Hypomania (Ma). Taking into account the elevated F-scale as a possible indicator of malingering on the part of the Navy DA group, the peaks for this group on Hs, Pd, Pa, Ma and Sc suggest a preponderance of antisocial or dyssocial traits, possibly with considerable focussed hostility (High Pd and Pa) and with some evidence for rather immature "acting out" behavior (High Hs and Ma) as part of this group's life style. The fact that the civilian DA groups showed higher mean scores on D and Pt suggests a more significant neurotic or emotional component in this group. The finding that the Navy DA group has a "strong" sociopathic component with possibly less intense emotional (depression and anxiety) involvement than the civilian DA groups suggests that the former group may be quite resistive to rehabilitative effort. The study further suggests the likelihood that a usefully valid MMPI profile analytical procedure could be developed for the purpose of identifying those DA cases most (and least) likely to respond favorably to treatment and rehabilitation. (Authors' abstract)

1987.
WEYBREW, B.B. and E.M. Noddin.
Factors related to drug abuse in the submarine service.
U.S. Nav. Submar. Med. Res. Lab., Rep. NSMRL 764, 33p. Sept. 24, 1973.

Involving two drug abuse (DA) samples (N=200 and 41), this study was designed to re-examine certain of the findings reported in earlier reports of this series and to investigate the relationships of selected sociological, personality and background factors to propensity for DA in the submarine service. As compared to appropriate control groups, the DA cases tended: (1) to be younger, (2) to have an inferior academic record, (3) to more frequently have a history of treatment for emotional conditions, (4) to have negative attitudes toward both their civilian and Navy instructors, and (5) to have more often a history of adjudicated crime. However, the DA group's paygrade level (corrected for time in service) was not different from the control group and their motivation for volunteering for submarines and their goal orientation generally were appropriate. Their below-average performance in "Sub" School appeared to result from low verbal aptitude and/or emotional instability. While more DA cases came from homes in metropolitan areas, the socioeconomic level, the marital stability and the geographical location of these homes were not significantly different between the two groups. Though the mechanisms are unknown, there appears to be a non-chance correlation between submarine School output and incidence of DA during equal time segments. A gross estimate of the incidence of DA in the submarine service for FY71 was comparatively low, of the order of 25 per 1000 enlisted men across all submarine classes, but possibly slightly higher for men in attack class as compared to those in either fleet type or Fleet Ballistic Missile billets. (Authors' abstract)

1988.
WEYNE, J., F. Van Leuven and I. Leusen.
Glutamate and glutamine in the brain: Influence of acute PCO_2 changes in normal rats and in rats under sustained hypercapnia or hypocapnia.
Life Sci. 12(Pt. II):211-218; 1973.

The effect of PCO_2 on the concentration of glutamate and glutamine in the brain was studied in anesthetized and curarized rats. Brain glutamate was found to decrease gradually as a function of increasing PCO_2 while glutamine showed the inverse relationship. Identical observations were made in rats maintained 24 hours in an atmosphere of 13% CO_2 in air (hypercapnia) or 10% O_2 in nitrogen (hypoxemic hypocapnia) before the experiment. (Authors' summary)

1989.
WHITE, F.N., M. Ikeda and R.W. Elsner.
Adrenergic innervation of large arteries in the seal.
Comp. Gen. Pharmacol. 4(15):271-276; 1973.

Radiological evidence for arterial constrictor responses during diving in the seal, Phoca vitulina, is presented. A pattern of penetration of sympathetic fibers to the muscular media of supply arteries to vascular beds, subject to constriction during diving, is described. In a comparison study the cat was typified the more general case in which sympathetic fibers terminate at the muscularis-adventitial border. The penetration of sympathetic terminals into the muscularis of supply arteries provides a mechanism for maximal "recruitment" of smoth muscle allowing constriction of a vascular bed at a site proximal to the competitive influence of metabolically produced vasodilator materials which act in non-diving forms such as the cat, at the arteriolar level. The cellular and peripheral neurophysiological organization which allows the selective distribution of blood flow and O_2 reserves in the seal and in other diving species is discussed. (© BA)

1990.
WHITE, P.E.
North Sea diving — some special problems.
Petrol. Rev. 24:406-408;Dec. 1970.

The special problems of North Sea diving are chiefly those imposed by the weather conditions. In order to allow for a certain proportion of the decompression time being spent under water, before returning to the surface decompression chamber, the weather conditions must be very carefully monitored. The variation in hydrostatic pressure caused by high wave heights has in itself been known to cause decompression sickness. Also, severe currents in tidal waters limit the useful work time to 15 minutes each side of slack water, four times within each 24 hour period. The use of a submersible work chamber under these conditions enable the diver to submerge at surface pressure, pressurize the chamber before starting his underwater task, then return to the surface within the chamber at the end of the operation without having to spend time in the water. This makes possible a more efficient use of the available work time. (MFW/BSCP)

1991.
WHITTON, J.T.
Calculations of whole body dose from absorption of an inhaled noble gas.
Health Physics 23:573-575;Oct. 1972.

When radioactive noble gases are released into the atmosphere whole body doses resulting from immersion in the gas are usually calculated by considering only external irradiation. The results ignore any contributions to dose resulting from the absorption of inhaled gas in the blood and its subsequent diffusion into other tissues. In this note the method of calculating the contribution to whole body dose from inhalation is described, and, using ^{85}Kr as an example, this dose is compared to that from external irradiation. Radioactive noble gases are not entirely insoluble in body fluids and hence for a man immersed in a cloud of noble gas the whole body dose from the gas absorbed by the body tissues following inhalation should be considered in addition to the dose from the radiations external to the body. A method of calculating the contribution to the whole body dose from the inhaled gas has been described and the doses compared with those from external irradiation. For a short term exposure of 1 min and a long term exposure of several hours to a cloud of ^{85}Kr the dose to most body tissues arising from absorption of the inhaled gas represents about 1% of the dose received from irradiation by the gammas and bremsstrahlung external to the body. The corresponding fraction for the fatty tissues is 10% as inert gases generally have an increased solubility in these tissues. (Author)

1992.
WICKIZER, C.L.
Subsea system has standard equipment.
Offshore 33:278,280,282-284;May 1973.

Late in 1971, Shell Oil Co. and Lockheed Petroleum Services joined efforts to develop and field test an ocean-floor system for completing and producing wells. The system is based on housing more-or-less standard equipment in one-atmosphere chambers. The chambers can then be linked together with subsea pipelines to form a complete producing system. . . . Men can perform oilfield operations very effectively in a normally pressured air environment on the sea floor. This was demonstrated by a total of 38 dives to the cellar lasting some 300 hours (1,100 man-hours). Forty-four non-crew members made dives for various reasons during this period. The flowline technique to a subsea chamber performed well enough to offer significant potential for future diverless connections. The operation has confirmed the practicality of the one-atmosphere system, and added emphasis to the next two phases of the program. Having demonstrated the feasibility of the wellhead cellar as the first building block, the next step to a viable subsea system is gathering the production from a number of wells to a surface facility for further handling. . . . The third phase is intended to accomplish the basic function of adding energy to the produced fluids. This function is conceived to be a vital building block for subsea development of fields greater than five miles away from a platform or shore facilities. (Author)

1993.
WIDE, P.
N_2-O_2 diving in the Swedish Navy.
In: The working diver, 1972, Symposium proceedings, February 1972, Columbus, Ohio, p.251-255; Washington, D.C., Marine Technology Society, 1972.

The paper outlines the Royal Swedish Navy's philosophy concerning the development of nitrox systems and also discusses diving experiments carried out in Sweden during recent years, giving an outlook on future development of nitrox systems in Sweden both commercially and militarily. Specific design parameters of fundamental concern to nitrox diving equipment are reviewed. . . . The key problem in nitrox diving is avoidance of oxygen poisoning from high PO_2 and decompression sickness from high PN_2 by striking a balance between the two extremes. . . . In September and October 1971, a test series was carried out to learn if three hours of total diving time in cold water could be withstood by the divers. Thirty-two nitrox dives were carried out at 20, 30, and 40 m in the Swedish Navy test facility. Water temperature was a steady 4°C, with heavy work on an ergometric bicycle carried out in a sequence that went on for three hours with ten minutes of work and ten minutes of rest alternately. Equipment used was the standard Swedish Navy hard-hat rig, modified Beckman helmet and suit, modified Drager mixed-gas helmet and Dragersuit. During these physically strenuous dives, no sign of oxygen intoxication was shown. Carbon dioxide that built up in the hard hats was felt less than with air, and all divers had the subjective feeling of a higher "octane" in the gas they were breathing; this was proven out by better results with work on the ergometric bicycle. (Author)

1994.
WIDELL, P.J., A.A. Pilmanis, L.W. Chapman, V.M. Plinanis and R.R. Given.
Physiological effects of saturation diving: oxygen toxicity, stress and fluid volume regulation.
Hydro-Lab J. 2(1):58-72; 1973.

The findings of the three physiological studies made during a 7-day 50-foot saturation dive in Hydro-Lab were briefly as follows: (1) Pi O_2 of 362 mm Hg resulted in a decrease in hematocrit and erythrocyte count, unchanged serum enzyme levels, and an absence of oxygen toxicity signs. (2) Measurement of serum enzyme, plasma cortisol, and aldosteron levels indicated that stress was minimal. (3) As to fluid volume regulation, an average weight loss of 4 pounds per person occurred, probably resulting from the 5 hour daily immersion, the low fat diet, and physical exertion. Negative ortho-static intolerance tests indicated no significant reduction in blood volume. It is important that adequate salt and water intake be maintained during saturation dives in order to compensate for diuresis. (MFW/UMS)

1995.
WIEDERHORN, S.M. and H. Johnson.
The effect of pressure on the static fatigue of glass.
J. Amer. Ceramic Soc. 54:585;Nov. 1971.

The static fatigue behavior of glass at elevated pressures was studied using fracture mechanics techniques. Stress time-to-failure data was obtained on three different glass compositions exposed to high pressure water, 7 kbar. The fracture behavior of glass in water was observed to be insensitive to pressure. It is suggested that this insensitivity resulted from compensating mechanisms in which the increase in fracture resistance arising from a positive activation volume for stress corrosion cracking is balanced by a decrease in fracture resistance due to increased hydroxyl ion concentration at the crack tip. (Authors) (GRA)

1996.
WIEMER, W. and P. Kiwull.
The role of the vagus nerves in the respiratory response to CO_2 under hyperoxic conditions.
Pfluegers Arch. 336:147-170; 1972.

In anesthetized rabbits rebreathing oxygen the respiratory and circulatory responses to increased $PACO_2$ were determined repeatedly in the same animal before and after inactivation of the vagus nerves by cold blocking and finally sectioning. In some animals responses were also obtained by blocking the vagi during respiration of constant mixtures of CO_2 and O_2. With intact vagi the $\dot{V}/PACO_2$ response curve was, on the average, practically linear up to an increase of the $PACO_2$ by 27 Torr. Inactivation of the vagi caused a small increase of the resting ventilatory minute volume during the initial breathing of pure oxygen, and a corresponding decrease of the resting $PACO_2$. In the range of small increases of $PACO_2$ the $\dot{V}/PACO_2$ response curve was significantly steepened and shifted to higher ventilatory values by the inactivation. With greater increases, the slope of the response with inactivated vagi was flatter and shifted to lower ventilatory values as compared with intact vagi. These effects were the result of corresponding changes of the response curves for tidal volume and respiratory rate: Inactivation considerably steepened the $V_T/PACO_2$ response at low values of $\Delta PACO_2$ while flattening the response at high values, whereas the $f/PACO_2$ curve was only depressed at all stages of hypercapnia. The results were principally the same whether the carotid sinus nerves were intact or sectioned. Vagal inactivation had only little influence on the reactions of systemic blood pressure and heart rate to the increase of $PACO_2$. It is concluded that vagal reflexes, possibly from stretch receptors of the lungs, modify the ventilatory efficacy of the central chemosensitive drive of respiration in the rabbit. (Authors' abstract)

1997.
WILCOX, R.H.
The squirrel monkey electroencephalogram in hyperbaric conditions.
In: Aerospace Medical Association, 1973 annual scientific meeting, Las Vegas, Nevada, May 1973. Preprints, p.269-270. Published by the Association, 1973.

EEG technology has recently been employed as a tool by which the condition of the diver at depth can be determined. In recent deep dives in France and England, increases in theta activity (4-8 Hz) caused the experiments to be shortened. Because of the involvement of various factors, depth, breathing mixture, degree of adaption and amount of individual experience, the meaning of the EEG anomalies is somewhat obscured. A systematic analysis of EEG changes in primate subjects in repeated dives with different gas mixtures was undertaken. Dives were made with air, N_2O_2, and HeO_2, to depths of from 20 to 200 feet. Behavioral adaptation was observed. EEG changes were not pronounced, theta activities actually decreased. Between-dive differences were more apparent, and appeared to be more sensitive to the number of previous dives (or, in other words, the degree of experience) than to breathing mixtures. A possible explanation for the paucity of EEG changes is the slow compression rate. (MFW/BSCP)

1998.
WILFONG, R.G. and J.F. Mullane.
Oxygen toxicity and the stomach.
Clin. Res. 20:873;Dec. 1972.

Abstract only. Entire item quoted: Prolonged exposure to high oxygen concentrations is toxic to heart, brain, lung, and several metabolic systems. We have studied the effects of breathing 100% O_2 for 48 hours on the stomachs of female albino rats weighing 60-100 gm by evaluating the following: (1) gastric acid production, (2) number of gastric erosions and ulcers induced by placing the rats in wire mesh restraint at hour 41 for the next seven hours, (3) in vitro tissue respiration of mucosal slices of gastric fundus, and (4) % gastric tissue water. Compared to controls, rats breathing 100% O_2 had no change in total gastric acid production (48 vs 38 μEq/four hours, $p > .05$) or in vitro tissue respiration without ($p > .4$) or with sodium succinate ($p > .5$) in the bath solution. When subjected to wire mesh restraint, rats breathing 100% O_2 had increased gastric erosions (6.8 vs 13.8 lesions/stomach, $p < .01$) and ulcers (0.1 vs 1.4 lesions/stomach, $p < .05$). Gastric tissue water was unchanged (79.0 vs 80.3%, $p > .05$) after 48 hours of 100% O_2 while lung water was increased (80.6 vs 82.9%, $p < .001$). 100% O_2 had no major effect on gastric histological structure while lesions typical of oxygen toxcity were present in the lung. The present study has demonstrated an increased susceptibility of the rat stomach to ulcer formation in the presence of 100% O_2.

1999.
WILHELM, J.
Data management procedures.
In: Miller, J.W., J.G. Van Derwalker, and R.A. Waller, eds. Tektite 2: Scientists-in-the-sea, p.VIII-27. Washington, D.C., U.S. Department of the Interior, August, 1971.

Two major types of data were collected in the Virgin Islands. Observational data were punched on site by University of Texas behavior observers onto IBM portapunch cards. Other measures were collected before and during each mission on questionnaires and mailed to Austin or California for keypunching. . . Due to the large volume of data generated during each mission, four preliminary data reduction programs were written. STATDAY gives daily totals on each variable for each diver form Status Record; MEALDAY, COMMDAY, and DIVEDAY similarly combine data from the Meal Record, Communication Record, and Dive Record to give daily summaries. All data reduction programs compute values for either a complete day or for a whole mission and print and punch these summaries for inspection and further statistical analyses. (Author)

2000.
WILKS, S.S.
Growth responses of paramecium caudatum to hypo- and hyperbaric oxygen environments: induction of high oxygen tolerance.
In: Aerospace Medical Association. 1971 annual scientific meeting. Houston, Texas, April 1971. Preprints, p.67-68. Published by the Association, 1971.

These experiments were begun in an effort to observe some of the physiological and biochemical responses of Paramecia, a single celled animal, to hypo- and hyperbaric stresses; and, from these observations elucidate, if possible, some of those mechanisms involved in protoplasmic inactivation by high partial pressures of oxygen. . . The optimum PO_2 for maximum growth rate in Paramecia appears to lie between 20 and 90 mm Hg. It has also been shown that oxygen tolerance can be induced in paramecia by culturing air-grown cultures for several generations under an atmosphere of oxygen. This high tolerance is maintained indefinitely after the organisms are returned to air. Further investigations are necessary in elucidating the basic mechanism of oxygen poisoning and increased oxygen tolerance in Paramecia. This may provide for a better understanding of oxygen poisoning in higher animal and plant forms including man himself. (Author)

2001.
WILKS, S.S.
Growth responses of paramecium caudatum to hypo- and hyperbaric environments: Induction of cellular tolerance to hyperbaric oxygen pressures.
In: Aerospace Medical Association. 1972 annual scientific meeting, Bal Harbour, Florida, May 1972. Preprints, p.124-125. Published by the Association.

In the present study an effort is made to observe and measure some of the physiological and biochemical responses of the protozoan ciliate Paramecium caudatum, a single-celled animal, to hypo- and hyperbaric stresses and, from these observations elucidate, if possible, some of the mechanisms involved in protoplasmic inactivation of this species, by HOP. Results of this investigation indicate that there are many factors which determine the tolerance of organisms to HOP. One of the primary factors appears to be the composition and architecture of the plasma membrane, the gateway of flux equilibra of materials passing between the cell and its environment. The membrane potential (electrical) may be the primary factor governing the flux equilibrium between the cell and its environment. Any alteration of the membrane architecture would bring about a shift in the flow pattern of materials between the cell and its environment. The altered membrane would thus behave differently at different oxygen pressures. (Author)

2002.
WILLIAMS, K.G.
Investigation of the feasibility of an NDIR technique to detect CO_2 in a hyperbaric gaseous environment.
Berkeley, Cal., Andros Inc., Rep. ARFR-56, 92p. Sept. 1972.
(AD 767-078/9GA)

A nondispersive infrared (NDIR) technique for monitoring CO_2 has been thoroughly evaluated to determine its suitability for use in a hyperbaric environment. The technique used is to subject a known volume of sample gas to a periodic density modulation and to measure the amount of CO_2 present by observing the fractional change in a beam of infrared radiation transmitted through that volume. Experimental results indicate the validity of the technique for total pressures up to 1200 psia, in He containing up to 15 psia of O_2/N_2, and CO_2 partial pressures up to 30 mm. A single point calibration with CO_2 span gas at any pressure should be necessary only infrequently. Response times of the order of a few seconds are possible. It is anticipated that this technique can be used in a CO_2 alarm sensor for inclusion in a saturation diver's breathing apparatus, as well as in hyperbaric habitats and Personnel Transfer Capsules. (Author's abstract modified by GRA)

2003.
WILLIAMSON, R.A.
A survey of the biologic effects of pressure.
Houston, Tex., Baylor Coll. Med., Thesis, June 1971. 146p.

Increasing pressure was associated with increasing weight loss in Ball/c+ and CBA mice; 300 to 750 psig produced lymphocytopenia. Lymphatic tissues showed progressive loss of lymphoid elements under high pressure, indicating that pressure had a stressful effect, activating the adrenal gland. Thymic weight was particularly susceptible; 300 psig the thymus underwent atrophy and subsequent regeneration. These changes occurred after 2-day exposures. Two days at 0 psig followed by compression to 500 psig for one minute produced negligible alterations. The liver of an animal exposed to 300 psig for two days showed an increase of glycogen and lipid. At 100 psig liver tissue showed a decrease in lipid. A pressure of 300 psig for two days boosted antibody titers. However, a cyclic pressure of 500 psig did not influence the skin graft rejection threshold of one species to the other. (MFW/UMS)

2004.
WILLIAMSON, R.A., R. Liebelt and K. Doener.
Hemolysin and hemagglutinin titers in mice exposed to pressure.
In: Aerospace Medical Association. 1973 annual scientific meeting, Las Vegas, Nevada, May 1973. Preprints, p.294. Published by the Association, 1973.

Hemolysin and hemagglutinin antibody titers were determined one week and two weeks following injection of sheep red blood cells into five groups of mice. The mice were subjected to 300 psig for two to two and one-half days and decompressed at 2 psig/minute. The variable was the interim of time between challenge and pressurization. Group I was the control group; Group II was compressed immediately after injection; Group III, two days after injection; Group IV four and one-half days after injection; Group V was injected five minutes after decompression following a compression period. After one week there was enhancement of hemolysin titers in Groups IV and V; there were no significant changes in agglutinin titers but a near-significant change for Group V; after two weeks there were no significant differences in the titers. The authors concluded that stress and resulting increased plasma steroid levels enhanced Group IV hemolysin titers, due to lympholytic activity and the release of antibody molecule. Increase of Group V hemolysin titers is thought to be related to the regenerative activity of the lymphoid systems following pressure exposure. Also it is possible that adaptation to pressure is accompanied by increased activity of the reticulo-endothelial systems, as has been observed during adaptation to hypoxia. (MFW/BSCP)

2005.
WILLIS, R.J. and C.C. Kratzing.
Effect of hyperbaric oxygen and norepinephrine on the level of lung ascorbic acid.
Amer. J. Physiol. 222:1391-1394;June 1972.

Rats were exposed to either hyperbaric air or oxygen at 3.5 atm absolute (Ata) in a pressure chamber for periods up to four hours. Lung ascorbic acid (AH_2) levels were decreased by 40% with this procedure within one hour. Norepinephrine administration was also found to produce decreases in lung AH_2. Prior treatment of rats with reserpine eliminated changes in lung AH_2 due to hyperbaric air treatment and reduced those due to hyperbaric oxygen exposure. The results suggest that part of the AH_2 store in lung is under sympathetic control, while the remainder may be acting as an antioxidant in vivo. (Authors' abstract)

2006.
WILLIS, R.J. and C.C. Kratzing.
Changes in levels of tissue nucleotides and glutathione after hyperbaric oxygen treatment.
Aust. J. Exp. Biol. Med. 50:725-729;Dec. 1972.

Rats were exposed for four hours to either hyperbaric air or oxygen at 3.5 atmospheres absolute in a pressure chamber. Oxygen treatment decreased the $NADPH_2$ content of lung by 43% and increased its GSSG level by a quarter. These results are consistent with the concept that the autoxidation of tissue constituents is a contributing factor in oxygen poisoning. (Authors' summary)

2007.
WILLIS, S.
Diver support of a large oceanographic instrument.
In: Diving applications in marine research. Proceedings of a seminar, National Institute of Oceanography, Godalming, Surrey, U.K., December 1971, p.14-37. Published by the Institute. 1972.

This paper describes the launch and recovery of a towed system comprising a 32ft long 7 ton torpedo shaped sonar vehicle which is suspended from a 2 ton float by a heavy armoured towing cable. It has been found possible to use a three man team equipped with snorkels for the majority of the routine work, with 10 cu.ft. aqualungs for working in choppy conditions near the surface at the normal working speed of 1.5 knots. 56 cu. ft. aqualungs have been used to advantage at this speed in rougher weather, particularly for longer intricate jobs. The methods of recovery in partial and total failure conditions are discussed with particular reference to the safety precautions necessary for deep diving in the deep ocean, from a moving ship which cannot stop, and which carries no recompression chamber. It has been found possible to launch an inflatable dinghy from a 2,000 ton ship at 4.5 knots in glass calm and at 1 knot in sea state six by making minor modification to the dinghy, which also enable it to perform well as a tug, even under static tow conditions. (Author's abstract)

2008.
WILSON, H.L.
Otolaryngologic problems of skin and scuba diving.
Arch. Otolaryngol. 96:407-411;Nov. 1972.

Skin and scuba diving are increasing rapidly in popularity. Both involve occasional injury. Most of these injuries fall into the realm of the otolaryngologist. The causes are pressure, prolonged immersion, and temperature change. The most frequent injuries involve the ears. Otitis externa, tympanic membrane perforation, and inner ear damage can result. Severe epistaxis is at times a complication. (Author's abstract)

2009.
WILSON, R.H. and F.R. O'Brien.
Bioengineering and physiologic mammalian research in high pressure environments.
In: Abstracts of BuMed-ONR sponsored Navywide workshop in high pressure biomedical research, U.S. Submarine Base, Groton, Conn., May 1971, p.34. Published by the Naval Submarine Medical Research Laboratory, 1971.

Abstract only. Excerpts quoted: An interdisciplinary group at the University of North Dakota has designed and is constructing a computer controlled deep sea simulator to study mammalian learning, memory, behavior and cellular physiology in simulated ocean environments and in the transition to and from normal environment. The hyperbaric physiology research projects cover (1) oxygen toxicity, (2) chick embryonic development, and (3) biochemical and neurophysiologic studies related to brain synthesis and degradation of gamma-aminobutyric acid in mice brains, in atmospheres of helium and oxygen with the oxygen partial pressure being maintained at 150 mm Hg. Studies related to subclinical and subtle changes in cells in high pressure atmospheres of $He\text{-}O_2$ were manifested by the leakage of enzymes such as lactic dehydrogenase, serum glutamicoxalacetic transaminase, and alkaline phosphatase, from the cells into the blood plasma. Research concerning the effects of high pressure helium (20-60 atm) with a partial pressure of oxygen on the activity of the erythrocyte carbonic anhydrase had been completed. There was no adverse effect on the biochemical function of erythrocyte carbonic anhydrase. Research has been done concerning the effects of helium at 60 atmospheres with a partial pressure of oxygen of 150 mm Hg on the activity of hepatic glucose-6-phosphatase and glucose-6-phosphate dehydrogenase in the mouse which revealed an increase in the microsomal activity in the livers of all mice. It was postulated that the stress of the high-pressure atmosphere caused an increase of the glucorticoid level and/or catecholamine in the blood, and this could have caused an increase in the activity of this enzyme in the liver.

2010.
WINSTON, J.M. and R.J. Roberts.
The effect of drug pretreatment on lethality of mice exposed acutely to carbon monoxide or 7.5% oxygen environments.
Pharmacologist 15(2):239; 1973.

Abstract only. Entire item quoted: Mice were treated with phenobarbital (PB), 80 mg/kg, i.p., chlorpromazine (CPZ), 20 mg/kg, i.p., or ethanol, 7.5 g/kg, p.o., 1 hr., 24 hrs., or for 3 days prior to exposure to 1900-1958 ppm carbon monoxide (CO) or nitrogen containing 7.5% oxygen (O_2). PB pretreatment for 3 days decreased the CO lethality (17/40 vs 27/43) but did not affect 7.5% O_2 lethality (6/29 vs 7/27). CPZ pretreatment for 3 days increased the lethality of mice exposed to CO (26/39 vs 21/42) but did not [?] affect 7.5% O_2 lethality (4/27 vs 8/28). Ethanol pretreatment for 3 days had no significant effect on either CO or 7.5% O_2 lethality. PB or CPZ pretreatment 24 hrs. prior to exposure to either CO or 7.5% O_2 had no effect on lethality. One hour pretreatment with CPZ increased the lethality of both CO (29/32 vs 17/30) and 7.5% O_2 (11/11 vs 5/12), while PB did not modify OC lethality (19/32 vs 17/30) but increased the lethality of exposure to 7.5% O_2 (11/12 vs 5/12). These data indicate that drug pretreatment can produce distinct modifications of lethality associated with both CO and 7.5% O_2 exposure.

2011.
WINTER, D.C., L.O. Heflinger and C. Knox.
Acoustic bubble detection: Acoustic-optical imaging techniques for decompression studies.
Redondo Beach, Calif., TRW Systems, Inc., Final Rep. on contract N00014-69-C-0231, 45p. Sept. 30, 1972.
(AD 749 087)

The acoustic-optical imaging process utilizes Bragg diffraction of light by a beam of sound to produce an optical image of an acoustically irradiated object. Inasmuch as many materials which are quite opaque to light are, to varying degrees, transparent to certain acoustic frequencies, the technique offers the possibility of visually examining the internal structure of optically opaque bodies. The imaging of internal features is made possible by the fact that different materials and structures often have different acoustic characteristics, thus causing the sound to be reflected, scattered, absorbed, and diffracted. These factors cause perturbation in the acoustic wavefronts which are transformed in the light-sound interaction into a visual image, in real time, which may be observed by eye, photographed by a camera, or processed by other conventional optical methods. This program was directed toward an evaluation of the acoustic-optical imaging technique as a means of detecting bubbles formed in the circulatory system during decompression. (DCD abstract)

2012.
WINTER, P.M., F.T. Oliver and E.A. Jacobs.
Alterations of systemic oxygen content-pressure relationships in the production of oxygen toxicity.
In: Wada, J. and I. Takashi, eds. Proceedings of the fourth international congress on Hyperbaric medicine, Sapporo, Japan, Sept. 1969, p.29-31. Baltimore, Williams and Wilkins, 1970.

Experiments were performed on rats breathing 100% O_2 at 2 ATA. A control group was exposed until death. The experimental group breathed a gas mixture containing 0.2% carbon monoxide and 99.8% oxygen. . . . Thus, while the two groups had very similar oxygen tensions, the production of high carboxyhemoglobin levels produced a large difference in arterial oxygen content between them. Contrary to expectation, rats with a lowered oxygen content succumbed more quickly to pulmonary oxygen toxicity: control groups — 18 hours 12 min + 1 hr 52 min; experimental group — 14 hrs 38 min + 1 hr 53 min. The authors feel that hypoxia is the ultimate cause of death in oxygen toxicity. (Authors)

2013.
WINTER, P.M., B.T. Williams, B. Roding and W.G. Schenk.
Coronary artery blood flow and oxygen transport under hyperbaric oxygenation.
In: Wada, J. and I. Takashi, eds. Proceedings of the fourth international congress of hyperbaric medicine, Sapporo, Japan, Sept. 1969, p.228-230. Baltimore, Williams and Wilkins, 1970.

It is often assumed that an increase in CaO_2 will result in a similar increase in oxygen delivery to tissue. This assumption implies a relatively stable blood flow under the various conditions of oxygenation. It has been demonstrated by many authors and confirmed by this study that blood flow does not remain unchanged, but decreases as arterial oxygen levels increase. On this basis some have suggested that oxygen transport might not be improved by increases in inspired oxygen tension. This study emphasizes the importance of looking beyond blood flow changes alone. Oxygen transport appears to be autoregulatory, and is held relatively constant by simultaneous and opposite changes in content and flow. It will be of considerable importance to determine the source of the feed-back mechanism responsible for the autoregulation. If it is a direct response of the arterial bed to increases in oxygen levels, then one may expect that auto-regulation of flow would be independent of tissue demand. The more likely alternative is that oxygen transport is determined by tissue demand for oxygen. If the latter is true the study of normal animals will tell us little about the response of the vessel to varying oxygen tension when there is vascular insufficiency to the end-organ. Since oxygen therapy is frequently directed at such situations, it is important, as a next step, that the vascular response to oxygen be studied under conditions of experimental tissue ischemia. (Authors' discussion)

2014.
WINTER, P.M. and G. Smith.
The toxicity of oxygen.
Anesthesiology 37:210-241;Aug. 1972.

The authors are mainly concerned with the pulmonary forms of oxygen toxicity. The article contains sections on human tolerance to oxygen; pathology and histology, as revealed in both animal and human studies; pathophysiology; mechanisms of pulmonary oxygen toxicity, including absorption collapse, effects of pulmonary surfactant, myocardial failure, the role of inert gas and carbon dioxide, and the role of the endocrine system. This comprehensive review is illustrated by charts, diagrams and tables drawn from the literature or complied by the authors. It is directed primarily toward the clinical use of hyperbaric oxygen. The authors note that CNS oxygen toxicity occurs in hyperbaric environments, either in chambers or in deep sea diving or caisson work. (MFW/BSCP)

2015.
WISCHHOEFER, L.L.
Experimental investigation of recompression chamber ventilation analysis.
In: Battelle Columbus Laboratories. Proceedings, 1973 divers' gas purity symposium, November 27-28, 1973, p.XIII-1-XIII-30. U.S. Navy Supervisor Diving, Nav. Ships Syst. Comm., Rep. 2-73, 1973.

Studies have been conducted on various aspects of ventilation of divers' decompression chambers. Of primary concern were levels of carbon dioxide (CO_2) occurring in the chamber as a function of CO_2 generated by chamber occupants, of ventilation rates, and of chamber pressures. Chamber oxygen (O_2) levels attained when chamber occupants breathed pure O_2 (using the chamber's oxygen system) were also of interest. The studies were carried out in two parts. First, an analytical model of an open circuit recompression chamber system was constructed employing the parameters of interest. Second, experiments were conducted using a standard Navy recompression chamber system. The experiments were designed to test the hypothesis upon which the mathematical model was based as well as to gain information about how the Navy's practice of chamber ventilation relates to their available facilities. (Author's abstract)

2016.
WITTNER, M. and R.M. Rosenbaum.
Inhibition and reversal of intranuclear RNA synthesis by hyperatmospheric oxygen.
J. Appl. Physiol. 33:820-824;Dec. 1972.

The effects of hyperbaric O_2 on macromolecular synthesis were studied in HeLa cells. Nucleolar, nucleoplasmic and cytoplasmic RNA processing was studied utilizing uridine-^{14}C pulse labeling techniques, followed by ultracentrifugation on sucrose gradients, fractionation of the gradient and scintillation spectroscopy. 45S RNA synthesis seemed relatively unaffected by 100% O_2. Cleavage of the 45S $\rightarrow$ 32S $\rightarrow$ 28S preribosomal RNA was inhibited, while the 45S $\rightarrow$ 18S RNA cleavage reaction remained relatively intact and appeared in the cytoplasm in about the usual fashion. If the cells were kept at elevated O_2 atmospheres, the O_2 block in rRNA synthesis eventually led to cell death. The block was reversible if the cells were returned to air. (© BA)

2017.
WOLFE, W.G., P.A. Ebert and D.C. Sabiston, Jr.
Effect of high oxygen tension on mucociliary function.
Surgery 72(2):246-252; 1972.

Mucociliary clearance was studied in dogs by ventilating the lungs for periods up to 72 hr through a divided tracheal tube with one lung receiving 100% O_2 and the other receiving room air. Ventilation with high concentrations of O_2 significantly decreased mucociliary clearance. From previous studies and observations on cilia grown in tissue culture, the effect of high O_2 tension is thought to be on the mucociliary blanket or on the mucous glands rather than on cilia directly. Available alveolar surfactant and the ability of the lung to produce surfactant were normal. Histologically, the early pulmonary lesion following ventilation with 100% O_2 is perivascular edema which appeared between 48 and 72 hr and is present in the absence of significant atelectasis or congestion. (DTA) (© BA)

2018.
WOLFE, W.G. and D.C. Sabiston, Jr.
Lung function in spontaneously breathing and mechanically ventilated dogs exposed to ninety-five per cent oxygen.
Surg. Gynecol. Obstet. 137:763-768;Nov. 1973.

The effect of high oxygen concentrations for prolonged periods in the inspired air have been evaluated both in dogs breathing spontaneously and in those with mechanical endotracheal ventilation. An environment of 95 per cent oxygen with spontaneous breathing produced marked deterioration of pulmonary function within 72 hours which was characterized by perivascular edema, atelectasis, and liquid-filled alveoli. These changes also occurred in the dogs with mechanical ventilation but were less severe. Following removal from the high oxygen concentrations, pulmonary function gradually improved, and the microscopic anatomy returned to normal in about ten days. Evidence is presented which suggests that the primary lesion in pulmonary oxygen toxicity is development of perivascular edema which then progresses to intra-alveolar collection of fluid. These changes then produce atelectasis, diminished pulmonary function, and may ultimately end fatally. (Authors' summary)

2019.
WOOD, C.D. and A. Graybiel.
The effectiveness of benactyzine hydrochloride and other antimotion sickness drugs in new combinations.
U.S. Nav. Aerosp. Med. Res. Lab., Rep. NAMRL 1152, 4p. 1971.

Different drug preparations (5) are compared for their effectiveness in preventing motion sickness in humans with the effectiveness found for the combination of scopolamine 0.6 mg with a d-amphetamine 10 mg in previous studies. Promethazine 25 mg plus d-amphetamine 10 mg was essentially equal to the base line drug in range of effectiveness. Halving the doses of the baseline combination did not provide the protection that it did in an earlier study.

Benactyzine 3 mg was only slightly effective and when combined with d-amphetamine 10 mg was only moderately so. Promethazine 25 mg plus ephedrine 25 mg was about 1/4 less effective than the baseline preparation. The unexpected finding of the efficacy of small doses (25 mg) of promethazine plus ephedrine is pointed out, and the benefits from the relatively great reduction in side effects found with this drug combination are stressed. (© BA)

2020.
WOOD, C.D., G.F. Perkins, A.G. Smith and J.M. Reaux.
Response of the cardiovascular system in oxygen toxicity.
Aerosp. Med. 43:162-167;Feb. 1972.

The pulmonary edema resulting from exposure to hyperbaric oxygen (O_2) was found to be secondary to a systematic hypertension which produced left ventricular failure. Elevated pulmonary venous pressures resulted which caused edema fluid to pass into the alveoli along with some intact red blood cells. Microscopic and gross changes in the lungs with pulmonary edema resulting from exposure to hyperbaric O_2 were identical to lungs with pulmonary edema resulting from preoptic hypothalamic injections of aconitine. These changes also were similar to those seen in clinical cases of pulmonary edema resulting from hypertensive heart failure. Exposure to 100% O_2 ambient atmospheric pressures resulted in circulatory failure. A decrease of 15.7% in the A.T.P. of the heart muscle was observed and this could have been responsible for the weakening of the heart and the development of pulmonary edema. Our results indicate that much of the major pulmonary pathology seen in oxygen toxicity could be accounted for by cardiovascular effects. (Authors' abstract)

2021.
WOOD, G.A. and B. Ricci.
Respiratory nitrogen elimination: a potential source of error in closed-circuit spirometry.
Aerosp. Med. 44:961-962;Aug. 1973.

Breathing pure oxygen from a closed respiratory system results in the gradual elimination of nitrogen from the lungs, body tissues and fluids, representing a potential source of error in conventional closed-circuit spirometry, unless the loss of nitrogen is paralleled by bodily storage of an equal volume of oxygen. Nitrogen elimination was studied in six males during a 10-min period by breathing pure oxygen from a closed-circuit spirometry system. Significant volumes of nitrogen were found to be expelled, but were less than that considered to be residual within the lungs alone prior to oxygen breathing. Statistical trend analysis demonstrated a highly significant linear trend of nitrogen elimination, further attesting to the single source of nitrogen, namely the lungs. No change in lung end-expiratory volume was observed, and it was concluded that the nitrogen eliminated during the testing period was replaced with an equal volume of oxygen and, therefore, does not represent a source of error in the closed-circuit technique. (Authors' abstract)

2022.
WOOD, J.D. and S.J. Peesker.
The effect on GABA metabolism in brain of isonicotinic acid hydrazide and pyridoxine as a function of time after administration.
J. Neurochem. 19:1527-1537; 1972.

The effects of intramuscularly administered isonicotinic acid hydrazide (INH) on brain levels of gamma-aminobutyric acid (GABA) in chicks was dependent on the amount injected. A subconvulsant dose of INH (1.1 mmol/kg) produced a slow steady decline in the level of GABA, whereas a convulsant dose (2.19 mmol/kg) brought about a sequential fall and rise in GABA level. This sequence of events reflected changes in the relative activities of glutamic acid decarboxylase (GAD) and α-oxoglutarate aminotransferase (GABA-T) brought about by the hydrazide the administration of pyridoxine together with the INH (2·19 mmol/kg) prevented the onset of seizures and lessened the effect of the INH on GABA levels and GAD activity but not on GABA-T activity. The possibility that a deranged GABA metabolism is responsible for hydrazide-induced seizures is discussed. (Authors' abstract)

2023.
WOOD, J.D. and S.J. Peesker.
The effect of hydrazides on hyperbaric oxygen-induced seizures and the possible role of gamma-aminobutyric acid.
Proc. Can. Fed. Biol. Sci. 16:107; 1973.

Abstract only. Entire item quoted: The intramuscular administration of isonicotinic acid hydrazide (INH) to chicks induces seizures during the period 40-80 min after the injection but these seizures can be prevented by the simultaneous administration of phridoxine. The administration of the hydrazide, with or without the B6 vitamer, produces a relatively long lasting anticonvulsant action against hyperbaric oxygen-induced seizures. Other hydrazides such as thiosemicarbazide and semicarbazide provide little or no protection under similar conditions. The hydrazides alter GABA metabolism and a possible relationship between brain GABA level and the anticonvulsant action of INH will be discussed.

2024.
WOOD, S.C., J.D. Bloom and A.A. Messier.
Methemoglobin formation in humans during exposure to hyperbaric oxygen in a standard Navy decompression treatment table.
U.S. Nav. Submar. Med. Res. Lab., Rep. NSMRL 676, 6p. July 30, 1971.

[The problem was] to test the hypothesis that hemoglobin oxidation (ferro-to-ferrihemoglobin) will occur at an increased rate if erythrocytes are exposed in vivo to hyperbaric oxygen at the level encountered while breathing O_2 during Standard Navy Decompression Treatment Tables. The hypothesis was accepted on the basis of two subjects exposed to hyperbaric oxygen in accordance with decompression treatment Table 6. Both subjects developed methemoglobin concentrations ranging from 6 - 9% of total hemoglobin during decompression from 60 FSW. Pre- and post-dive values were 1 to 4% methemoglobin. The significance of these changes is that oxygen transport to tissues is compromised in the presence of methemoglobin by (a) decreased O_2 content of arterial blood and (b) increased oxygen affinity of arterial blood. These findings, while preliminary, deserve consideration by submarine medical officers dealing with decompression treatment or experimental compression of subjects breathing oxygen. Persons susceptible to methemoglobinemia, e.g., those taking antimalarial and certain other drugs and glucose-6-phosphate dehyodrogenase deficient individuals, should be identified before being exposed to OHP. (Authors' abstract)

2025.
WOOD, S.C. and K. Johansen.
Respiratory adaptations to diving in the Nile monitor lizard, Varanus Niloticus.
Physiologist 16:489;Aug. 1973.

Abstract only. Entire item quoted: The objectives of this study included direct in vivo measurements of circulating blood gases, pH, heart rate, and blood pressure during voluntary dives of unrestrained Nile monitor lizards. A radiometer flow-through cuvette was employed for continuous recording of arterial PO_2, PCO_2 and pH. The morphological properties of the blood revealed no particular adaptations for diving. Mean values were: hematocrit = 24%; hemoglobin concentration = 7.1 g %; oxygen capacity = 9.3 vol %; red cell dimensions = 22 x 12μ; red cell count = 0.67 million/μ l. The respiratory properties of the blood, studied in vitro and in vivo, show distinct adaptations to habitual diving. Oxygen affinity of blood is low (P_{50} = 42.4 at pH 7.45, 25°) and the dissociation curves is markedly sigmoid (n = 3.1). These features, coupled with a Bohr factor ($\Delta \log P_{50}/\Delta$ pH) of -0.48, ensure increased utilization of oxygen while maintaining relatively high tissue PO_2. Arterial pH decreases during diving from about 7.5 to 7.1 due to combined respiratory and metabolic acidosis. High plasma bicarbonate (30 mM/l at PCO_2 = 25 mmHg) and a buffering capacity of $\Delta HCO_3/\Delta$ pH = 18.9 mM/l increase the tolerance to this acidosis and prolong diving time. The in vivo oxygen dissociation curve shows a 90% depletion of arterial oxygen content during typical dives. Diving elicited a rapidly developing bradycardia with maximum of 85% reduction in heart rate. The temperature sensitivity of HbO_2 binding was very low (ΔH = -3 kCal). This would minimize the HbO_2 affinity increase accompanying the decrease in body temperature likely to occur in lizards going from sun basking to submergence in water.

2026.
WOODHALL, B., R.S. Kramer, W.D. Currie and A.P. Sanders.
Brain energetics and neurosurgery. A review of recent studies done at Duke University.
J. Neurosurg. 34(1):3-14; 1971.

Consecutive studies of brain energetics undertaken at Duke University during a period of five years are described. Various forms of stress such as hypoxia, hyperbaric oxygenation, and selected drugs were used to depict quantitative adverse effects upon the brain's basic energy system, and protectant measures evaluated including hypothermia and appropriate substrates. A systematic survey of substrate protectants was carried out in laboratory animals, and the theory and practice of preserving brain energy levels explored. A foundation for clinical application has been established. (Authors' abstract)

2027.
WOODRUFF, J.J.
What every girl should know about diving.
Skin Diver 21:38-39, 76;Mar. 1972.

The author points out the underwater accomplishments of women, citing the Tektite II experiment and the long-established commercial diving history of the ama. Women are more buoyant than men, and lose heat less readily, due to the more favorable distribution of subcutaneous fat. It is stated that there should be no fear of diving during menstruation, provided that general health is good at this time. There is possible danger for women who are on oral contraceptive medication, because of some indications that this medication has a sludging effect on some women which would make them more susceptible to decompression sickness. While this would make it undesirable for women on this medication to participate in saturation diving projects, it should have no effect in cases of shallow no-decompression dives. There is apparently no reason why women should not dive during pregnancy: it is a matter of record that the amas have given birth in the boat immediately upon completing a dive. Pregnant women must make allowances for increased buoyancy, as well as for increased girth. If a woman is subject to nausea or to vestibular dysfunction during pregnancy, she should, of course, not dive. There are known cases of female underwater research scientists and photographers, other than amas, who have undertaken dives up to the last stage of pregnancy, with no ill effects. (MFW/BSCP)

2028.
WOODS, J.D. and J.N. Lythgoe.
Apparatus and methods for the diving scientist.
In: Woods, J.D. and J.N. Lythgoe, eds. Underwater science: An introduction to experiments by divers, p.1-31. London, Oxford University Press, 1971.

The authors describe the techniques and equipment by which the underwater scientist can make himself more efficient, comfortable and safe. After a brief section on training and safety, the various types of breathing apparatus are described — open circuit, surface supply, and closed circuity. The last-named is at present used primarily by military and commercial divers, rather than by scientists. The Starck-Kanuisher electrolung developed by Oceanic Equipment Corporation, designed specifically for scientific diving, is at time of writing (1971) being tested. It is silent, has several hours endurance, and a depth capability of 300m. Heated suits and dry suits such as the Poseidon Unisuit are briefly described. Habitats and their uses are discussed. Their most important function is in support of saturation diving projects. These at present are chiefly in the commercial field, but after the successful Tektite experiments, habitats for scientific use will probably become more general. Small shelters for use at shallower depths for various purposes, including decompression, are discussed. Various towed vehicles for diver transport are discussed and illustrated, as are self-propelled vehicles. The Irving glider, a winged vehicle designed to utilize the buoyancy control possible with compressed air cylinders, is described and illustrated. The manifold problems of communication consists, first, of the difficulties brought about by the equipment itself, then, at greater depths, the effects of helium on speech intelligibility. Types of masks which permit clearer speech are illustrated. It is important that the mask enclose a maximum volume of air. In communication, training is most important; the diver must learn how to enunciate most effectively, and also which sounds are most easily understood. A table lists and describes the causes of transmission loss for sound underwater: absorption, scattering, refraction and multiple path distortion. There is a somewhat detailed technical discussion of modulated carrier wave systems, and telephones for hookah, or surface-demand diving. Very useful where a permanent experimental site is being used in a small airfield shelter, which is the simplest, cheapest and most effective aid to on-site communication between divers. The simplest method of recording underwater observations consists of a plastic board and graphite or waxed pencil. Tape recorders have not become widely used, but have some potential. Photography is the most satisfactory means of recording, and photographic equipment is described and illustrated. (MFW/BSCP)

2029.
WOODS, J.D. and J.N. Lythgoe.
Underwater science. An introduction to experiments by divers.
London, Oxford University Press, 1971. 320p.

The chief purpose of this book is to inform the underwater scientist as to the present state-of-the-art in diving technology, and the problems confronting the administrators of underwater projects requiring the use of divers and diving equipment. Chapters on diver performance and on vision and spatial perception contain much valuable data. Other chapters deal with branches of underwater science. The chapters on diver-related problems will be found under the following author entries: Baddely, A.D.; Lythgoe, J.N.; Ross, H.E.; Woods, J.D. and J.N. Lythgoe. (MFW/BSCP)

2030.
WOODS, J.D.
The diver in physical oceanography.
In: Diving applications in marine research. Proceedings of a seminar, National Institute of Oceanography, Godalming, Surrey, U.K., December 1971, p.39-44. Published by the Institute. 1972.

The diver's contribution to physical oceanography is determined by the following scale limitations: *Space Scale* — (a) his range of movement through the water is about 1 km; (b) his visual range is up to about 5 metres; (c) his visual acuity is about 1 millimetre. *Time Scale* — (a) his maximum endurance is about one hour; (b) he can time motions (e.g., with a stopwatch) down to about 1 second. Within these scales, lies a range of fluid motions and structures which are usually given the name *micro-oceanography*, by analogy with the term *micro-meteorology*. Micro-oceanography is concerned with mixing motions in the sea. . . [The diver] can identify and study in detail the various small-scale motions that are responsible for local mixing, but he cannot obtain statistical information concerning their distribution. Thus the contributions of the diver and the conventional oceanographer are complementary; each needs the other. (From author's abstract)

2031.
WOODWARD, D.
The Shark Hunter.
Skin Diver 20:58;Apr. 1971.

The Perry Shark Hunter is a two-man submersible with a depth capability of 150 feet. It is 14 feet long, 5 feet high and 8 feet wide, made mostly of fiberglass, and weighs about 1300 pounds. The submersible has a duration capability of two and one half hours at two knots and one and one-half hours at three knots. This range can be doubled by use of additional batteries. It can be anchored to the bottom while its passengers perform their underwater tasks. It is highly manoeuverable, with two speeds forward and two speeds back. (MFW/BSCP)

2032.
WOZNIAK, J., C.K. Raft and R.W. Alperi.
"Wake steering" — a new approach to propulsion and control.
In: Applications of marine technology to human needs. Preprints, 8th annual conference and exposition, Marine Technology Society, September, 1972, Washington, D.C., p.681-698. Published by the Society, 1972.

A new means of developing propulsions and steering forces for submersible vehicles is presented. The concept, termed wake steering, utilizes a propeller in a converging-diverging nozzle. The nozzle has four slots through the surface which may be closed or opened mechanically. By selectively opening these slots radial thrust for vehicle maneuvering is produced. An experimental model of the wake steering device was fabricated and tested. Internal wall static pressure measurements were made and forces were measured. A theoretical model of the nozzle is developed and the results of the model are compared to the experimental data. (Authors' abstract)

2033.
WRIGHT, W.B., A.B. Fisher, P.L. Hendricks, J.S. Brody and C.J. Lambertsen.
Effects on pulmonary function of a two-week exposure to 94.8% nitrogen-5.2% (normal) oxygen at a pressure equivalent to 100 feet of sea water.
In: Aerospace Medical Association. 1971 annual scientific meeting. Houston, Texas, April 1971. Preprints, p.76-77. Published by the Association, 1971.

This study represents one phase of an integrated investigation designed to determine the physiological limits of saturation exposures to increased nitrogen pressures. . . . These studies show that a two-week exposure to a gas pressure of 4 Ata produced no progressive deterioration in pulmonary function. The decreased inspiratory and expiratory flow rates and MVV's and the increased pulmonary resistance and flow resistive work during the exposure phase are consistent with the increased density of the respired gas. These changes were not large enough to produce any subjective sensation of respiratory disability even during moderate exercise, and the decrement in performance was reversible upon return to sea level. The increase in vital capacity was accompanied by a more negative maximal inspiratory esophageal pressure. This should represent an increase in muscular strength of the chest cage. (Authors)

2034.
WRIGHT, W.B.
Use of the University of Pennsylvania, Institute for Environmental Medicine procedure for calculation of cumulative pulmonary oxygen toxicity.
U.S. Navy Exp. Diving Unit, Rep. NEDU-2-72, 45p. 1972.

The use of elevated oxygen pressures in diving, treatment of decompression sickness, and hyperbaric oxygen therapy exposes the subject to the risk of oxygen toxicity of the lungs. At present no adequate guidelines exist to assist the physician in planning an oxygen exposure which will be safe from this hazard. An extensive multi-year research series recently completed by the University of Pennsylvania, Institute for Environmental Medicine has allowed the development of a method of calculating an estimated rate of onset and severity of pulmonary oxygen toxicity in man for any oxygen exposure. This report explains that method and provides tables that may be used to rapidly estimate the severity of pulmonary toxicity which may be incurred by an oxygen exposure. Recommendations as to safe limits of oxygen exposures for various procedures are included. . . . During decompression and for treatment of mild decompression sickness, the total oxygen exposure should be limited to that which yields a unit pulmonary toxic dose (UPTD) of 615 or less. In the use of oxygen for medical therapy or treatment of serious decompression sickness, which is responding poorly, an extreme limit of oxygen exposure which yields a UPTD of 1425 or less should be planned. (Author's abstract, conclusions and recommendations)

2035.
WRIGHT, W.B., Y. Seki and C.J. Lambertsen.
The role of the bronchial arteries in pulmonary oxygen toxicity.
In: Aerospace Medical Association. 1972 annual scientific meeting, Bal Harbour, Florida, May 1972. Preprints, p.178. Published by the Association.

Dynamic pulmonary compliance reflects the general status of lung elastic tissue and surfactant. The changes in compliance caused by oxygen poisoning appear to be related to the direct action of oxygen in the airways. Changes in nonelastic work of ventilation reflect damage to the bronchiolar tissue causing increased airway resistance. These changes are apparently caused by the high levels of oxygen in the bronchial arterial blood. . . This study emphasizes the fact that pulmonary oxygen toxicity is a complex syndrome. Although each cell in the lung is probably damaged by oxygen, certain cells, anatomical structures and pulmonary functions are damaged at different rates and in different ways. (From authors' conclusions)

2036.
WRIGHT, W.B., R. Peterson and C.J. Lambertsen.
Pulmonary mechanical functions in man breathing dense gas mixtures at great depths. Preliminary summary.
U.S. Navy Exp. Diving Unit, Rep. NEDU-14-72, 9p. July 1972.

The high density of breathing gas at great depths may impair a diver's performance by mechanical overload of his respiratory system. In order to describe this phenomenon and to search for a respiratory limit to deep diving we measured pulmonary mechanical functions at 19 different breathing gas densities ranging from 0.4 to 25 gms/L. (equivalent to helium at sea level to helium to 150 Ata). The results of these studies showed that function at rest is not severely affected by the great density increase. Respiratory limits to forced or exercising ventilation do appear, but useful function persists even to the maximum density studied and can be predicted to persist to even much greater densities. (Authors' abstract)

2037.
WRIGHT, W.B. and J.R. Crothers.
Effects of immersion and high pressures on pulmonary mechanical functions in man.
In: Aerospace Medical Association. 1973 annual scientific meeting, Las Vegas, Nevada, May 1973. Preprints, p.39. Published by the Association, 1973.

The purpose of this experiment was to determine to what extent the additional stress of actual submersion in water, as compared to subjection to high pressure in a chamber, would affect lung function. It was found that at sea level, maximum voluntary ventilation (MMV) was 11% less than that in the chamber. As pressure increased, the two values came closer together, until at 1000 fsw the MMV of the submerged diver was only 5% less than that of the dry subject. The insignificance of this difference would indicate that extrapolation of dry studies to open water conditions is valid, and also, that the chief limiting factor in underwater respiration is the breathing apparatus rather than the pulmonary system as affected by submersion. (MFW/BSCP)

2038.
WRIGHT, W.B., A.B. Fisher, P.L. Hendricks, J.S. Brody and C.J. Lambertsen.
Pulmonary function studies during a 14-day continuous exposure to 5.2% O_2 in N_2 at pressure equivalent to 100 fsw (4 ata).
Aerosp. Med. 44(7,Sec.II):837-848;July 1973.

To determine the immediate changes in pulmonary function induced by a four-fold increase in density of respired gas, subjects were exposed to nitrogen-oxygen breathing at 4 ata. Then to follow adaptations or deteriorations in pulmonary function during sustained increase in respiratory resistance, the studies were repeated during a two-week, uninterrupted exposure to the increased ambient pressure. While predictable increases in respiratory resistance and work of breathing accompanied the acute exposure to elevated ambient nitrogen pressure, no deleterious effects of either acute or chronic exposure to the 4 ata pressure were encountered. (Authors' abstract)

2039.
WUNSCHE, O. and G. Scheele.
Knochencysten bei Albinoratten nach Dekompression aus Uberdruck.
[Bone cysts in albino rats following decompression from high pressure].
Arch. Orthop. Unfall-Chir. 77:7-16; 1973.

In a series of experiments albino rats were subjected to repeated decompressions from high pressure. After 274 days cysts were demonstrated in bone segments close to the joints. These findings are the unequivocal consequence of the experimentally induced decompression sickness. Hence a model follows for skeletal alterations after high pressure exposure. (English abstract)

2040.
YAMADA, H.
[Experimental studies on effects of hyperventilation on cerebrospinal fluid pressure and oxygen tension in the cerebral cortex].
Acta Sch. Med. Univ. Gifu 20(1):52-87; 1972.

In performing human intracranial surgery, especially in the presence of a high intracranial pressure, reduction of the brain volume or shrinkage of the brain to reduce high intracranial pressure is essential. These procedures may make intracranial surgery easy and operative damage to the brain tissue minimal. Hyperventilation during anesthesia is one of the effective procedures. The problems of performing hyperventilation by the method of intermittent positive pressure breathing was investigated in adult mongrel dogs. An optimal condition of hyperventilation, under which there is little influence on the arterial and venous pressure and under which lowest cerebrospinal fluid pressure (CSFP) can be obtained, was sought. Various combinations of respiratory rate per min and respiratory tidal volume was investigated. The most suitable combination of respiratory rate and volume was 20/min respiration combined with a tidal volume twice as large as normal one (about 400 ml). The effects of such respiratory gases as air, 100% O_2, 3% $CO_2 + O_2$, 4% $CO_2 + O_2$ and 5% $CO_2 + O_2$ were investigated. The effects of hyperventilation by the method of intermittent positive pressure breathing with these gases on CSFP, cerebral cortical PO_2 [oxygen tension] and arterial and venous pressure were also investigated. (JAL) (© BA)

2041.
YANG, W.J., R. Echigo, D.R. Wotton, J.W. Ou and J.B. Hwang.
Mass transfer from gas bubbles to impinging flow of biological fluids with chemical reaction.
Biophys. J. 12(11):1391-1404; 1972.

The rates of mass transfer from a gas bubble to an impinging flow of a biological fluid such as whole blood and plasma are investigated analytically and experimentally. Gases commonly found dissolved in body fluids are included. Consideration is given to the effects of the chemical reaction between the dissolved gas and the liquid on the rate of mass transfer. Through the application of boundary layer theory the over-all transfer is found to be Sh/(Re) 1/2 = 0.845 Sc 1/3 in the absence of chemical reaction, and Sh/(Re) 1/2 = F'(0) in the presence of chemical reaction, where Sh, Re, and Sc are the Sherwood, Reynolds, and Schmidt numbers, respectively, and F'(O) is a function of Sc and the dimensionless reaction rate constant. Analytical results are also obtained for the bubble lifetime and the bubble radius-time history. These results, which are compatible with experimental results, can be applied to predict the dissolution of the entrapped gas emboli in the circulatory system of the human body. (© BA)

2042.
YANG, W.J. and C.Y. Liang.
Dynamics of dissolution of gas bubbles or pockets in tissues.
J. Biochem. 5(4):321-322; 1972.

A mathematical model is developed which describes the dynamic characteristics of gas bubbles in subcutaneous tissues. Consideration is given to both inert and reacting gases. The effects of blood perfusion (or O_2 consumption in the tissue in dead animals), diffusion of the dissolved gases, a creep process occurring in the tissue, and thermodynamic behavior of the gases in the cavity on the dissolution of the gas bubbles are taken into account. The stress-strain relation of the tissues in creep is described by the standard linear model of visco-elasticity. The theoretical analysis is presented in three categories: tissue creep controlled, mass transfer controlled, and the intermediate case where both mechanisms are of comparable importance. A close agreement is obtained between the theoretical predictions and the existing experimental data for subcutaneous inert gas pockets in air breathing rats. (© BA)

2043.
YASTREBOV, V.
The 'crab' remote-controlled underwater craft.
Underwater J. 5:117-119;June 1973.

The 'Crab' remote-controlled underwater craft is intended to carry out simple operations for collecting sea-bed material and animal specimens from the ocean floor at depths of up to 3600 m. It carries a TV-system, a manipulator, a hydraulic power system, a remote-control system and an autonomous storage battery supply. The entire electronic section of the equipment is housed in the front part of the 'Crab' in spherical boxes which are provided with portholes through which observations are conducted with the aid of television and a photographic camera. The boxes carry a hinged telescopic manipulator, the gripping part of which is adjusted for picking up objects of any shape as well as loose ground samples. The manipulator has a range, relative to the immobile craft, 0.4 m. The whole craft is positioned on a three-bearing flat platform and may revolve, relative to the platform, around its vertical axis, for 320°, allowing scanning of the area when the craft is on the ocean floor. The spherical boxes with the manipulator may be inclined to 30° giving the craft the facility for scanning, and the manipulator the possibility of servicing, a circular zone with an inner diameter of 2.2 m and outer diameter of 3 m. The craft itself is 1.4 m long, 1 m. wide and 0.4 m high and weighs 620 kg in air. After scooping the sample, the manipulator turns back and stops in its extreme rear position over a bin into which the scooped materials are placed. (Author)

2044.
YASUDA, K., H. Takeya, T. Yoshida and K. Furukawa.
Analysis of the cardiovascular function under a hyperbaric environment using an analog computer.
In: Wada, J. and I. Takashi, eds. Proceedings of the fourth international congress of hyperbaric medicine, Sapporo, Japan, Sept. 1969, p.185-190. Baltimore, Williams and Wilkins, 1970.

In order to investigate the influence of hyperbaric oxygen on the cardiovascular function, the ventilatory conditions and the depth of anesthesia must be kept constant throughout the experiment. In this experiment, both the intratracheal pressure and the minute volume under 3 ATA were held at values equal to that under 1 ATA. Further, the fluctuation of halothane concentration in the arterial blood, brought about by changes in the environmental pressures, were slight and may be surmised to have little or no influence on the cardiovascular system. By our preliminary experiments it was shown that the changes in environmental pressure had little or no influence on the pressure transducer and flo-probe. Thus, it was concluded that the deviation of the measured values were negligible. In the state of 3 ATA compression, the changes in cardiovascular parameters showed a 15% to 20% decrease from the control values in the first derivative of aortic blood flow, in the left ventricular work and in the contractile force which seems to be suggestive of the decrease in the cardiac function. On the other hand, the total peripheral resistance showed a 20% increase which is suggestive of a contraction of peripheral blood vessels. (From authors' summary and conclusions)

2045.
YAYANOS, A.A.
Molecular effects of pressure.
In: Abstracts of the Twenty-fifth Congress of Physiological Sciences Satellite Symposium. Recent progress in fundamental physiology of diving. Marseille, France, July 1971, p.22. (Proceedings unpublished)

Abstract only. Entire item quoted: The values of partial molal volumes and their pressure dependence are central to the interpretation of high pressure biological phenomena from the point of view of thermodynamics. The effects of pressure on the partial molal volume of some amino acids are discussed. The increase with pressure of the partial molal volume of an amino acid will be considered from the point of view of a pressure effect on the electrostriction of water. A concise review of the physico-chemical basis for the effects of pressure is given. The topics to be reviewed include chemical equilibria, reaction rates and phase changes. Topics from the recent literature will be discussed which include the effects of pressure on protein structure, nucleic acid structure and on micelles.

2046.
YOKOYAMA, T.
The limiting factors affecting the depth of breath-hold diving on the ama in Japan.
In: Abstracts of the Twenty-fifth Congress of Physiological Sciences Satellite Symposium, Recent progress in fundamental physiology of diving. Marseille, France, July 1971. p.18-19. (Proceedings unpublished)

Abstract only. The author summarizes some of the data collected during a series of observations made of amas. Unassisted, the ama reached only 10 meters, assisted (presumably by a co-worker in a boat with a line) the ama could reach 28 meters. This is markedly less than depths reached by sports divers using modern equipment. The swimming fin increased the maximum depth by improving the efficiency of their energy expenditure. The unclothed ama could reach greater depths than the clothed ama, but lost this advantage during repeated dives because of the lack of cold protection. Increased oxygen consumption due to loss of body heat decreased the oxygen available for energy expenditure. Wet suits are now beginning to be used. (MFW/BSCP)

2047.
YOUDIN, M.and T. Reich.
Biomedical research instrumentation for a 6 ATA hyperbaric chamber.
In: Wada, J. and I. Takashi, eds. Proceedings of the fourth international congress of hyperbaric medicine, Sapporo, Japan, Sept. 1969, p.116-120. Baltimore, Williams and Wilkins, 1970.

The following seven requirements are listed as being most essential in designing a hyperbaric chamber: (1) unobstructed space around the hull for at least four to six feet; (2) as large a number of access ports as possible; (3) a maximum number of viewing ports; (4) a six-inch usable diameter for all access ports; (5) a versatile means for supporting instrumentation from the ceiling of the chamber; (6) raceways or troughs outside the chamber for tubing and cables; (7) electric power outlets close to the access ports on the outside of the chamber, to be supplied from an isolation transformer. (MFW/BSCP)

2048.
YU, C.J., B. Lutherer, A.R. Guyatt and A.B. Otis.
Comparison of blood and alveolar gas composition during rebreathing in the dog lung.
Resp. Physiol. 17(2):162-177; 1973.

In ten dogs, one lung was connected to a rubber bag and made to rebreathe while the other lung was allowed to breathe freely. Blood samples were taken from a pulmonary vein of the rebreathing lung and from the pulmonary artery. Gas samples were taken from the rebreathing bag. PCO_2 [CO_2 tension] and PO_2 [O_2 tension] of the gas phase were higher than the corresponding partial pressures in either blood sample. PCO_2 of pulmonary venous blood was higher than that of pulmonary arterial blood, but there was no significant difference between the values for PO_2 of the two samples. Pulmonary venous blood had a slightly lower pH than pulmonary arterial blood, but the difference was not statistically significant. Over a period of two hours plasma bicarbonate decreased slightly, and negative base excess increased by a similar magnitude. The experiments confirm but do not explain the results of other investigators in demonstrating the presence of positive gradients for CO_2 between gas and blood phases during rebreathing. (© BA)

2049.
YU, M.C., L. Bakay and J.C. Lee.
Effects of hypoxia and hypercapnic hypoxia on the ultrastructure of central nervous synapses.
Exp. Neurol. 40:114-125;July 1973.

Pronounced ultrastructural changes in the presynaptic terminals of central nervous tissues of rats were observed after various durations of sustained hypoxia and hypercapnic hypoxia. Two distinct types of morphological alterations were found. In the first type, the presynaptic terminal was greatly enlarged, measuring 3-10 μ m in the greatest diameter. These terminals contained unusual multilamellar bodies in the form of compact lamellae. The second type of terminal changes consisted of aggregated or clumped vesicles, often surrounded by attenuated glial processes. The first type of altered terminals occurred predominantly in the deep cerebellar nuclei, while the second type was present in all regions of the central nervous system examined. (Authors' abstract)

2050.
YUKHIMETS, A.D. and N.G. Trinyak.
Functsional'noe sostoyanie shchitovidnoi zhelezy pri giperbaricheskoi oksigenatsii.
[Functional state of the thyroid gland in hyperbaric oxygenation].
Patol. Fiziol. Eksp. Ter. 17:76-78;Mar./Apr. 1973.

Hyperbaric oxygenation (3 atm for 2 hr), acute hypoxic hypoxia and also hyperbaroxia against the background of acute hypoxia were characterized by increased thyroid gland activity (determined by blood-protein-bound iodine and by morphological picture of the gland). There was established a direct correlation between the initial level of thyroid hormones circulating in the blood and the toxic action of oxygen on the animal organism. (English summary)

2051.
ZAGRYADSKII, V.P.
Izmenenie dykhaniya pri narastayushchei giperkapnii.
[Respiratory changes in growing hypercapnia].
Fiziol. Zh. SSSR Sechenova 57(12):1820-1822; 1971.

Compensatory reactions of external respiration in man during hypercapnia, consisted of initial adaptation to CO_2, the further adaptation being connected with decrease of metabolic activity. On the contrary, during hypocapnia, metabolic activity increases with the growth of CO_2 production. (SB) (© BA)

2052.
ZALTSMAN, G.L.
Means of penetrating the ocean.
Priroda 10:28-37; 1971.
(Translation JPRS 54789)

The principal factor directly affecting the human organism under conditions of underwater descents is the increased pressure of the gas medium. From a physiological standpoint, the pressure rise is manifested as a complex irritant evoking numerous changes and response reactions, both adaptive and pathological. In analyzing these processes, one should differentiate the various types of effect exerted by increased pressures of the gas medium on the organism. The mechanical effect of increased pressures is manifested in the form of a general volumetric compression of the organism — its systematic compression as a result of the transfer of compressed gas molecules' energy to all the body surfaces. Such a compression causes a specific pathological reaction, termed 'mechano-narcosis' by many authors. An additional form of the mechanical effect of increased pressures is the local compression of an organism's tissues, surrounding the internal gas cavities. As a result of the variation in the gas volume, there occurs a deformation and displacement of tissues surrounding the gas cavity, while in case of exceeding their elasticity, we get tissue trauma, said to be barotrauma. An additional resistance is offered to the active movement of gas in the human respiratory tracts which leads to a disruption in the functioning of breathing and to the development of hypoxia. Another mandatory component of breathing mixtures is represented by the inert gases, nitrogen, or helium, hydrogen, argon etc., in the manmade gas mixtures. Saturating an organism under pressure, these gases cease to be inert and exert a narcotic effect. Finally, the last type of influence of the increased pressures from a gas medium is represented by the phase transformations of excess dissolved inert gas in an organism. Gas emboli develop in the blood in the form of bubbles at rapid transfer from high atmospheric pressure to a lower pressure. (GRA)

2053.
ZANDER, R.
Solubility of oxygen in fluorocarbon liquids.
Pfluegers. Arch. (Suppl.) 343:R5; 1973.

Abstract only. Entire item quoted: Fluorocarbons are perfluorinated organic liquids, inert, colorless, nearly nontoxic, insoluble in water, and of high density and extremely low surface tension. Due to their high gas solubility capacities fluorocarbons have gained intensive interest in medical and biological research, e.g. liquid-liquid-oxygenators, whole animal perfusion, synthetic blood, in vivo and extracorporal organ perfusion, and storage of isolated organs. The bibliographical data for oxygen solubility, however, differ between 0.16 and 0.6 ml O_2/ml atm, there is also great difference in the temperature behavior of the oxygen solubility coefficients. This is the reason why we measured the oxygen solubility coefficients of one fluorocarbon (FC 43, e-M-Comp.), a perfluorotributylamine (C_{12} $F_{27}N$) at temperatures from 10 to 50°C at different oxygen partial pressures between 100 and 700 mmHg. After equilibration of the fluorocarbon in a LAUE tonometer with gas of known oxygen partial pressure (determination of oxygen concentration by the apparatus) the oxygen content was measured in the classical manometric apparatus at constant temperature (sample: 0.2 ml, constant gas volume: 0.16 ml). The results show that 1. the solubility coefficient for oxygen at FC 43 at 37°C amounts to 0.362 + 0.007 ml O_2/ml atm, 2. HENRY-DALTON-s law is not completely fulfilled in a range between 100 - 700 mmHg, 3. with increasing temperature, the solubility coefficient decreases linearly.

2054.
ZANDER, R.
Die Sauerstoff-Abgabe menschlicher Erythrocyten unter Hyperoxie.
[Effect of hyperoxia on the oxygen release from human erythrocytes].
Pneumonologie 149:83-86;Oct. 31, 1973.

Oxygen release from packed erythrocytes was measured under conditions of rest and quick flow (cone-plate viscosimeter) after saturation with oxygen partial pressures ranging from 50 to 600 mmHg. Under these experimental conditions oxygen release reaches its maximum value at an initial oxygen partial pressure of about 300 mmHg in resting cells and about 100-200 mmHg in flowing cells. Therefore, co-operation of the four possible intracellular oxygen transport mechanisms, i.e. oxygen and oxyhemoglobin diffusion and convection is essential for optimum efficient oxygen release from human erythrocytes. (English abstract)

2055.
ZANNINI, D. and D. Bonsignore.
Pneumoperitoneo e pneumomediastino da risalita a rapida in subacqueo.
[Pneumoperitoneum and pneumomediastinum resulting from rapid ascent while diving].
Ann. Med. Nav. 78:5-10;Jan.-Mar. 1973.

A diving accident involving gastrointestinal distention and pulmonary hypertension was the result of a rapid ascent from 30 meters necessitated by failing breathing apparatus. Therapeutic recompression according to the U.S. Navy Table 1A relieved the symptoms (loss of consciousness, cyanosis, tachycardia, hypertension, abdominal distension). It is described here as "a case of gastrointestinal distension and probably cerebral gas embolism resulting from pulmonary hypertension with pneumoperitoneum and pneumomediastinum." The puzzling aspect of this case is the origin of the air in the peritoneal cavity and the mediastinum, since no air was found in the pleural cavity. Various hypotheses are put forward regarding the route by which the air traveled into the mediastinum and peritoneum: (1) via the pulmonary portion of the pleural retrocardial bursa; (2) via the peritronchial and peritracheal connective tissue; (3) via the digestive tract and a stomach lesion. The lower fever and leukocytosis which followed the recompression and persisted for several days is attributed to "a reaction of the pulmonary parenchyma at the point of the penetration of the air." (MFW/BSCP from translation of MEMH/SCD)

2056.
ZEHL, D.N., A.T.K. Cockett, J. Hanley, W.R. Adey, A.P. Roberts and R. Zweizig.
Bubble-emboli formation and neurocirculatory changes in decompression sickness.
In: Aerospace Medical Association, 1973 annual scientific meeting, Las Vegas, Nevada, May 1973. Preprints, p.200. Published by the Association, 1973.

The purpose of this report is threefold: (1) to report emboli formation with pupillary and eye ground changes, (2) to document bubble formation with changes in the EEG and (3) to report slow wave changes in the EEG of a patient undergoing treatment for bends in a recompression chamber. The experimental changes seen in the animals' eyes have not been previously correlated with brain wave changes. We believe that bubbles and lipid emboli are probably responsible for these changes. One of two divers undergoing treatment in the recompression chamber also had slow wave changes on the EEG from the occipital-parietal region. We believe that these changes are probably secondary to embolic phenomena. (Authors)

2057.
ZHIRONKIN, A.G., L.A. Isaakyan and G.V. Troshikhin.
Vliyanie povyshennogo atmosferiogo davleniya ma dinamiku codeizhaniya svobodnogo kisloroda v. myshechnoi tkani u zhivotnykh.
[The effect of high atmospheric pressure on the dynamics of free oxygen concentration in the muscle tissue of animals].
Fiziol. Zh. SSSR 58:1109-1114;July 1972.

These experiments were carried out on 70 rats in a 300 liter compression chamber. The animals were exposed to helium-oxygen and the nitrogen-oxygen under various pressures, and the free oxygen in the musculus quadriceps femoris was measured by polarography. It was found that five hours of helium-oxygen at 20 kgs/cm^2 and at 40 kgs/cm^2, the oxygen level was also lowered, probably due to the compression of the inhaled air, or to the narcotic effect of nitrogen. It is noted that further studies are necessary for a better understanding of the mechanisms involved. (OLC/BSCP)

2058.
ZHUKOV, R.F., A.A. Kondratovich, S.D. Mogilnyi and B.I. Tsipko.
Sistemy, pribory i ustroistva podvodnogo poiska.
[Underwater search systems, instruments and devices].
Moscow 1972, 182p.
(Translation JPRS 58916)

A study was made of the physical principles of constructing underwater search systems, their instruments and devices. Underwater search systems are described, the operation of which is based on various physical principles, and methods of utilizing them. The description of the systems, instruments, devices, physical principles and the principles of the construction and operation of them and also methods of utilizing them and determining the efficiency are presented from froeign publications. There is a brief discussion of the principles of determining the efficiency of various underwater search systems. Examples are presented of the organization of underwater search operations — the search for the sunken Affray, Thresher and Scorpion submarines, the American hydrogen bomb lost off the coast of Spain and other objects. (GRA)

2059.
ZIDER, R.B.
A perfect pair.
Sea Frontiers 19:72-77;Mar./Apr. 1973.

The Johnson-Sea-Link is unique in that while divers can lock-out at 1500 fsw, pilot and observers remain in a one-atmosphere environment with 360° visibility. This article gives a detailed drawing of the submersible. The pressure in the diver's chamber can be controlled either from the pilot's position in the acrylic sphere, or from within the chamber itself. Lock-out procedures are sufficiently simple for inexperienced divers to master with an hour's instruction. Safety features include the pneumatic blowing of ballast, and the ability to ditch the battery pod. Formerly handled by Sea Diver, designed for the purpose, Sea-Link has recently been handled by the research vessel Researcher, which has greater depth capability and is better equipped to handle submersibles in rough seas. Tests were made successfully launching and recovering Sea-Link from Researcher to a depth of 1000 ft with one delay which occurred at 500 ft when two motors shorted out due to the failure of the seals at high pressure. At present the sub does not carry manipulators, but as dives become deeper, these will be added. The diving chamber is kept at one atmosphere until the object of the search is located by the pilot, then it is pressurized to ambient pressure. When ambient pressure is reached, the hatch opens. At less than 150 feet, compressed air is the breathing mixture, and conventional scuba gear is used. Beyond this depth, helium-oxygen is used, with closed circuit breathing apparatus. Decompression is carried out in the diving chamber at present, but its small size makes it undesirable for long decompressions. A larger chamber will be constructed aboard the support vessel. Several search and recovery methods have been carried out successfully with inexperienced divers, thus proving the safety and practicability of the design. (MFW/BSCP)

2060.
ZILLIOUX, E.J.
Diver-operated versus remote-controlled chambers used in underwater tracer experiments.
Helgolander Wiss. Meeresunters. 24:112-119; 1973.

Two chambers, one diver-operated and the other remote-controlled, were developed for in situ feeding experiments. Both chambers have been used effectively in numerous experiments with vertically migrating copepods fed ^{65}Zn-labeled microzooplankton. Laboratory results demonstrated no significant difference in recovered radioactivity due to differences in material or design of the two chambers. Diver-operated chambers are initially much less expensive and are generally more adaptable to changes in experimental design. Remote-operated chambers require less personnel and are necessary when determining effects of depth within the entire range common for vertically migrating zooplankton. (Author's summary)

2061.
ZIMIN, A.B. and N.S. Malinovskaya.
Potreblenie pishchi i morfologicheskie pokazateli krovi u belykh myshei pri zamene azota vozdukha inertnymi gazami v usloviyakh germeticheskoi kamery.
[Food intake and morphological indices of the blood in white mice in a sealed atmosphere in substitution of inert gases for nitrogen].
Kosm. Biol. Med. 7(4):21-26; 1973.

White male mice were exposed for 5 days to $Ar\text{-}O_2$, $He\text{-}O_2$ and $N\text{-}O_2$ atmospheres. Food intake was measured. Significant variations in the amount of the food intake were noted and correlated with the gas composition and temperature of the enclosed atmosphere. Changes in the blood morphological composition were within the physiological limits for laboratory mice, although they indicated certain relationship with thermal and physical properties of the atmosphere. The greatest deviations were noted in a $He\text{-}O_2$ atmosphere at relatively low temperatures. (MH) (© BA)

2062.
ZIMMERMAN, A.M.
Effects of pressure on cellular and subcellular structures and systems.
In: Abstracts of the Twenty-fifth Congress of Physiological Sciences Satellite Symposium. Recent progress in fundamental physiology of diving. Marseille, France. July 1971, p.22-24. (Proceedings unpublished)

Abstract only. The author discusses the effects of high hydrostatic pressure on cellular systems, primarily with regard to morphological, physiological and biochemical changes. The structural and physiological effects are probably a result of biochemical changes. Macromolecular alterations are probably the cause of cellular effects which in turn bring about physical and structural changes. It is stated that "macromolecular synthesis. . . is inhibited by 5,000 to 7,000 psi in protozoa and marine eggs. . . Ribosomes isolated from pressure treated protozoa retain the ability to synthesize protein and that their translational efficiency is comparable to atmospheric control cells." (MFW/BSCP)

2063.
ZINKOWSKI, N.B.
Commercial oil-field diving.
Cambridge, Maryland, Cornell Maritime Press, Inc., n.d. 372p.

The author is a diving veteran of wide experience in the U.S. Navy and in commercial diving. This book is filled with practical suggestions that could greatly add to the comfort and efficiency of underwater work. The chapter headings are: Diving as a career; Physics and physiology; Tending and breaking out; Diving equipment; Decompression and treatment tables for air diving; Rigging; Burning and welding underwater; Use of explosives; Diving from a pipelay barge; Diving froma pipeline barge, or jet barge; Miscellaneous diving applications in the oil field; Diving from a drilling rig; Mixed gas diving; Diving from a bell, saturation diving, dry-atmosphere welding huts; Diver's pay unions, summary of safety precautions; and an appendix on manufacturers and distributors. (MFW/BSCP from a review by R. Barton in Hydrospace 5:31;June 1972)

2064.
ZOBELL, C.E. and J. Kim.
Effects of deep-sea pressures on microbial enzyme systems.
In: The effect of pressure on organisms. Symposia of the Society for Experimental Biology, No. 26, p.125-246. Cambridge, University Press, 1972.

Deep-sea pressures, say 50-1200 atm, have measurable effects on the stability and activity of microbial enzyme systems. A good many enzyme reaction rates are inhibited by such pressures. In most cases, pressure inhibition is attributable to the inactivation of enzyme systems. Deep-sea pressures accelerate certain enzymatically catalysed reactions by producing molecular volume changes which influence absolute chemical reaction rates. Several other mechanisms also help to account for the effects of hydrostatic pressure. The barotolerance of enzymes is influenced by temperature, duration of compression, and the chemical composition of the medium, especially pH, salinity, bivalent cations, concentration of substrate, and free or dissolved oxygen. Marked differences occur in the barotolerance of the same kinds of enzymes produced by different organisms. There seems to be a relationship between the molecular weights and structure of enzymes and their barotolerance. . . . A large variety of microbial enzymes have been shown to be produced, quite stable and active at the greatest known oceanic depths. It is particularly significant that such complex polymers as agar, cellulose, starch, chitin and various proteins undergo enzymatic hydrolysis at deep-sea pressures and temperatures. (Authors' summary and conclusions).

2065.
ZUIKHIN, D.P. and V.M. Strogapov.
Ob intensivnosti fizichkoi podgotovki podvodnikov v pokhodakn.
[Intensity of physical activity of submarine crews during voyages].
Voennomed. Zh. (2):67-69;Feb. 1971.

Physical activity of submarine crews during prolonged expeditions is extremely limited. Measured by individual pedometers the performance of crew members ranges between 10,000 and 700 steps in a 24 hrs. period. In a comparative study the authors evaluated the performance and endurance of three groups of men during two expeditions. The three groups performed heavy (1), medium (2) and light (3) physical tasks; all of them had previous physical training. The effect of physical exercise on their well-being was evaluated by cardiovascular tests as well as individual questionnaires. The first two groups complained of fatigue and pain, while the third, with the lightest load, did not report any change in physical well-being. On the other hand, the cardiovascular tests showed considerably more improvement in the physical condition of the first two groups, with heavy to medium load, than in the third, with the lightest load. Thus the subjective findings (questionnaire) were not in accordance with the results of the objective (physiological) tests. The authors conclude that more tests and studies are needed to establish the effects of hypodynamia and exertion on the human organism. (OLC/BSCP)

2066.
ZWEIZIG, J.R., W.R. Adey, J. Hanley, P.M. Hahn, A.A. Pilmanis, R.R. Given and A.T.K. Cockett.
EEG monitoring of a free-swimming diver at a working depth of 15 meters.
Aerosp. Med. 43:403-407;Apr. 1972.

Feasibility has been shown for underwater transmission of physiological signals, using frequency modulation of carriers transmitted by return-current-density methods, as part of a personal biotelemetry system. In the prototype system, a standard IRIG subcarrier frequency (2300 Hz) was used. Power requirements, antenna design and signal attenuation are compatible with free-ranging diving activity at distances up to 15 meters from the receiver. Extrapolation from this study and further developments are expected to substantially increase the range. Advantages of this system include subcarrier compatibility with standard IRIG demodulators using Channels 1 through 10, the absence of highly specialized antenna requirements, and reasonable attenuation characteristics for transmission through the turbidity of typical seawater. Moreover the system would not apear to be depth limited, and to be compatible with use of high-powered transponders of the same type for long-distance transmission, with or without further encoding. (Authors' abstract)

MICROTHESAURUS

This is a condensed and refined version of the microthesaurus presented in the preceding bibliography. An attempt has been made to avoid duplication and to work out a word list which will most accurately reflect current terminology. This list is by no means frozed or static; from time to time, words are added as they become prevalent in the literature. In order to prevent the index from becoming impossible unwieldy, we have not used words indicating source or type of document, although these words do in fact occur in the retrieval system which contains and makes available material from all three of our bibliographies. The words which comprise the index are in capital letters. Related words are in lower case.

ACCIDENT
acclimatization: see ADAPTATION
ACID-BASE BALANCE
acidosis: see ACID-BASE BALANCE
ACOUSTICS
ADAPTATION
ADENOSINE TRIPHOSPHATE
ADIPOSE TISSUE
ADRENAL
AEROSOLS
AGE
agglutination: see SLUDGING
AIR AMBOLISM
air purity: see BREATHING MIXTURES, CONTAMINANTS, ATMOSPHERE CONTROL
AIRWAYS
alcohol: see PRE-DIVE CONDITIONS
ALERTNESS
ALGAE
ALTITUDE
ALVEOLAR
ama: see WOMEN
AMINES
AMINO ACIDS
ANESTHESIA
ANIMAL (LABORATORY)
ANTHROPOMETRY
ANTIBIOTICS
ANTICOAGULANTS
ANTITOXIN
ANXIETY
APNEA
APTITUDE
aqualung: see BREATHING APPARATUS
argon: see INERT GAS, BREATHING MIXTURES
AROUSAL
ARRHYTHMIA
arteries: see VASCULAR SYSTEM
ARTHRALGIA
ARTIFICIAL RESPIRATION
ASCENT
aseptic bone necrosis: see OSTEONECROSIS
ASPHYXIA
aspirin: see DRUGS
ATELECTASIS
ATMOSPHERE CONTROL
ATOMIC ENERGY
AUDIOMETRY
auditory acuity: see HEARING
auditory evoked responses: see EVOKED RESPONSES
bacteria: see MICROORGANISMS
BAROTRAUMA
Barylime: see ATMOSPHERE CONTROL
BEHAVIOR
BELL (DIVING)
belt: see PERSONAL EQUIPMENT
bends: see DECOMPRESSION SICKNESS
BIBLIOGRAPHY
BIOCHEMICAL
BIOENGINEERING
BIOLOGICAL RHYTHMS
BLACKOUT
BLAST
BLOOD
blood flow: see CIRCULATION
BLOOD PRESSURE
body measurement: see ANTHROPOMETRY
BONE
bone conduction: see HEARING
BONE MARROW
BOREDOM
BOUNCE DIVING
BRADYCARDIA
BRAIN
BREATH-HOLD DIVING
breathing: see RESPIRATION
BREATHING APPARATUS
BREATHING MIXTURES
BUBBLES
BUOYANCY
buoyant ascent: see ASCENT
caisson sisease: see DECOMPRESSION SICKNESS
caisson workers: see COMPRESSED AIR WORKERS
CANADA
CAPILLARY
carbohydrates: see NUTRITION
CARBON DIOXIDE
CARDIAC OUTPUT
CARDIORESPIRATORY
CARDIOVASCULAR
CASE HISTORY
CAVE DIVING
cavitation: see BUBBLES
CELLS
central nervous system: see CNS
CERTIFICATION
cerebrospinal fluid: see CSF
chamber: see HYPERBARIC CHAMBER
CHEMICAL
cholesterol: see LIPIDS
circadian rhythms: see BIOLOGICAL RHYTHMS
CIRCULATION
closed circuit breathing apparatus: see BREATHING APPARATUS
CLOSED ENVIRONMENT
CNS
COAGULATION
cognitive processes: see MENTAL FUNCTION
COLD
COLOR
color vision: see VISION
combustion: see FIRE
COMMUNICATION
COMMUNICATION EQUIPMENT
compressed air: see BREATHING MIXTURES
compressed air illness: see DECOMPRESSION SICKNESS
COMPRESSED AIR WORKERS
COMPRESSION RATE
COMPRESSORS
computers: see DATA PROCESSING
CONFINEMENT
CONTAMINANTS
CONVULSIONS
CORROSION
COUNTERDIFFUSION
CSF
CUTANEOUS
cycles: see BIOLOGICAL RHYTHMS
cytology: see CELLS
dangers: see HAZARDS
data book: see HANDBOOK
DATA COLLECTION
DATA PROCESSING
DEAFNESS
DEATH
decanting: see DECOMPRESSION
deck decompression chamber: see DIVING SYSTEMS
DECOMPRESSION
decompression chamber: see HYPERBARIC CHAMBER
decompression schedules: see DECOMPRESSION TABLES
DECOMPRESSION SICKNESS
DECOMPRESSION TABLES

PERMUTED SUBJECT INDEX

This index lists in alphabetic order all of the key words which appear in the title of the article, plus those which denote the subject matter. Words not in the title are in brackets. As has previously been explained, the only key words used are those which appear in the microthesaurus. The number at the right indicates the number of the entry in the bibliography. Lines are necessarily limited in length, so that long titles do not appear in full. A painstaking attempt has been made to select key words that will describe the article as fully as possible.

The following is an example of a citation and abstract as it appears in the text, with the lines from the index that refer to it.

211.
BENNETT, P.B.
Review of protective pharmacological agents in diving.
Aerosp. Med. 43:184-192; Feb.1972.

From 89 references the effects of a large number of pharmacological agents capable of ameliorating or preventing the major physiological hazards in diving of decompression sickness, oxygen toxicity and inert gas narcosis are reviewed. The indications, which the use of these compounds give, of the possible mechanisms for the production of these hazards is discussed and the direction of contemporary research on the use of drugs indicated. (Author's abstract)

Made in United States
North Haven, CT
17 October 2026

20527446R00370